Interventional Radiology

Volumes of
Golden's Diagnostic Radiology Series

*Out of print.

Interventional Radiology

Edited by

Wilfrido R. Castañeda-Zuñiga, M.D., M.Sc.

Professor of Radiology
Department of Radiology
University of Minnesota Hospital and Clinic
Minneapolis, Minnesota

S. Murthy Tadavarthy, M.D.

Clinical Assistant Professor of Radiology
University of Minnesota Hospital and Clinic
Chief Section of Cardiovascular
Interventional Radiology
Abbott Northwestern Hospital
Minneapolis, Minnesota

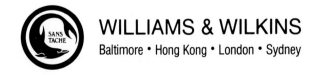

WILLIAMS & WILKINS
Baltimore • Hong Kong • London • Sydney

GOLDEN'S DIAGNOSTIC RADIOLOGY
JOHN H. HARRIS, JR., M.D., SERIES EDITOR

Editor: Timothy H. Grayson
Associate Editor: Carol Eckhart
Copy Editor: Deborah Tourtlotte
Design: JoAnne Janowiak
Illustration Planning: Wayne Hubbel
Production: Raymond E. Reter

Copyright © 1988
Williams & Wilkins
428 East Preston Street
Baltimore, MD 21202, U.S.A.

Accurate indications, adverse reactions, and dosage schedules for drugs are provided in this book, but it is possible that they may change. The reader is urged to review the package information data of the manufacturers of the medications mentioned.

Printed in the United States of America

Library of Congress Cataloging-in-Publication Data

Interventional radiology.

  (Golden's diagnostic radiology)
  Includes bibliographies and index.
  1. Radiology, Interventional. I. Castañeda-Zuñiga, Wilfrido R.   II. Series: Golden's diagnostic radiology series.   [DNLM: 1. Radiography.   2. Technology, Radiologic.   WN 160 I612]
RD33.55.I58   1988   616.07′57   87-23039
ISBN 0-683-01475-7

88 89 90 91
10 9 8 7 6 5 4 3 2 1

Foreword

It is with immense pride and pleasure that the officers and Editorial Board of Williams & Wilkins join me in introducing you, the reader, to Wilfredo R. Castañeda-Zúñiga, M.D., and S. Murthy Tadavarthy, M.D., the newest members of the distinguished group of authors in the Golden's Diagnostic Radiology Series.

Golden's Diagnostic Radiology Series was created to present authoritative, comprehensive, timely reference texts on clearly defined aspects of diagnostic radiology specifically intended for radiologists and those nonradiologists with major interest in the imaging aspects of their area of specialization.

Fulfillment of that goal demands authors and/or editors of proven stature and reputation in their field of diagnostic radiology. Candidates for authorship in the Series are identified from a rigorous selection process and are invited to become contributors to the Series. Thus, not only is the intent of the Golden's Series met and its purpose for the reader assured, but the authors are afforded an accolade available to a very select few. The unique prestige of the Golden's Series, continually enhanced by the character of its authors, has persisted for over a decade.

Drs. Castañeda-Zúñiga and Tadavarthy are uniquely qualified to author and edit *Interventional Radiology*. Both are academicians (teachers) in the true sense of the word, having spent their professional careers at the University of Minnesota. Both are direct professional descendants—or disciples—of one of the first American angiographers to expand into intervention, namely Kurt Amplatz, M.D., under whose direction both have studied, performed original bench and clinical research, and matured into respected teachers and clinicans. As disciples of Dr. Amplatz, Drs. Castañeda-Zúñiga and Tadavarthy represent the current generation of traditional angiographer-interventionists in contradistinction to modality-oriented radiologists who perform intervention within the scope of their modality interest or radiologists who limit their intervention to the organ system of their interest. Thus, this work is the statement of the years of experience of the authors and their carefully selected contributors.

Interventional Radiology is a superb example of the intent of the Golden's Series. It is timely and comprehensive in scope yet not overbearingly encyclopedic. Its organization is logical, and the text is interesting, entirely practical, and scholarly. The volume is replete with carefully selected radiographs of excellent quality, photographs, and clean, informative drawings.

Gilbert Fletcher, M.D., in his Foreword for another Golden's Series text stated, "Writing has meaning and substance only if the authors have knowledge and conviction of the usefulness of their writing." Certainly, Drs. Castañeda-Zúñiga and Tadavarthy and their contributors have satisfied Dr. Fletcher's criteria of excellence and are to be congratulated for preparing a text that is destined to become the standard in its field.

Finally, it is an extraordinarily wonderful coincidence that *Interventional Radiology*, authored and edited by two of his students, has been published in the same year that Dr. Amplatz received the Gold Medal of the American College of Radiology for his enormous contributions to the development of interventional radiology.

John H. Harris, Jr., M.D., D.Sc.
Editor, *Golden's Diagnostic Radiology*

Preface

Interventional radiology is a complex discipline in continuous expansion at the expense of formerly classic operations. Its breadth and importance seemed to justify a text, yet its complexity and rapid evolution make the writing and publication of a reference textbook a nearly impossible task; the instruments and techniques risk obsolescence by the publication date.

To reduce the speed with which this text becomes obsolete, the emphasis has been placed on the general philosophy of the indications, contraindications, approaches, and instrumentation rather than on specific techniques. Extensive drawings and radiographic illustrations provide a review of techniques and technical problems. In this way, we hope to prepare the readers for what will be current in practice when they read this book, not simply to portray the field as it was when we wrote it. Each chapter has extensive references for those who wish more theoretical background or a deeper understanding of the history of this field.

Even as this book goes to press, we are seeing spinoffs of established interventional radiologic techniques for new indications—*e.g.* the use of dilating balloons, once used primarily for vascular narrowings, to relieve urinary obstruction by prostatic hyperplasia. What might be available by the time the second edition of this book comes out can only be imagined—and in some cases, no doubt, has not yet been.

Acknowledgments

Interventional radiology has become a complex discipline. The knowledge of all the pertinent information in this field cannot be served by one or two authors; therefore, the help of a large number of contributors has been solicited. We are most grateful to these nationally and internationally known experts for their willingness to contribute, in spite of their busy professional commitments and teaching schedules.

We are indebted to our teacher, Dr. Kurt Amplatz, affectionately known as "Kurt," for training us and serving as a constant stimulus throughout our lives. His teachings, wisdom, vision, and enthusiasm in the field of cardiovascular and interventional radiology have been carried over to his residents and fellows who have directly or indirectly contributed to this book. It is difficult to find enough praise and gratitude for the excellence and motivation he has created for us.

Many of the interventional radiological procedures that we perform today were envisioned by the late Charles T. Dotter. Though we have not had the privilege or the honor to work with this "legend," we acknowledge his pioneering principles, which have led to the explosion of the current interventional techniques in radiology.

We thank the present and past residents and fellows for the case material included in this book. It was the result of their hard work while undergoing training at the University of Minnesota Hospitals.

The excellent quality of the artwork depicting the technicalities of the various procedures is the result of innumerable hours put in by Mr. Martin Finch, head of biomedical graphics at the University of Minnesota Hospital. We feel his artwork is second to none.

The publication of this book was only possible with the dedication and patience of Ms. Judith Gunn Bronson, who has revised and edited the manuscript. We also acknowledge the efforts of Mr. Kevin Sitter and Ms. Carla J. Nelson for typing innumerable revisions to the chapters in this book.

Last but not least, we would like to acknowledge our wives (Sylvia and Prameela) and children. While we prepared this book, they created an atmosphere that allowed us the peace of mind to complete this project.

Contributors

Kurt Amplatz, M.D.
(Chapters 3, 6, 12, 21–24, 27, 32)
Professor, Department of Radiology, University of
Minnesota Hospital and Clinic, Minneapolis,
Minnesota

Klemens H. Barth, M.D.
(Chapter 4)
Professor, Department of Radiology, Georgetown
University Hospital, Washington, D.C.

John L. Bass, M.D.
(Chapter 18)
Associate Professor, Pediatric Cardiology, University of
Minnesota Hospital and Clinic, Minneapolis,
Minnesota

Gary J. Becker, M.D.
(Chapters 5, 20, 30)
Professor, Department of Radiology, Indiana University
School of Medicine, Indianapolis, Indiana

T. J. Bowker, M.A., M.R.C.P.
(Chapter 19)
Medical Registrar, The National Heart Hospital and
University College Hospital, London, England

Werner Brüehlman, M.D.
(Chapter, 27)
Chairman, Department of Radiology, Stadtspital
Triemli, Institute fur Rontgendiagnostik, Zurich,
Switzerland

Peter Bub, M.D.
(Chapter 26)
Katharinen Hospital, Urologische Ab Teilung, Stuttgart,
West Germany

Dana R. Burke, M.D.
(Chapter 29)
Assistant Professor, Staff Angiographer, Department of
Radiology, Hospital of the University of Pennsylvania,
Philadelphia, Pennsylvania

John F. Cardella, M.D.
(Chapters 3, 9)
Clinical Assistant Professor, Department of Radiology,
University of Minnesota Hospital and Clinic, Staff
Radiologist, Department of Radiology, Metropolitan
Medical Center, Minneapolis, Minnesota

Flavio Castañeda, M.D.
(Chapters 3, 6, 9, 21–24, 27, 32)
Instructor, Department of Radiology, University of
Minnesota Hospital and Clinic, Minneapolis,
Minnesota

Wilfrido R. Castañeda-Zuñiga, M.D., M.Sc.
(Chapters 1, 3, 6, 9, 12, 21–25, 27, 28, 32)
Professor, Department of Radiology, University of
Minnesota Hospital and Clinic, Minneapolis,
Minnesota

Ralph V. Clayman, M.D.
(Chapter 26)
Associate Professor, Division of Urology, Washington
University, St. Louis, Missouri

Carol C. Coleman, M.D.
(Chapters 3, 6, 9, 21–23, 27)
Associate Professor, Department of Radiology, Veterans
Administration Medical Center. Associate Professor,
Department of Radiology, University of Minnesota
Hospital and Clinic, Minneapolis, Minnesota

Frank Comhaire, M.D., Ph.D.
(Chapter 7)
Department of Internal Medicine, Section of
Endocrinology, Academisch Ziekenhuis, Ghent, Belgium

Dewey J. Conces, Jr., M.D.
(Chapter 30)
Assistant Professor, Department of Radiology, Indiana
University School of Medicine, Indianapolis, Indiana

Constantin Cope, M.D.
(Chapter 17)
Professor, Department of Radiology, Hospital of the
University of Pennsylvania, Philadelphia, Pennsylvania

Andrew H. Cragg, M.D.
(Chapters 3, 6, 9, 12, 21–23, 27, 32)
Assistant Professor, Department of Radiology,
University of Iowa Hospitals and Clinics, Iowa City,
Iowa

Michael D. Darcy, M.D.
(Chapters 3, 6, 9, 21–23, 27, 32)
Assistant Professor, Department of Radiology, Medical
University of South Carolina, Charleston, South
Carolina

Morteza K. Elyaderani, M.D.
(Chapters 23, 32)
Professor, Department of Radiology, St. Joseph's
Hospital, Omaha, Nebraska

Cesar Ercole, M.D.
(Chapter 6)
Assistant Professor, Division of Urology, University of
Minnesota, Minneapolis, Minnesota

Wilson Greatbatch, Ph.D., F.I.E.E.E.
(Chapter 19)
Greatbatch Enterprizes, Inc., Clarence, New York

Carlos Guerra, M.D.
(Chapter 28)
Department of Radiology, Hospital Nuestra Senora del
Pino, Islas Canarias, Spain

Robert W. Holden, M.D.
(Chapters 5, 20)
Associate Professor, Department of Radiology, Indiana
University School of Medicine, Indianapolis, Indiana

John C. Hulbert, M.D.
(Chapters 23, 24)
Associate Professor, Department of Urologic Surgery,
University of Minnesota Hospital and Clinic,
Minneapolis, Minnesota

David W. Hunter, M.D.
(Chapters 3, 6, 9, 12, 13, 16, 21–24, 27, 32)
Associate Professor, Department of Radiology,
University of Minnesota Hospital and Clinic,
Minneapolis, Minnesota

Charles D. Kellum, M.D.
(Chapter 15)
Assistant Professor, Attending for Special Procedures,
Department of Radiology, University of Virginia
Medical Center, Charlottesville, Virginia

Eugene C. Klatte, M.D.
(Chapter 5)
Professor and Chairman, Department of Radiology,
Indiana University School of Medicine, Indianapolis,
Indiana

Donald L. Kreipke, M.D.
(Chapter 30)
Associate Professor, Department of Radiology, Indiana
University School of Medicine, Indianapolis, Indiana

Marc Kunnen, M.D., Ph.D.
(Chapter 7)
Department of Radiodiagnostics, Academisch
Ziekenhuis, Ghent, Belgium

Paul Lange, M.D.
(Chapter 23)
Professor, Department of Urologic Surgery, University of
Minnesota Hospital and Clinic, Minneapolis,
Minnesota

Bert W. Larson, M.D.
(Chapter 24)
Staff Physician, Department of Radiology, Veterans
Administration Medical Center, Minneapolis,
Minnesota

Won Lee, M.D.
(Chapter 23)
Associate Professor, Director, Division of Uroradiology,
Department of Radiology, Long Island Jewish Hospital,
New Hyde Park, New York

Janis Gissel Letourneau, M.D.
(Chapters 23, 24, 27, 31, 32)
Associate Professor, Department of Radiology,
University of Minnesota Hospital and Clinic,
Minneapolis, Minnesota

Gunnar Lund, M.D.
(Chapters 3, 6, 9, 21–23, 27, 32)
Associate Professor, Department of Radiology,
University of Nebraska Medical Center, Omaha,
Nebraska

Francisco Martinez, M.D.
(Chapter 28)
Department of Radiology, Hospital Nuestra Senora del
Pino, Islas Canarias, Spain

Manuel Maynar-Moliner, M.D.
(Chapter 28)
Director, Vascular and Interventional Radiology,
Hospital Nuestra Senora del Pino, Islas Canarias, Spain

Gordon K. McLean, M.D.
(Chapter 29)
Associate Professor, Chief, Angiography/Interventional
Section, Department of Radiology, Hospital of the
University of Pennsylvania, Philadelphia, Pennsylvania

Steven G. Meranze, M.D.
(Chapter 29)
Assistant Professor, Staff Angiographer, Department of
Radiology, Hospital of the University of Pennsylvania,
Philadelphia, Pennsylvania

Richard L. Morin, Ph.D.
(Chapter 2)
Senior Associate Consultant, Department of Radiology,
Mayo Clinic. Associate Professor, Department of
Radiology, Mayo Medical School, Rochester, Minnesota

Pratab K. Reddy, M.D.
(Chapters 23–25)
Assistant Professor, Department of Urologic Surgery,
University of Minnesota Hospital and Clinic,
Minneapolis, Minnesota

Masao Sako, M.D.
(Chapter 8)
Associate Professor, Department of Radiology, Kobe
University School of Medicine, Kobe, Japan

Erich K. Salomonowitz, M.D.
(Chapters 23, 27, 32)
Associate Professor, General Roentgen, University of
Vienna, Vienna, Austria

Donald E. Schwarten, M.D.
(Chapter 14)
Director of Cardiovascular Services, Department of
Radiology, St. Vincent's Hospital and Health Care
Center, Indianapolis, Indiana

Tony P. Smith, M.D.
(Chapters 3, 6, 9, 21–23, 27, 32)
Assistant Professor, Department of Radiology,
University of Iowa Hospitals and Clinics, Iowa City,
Iowa

Samuel K. S. So, M.B., B.S.
(Chapter 16)
Transplant Fellow in Surgery, Department of Surgery,
University of Minnesota Hospital and Clinic,
Minneapolis, Minnesota

S. Murthy Tadavarthy, M.D.
(Chapters 3, 9, 21–23, 27, 32)
Clinical Associate Professor, Department of Radiology,
University of Minnesota Hospital and Clinic. Chief,
Cardiovascular Section, Department of Radiology.
Abbott-Northwestern Hospital. Cardiovascular
Radiologist, Minneapolis Heart Institute, Minneapolis,
Minnesota

Robert D. Tarver, M.D.
(Chapter 30)
Assistant Professor, Department of Radiology, Wishard
Memorial Hospital, Indiana University School of
Medicine, Indianapolis, Indiana

Charles J. Tegtmeyer, M.D.
(Chapter 15)
Professor of Radiology, Associate Professor of Anatomy,
Director of Angiography, Interventional Radiology, and
Special Procedures, Department of Radiology,
University of Virginia Medical Center, Charlottesville,
Virginia

Ivan Vujic, M.D.
(Chapters 10, 11)
Professor, Department of Radiology, Temple University
Hospital, Philadelphia, Pennsylvania

Antony T. Young, M.D.
(Chapters 3, 27)
Attending Radiologist, Department of Radiology,
Christchurch Hospital, Christchurch, New Zealand

Heun Y. Yune, M.D.
(Chapter 5)
Professor, Department of Radiology, Indiana University
School of Medicine, Indianapolis, Indiana

Robert M. Zeit, M.D.
(Chapter 17)
Clinical Associate Professor, Department of Radiology,
Temple University Hospital. Staff Radiologist, Albert
Einstein Medical Center, Philadelphia, Pennsylvania

Christoph L. Zollikofer, M.D.
(Chapters 12, 23, 27)
Chairman, Department of Radiology, Winterthur
Kantonspital, Switzerland

Contents

1

Interventional Radiology: Yesterday, Today, Tomorrow[a]

WILFRIDO R. CASTAÑEDA–ZUÑIGA, M.D., M.Sc.

The origins of interventional radiology are in the angiographic Seldinger techniques developed by cardiovascular radiologists in the late 1950s and early 1960s. Using these angiographic principles, one can gain access to many organ systems by percutaneous puncture. Performance of such percutaneous radiologic procedures has been facilitated by the development of high-resolution image-intensified fluoroscopy, ultrasound (US), and computed tomography (CT). Moreover, interventional radiology has benefited from rapid developments in materials science and biotechnology.

In this brief introduction, the author reviews the development of interventional radiology and speculates about its future and the preparation we need to make for it. In doing so, he cautions that it is difficult to predict the future of such a rapidly changing field as interventional radiology.

INTERVENTIONAL CARDIOVASCULAR RADIOLOGY

As interventional radiology has its foundations in cardiovascular procedures, it is appropriate that this survey begins there.

The nonsurgical hemodynamic correction of occlusive atherosclerotic disease with the aid of coaxial Teflon dilators was first reported by Dotter and Judkins in 1964. This trial followed Dotter's incidental observation of recanalization of a totally occluded right common iliac artery by an angiographic catheter during conventional diagnostic angiography.

Because of the excessive shearing and the "snowplowing" effect produced by Dotter's coaxial techniques, modifications were devised by Staples and subsequently by Van Andel. The main disadvantage of the Teflon dilators persisted, however; their small size limited their use to arteries no more than 4 mm in diameter, because larger dilators were associated with an unacceptably high frequency of local complications. To overcome these technical limitations, Portsmann described a "caged" or "corset" balloon catheter in 1973. This catheter system employed a latex balloon enclosed in a Teflon dilator with strips cut out from the area overlying the balloon to minimize the propensity of the latex to deform with inflation in the atherosclerotic lesion. However, because of the large size of the caged catheter and its high thrombogenicity, these modifications did not change the prevailing attitude of U.S. surgeons and radiologists to the Dotter technique. In contrast, in Europe, thousands of Dotter procedures were performed at leading academic institutions, with excellent immediate and long-term results being reported by Zeitler, Portsmann, Schoop, Van Andel, and many others.

It was not until 1974 that one of Zeitler's former students, the late Andreas Grüntzig, and his colleague, Hopff, developed a nonexpandable dual-lumen balloon that produced safe, fast dilatation of narrowed vessel segments by applying radial forces against the plaque and arterial wall. In addition, the wide variety of balloon sizes available for Grüntzig catheters allowed dilatation of vessels as large as the aorta while minimizing the size of the puncture needed for catheter insertion. This catheter and its progeny are now used for dilatation procedures in many different groups. The physiopathologic changes produced by balloon angioplasty were studied extensively by University of Minnesota researchers including, Amplatz, Formanek, Edwards, Zollikofer, and Laerum, who described the "controlled vascular injury" that is produced.

Cragg enriched and expanded this theory with his meticulous evaluation of the physiologic changes occurring at the cellular level. With this understanding of the physiopathologic phenomena, it has been possible to formulate more rational pharmacologic management of the acute complications of the procedure and to enhance the long-term patency rates of dilated vessels. The long-term results of transluminal angioplasty in properly selected patients are equivalent to the results achieved with the traditional surgical methods, often with a lower morbidity. Moreover, in most cases angioplasty can easily be repeated if the first procedure is a failure or if the narrowing recurs. As a result, angioplasty is supplanting sur-

---

[a]Excerpted from the Malcolm B. Hanson Memorial Lecture. University of Minnesota Continuing Medical Education. Radiology Annual Course, September 1986.

gery for some diseases, such as peripheral vascular obstructions, which traditionally would be treated by the femoropopliteal bypass technique.

Five-year patency rates in peripheral angioplasty range from 90% in the iliac vessels to 60%–70% for long-segment recanalization of superficial femoral artery lesions. Transluminal angioplasty is particularly useful in patients with renovascular hypertension, where the best results are obtained in patients with fibromuscular dysplasia, with patency rates between 80%–90% at 5 years. Lower patency rates are obtained for atherosclerotic lesions, depending on location and bilaterality of the lesion. The technique is complementary to operation in other settings such as coronary artery disease. Given these promising results, the time may have come for a more aggressive approach to patients with early symptoms of atherosclerotic vascular disease who might not be considered surgical candidates.

Perhaps in the near future, one can consider removing some of these obstructive lesions rather than remodeling and displacing them, as is done with transluminal angioplasty. Several investigative groups are attempting to resolve the many problems involved with the intravascular use of laser radiation to ablate atherosclerotic lesions. Several types of lasers are currently under clinical and laboratory investigation for intravascular uses. The one with most potential is the CO_2 laser, because its energy is absorbed at the surface site of impact, with very little tissue penetration and therefore less chance of causing perforation or secondary thermal tissue injury. Its main disadvantage has been the lack of adequate fiberoptics to deliver the beam at a distance. The argon laser has more tissue penetration than the CO_2 laser and also produces forward and back scatter. The neodymium:YAG laser has the greatest potential for vascular perforations and thermal tissue injury. Great hopes lie with the excimer lasers, which at shorter wavelengths (193 nm) disrupt molecular bonds. Their potential lies in their nonthermal effect and their great precision.

Two delivery approaches for the laser are being studied. One uses a modified angioplasty-balloon catheter as the conduit for the optic fiber, which is used under fluoroscopic control to remove tissue, thus creating a pathway for advancement of the dilating balloon across atherosclerotic lesions. After removal of plaque by the laser, the balloon is advanced and inflated as in traditional angioplasty. The advantage of this technique is said to be the removal of tissue, leaving a smoother arterial lumen than after traditional angioplasty. The other technique uses angioscopes to remove tissue under direct vision, thus (it is hoped) decreasing the chances of perforation. The disadvantage of this technique is the large size of the angioscopes currently available and their short depth of field.

A different approach has been used by Cumberland et al in England. A metallic tip, heated to between 400° and 1000° C using a laser beam, is advanced under fluoroscopic control through the vascular obstruction to ablate tissue thermally. It is unknown if this extreme heat will produce long-term damage.

The hope is that the result of laser angioplasty with a smoother lumen will be better than the postangioplasty result, which creates a more irregular lumen because of the continued intraluminal presence of the plaque. Formidable problems remain; nonetheless, the rapid progress to date is promising.

Another approach uses a drill or a blade mounted on an angiographic catheter and powered by an external source to remove atherosclerotic or thrombotic material at the site of vascular occlusion. These techniques are in the process of development and will probably become an important part of the percutaneous revascularization techniques, together with the vascular stents recently described by Gianturco, Palmas, Cragg, and Mass.

THROMBOLYSIS

Of course, not all vascular obstructions are plaques or stenoses. Some are thrombi or emboli. These, too, can be managed by the interventional radiologist. The discovery of streptokinase by Tillett and Garner in 1933 and of urokinase by McFarlane in 1946, and the subsequent understanding of the interactions of these substances with the human fibrinolytic system, resulted in a wide variety of clinical applications. In 1959, Johnson and McCarthy reported clinical lysis of clot by the intravenous administration of streptokinase. This report initiated the use of high-dose intravenous systemic infusion of thrombolytic agents to lyse thrombi and thromboemboli. In 1973, a large therapeutic trial for pulmonary embolism showed greater resolution of thrombi and a more significant improvement in pulmonary artery pressures and clinical status in those patients treated with thrombolytic agents rather than with heparin. Nonetheless, the use of thrombolytic agents fell into disfavor, mainly because of the fear of systemic complications, particularly hemorrhage.

In order to avoid the hemorrhagic complications, Dotter, in 1974, suggested delivering streptokinase locally to peripheral vascular occlusions at approximately 1/20 the systemic dose. Despite good results, this new method did not become popular. Renthrop subsequently described the use of high-dose, short-duration infusion in the coronary arterial tree in 1979, and Katzen described the use of local low-dose infusions in the peripheral vasculature in 1981. These and subsequent reports attest to the efficacy and increased popularity of local thrombolytic therapy. However, one should remember Dotter's words of caution: "Thrombolysis is not curative; it merely restores patency and helps identify a local anatomical obstruction which requires treatment" and that "even in small doses thrombolysis can cause distal systemic complications." Moreover, several challenging problems associated with thrombolytic therapy remain, including the incidence of local complications, the high cost of the drugs, and the lengthy hospitalization required for complete resolution of clots.[1]

Some of these problems may be resolved by the development of a new generation of thrombolytic substances, particularly tissue-type plasminogen activator (tPA), which can now be abundantly produced by recombinant genetic techniques. This agent acts only on clots and thus avoids the systemic fibrinolytic effects and their associated hemorrhagic complications. Nursing demands and specialized care are markedly reduced for the management of thrombolysis with this agent compared with other techniques because of its local action. Some even foresee the prophylactic use of tPA by emergency medical technicians during ambulance transport of patients suffering myocardial infarction.

EMBOLOTHERAPY

Whereas angioplasty and thrombolysis have been developed to resolve vascular occlusion, embolotherapy has been developed to produce vascular occlusion. As technical advances in transcatheter vascular embolization have been made, the indications for the procedure have been more clearly defined. In many situations, embolotherapy is now an alternative to the more conventional techniques of surgery, radiation, and drugs. Without the availability of controlled clinical trials, however, it is difficult to define precisely the role of embolotherapy for any given clinical situation.

Although interest in embolotherapy has been greatest in the past decade, the principle of vascular embolization dates to 1904, when Dawbain described the preoperative injection of melted paraffin (Vaseline) into the external carotid arteries of patients suffering head and neck tumors. Brooks, in 1930, introduced particulate embolization with the occlusion of a traumatic carotid cavernous fistula by the injection of a muscle fragment attached to a silver clip into an internal carotid artery. Embolotherapy was influenced greatly by a landmark 1963 paper by Nusbaum and Baum, who demonstrated the angiographic detection of gastrointestinal bleeding at 0.5 ml/min. Transcatheter managment of hemorrhage followed soon after, first achieved with intraarterial infusions of vasopressin. This pharmacologic success was soon followed, in 1972, by Rosch's report of control of acute gastric hemorrhage by embolization of the gastroepiploic artery using autologous clot.

An upsurge of interest in embolization began in the 1970s, fostered by parallel developments in catheter technology and embolic agents. The availability of a wide range of preshaped catheters and the introduction of coaxial systems allowed relatively routine superselective catheter placement and embolic agent delivery. In 1972, the tissue adhesive isobutylcyanoacrylate was described by Zanetti and Sherman. The use of Gelfoam particles as an embolic agent was first reported by Carey in 1974, as was the use of the permanent embolic agent Ivalon in its particulate form by Tadavarthy at the University of Minnesota.

Detachable balloons were first described by Serbinenko in the USSR in 1974 for the embolization of vascular malformations and aneurysms in the cerebral circulation and subsequently perfected by Debrun, Kerber, and White. The concept of tissue ablation by absolute ethanol was introduced by Ellman in 1980. Klatte, also in 1980, reported its efficacy for the embolization of renal tumors.

In 1982, Amplatz illustrated the efficacy of boiling contrast medium to occlude veins in laboratory animals. Because of difficulty in finding human volunteers to test the technique, he eventually had to volunteer a vein in his forearm for hot-contrast injection. The vein was subsequently removed, and light microscopy confirmed what angiography had already shown: the complete obstruction of the venous channel.

For the occlusion of larger vascular structures, Gianturco created the wool coil, a current modification of which is nowadays in widespread use, mainly for renal artery occlusion in patients with large renal cell carcinomas. Because of the risk of pulmonary or systemic embolization in patients with large arteriovenous fistulae (AVFs), self-retaining devices to prevent pulmonary embolization were described by Castañeda and Amplatz: a barbed coil was used safely to embolize a large postnephrectomy AVF in a patient with congestive heart failure and renal allograft. For the same purpose, a spider-like device was also described by the same investigators in 1981. Large AVFs have been safely obliterated since then, not only in the abdominal area but also in the pulmonary circulation. A detachable spider was developed since then by Lund to obtain better control of the spider's release.

ABSCESS DRAINAGE

The technical advances made in diagnostic and interventional cardiovascular radiology have been easily transferred to the percutaneous management of diseases in other organ systems. For many radiologists, this means the percutaneous management of infection.

Despite the widespread use of antibiotics, untreated abdominal abscesses carry a mortality rate of 80%. Traditional surgical treatment is associated with a mortality rate of 20%–43%. Cross-sectional imaging allows earlier detection of abdominal abscesses and provides a means for guidance of percutaneous drainage procedures. With accurate detection and guidance by US and CT, percutaneous catheter drainage of abdominal abscesses can be associated with a success rate of 80%–85%. Certainly, the periprocedural mortality rate of catheter drainage, 6%, compares very favorably with that of operative drainage. In addition, percutaneous drainage is less traumatic and disruptive of the normal anatomy.

Failures of percutaneous abscess drainage usually occur in patients who are not suitable candidates; for example, unsuitable collections include multiple and multiloculated abscesses with central necrosis and poorly defined parenchymal margins, necrotic tumors, those with communications to the gastrointestinal tract, and diffuse microabscesses or inflammatory phlegmons. The precise role of percutaneous abscess drainage must be defined by the use of randomized trials with rigidly prescribed protocols. These trials must segregate the results of drainage in immunocompromised and nonimmunocompromised patients, since results of treatment are different in these two groups. Until the results of these studies are available, continued significant controversy about the virtues and defects of percutaneous drainage of abdominal abscesses can be expected. Unfortunately, patient selection cannot always be ideal; many percutaneous drainages will have to be performed on patients in poor physical and hemodynamic conditions because they present an unacceptably high surgical risk. These patients cannot be denied the procedure, as it may represent their only hope for survival.

PERCUTANEOUS BIOPSIES

Percutaneous biopsy of lesions has become very popular with the advent of CT and US. A wide variety of different needle designs have been developed in an attempt to obtain better samples for tissue diagnosis, rather than simply obtaining cells for cytologic diagnosis. The latter is not always available because of the pathologist's dislike for cell in place of tissue diagnosis.

RENAL INTERVENTION

Another target for percutaneous interventional techniques is the kidney. Percutaneous nephrostomy has been refined remarkably since its original description 30 years ago by Goodwin and his colleagues as a treatment of last resort. It is currently the preferred method of relieving supravesical ureteral obstruction because of its ease of performance, its low morbidity, and its minuscule mortality rate. Moreover, percutaneous nephrostomy now is often but a prelude to other interventional procedures, such as dilation of ureteral strictures, incision of infundibular stenoses and ureteropelvic junction obstructions, stenting of ureteral fistulae, retrieval of fractured or blocked stents, local infusion of various chemotherapeutic agents, and even laser ablation of renal pelvic tumors. The introduction of catheters in and around the renal pelvis is easily accomplished with the use of fluoroscopy. Cross-sectional imaging elucidates basic anatomic relations, knowledge of which helps avoid complications such as colonic, hepatic, and splenic perforations.

The feasibility of removing renal stones through a percutaneously created nephrostomy tract was initially reported by Fernström and Johannson in 1976. In 1978, Smith et al from the University of Minnesota reported the extraction of ureteral calculi through a percutaneous nephrostomy tract from a patient with an ileal loop. The development of nephrostomy tract dilators by Amplatz in 1982 led to the development of the percutaneous techniques for the removal of retained urinary stones. Since then, many reports, both from Europe and from this country, have documented the success and safety of percutaneous nephrolithotomy in thousands of patients. The success rate of percutaneous nephrostomy is 95%–98% for simple decompression of obstructive uropathy, with similar success rates reported for the establishment of the more complicated nephrostomy tracts sometimes needed in patients with retained urinary stones. High success rates (98%) in the removal of retained urinary stones have been reported using a combination of techniques including ultrasonic lithotripsy and stone basketing or grasping with additional endoscopic guidance.

The University of Minnesota approach to endourology has depended on the cooperation between the radiology and urology services. Such a team utilizes the anatomic background of the radiologist in selecting a suitable puncture site in an appropriate calix by formulating a three-dimensional image from multidirectional fluoroscopic capabilities. Catheter and guidewire manipulations are also the responsibility of the radiologist. On the other hand, the urologist is primarily responsible for the management of the patient. His or her experience with rigid and flexible endoscopes and their auxiliary instruments permits stone removal. Thus, successful percutaneous nephrolithotomy is accomplished using the combined skills of radiologists and urologists.

The present technique of nephrolithotomy is associated with little postoperative morbidity and no mortality. It allows the patient to resume normal activities within several days after hospital discharge. At the University of Minnesota the procedure has even been performed on several asymptomatic patients who had compelling reasons for having their stones removed.

However, while percutaneous stone extraction techniques were being perfected, extracorporeal shock wave lithotripsy (ESWL) was being developed. This technique uses radiographic localization of the calculus and a high-wave ultrasound beam for fragmentation. ESWL has restricted the use of endourologic procedures to places where ESWL is not available, those cases in which ESWL has failed, many with ureteral stones, and to those with any of several particular types of stones, such as those trapped behind an obstruction, those which are radiolucent, and those which fill much of the collecting system or are infected. Therefore, percutaneous stone extraction will continue to be a significant means of management of patients with urinary tract calculi. One warning has to be given, however, concerning the long-term effects of ESWL on the kidney. We do not know what effects ESWL may have, because CT or magnetic resonance imaging studies are not routinely obtained. Carefully controlled studies are a necessity!

BILIARY INTERVENTION

Diagnostic and therapeutic biliary intervention can be carried out in a fashion analogous to that in the urinary tract.

The diagnostic technique of percutaneous transhepatic cholangiography was originally described by Burkhardt and Mueller in 1921 with injections of the gallbladder through a needle introduced through the liver. In 1937, this technique was modified by Huard and Do-Xuanhuop, who injected Lipiodol into the bile ducts. However, direct cholangiography was not routinely performed until 1952, following the reports by Carter and Leger and their coworkers, who used a large needle. In 1974, Okuda popularized transhepatic cholangiography by using a long, thin, flexible needle in 114 patients, modifying a technique earlier described by Ohto and Tsuchiya. This fine-needle technique eliminated the need for operation immediately after the procedure. Compared to techniques that utilized a large needle, there was a reduction in the rate of intraperitoneal hemorrhage by a factor of 6, of bile leakage by a factor of 3, and of the procedure-associated mortality by a factor of 2.6.

In 1966, Seldinger reported his experience with transhepatic cholangiography by a right costal approach using a sheathed needle that allowed decompression of the biliary system at the time of cholangiography. Ferrucci and Ring refined and popularized the technique in this country. Decompression of biliary obstruction in now performed in patients with either primary or metastatic liver tumors and in those with benign biliary strictures and fistulae. Percutaneous biliary drainage also allows access for removal of retained biliary calculi. Specialized guidewires and catheters have been developed to pass through areas of stricture or obstruction; with their aid, indwelling catheters can be placed and combined external–internal drainage with antegrade flow of bile into the bowel can be achieved.

The principal application of percutaneous biliary decompression has been in the nonsurgical palliation of malignant biliary obstruction. The traditional treatment has been the surgical creation of a biliary–enteric anastomosis, which is associated with significant morbidity and an operative mortality rate of 5%–15%. Percutaneous drainage thus permits relief of cholestasis and its sequelae with relatively low risk. The criteria that determine whether a particular patient will undergo a surgical or a percutaneous decompression are both anatomic and physiologic. Patients with high or multiple branch obstructions are also candidates for percutaneous drainage. In contrast, patients with lower common duct or periampullary obstruction presenting in stable hemodynamic condition early in the course of their disease will typically undergo surgical palliation. This preselection of patients for operation has led to statements in the surgical literature that open palliation is more effective than percutaneous biliary drainage in the management of biliary obstruction. However, when similar groups of patients are treated, or when correction is made by statistical analysis, similar morbidity and mortality are found.

THE FUTURE

New techniques currently being developed and evaluated include percutaneous gastrostomies, enterostomies, cecostomies, and cholecystostomies; percutaneous gallstone dissolution; transgastric drainage of pseudocysts of the pancreas; retrograde balloon dilatation of the prostate; and vascular endoprostheses. Randomized prospective studies with statistical analysis and long-term follow-up will be required to establish the role of each of these new interventional radiologic procedures.

Undoubtedly, the introduction of prospective pricing systems and Diagnosis-Related Groups (DRGs) will have a strong influence on the future development and utilization of interventional radiology. Under the DRG prepayment plan, hospitals receive a fixed reimbursement for inpatient care for a given diagnosis regardless of the length of hospitalization or the complexity of diagnostic evaluation and subsequent treatment. Moreover, if the interests of society are to reduce medical care costs, the most effective route is to minimize hospitalization expenses. DRG reimbursement thus encourages the use of percutaneous radiologic procedures, because they typically decrease the length of hospital stay and, therefore, minimize hospitalization expenditures.

Radiologists can well rejoice in these indirect benefits but must recognize the possibility of profound alterations in practice. For example, radiologists must assume a consultative role with their clinical colleagues, provide diagnostic algorithms for the work-up of clinical problems, and establish utilization guidelines for the many new radiologic services. They must, therefore, become more directly involved in the day-to-day care of patients. *A dedicated commitment is necessary!* This approach to interventional radiology provides great rewards, because the therapeutic effects of radiologic procedures are often immediately apparent. In sum, one must leave behind the more contemplative attitude with which radiology was approached in the past.

Interventional radiology has come of age. It is here, and it should be embraced, developed, and advocated. The future is bright if technical excellence is sought. Radiologists today have been given opportunities far exceeding those granted most of their predecessors; let us use those opportunities well.

Reference

1. Dotter CT, Judkins MP: Transluminal treatment of arteriosclerotic obstruction. *Circulation* 1964;30:654–670

2

Radiation Protection in Interventional Radiology

RICHARD L. MORIN, Ph.D.

Interventional radiology procedures can require substantial amounts of ionizing radiation and therefore necessitate particularly close attention to radiation protection. In this chapter, radiation units, regulations, and the fundamental principles of radiation protection are reviewed. Then the procedures and devices designed to reduce patient and staff exposure in interventional radiology are examined.

RADIATION UNITS

The fundamental interactions of x-rays with matter produce ion pairs via photoelectric and Compton interactions.[1] The *Roentgen* (SI unit: coulomb (C) per kilogram) is the unit used to measure the number of ion pairs produced by x- or gamma radiation in a standard volume of air. The process of ion pair production is formally termed *radiation exposure* and is fundamental in radiation protection.

The number of ion pairs produced in air does not directly measure the amount of energy deposited in another medium because of the differences in x-ray absorption by different materials.[1] The *rad* is used as a measure of the radiation *absorbed dose* (energy deposited per unit mass). A rad is equal to 100 ergs/g (SI unit: joule per kilogram or Gray (Gy)). This unit is of fundamental importance in patient dosimetry.

Ionizing radiations other than x- and gamma rays, such as alpha particles or neutrons, may induce a greater biologic effect for a given absorbed dose. To quantitate this observation, the *rem* (SI unit: Sievert (Sv)) is used to measure the *dose equivalent*. The rem is equal to the number of rads multiplied by a quality factor ranging from 1 to 20 that expresses the degree of biologic insult for equal amounts of different types of ionizing radiation. The quality factor for x- and gamma radiation is equal to 1. This unit is most often utilized in health physics and personnel exposure measures. These radiation units are summarized in Table 2–1.

RADIATION PROTECTION FUNDAMENTALS

In order to decrease the absorbed dose to the patient and the exposure of the staff, the radiation protection principles of *time*, *distance*, and *shielding* must be considered. Radiation exposure is directly related to exposure *time*, so by halving the exposure time, one halves radiation dose. Because an x-ray beam diverges as it passes through *space*, radiation intensity decreases as the inverse square of the distance from the radiation source:

$$\frac{I_2}{I_1} = \frac{d_1^2}{d_2^2}$$

Hence, if the distance from a radiation source is doubled, the radiation intensity decreases to one-fourth its original value (Fig. 2–1). Although this relation holds strictly only for a point source, the distance principle is useful in reducing clinical radiation exposure when the patient is

Table 2–1
Radiation Units

Radiation Quantity	Traditional Unit	SI Unit	Conversion
Exposure	Roentgen	Coulombs/kg	2.6×10^{-4} C-kg^{-1} = 1 R
Absorbed dose	Rad	Gray (Gy)	10 mGy = 1 rad
Dose	Rem	Sievert (Sv)	10 mSv = 1 rem

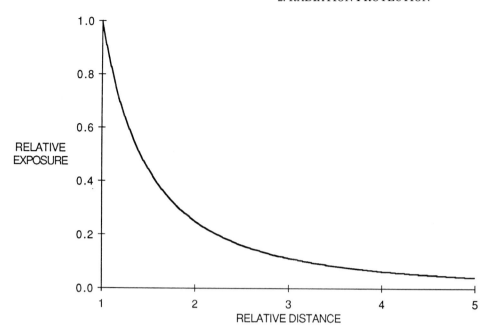

Fig. 2-1 Reduction of radiation intensity according to the inverse-square law.

the principal source. The attenuation of an x-ray beam (loss of intensity as it passes through matter) is exponential ($I = I_o e^{-ux}$, where I and I_o are the initial and transmitted radiation, respectively, u is the attenuation coefficient of the material (which depends on the atomic number and density and on the energy of the photons), and x is the thickness of the attenuating material). Therefore, small amounts of attenuating (*shielding*) material can greatly reduce the intensity of an x-ray beam. For example, a 99% reduction of a diagnostic x-ray beam is obtained by using a 0.5-mm Pb-equivalent material. Examples of exponential attenuation for diagnostic radiology x-ray beams are shown in Figure 2-2.

Because fluoroscopy is utilized extensively during some interventional radiology procedures, the continual observation of these fundamental principles is of far greater importance than in most areas of diagnostic radiology.

RADIATION PROTECTION REGULATIONS

Unlike other areas in medicine in which ionizing radiation is used to diagnose or treat disease (*e.g.*, therapeutic radiology, nuclear medicine), x-ray protection and use are not regulated at the federal level. No federal body analogous to the Nuclear Regulatory Commission exists to supervise the medical use of x-rays. Instead, except for the regulations concerning equipment construction,[2] this regulatory function is administered at the state level,

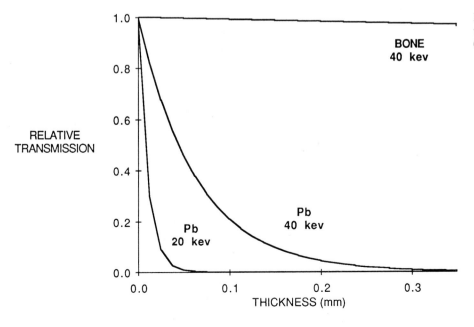

Fig. 2-2 Reduction of radiation intensity with increasing thickness of lead and bone at 60 kVp (20 kev) and 120 kVp (40 kev).

Table 2–2
Maximum Permissible Dose Equivalent (rem)[3]

Area	13 Weeks	Yearly	Cumulative
Whole body, gonads, blood-forming organs, lens of eye	3		5 (N-18)*
Skin	10	30	
Hands and forearms, head, neck, feet, ankles	25	75	

*N = Age in years

Table 2–3
Eye Exposure Limits

Regulatory/Advisory Body	Limit (Rem/qtr)	Reference
ICRP	7.5	6
NCRP	3.0	3, 7
OHSA	1.25	8
NRC	1.25	9

most often within a state's department of health and human services. Although one might expect this arrangement to engender a morass of disparate regulations, the state-to-state variation actually is not great, since most states have patterned their regulations after the recommendations of the National Council on Radiation Protection and Measurements (NCRP). This body has developed an extensive set of regulatory guidelines that have become *de facto* standards for the safe and proper use of ionizing radiation (summarized in Table 2–2). Other sources give further details of the general philosophy of radiation protection, as well as specific recommendations for particular situations.[3–5]

Two other bodies also publish recommendations for radiation protection: the International Commission on Radiation Protection (ICRP) and the International Council on Radiation Protection and Units (ICRU). Additionally, in some instances, the regulations of the Occupational Safety and Health Administration (OSHA) govern the operation of x-ray equipment in a particular diagnostic radiology department.

The presence of these diverse recommendations is particularly important in interventional radiology, since the maximum quarterly exposure to the eyes permitted by the various recommendations differs by a factor of 6 (Table 2–3). These quarterly allowances are intended to account for sporadic or variable, not continual, exposure. Exposures should always be kept "as low as reasonably achievable" (ALARA). Although the operator's hands and forearms may be exposed during interventional radiology procedures, in general, exposure of the eyes and thyroid is of greater concern and therefore most closely monitored.

Concern is often expressed about the absorbed dose to the eye because of the risk of radiation-induced cataracts. This biologic effect appears to have a threshold, in that about 600 rads of diagnostic x-irradiation over several weeks are necessary to produce cataracts in humans.[3,10,11] It may be that absorbed doses of about 1500 rads are necessary to induce cataracts in the diagnostic radiology setting.[6,10] Nonetheless, it is prudent to monitor the staff and use all reasonable means to decrease head and neck exposures in interventional radiology. These concerns often prompt the use of helmet-like protective devices (Moti X-ray Mask; Nuclear Associates), lead-acrylic eyeglasses, and thyroid shields.

STAFF RADIATION EXPOSURE MONITORING

In general, monitoring devices must be worn if it is reasonably likely that a person could receive 25% of the maximum permissible exposure in the discharge of his or her duties. This rule most assuredly mandates exposure monitoring of the interventional radiologist, the clinical colleagues routinely involved in procedures, and the usual support staff.

The most popular method of monitoring is the film badge because it is practical and economical. Usually, each person wears one film badge beneath the lead apron and another at collar level outside the lead apron. If only one film badge is available, it can be worn at either location provided that all persons adopt the same convention. The radiation protection officer must be informed of the convention so the reports of radiation exposure can be properly interpreted. The choice of location hinges on whether the maximum exposure or the whole-body exposure is more important, a matter which has for some time been controversial in the health physics community. Usually, the choice is made by the radiation protection officer at a particular facility.

Ring badges containing thermoluminescent dosimeters (TLD) may be worn to monitor hand radiation exposure.[10] This practice has not received overwhelming support because of technical problems with the dosimeters and the resistance of some radiologists.

A possible disadvantage of film badges and rings lies in the fact that the actual radiation exposure is not known until perhaps 2 months later, when the film is developed. The use of the personal ionization chamber ("pocket chamber") avoids this problem,[10] but these devices are expensive and fragile.

RADIATION PROTECTION IN FLUOROSCOPY

Radiation protection in interventional radiology using both conventional and C-arm fluoroscopy is discussed in this section. The radiation exposure of the operator is heavily dependent on imaging geometry. Typical isoex- posure lines for several imaging configurations are shown in Figure 2–3; note the tremendous increase in operator exposure with configurations in which the x-ray tube is above the patient. This increase occurs for two reasons:

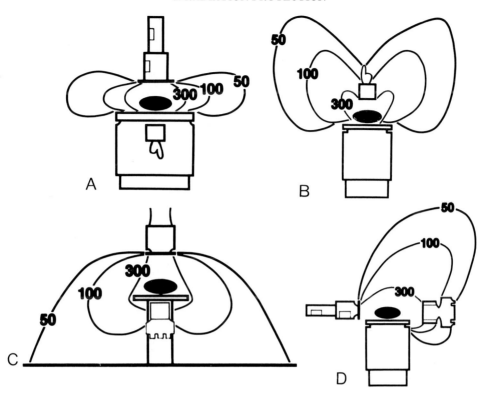

Fig. 2–3 Scatter radiation from several equipment configurations. Isoexposure lines are given in mR/hr. A. Conventional fluoroscopy. B. Overhead tube. C. Posteroanterior fluoroscopy with C- or U-arm. (Courtesy of General Electric Medical Systems Division.)

the overall intensity of the scattered radiation beam is approximately 98% greater at the patient entrance site compared to the patient exit,[1] and there is less attenuating material (e.g., image intensifier) between the patient and the operator. As a rule of thumb, the maximum operator exposure at a given distance occurs when there is an unobstructed path between an object and the location at which the x-ray beam enters the patient. For example, maximum operator eye exposure occurs when the operator can see the beam entrance site. The "see it-beat it" radiation protection procedure consists of changing one's position if it is possible to see the beam entrance area directly. In addition to the amount of time spent in a particular area during a procedure, overall distance from the patient is also important and indeed may be a primary consideration for some staff members. For example, anthropomorphic-phantom measurements of eye exposures for individuals 5'10" and 6'4" tall demonstrated an exposure increase of approximately 70%–115% for the shorter individual.[2] Different radiation protection considerations therefore may be necessary depending on staff members' heights. Because it is not always possible to change one's position relative to the beam, many devices have been suggested to reduce staff exposure during interventional radiology procedures.[12–17] Unfortunately, effective devices are often somewhat awkward given the usual time and space demands of interventional radiology.

In addition to time, distance, and shielding, another important radiation protection parameter is x-ray beam size. The amount of scattered radiation exposure is directly related to beam size. In addition, the patient dose and image quality are affected by changes in collimation.

Hence, by limiting the beam size to the smallest necessary area, the fluoroscopist can decrease both personnel and patient exposures while improving image quality.

The recent concept of surface shielding consists of shielding the operator's line of sight from the patient's surface rather than the operator's level.[12,19] The shielding may be fabricated in strips or solid pieces from lead aprons and therefore may be sterilized for reuse. Typical radiation exposure reductions with a 0.77-mm surface shield can range from 33%–75% (Fig. 2–4). The use of such devices is important to minimize staff radiation exposures and comply with regulations.

To provide perspective on the radiation exposures encountered in interventional radiology, consider the following example:

If   Radiation exposure = 300 mR/hr, fluoroscopy time = 0.5 hr/exam, and maximum permissible exposure = 1.25 R/quarter,

then   Allowable procedures = 8 exams/quarter!

The importance of attention to radiation protection during these procedures is apparent (Table 2–4).

In summary, to minimize personnel exposure during fluoroscopic interventional radiology, the lowest acceptable exposure rate and smallest acceptable field size should be used with the most efficacious equipment configuration.[20–22] Additionally, although the inverse-square law is not strictly maintained in fluoroscopy,[20] distance from the patient should be maximized, and when possible shielding material should be placed between the patient and personnel.

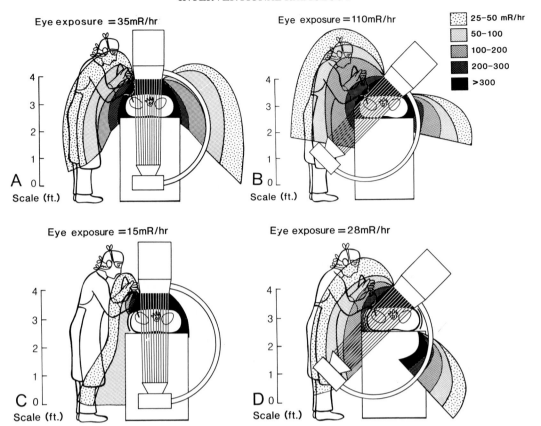

Fig. 2–4   Scatter radiation reduction with surface shielding (2.8 R/min patient skin entrance exposure). A. Vertical fluoroscopy without shielding. B. Oblique (45°) fluoroscopy without shielding. C. Vertical fluoroscopy with a 25 × 15-cm (0.75-mm lead equivalent) surface shield. D. Oblique (45°) fluoroscopy with surface shielding in place.

(Reprinted from Young AT, Morin RL, Hunter DW, et al: Surface Shield: device to reduce personnel radiation exposure. *Radiology* 1986;159:801–803 with permission of the Radiological Society of North America, Inc.)

RADIATION PROTECTION IN CINEFLUOROGRAPHY

Because cinefluorography (cine) is an extension of fluoroscopy, all of the previous radiation protection considerations apply; however, radiation exposure is significantly higher for the patient as well as the staff. Typical patient skin entrance exposures can range from 20–90 R/min,[23–25] depending on the system and image acquisition parameters—substantially higher than the typical 2–3 R/min[24,25] skin entrance exposures in fluoroscopy. The scattered radiation levels shown in Figure 2–4 were obtained with a skin entrance exposure of 2.8 R/min; to depict the cine scattered radiation exposure, the values in the figure should be multiplied by a factor of 7 to 32! Eye exposures for cine without shielding would range from 245–3520 mR/hr. The use of surface shielding would decrease these eye exposures to 105–896 mR/hr. Additionally, measurements indicate that eye exposure reductions of 84% are possible by changing the operator's position from table-side to 30 cm from the table.[26] Such reductions are system dependent and should be verified for a particular radiology suite.

From these observations, it is apparent that distance and shielding radiation protection techniques should receive increased attention when cine is used during interventional radiology procedures.

RADIATION PROTECTION IN COMPUTED TOMOGRAPHY

The scatter radiation distribution surrounding a computed tomography (CT) scanner is, of course, quite different from the exposure levels found in fluoroscopy, both because the beam area is much smaller during slice acquisition and because the x-ray tube gantry surrounds the patient, thereby providing shielding. Typical isoexposure lines for a CT scanner are shown in Figure 2–5.[10,27] Head and neck exposures could range from approximately 300–900 mR for an interventional procedure involving a table-side position for 10–20 exposures. Note that movement to the side of the gantry reduces exposure greatly in comparison to that received when one stands in front of or behind the gantry. In this case, a small step dramatically reduces radiation exposure.

SUMMARY

Interventional radiology demands an increased awareness of the fundamental radiation protection principles of time, distance, and shielding. Staff exposures can be reduced through the proper use and configuration of the imaging system, as well as through the use of ancillary shielding materials such as surface shielding. These considerations should be strongly reinforced when cine is utilized. Typical patient exposures are on the order of 3 R/min during fluoroscopy and 50 R/min during cine. Staff eye exposures can range from approximately 10–100 mR/hr during fluoroscopy and from approximately 100–2500 mR/hr during cine. In general, staff exposure is markedly decreased for interventional procedures that utilize CT, with the greatest reduction if staff members step to the side of the gantry or leave the room during the slice acquisition.

Table 2–4
Maximum Number of Fluoroscopic Procedures in a 3-Month Period without Exceeding Eye Exposure of 1.25 R/Quarter

Fluoroscopic Time per Procedure (hr)	Radiation Exposure at Eye Level (mR/hr)					
	10	25	50	100	200	300
0.10	1250	500	250	125	62	41
0.25	500	200	100	50	25	16
0.50	250	100	50	25	12	8
0.75	166	67	33	16	8	5
1.00	125	50	25	12	6	4
1.50	83	33	16	8	4	2
2.00	62	25	12	6	3	2

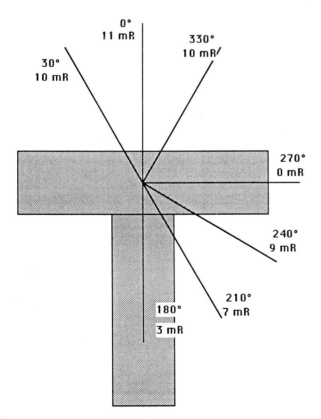

Fig. 2–5 Approximate scattered radiation exposures about CT scanner. Exposures are derived from reference 27 for a 130-kVp, 50-mA, 10-s, 10-mm scan at a distance of 1 m and a height equal to the isocenter.

References

1. Curry TS, Dowdy JE, Murry RC: *Christensen's Introduction to the Physics of Diagnostic Radiology.* Philadelphia, Lea & Febiger, 1984
2. Code of Federal Regulations, Title 21, parts 1000–1050, U.S. Government, 1985. Revision of the Radiation Control for Health and Safety Act of 1968
3. National Council of Radiation Protection and Measurements: *Basic Radiation Protection Criteria.* NCRP Report No. 39. Washington, DC, 1971
4. National Council on Radiation Protection and Measurements: *Medical X-Ray and Gamma Ray Protection for Energies up to 10 Mev.* NCRP Report No. 33. Washington, DC, 1968
5. National Council on Radiation Protection and Measurements: *Structural Shielding Design and Evaluation for Medical Use of X-Rays and Gamma Rays of Energies up to 10 Mev.* NCRP Publication No. 49. Washington, DC, 1976
6. Recommendations of the International Commission on Radiological Protection: *Radiation Protection.* ICRP Publication 26. Oxford, Pergamon Press, 1977
7. National Council on Radiation Protection and Measurements: *Review of the Current State of Radiation Protection Philosophy.* NCRP Report No. 43. Washington, DC, 1975
8. Code of Federal Regulations, Title 29, part 16, chapter 17, section 1910.96. Washington, DC, US Government Printing Office, 1971
9. Code of Federal Regulations, Title 10, part 20, chapter 1, section 20.102. Washington, DC, US Government Printing Office, 1971
10. Bushong SC: *Radiologic Science for Technologists: Physics, Biology, and Protection.* St. Louis, CV Mosby, 1984
11. Pizzarello DJ, Witcosfski RC: *Medical Radiation Biology.* Philadelphia, Lea & Febiger, 1982
12. Rusnak B, Castañeda–Zuñiga WR, Kotula F, et al: Radiolucent handle for percutaneous puncture under continuous fluoroscopic monitoring. *Radiology* 1981;141:538
13. Gertz EW, Wisneski JA, Gould RG, et al: Improved radiation protection for physicians performing cardiac catheterization. *Am J Cardiol* 1982;50:1283
14. Allsion JD, Teeslink CR: Special procedures screen. *Radiology* 1980;136:233
15. Thomson KR, Brammall J, Wilson BC: "Flagpole" lead-glass screen for radiographic procedures. *Radiology* 1982;143:557
16. Gilula LA, Barbier J, Totty WG, Eichling J: Radiation shielding device for fluoroscopy. *Radiology* 1985;147:882
17. Miotto D, Feltrin G, Calamosca M: Radiation protection device for use during percutaneous transhepatic examinations. *Radiology* 1984;151:799
18. Young AT, Morin RL, Hunter DW, et al: Surface shield: device to reduce personnel radiation exposure. *Radiology* 1986;159:801
19. Miller DL, Vucich JJ, Cope C: A flexible shield to protect personnel during interventional procedures. *Radiology* 1985;155:825

20. Linos DA, Gray JE, McIlrath DC: Radiation hazard to operating room personnel during operative cholangiography. *Arch Surg* 1980;115:1431

21. Jacobson A, Conley JG: Estimation of fetal doses to patients undergoing diagnostic x-ray procedures. *Radiology* 1976; 120:683

22. Bush WH, Jones D, Brannen GE: Radiation dose to personnel during percutaneous renal calculus removal. *AJR* 1985; 145:1261

23. Webster EW: Quality assurance in cineradiographic systems, in Waggener RG, Wilson CR (eds): *Quality Assurance in Diagnostic Radiology: Medical Physics Monograph No. 4.* New York, American Institute of Physics, 1980

24. Gray JE, Winkler NT, Stears J, Frank ED: *Quality Control in Diagnostic Imaging.* Baltimore, University Park Press, 1983

25. American Institute of Physics: *Evaluation of Radiation Exposure Levels in Cine Cardiac Catheterization Laboratories.* AAPM Report No. 12. New York, American Institute of Physics, 1984

26. Jeans SP, Faulkner K, Love HG, Bardsley RA: An investigation of the radiation dose to staff during cardiac radiological studies. *Br J Radiol* 1985;58:419

27. Picker International, Inc: *Typical Drawings and Specifications for Synerview 1200 SX/600S.* Cleveland, Picker International, Inc, 1982

3

Embolotherapy: Agents, Equipment, and Techniques

ANTONY YOUNG, M.D., S. MURTHY TADAVARTHY, M.D., CAROL C. COLEMAN, M.D., GUNNAR LUND, M.D., DAVID W. HUNTER, M.D., ANDREW H. CRAGG, M.D., JOHN F. CARDELLA, M.D., MICHAEL D. DARCY, M.D., TONY P. SMITH, M.D., FLAVIO CASTAÑEDA, M.D., AND KURT AMPLATZ, M.D., WILFRIDO R. CASTAÑEDA–ZUÑIGA, M.D., M.Sc.

Transcatheter vascular embolization has become an important aspect of the burgeoning field of interventional radiology and promises to increase in popularity as the indications for embolization are clarified and the techniques refined. Nonetheless, at present, when examining the considerable volume of literature on the subject, it should be recognized that many of these reports are anecdotal and written to demonstrate that a certain technique might be possible rather than to show the technique to be safe or as effective as traditional therapy by comparison with an adequate control group. Because of this failing, it is difficult to define the relative roles of embolotherapy and the conventional techniques of surgery, radiotherapy, drugs, and endoscopy for any given clinical situation. However, it seems likely that, although embolotherapy is now often used as a last resort when conventional therapy has failed, it eventually will assume a more prominent place in the treatment of hemorrhage and neoplasia. The challenge is to continue developing new techniques, to demonstrate the efficacy of embolotherapy, and to show that it can be reliable and safe.

HISTORICAL ASPECTS

Although it has been only in the last decade that there has been much interest in embolotherapy, the principle of vascular embolization is not new; it dates back to 1904, when Dawbain described preoperative injection of melted paraffin–petrolatum into the external carotid arteries of patients suffering head and neck tumors.[1] Brooks, in 1930, introduced particulate embolization when he described occluding a traumatic carotid–cavernous fistula by injecting a fragment of muscle attached to a silver clip into the internal carotid artery.[2] Similarly, Lussenhop and Spence, in 1960, injected spheres of methylmethacrylate into the surgically exposed common carotid artery of a patient suffering from an arteriovenous malformation (AVM) fed by the middle cerebral artery, achieving clinical improvement.[3]

In 1963, Baum and Nusbaum, in a landmark paper, demonstrated that bleeding at rates as low as 0.5 ml/min could be detected angiographically.[4] This report set the stage for the transcatheter management of hemorrhage, which was first achieved with selective infusions of vasopressin. In 1972, Rosch, Dotter, and Brown reported controlling acute gastric hemorrhage by embolization of the gastroepiploic artery with autologous clot.[5]

The tremendous upsurge of interest in embolization that began in the 1970s was fueled by parallel developments in catheter technology and embolic agents. The availability of a wide range of preshaped catheters and the introduction of coaxial systems allowed radiologists to place catheters subselectively, making possible highly selective delivery of embolic agents. Lin et al, in 1974, introduced the concept of injecting soft silicone tubing through lumens only slightly larger than itself,[6] and this was followed in 1974 by the report of Serbinenko from the Soviet Union of the use of detachable balloon catheters for embolization.[7] White and Debrun and their colleagues borrowed from these researchers and produced an injectable flow-directed catheter with a detachable silicone balloon for permanent vascular occlusion.[8,9] Similarly, Kerber developed a silicone calibrated-leak balloon that allows highly selective flow-directed placement and then balloon occlusion angiography or embolization using the low-viscosity tissue adhesives.[10]

The tissue adhesive isobutyl-2-cyanoacrylate (IBCA; Bucrylate) was introduced as an embolic agent in the United States by Zanetti and Sherman in 1972.[11] The use of Gelfoam particles as a medium-term embolic agent was first described by Carey and Grace in 1974.[12] For long-term results, polyvinyl alcohol (Ivalon) was used as a plug for closure of a patent ductus arteriosus by Portsmann et al in 1971,[13] and this led to research on its use in particulate form by Tadavarthy and coworkers.[14,15] In 1975, Gianturco and his colleaques created the wool coil, a modification of which is currently in widespread use.[16]

The concept of tissue ablation with absolute ethanol was introduced in 1981 by Ellman et al, who used it for infarction of kidneys.[17] In 1982, Amplatz and his colleagues demonstrated the efficacy of boiling contrast medium by publishing photomicrographs of an occluded vein from his own forearm.[18,19] Sodium tetradecyl sulfate (Sotradecol) has been similarly used as a visceral sclerosing agent.[20]

It is difficult to predict developments in a rapidly changing field such as interventional radiology. It may well be that the authors have overlooked what will turn out to be milestones, and for that, they apologize. Transcatheter electrocoagulation,[21,22] the guidance of emboli by external magnetic forces (Chapter 8),[23] and embolization with capsules of drugs or radioactive particles[24] may well be such milestones.

PATIENT CARE

Preoperative Management

Embolization is a major procedure, and it is imperative that the radiologist be fully aware of the clinical status of the patient. When taking the history, inquiry should be made into any previous operations. For example, previous surgery around the stomach may have destroyed the rich collateral blood supply to this organ, so that left gastric artery embolization, which is normally a relatively benign procedure, may lead to severe gastric ulceration or infarction.[25] Informed consent is obtained after a full and frank discussion of the benefits and the risks of the procedure, including the possibility of unintentional embolization of nontarget areas and pain both during and after the procedure. Relevant laboratory values and previous radiologic studies should be reviewed.

Before embolization, the patient should be well hydrated, both because of the potential need for large volumes of contrast medium and because of the possibility of acute renal failure, which has followed embolization of large soft tissue tumors as a result of hyperuricemia. Antibiotics are used preoperatively and for 2 or 3 days after embolization. A cephalosporin is a common choice. Other premedication consists of an intramuscular sedative such as secobarbital and a narcotic analgesic such as meperidine (Demerol), or midazolam (Versed) given intravenously during the procedure.

The intended puncture site should be shaved immediately before the procedure, preferably in the radiology suite, in order to reduce the superficial skin irritation with infection caused by shaving.

Intraoperative Care

During embolization procedures, the authors prefer to have a nurse anesthetist monitor the patient and administer drugs as necessary. Most embolizations are performed using local anesthesia and intravenous sedation. However, in children, when embolization is likely to be painful (for example, during embolization in a limb), general anesthesia may be chosen. Oxygen is delivered by nasal prongs; this may help to protect any tissues unintentionally embolized until collaterals develop. In all patients, proper fluid balance must be maintained.

Postoperative Care

Postoperatively, a high fluid input is important to reduce the likelihood of acute urate nephropathy. This is particularly true after embolization for liver tumors. Adequate analgesia should also be given, not only for the patient's comfort but also to reduce the risk of complications.[5] For example, abdominal pain may impair breathing motion, which may, in turn, lead to atelectasis and pneumonia. Antibiotics are continued for 2–3 days in most cases, and for up to 1 week after splenic embolization to decrease the risk of splenic abscess. Postembolization measurement of serum creatinine concentration is advisable as an assessment of renal function.

GENERAL PRINCIPLES OF EMBOLIZATION

The effects of embolization on any organ are specific to that organ, and this fact makes generalization about the techniques of embolization difficult. For example, proximal occlusion of the main renal artery is likely to cause infarction of the kidney, whereas occlusion of the common hepatic artery rarely results in hepatic necrosis because of the collateral blood supply of the liver and of the portal circulation, which provides approximately 75% of the blood flow to the liver and 50% of its oxygen requirement. The effects of embolization also depend on the clinical status of the patient. For example, hypotensive shock and infusions of vasopressin reduce portal venous flow and render the liver more susceptible to ischemic necrosis. Previous operations around the stomach and vasopressin infusion reduce the collateral supply, again increasing the susceptibility of the organ to necrosis following embolization. Concurrent disease such as atherosclerosis or vasculitis may also leave an organ more susceptible to ischemic necrosis. Age is another factor: occlusion of the common femoral artery in a child is usually well tolerated, although it often leads to later growth disturbance in the limb, whereas occlusion of the common femoral artery in an adult often leads to severe ischemia.

Proximal occlusion of an artery carries less chance of tissue necrosis because of the potential for collateralization into the distal circulation. Such occlusion may alter the hemodynamics sufficiently to stop a hemorrhage. Inducing the development of collaterals may be the purpose of the procedure. For example, when infusion of chemotherapy into the liver is complicated by the existence of an anomalous arterial supply to the right or left lobes, embolization of one of the major arteries results in the blood supply to the entire liver arising from the other vessel via existing collaterals that open up almost immediately.[26] Chemotherapy may then be given more efficiently.

Distal occlusion of vessels with minute particles or liquid agents carries a higher likelihood of tissue necrosis, which may well be the purpose of the procedure—for example, in renal ablation with ethanol.[17] Distal embolization reduces the possibility of blood being supplied to the tissues from collaterals, which may be desired, e.g., in embolization of an arteriovenous malformation (AVM). Such lesions almost invariably recur unless embolization is performed beyond the inflow from any collateral branches.

Generally, catheters should be placed as selectively as possible in order to avoid embolization of normal tissues. Reliance on the increased flow in a bleeding artery to guide the emboli is not only unsafe but particularly dangerous.

Reflux of emboli from the catheterized artery must be avoided. Delivery of particulate materials should be stopped once flow is severely reduced; no attempt should be made to occlude the vessel totally just distal to the catheter with particulates, as these are likely to reflux. Balloon occlusion catheters have been advocated to avoid reflux, although their value for this task is unproved.

Where a large organ or lesion is to be embolized, performing the procedure in separate stages is advisable in order to prevent widespread tissue necrosis, to allow time for normal tissues to recover, and to permit early detection of complications. Great care must be taken when embolizing with liquids such as silicone, IBCA, or absolute ethanol, because neurologic damage, both of peripheral nerves and of the spinal cord; necrosis of the bile ducts and of bronchi; and gastrointestinal perforation have all occurred.

MATERIALS FOR EMBOLIZATION

The radiologist performing embolization procedures should know well the physical, chemical, and biologic characteristics of the different embolic agents and devices currently available, as well as the best technique for their delivery. The embolic agent is selected on the basis of whether temporary or permanent occlusion is wanted; whether proximal or peripheral occlusion is desirable; and the individual vascular anatomy. Only if the proper choice is made will permanent success be achieved.

Embolic materials can be classified as absorbable (used for temporary occlusion) and nonabsorbable (used for permanent occlusion):

1. Absorbable materials:
   a. Autologous blood clot;
   b. Modified autologous blood clot;
   c. Oxycel (oxidized cellulose);
   d. Gelfoam (surgical gelatin sponge).
2. Nonabsorbable materials:
   a. Particulate agents:
      —Autologous fat or muscle;
      —Ivalon (polyvinyl alcohol (PVA) sponge);
      —Silastic spheres and Silastic with steel balls;
      —Stainless-steel pellets;
      —Ferromagnetic microspheres;
      —Acrylic spheres;
      —Methylmethacrylate spheres.
   b. Injectable (fluid) embolic agents:
      —IBCA;
      —IBCA modifications (tissue glues);
      —Silicone rubber;
      —Ethibloc (amino acid occlusion gel).
   c. Sclerosing agents:
      —Absolute ethanol;
      —Boiling contrast medium;
      —Sodium morrhuate;
      —Sotradecol.
   d. Nonparticulate agents:
      —Stainless-steel coils;
      —Stainless-steel coils with barbs;
      —Silk streamers;
      —Plastic brushes;
      —Detachable balloons.
3. Electrocoagulation (endovascular diathermy).

Embolic materials can either be radiopaque by themselves or be made radiopaque by the addition of various chemical compounds containing barium, tantalum, bismuth, tin, or other metals. However, with good fluoroscopy, even nonopaque emboli such as Ivalon can be seen if suspended in dilute contrast medium, particularly Pantopaque. Recently, techniques for radionuclide labeling of Gelfoam have been described that allow nonradiographic external location of the emboli with a gamma camera.[27,28]

Specific Embolic Agents and Techniques

AUTOLOGOUS MATERIALS

Various autologous materials, such as fragments of skeletal muscle, dura, and fat, have been used for embolization.[3,29,30] The duration of vessel occlusion with these agents is not known for certain but is probably several weeks to several months. The main disadvantage of these materials is that they need to be harvested from the patient, which necessitates a further procedure.

The most widely used autologous material has been blood clot (Fig. 3–1). The duration of vessel occlusion in swine, which have a fibrinolytic system similar to that of human beings, is >48 hr. After 2 weeks, approximately half of the vessels will be recanalized.[5]

The technique of injecting blood clot is as follows. Blood is drawn from the patient and allowed to clot in a sterile container. Once a solid clot has formed, some of it is aspirated into a 1-ml syringe and injected into the catheter. Because the clot conforms to the size of the catheter, it is easy to inject. Mixing the clot with additives has been

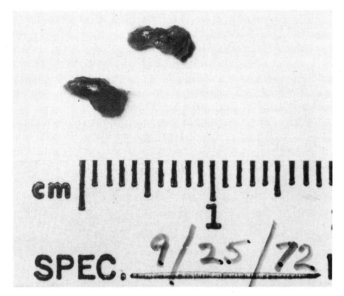

Fig. 3–1   Autologous blood clot.

proposed as a way to prolong vessel occlusion,[31] but the addition of thrombin or ε-aminocaproic acid to clot does not retard fibrinolysis, although it will help produce a firmer clot in patients with coagulation abnormalities.[31–33] Oxycel, which is made from oxidized cellulose, has also been added to clot; in dogs, this significantly retards clot lysis.[31,33,34] Because patients undergoing embolization for hemorrhage have impaired coagulation as a result of either their underlying disease or multiple transfusions, platelets and thrombi have been added to clots.

The advantages of autologous clot are its low cost and lack of toxicity. Its major disadvantage is its rapid lysis, which makes it unsuitable for uses other than treatment of hemorrhage and fistulae. Autologous clot has been said to be the embolic material of choice for severe bleeding after biopsy of the kidney, because the rapid dissolution may prevent renal infarction.[32]

Autologous blood clot is increasingly being superseded by Gelfoam and the more permanent embolic materials.

GELFOAM

Gelfoam (Upjohn Co.; Kalamazoo, MI) is an absorbable sponge derived from gelatin that was introduced in 1945 as an aid to hemostasis in surgical procedures. Light and Prentice showed that when Gelfoam is implanted in various locations in the cranium, the maximum tissue reaction is reached within 12 days, with complete disappearance of the material by 45 days.[35] In 1967, Ishimori introduced pledgets of Gelfoam into the surgically exposed internal carotid artery for embolization of carotid–cavernous fistulae.[36] Carey and Grace, in 1974, controlled hemorrhage from a duodenal ulcer.[12]

Gelfoam embolization causes a severe form of panarteritis characterized by infiltration of leukocytes into all layers of the vessel wall, as well as by disruption of the intima and elastic tissues. This panarteritis usually resolves completely within 4 months.[34,37,38] The occlusion lasts from a few days to a few weeks.

Gelfoam is commercially available in sheets or in powder. The sheets may be cut into suitable sizes with a scalpel or scissors (Fig. 3–2). The powder form consists of particles of 40–60 μm in diameter.

To prepare Gelfoam for injection, appropriate size particles are mixed thoroughly with 30% iodinated contrast medium. The Gelfoam is ready when it is clear and jellylike. A 10-ml syringe is used to aspirate one or several particles, depending on the target vascular bed. Because Gelfoam floats, the syringe should be held nozzle up while the particles are injected into a transparent tube connected to the angiographic catheter after the stopcock is removed. The loaded syringe is replaced with a syringe containing normal saline, and the contents of the connecting tube are carefully injected into the catheter. It is important not to inject too fast to avoid causing reflux of emboli from the target artery. The particles of Gelfoam usually can be seen as filling defects within the half-strength column of contrast medium.

After the emboli have been injected, careful test injections of full-strength contrast medium are made to determine the flow patterns. Once all the branch arteries have been occluded and blood flow is severely reduced, no more emboli should be injected. No attempt should be made to fill the main artery with Gelfoam, as there is a high risk of reflux of particles because of the turbulence produced by fast injection of additional emboli into the stagnant column of blood.[39] Greenfield et al advocate Gelfoam embolization with the aid of balloon occlusion to prevent reflux.[40] Even if balloon occlusion is used, however, the parent artery still should not be filled with Gelfoam because of the risk of reflux once the balloon is deflated. Test injections into the artery should be gentle, because otherwise they may dislodge fragments.

Fragments of Gelfoam as large as 4 mm in diameter can be injected through standard angiographic catheters as small as 3F. There is evidence that Gelfoam fragments in the catheter, making the injected particle smaller than intended.[40,41]

Gelfoam powder occludes vessels of 100–200 μm. As the particles measure 40–100 μm, they apparently clump to some extent. These particles travel more distally than do the larger fragments of Gelfoam, so there is a much higher incidence of ischemic complications when Gelfoam

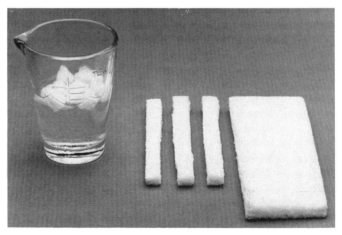

Fig. 3–2   Gelfoam emboli cut with scissors into small fragments.

powder is used, particularly with embolization of the gastrointestinal tract.[24] Gelfoam powder should not be used for embolization of large arteriovenous communications, because the particles may pass into the lung.

Gelfoam promotes clot formation, so thrombosis commonly propagates distal to the embolization site, but intact Gelfoam fragments are seldom found more than 24–48 hr postembolization. The duration of vascular occlusion averages 3–4 months, and recanalization usually follows.[34,37]

Gelfoam is commonly used for one of two purposes: nonpermanent occlusion, such as for preoperative embolization or control of hemorrhage,[43,44] and, in combination with a nonabsorbable substance such as a coil or tissue adhesive, for complete permanent vascular occlusion. A minor disadvantage of Gelfoam is its rapid contamination with bacteria when left exposed to room air, even in the operating room.[41]

Conroy et al label Gelfoam with radionuclides so that the destination of the emboli can be determined.[27] The present authors have also found this useful.

OXYCEL

This cotton-like material is made from oxidized cellulose (Parke–Davis; Detroit, MI). When added to blood, it makes a clot firmer. For introduction, the Oxycel–clot preparation is cut into small fragments with a blade or scissors. The fragments are aspirated with a 10-ml syringe, injected into the clear plastic tubing connected to the angiographic catheter, and flushed into the vessel with dilute contrast medium. Because of the harder nature of this embolic agent and the fact that recanalization commonly occurs within 4 months,[34] it is seldom if ever used now.

IVALON

Ivalon (Unipoint Industries) is a biologically inert PVA sponge with the unique property of being compressible when wet and of re-expanding to its original shape and size when a dried piece is placed in an aqueous solution such as blood (Fig. 3–3).[15] This property makes Ivalon particularly attractive for the occlusion of large vessels,[13,14,45] in which it produces a permanent occlusion.[15,45,46] Histologically, Ivalon is initially invaded by fibroblasts, with subsequent dense fibrous connective tissue formation around the sponge and a moderate inflammatory reaction around the area of thrombosis that involves the wall of the arteries. Organization of the thrombus then takes place, with fibrosis of the arterial wall and disappearance of the inflammatory infiltrate (Fig. 3–4). Recanalization of the thrombus does not occur, and partial occlusion of the vessel wall by an organized thrombus is commonly found beyond the site of the initial occlusion.[46]

Delivery Materials

Plug delivery via a catheter. From compressed Ivalon sponge, plugs of the proper size are cut and placed in plastic tubing connected to the catheter, from which they are flushed into the vessel.[15,47,48] Catheters should not have tapered tips and so require introduction through a sheath.

Delivery with a wire. Ivalon plugs also can be delivered by means of a wire.[45] The Ivalon is compressed around a stainless-steel mandrel in a vise (Figs. 3–5 and 3–6), and the resulting plugs are delivered through the catheter to a preselected site (Fig. 3–7). The plug and wire are left in place until the sponge re-expands to its original size. The plug is then stripped off either against a stainless-steel spring coil that fits over the mandrel or against the catheter tip. Small and medium-sized vessels can be occluded with one plug (Fig. 3–8). Some flow through the meshwork of the expanded plug may occur during the first 10–20 min until all pores become filled with fibrin. If flow is still apparent after 20 min, a second plug can be placed to complete the obliteration. Since it is friction against the vessel wall which holds the swollen plug in place, the plug should always be larger than the lumen of the vessel to be embolized, particularly in high-flow arteries, to prevent distal dislocation.

This method is especially helpful for exact placement of the plug at a predetermined site. Also, the site can be tested by advancing a similar wire without an attached plug. The main advantage of this technique is that the plug is passed rapidly through the catheter lumen, eliminating the intracatheter expansion of the plug that is so often a problem with transcatheter delivery of compressed Ivalon plugs because of their high friction coefficient. To retard the re-expansion of the compressed sponge, it is coated with a thin layer of 75% dextran solution, which keeps the plug in its compressed state for 60–90 sec after it makes contact with blood. This period is adequate for safe positioning of the plug at the desired site in the vessel. The 4- or 5-mm diameter plugs can be introduced through a 7F nontapered catheter; 9-mm plugs need a 9F thin-wall catheter (Formocath; Becton–Dickinson).

Shavings. Ivalon shavings are small particles produced from an uncompressed block (Fig. 3–9) with a metal saw blade (Fig. 3–10), blender,[49] or motor-driven rotating grasp (Fig. 3–11).[49,50] After the particles have been separated by size in a vibrating sieve (Fig. 3–12), shavings of similar size (0.25 mm, 0.5 mm, 1 mm, and

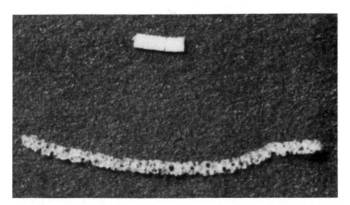

Fig. 3–3　Ivalon plug in compressed (top) and re-expanded (bottom) forms.

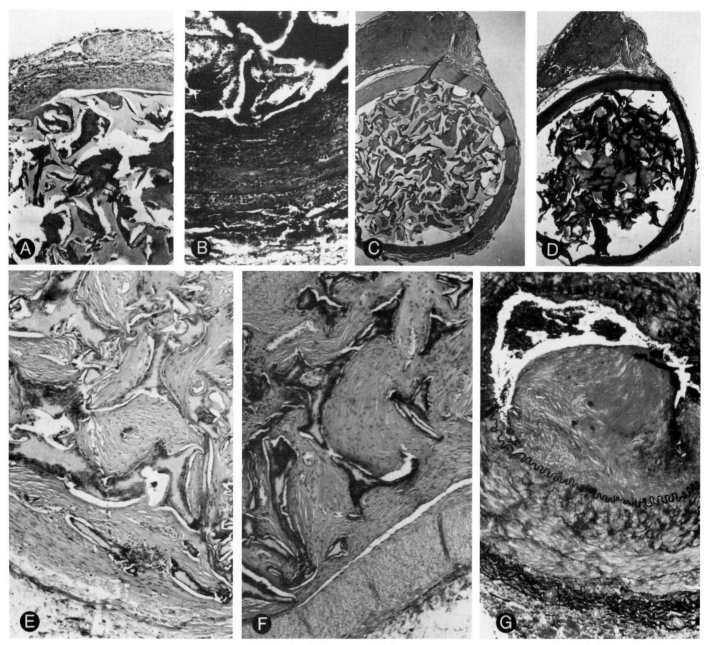

Fig. 3–4   Consequences of embolization. A. Canine splenic artery 3 days after embolization. Ivalon fragments fill vessel lumen, and clotted blood is present between fragments. Arterial wall is unremarkable. H & E; × 40. B. Splenic artery soon after embolization. Plastic fragments fill lumen. Note blood clot between fragments. Wall of artery is intact. × 250. C. Splenic artery of dog sacrificed 15 days after embolization. Thrombus has a histologic appearance similar to that in previous figure panel, but wall of artery appears to be infiltrated by polymorphonuclear leukocytes. Intimal division has disappeared. H & E; × 80. D. Artery 15 days after embolization, showing disruption of intima, disarranged elastic tissue, and wall with marked inflammatory infiltrate. Elastic tissue stains black with van Gissen stain. × 44. E. Nine months after embolization, thrombus appears fibrous and seems to be in continuity with vessel wall. Plastic fragments appear partially coated by calcium (dark areas). H & E; × 100. F. Arterial wall appears detached from thrombus and well preserved. H & E; × 100. G. Organized thrombus distal to main embolus does not contain plastic fragments. Note that lamina elastica is fragmented in one small area. van Gissen stain; × 125. (Reproduced from Castañeda–Zuñiga WR, Sanchez R, Amplatz K: Experimental observations on short- and long-term effects of arterial occlusion with Ivalon. *Radiology* 1978;126:783–785.)

larger) are packaged in plastic bags and sterilized with ethylene oxide (Fig. 3–13).

The Ivalon suspension is prepared at the beginning of the procedure by mixing 20 ml of Rheomacrodex (dextran 40,000; Pharmacia, Piscataway, NJ), 10 ml of 60% diatrizoate, and 5 ml of albumin with 1 teaspoonful (about 5 ml) of Ivalon particles in a glass beaker (Fig. 3–14A). This mixture prevents aggregation of the Ivalon particles resulting from their surface charge (Fig. 3–14B). That is, albumin, because of its bipolar charge, probably is adsorbed onto the surface of the particles, so that each Ivalon particle exerts a repellent force. Dextran probably

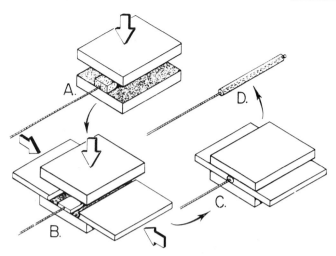

Fig. 3–5 Schematic representation of compression of Ivalon plug around a wire. (Reproduced from Zollikofer C, Castañeda–Zuñiga WR, Galliani C, Rysavy JA, Formanek A, Amplatz K: Therapeutic blockade of arteries using compressed Ivalon. *Radiology* 1980;136:635–640.)

increases the viscosity, delaying sedimentation of the particles. To facilitate delivery, a special cone-shaped syringe is used for injection (Fig. 3–15). This design eliminates peripheral stagnation of the particles at the distal end of the syringe.[49]

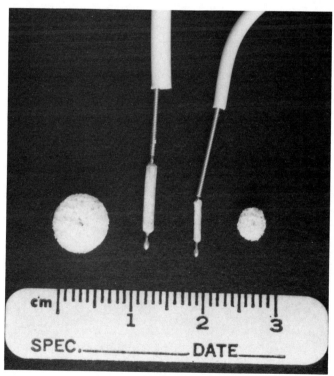

Fig. 3–6 Ivalon plugs of 8- and 3-mm diameter in expanded and compressed form around stainless-steel wire. The 8-mm compressed plug passes through 9F thin-wall Formocath nontapered catheter; the 3-mm compressed plug passes through 7F wire-mesh catheter with tapered tip cut off. (Reproduced from Zollikofer C, Castañeda–Zuñiga WR, Galliani C, Rysavy JA, Formanek A, Amplatz K: Therapeutic blockade of arteries using compressed Ivalon. *Radiology* 1980;136:635–640.)

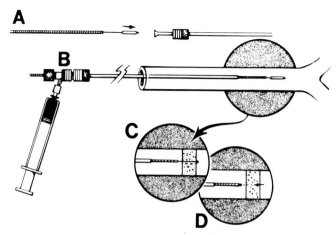

Fig. 3–7 Schematic representation of mechanism of delivery of compressed Ivalon plugs over wire. A. Compressed Ivalon plug on wire is advanced through angiographic catheter after removal of Tuohy–Borst adapter. B. Compressed Ivalon plug on wire is advanced to preselected site for arterial occlusion; Tuohy–Borst adapter has been tightened around wire to prevent blood loss during wait for Ivalon re-expansion. Flushing can be performed through sidearm of adapter. C. Ivalon plug has re-expanded to its original dimensions after contact with blood. D. Stainless-steel wire is pulled back gently from within re-expanded, slightly oversized Ivalon plug, which remains in place without migration because of pressure it exerts on arterial wall. (Reproduced from Zollikofer C, Castañeda–Zuñiga WR, Galliani C, Rysavy JA, Formanek A, Amplatz K: Therapeutic blockade of arteries using compressed Ivalon. *Radiology* 1980;136:635–640.)

A simpler preparative method has been described by Kerber et al.[48] After being sorted by size, particles are placed in 50-ml bottles with saline and sterilized. For injection, the particles are passed back and forth between two syringes connected by plastic tubing through a partially closed stopcock after the air has been expelled. When the particles are uniformly suspended, they are transferred to a syringe containing contrast medium for injection through the angiographic catheter.[48]

Uses

The disadvantage of Ivalon is that it is cumbersome to prepare and introduce. Furthermore, a relatively high injection pressure is needed to eject the particles into the blood vessel, increasing the risk of reflux of the embolus. Therefore, delivery of shavings through balloon occlusion catheters has been recommended.[39,40] On the other hand, because of the readily adjustable size of this material, practically all types of embolization can be performed. The small particles are ideal for peripheral embolization of AVMs and for tumor ablation,[15,49,51] while, in combination with metal devices that secure it in the lumen, an Ivalon plug can be used for occlusion of larger arteries.[52,53] For example, compression in a vise of the Ivalon plug around the straightened end of a stainless-steel spring coil (coilon) (Fig. 3–16A,B) or on a wire attached to a spider (spiderlon) (Fig. 3–17A,B) was reported by Zollikofer and Castañeda and their coworkers.[52,53] The advantages of these devices are, first, that total occlusion is achieved in one stage at the chosen site and, if needed,

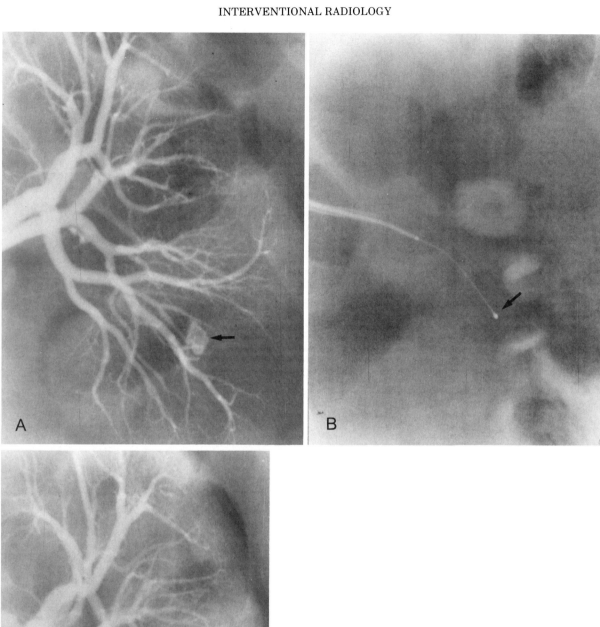

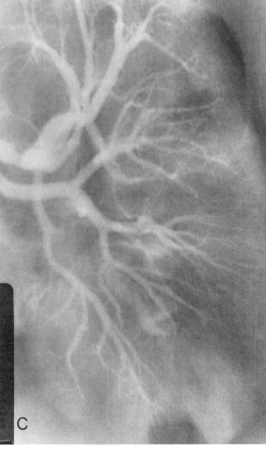

Fig. 3–8 Management of AV fistula. A. Left renal arteriogram in patient with postbiopsy AV fistula and recurrent hematuria; false aneurysm of branch of anterior division of artery (arrow). B. A 3-mm compressed Ivalon plug has been advanced beyond tip of catheter into branch with abnormality (arrow). C. Complete obliteration of lower branch is noted 10 min after release of plug.

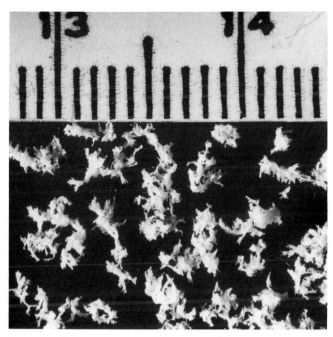

Fig. 3–9 High-power view of Ivalon particles produced by saw blade. Observe extreme variability in size, which makes separation of the particles by graduated sieves a necessity.

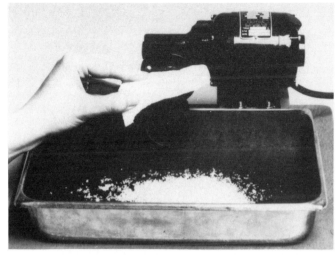

Fig. 3–11 Rotating grasp for mechanical production of Ivalon particles. (Reproduced from Herrera M, Rysavy J, Kotula F, Castañeda–Zuñiga WR, Amplatz K: Ivalon shavings: a new embolic agent. *Radiology* 1982;144:638–640.)

an additional Ivalon plug can be safely placed behind the coilon or spiderlon. In addition, a large Ivalon plug occludes the vessel more rapidly than does a woolly or Dacron-tailed coil. Finally, the same technique can be used in the venous system simply by changing the location of the Ivalon plug: pulmonary embolization is prevented by placing the steel coil upstream from the plug (Fig. 3–18A). For placement, the coilon is mounted over a special introducer from which it is stripped by advancing the spring coil over the mandrel (Fig. 3–19).

Attempted occlusion of large AV fistulae with Gianturco coils, Gelfoam, Ivalon, or other embolic agents can lead to pulmonary embolization (Fig. 3–20) because of the larger caliber and rapid flow in the vessel.[54] To prevent this complication, two devices have been developed. The first is a barbed stainless-steel coil, whose sharp barbs are embedded in the vascular wall upon leaving the catheter (Fig. 3–21), so that the coil forms a baffle behind which additional Gianturco coils or Ivalon plugs can be deposited (Fig. 3–22).[55] On the venous side, dislodgment of the embolic agent may result from pressure changes such as coughing or because the veins become larger toward the heart. The other device is a stainless-steel spider with a design similar to the Mobin–Uddin-type vena caval filter (Fig. 3–23).[56] The spider can be modified by attaching a piece of stainless-steel wire to its cone head, over which an Ivalon plug is compressed.[53] For introduction, the spider is mounted on an introducer wire (Fig. 3–24) and placed in the catheter with the prongs oriented

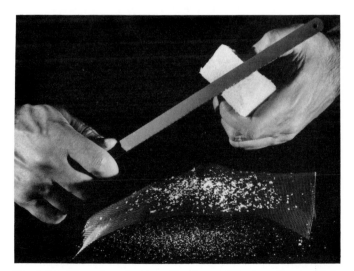

Fig. 3–10 Manual production of Ivalon particles by using saw blade to shave surface of block. A wire mesh of known dimension is used to separate particles.

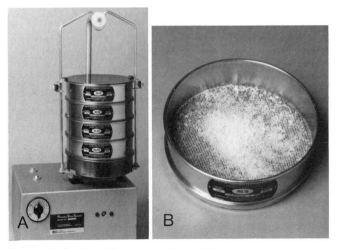

Fig. 3–12 Sorting of Ivalon particles. A. Vibrating sieve used to sort Ivalon particles by size. B. Individual container from sieve, showing collected particles.

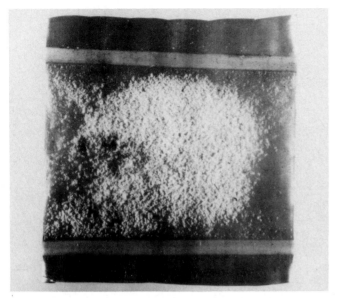

Fig. 3–13 Ivalon particles packed in sterile plastic container for storage. (Reproduced from Herrera M, Rysavy J, Kotula F, Castañeda–Zuñiga WR, Amplatz K: Ivalon shavings: a new embolic agent. *Radiology* 1982;144:638–640.)

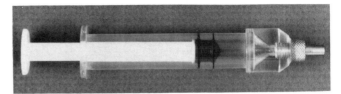

Fig. 3–15 Cone-shaped syringe for injection of Ivalon particles facilitates central flow.

in the direction of the blood flow and the Ivalon plug trailing. As the prongs emerge from the catheter tip, they open immediately, piercing the vessel wall and preventing migration and pulmonary embolization (Fig. 3–25). Once the prongs engage the vessel wall, the introducing wire is removed.[53,56]

Ivalon has been used as a plug after percutaneous splenoportography to tamponade the tract,[57] as well as for occlusion of any other tubular structure. Generally, Ivalon is used in diluted contrast medium, but the particles also can be made radiopaque by adding 60% barium sulfate or tantalum powder.[47,48]

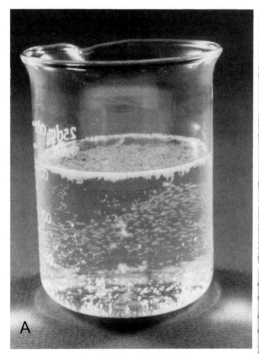

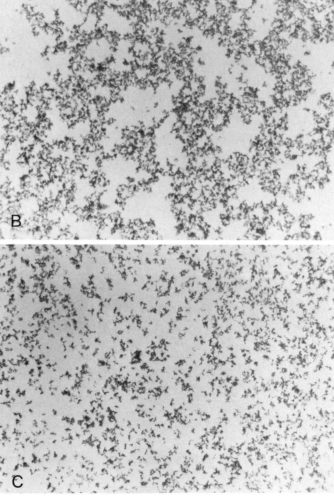

Fig. 3–14 Preparation of Ivalon particles for injection. A. Ivalon suspension in crystal container ready for injection. B. Particles suspended in contrast medium; note agglutination. C. Particles suspended in solution of contrast medium and Rheomacrodex; note lack of agglutination. (Reproduced from Herrera M, Rysavy J, Kotula F, Castañeda–Zuñiga WR, Amplatz K: Ivalon shavings: a new embolic agent. *Radiology* 1982;144:638–640.)

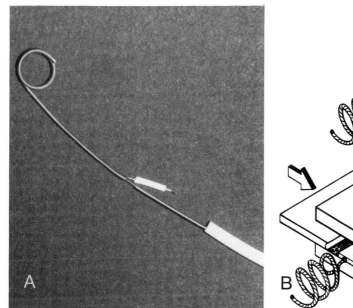

Fig. 3–16 Embolization devices. A. Coilon for arterial embolization loaded over coil introducer. B. Ivalon plug mounted over wire attached to spring coil during compression in a vise. (Reproduced from Zollikofer C, Castañeda–Zuñiga WR, Galliani C, et al: A combination of stainless steel coil and compressed Ivalon: a new technique for embolization of large arteries and arteriovenous fistulas. *Radiology* 1981;138:229–231.)

OTHER NONABSORBABLE PARTICULATE MATERIALS

Microspheres of different materials such as stainless[58] or ferromagnetic[23,59] steel, acrylic,[60] methylmethacrylate,[3] Silastic, and silicone[61–63] are inert and available in a great variety of sizes. Most of them are radiopaque, allowing detection by radiography. Microspheres are commonly used to occlude AVMs of the nervous system.

One of the specific advantages of Silastic or silicone spheres is a specific gravity that lets them float and consequently have a flow-guided distribution. This makes them advantageous for occluding lesions with strong flow, such as hypervascular tumors or AVMs.[64]

ISOBUTYL-2-CYANOACRYLATE

IBCA (Ethicon; Braum–Melsungen, etc.) is a rapidly hardening plastic adhesive chemically similar to Superglue. It has been used surgically since the 1960s[65] and radiologically since 1972.[11] The rationale behind its use is the possibility of directly and selectively depositing the embolic agent in the desired location. The liquid plastic is readily injectable, even through very small (3F) catheters, and polymerizes almost immediately upon contact with ionic fluids such as blood or vascular endothelium. This polymerization leaves the plastic solid.[66] By modifying the introducing technique or the polymerization process, localized obstruction or casts of the vascular tree can be obtained (Fig. 3–26).

A coaxial technique is used, utilizing a 6.5F or 7F catheter for catheterization of the desired vessel. Once a suitable position has been reached, a 3F Teflon catheter is introduced through the larger catheter and advanced beyond its tip. The inner catheter is then flushed with glucose solution through a 3-way stopcock to clear it of blood or contrast medium. The previously opacified IBCA is injected through the inner catheter after changing the position of the stopcock. The forward progress of the adhesive should be carefully monitored so the injection can be stopped as soon as the desired occlusion has been obtained; at this moment, the stopcock is switched and the inner catheter is flushed with glucose solution, to prevent the catheter tip from being glued to the blood vessel.[67,68] Balloon occlusion of the vessel has been recommended to help localize the obstruction.[67]

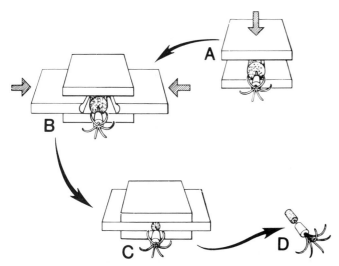

Fig. 3–17 Ivalon plug mounted over wire attached to a spider during compression in a vise (A, B, C). Spiderlon (D). (Reproduced from Castañeda–Zuñiga WR, Galliani CA, Rysavy J, Kotula F, Amplatz K: "Spiderlon": a new device for simple, fast arterial and venous occlusion. *AJR* 1981;136:627–628. © by American Roentgen Ray Society, 1981.)

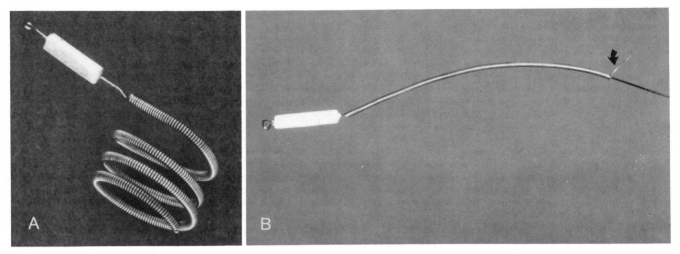

Fig. 3–18 Coilons. A. Spring embolus with compressed Ivalon plug on wire for venous obliteration. B. Coilon for venous embolization loaded over introducer. Observe modification of proximal end of spring by straightening to facilitate fixation of device in vein and so prevent migration (arrow).

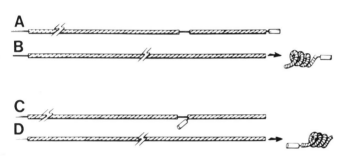

Fig. 3–19 Schematic representation of delivery of venous (A, B) and arterial (C, D) coilon using coil introducer.

Modification of the polymerization process is required when a cast of the vascular tree is desired, as for AVMs or for organ ablation. Goldman et al recommend mixing the adhesive with Ethiodol.[67]

Abroad, IBCA is the most popular tissue adhesive. In the United States, however, it is not approved for clinical use except for experimental purposes.

Because of the rapid polymerization of the plastic upon contact with ionic substances, a coaxial catheter technique and considerable skill are required for IBCA use.[67,69] It is not radiopaque by itself, but it can be readily mixed with tantalum powder,[67,70] ethiodized oils,[70] or

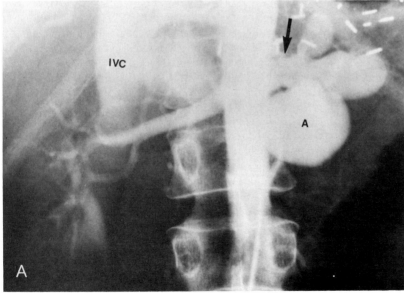

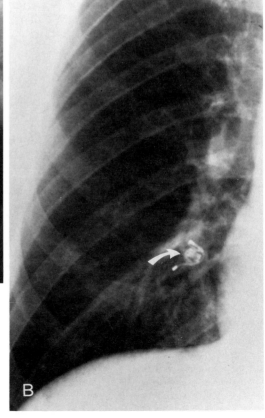

Fig. 3–20 Inappropriate embolization of occluding device in high-flow fistula. A. Abdominal aortogram reveals extensive AV shunting through stump of left renal artery postnephrectomy (arrow). IVC = inferior vena cava; A = aneurysm. B. Attempts to obliterate fistula with Gianturco-Wallace-Chuang (GWC) spring coil resulted in pulmonary embolization of occluding device (arrow). (Reproduced from Mazer MJ, Baltaxe HA, Wolf GL: Therapeutic embolization of the renal artery with Gianturco coils: limitations and technical pitfalls. *Radiology* 1981;138:37–46.)

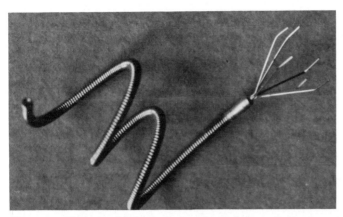

Fig. 3–21 Spring coil with barbed ends used for embolization of large AV fistulae. (Reproduced from Castañeda–Zuñiga WR, Tadavarthy SM, Beranek I, Amplatz K: Nonsurgical closure of large arteriovenous fistulas. *JAMA* 1976;236:2649–2650. Copyright 1976, American Medical Association.)

iophendylate.[71] Addition of these oily substances or of nitrocellulose[72] also slows the polymerization of the plastic, making it easier to handle. Prefilling of the catheter and flushing of the entire system with 50% glucose solution permit clinical application without risk of the catheter tip becoming glued to the vessel.[68]

This occlusive material can be introduced through small catheters, yet larger vessels can be occluded.[67] One of the principal applications is in AVMs because the instant hardening of the plastic can prevent the pulmonary embolization that is often a problem in such lesions with other agents.[47,69] A disadvantage of IBCA is the severe inflammatory local reaction it engenders, which is predominantly a foreign body-type reaction with multinucleated giant cells migrating around the particles.[65,73] Use of IBCA should be undertaken with great caution in

the gastrointestinal tract, since peripheral embolization of the adhesive can cause ischemic changes.[73,74] The use of IBCA is discussed further in Chapter 7 on embolotherapy in the treatment of male subfertility.

SILICONE RUBBER

Silicone rubber (Dow–Corning) is a convenient biocompatible material for vascular embolization. The substance can be made radiopaque by adding tantalum powder but is also available from the manufacturer as a radiopaque preparation. A silicone rubber mixture consists of Silastic elastomers that are vulcanized by catalysts.[75] The catalysts are mixed with liquid prior to injection, and the amount of catalyst can be altered in order to control the speed of polymerization.[75,76] To decrease the viscosity of the silicone rubber mixture, a specific fluid can be added in various proportions.[76] Thus, selective injection of vessels of any size can be achieved.

Silicone rubber seems to be an ideal substance for creating complete vascular casts.[75,76] Cessation of blood flow facilitates the injection, so the use of double-lumen balloon catheters is advantageous.[76] For safe delivery of the substance and to prevent spillover, a highly selective injection is desired. The disadvantage of silicone rubber is that it does not have adhesive properties. Thus, the vascular bed must be completely filled to keep the substance in place (Fig. 3–27). No reaction between the elastomer and the vessel wall is apparent macroscopically or microscopically.[75]

ETHIBLOC

Ethibloc (Ethicon) is an amino acid occlusion gel said to be specifically appropriate for preoperative emboliza-

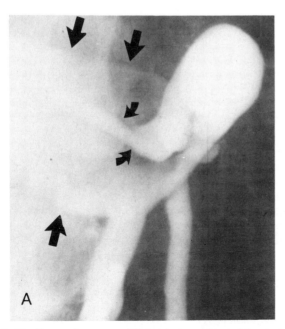

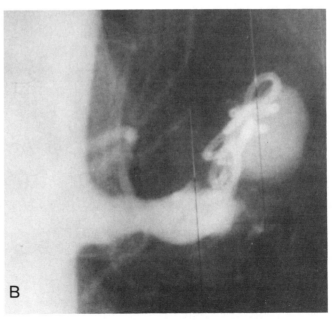

Fig. 3–22 Postnephrectomy AV fistula in patient with renal allograft and severe high-output congestive heart failure. A. Selective injection of stump of left renal artery (small arrows) reveals extensive AV shunting through stump of renal vein, which is severely dilated (large arrows). B. After placement of barbed coil, additional GWC spring embolus and silk streamers were placed to cause complete thrombosis of fistula. (Reproduced from Castañeda–Zuñiga WR, Tadavarthy SM, Beranek I, Amplatz K: Nonsurgical closure of large arteriovenous fistulas. *JAMA* 1976;236:2649–2650. Copyright 1976, American Medical Association.)

Fig. 3–23 Stainless-steel spider. A. Spider mounted on introducer. B. Tip of introducer is of smaller diameter than the remainder of stylet to allow its placement through hollow core of spider.

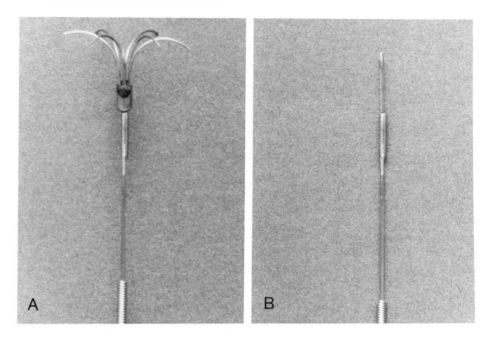

tion of renal tumors.[77] The substance is made radiopaque with iodine. Ethibloc has a low viscosity and comes premixed in a plastic syringe. It penetrates deep into the vascular tree, apparently without risk of pulmonary embolization.[77,78]

MICROFIBRILLAR COLLAGEN

Microfibrillar collagen (MFC) is a hemostatic agent derived from bovine hide. Its mechanism of action is thought to involve platelet aggregation and activation.[79]

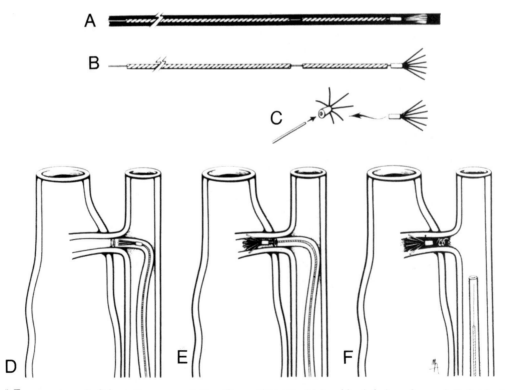

Fig. 3–24 Spider delivery system. A. Schematic representation. B. Folded spider is being advanced with legs forward through angiographic catheter. C. Upon exiting from angiographic catheter, legs of spider expand and engage arterial wall. D. Diagram of AV communication between stump of renal artery and inferior vena cava with selective catheterization of arterial stump by angiographic catheter, through which spider is being advanced. E. Spider has been released beyond catheter tip. F. With spider secured, angiographic catheter has been removed. (Reproduced from Castañeda–Zuñiga WR, Tadavarthy SM, Galliani C, Laerum F, Schwarten D, Amplatz K: Experimental venous occlusion with stainless steel spiders. *Radiology* 1981;141;238–241.)

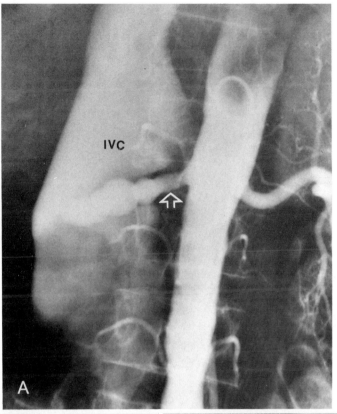

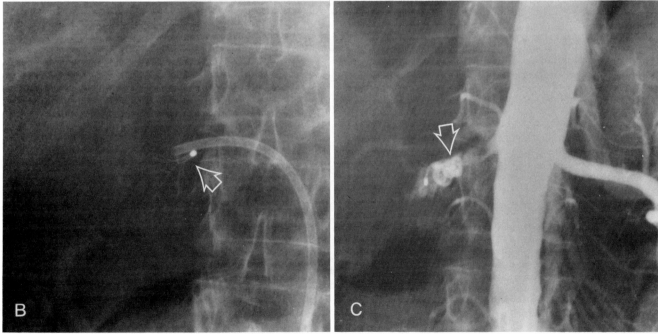

Fig. 3–25 Postnephrectomy AV fistula of left kidney. A. Abdominal aortogram shows large fistula between stump of right renal artery (open arrow) and inferior vena cava (IVC). B. A spider has been placed within stump of artery (arrow). C. Aortogram reveals complete thrombosis of arterial stump (arrow) after placement of two GWC spring emboli behind spider. (Reproduced from Castañeda-Zuñiga WR, Tadavarthy SM, Galliani C, Laerum F, Schwarten D, Amplatz K: Experimental venous occlusion with stainless steel spiders. *Radiology* 1981:141;238–241.)

When mixed with methylglucamine diatrizoate, MFC forms a radiopaque suspension that can be injected easily through an angiographic catheter as small as 3F. Two weeks after embolization, there is a severe granulomatous arteritis, which subsides by 3 months, with fibrosis replacing inflammation. Histologically, MFC occludes large and medium vessels as well as small end arteries. This last feature, although desirable in the preoperative or palliative embolization of tumors or in the nonsurgical management of AVMs, where a distal occlusion is impor-

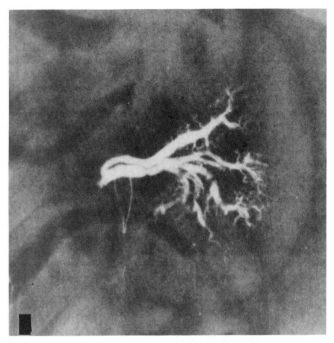

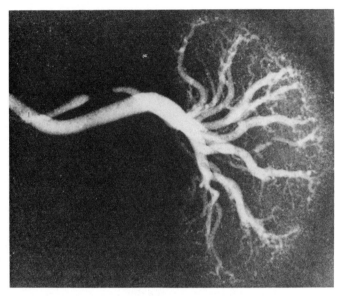

Fig. 3–27   Cast of renal artery has been formed with silicone mixture made radiopaque by addition of heavy metals.

Fig. 3–26   Cast of renal artery produced with IBCA made radiopaque by addition of tantalum powder.

tant to prevent recurrences,[80] is undesirable in other applications such as control of bleeding in the gastrointestinal tract, where it could cause tissue necrosis by reducing collateral flow.[81]

MFC is available in sterile 1-g and 5-g containers as a dry, finely shredded substance that is mixed with contrast medium to produce a suspension. Small amounts of the suspension are injected, and the catheter is immediately flushed with 3–5 ml of saline to prevent blockage. The use of an introducer sheath is recommended for catheter exchange purposes. A coaxial technique has also been used for delivery, as has a balloon occlusion method to prevent reflux of the embolic agent into peripheral vessels, which has been one of the complications of MFC use.[80]

ABSOLUTE ETHANOL

Recently, absolute ethanol was added to the list of sclerosing agents for transvascular embolization. It has aided in the obliteration of gastroesophageal varices and is able to produce organ ablation.[17,82] Absolute ethanol is presumed to have a direct toxic effect on the endothelium that activates the coagulation system on the dehydrated endothelial layers. Vascular occlusion, therefore, is not achieved instantly but rather in days to weeks.[17] The toxic effect extends into the perivascular tissues, and use of absolute ethanol has caused perivascular necrosis.[83]

Depending on the size of the vessel to be occluded and on the velocity of blood flow, the amount of absolute ethanol needed differs. Several injections may be required to occlude major feeders. The use of double-lumen balloon catheters is recommended. Absolute ethanol can also be delivered through tiny flow-guided balloon catheters, which is a distinct advantage of this substance. It is naturally sterile and is diluted quickly after injection, which reduces the direct toxic effect. No clinically important systemic toxic effects have been reported. Use of this agent is discussed in more detail in later chapters.

HOT CONTRAST MEDIUM

Contrast medium heated to 100° C has been successful at the University of Minnesota in experimental animals for obliteration of spermatic veins.[18,19] Both toxic[84] and heat[18,19] damage was seen in the vessels, and permanent occlusion of veins was achieved after injection of as little as 2 ml (Fig. 3–28A–C). Thrombosis was not immediate; thrombi usually appeared in the lumen and vasa vasorum after 1–5 days. In all cases, the thrombi were well organized at the end of 2 weeks, with no evidence of perivascular damage.[18] The occlusion becomes permanent by the invasion of fibroblasts, which turn the vessel into a fibrous cord (Fig. 3–28D).

The technique requires transmission of heat through an angiographic catheter 80–100 cm long. Fortunately, minimal heat loss occurs during transit through the catheter, probably due to the poor thermal conduction properties of plastics and the high specific heat of the contrast medium. Heated contrast medium is preferred to heated saline or glucose solutions for two reasons: first, contrast medium can be seen fluoroscopically, so the length of the thermal injury can be controlled. Second, the hypertonicity of contrast medium may cause cumulative damage to the vascular endothelium. An advantage of heated contrast medium over other sclerosing agents is that heat is rapidly dissipated by mixing with blood, whereas thrombosis caused by the effects of other sclerosing agents cannot be prevented by blood.[85] Thus, the extent of thermal injury is governed by heat dissipation, the capacity of the treated vessel, and the diluting effect of blood flow.

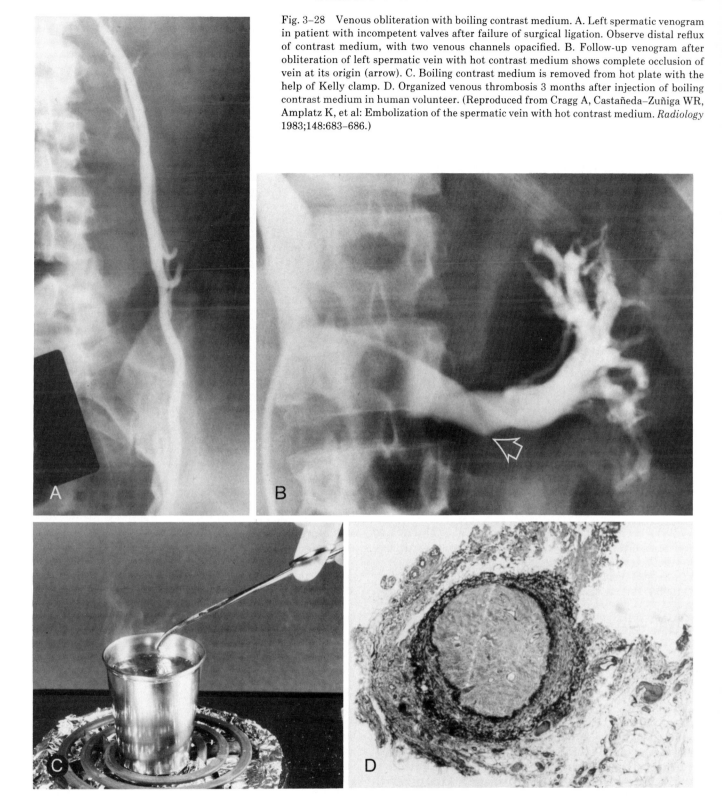

Fig. 3–28 Venous obliteration with boiling contrast medium. A. Left spermatic venogram in patient with incompetent valves after failure of surgical ligation. Observe distal reflux of contrast medium, with two venous channels opacified. B. Follow-up venogram after obliteration of left spermatic vein with hot contrast medium shows complete occlusion of vein at its origin (arrow). C. Boiling contrast medium is removed from hot plate with the help of Kelly clamp. D. Organized venous thrombosis 3 months after injection of boiling contrast medium in human volunteer. (Reproduced from Cragg A, Castañeda–Zuñiga WR, Amplatz K, et al: Embolization of the spermatic vein with hot contrast medium. *Radiology* 1983;148:683–686.)

Clinically, this method has been successful for obliterating the spermatic vein in subfertile men with varicoceles.[86] The method has been unsuccessful in obliterating AVMs, probably due to too rapid dissipation of heat by the inflow of blood from additional feeding vessels during contrast injection into the main vessel.

GIANTURCO COILS

Gianturco and Wallace introduced steel coils for permanent vascular occlusion of major arteries.[16,87] The devices have been used mainly for preoperative embolization of renal cell carcinomas and bleeding tumors. They

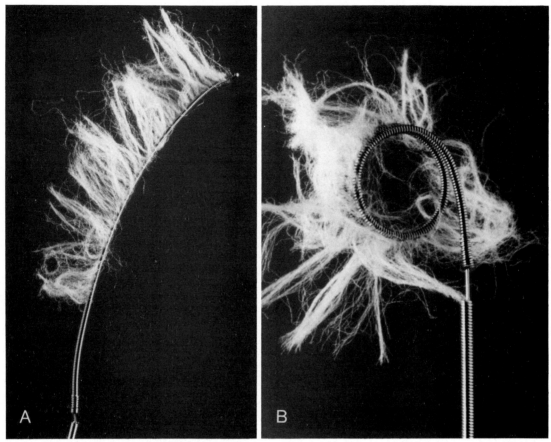

Fig. 3–29 GWC minicoil. A. Mounted over introducer wire. B. Partially extruded from introducer wire. (Reproduced from Castañeda–Zuñiga WR, Zollikofer C, Barreto A, Formanek A, Amplatz K: A new device for the safe delivery of stainless steel coils. *Radiology* 1980;136:230–231.)

also have been used for complete organ ablation as an alternative to surgical intervention, although, because of the persistence of distal flow beyond the coil from collateral parasitic vessels, particulate or fluid embolic agents generally are preferred for palliative purposes when no operation is contemplated.

There is experimental as well as clinical evidence that permanent vascular occlusion occurs after coil placement.[73] The coils do not occlude the vessel lumen completely but rather induce thrombosis. To increase thrombogenicity, wool strands ("tails") were attached to the coils, but because of the severe granulomatous arteritis induced by these woolly tails, which extended into and beyond the adventitia, the wool was replaced by Dacron in subsequent designs. The result of embolization with these devices is similar to surgical ligation, although if complete control of hemorrhage or complete organ infarction is desired, combined use of a more peripheral occluding agent plus a coil placed more proximally is recommended. The principal indications for the use of spring coils currently are obliteration of large AV fistulae,[88] occlusion of large vessels after trauma,[89] preoperative embolization of renal tumors,[16,87] obliteration of esophageal varices,[90] and occlusion of systemic–pulmonary shunts accompanying congenital heart disease.[91] Steel coils are available in many sizes (Fig. 3–29) and may be introduced through small catheters—*e.g.*, the 4-mm diameter coil through an untapered 5F polyethylene catheter.[92]

The complications of steel coil use, both immediate and delayed, have been discussed in detail by Mazer and coworkers[54] and will be summarized here.

Immediate Complications of Coil Use

Misplacement during insertion of the coil through a noncustomized catheter. Minicoils are designed for insertion through a 5F polyethylene, tapered-tip, nontorquable catheter with a floppy-tip 0.035-inch guidewire as a pusher. A common mistake is attempting to pass a minicoil through a 6F or 7F preshaped torque-control catheter; but when this is done, the minicoil tends to buckle inside the larger lumen (Fig. 3–30), allowing the pusher to wedge through it and hinder coil advancement. Switching to a more rigid mechanical pusher may only produce additional complications such as proximal catheter perforation.[54] A coil wedged within a catheter can be safely withdrawn by removing the catheter, but a coil that is partially dangling outside the catheter and cannot be extruded further is a more difficult dilemma. If the coil is not washed off the catheter by the blood current, it is likely to be expelled from the tip as the catheter is withdrawn from the puncture site. Thus,

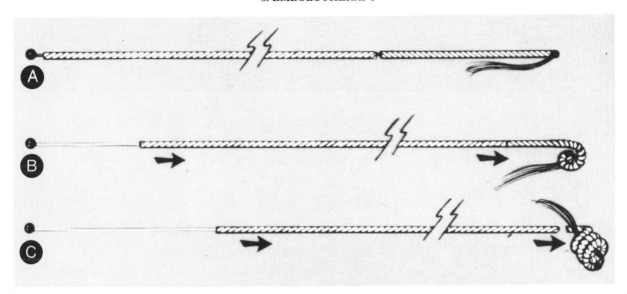

Fig. 3–33 Introduction of coil. A. Introducer with GWC coil loaded, ready for advancement through angiographic catheter. B. In order to release spring embolus, movable core of introducer is pulled back while keeping outer sheath in place. C. After stylet has been completely removed from spring embolus, this resumes its coiled shape and is released.

migration of GWC spring embolus after spermatic embolization, the coils can be modified by straightening their distal end, to form a sharp prong which can engage the venous wall, anchoring the device (Fig. 3–35).

Delayed Complications of Coil Use

Failure of vessel occlusion. The occlusive action of coils is dependent on the patient's clotting mechanism. Therefore, in patients with poor clotting, including those receiving anticoagulants, the use of cast-forming embolic agents (silicone, IBCA) is preferable to the use of coils.[98]

SILK TUFTS ("STREAMERS")

Silk has been used extensively in surgery, and its biocompatibility has been proved. Since the original report,[55] it has been used in combination with coils for rapid, permanent occlusion of large vessels and malformations and of post-traumatic (including postbiopsy) AV communications and for tumor ablation (Fig. 3–36A,B).

BRISTLE BRUSHES

Small nylon brushes are safe and effective for transcatheter occlusion of large arteries both experimentally and clinically. They are particularly suitable for occlusion of larger AV communications. Brushes rapidly occlude the artery by mechanical blockage and induce secondary formation of a firmly adherent thrombus.[99] Histologic examination of the artery wall reveals only a mild inflammatory reaction in all three layers without destruction. Brushes create a less obvious density on x-ray films than do coils but have no other particular disadvantages.

DETACHABLE BALLOONS

Detachable balloons (Becton–Dickinson; Surgimed; Ingenoor; and others) are available for occlusion of vessels as large as 6 mm in luminal diameter (Fig. 3–37).[8] They have the advantage of being carried by the blood to a superselective location, where they can be detached.[7–10,100] The effect of vessel occlusion can be tested before detaching the balloon. For the occlusion of AVMs, detachable balloons appear ideal; there is no danger of influx or reflux leading to pulmonary embolism. The disadvantages are the considerable cost of these devices and their tendency to deflate after several weeks, which may lead to recanalization and migration. Also, the introduction system can be difficult to handle.

ELECTROCOAGULATION (DIATHERMIC VASCULAR OCCLUSION)

Blood clots can be produced *in vivo* by electrocoagulation with an indifferent electrode applied to the body, a conducting wire extending through a selectively placed catheter, and a direct current.[21] The method is the same as that of the electrocautery used in surgery. The blood coagulates at the intravascular electrode, but this takes as long as 30 min or even 1 hr. With an electrode designed primarily to cauterize the vascular wall with a diathermic current, there is higher probability of vascular occlusion.[22] Because of the high current density at the electrode, localized heat is produced, resulting in thrombus formation and local necrosis of the vascular wall. With an endothelial lesion, the thrombi cause permanent vascular occlusion. At present, this technique is experimental.[22]

ANGIOGRAPHIC TECHNIQUES AND CATHETER SELECTION

The appropriate catheters for angiography and embolization depend on the embolic substance that will be used and on the vascular structure that will be embolized.

Introducer Sheaths

An introducer sheath is almost invariably used during transcatheter embolization, principally because it per-

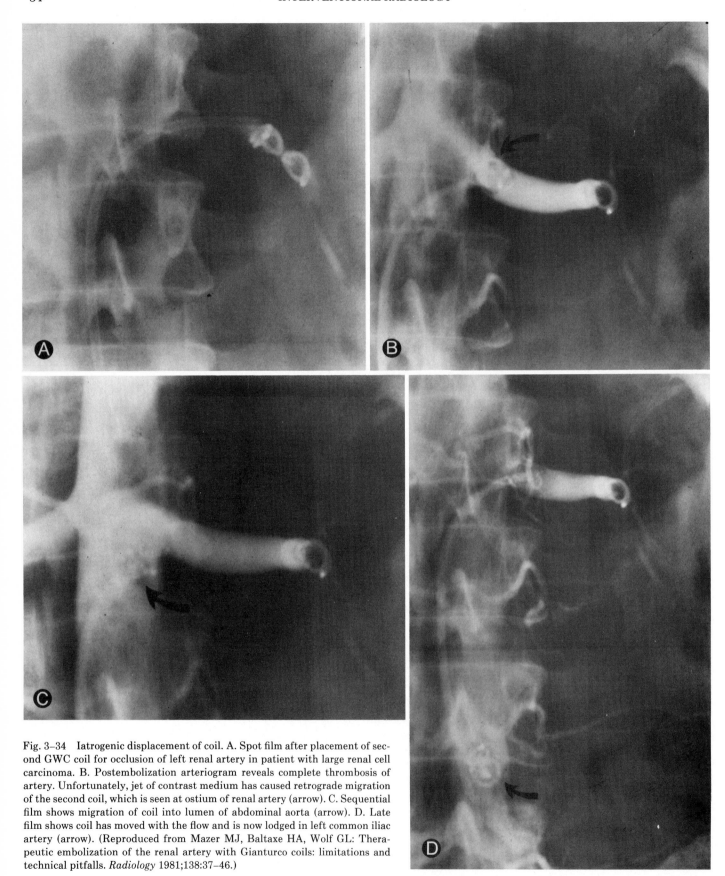

Fig. 3–34 Iatrogenic displacement of coil. A. Spot film after placement of second GWC coil for occlusion of left renal artery in patient with large renal cell carcinoma. B. Postembolization arteriogram reveals complete thrombosis of artery. Unfortunately, jet of contrast medium has caused retrograde migration of the second coil, which is seen at ostium of renal artery (arrow). C. Sequential film shows migration of coil into lumen of abdominal aorta (arrow). D. Late film shows coil has moved with the flow and is now lodged in left common iliac artery (arrow). (Reproduced from Mazer MJ, Baltaxe HA, Wolf GL: Therapeutic embolization of the renal artery with Gianturco coils: limitations and technical pitfalls. *Radiology* 1981;138:37–46.)

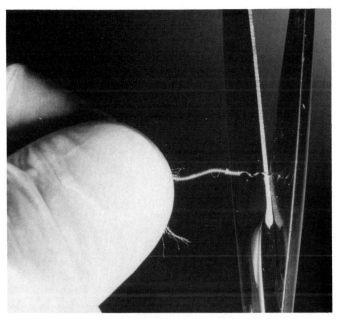

Fig. 3–35 GWC coil being modified by partial straightening of distal spring, which is subsequently trimmed with scissors.

mits catheter exchange. Catheters may become blocked during injection of particulate materials, especially Ivalon, or of tissue adhesives or Gianturco coils. In this last situation, the presence of the sheath may allow a partially extruded coil to be removed safely from the artery, whereas without a sheath, it probably would pull free as the catheter is pulled back through the arteriotomy. Sheaths also simplify routine catheter exchanges and allow insertion of balloon catheters (Fig. 3–38).

Sheaths are available with and without a sealing diaphragm. The advantage of a diaphragm is that there is no blood loss once the catheter has been removed. The disadvantage is that balloons may be dislodged by the diaphragm, as may partially extruded coils. Sheaths without diaphragms may be fitted with adapters such as the Tuohy–Borst, which may be tightened to provide a water tight seal around a smaller catheter yet be loosened to allow safe withdrawal of balloon catheters.

Catheters

Depending on the embolizing agent selected and the vascular structure to be embolized, the available angiographic catheters include:

Fig. 3–36 Silk streamers. A. Streamers with different numbers of silk threads. B. Streamer loaded in Teflon tubing and connected to syringe loaded with dilute contrast medium for flushing.

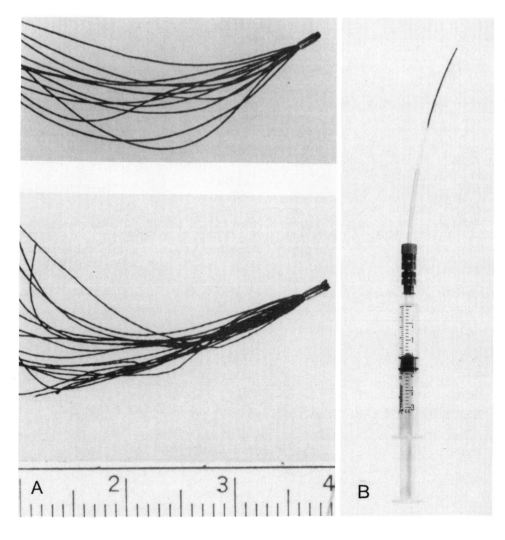

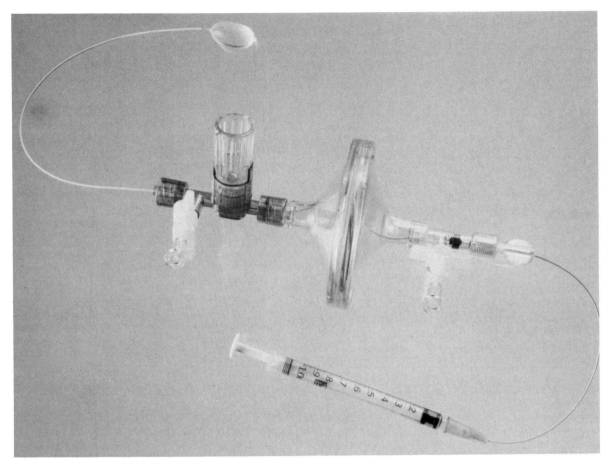

Fig. 3–37   Detachable balloon with delivery system.

A tapered catheter with an end hole (used for spring coils, Gelfoam, Ivalon particles, and fluid embolic agents);

Coaxial systems (used for fluids such as IBCA or MFC or for small particulate agents);

Nontapered Teflon catheters (used for spider placement or delivery of compressed Ivalon);

A balloon catheter (used to prevent reflux during delivery of particulate media and fluid agents).

Each of these will be reviewed.

TAPERED CATHETERS

Most embolization techniques can be performed through regular tapered angiographic catheters. The authors prefer the 5F polyethylene catheter with a 45° curve at the tip, which can easily be reshaped with steam, and the 6.5F reinforced polyethylene and 7F reinforced polyurethane catheters, which have much better torque control than does the 5F polyethylene catheter.

COAXIAL CATHETERS

Coaxial systems are becoming increasingly popular, particularly when highly selective catheter placement is required. The catheters that accept a 0.038-inch guide-wire also accept a 3F Teflon catheter (Massachusetts General Catheter) suitable for embolization with liquid agents such as IBCA and MFC and with Gelfoam particles.

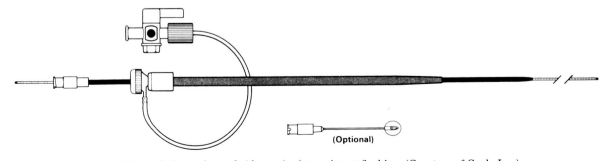

(Optional)

Fig. 3–38   Introducer sheath with check-flow valve and sidearm for intermittent flushing. (Courtesy of Cook, Inc.)

NONTAPERED CATHETERS

Nontapered wide-lumen catheters are useful as guiding catheters in the coaxial systems for introduction of large baffle-forming devices such as barbed coils[55] and spiders[56] and for the introduction of one-step occluding devices such as coilons,[52] spiderlons,[53] detachable balloons,[7–10,100] and compressed Ivalon.[45]

BALLOON OCCLUSION CATHETERS

The balloon occlusion catheters in current use are constructed with either double or single lumens.

Double-Lumen Balloon Catheters

The double-lumen balloon occlusion catheters have the advantage of allowing distal injection after occlusion of an artery. They are used to prevent reflux during embolization with particulate materials, such as Gelfoam and Ivalon, or with liquids such as ethanol. Proximal occlusion of the vessel allows the introduction of polymerizing plastics, because the control of blood flow by the balloon prevents passage of the material into the capillaries or the venous circulation before it polymerizes. The injection of contrast medium prior to the injection of liquid embolic agents provides a measure of the total capacity of the arterial circulation distal to the inflated balloon. By eliminating dilution with unopacified blood, balloon occlusion arteriography provides exquisite detail, even in the presence of torrential flow through an AV fistula.

These catheters are available in sizes of 5F to 8F with balloons up to 4 cm in diameter fully inflated. They are available preshaped (Fig. 3–39) or may be custom shaped using steam. Care should be taken not to heat the junction between catheter and balloon for fear of weakening this area.

Single-Lumen Balloon Catheters

The simplest single-lumen balloon catheter is the Fogarty, which is commonly used for arterial embolectomy and for temporary intraoperative occlusion—for example, occlusion of a carotid–cavernous sinus fistula[101] or traumatized pelvic vessels.[102] These catheters are made of polyvinyl chloride and require insertion through a coaxial catheter.

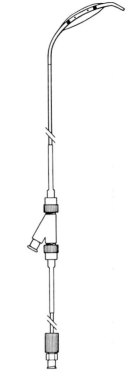

Fig. 3–39 Angiographic cobra balloon catheter.

In 1976, Kerber described an elegant single-lumen catheter with a controlled-leak balloon[10] that allows occlusion of the vessel with a balloon and distal injection of contrast medium or embolic material. The shaft of the catheter and the balloon are both made from silicone, which creates a very soft flexible catheter. Silicone catheters may be passed through a larger coaxial catheter and are excellent for flow direction. Similarly, Pevsner developed a controlled-leak balloon mounted on a polyethylene shaft.[103] This catheter is not propelled by injection as in the Kerber system, but it does allow a degree of flow direction.

The other single-lumen balloon catheters are used solely for embolization. Contrast medium must be injected either through a separate catheter or through the larger coaxial guiding catheter. Such catheters were described by Debrun et al in 1975,[9] Pevsner in 1977,[103] DiTullio et al in 1978,[104] and White et al in 1979[105] and will be discussed more specifically in a subsequent section.

X-RAY EQUIPMENT

High-quality fluoroscopy is a *sine qua non* of most interventional radiologic procedures, and this is particularly true of transcatheter embolization. Facilities for video recording and playback are also desirable. For embolization in the central nervous system, including the spinal cord, high-quality photographic subtraction is essential. This is also true of embolization of intercostal or lumbar arteries, the reason being that small reticular branches may not be seen on the regular films, and embolization in such a situation has led to disastrous complications. Digital subtraction angiography has similar advantages, although it is often time consuming.

The portable gamma camera has been useful in determining the destination of injected emboli. Conroy and Endert and their colleagues labeled Gelfoam particles with radionuclide and were then able to pinpoint their final resting place.[27,28]

ARTERIOVENOUS MALFORMATIONS: AN OVERVIEW

Adequate management of AVMs remains a most challenging problem. Numerous treatments have been tried, including primary excision, ligation of the feeding vessels, injection of sclerosing agents, and radiation; but all of them, with the exception of total excision, have the shortcoming of allowing recurrence due to development of collateral vessels. Further, complete excision often is not possible or has unacceptable cosmetic results. Because of these problems, interest arose in developing embolization techniques for the management of AVMs. The success of these endeavors has further reduced the use of simple ligation of arterial feeders, which commonly results in early recurrence and makes future management by embolization more difficult.[106–108]

Therapeutic arterial embolization was first utilized by neurosurgeons in the managment of AV fistulae of the brain. Small emboli of autogenous muscle were placed directly in the feeding artery exposed by an arteriotomy.[2] With the advent and development of percutaneous selective and superselective vascular catheterization techniques, the open operation was replaced by the more selective and simpler percutaneous approach, which has been widely applied to AVMs throughout the body. Better and more readily available synthetic embolic materials have replaced the autologous fat, muscle, or clots originally used.

Embryologic Basis of Arteriovenous Malformations

Early in embryologic development, the vascular system is a meshwork of endothelial lakes usually referred to as the "endothelial stage." These lakes later coalesce into intercommunicating capillary channels, some of which develop muscular coats ("reteform stage"). Finally, during further differentiation, mature arteries and veins are formed. A lack of differentiation in the endothelial stage results in the formation of hemangiomas of the capillary or cavernous type, whereas arrested development at a subsequent stage may create large AV fistulae with or without associated hemangiomas and various degrees of AV shunting.[109]

Anatomy and Physiology

PATHOLOGIC ANATOMY

Arteriovenous communications can be classified as congenital or acquired. The congenital AVM can be localized or diffuse and can be classified as capillary, juvenile, or cavernous hemangiomas. Capillary hemangiomas are characterized by a proliferation of capillary-sized vessels, which often show considerable active growth evidenced by mitotic activity. The juvenile hemangioma, formed in infants and children, is a variant of the capillary hemangioma. Microscopically, there is a much greater degree of cellularity. The capillary channels are not well formed, and many of the proliferating endothelial cells are plump and arranged in solid sheets. Because of these microscopic characteristics, juvenile hemangioma is also termed hypertrophic hemangioma. It is common for this lesion to be less circumscribed and to infiltrate more into adjacent structures. Cavernous hemangiomas are composed of prominent, dilated, blood-filled spaces lined by inconspicuous flattened endothelial cells with little evidence of active growth or proliferation. In any hemangioma, there may be a mixture and transition of various histologic types, which has led some investigators to believe that these malformations mature, with a transition from the capillary type to the more complex hypertrophic angiomatous variants found in adults.[110]

Acquired communications are commonly referred to as AV fistulae and are usually secondary to trauma or surgery. A single large communication is generally found between the artery and the vein.

PATHOPHYSIOLOGY

An AVM represents a bypass of the capillary bed, with a marked decrease of peripheral resistance. Blood flows preferentially into this low-resistance system, resulting in a steal phenomenon and decreased pressure in the adjacent normal circulation. Cardiac output and blood volume increase to maintain the systolic blood pressure. Cardiac output increases primarily by an increase in the stroke volume, as the pulse remains normal initially; but with extensive shunting, tachycardia develops.[111] The feeding arteries dilate, and the arterial wall begins to degenerate, with atrophy of the muscular and elastic coats.[111] The shunting of blood also provides a powerful stimulus for the development of an extensive collateral circulation (Fig. 3–40), whereas the peripheral tissues are

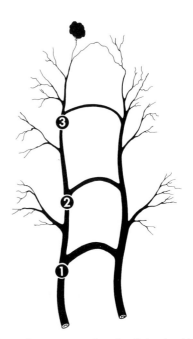

Fig. 3–40 Schematic representation of collateral pattern in peripheral AVM. Occlusion of afferent vessel at level 1, 2, or 3 would result in recurrence of lesion due to development of collateral flow. Cast-like occlusion of nidus of malformation would be needed for permanent obliteration.

deprived of blood.[112] Arteriovenous malformations occur predominantly in the head and neck area (50% of cases)[113] and the legs.

Characteristics of Lesions

CLINICAL FINDINGS

Congenital AVMs commonly are asymptomatic until puberty, when pain, bleeding, ulceration, or enlargement of the limb may appear. Not infrequently, cardiac decompensation with high-output failure is the principal presenting symptom.

DIAGNOSTIC EVALUATION

Evaluation by Doppler ultrasound and plethysmography is useful initially, and also provides a noninvasive way to assess the progression, regression, or recurrence of the lesion after therapy. Hemodynamic evaluation (for example, of cardiac output), as determined by thermodilution and radionuclide techniques, and determinations of regional blood flow near the AVM[114] are most useful in treatment planning. Selective arteriography provides anatomic information and is carried out principally as a preliminary step in the nonsurgical obliteration of the lesion. Informed consent for both angiography and embolization is obtained, since both procedures can be carried out in one sitting.

Because of the rapid blood flow and consequent dilution of contrast medium, angiography must be carried out selectively with balloon occlusion techniques with comparatively large-bore catheters and rapid injection. Any collateral feeders must be opacified. The most common angiographic findings are:

Dilation and tortuosity of the efferent vessels;
Early preferential flow of contrast medium into the AVM;
Delayed and poor filling of the arteries supplying adjacent tissue that has normal vasculature (hemodynamic steal);
Early opacification of the draining veins.

Treatment of Arteriovenous Malformations by Arterial Embolization

The therapeutic embolization of AVMs requires experience, judgment, and skill. If a nonabsorbable embolic agent of the proper size is used and all feeding arteries are embolized, AVMs may be permanently cured (Fig. 3–41). If such lesions are too extensive or have too many peripheral feeders to be cured, they still can often be controlled, stabilizing the patient's hemodynamic status (Fig. 3–42). Although recurrences may develop, they can be treated by a repeat embolization should cardiac failure recur.

BASIC PRINCIPLE

An AVM is a hemodynamic runoff lesion, usually supplied by a diffuse network of feeders with many anastomoses (Fig. 3–40). Therefore, occlusion of proximal feeding arteries obviously will result in recurrence by collateral flow through an adjacent communicating branch just as after surgical ligation of feeders, which results in recurrence in a short time.

The main advantage of embolization over operation is the possibility of delivering occluding nonabsorbable emboli toward the periphery of the malformation, bypassing larger collateral channels. Ideally, an embolus will be small enough to occlude the finer branches without passing through the malformation into the venous circulation. It is important, therefore, to have an assortment of particle sizes of the embolic material at hand. The proper-size embolus is chosen empirically by careful analysis of the angiogram. Passage of minute (0.1–0.5-mm) emboli through the AVM into the venous circulation has not occurred in the authors' experience. In spite of a large shunt through the malformation, the communications are anatomically small (Fig. 3–41), unlike the situation in pulmonary AV fistulae, where there commonly are large communicating channels. (In spite of these large communications, the AV shunt is usually not great in the lung because of the much smaller pressure gradient between the pulmonary artery and pulmonary vein than in a systemic artery and vein. This subject is discussed later in this chapter.) Passage of emboli through AVMs can be detected by isotopic tagging,[27,28] but this is seldom necessary. The blood flow across the AVM usually decreases immediately after injection of the test dose of emboli, confirming selection of the proper size.

The success rate of embolic treatment of AVMs depends largely on the size of the lesion and the number of major feeding branches. Obviously, all feeders must be embolized, which is sometimes not feasible (Fig. 3–41). Therefore, AVMs with a few large arterial feeders (Fig. 3–42), particularly traumatic (Fig. 3–43) and iatrogenic (Fig. 3–44) malformations, are easier to obliterate.

TECHNICAL CONSIDERATIONS

An AVM can be treated or cured only if all feeding branches are occluded as far peripherally as possible. This requires thorough angiographic imaging of all arteries participating in the malformation. Because of the low resistance in the malformation, several adjacent vascular beds may give off feeders. Generally, it is useful to inject one of the larger distant arteries for identification of the various participating vascular beds (Fig. 3–45A). With a mapping angiogram in hand, it becomes possible to catheterize various branches and inject embolic material selectively (Figs. 3–45B–F). Emboli suspended in 30% contrast medium are injected under fluoroscopic control into a smaller feeding branch to make sure the emboli are not so small that they pass into the venous side. Because of the rapid blood flow, the injection is hardly visible on fluoroscopy, but the contrast density will increase rapidly because of the progressive obstruction of the AV shunt in the particular branch.

After the rapid forward flow of emboli during the early phase of administration, the flow in the feeding artery decreases, and stagnation finally occurs. Therefore, injec-

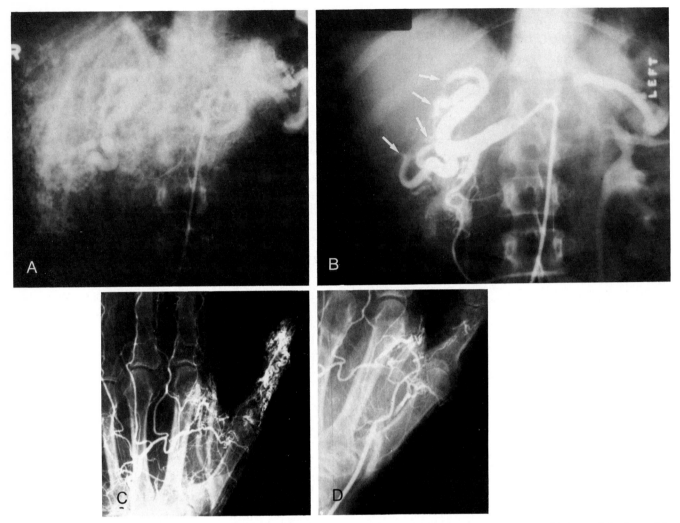

Fig. 3–41 Patient with hereditary hemorrhagic telangiectasia (Rendu–Osler–Weber syndrome) with severe AV shunting through liver causing chronic congestive heart failure. A. Selective celiac axis injections show severe AV shunting throughout liver. B. Selective common hepatic arteriogram after second stage of embolization of hepatic branches shows complete obliteration of intrahepatic arteries (arrows). C. AVM of left thumb; note multiple small feeders arising from palmar arches. D. After embolization with Ivalon particles. Note persistence of flow even though significant improvement has been obtained. It was considered too dangerous to embolize all feeders completely (risk of gangrene of thumb).

tion speed must be carefully gauged in order to prevent backflow of emboli into the proximal arteries supplying various organs. The spillover of emboli into the abdominal aorta is usually of no clinical consequence, but spillover into the carotid artery is much more dangerous, as it may result in stroke. Backflow of material can be eliminated by balloon occlusion of the feeding artery, but this is not usually necessary if the catheter can be advanced deep into the feeding artery and if the injection is made cautiously under fluoroscopic control.

The addition of 30 mg of papaverine to the suspension induces maximum vasodilation and eliminates vasospasm, a condition that decreases flow and increases the risk of reflux. One should not continue embolizing until forward flow ceases completely; it is adequate, indeed wise, to terminate the injection when the flow in the artery has become sluggish. With this approach, retrograde reflux of embolic material is less likely, and, in the authors' experience, complete thrombosis occurs spontaneously around the emboli. Use of a 2-ml syringe is helpful in controlling the injection.

It is not prudent to introduce large obstructive devices such as an Ivalon plug or a spring coil into major feeding branches, because this would make repeat embolization impossible and would necessitate the catheterization of smaller collateral branches. The same technical difficulty exists if large arterial branches of the lesion have previously been ligated.

On rare occasions, such as in malformations in the foot, feeding arteries are not accessible by indirect catheterization. Under these circumstances, surgical exposure of the major feeders is indicated. However, the feeding branches should not be ligated but rather embolized. Also, malformations with very short feeding branches which do not allow deep introduction of catheters into the artery are best exposed by the surgeon and then embolized to eliminate backwash of embolic material.

The actual procedure requires excellent fluoroscopic facilities, since the risk is greater if the imaging is poor. Embolization is best carried out by two experienced angiographers. The embolic suspensions are prepared by one angiographer on a separate table (to prevent contam-

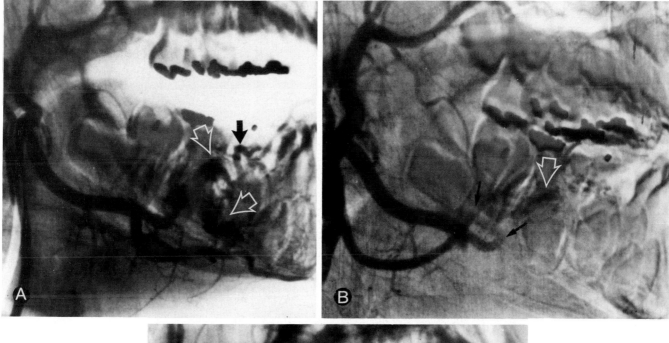

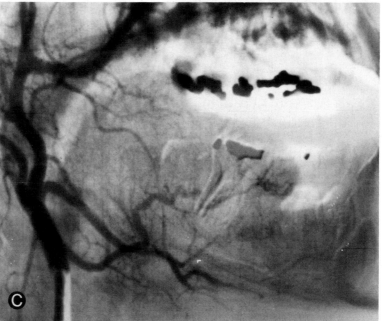

Fig. 3–42 Eight-year-old boy with severe bleeding during dental examination for loose teeth. A. Selective left external carotid arteriogram shows large areas of pooled contrast medium (open arrows) with early draining of large veins (black arrows). B. Angiogram after embolization with small Ivalon particles reveals obstruction of two major arterial feeders (long arrows) with forward flow through lingual artery and little pooling of contrast medium (open arrow). C. Follow-up left carotid arteriogram 3 months after embolization reveals continued occlusion of embolized arteries with no evidence of AV shunting through lingual artery and no evidence of crossover from right side. (Reproduced from Castañada–Zuñiga WR, Lehnert M, Nath PH, Zollikofer C, Velasquez G, Amplatz K: Therapeutic embolization of facial arteriovenous fistulas. *Radiology* 1979;132:599–602.)

ination of the flushing solution) and loaded in several small injection syringes, which are handed to the other angiographer who performs the actual injections.

EMBOLIZATION MATERIALS

In the ideal situation, the feeders of an AVM are occluded with permanent embolic agents at the precapillary level. Otherwise, early bypassing collaterals develop, the malformation recurs, and, importantly, the management of the new collateral communication is more difficult. Consequently, suspensions of tiny emboli carried by the bloodstream are most effective. Mechanical obstructing devices are useful in traumatic AVMs (Fig. 3–43) or in the lung, where there are larger single feeders. It is of paramount importance that the angiographer be entirely familiar with the physical, chemical, and biologic characteristics of various emboli, since only if the proper agent is used can permanent success be expected.

Embolic materials can be made radiopaque by the

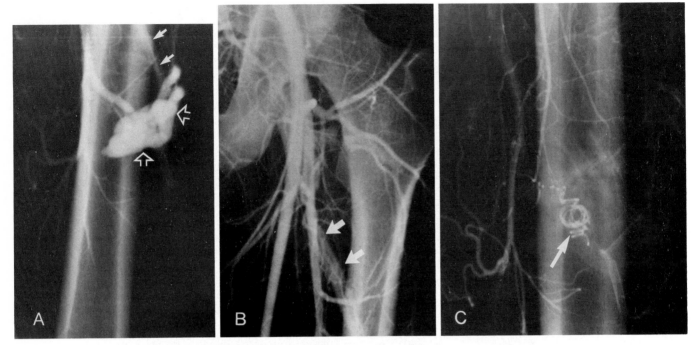

Fig. 3–43 Stab wound in upper left thigh 8 days earlier resulted in AV fistula with audible bruit. A. Selective left deep femoral arteriogram reveals traumatic AV communication from branches of deep femoral artery (open arrows). Note early opacified veins (white arrows). B. Early venous opacification can be seen (arrows). C. After selective catheterization of feeding artery, occlusion with GWC spring coil (arrow) eliminated AV communication.

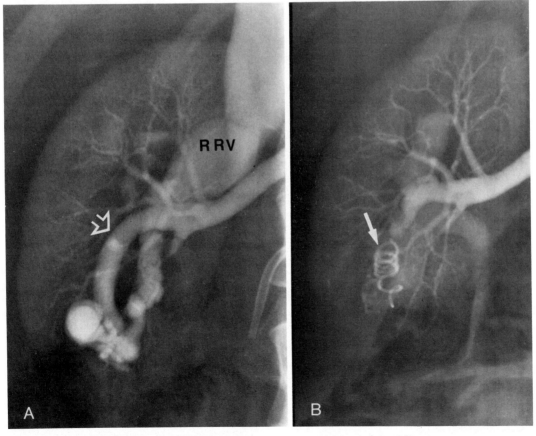

Fig. 3–44 Postbiopsy AV fistula of right kidney. Attempts to ligate main feeder were unsuccessful. A. Selective right renal arteriogram reveals stump of surgically ligated artery and large AV fistula (arrow) supplied by one of the lower branches of the anterior division, with extensive AV shunting. RRV = right renal vein. B. After embolization of main feeder with GWC spring embolus (arrow), there is complete thrombosis of vessel with no evidence of residual AV shunting.

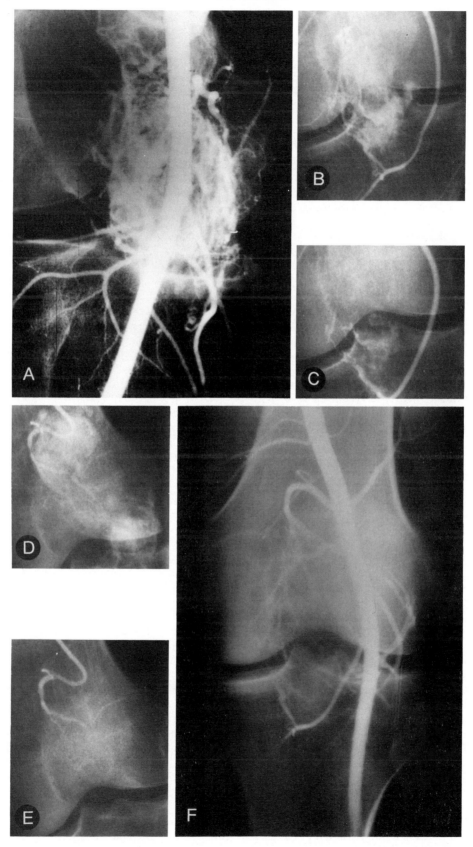

Fig. 3–45 Embolization with fine Ivalon particles. A. Large AVM in soft tissue of right knee fed by multiple genicular branches. B.–F. Selective catheterization followed by embolization with fine Ivalon particles completely obliterated malformations.

addition of various heavy metal compounds containing barium, bismuth, tin, etc. However, with good fluoroscopy, even nonopaque emboli, such as Ivalon, can be seen if suspended in dilute contrast medium. Recently, a technique for radionuclide labeling of Gelfoam emboli was described that allows their nonradiographic external location by a gamma camera.[27,28]

Nonabsorbable or Permanent Embolic Materials

Ivalon. Ivalon, which is nonabsorbable, is an ideal agent for the embolization of AVMs. Its principal disadvantage is its high friction coefficient, which makes delivery difficult. Selection of the proper particle size is vital. If the particles are too large, they will lodge upstream of larger collaterals, thus leading to recurrence, as after surgical ligation of feeding arteries; if the particles are too small, they may pass through the arteriovenous anastomoses and embolize into the lungs. If the particles are of proper size they will occlude the precapillary vessels downstream from the large collaterals, and embolization may indeed be curative (Fig. 3–42).[14,46,47–50,115]

Distal embolization commonly results in local increased temperature, redness, tenderness, and swelling of the skin over the AVM. The patient may have a fever for a few days, but symptoms subside without treatment. After this transient inflammatory reaction, the open-pore sponge is invaded by fibroblasts.[46] Organization and permanent incorporation lead to permanent vascular occlusion.

Nonabsorbable particulate materials. Spheres of stainless-steel pellets,[58] acrylic,[60] methylmethacrylate,[3] Silastic, and silicone[61–63] are inert and nonantigenic and are available in a variety of sizes. They are radiopaque, allowing detection by radiography. Spheres are popular with neuroradiologists for treatment of AVMs of the nervous system.

Silicone spheres are available in diameters of 0.5–3 mm and can be made radiopaque with barium sulfate. Silastic spheres were introduced for embolization of cerebral angiomas through the surgically exposed carotid artery by Lussenhop and Spence and through percutaneously introduced catheters by Kricheff et al.[3,64] The silicone spheres are distributed according to blood flow through the malformation, and bigger spheres are then injected to occlude larger feeding arteries.[47,116] The advantage of spheres is their flotation and consequent flow-guided distribution. However, spheres tend to obstruct the catheter, since they are not compressible. Small particles may pass through AV fistulae and produce pulmonary emboli, which are of no clinical importance because the pulmonary vascular bed is so large. Silastic spheres have also been used to embolize carotid–cavernous sinus fistulae[117] and large juvenile angiofibromas.[118]

Liquid embolic agents. The rationale for the use of liquid or semiliquid agents is the possibility of selectively depositing them directly in smaller peripheral branches. With liquid agents such as IBCA and silicone-rubber mixtures, the occluding agent flows as long as it is injected. However, IBCA hardens rapidly and may occlude only larger vessels. Another disadvantage of these agents is the risk of pulmonary embolization when they are introduced into malformations with larger AV shunts. This risk can be minimized by slowing the blood flow by balloon occlusion or by preliminary infusion of vasopressin. The handling of tissue glues requires extensive experience; it is not as simple as the injection of emboli, since the catheter may become glued to the blood vessels.

Isobutyl-2-cyanoacrylate. This agent is a fast-hardening plastic adhesive used primarily as a cement for orthopaedic prostheses.[119] The plastic is cured by contact with ionic fluids such as blood, so it is delivered through catheters by nonionic liquids such as glucose solution. If IBCA is injected intravascularly, it hardens rapidly and creates a permanent occlusion. Because of this rapid hardening, the injection is best made through a coaxial catheter system. IBCA has been used to obliterate intracranial AVMs.[11,66,120,121]

Silicone rubber mixtures. Silicone rubber is a permanent biocompatible agent that can be made radiopaque with tantalum powder. The mixture consists of the Silastic elastomer 382R, which is vulcanized by catalysts. To decrease the viscosity, silicone fluid 360rs can be added. The Silastic and silicone fluid are thoroughly mixed in various proportions, depending on the desired viscosity. Two catalysts are required for vulcanization: Dow–Corning catalyst M (stannous octate) and the co-linker tetraethyl silicate.[75,122]

Complete stasis of blood flow facilitates the injection of silicone and may be accomplished with a double-lumen balloon catheter. Superselective injection is advisable to ensure safe delivery. Injection of the silicone results in a complete cast of the vascular bed, which is necessary to prevent distal migration, since silicones have no adhesive properties.

Ethibloc. Ethibloc, an amino acid gel, has recently been introduced in Europe as an embolic agent. Because of its low viscosity, Ethibloc penetrates deeply into the vascular tree, apparently without risk of systemic or pulmonary embolization.[78] If balloon occlusion is used, embolization of capillaries results in tissue necrosis.

Sclerosing Agents

Absolute ethanol. Recently, absolute ethanol has been used effectively in the obliteration of tumors and gastroesophageal varices and for organ ablation.[17,82] It can be mixed with nonionic contrast medium for radiopacity. The mechanism of vascular occlusion is probably a direct toxic effect on the endothelium, resulting in activation of the coagulation system.[17] This toxic effect extends into the perivascular tissues, causing necrosis.[123] The amount of ethanol injected depends on the size of the vessels to be occluded and on the velocity of blood flow. Multiple injections may be required to occlude major feeders. The ability to deliver ethanol through tiny flow-directed balloon catheters is a distinct advantage, and the vascular occlusion by the inflated balloon reduces the amount of ethanol needed.

Alcohol has been used for the obliteration of AVM. A slow infusion rate (0.1 ml/sec) is used to minimize perivascular damage.

Boiling contrast medium. Contrast medium heated to 100° C has been successful experimentally for

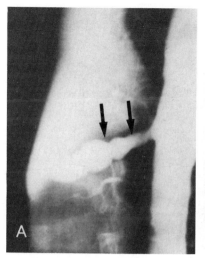
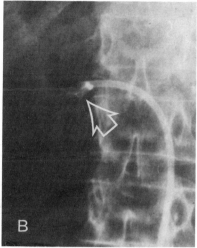
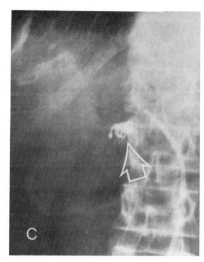

Fig. 3–46 Large AV fistula postnephrectomy. A. Aortogram shows large communication between stump of right renal artery and vein (arrows). B. Two spiders have been placed in stump of renal artery (arrow). C. Two GWC coils have been placed behind spiders to com- plete the obliteration (arrow). (Reproduced from Castañeda–Zuñiga WR, Tadavarthy SM, Galliani C, Laerum F, Schwarten D, Amplatz K: Experimental venous occlusion with stainless steel spiders. *Radiology* 1981;141:238–241.)

obliteration of human veins. A permanent occlusion is achieved by means of direct endothelial damage that causes endothelial necrosis with activation of clotting mechanisms. The thrombus becomes organized, and there is no apparent perivascular damage. This agent has not been successful in the treatment of AVMs.[18]

Nonparticulate Permanent Agents

Gianturco steel coils. Steel coils were first used by Gianturco et al to produce permanent vascular occlusion of major arteries, primarily for preoperative embolization of renal cell carcinomas and bleeding tumors.[16,87] Experimental and clinical experience confirms the prompt sustained vascular occlusion.[16,73]

Generally, coils should not be used in the primary treatment of congenital AVMs, because they will occlude only large proximal feeding vessels, causing development of bypassing collaterals with recurrence of the lesion. They can, however, be used in the obliteration of pulmonary AVMs, which are usually fed by a single artery, and for closure of AV fistulae with a single large feeder (Figs. 3–43 and 3–44). The diameter of the coil should be slightly larger than that of the vessel to prevent passage through the fistula and systemic embolization. If such large AVMs are to be occluded, a firm baffle is formed first with barbed coils or spiders (Fig. 3–46).[55,56] The barbs immediately engage the arterial wall, preventing passage of the device through the malformation. This sys- tem has been successful for the occlusion of large AV communications of the pulmonary artery (Fig. 3–47A).[55,56] Once a baffle is in place, additional coils or other embolic material such as silk can be injected safely to complete the occlusion (Fig. 3–47B). Gelfoam should not be used, because it passes through the coils.

Summary of the Treatment of Arteriovenous Malformations

1. The current treatment of choice for AVMs is emboli- zation; surgery is indicated only if the lesion is small and can be excised with cosmetically acceptable results.
2. Surgical ligation of major feeding arteries alone or per- cutaneous occlusion of large arteries alone results in recurrence.
3. If feeding arteries cannot be catheterized, they should be surgically exposed for embolization.
4. All feeding vessels must be occluded; this may result in permanent cure.
5. Extensive AVMs resulting in intractable heart failure can be controlled, but seldom cured, by embolization.
6. The best results are obtained if emboli of the proper size are used to occlude feeding branches as peripher- ally as possible.
7. Many agents and methods are available for vessel occlusion, and no single technique is applicable to all cases.

PULMONARY ARTERIOVENOUS FISTULAE

Pulmonary AV fistulae appear most frequently as part of hereditary hemorrhagic telangiectasia (60%) but may be an isolated anomaly. The patients may be completely asymptomatic or may manifest cyanosis, dyspnea, poly- cythemia, hemoptysis, or pulmonary osteoarthropathy. The extent of these findings does not necessarily correlate with the size or number of the vascular malformations; indeed, not all large or multiple malformations are symptomatic.[124,125]

It has been stated that the presence of a pulmonary AVM, even in the absence of symptoms, should be cor- rected surgically because of the possibility of paradoxical

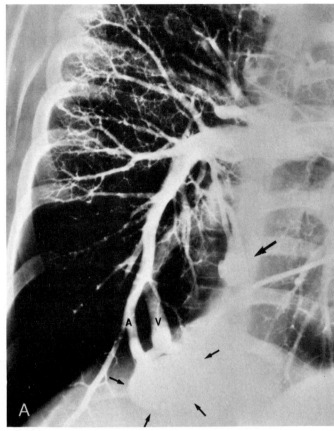
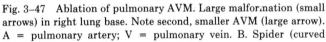
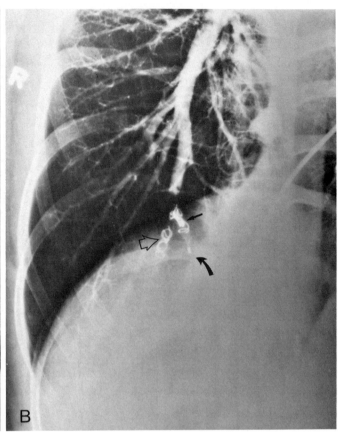

Fig. 3–47   Ablation of pulmonary AVM. Large malformation (small arrows) in right lung base. Note second, smaller AVM (large arrow). A = pulmonary artery; V = pulmonary vein. B. Spider (curved arrow) was placed to form baffle in arterial feeder and could have been placed to complete the obliteration (small arrow). Coils have also been placed in additional AVMs to lower lobe (open arrow).

embolism, infection, and spontaneous rupture with severe bleeding.[126] Serious complications or death occurred in 20% of the patients with pulmonary artery fistulae reported by Stringer et al.[126] However, the high incidence of multiplicity of these lesions (35%–40%)[125,126] makes traditional surgical treatment difficult. Lobectomy or pneumonectomy may be required. Further, although clinical improvement has followed surgical resection of larger fistulae,[127] the widespread nature of the malformations in some cases would necessitate extensive resection. Operation eliminates some of the larger communications, but numerous other shunts often remain and enlarge with time. Such potential shunts can be identified angiographically by wedging the catheter into the mature fistula.

Therapeutic embolization offers more effective treatment.[128] Histologically, no communications exist proximal to the malformations unless multiple feeders are present,[126] so occlusion of the pulmonary artery branch leading to the fistula should totally obstruct the corresponding shunt. In patients with multiple bilateral AV communications, selective obliteration of the largest communications in both lungs is a preferable therapeutic approach, because no lung tissue is sacrificed (Fig. 3–48A).[129] Some of the remaining fistulae may slowly enlarge,[125,126] leading to increased shunting and cyanosis, at which time re-embolization can be carried out, preserving functioning lung tissue (Fig. 3–48B). Occlusion of

multiple AV fistulae leading to improvement in the condition of a patient with diffuse pulmonary involvement was first reported by Taylor et al.[128] Several later reports of embolization have stressed the use of spring coils[130–133] and detachable balloons.[134–136]

Anatomy

A classification of pulmonary AV fistulae on the basis of the angiographic appearance has been proposed by White et al.[135] The simple type is the most common (79%) and consists of a single pulmonary artery–pulmonary vein communication, usually aneurysmally dilated and nonseptated. The complex type in the remaining 21% of the cases consists of multiple feeding arteries and draining veins; the connection between them is commonly aneurysmic and septated. Sometimes, the communication is through a network of small vessels.[135] A similar classification was proposed by Higgins and Wexler for lesions in children.[137] Here, there are four subgroups: solitary, multiple of uniform size, multiple of various sizes, and diffuse (telangiectatic).[137] The anatomic–pathologic basis of these classifications was provided by Moyer and colleagues, who described similar findings in surgical specimens.[138,139] The diameters of the feeding arteries range from 2–8 mm; the draining veins are larger.[126] In 96% of the cases, the feeding vessel is a

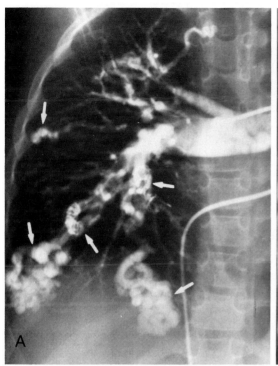
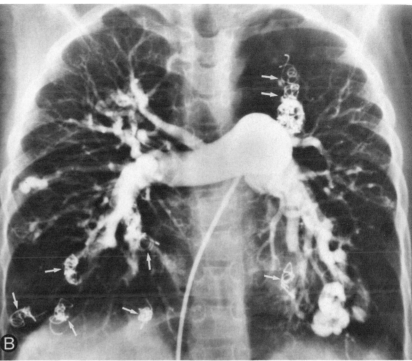

Fig. 3–48 Multiple AVMs in both lungs appearing as isolated anomaly in 6-year-old girl whose main complaint was shortness of breath with deep cyanosis; hemoglobin was 23.5 g/dl and hematocrit 66% at the time of catheterization. A. Pulmonary arteriogram after embolization with GWC spring coils in both lungs (arrows). The patient's oxygen saturation rose from 73% to 94%, with a significant increase in her exercise tolerance. B. Pulmonary arteriogram after repeat embolization shows multiple occluded AVMs with enlargement of residual lesions. (Reproduced from Castañeda–Zuñiga WR, Epstein M, Zollikofer C, et al: Embolization of multiple pulmonary artery fistulae. *Radiology* 1980;134:309–310.)

branch of the pulmonary rather than the systemic circulation.[125] Most fistulae are subpleural and are found in the lower lobes.[126]

Technique

Angiography provides precise information on the size, number, and location of the lesions. Biplane fluoroscopy is needed for the often technically difficult selective catheterization of the feeding arteries. During the angiographic study, arterial gas values are determined, since they are the single most important piece of baseline information for assessing physiologic improvement during therapeutic maneuvers. The diameter of the feeding pulmonary artery branch is measured on the angiogram, with correction for magnification, for proper selection of the coil or detachable balloon.

A superselective position of the catheter tip near the communication with the draining vein should be obtained for spring coil embolization, since the coil should be delivered precisely at the site of the AVM. Such precise catheterization is not necessary for detachable balloon embolotherapy, since balloons can be flow directed to the fistula once the introducer catheter has entered or is aimed at the proximal segment of the feeding artery (Fig. 3–49).

The diameter of the embolic device should be greater than that of the feeding artery to prevent migration with systemic embolization. For the same purpose a device, described by Castañeda et al[56] and later modified by Lund et al,[140] can be used for more precise release at the chosen site (Fig. 3–50). Behind this device, coils or other embolic agents can be safely introduced (Fig. 3–51). The use of modified detachable coils (Cook, Inc.) is highly recommended, because if the coil is smaller than the lumen of the vessel being embolized, the coil can easily be withdrawn through the introducing catheter. If the coil proves to be slightly larger than the vessel and a tight fit is obtained that can be expected to prevent migration of the device, it can then be released simply by unscrewing the coil introducer.

The simplicity, availability, and low cost of the spring coils make them the most popular agent for the embolization of pulmonary AV communications.

BRONCHIAL ARTERY EMBOLIZATION

Hemoptysis is one of the most impressive and alarming manifestations of tracheobronchial or pulmonary disease. In most acute episodes, the blood loss is of moderate volume and ceases spontaneously. The less common cases of severe hemoptysis are life-threatening emergencies, not because of the volume of blood lost (500–600 ml) but because the continuous bleeding floods the tracheobronchial tree, with subsequent asphyxiation, which accounts

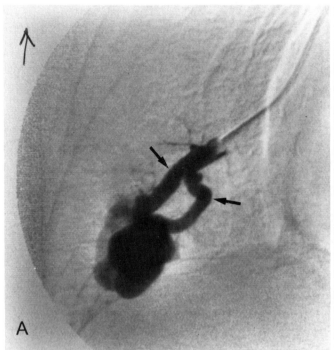

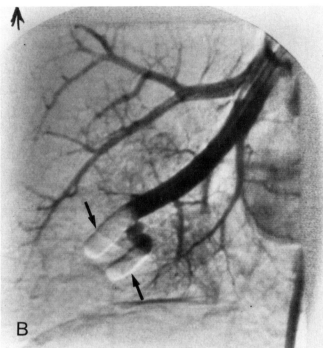

Fig. 3–49   Ablation of pulmonary AVM. A. AVM fed by right lower lobe pulmonary artery branches (arrows). B. Two detachable bal-loons (arrows) have been used to occlude feeding arteries. (Courtesy of RJ White, M.D., Johns Hopkins University.)

for as many as 80% of the deaths.[141–143] Common causes of significant hemoptysis in the United States include cystic fibrosis, neoplasm, and bronchiectasis. In most other countries, pulmonary tuberculosis accounts for a larger percentage of cases.[144]

Anatomy

The bronchial arteries usually originate from the aorta at the level of the T_5 and T_6 vertebrae, although there is considerable variation. The classic work of Caldwell et al in 1948 described four major vascular patterns[145]:

1. Two arteries on the left and one on the right as a common trunk with the intercostal suprema;
2. One artery trunk on the left and one on the right;
3. Two arteries on the left and two on the right;
4. One artery on the left and two on the right.

First-class bronchial arteriography is a must, with subtraction or digital subtraction films to study the anterior and posterior radicular arteries, which can originate from the intercostal arteries and supply collaterals to the spinal cord. Therefore, the presence of an anterior spinal artery arising from the cervicointercostal trunk,[146] from an intercostal artery,[147] or from the common intercosto-bronchial trunk[148] should be considered an absolute contraindication to therapeutic embolization; several instances of transverse myelitis have followed intercostal or bronchial arteriography[147–149] or embolization in such cases.[144,147,150,151]

Extensive collateralization from mediastinal arteries and transpleural collaterals may be found, particularly after thoracotomy or in chronic inflammatory processes of the lung. Collateralization can be so strong as to

reverse blood flow in the pulmonary artery (Fig. 3–52).[152] Consequently, a complete study of the bronchial circulation should include a thoracic aortogram to exclude the presence of this type of collaterals, particularly in

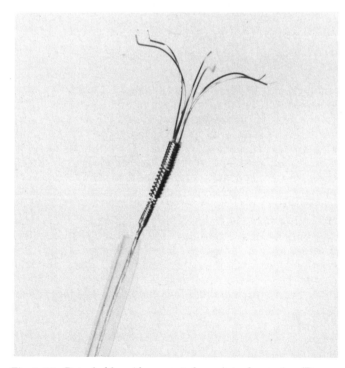

Fig. 3–50   Detachable spider mounted over introducer wire. (Reproduced from Lund G, Rysavy J, Kotula F, Castañeda–Zuñiga WR, Amplatz K: Detachable spring coils for vessel occlusion. *Radiology* 1985;155:530.)

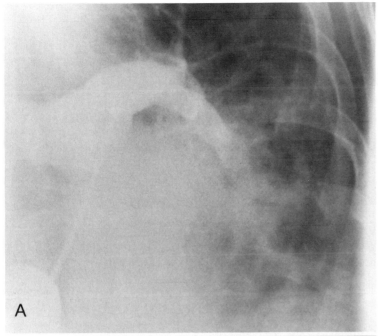

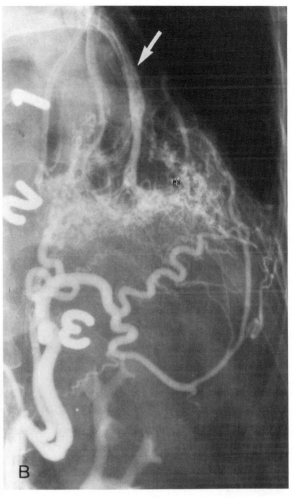

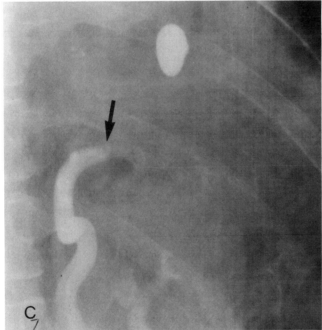

Fig. 3–51 Patient with recurrent bouts of pulmonary infections over 15 years. A. Left pulmonary arteriogram shows apparent obstruction. On cine pulmonary arteriogram, retrograde flow was evident. B. Selective phrenic arteriogram reveals extensive transpleural communications between branches of phrenic artery and left pulmonary artery. Oxygen saturation in left pulmonary artery was 95%, with retrograde flow from left pulmonary artery into right lung. C. After embolization of phrenic artery with small Ivalon shavings, there was complete thrombosis (arrow). (Reproduced from Tadavarthy SM, Klugman J, Castañeda–Zuñiga WR, Nath PH, Amplatz K: Systemic to pulmonary collaterals in pathologic states: a review. *Radiology* 1982;144:75–76.)

patients with recurrent bleeding after successful embolization of bronchial arteries.

Technique

Except in patients with cystic fibrosis, bronchial arteriography is performed first on the side where there is bronchoscopic evidence of bleeding. Catheterization is usually performed with a Simmons catheter. Digital subtraction arteriography is particularly useful, because it allows evaluation of the existence of radicular branches while minimizing the amount of contrast medium needed, thus decreasing the risk of neurotoxicity.

After the presence of radicular branches has been ruled out, the catheter tip is advanced deeper into the artery, and embolization is performed, usually with Gelfoam or Ivalon particles. Embolization should be as distal as possible to reduce the chances of recurrence due to distal collateralization. Care should be taken, however, to avoid reflux of the embolic agent into the aorta.

A postembolization angiogram is obtained to assess the results. If the opposite side was considered to be free of problems, a thoracic aortogram is performed to evaluate the existence of other systemic influx into the bronchial circulation. If other sources of collateral inflow are present, they also are embolized (Fig. 3–53). This is particularly important in the patient with recurrent bleeding after an initially successful embolization.

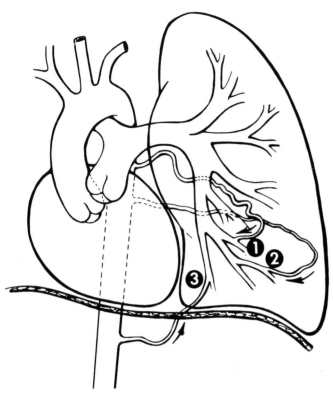

Fig. 3–52   Diagram of sources of transpleural collateralization of left pulmonary artery in patient in Fig. 3–51. (Reproduced from Tadavarthy SM, Klugman J, Castañeda–Zuñiga WR, Nath PH, Amplatz K: Systemic to pulmonary collaterals in pathologic states: a review. *Radiology* 1982;144:75–76.)

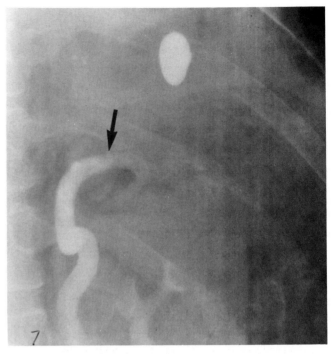

Fig. 3–53   After embolization of phrenic artery with small Ivalon shavings, there was complete thrombosis (arrow). (Reproduced from Tadavarthy SM, Klugman J, Castañeda–Zuñiga WR, Nath PH, Amplatz K: Systemic to pulmonary collaterals in pathologic states: a review. *Radiology* 1982;144:75–76.)

In patients with cystic fibrosis, selective bronchial arteriography and embolization are performed bilaterally.

Indications

The marked improvement in the diagnosis and pharmacotherapy of pulmonary tuberculosis and of other granulomatoses and infectious diseases that used to be the cause of bronchiectasis has left cystic fibrosis as the leading cause of hemoptysis in the teenager and young adult. Malignant tumors are the most common cause in the elderly.

CYSTIC FIBROSIS

Among the many factors that contribute to the production of hemoptysis in cystic fibrosis are:

Destruction of lung parenchyma;
Erosion of blood vessels;
Hyperemia with enlarged, tortuous bronchial arteries in the areas of bronchiectasis[153,154];
The existence of bronchopulmonary arterial anastomoses, with concomitant development of a systemic–pulmonary shunt[155];
Development of pulmonary hypertension.[155]

Fellows and coworkers treated 13 patients with cystic fibrosis by embolization. Seven patients had no recurrence of hemoptysis, and five had only a minor recurrence (loss of 60 ml or less). One of the main advantages of embolization is that vigorous treatment for cystic fibrosis can be reinstated within 24–48 hr, with consequent shortening of the hospital stay.[156]

UNRESECTABLE MALIGNANT TUMORS, EITHER PULMONARY OR METASTATIC

Embolization can be used for palliation while more conventional therapy controls the primary disease.[144,157]

TUBERCULOSIS AND OTHER GRANULOMATOUS OR OCCUPATIONAL DISEASES (PNEUMOCONIOSES)

Embolization can be used for palliation while more conventional therapy controls the primary disease.[144,157]

TRAUMA

In the polytraumatized patient, embolotherapy of a bleeding bronchial artery can be a life-saving maneuver.[157] The other traumatic indications are:

Post-thoracotomy bleeding; in these patients, reoperation has a high mortality rate due to associated complications such as sepsis and renal failure;
Bilaterally for advanced bronchopulmonary disease when no bleeding site can be identified by bronchoscopy[158];
Patients who refuse operation.

VASCULAR TRAUMA

The recognition of serious vascular trauma in a wound from which blood is spurting is simple, but recognition of the same problem in the chest, abdomen, or extremities when there is no blood visible, particularly after blunt trauma, is sometimes difficult. Any patient who is in shock or who has a penetrating injury or severe blunt trauma must be considered to have a serious vascular injury until proved otherwise.

Blunt abdominal trauma may cause particularly difficult diagnostic problems. The principal findings are shock and hemoperitoneum, which may be confirmed by peritoneal tap. Retroperitoneal hemorrhage is particularly difficult to diagnose and requires extensive evaluation.

Proper assessment of the severely injured patient requires a complete fast diagnostic evaluation. Abdominal computed tomography and angiography provide the most accurate and precise diagnostic information on the location and extent of injury. However, proper surgical care should not be delayed in the unstable patient in whom major vascular or organ injury is suspected.[159] Frequently, it is in the care of the postoperative complications—delayed bleeding, abscess, etc.—that the interventional radiologist is particularly important.

Extremities

Vascular injury in the extremities is commonly caused by penetrating injuries, rarely by blunt trauma. Preoperative evaluation is commonly performed only where a stable lesion is suspected since if the patient is bleeding severely, immediate operation is indicated. Significant arterial injury can be present even when peripheral pulses are present.[160,161]

Adequate angiographic evaluation can prevent delays in surgical repair. It demonstrates to best advantage the precise location and extent of the vascular injury, providing a road map for surgical repair or for therapeutic embolization, particularly in patients in critical condition or in injuries where surgical hemostasis is difficult, as in the thigh or buttocks.[162] Catheterization should be as selective as possible without extending the exploration time unduly. Steel coils are commonly used, since they produce a fast and permanent occlusion, but agents such as Gelfoam or Ivalon also can be used. Embolization should not be attempted when the vascular lesion is in such a location that arrest of blood flow would endanger limb viability.

If untreated, these vascular lesions can lead to the formation of post-traumatic AV fistulae (Fig. 3–54), 85% of which occur in the extremities.[163]

Pelvis

Deaths after pelvic fracture are due to blood loss in 60% of cases.[164] Ligation of the hypogastric artery has been used to control bleeding.[160] Selective catheterization to demonstrate the source of bleeding, followed by embolization of the hypogastric artery with autologous blood clot, was used by Kerr et al to stop the bleeding in three patients.[161,165]

Due to the extensive pelvic collateral arterial network, a proximal occlusion of the hypogastric artery crossing the midline can help maintain extravasation at the site of vascular injury distal to the proximal occlusion. This leakage can be prevented by using Gelfoam or Ivalon particles to accomplish a distal embolization beyond the bleeding point. In addition, bleeding following pelvic trauma is frequently diffuse due to the transection of innumerable small peripheral vessels (Fig. 3–55). Often, this type of bleeding can be stopped only by bilateral peripheral embolization of the hypogastric artery. In one study, branches of the anterior division of the hypogastric artery were involved in 66% of the cases, whereas posterior division branches were involved in only 33%. Many patients had only one site of bleeding in spite of multiple fractures.[166] The early angiographic evaluation in patients with major pelvic trauma prevents the development of serious renal, pulmonary, and hepatic complications of shock and of multiple transfusions.

Retroperitoneum

RENAL TRAUMA

Renal vascular injuries are due to iatrogenic trauma in almost 50% of the cases, with renal biopsy accounting for the largest percentage.[105,167–177] Recently, injuries secondary to percutaneous nephrostomy also have become important.[178–180] Penetrating wounds account for a smaller percentage of cases.[181]

Arteriovenous fistula formation is a relatively common complication of percutaneous renal biopsy, occurring in as many as 36% of hypertensive patients.[147] Hypertension and nephrosclerosis are the most important predisposing factors.[182–184] The use of large-bore cutting needles and the performance of the biopsies without radiologic guidance (fluoroscopy, ultrasound, CT) to minimize the number of attempts have also been blamed for the relatively high incidence of postbiopsy fistulae (Fig. 3–56).[185–188]

Approximately 70% of these fistulae close spontaneously. Therefore, in the absence of life-threatening symptoms, conservative management is generally followed.[182–184] The most common complications are hematuria, hypertension, decreased renal function, and congestive heart failure.[55,182–184] Percutaneous obliteration of a post-biopsy renal AV fistula was reported by Bookstein and Goldstein.[167] Subsequently, several reports of successful embolization confirmed the benignity of the procedure.[105,168–175] Various embolic agents have been used: autologous clot, fat, Gelfoam, IBCA, and spring coils. Short-acting, absorbable embolic agents are preferred to minimize the size of the areas of ischemia produced by the vascular occlusion, since too extensive ischemia could lead to hypertension.

Nephrostomy-induced vascular trauma is usually associated with arteriovenous lacerations (Fig. 3–57A), false-aneurysm formation (Fig. 3–58), or an AV fistula.[178–180]

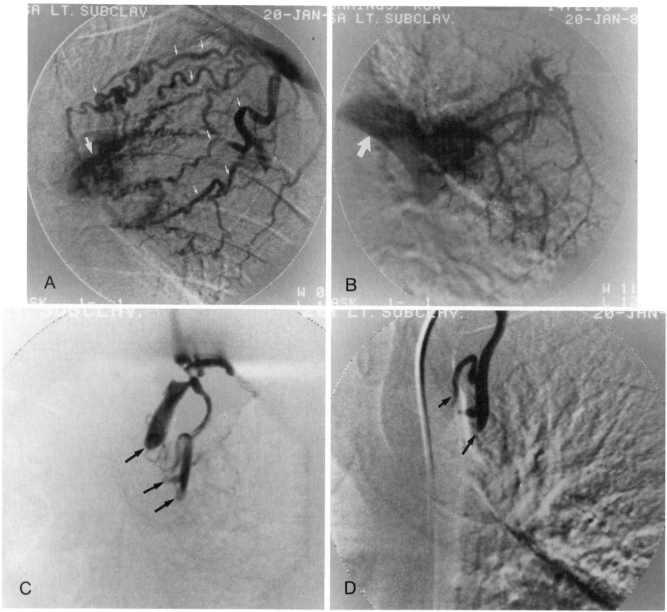

Fig. 3–54 A 21-year-old man with left-sided sternal murmur and hemoptysis after motor vehicle accident. A. Selective left subclavian arteriogram shows numerous fistulous communications between branches of intercostal arteries (small arrows) and right upper pul-monary artery (large arrow). B. Opacification of pulmonary veins on late films (arrow). C, D. After embolization with Ivalon and Gelfoam plugs, complete thrombosis of feeding arteries is apparent (arrows).

Many of these vascular lesions heal spontaneously after tamponade of the nephrostomy tract with a large-bore drainage catheter. The remaining cases require selective arterial embolization to obliterate the bleeding site (Fig. 3–57). The lower incidence of vascular complications after percutaneous nephrostomy in comparison with that of renal biopsy is probably due to the use of an approach through the relatively hypovascular posterolateral margin of the kidney for nephrostomy and to the use of fluoroscopy.

The choice between conservative *versus* surgical treatment in patients with noniatrogenic renal trauma is a difficult one. In general, the treatment is conservative. In the patient with multiple injuries and hematuria, renal evaluation is commonly limited to an intravenous urogram (IVU). Occasionally, ultrasound or CT is performed just prior to an emergency surgical exploration. Exploration of the renal fossa is usually performed in those patients with gross hematuria with a large retroperitoneal hematoma or nonfunctioning kidneys on IVU.[189]

More definite diagnostic information is provided by selective renal arteriography to demonstrate the source of bleeding.[190–195] Therapeutic embolization is an excellent alternative in the management of renal trauma, because bleeding commonly is from a single lobar branch (Fig. 3–59).[191] Furthermore, the absence of a dual vascular sup-

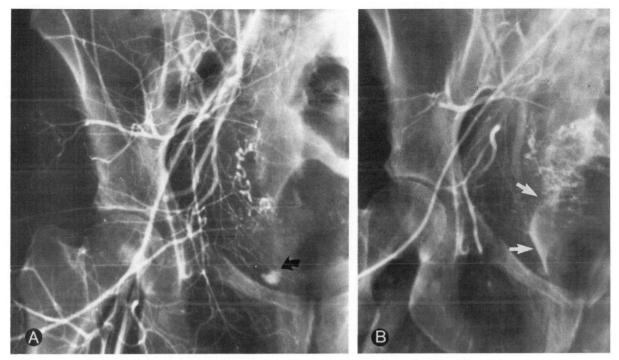

Fig. 3–55 Post-traumatic bleeding. A. Right common iliac arteriogram in patient with history of pelvic trama and falling hematocrit. Observe extravasation of contrast medium from branches of anterior division of hypogastric arteries (arrow) and fracture of ischion. B. Late phase shows extensive extravasation of contrast medium (arrows). Because of midline location of extravasation, bilateral occlusion would probably be necessary for adequate control.

ply enhances the success rate of embolization. Superselective embolization is recommended to minimize ischemic damage.

Angiography is superior to surgical exploration both as a diagnostic and as a therapeutic modality, since during surgical exploration, the presence of a large retroperitoneal hematoma and the continuous extravasation of blood make examination of the surgical field extremely difficult. Not uncommonly, heminephrectomy or total nephrectomy is the only answer to the problem, yet with arteriography some of these kidneys or parts thereof might be salvaged.

OTHER RETROPERITONEAL VASCULAR TRAUMA

If renal injuries are excluded from this group, the most commonly affected vascular structures are the lumbar

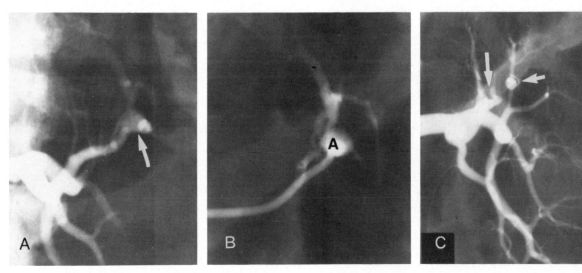

Fig. 3–56 Control of postbiopsy AV fistula. A. Selective left renal arteriogram in patient with postbiopsy fistula and persistent hematuria reveals AV communication from a branch of upper pole (arrow). B. Superselective catheterization of involved arterial branch with tip of catheter within false aneurysm (A). C. After release of GWC spring coil (small arrow) within false aneurysm, observe complete thrombosis of branch artery (large arrow).

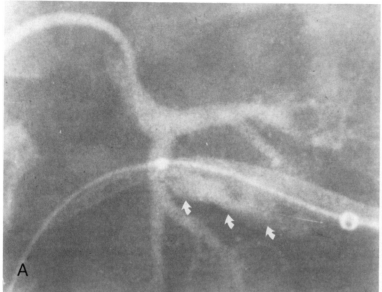

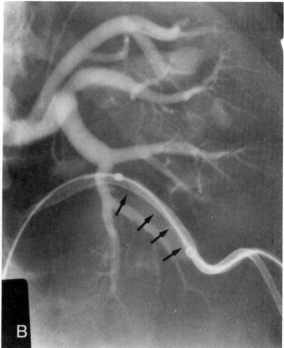

Fig. 3–57 Hemorrhage during tract creation for nephrostolithotomy. A. Selective renal arteriogram shows extensive extravasation of contrast medium from lobar branch (arrows). B. Angioplasty balloon in tract tamponades bleeding site (arrows).

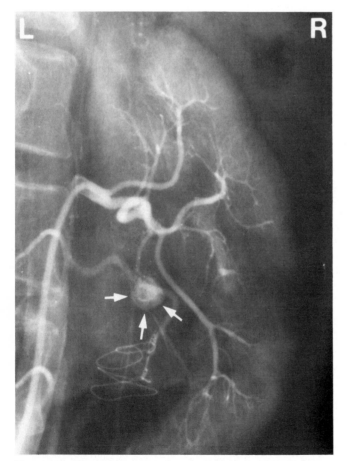

Fig. 3–58 Hemorrhage 2 weeks after percutaneous renal stone removal. Selective renal arteriogram shows large false aneurysm of lobar artery (arrows).

arteries[194,196–199] and, less often, the duodenal and pancreatic arteries.[200] Angiography with selective embolization of the injured vessel commonly controls the problem (Fig. 3–60).

Liver Trauma

Liver injuries caused by blunt or penetrating trauma are second only to small bowel injuries in incidence.[201] Liver trauma is commonly associated with severe injuries to the pancreas, spleen, stomach, bowel, or diaphragm.[202]

Liver injuries can be divided anatomically into three categories: lacerations, linear fractures, and deep stellate fractures.[202] Many (70%) injuries stop bleeding spontaneously and require surgical drainage and debridement of devitalized structures.[201] The remaining 30% of cases require extensive surgical manipulation for control of bleeding and bile leakage, resection of devitalized tissues, etc. Angiography is usually required only in the stable patient with persistent hemobilia,[202–205] AV fistula, or extravasation of blood.[206–208] It is also indicated postoperatively for recurrent bleeding causing subcapsular or intrahepatic hematomas[209,210] or severe hemobilia[204–207] or for the control of large hepaticosystemic fistulae causing hemodynamic disturbances.[211]

The angiographic evaluation of these patients includes imaging of the hepatic arterial and portal circulation, commonly by aortography and celiac and hepatic artery injections. Superior mesenteric artery (SMA) injections are needed to study the replaced right hepatic artery arising from the SMA. Adequate confirmation of an intact, physiologically normal portal circulation is needed before attempting embolization of the hepatic artery, inasmuch as 80% of hepatic perfusion is provided by this system

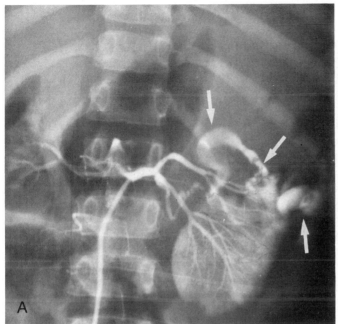

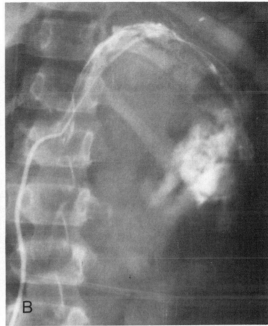

Fig. 3–59 An 18-year-old victim of motor vehicle accident. A. Selective left renal arteriogram shows fracture of kidney with extensive extravasation from branches of renal artery (arrows). B. After embolization of artery with Gelfoam plugs, persistence of extravasation of contrast medium was noted on an aortogram. Selective injection of capsular artery slows extravasation of contrast medium. Observe displacement of capsular branches by large hematoma. (Courtesy of A. Waltman, M.D., Massachusetts General Hospital.)

and embolization of the hepatic artery in a patient with an occluded portal vein or in the presence of portal hypertension would be catastrophic.[211–213]

Superselective catheterization of the injured hepatic artery branch is ideal, although a more central embolization is acceptable if selective catheterization is difficult or if the bleeding is life threatening (Fig. 3–61). In these instances, embolization of the cystic artery may result in gallbladder necrosis.[214,215] Different embolic agents have been used, including Gelfoam, Ivalon, IBCA, and coils.

Iatrogenic injuries are commonly caused by percutaneous liver biopsy or percutaneous biliary drainage pro-

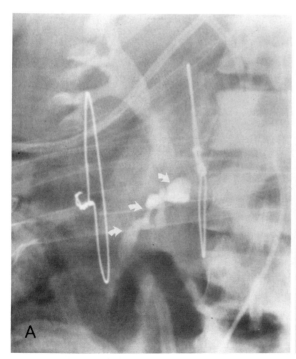

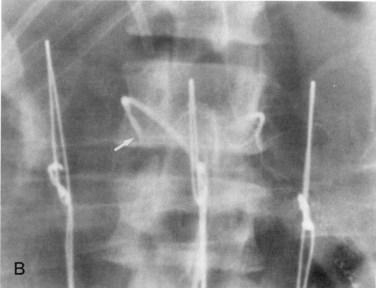

Fig. 3–60 A 16-year-old boy with severe retroperitoneal bleeding 3 weeks after gunshot injury. A. Selective lumbar arteriogram shows extensive extravasation from second right lumbar artery (arrows). B. Arteriogram after embolization of bleeding artery with Gelfoam shows complete thrombosis (arrow). (Courtesy of A. Waltman, M.D., Massachusetts General Hospital.)

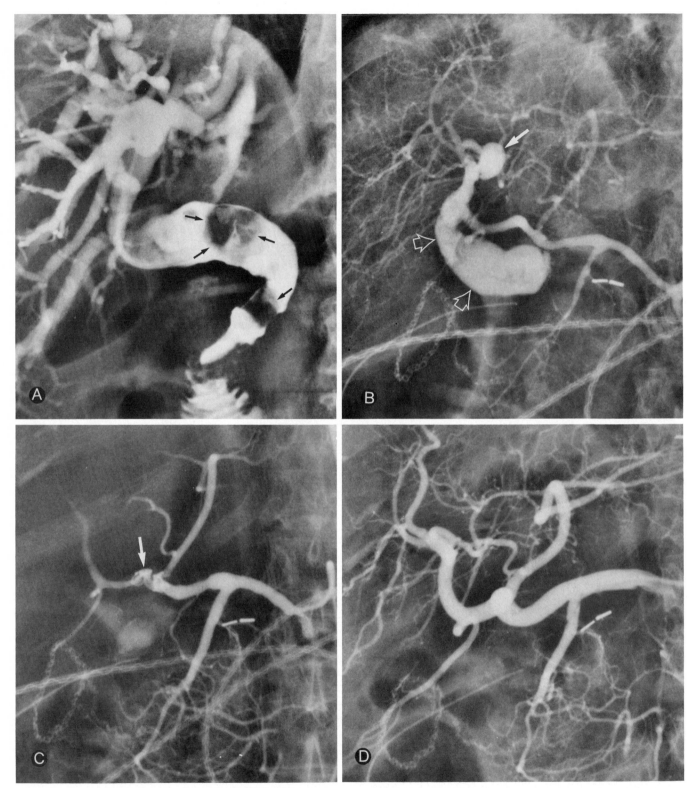

Fig. 3–61   Seventy-seven-year-old woman with massive hemorrhage from a percutaneous transhepatic tract, manifested by hemobilia and hematemesis. A. Transhepatic cholangiogram demonstrates marked dilatation of the biliary tree with multiple stones in the common bile duct (arrows). B. Selective celiac arteriogram because of persistent hemobilia reveals the presence of a large arterial biliary fistula (white arrow) in central part of the right lobe of the liver with massive opacification of the common bile duct (open arrows). Diffuse vasoconstriction of the arterial system is due to hypovolemic shock. C. Follow-up hepatic arteriogram 15 min after the placement of two GWC spring coils in the origin of the right hepatic artery (arrow) demonstrates minimal flow through the right hepatic artery with no evidence of opacification of the fistula. D. Follow-up hepatic arteriogram 6 days after transcatheter embolization reveals good flow in the right hepatic artery with no evidence of opacification of the false aneurysm. (Courtesy of J. Rosch, University of Washington.)

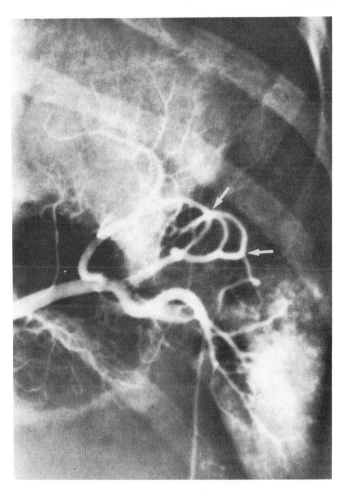

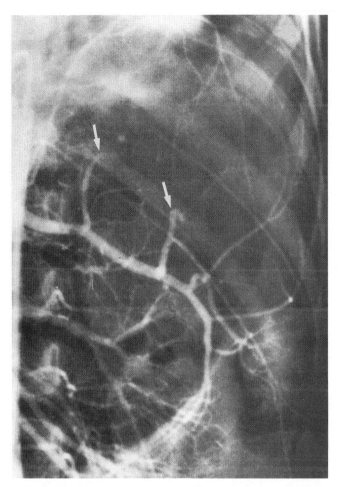

Fig. 3–62 Fragmentation pattern: selective splenic arteriogram 3 days after blunt abdominal trauma. The spleen is fragmented at the center, with the two parts being held together by a large clot. The arterial branches are patent and are seen embedded in the clot (arrows). There is no evidence of active bleeding. Punctate hemorrhages are also present in the lower pole (regional snowstorm pattern). (Reproduced from Fisher RG, Foucar K, Estroda R, Ben-Menachem Y: Splenic rupture in blunt trauma. *Radiol Clin North Am* 1981;19:141–166.)

Fig. 3–63 Transection of the major arterial branches: detail of the early arterial phase of a celiac arteriogram shows absence of blood flow in the major branches of the splenic artery (arrows). Note splaying of parenchymal branches around large hematoma. (Reproduced from Fisher RG, Foucar K, Estroda R, Ben-Menachem Y: Splenic rupture in blunt trauma. *Radiol Clin North Am* 1981;19:141–166.)

cedures. The most common lesions are AV fistulae[216–226] and hemobilia.[204–207] Small peripheral AV communications and arteriobiliary communications tend to close spontaneously.[227] When bleeding persists or when systemic manifestations of the hepatic shunt such as congestive heart failure are evident, therapeutic embolization can be accomplished easily. Again, a superselective embolization of the involved hepatic artery branch is desired to minimize parenchymal damage.

Splenic Trauma

The spleen is the organ most frequently injured in blunt abdominal trauma.[228] An angiographic classification of splenic trauma was developed by Fisher et al[229] with therapeutic implications. According to this study, severe splenic injuries, including fragmentation of the parenchyma (Fig. 3–62) and transection of major arterial branches (Fig. 3–63), mandate emergency splenectomy.

Patients in the intermediate group (major injuries including parenchymal lacerations (Fig. 3–64) and intraparenchymal, subcapsular, and extrasplenic hematomas (Figs. 3–65 and 3–66)) may require splenic operation. This is the group in which therapeutic embolization can be useful, either to help stabilize the patient or to control extravasation. Patients with minor injuries, including small lacerations and small intraparenchymal hematomas (Fig. 3–67), can usually be managed conservatively.[229]

The late sequelae of splenectomy, particularly in children, namely overwhelming infection and rapid death, are well documented.[230–234] Because of these problems, there is a growing consensus in favor of splenic preservation. To preserve splenic function, a central embolization has been advocated by Sclafani[232,233]; this technique avoids the extensive infarction commonly caused by peripheral particulate embolization.[51,235] The rationale of Sclafani's technique is that the decrease in splenic artery flow and pressure allows thrombus to form around the site of injury, stopping the extravasation, while at the same time flow to the remainder of the spleen is preserved via collaterals beyond the site of occlusion.[232,233]

ORGAN ABLATION

Spleen

Surgical removal of the spleen is a well-established procedure in a number of hematologic disorders, including various types of hemolysis and thrombocytolysis, when splenic destruction of peripheral blood cells is especially rapid and replacement and drug therapy prove inadequate. On the other hand, the absence of the spleen impairs the body's ability to produce antibodies[234] and to eliminate encapsulated microorganisms from the bloodstream[236] and increases the susceptibility to fulminant sepsis.[237] From studies on laboratory animals, Van Wyck and Witte suggested that a critical mass of spleen (more than one-third) is needed to maintain host resistance to lethal blood-borne infection from encapsulated microorganisms.[238] Although these problems have been more common in children, overwhelming infection apparently can appear in all patients, regardless of age.[239] Vulnerability to infection seems to be higher in children under 5 years of age and in patients undergoing splenectomy for secondary hypersplenism caused by disease affecting the reticuloendothelial system such as Hodgkin's disease, Cooley's anemia, Gaucher's disease, and histiocytosis[239-241] as well as in renal allograft recipients.[242]

INDICATIONS

The indications for splenic embolization are:

Post-traumatic splenic bleeding[33,243];
Control of variceal bleeding in portal hypertension[244-248];

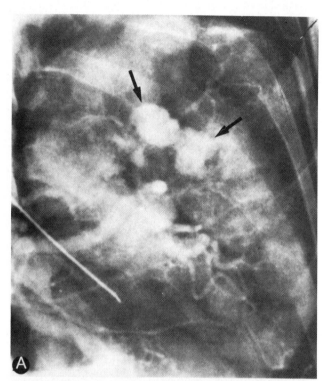

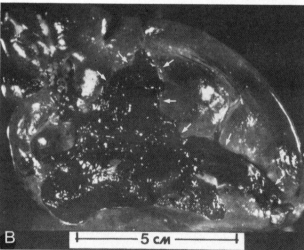

Fig. 3–64 Large intrasplenic bleeding in the upper portion of the splenic hilum is evident (arrows) without angiographic indication of a laceration. B. A specimen of the spleen of another patient shows a large hematoma (arrows). The hematoma occupies the entire splenic hilum. (Reproduced from Fisher RG, Foucar K, Estroda R, Ben-Menachem Y: Splenic rupture in blunt trauma. *Radiol Clin North Am* 1981;19:141–166.)

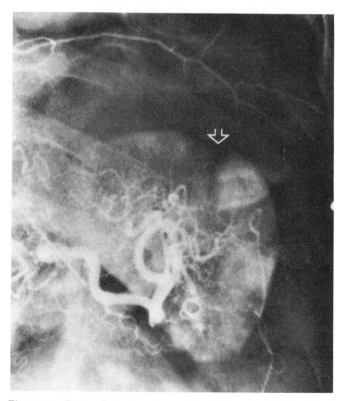

Fig. 3–65 Extrasplenic hematoma. The hallmark of this splenic injury is the displacement of the spleen from the diaphragm and abdominal wall by a massive extrasplenic clot. A cleavage point on the surface of the spleen (arrow) is part of a fetal lobulation. A relatively avascular line can be traced from this point downward representing the continuation of the cleavage line of the lobulation. Slight arterial irregularity and small branch occlusions along this line, as well as the presence of an extrasplenic hematoma, indicate laceration of the spleen along the line. (Reproduced from Fisher RG, Foucar K, Estroda R, Ben-Menachem Y: Splenic rupture in blunt trauma. *Radiol Clin North Am* 1981;19:141–166.)

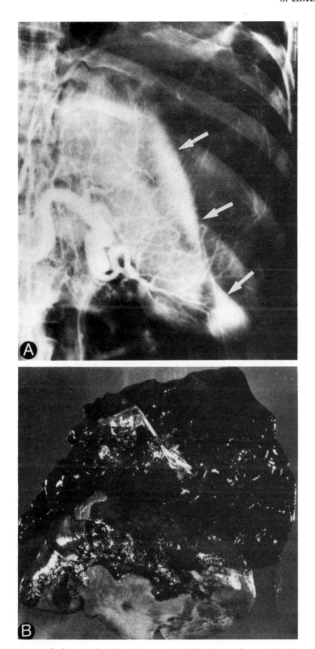

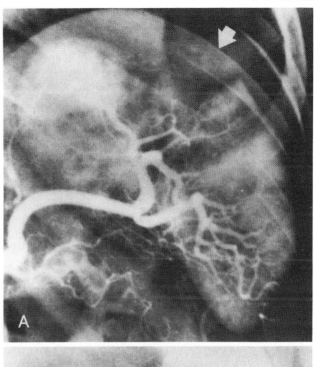

Fig. 3–66 Subcapsular hematoma. A. Massive subcapsular hematoma is indicated by the severe compression of the splenic pulp (arrows), the concavity of the splenic outline, and extension of the stretched branches of the splenic artery well beyond the visible splenic parenchyma. These three findings should help to distinguish subcapsular hematomas from extrasplenic ones. B. The massive size of this subcapsular clot is clearly depicted; the capsule has been partially sliced to show the contents of the hematoma. Subcapsular hematomas are not necessarily as large as this one, and are sometimes discernible only on microscopic examination. (Reproduced from Fisher RG, Foucar K, Estroda R, Ben-Menachem Y: Splenic rupture in blunt trauma. *Radiol Clin North Am* 1981;19:141–166.)

Hypersplenism in portal hypertension[50,235];
Thalassemia major[235];
Variceal bleeding in splenic vein thrombosis[235];
Thrombocytopenia[50,248,249];
Gaucher's disease[249];
Hodgkin's disease.[249]

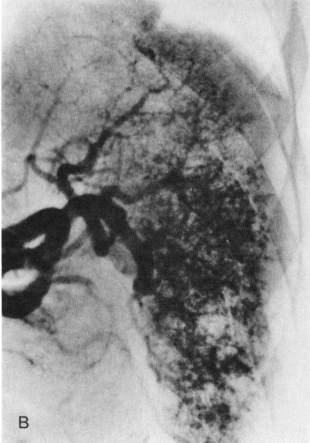

Fig. 3–67 A. Large avascular areas as in this patient can be interpreted as clots filling the base of a laceration, with or without a capsular tear (arrow). B. Widespread snowstorm extravasation. Typical fluffy appearance of snowstorm hemorrhages. This is a fairly benign injury. (Reproduced from Fisher RG, Foucar K, Estroda R, Ben-Menachem Y: Splenic rupture in blunt trauma. *Radiol Clin North Am* 1981;19:141–166.)

METHOD

Initial attempts to embolize the spleen by proximal occlusion of the splenic artery were unsuccessful because of the inadequate hemodynamic response produced. The failure to respond was attributed to the abundant collateral circulation available through the short gastric and gastroepiploic arteries, which re-establish the blood supply to the spleen around the occluded segment of the splenic artery (Fig. 3–68).[50,250,251] Nevertheless, the hemodynamic effects of embolization in the patients with thrombocytopenia, although temporary, improve the patient's status sufficiently to permit surgical splenectomy with a lower risk.[252]

Because of the need for a more enduring and effective hematologic or hemodynamic reponse, total infarction of the organ was attempted with particulate materials in either one or two steps (Fig. 3–69) with adequate hemodynamic results.[50,249,253] Unfortunately, in a high percentage of patients, severe complications developed, including severe unrelenting bronchopneumonias,[235,248,254] splenic abscess,[50,235,248,253–255] and splenic vein thrombosis.[255] This high incidence of complications reflects experimental data in animals, where the larger the infarcted splenic mass, the more serious the complications and secondary effects of the procedure.[50]

It has been suggested that widespread infarction of splenic parenchyma predisposes to growth of anerobic microorganisms in the hypoxic, devitalized tissues. Other factors mentioned include a decrease in the immunologic response of the patient, introduction of exogenous bacteria with the catheter[219] or embolic agents,[235] and contamination of the ischemic vascular bed with intestinal organisms by retrograde flow of portal blood secondary to an inversion of portal vein flow due to the splenic ischemia.[235,249,251,256]

Because of these overwhelming complications, Spigos et al adopted a modified strict protocol including the use of local and systemic antibiotics, careful aseptic techniques, and effective pain control, and accomplished a 30%–70% partial embolization of the organ in 87% of their patients, with a remarkably low incidence of complications: one case each of splenic abscess and pancreatitis, pleural effusion in two, and pneumonia in five, with no deaths.[235] However, other investigators who followed a similar protocol have not been able to reproduce the results. In one series, three abscesses were the result of partial splenic embolization in three patients.[253] It is conceivable that patients with terminal liver disease react differently to splenic embolization[253,255] than do patients in better hemodynamic condition such as those in the Spigos series, virtually all of whom were transplant recipients or were in chronic renal failure.

Spigos Protocol

The steps of the Spigos technique are as follows[235]:

1. Systemic antibiotics: broad-spectrum antibiotics (gentamicin–penicillin G–cefoxitin) are started 8–12 hr before the procedure and continued for 1–2 weeks;
2. Local antibiotics: a suspension of 32,000 units of penicillin G and 12 mg of gentamicin in 100 ml of normal saline is used for suspending the embolic particles (Ivalon or Gelfoam) and for flushing the embolic agent toward the spleen;
3. Local care: either wide scrubs or whole-body baths with povidone–iodine;

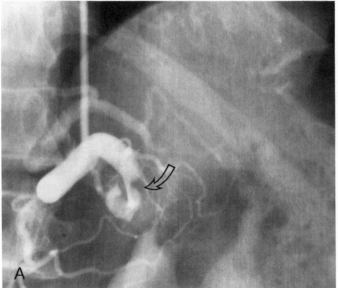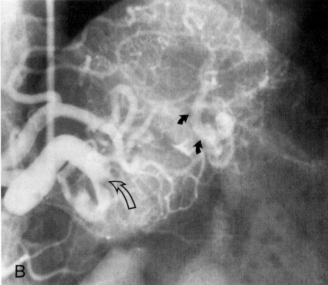

Fig. 3–68 A 50-year-old man with immune thrombocytopenia and platelet count of 44,000/ml. A. Splenic angiogram after proximal occlusion of splenic artery with large Ivalon plugs; observe complete thrombosis of vessel in its midsegment (arrow). B. Repeat splenic arteriogram 4 days later shows complete thrombosis of medial segment of vessel (open arrow). However, left gastric artery is markedly enlarged, with extensive collateralization to distal splenic artery and to peripheral splenic artery branches (black arrow). Initially, transient rise in platelet count to 104,000/ml occurred, but count returned to 74,000/ml within 24 hr because of the extensive collateralization through left gastric artery as a consequence of proximal occlusion of splenic artery. Surgically removed spleen showed only segmental infarct with peripheral organization despite splenic artery thrombosis. (Reproduced from Castañeda–Zuñiga WR, Hammerschmidt DE, Sanchez R, Amplatz K: Nonsurgical splenectomy. *AJR* 1977;129:805–811. © by American Roentgen Ray Society, 1977.)

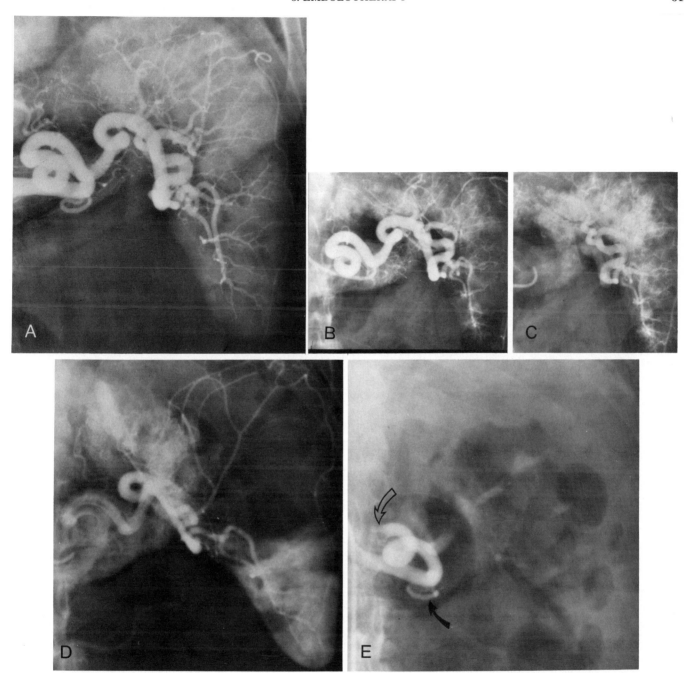

Fig. 3–69 A 49-year-old man admitted for renal transplant with diagnosis of immune thrombocytopenic purpura. A. Splenic arteriogram reveals markedly enlarged spleen. B, C. After partial distal embolization of spleen with small Ivalon particles, multiple peripheral infarcts are seen throughout the organ. D. Angiogram 10 days after first embolization reveals extensive infarction of spleen, with slow clearance of contrast medium and large capsular arteries. E. Angiogram after second embolization shows complete infarction of spleen, with complete occlusion of splenic artery (open curved arrow) and persistence of large pancreatic branch of splenic artery (black arrow).

Adequate platelet response followed procedure, reaching maximum of 511,000/ml on 16th day. Patient was discharged 8 days after second procedure with normal platelet count. Two months later, fever and left upper quadrant abdominal pain developed, and on admission large, tender, nonpulsatile, left upper quadrant mass was palpable. Cardiac arrest occurred, and during resuscitation attempts, the abdominal mass disappeared. The patient died. At autopsy, abscess of lesser omental sac and splenic necrosis were found. (Reproduced from Castañeda–Zuñiga WR, Hammerschmidt DE, Sanchez R, Amplatz K: Nonsurgical splenectomy. *AJR* 1977;129:805–811. © by American Roentgen Ray Society, 1977.)

4. Superselective catheterization, preferably with the tip of the catheter beyond the dorsal pancreatic artery, to decrease the chances of pancreatitis. Careful fluoroscopic control of the extent of infarction is a must to limit the total to approximately 60%;

5. Effective pain control with narcotics, or, as Spigos has

done, with epidural block for 48 hr to prevent splinting of the hemidiaphragm and pleuropulmonary complications;

6. If needed, repeat embolization at a subsequent date;

7. Postembolization white blood cell and platelet count to evaluate the hematologic response.

Kidney

INDICATIONS

In patients with end-stage renal disease or renovascular hypertension and in renal allograft recipients with native kidneys *in situ*, for whom unilateral or bilateral nephrectomy has been chosen as an elective treatment, renal ablation is a useful alternative. Its principal advantage is the substantially lower morbidity and mortality rates for the percutaneous method in comparision with the surgical technique.[257,258]

Renal ablation as a treatment for severe, uncontrollable hypertension was first described by Goldin et al in 1974.[259] Subsequently, the technique has been successful in ablating kidneys in patients with end-stage renal disease on dialysis,[259,260] the native kidneys in allograft recipients,[261] and in nephrotic syndrome.[262] The rationale

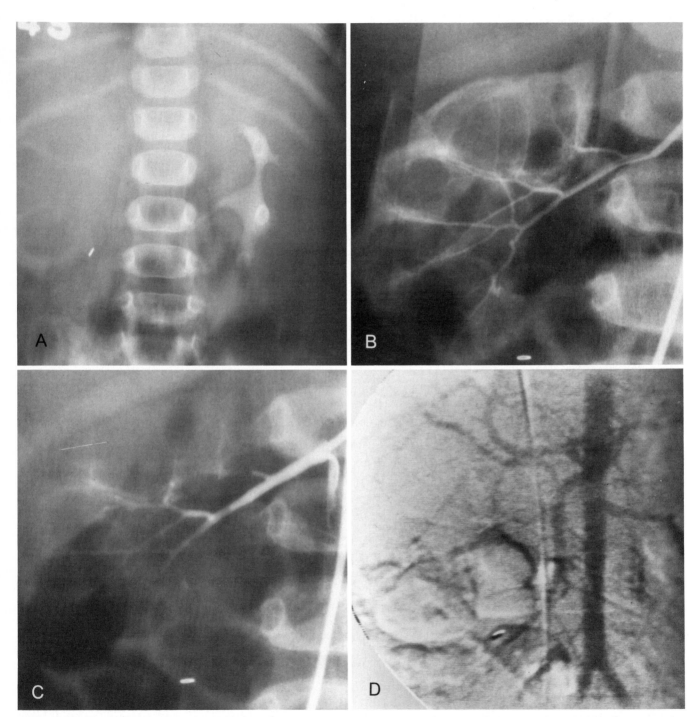

Fig. 3–70   Five-year-old boy with hypertension. A. Intravenous urogram reveals normal collecting system on left and excretion of contrast medium from hydronephrotic right kidney. B. Selective right renal arteriogram reveals marked hydronephrosis of kidney with splaying of renal artery branches around hydronephrotic sacs. C. Arteriogram after injection of 1.5 ml of absolute ethanol shows marked reduction in flow through right kidney. D. Intravenous digital subtraction study 3 months after embolization shows no flow through right renal artery. Blood pressure normalized.

behind both surgical nephrectomy and percutaneous renal ablation in patients with drug-resistant hypertension is that the ischemic renal parenchyma continues to produce renin; the function of the renin–angiotensin system is preserved long after the diseased kidneys have lost all their excretory capacity.[263]

TECHNIQUE

Abdominal aortography is the initial screening procedure, with either standard or digital intra-arterial technique (Fig. 3–70A,B). In patients with an occluded renal artery, delayed films are taken to evaluate the degree of reconstitution of the renal circulation via collaterals. Selective renal arteriography is commonly needed for a more precise delineation of the renal artery anatomy and the number of vessels and their contribution to total blood flow.

In subjects with nonoccluded renal arteries, a Simmons I or II catheter is preferred for selective catheterization, because it can easily be wedged into the renal artery for embolization (Fig. 3–70C). For patients with occluded renal arteries, a technique of recanalization angioplasty of the occluded segment with subsequent embolization was described by Eliscu et al[264] and Denny et al.[265] Embolization can be done in the same sitting or it can be delayed to evaluate the function in the involved kidney and the effects of reperfusion on blood pressure.[265]

The purpose of embolization in these patients is to ablate the juxtaglomerular apparatus and therefore prevent renin production. This can be accomplished only by performing a distal embolization at the arteriolar level or beyond.[78] Small particulate agents such as Gelfoam powder and Ivalon shavings (250–500 μm) or liquid agents such as ethanol or IBCA should be used (Fig. 3–70D). The catheter is wedged in the renal artery, and, under fluoroscopic control, small amounts of the particulate embolic agent suspended in contrast medium are injected, with great care to avoid reflux into the aorta. If a liquid embolic agent is to be used, the total capacity of the renal vascular bed is determined by injecting contrast medium through the catheter until complete opacification of the vascular bed is documented fluoroscopically. Subsequently, an equal amount of the embolic agent is injected through the wedged catheter, and this is repeated until the flow is decreased significantly. Embolization beyond this point would predispose to reflux into the aorta and concomitant complications. The completeness of embolization is verified by follow-up selective arteriography (Fig. 3–70C). If residual renal parenchyma is detected, it is embolized.

Postinfarction syndrome with severe pain is common after the percutaneous procedure and may be attributable in part to an immunologic response to the necrosing tissue. It is managed by the administration of narcotics and subsides in 48–72 hr. No infectious complications have been reported. Delayed reperfusion of segments or of the entire kidney has been seen after apparently complete embolizations.[262] Embolization can easily be repeated, usually with a long-lasting result.[262]

Selective segmental infarction of the kidney was proposed by Reuter et al for patients with segmental renal artery stenosis causing hypertension.[266] Today, these lesions can best be treated by transluminal angioplasty.

EMBOLIZATION IN CANCER

Embolotherapy has been used for both primary and metastatic tumors. The reasons for embolization can be classified into two large groups:

1. Preoperative embolization of primary tumors;
2. Palliative embolization of unresectable tumors to:
   a. Alleviate symptoms, *e.g.*, pain, bleeding, fever, hypercalcemia;
   b. Minimize further dissemination;
   c. Enhance the response to chemotherapy or radiation.

Kidney Tumors

Renal carcinoma is the most common malignancy of the urinary tract, accounting for approximately 3% of all malignancies. The tumor occurs with a 3:1 male:female ratio. In adults, 85%–90% of renal tumors are adenocarcinomas (renal cell carcinomas), with the remainder being sarcomas and lymphoblastomas. Most tumors of the renal pelvis are transitional cell carcinomas.[267,268] Approximately one-fourth (25%–27%) of the patients have metastases at the time of diagnosis.[269,270] Renal cell carcinoma is characterized by a remarkably extensive variety of presentations, systemic effects, and prognoses.[271] Radical nephrectomy has been the conventional therapy, particularly for relatively localized disease (Stages I–III).[272,273]

Attempts to modify the progression of renal carcinoma by embolization were initially reported by Lang, who used radioactive gold grains in 20 patients, reportedly with a decrease in the size of the tumor.[273] Almgard et al reported reduced tumor vascularity, widespread necrosis, shrinkage, and easier resection after tumor embolization with autologous muscle.[274] In a prospective study in 1981, Wallace et al reported a 36% response rate in patients with known metastases.[275] In a similar study, Kaisary et al confirmed that surgery is technically easier, but they could not confirm any changes in the response to delayed hypersensitivity skin testing or any significant regression of the primary or metastatic tumor after embolization alone or with nephrectomy and hormonal/chemotherapeutic treatment. However, in those patients who underwent embolization alone,[276] Sandoval Parra et al obtained an average of 78.2% tumor necrosis with dextran and 53%–64% with Gelfoam and Gelfoam–aluminum. Only 5 of the 81 patients required a second embolization.[277]

INDICATIONS

The principal indications for embolization are:

1. Preoperative: Dilated, tortuous veins commonly cover the surface of large hypervascular tumors. Regional tumor extension into the renal hilum can make dissection of this area difficult. Embolization in these cases

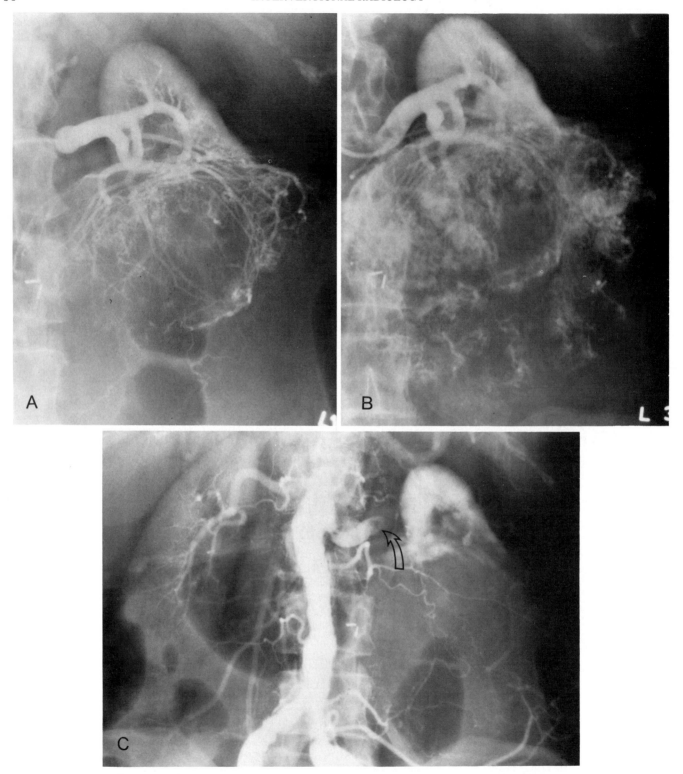

Fig. 3–71   Large renal cell carcinoma of left kidney. A. Early phase of balloon occlusion selective left renal arteriogram shows large vascular mass in lower pole. B. Late phase of balloon occlusion arteriogram after deflation of balloon shows to better advantage the large mass with irregular margins. It is highly vascular but with areas of hypovascularity, probably representing areas of necrosis within tumor. C. Aortogram after embolization of left renal artery with Gelfoam plugs during balloon occlusion of artery. Observe complete thrombosis (arrow).

will shrink the tumor and minimize blood loss, facilitating the operation. Tumors unresectable because of their size and local extension can be made operable by tumor embolization (Fig. 3–71).[275,276] Preoperative embolization is not indicated for small tumors, oncocytomas, or cancers of the renal pelvis.[277]

2. Palliation: In patients with metastatic disease, mean survival is 6 months if there are pulmonary metasta-

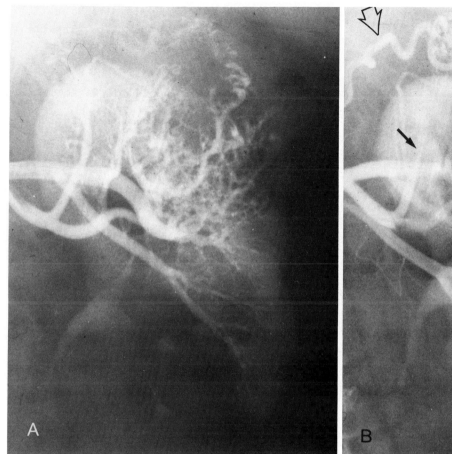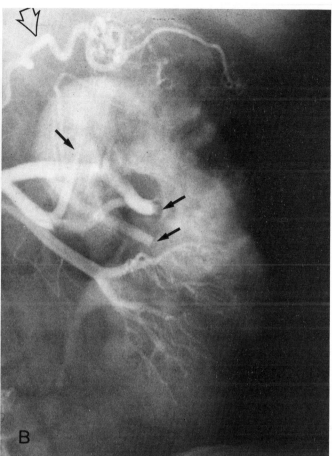

Fig. 3–72 Tumor embolization for palliation in patient with extensive metastatic disease. A. Selective left renal arteriogram shows large hypervascular mass lesion in upper pole with perirenal extension. B. After distal embolization of branches feeding tumor with small Ivalon fragments (arrows), observe increase in diameter of capsular artery providing parasitic blood supply (open arrow). This vessel was selectively embolized.

ses, 15 months with bone metastases, and 2–3 months with cerebral and hepatic metastases. Because of this dismal prognosis, embolization is used only as a palliative measure for control of pain and hematuria (Figs. 3–72 and 3–73).[275]

TECHNIQUE

Because of the severe pain commonly induced by the procedure, premedication with atropine and morphine is useful. These drugs are commonly supplemented by the administration of additional narcotics during and after the procedure.

Because of the frequent presence of a parasitic blood supply to the tumor, an extensive angiographic evaluation, including aortography and selective hepatic and bilateral selective renal arteriography, is performed to delineate the tumoral vascular anatomy. Peripheral obliteration of as many vascular sources as possible is necessary for successful tumor ablation; a proximal or partial vascular embolization will not sufficiently reduce the tumor's blood supply. A distal obliteration is particularly important in patients in whom embolization is planned as the sole treatment because they have extensive metastatic disease or medical contraindications to surgery (Fig. 3–74).

Several embolic agents have been used: radioactive gold seeds, emulsified autologous muscle, Gelfoam, IBCA, spring coils, and ethanol. Of these, distal Gelfoam embolization complemented with spring coils for proximal occlusion[275] and ethanol[278] are most commonly used at present. Gelfoam is cut into small (2 × 2-mm) pieces that are suspended in contrast medium for small vessel embolization. Larger pieces (2 × 3 × 20-mm) are used for more proximal occlusion.[275] Once a substantial decrease in blood flow is visible angiographically, one or two spring coils are deposited in the renal artery to complete the obliteration, preventing the vascular recanalization that occurs 1 week to 4 months after deposition of Gelfoam alone.[31]

Balloon occlusion of the renal artery has been recommended during embolization with Gelfoam[39] and ethanol[278] to prevent reflux of the embolic agent and systemic embolization.

COMPLICATIONS

The most common complications are the postembolization syndrome, consisting of fever, nausea, vomiting, and pain, which occurs in nearly all patients and can last 1–5 days. Narcotics and intravenous fluids are needed for pain control and fluid replacement.[275] Transient hyper-

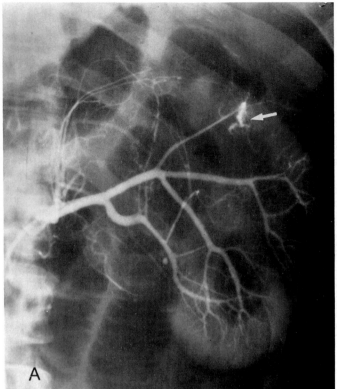

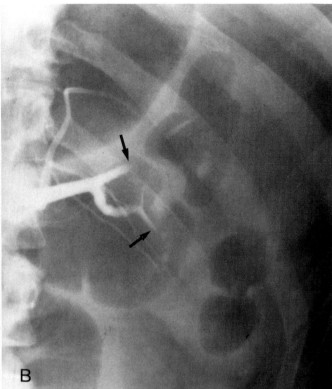

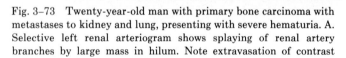

Fig. 3–73   Twenty-year-old man with primary bone carcinoma with metastases to kidney and lung, presenting with severe hematuria. A. Selective left renal arteriogram shows splaying of renal artery branches by large mass in hilum. Note extravasation of contrast medium from peripheral branch of renal artery (arrow). B. Arteriogram after embolization of the left renal artery with Gelfoam shows complete occlusion (arrow) with cessation of extravasation. (Courtesy of A. Waltman, M.D., Massachusetts General Hospital.)

tension has been reported by Wallace et al, and prolonged hypertension (4–7 days) was reported by Mazer et al in patients who underwent palliative embolization for inoperable tumors.[54,275] This condition probably is related to high plasma renin levels after renal parenchymal embolization, as reported by Cho et al.[279] Renal failure is commonly related to the use of large amounts of contrast medium.[275] Undetected coil embolization to the contralateral kidney has been reported by Mazer et al as an unusual cause of renal failure after preoperative renal embolization.[54]

Because of the possible development of a renal abscess after embolization, patients with chronic calculous disease or recurrent or concurrent urinary infections should receive antibiotics before, during, and after embolization.[54,275]

Poor technique and lack of understanding of blood flow characteristics are the common denominators in all systemic complications involving embolization of the agent to undesired sites. Although this complication most commonly occurs with particulate or liquid embolic agents, it has also been reported with coils.[54] A good-quality image intensifier and proper positioning of the catheter are the first steps in prevention. Injection of particulate and liquid embolic agents should be interrupted immediately when the blood flow can be seen to have slowed markedly; insisting on completing the obliteration beyond this point will only cause reflux of the embolic agent. The use of occlusion balloons has been recommended to prevent reflux.[39]

Pelvic Malignancy

As in other parts of the body, therapeutic embolization is frequently indicated in patients with neoplasia of the pelvic organs. Common indications include control of bleeding, palliation of pain, shrinkage of the tumor, and minimizing of blood loss during resection of large vascular tumors.

Typically, in bleeding from genital or vesical tumors, bilateral embolization of the hypogastric artery is performed, because unilateral occlusion is not sufficient to control the hemorrhage due to the crossover circulation from the contralateral hypogastric artery.

BLADDER HEMORRHAGE IN RADIATION CYSTITIS

Control of intractable hemorrhage from the bladder by embolization was first reported in 1974 by Hald and Mygind, who used fragments of muscle.[280] Commonly, the pre-embolization angiographic study fails to demonstrate extravasation of contrast medium (Figs. 3–75A,B). Bilateral embolization of the anterior division of the hypogastric artery is usually needed to accomplish hemostasis (Fig. 3–75C). The excellent collateral network in

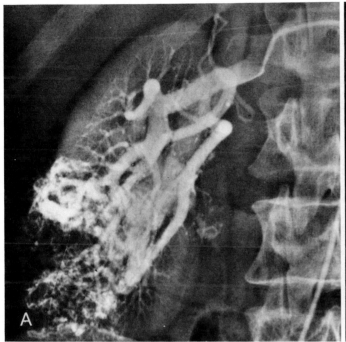 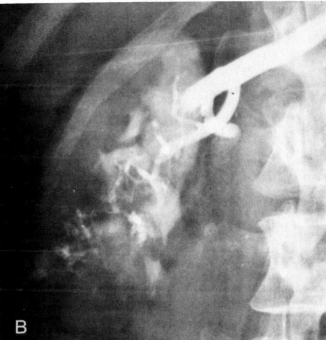

Fig. 3–74 Palliative embolization in metastatic renal cell carcinoma. A. Hypervascular mass in lower pole of right kidney. B. Selective right renal arteriogram after embolization with ethanol shows occlusion of the renal artery. (Reproduced from Becker GJ, Holden RW, Klatte EC: Therapeutic embolization with absolute ethanol. *Semin Intervent Radiol* 1985;1:118–129.)

the bladder muscularis assures an acceptable capillary blood flow to the areas where the main vascular blood supply has been obliterated, thus preventing tissue necrosis. In spite of this collateral flow, the procedure is effective, because the reduced pressure gradient in the embolized vascular system permits clot formation at the level of the diffuse mucosal bleeding.[281]

BLADDER TUMORS

Adequate staging and topographic localization of the tumor by CT and arteriography are important factors in determining whether unilateral or bilateral embolization should be undertaken in patients with primary or metastatic tumors of the bladder.[281] As with hemorrhagic cystitis, the bleeding site is frequently not identified in these cases; and in those patients in whom the tumor is not lateralized, both hypogastric arteries have to be embolized to control the bleeding.[281,282] Unilateral embolization can, however, control the bleeding from bladder carcinoma, as in two patients in Lang et al's series.[281] When possible, superselective catheterization of the vesical arteries should be attempted to limit embolization to the affected area. An axillary or brachial artery approach is particularly suitable for bilateral superselective catheterization. In emergencies due to severe bleeding or in critically ill patients, central occlusion of the anterior division is adequate to control the hemorrhage.

GYNECOLOGIC TUMORS

Ligation of the hypogastric arteries is the established surgical approach for control of hemorrhage in gynecologic and small malignant genital tumors. Embolization of the hypogastric artery, usually bilaterally, provides a more than satisfactory alternative (Fig. 3–76).[281–284] Other indications for embolization include pain control, tumor shrinkage, and reduction of intraoperative blood loss.[282] As is the case with bladder tumors, the bleeding site may not be identified. Nonetheless, hemorrhage is almost immediately controlled by bilateral embolization of the hypogastric artery.[282] Lack of extravasation in the presence of active bleeding has been explained as chronic capillary bleeding from a broad surface of hypervascular granulation tissue formed in response to radiation or from hypervascular neoplastic tissue.[285]

Severe bleeding from the prostate postoperatively in three patients and after biopsy with a Vim–Silverman needle in another was controlled by unilateral or bilateral embolization of the hypogastric artery. Unilateral embolization was performed only when the arteriogram demonstrated localized bleeding. Frequently, bilateral hypogastric embolization would be required due to the extensive collateral network from the external iliac, common femoral, and inferior mesenteric arteries.[286]

Bone Tumors

Preoperative embolization has been used to reduce blood loss from vascular bone tumors, which can total 1–3 liters,[287–292] during resection of the tumor or during orthopaedic maneuvers such as hip replacement[292] or internal fracture fixation.[293] Embolization should be performed as close to the time of the operation as possible to prevent development of collateral circulation that bypasses the occlusion site.[292] There is no evidence that

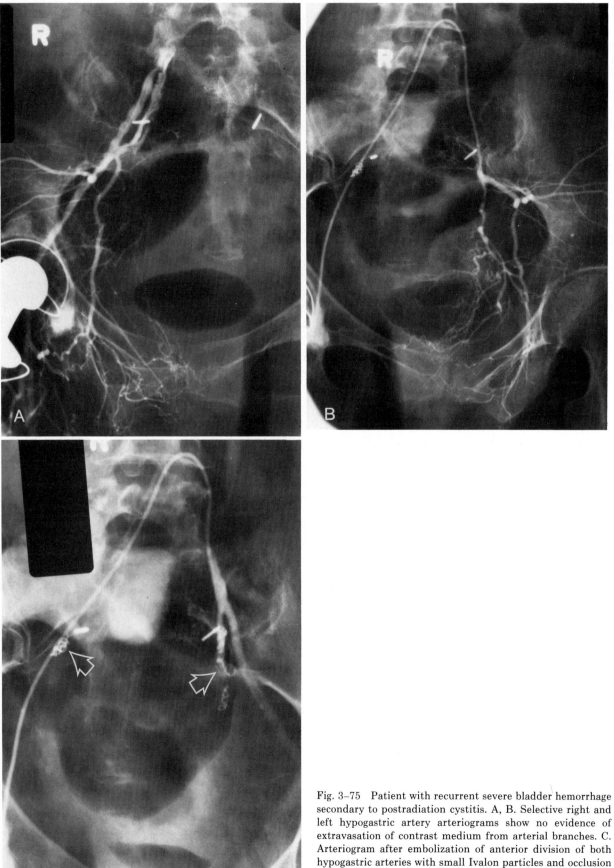

Fig. 3–75 Patient with recurrent severe bladder hemorrhage secondary to postradiation cystitis. A, B. Selective right and left hypogastric artery arteriograms show no evidence of extravasation of contrast medium from arterial branches. C. Arteriogram after embolization of anterior division of both hypogastric arteries with small Ivalon particles and occlusion of proximal trunk with GWC coils shows complete occlusion of both arteries (arrows).

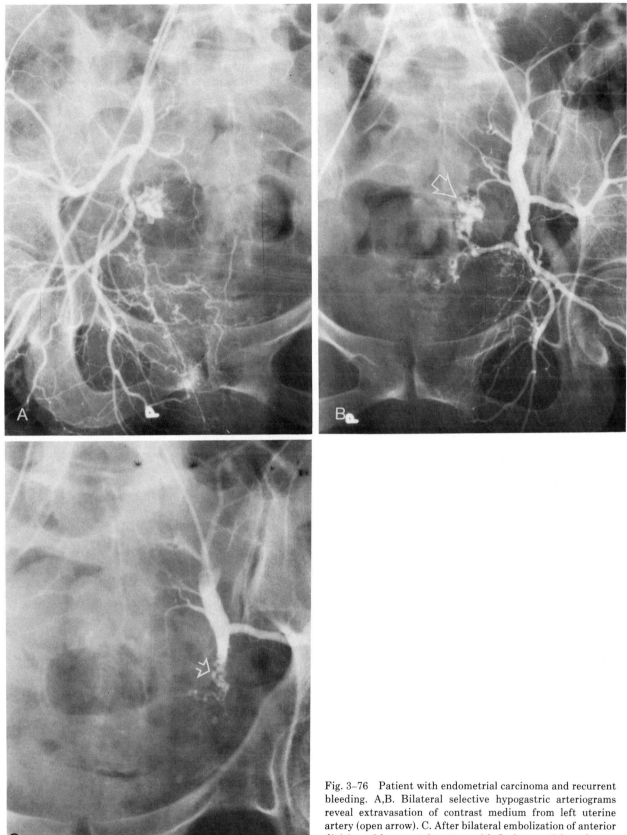

Fig. 3–76 Patient with endometrial carcinoma and recurrent bleeding. A,B. Bilateral selective hypogastric arteriograms reveal extravasation of contrast medium from left uterine artery (open arrow). C. After bilateral embolization of anterior division of hypogastric artery with Ivalon particles, observe complete thrombosis of this vessel (arrow).

embolization retards healing at the fracture site; callus formation, restoration of function, and resolution of pain were observed within the first 2 weeks after embolization in a series reported by Rowe et al.[293] Embolization has also been used as the primary treatment for benign tumors, particularly when resection would require a crippling major operation or when the tumor is in a poorly accessible part of the body such as the spine. Such use was reported by Keller et al in two patients with aneurysmal bone cysts and another with a giant cell tumor of the sacrum.[292,294,295]

Embolization of bone tumors has been applied primarily for relief of pain.[287,291,292,294,296] The mechanism by which the procedure relieves pain is unknown, although Wallace and Chuang have hypothesized that the fastest growing portion of the tumor is the more vascular area and that vascular occlusion thus decreases the tumor growth rate, thereby reducing the pressure on the periosteum, with consequent decrease or disappearance of pain.[291,294] An additional beneficial side effect of a successful embolization is the shrinkage of tumor mass, particularly when nonabsorbable embolic agents are used (Fig. 3–69).

Embolic Agents

Depending on whether embolization will be followed immediately by surgical resection, an absorbable embolic agent, such as Gelfoam, or a nonabsorbable agent, such as Ivalon particles or IBCA, should be used. Gelfoam produces a temporary occlusion, with subsequent recanalization of the vessels, so proximal vascular occlusion with 2–3-mm Gelfoam pieces might be adequate as an immediate preoperative measure occlusion designed to minimize blood loss.[287–291] However, if the surgical procedure is delayed, recanalization of the occluded vessel, development of parasitic peripheral blood flow, or both will ensue if Gelfoam is used, negating the embolization procedure. If embolization is carried out for palliation (*e.g.*, pain relief, tumor shrinkage, fracture fixation) or as the primary treatment for benign tumors, permanent embolic agents should be used. The agent used in these cases should be able to inhibit the development of collaterals beyond the site of vascular occlusion to prevent revascularization of the tumor. Embolic fluid agents, with the possible exception of ethanol (because of the ischemic complications it can cause[293]), and Ivalon microparticles are the best agents to create this type of embolization.

Superselective catheterization is desirable to confine infarction to the tumor. If an ideal superselective catheter position is not attainable, protection of the noninvolved distal vessels with coils has been used in the pelvic area.[292]

Complications

A postembolization syndrome of pain, fever, numbness, and parasthesia of the affected area has been described[291,296]; it usually subsides within 48–72 hr.

Unintentional embolization of normal vessels is the greatest risk, and skin breakdown[293] and ischemic neuropathy[292] have been reported after otherwise successful embolizations. Protection by occlusion of noninvolved contiguous vessels[292] with Gianturco-Wallace-Chuang (GWC) coils, particularly careful angiographic evaluation before the embolization to select the target vessels, superselective distal catheterization, and avoidance of overzealous injections of the embolic agent are the best means of avoiding these complications.

References

1. Dawbain G. In Lussenhop AJ, Spence WT: Artificial embolization of cerebral arteries: report of use in a case of arteriovenous malformation. *JAMA* 1960;172:1153–1155
2. Brooks B: The treatment of traumatic arteriovenous fistula. *South Med J* 1930;23:100–106
3. Lussenhop AJ, Spence WT: Artificial embolization of cerebral arteries: report of use in a case of arteriovenous malformation. *JAMA* 1960;172:1153–1155
4. Baum S, Nusbaum M: The control of gastrointestinal hemorrhage by selective mesenteric arterial infusion of vasopressin. *Radiology* 1971;98:497–505
5. Rosch C, Dotter CT, Brown MJ: Selective arterial embolization. *Radiology* 1972;102:303–306
6. Lin SR, LaDow CS, Tatoian JA, Go EB: Angiographic demonstration and silicone pellet embolization of facial hemangiomas of bone. *Neuroradiology* 1974;17:201–204
7. Serbinenko FA: Balloon catheterization and occlusion of major cerebral vessels. *J Neurosurg* 1974;41:125–145
8. White RI, Barth KH, Kaufman SL, DeCaprio V, Strandberg JD: Therapeutic embolization with detachable balloons. *CardioVasc Intervent Radiol* 1980;3:229–241
9. Debrun G, Lacour P, Caron JP, Hurth M, Comoy J, Keravel Y: Inflatable and released balloon technique experimentation in dog: application in man. *Neuroradiology* 1975;9:267–271
10. Kerber C: Balloon catheter with a calibrated leak. *Radiology* 1976;120:547–550
11. Zanetti PH, Sherman FE: Experimental evaluation of a tissue adhesive as an agent for the treatment of aneurysms and arteriovenous anomalies. *J Neurosurg* 1972;36:72–79
12. Carey LS, Grace DM: The brisk bleed: controlled by arterial catheterization and Gelfoam plug. *J Can Assoc Radiol* 1974;25:113–115
13. Portsmann W, Wierny L, Warnke H, Gerstberger G, Romaniuk PA: Catheter closure of patent ductus arteriosus: 62 cases treated without thoracotomy. *Radiol Clin North Am* 1971;9:203–218
14. Tadavarthy SM, Knight L, Ovitt TW, Snyder C, Amplatz K: Therapeutic transcatheter arterial embolization. *Radiology* 1974;112:13–16
15. Tadavarthy SM, Moller JH, Amplatz K: Polyvinyl alcohol (Ivalon): a new embolic material. *AJR* 1975;125:609–616
16. Gianturco C, Anderson JH, Wallace S: Mechanical devices for arterial occlusion. *AJR* 1975;124:428–435
17. Ellman BA, Parkhill BJ, Curry TS, Marcus PB, Peters PC: Ablation of renal tumors with absolute ethanol: a new technique. *Radiology* 1981;141:619–626
18. Rholl KS, Rysavy JA, Vlodaver Z, Cragg AH, Castañeda-Zuñiga WR, Amplatz K: Transcatheter thermal venous occlusion: a new technique. *Radiology* 1982;145:333–337
19. Cragg AH, Rosel P, Rysavy JA, Vlodaver Z, Castañeda-Zuñiga WR, Amplatz K: Renal ablation using hot contrast medium: an experimental study. *Radiology* 1983;148:683–686
20. Cho KJ, Williams DM, Brady TM, et al: Transcatheter embolization with sodium tetradecyl sulfate: experimental and clinical results. *Radiology* 1984;153:95–99
21. Thompson WM, Johnsrude IS: Vessel occlusion with trans-

catheter electrocoagulation. *CardioVasc Intervent Radiol* 1980;2:244–255

22. Cragg AH, Galliani CA, Rysavy JA, Castañeda–Zuñiga WR, Amplatz K: Endovascular diathermic vessel occlusion. *Radiology* 1982;144:303–308

23. Fingerhut AG, Alksne JF: Thrombosis of intracranial aneurysms: an experimental approach utilizing magnetically controlled iron particles. *Radiology* 1966;86:342–347

24. Lang EK: Superselective arterial catheterization as a vehicle for delivering radioactive infarct particles to tumors. *Radiology* 1971;98:391–399

25. Prochaska JH, Flye MW, Johnsrude IS: Left gastric artery embolization for control of gastric bleeding: a complication. *Radiology* 1973;107:521–522

26. Chuang VP, Wallace S: Hepatic arterial redistribution for intraarterial infusion of hepatic neoplasms. *Radiology* 1980;135:295–299.

27. Conroy RM, Lyons KP, Kuperus JH, Juler GL, Joy I, Pribram HFW: New technique for localization of therapeutic emboli using radionuclide labeling. *AJR* 1978;130:523–528

28. Endert G, Ritter H, Schumann E: ^{99m}Tc-Markierung von Gelantineschwamm für die Katheterembolisation. *Fortschr Röntgentstr* 1979;131:600–603

29. Cunningham DS, Paletta FX: Control of arteriovenous fistula in massive facial hemanginoma by muscle emboli. *Plast Reconstr Surg* 1970;46:305–308

30. Bryan WM, Maull KI: Arteriovenous malformations of the mandible. *Plast Reconstr Surg* 1975;55:690–696

31. Bookstein JJ, Cholasta EM, Foley D, Walters JS: Transcatheter hemostasis of gastrointestinal bleeding using modified autogenous clot. *Radiology* 1974;113:227–231

32. Meaney TF, Chicatelli PD: Obliteration of renal arteriovenous fistula by transcatheter clot embolization: case report and experimental observations. *Cleve Clin Q* 1974;41:33–38

33. Chuang VO, Reuter SR: Experimental diminution of splenic function by selective embolization of the splenic artery. *Surg Gynecol Obstet* 1975;140:715–720

34. Barth KH, Strandberg JD, White RI Jr: Long-term follow-up of transcatheter embolization with autologous clot, Oxycel, and Gelfoam in domestic swine. *Invest Radiol* 1977;12:273–280

35. Light RU, Prentice HR: Surgical investigation of a new absorbable sponge derived from gelatin for use in hemostasis. *J Neurosurg* 1945;2:435–445

36. Ishimori S: Treatment of carotid–cavernous fistula by Gelfoam embolization. *J Neurosurg* 1967;27:315–319

37. Goldstein HM, Wallace S, Anderson JH, Bell RL, Gianturco C: Transcatheter occlusion of abdominal tumors. *Radiology* 1976;120:539–545

38. Page RC, Larson EJ, Siegmund E: Plastic sponge occludes arteriovenous defect. *JAMA* 1976;236:1335–1338

39. Levin DC, Beckmann CF, Hillman B: Experimental determination of flow patterns of Gelfoam emboli: safety implications. *AJR* 1980;134:525–528

40. Greenfield AJ, Athanasoulis CA, Waltman AC: Transcatheter embolization: prevention of embolic reflux using balloon catheters. *AJR* 1978;131:165–168

41. Greenfield AJ: Transcatheter vessel occlusion: selection of methods and material. *CardioVasc Intervent Radiol* 1980;3:222–228

42. Rosch J, Keller FS, Kozak B, Niles N, Dotter CT: Gelfoam powder embolization of the left gastric artery in treatment of massive small gastric bleeding. *Radiology* 1984;151:365–370

43. Jander HP, Russinovich NAE: Transcatheter Gelfoam embolization in abdominal, retroperitoneal, and pelvic hemorrhage. *Radiology* 1980;136:337–344

44. Richman SD, Green WM, Kroll R, Casarella WJ: Superselective transcatheter embolization of traumatic renal hemorrhage. *AJR* 1977;128:843–844

45. Zollikofer C, Castañeda–Zuñiga WR, Galliani C, Rysavy JA, Formanek A, Amplatz K: Therapeutic blockade of arteries using compressed Ivalon. *Radiology* 1980;136:635–640

46. Castañeda–Zuñiga WR, Sanchez R, Amplatz K: Experimental observations on short- and long-term effects of arterial occlusion with Ivalon. *Radiology* 1978;126:783–785

47. Berenstein A, Kricheff II: Catheter and material selection for transarterial embolization. Technical considerations II: materials. *Radiology* 1979;132:631–639

48. Kerber CW, Bank WO, Horton JA: Polyvinyl alcohol foam: prepacked emboli for therapeutic embolization. *AJR* 1978;130:1193–1194

49. Herrera M, Rysavy J, Kotula F, Castañeda–Zuñiga WR, Amplatz K: Ivalon shavings: a new embolic agent. *Radiology* 1982;144:638–640

50. Castañeda–Zuñiga WR, Hammerschmidt DE, Sanchez R, Amplatz K: Nonsurgical splenectomy. *AJR* 1977;129:805–811

51. Chuang VP, Soo CS, Wallace S: Ivalon embolization in abdominal neoplasms. *AJR* 1981;136:729–733

52. Zollikofer C, Castañeda–Zuñiga WR, Galliani C, et al: A combination of stainless steel coil and compressed Ivalon: a new technique for embolization of large arteries and arteriovenous fistulas. *Radiology* 1981;138:229–231

53. Castañeda–Zuñiga WR, Galliani CA, Rysavy J, Kotula F, Amplatz K: "Spiderlon": new device for simple, fast arterial and venous occlusion. *AJR* 1981;136:627–628

54. Mazer MJ, Baltaxe HA, Wolf GL: Therapeutic embolization of the renal artery with Gianturco coils: limitations and technical pitfalls. *Radiology* 1981;138:37–46

55. Castañeda–Zuñiga WR, Tadavarthy SM, Beranek I, Amplatz K: Nonsurgical closure of large arteriovenous fistulas. *JAMA* 1976;236:2649–2650

56. Castañeda–Zuñiga WR, Tadavarthy SM, Galliani C, Laerum F, Schwarten D, Amplatz K: Experimental venous occlusion with stainless steel spiders. *Radiology* 1981;141:238–241

57. Probst P, Rysavy J, Amplatz K: Increased safety of splenoportography by plugging the needle tract. *AJR* 1978;131:445–449

58. Doppman JL, DiChiro G, Ommaya A: Obliteration of spinal-cord arteriovenous malformations by percutaneous embolisation. *Lancet* 1968;1:477–486

59. Meyers PH, Cronic F, Nice CM Jr: Experimental approach in the use and magnetic control of metallic iron particles in the lymphatic and vascular system of dogs as a contrast and isotopic agent. *AJR* 1963;90:1068–1077

60. Loop JW, Foltz EL: Applications of angiography during intracranial operation. *Acta Radiol [Diagn]* 1966;5:363–376

61. Fleischer AS, Kricheff I, Ransohoff J: Postmortem findings following the embolization of an arteriovenous malformation. *J Neurosurg* 1972;37:606–609

62. Lin SR, LaDow CS, Tatoian JA, Go EB: Angiographic demonstration and silicone pellet embolization of facial hemangiomas of bone. *Neuroradiology* 1974;7:201–204

63. Longacre JJ, Benton C, Unterthiner RA: Treatment of facial hemangioma by intravascular embolization with silicone spheres. *Plast Reconstr Surg* 1972;50:618–621

64. Kricheff I, Madayag M, Braunstein P: Transfemoral catheter embolization of cerebral and posterior fossa arteriovenous malformations. *Radiology* 1972;103:107–111

65. Matsumoto T: *Tissue Adhesives in Surgery.* New York, Medical Examination Publishing Co, 1972

66. Dotter CT, Goldman ML, Rosch J: Instant selective arterial occlusion with isobutyl-2-cyanoacrylate. *Radiology* 1975;114:227–230

67. Goldman ML, Philip PL, Sarrafizadeh MS: Bucrylate, a liquid tissue adhesive for transcatheter embolization. *Appl Radiol* 1984; Nov/Dec:89–94

68. Thelen M, Bruehl P, Gerlach F, Biersack HJ: Katheteroembol-

isation von metastasierten Nierenkarzinomen mit Butyl-2-Cyanoacrylat. *Fortschr Röntgenstr* 1976;124:232–235

69. Freeny PC, Bush WH, Kidd R: Transcatheter occlusive therapy of genitourinary abnormalities using isobutyl-2-cyanoacrylate. *AJR* 1979;133:647–656

70. Papo J, Baratz M, Merimsky E: Infarction of renal tumors using isobutyl-2-cyanoacrylate and Lipiodol. *AJR* 1981;137:781–785

71. Cromwell LD, Kerber CW: Modification of cyanoacrylate for therapeutic embolization: preliminary experience. *AJR* 1981;137:781–785

72. Salomonowitz E, Gottlob R, Castañeda–Zuñiga WR, Amplatz K: Transcatheter embolization with pro-celloidin cyanoacrylate. *Radiology* 1983;149:445–448

73. White RI, Strandberg JV, Gross GS, Barth KH: Therapeutic embolization with long-term occluding agents and their effects on embolized tissues. *Radiology* 1977;125:677–687

74. Goldman ML, Land WC Jr, Bradley EL III: Transcatheter therapeutic embolization in the management of massive upper gastrointestinal bleeding. *Radiology* 1976;120:513–521

75. Doppman JL, Zapol W, Pierce J: Transcatheter embolization with a silicone rubber preparation: experimental observations. *Invest Radiol* 1971;6:304–309

76. Berenstein A: Flow-controlled silicone fluid embolization. *AJR* 1980;135:1213–1218

77. Buecheler E, Hupe W, Klosterhalfen J, Altenaehr E, Erbe W: Neue Substanz zur therapeutischen Embolisation von Nierentumoren. *Fortschr Röntgenstr* 1976;124:232–235

78. Kauffman GW, Rassweiler J, Richter G, Hauenstein HK, Rohrbock R, Friedburg H: Capillary embolization with Ethibloc: new embolization concept test in dog kidneys. *AJR* 1981;137:1163–1168

79. Abbott WM, Austen WG: The effectiveness and mechanism of collagen induced hemostasis. *Surgery* 1975;78:723–729

80. Diamond NG, Casarella WJ, Bachman DM, Wolff M: Microfibrillar collagen hemostat: a new transcatheter embolization agent. *Radiology* 1979;133:775–779

81. Kaufman SL, Strandberg JD, Barth KH, White RI: Transcatheter embolization with microfibrillar collagen in swine. *Invest Radiol* 1978;13:200–204

82. Mineau DE, Miller FJ, Lee RG, Nakashima EN, Nelson JA: Experimental transcatheter spenectomy using absolute ethanol. *Radiology* 1982;142:355–359

83. Ekelund L, Jonsson N, Trugut H: Transcatheter obliteration of the renal artery by ethanol injection: experimental results. *CardioVasc Intervent Radiol* 1981;4:1–7

84. Doppman JL, Popovsky M, Girton M: The use of iodinated contrast agents to ablate organs: experimental studies and histopathology. *Radiology* 1981;138:333–340

85. Seyferth W, Jecht E, Zeitler E: Percutaneous sclerotherapy of varicocele. *Radiology* 1981;139:335–340

86. Hunter DW, Castañeda–Zuñiga WR, Young A, et al: Spermatic vein embolization with hot contrast medium or detachable balloons. *Semin Intervent Radiol* 1984;1:163–169

87. Wallace S, Gianturco C, Anderson JH, Goldstein HM, Davis LJ: Therapeutic vascular occlusion utilizing steel coil technique: clinical applications. *AJR* 1976;127:381–387

88. Anderson JH, Wallace S, Gianturco C: Transcatheter intravascular coil occlusion of experimental arteriovenous fistulas. *AJR* 1977;129:795–798

89. Formanek A, Probst P, Tadavarthy SM, Castañeda–Zuñiga WR, Amplatz K: Transcatheter embolization in the pediatric age group. *Ann Radiol* 1979;22:150–158

90. Widrich WC, Robbins AJ, Johnson WC, Nasbeth DC: Pitfalls of transhepatic portal venography and therapeutic coronary vein occlusion. *AJR* 1978;131:637–640

91. Fuhrman BP, Bass JL, Castañeda–Zuñiga WR, Amplatz K, Lock JE: Coil embolization of congenital thoracic vascular anomalies in infants and children. *Circulation* 1984;70:285–289

92. Anderson JH, Wallace S, Gianturco C: "Mini" Gianturco stainless steel coils for transcatheter vascular occlusion. *Radiology* 1979;132:301–303

93. Castañeda–Zuñiga WR, Zollikofer C, Barreto A, Formanek A, Amplatz K: A new device for the safe delivery of stainless steel coils. *Radiology* 1980;136:230–231

94. Anderson JH, Wallace S, Gianturco C: Transcatheter intravascular coil occlusion of experimental arteriovenous fistulas. *AJR* 1977;129:795–798

95. Wallace S, Gianturco C, Anderson JH, et al: Therapeutic vascular occlusion utilizing steel coil technique: clinical applications. *AJR* 1976;127:381–387

96. Tisnado J, Beachley MC, Cho SR: Peripheral embolization of a stainless steel coil. *AJR* 1979;133:324–326

97. Chuang VP: Nonoperative retrieval of Gianturco coils from abdominal aorta. *AJR* 1979;132:996–997

98. Freeny PC, Busch WH Jr, Kidd R: Transcatheter occlusive therapy of genitourinary abnormalities using isobutyl-2-cyanoacrylate (Bucrylate). *AJR* 1979;133:647–656

99. Gomes AS, Rysavy JA, Spadaccini CA, Amplatz K: The use of the bristle brush for transcatheter embolization. *Radiology* 1978;129:354–360

100. Hieshima GBM, Grinnell VS, Mehringer CM: A detachable balloon for therapeutic transcatheter occlusion. *Radiology* 1981;138:227–228

101. Wholey MH, Kessler L, Boehnke M: A percutaneous balloon catheter technique for the treatment of intracranial aneurysms. *Acta Radiol [Diagn]* 1972;13:286–292

102. Paster SB, Van Houten FX, Adams DF: Percutaneous balloon catheterization. *JAMA* 1975;230:573–575

103. Pevsner PH: Micro-balloon catheter for superselective angiography and therapeutic occlusion. *AJR* 1977;128:225–230

104. DiTullio MC, Rand RW, Frisch E: Detachable balloon catheter: its application in experimental arteriovenous fistulae. *J Neurosurg* 1978;48:717–723

105. White RI, Kaufman SL, Barth KH, DeCaprio V, Strandbert JD: Embolotherapy with detachable silicone balloons: technique and clinical results. *Radiology* 1979;131:619–627

106. Gomes MMR, Bernatz PE: Arteriovenous fistulas: a review and ten year experience at the Mayo Clinic. *Mayo Clin Proc* 1970;45:81–102

107. Szilagyi DE, Elliot JP, DeRusso RJ: Peripheral congenital arteriovenous fistulas. *Surgery* 1965;57:61–73

108. Coursely C, Ivan JC, Barker NW: Congenital AVF in the extremities: an analysis of sixty-nine cases. *Angiology* 1956;7:201–206

109. Rappaport I, Yim D: Congenital AVF of the head and neck. *Arch Otolaryngol* 1973;97:350–353

110. Hoehn JF, Farrow GM, Devine KD, Masson JK: Invasive hemangioma of the head and neck. *Am J Surg* 1970;120:495–500

111. Reid MR: Studies on abnormal AV communication acquired and congenital: the origin and nature of AV aneurysms, cirsoid aneurysms and simple angiomas. *Arch Surg* 1925;10:996–1009

112. Devine KD: Congenital AV fistulas of the face and neck. *Plast Reconstr Surg* 1959;23:273–282

113. Watson WL, McCarty WD: Blood and lymph vessel tumors: a report of 1056 cases. *Surg Gynecol Obstet* 1940;71:569–578

114. Siegel ME, Grangiana FA, White RI: The use of nuclear medicine in the evaluation of peripheral arterial disease, in Strauss AW, Pitt B, James AE (eds) *Cardiovascular Nuclear Medicine.* St. Louis, CV Mosby Co, 1979, p 302

115. Castañeda–Zuñiga WR, Lehnert M, Nath PH, Zollikofer C, Velasquez G, Amplatz K: Therapeutic embolization of facial arteriovenous fistulas. *Radiology* 1979;132:599–602

116. Fleischer AS, Kricheff I, Ransohoff J: Postmortem findings following the embolization of an arteriovenous malformation: case report. *J Neurosurg* 1972;37:606–609

117. Mahalley MS Jr, Boone SC: External carotid–cavernous fistula

treated by arterial embolization. *J Neurosurg* 1974;40:110–114

118. Roberson GH, Biller J, Sessions DG, Ogura JH: Presurgical internal maxillary artery embolization in juvenile angiofibroma. *Laryngoscope* 1958;82:1523–1532

119. Kerber C: Intravascular cyanoacrylate: a new catheter therapy for AVM. *Invest Radiol* 1975;10:536–538

120. Sashin D, Goldman RL, Zanetti P, Heinz ER: Electronic radiography in stereotaxic thrombosis of intracranial aneurysms and catheter embolization of cerebral arteriovenous malformations. *Radiology* 1972;105:359–370

121. Kerber S: Experimental arteriovenous fistula: creation and percutaneous catheter obstruction with cyanoacrylate. *Invest Radiol* 1975;10:10–17

122. Hilal SK, Michelson WJ: Therapeutic percutaneous embolization for extra-axial vascular lesions of the head, neck, and spine. *J Neurosurg* 1975;43:275–287

123. Parkhill BJ, Ellman BA, Curry TS, Marcus PB, Peters PC: Mechanism of organ ablation by intraarterial ethanol. Presented at the Radiological Society of North America Annual Meeting, Chicago, IL, November 1981

124. Dines DE, Arms RA, Bernatz PE, et al: Pulmonary arteriovenous fistulae. *Mayo Clin Proc* 1974;49:460–465

125. Lindskog GE, Liebow AA, Kausel H, et al: Pulmonary arteriovenous aneurysm. *Ann Surg* 1950;132:591–606

126. Stringer CJ, Stanley AL, Bates RC, et al: Pulmonary arteriovenous fistula. *Am J Surg* 1955;89:1054–1080

127. Shumacker HB Jr, Waldhausen JA: Pulmonary arteriovenous fistulas in children. *Ann Surg* 1963;158:64:713–720

128. Taylor BG, Cockerill EM, Manfredi F: Therapeutic embolization of the pulmonary artery in pulmonary arteriovenous fistula. *Am J Med* 1978;64:360–365

129. Castañeda–Zuñiga W, Epstein M, Zollikofer C, et al: Embolization of multiple pulmonary artery fistulae. *Radiology* 1980;134:309–310

130. Jonsson K, Hellekant C, Olsson O, Holen O: Percutaneous transcatheter occlusion of pulmonary arteriovenous malformation. *Ann Radiol* 1980;23:335–337

131. Keller FS, Rosch J, Barker AF, Nath PH: Pulmonary arteriovenous fistulas occluded by percutaneous introduction of coil springs. *Radiology* 1984;152:373–375

132. Castañeda–Zuñiga WR, Epstein M, Formanek A, Amplatz K: Embolization of multiple pulmonary artery fistulas. *Radiology* 1980;134:309–310

133. Hatfield DR, Fried AM: Therapeutic embolization of diffuse pulmonary arteriovenous malformations. *AJR* 1981;137:861–863

134. Terry PB, Barth KH, Kaufman SL, White RI: Balloon embolization for treatment of pulmonary arteriovenous fistulas. *N Engl J Med* 1980;302:1189–1196

135. White RI, Mitchell SE, Barth KH, Kaufman SL, Kadir S: Angioarchitecture of pulmonary arteriovenous malformations: an important consideration before embolotherapy. *AJR* 1983;140:681–686

136. Barth KH, White RI Jr, Kaufman SL, Terry PB, Roland JM: Embolotherapy of pulmonary arteriovenous malformations with detachable balloons. *Radiology* 1982;142:559–606

137. Higgins CB, Wexler L: Clinical and angiographic features of pulmonary arteriovenous fistulas in children. *Radiology* 1976;119:171–175

138. Moyer JH, Ackerman AJ: Hereditary hemorrhagic telangiectases associated with pulmonary arteriovenous fistula in two members of a family. *Ann Intern Med* 1948;29:775–802

139. Moyer JH, Glentz G, Brest AN: Pulmonary arteriovenous fistulas. *Am J Med* 1962;32:417–435

140. Lund G, Rysavy J, Kotula F, Castañeda–Zuñiga WR, Amplatz K: Detachable spring coils for vessel occlusion. *Radiology* 1985;155:530–532

141. Wagner RB, Baeza OR, Stewart JE: Active pulmonary hemorrhage localized by selective pulmonary arteriography. *Chest* 1975;67:121–122

142. Garzon A, Cerruti M, Gourin A: Pulmonary resection for massive hemoptysis. *Surgery* 1970;67:633–638

143. Thoms NW, Wilson RF, Puro HE: Life-threatening hemoptysis in primary lung abscess. *Ann Thorac Surg* 1972;14:347–358

144. Remy J, Arnaud A, Fardou H, Giraud R, Voisin C: Treatment of hemoptysis by embolization of bronchial arteries. *Radiology* 1977;122:33–37

145. Caldwell EW, Siekert RG, Lininger RE: The bronchial arteries: an anatomic study of 150 human cadavers. *Surg Gynecol Obstet* 1948;86:396–415

146. Di Chiro G: Unintentional spinal cord arteriography: a warning. *Radiology* 1974;112:231–233

147. Kardjiev V, Symeonov A, Chankov I: Etiology, pathogenesis and prevention of spinal cord lesions in selective angiography of the bronchial and intercostal arteries. *Radiology* 1974;112:81–83

148. Botenga ASJ: *Selective Bronchial and Intercostal Arteriography.* Leiden, The Netherlands, HE Stenfert Kroses, 1970

149. Milne E: *Bronchial Arteriography,* ed. 2. Boston, Little, Brown & Co, 1971, pp 567–577

150. Remy J, Marache P, Lemaitre ML: Accidents de l'embolisation dans le traitement des hemoptysies. *Nouv Presse Med* 1978;7:4306–4310

151. Vujic I, Pyle R, Parker E, Mithoefer J: Control of massive hemoptysis by embolization of intercostal arteries. *Radiology* 1980;137:617–620

152. Tadavarthy SM, Klugman J, Castañeda–Zuñiga WR, Nath PH, Amplatz K: Systemic to pulmonary collaterals in pathologic states: review. *Radiology* 1982;144:75–76

153. Liebow AA, Hales MR, Lindskog GE: Enlargement of the bronchial arteries and their anastomoses with the pulmonary arteries in bronchiectasis. *Am J Pathol* 1949;25:211–225

154. Mack JF, Moss AJ, Harper WW, O'Loughlin BJ: The bronchial arteries in cystic fibrosis. *Br J Radiol* 1965;38:422–431

155. Moss AJ, Desilets DT, Higashino SM, Ruttenberg HD, Marcano BA, Dooley RA: Intrapulmonary shunts in cystic fibrosis. *Pediatrics* 1968;41:438–447

156. Fellows KE, Shaw KT, Schuster S, Shwachman H: Bronchial artery embolization in cystic fibrosis: technique and long-term results. *J Pediatr* 1979;95:959–963

157. Wholey MH, Chamorro HA, Gopal R, Ford WB, Miller WH: Bronchial artery embolization for massive hemoptysis. *JAMA* 1976;236:2501–2504

158. Harley JD, Killien FC, Peck AG: Massive hemoptysis controlled by transcatheter embolization of the bronchial arteries. *AJR* 1977;128:302–304

159. Ben-Menachem Y, Handel SF, Ray RD, Childs TL III: Embolization procedures in trauma: a matter of urgency. *Semin Intervent Radiol* 1985;2:107–117

160. Seavers R, Lynch K, Ballard R, Jernigan S, Johnson J: Hypogastric artery ligation for uncontrollable hemorrhage in acute pelvic trauma. *Surgery* 1964;55:516–525

161. Margolies MN, Ring EJ, Waltman AC: Arteriography in the management of hemorrhage from pelvic fractures. *N Engl J Med* 1972;287:317–321

162. Fisher RG, Ben-Menachen Y: Embolization procedures in trauma: the extremities—acute lesions. *Semin Intervent Radiol* 1985;2:118–124

163. Rich NM, Hobson RW, Collins GJ: Traumatic arteriovenous fistulas and false aneurysms: a review of 558 lesions. *Surgery* 1975;78:817–825

164. Hauser CW: Initial treatment of pelvic fractures. *Lancet* 1966;86:285–286

165. Kerr WS Jr, Margolies MN, Ring EJ, Waltman AG, Baum SN: Arteriography in pelvic fractures with massive hemorrhage. *J Urol* 1973;109:479–485

166. Matalon T, Athanasoulis CA, Margolies MN, Waltman AC, Novelline RA: Hemorrhage with pelvic fractures: efficacy of transcatheter embolization. *AJR* 1979;133:859–867

167. Bookstein JJ, Goldstein HM: Successful management of post biopsy arteriovenous fistula with selective arterial embolisation. *Radiology* 1973;109:535–536

168. Rizk GK, Atallah NK, Bridi GI: Renal arteriovenous fistula treated by catheter embolisation. *Br J Radiol* 1973;46:222–223

169. Chuang VP, Reuter SR, Walter J, Foley WD, Bookstein JJ: Control of renal hemorrhage by selective arterial embolization of renal arteriovenous fistula. *AJR* 1975;125:300–306

170. Goldman ML, Fellner SK, Parrott TS: Transcatheter embolization of renal arteriovenous fistula. *Urology* 1975;6:386–388

171. Silber SJ, Clark RE: Treatment of massive hemorrhage after renal biopsy with angiographic injection of clot. *N Engl J Med* 1975;292:1387–1388

172. Barbaric FL, Cutcliff WB: Control of renal arterial bleeding after percutaneous biopsy. *Urology* 1976;8:108–111

173. Kerber CW, Freeny PC, Cromwell L, Margolis MT: Cyanoacrylate occlusion of renal arteriovenous fistula. *AJR* 1977;128:663–665

174. Rosen RJ, Feldman L, Wilson AR: Embolization for post-biopsy renal arteriovenous fistula: effective occlusion using homologous clot. *AJR* 1978;131:1072–1073

175. McAlister DS, Johnsrude I, Miller MM, Clap J, Thompson WM: Occlusion of acquired renal arteriovenous fistula with transcatheter electrocoagulation. *AJR* 1979;132:998–1000

176. Pontes JE, Parekh N, McGuckin JT, Banks MD, Pierce JM: Percutaneous transfemoral embolization of arterio–infundibular–venous fistula. *J Urol* 1976;116:98–100

177. Maxwell DD, Frankel RS: Wedged catheter management of a bleeding renal pseudoaneurysm. *J Urol* 1976;116:96–97

178. Coleman CC, Kimura Y, Reddy P, et al: Complications of nephrostolithotomy. *Semin Intervent Radiol* 1984;1:70–74

179. Clayman RV, Surya V, Hunter DW, et al: Renal vascular complications associated with percutaneous removal of renal calculi. *J Urol* 1984;132:228–230

180. Clayman R, Castañeda–Zuñiga WR: Nephrostolithotomy: percutaneous removal of renal calculi. *Urol Radiol* 1984;6:95–112

181. Fisher RG, Ben-Menachem Y: Embolization procedures in trauma: the abdomen—extraperitoneal. *Semin Intervent Radiol* 1985;2:148–157

182. Silverberg DS, Dossetor JB, Eid TC, Mant MJ, Miller JDR: Arteriovenous fistula and prolonged hematuria after renal biopsy: treatment with epsilon aminocaproic acid. *Can Med Assoc J* 1974;110:671–672

183. Ekelund L, Gothlin J, Lindholm T, Lindstedt E, Mattsson K: Arteriovenous fistulas following renal biopsy with hypertension and hemodynamic changes. *J Urol* 1972;108:373–376

184. O'Brien DP, Parott TS, Walton KN, Lewis EL: Renal arteriovenous fistulas. *Surg Gynecol Obstet* 1976;118:1305–1311

185. Iverson P, Brun C: Aspiration biopsy of the kidney. *Am J Med* 1951;11:324–328

186. Bartels ED, Jorgensen HE: Experiences with percutaneous renal biopsy. *Scand J Urol Nephrol* 1972;15(suppl 6):57–65

187. Bolton WK: Localization of the kidney for percutaneous biopsy: a comparative study of methods. *Ann Intern Med* 1974;81:159–164

188. Zeis PM: Ultrasound localization for percutaneous renal biopsy in children. *J Pediatr* 1976;89:263–268

189. Morrow JW, Mendez R: Renal trauma. *J Urol* 1970;104:649–653

190. Kalish M, Greenbaum L, Silber SJ: Traumatic renal hemorrhage: treatment by arterial embolization. *J Urol* 1978;112:138–141

191. Grace DM, Pitt DF, Gold RE: Vascular embolization and occlusion by angiographic techniques as an aid or alternative to operation. *Surg Gynecol Obstet* 1976;143:469–482

192. White RI Jr: Arterial embolization for control of renal hemorrhage. *J Urol* 1976;115:121–122

193. Richman SD, Green WW, Kroll R, Casarella WJ: Superselective transcatheter embolization of traumatic renal hemorrhage. *AJR* 1977;128:843–844

194. Chang J, Katzen BT, Sullivan KP: Transcatheter Gelfoam embolization of post-traumatic bleeding pseudoaneurysms. *AJR* 1978;131:645–650

195. Blackwell JE, Potchen EJ, Laidlaw WW, Paul LH: Traumatic arteriocaliceal fistula: effective occlusion using homologous clot. *AJR* 1978;129:633–634

196. Haydu P, Chang J, Knox G, Nealson TF Jr: Transcatheter arterial embolization of a traumatic lumbar artery false aneurysm. *Surgery* 1978;84:288–291

197. Fankuchen EI, Martin EC, Karlson KB, Mattern RF, Casarella WJ: Small coils for large hemorrhages. *AJR* 1981;136:816–818

198. Stock JR, Athanasoulis CA: Musculoskeletal trauma: control of bleeding with transcatheter embolization, in Athanasoulis CA, Pfister RC, Greene RE, Roberson GH (eds): *Interventional Radiology*. Philadelphia, WB Saunders Co, 1982, pp 174–195

199. Scalfani SJA, Shaftan GW, Mitchell WG, Nayaranaswamy TS, McAuley J: Interventional radiology in trauma victims: analysis of 51 consecutive cases. *J Trauma* 1982;22:353–360

200. Ben-Menachem Y: Interventive and guidance procedures, in Ben-Menachem Y (ed): *Angiography in Trauma: A Work Atlas*. Philadelphia, WB Saunders Co, 1981, pp 411–452

201. Trunkey DD, Shires GT, McClelland R: Management of liver trauma in 811 consecutive patients. *Ann Surg* 1974;179:722–728

202. Heinbach DM, Ferguson GS, Harley JD: Treatment of traumatic hemobilia with angiographic embolization. *J Trauma* 1978;18:221–224

203. Hirsch N, Avinoach I, Keynan A: Angiographic diagnosis and treatment of hemobilia. *Radiology* 1982;144:771–772

204. Scenoy SS, Bergsland J, Cerra FB: Arterial embolization for traumatic hemobilia with hepatoportal fistula. *CardioVasc Intervent Radiol* 1981;4:206–208

205. Walter JF, Paaso BT, Cannon WB: Successful transcatheter embolic control of massive hematobilia secondary to liver biopsy. *AJR* 1976;127:847–849

206. Aldrete JS, Halpern NB, Ward S: Factors determining mortality and morbidity in hepatic injuries. *Ann Surg* 1979;189:466–474

207. Lambeth W, Rubin BE: Non-operative management of intrahepatic hemorrhage and hematoma following blunt trauma. *Surg Gynecol Obstet* 1979;148:507–511

208. Rubin BE, Katzen BT: Selective hepatic artery embolization to control massive hepatic hemorrhage after trauma. *AJR* 1977;129:253–256

209. Bass EM, Crosier JH: Percutaneous control of post-traumatic hepatic hemorrhage by Gelfoam embolization. *J Trauma* 1977;17:61–63

210. Jander HT, Laws HL, Kogget MS: Emergency embolization in blunt hepatic trauma. *AJR* 1977;129:249–252

211. Sclafani SJA, Shaftan GW, McAuley J: Interventional radiology in the management of hepatic trauma. *J Trauma* 1984;24:256–262

212. Struyven J, Krener M, Pirson P, et al: Post-traumatic bilhemia: diagnosis and catheter therapy. *AJR* 1982;138:746–747

213. Reuter SR, Palmaz JC, Berk RV: Hepatic artery injury during the portocaval shunt surgery. *AJR* 1980;134:349–353

214. Doppman JL, Girton M, Vermass M: The risk of hepatic artery embolization in the presence of obstructive jaundice. *Radiology* 1982;143:37–43

215. Kuroda C, Iwaski M, Tanaka T: Gallbladder infarction following hepatic transcatheter arterial embolization. *Radiology* 1983;149:85–89

216. Levinson JD, Olsen G, Terman JW, Cleaveland CR, Graham

CP, Breen KJ: Hemobilia secondary to percutaneous liver biopsy. *Arch Intern Med* 1972;130:396–400

217. Viranuvatti V, Plengvanit U, Kalayasiri C, Bhamarapravati N: Needle liver biopsy with particular reference to complications. *Am J Gastroenterol* 1964;42:529–536

218. Attiyeh FF, McSweeney J, Fortner JG: Hemobilia complicating needle liver biopsy. *Radiology* 1976;18:559–560

219. Walter JF, Paaso BT, Cannon WB: Successful transcatheter embolic control of massive hematobilia secondary to liver biopsy. *AJR* 1976;127:847–849

220. Terry R: Risks of needle biopsy of the liver. *Br Med J* 1952;1:1102–1105

221. Debray D, Leymarios E, Martin E, Hernandez CI, Carayon J, Coste F: Fistules arterioveineuses hepatico-portale consecutive a une ponctionbiopsie du foie. *Presse Med* 1968;76:737–740

222. Preger L: Hepatic arteriovenous fistula after percutaneous liver biopsy. *AJR* 1976;101:619–620

223. Walter JF, Paaso BT, Connon WB: Successful transcatheter emboli control of massive hematobilia secondary to liver biopsy. *AJR* 1976;127:847–849

224. Merino–de Villasante J, Alvarez–Rodriquez RE, Hernandez–Ortiz J: Management of post biopsy hemobilia with selective arterial embolization. *AJR* 1977;121:668–671

225. Perlberger RR: Control of hemobilia with angiographic embolization. *AJR* 1977;128:672–673

226. Dunnick NR, Doppman JL, Brereton HD: Balloon occlusion of segmental hepatic arteries: control of biopsy induced hemobilia. *JAMA* 1977;238:2524–2525

227. Scalfani SJA, Nayaranaswamy T, Mitchell WG: Radiologic management of traumatic hepatic artery–portal vein arteriovenous fistulae. *J Trauma* 1981;21:576–580

228. Fitzgerald JB, Crawford ES, DeBakey ME: Surgical considerations of nonpenetrating abdominal injuries: an analysis of 200 cases. *Am J Surg* 1960;100:22–41

229. Fisher RG, Foucar K, Estroda R, Ben-Menachem Y: Splenic rupture in blunt trauma. *Radiol Clin North Am* 1981;19:141–166

230. King H, Schumaker MB Jr: Splenic studies: susceptibility to infection after splenectomy performed in infancy. *Ann Surg* 1951;136:239–242

231. Robinette CD: Splenectomy and subsequent mortality in veterans of 1939–45 war. *Lancet* 1977;2:373–381

232. Sclafani SJA: Angiographic control of intraperitoneal hemorrhage caused by injuries to the liver and spleen. *Semin Intervent Radiol* 1985;2:138–147

233. Sclafani SJA: Angiographic hemostasis: its role in the salvage of the injured spleen. *Radiology* 1981;141:645–650

234. Rowley DA: The formation of circulatory antibody in the splenectomized human after injection of heterologous erythrocytes. *J Immunol* 1950;65:515–521

235. Spigos DG, Jonasson O, Mozes M: Partial splenic embolization in the treatment of hypersplenism. *AJR* 1979;132:777–782

236. Leung LE, Szal GJ, Drachman RH: Increased susceptibility of splenectomized rats to infection with *Diplococcus pneumoniae*. *J Infect Dis* 1972;126:507–515

237. Singer DB: Postsplenectomy sepsis, in Rosenberg JS, Bolande RP (eds): *Perspectives in Pediatric Pathology*. Chicago, Year Book Medical Publishers, 1973, p 285

238. Van Wyck DB, Witte MH: Critical splenic mass for survival from experimental pneumococcemia. *J Surg Res* 1980;28:14–17

239. Boles TE Jr. The spleen, in Ravich MM, Welch KJ, Benson CDM, Aberdeen E, Randolph JC (eds): *Pediatric Surgery*, vol 2, ed 3. Chicago, Year Book Medical Publishers, 1979, pp 878–883

240. Krivit W, Giebink GS, Leonard A: Overwhelming postsplenectomy infections. *Surg Clin North Am* 1979;59:223–235

241. Pearson JA: Disorders of the spleen, in Cellis SS, Kagan BM (eds): *Current Pediatric Therapy*, ed 9. Philadelphia, WB Saunders Co, 1980, pp 286–287

242. Schroter GPJ, West JC, Weil R: Acute bacteremia in asplenic renal transplant patients. *JAMA* 1977;237:2207–2208

243. Guilford WB, Scatliff JH: Transcatheter embolization of the spleen for control of splenic hemorrhage and in situ splenectomy: an experimental study using silicone spheres. *Radiology* 1976;119:549–553

244. Bucheler E, Thelen M, Schirmer G: Katheter Embolisation der Milzarterien zum Stop der akuten Varizenblutung. *Fortschr Röntgenstr* 1975;122:539–546

245. Günther R, Bohl J, Klose K, Anger J: Transkatheteremblisierung der Milz mit Butyl-2-Cyanoacrylat. *Fortschr Röntgenstr* 1980;133:158–163

246. Maddison F: Embolic therapy of hypersplenism. *Invest Radiol* 1973;8:280–295

247. Zannini G, Masciariello S, Pagano G, Sangiulo P, Zotti G: Percutaneous splenic artery occlusion for portal hypertension. *Arch Surg* 1983;118:897–900

248. Witte CL, Ovitt TW, Van Wyck DB, Witte MH, O'Mara RE: Ischemic therapy in thrombocytopenia from hypersplenism. *Arch Surg* 1976;111:1115–1121

249. Wholey MH, Chamorro HA, Rao G, Chapman W: Splenic infarction and spontaneous rupture of the spleen after therapeutic embolization. *Cardiovasc Radiol* 1978;1:249–253

250. Thanopoulos BD, Frimas CA: Partial splenic embolization in the management of hypersplenism secondary to Gaucher disease. *J Pediatr* 1982;101:740–742

251. Anderson JH, VuBan A, Wallace S, Hester JP, Burke JS: Transcatheter splenic arterial occlusion: an experimental study in dogs. *Radiology* 1977;125:95–102

252. Levy JM, Wasserman P, Pitha N: Presplenectomy transcatheter occlusion of the splenic artery. *Arch Surg* 1979;114:198–199

253. Vujic I, Lauver JW: Severe complications from partial splenic embolisation in patients with liver failure. *Br J Radiol* 1981;54:492–495

254. Alwmark A, Bengmark S, Gullstrand P, Joelsson BO, Lunderquist A: Evaluation of splenic embolization in patients with portal hypertension and hypersplenism. *Ann Surg* 1982;196:518–524

255. Owman T, Lunderquist A, Alwmark A, Borjesson B: Embolization of the spleen for treatment of splenomegaly and hypersplenism in patients with portal hypertension. *Invest Radiol* 1979;14:457–464

256. Tsapogas MJ, Peabody RA, Karmody AM: Pathophysiological changes following ischemia of the spleen. *Ann Surg* 1973;178:179–183

257. Matas AJ, Simmons RL, Buselmeier TJ, Najarian JS, Kjellstrand CM: Lethal complications of bilateral nephrectomy and splenectomy in hemodialized patients. *Am J Surg* 1975;129:616–620

258. Yarimizu SN, Susan LP, Straffon RA, Stewart BM, Magnusson MO, Nakamoto SS: Mortality and morbidity in pretransplant bilateral nephrectomy: analysis of 305 cases. *Urology* 1978;12:55–58

259. Goldin AR, Naude JH, Thatcher GN: Therapeutic percutaneous renal infarction. *Br J Urol* 1974;46:133–135

260. Powischer G, Wolf A, Eyre G: Kidney embolization with collagen fluids in malignant hypertension, in Anacker V, Burotta V, Rupp N (eds): *Percutaneous Biopsy and Therapeutic Vascular Occlusion*. Stuttgart, Georg Thieme, 1980, pp 169–172

261. Fletcher EWL, Thompson JF, Chalmers DHK, Taylor HM, Wood RFM, Morris PS: Embolization of host kidneys for the control of hypertension after renal transplantation: radiology aspects. *Radiology* 1984;57:279–284

262. McCarron DA, Rubin RJ, Barnes BA, Harrington JT, Millan

VG: Therapeutic bilateral renal infarction and end-stage renal disease. *N Engl J Med* 1976;294:652–660

263. Leenen FHH, Galla SJ, Geyshes GG, Murdaugh HV, Shapiro AP: Effects of hemodialysis and saline loading on body fluid compartments, plasma renin activity and blood pressure in patients on chronic hemodialysis. *Nephron* 1977;18:93–100

264. Eliscu EH, Haire HM, Tew FT, Newton LW: Control of malignant renovascular hypertension by percutaneous transluminal angioplasty and therapeutic renal embolization. *AJR* 1980;134:815–817

265. Denny DF, Perlmutt LM, Bettmann MA: Percutaneous recanalization of an occluded renal artery and delayed ethanol ablation of the kidney resulting in control of hypertension. *Radiology* 1984;151:381–382

266. Reuter SR, Pomeroy PR, Chuang VP, Kyung JC: Embolic control of hypertension caused by segmental renal artery stenosis. *AJR* 1976;127:389–392

267. Bennington JL, Beckwith JB: Tumors of the kidneys, renal pelvis and ureter, in *Atlas of Tumor Pathology,* 2nd series, fasc 12. Washington DC, Armed Forces Institute of Pathology, 1975, pp 25–29

268. Bennington JL: Cancer of the kidney—etiology, epidemiology, and pathology. *Cancer* 1973;32:1017–1029

269. Skinner DG, Colvin RB, Vermillion CD: Diagnosis and management of renal cell carcinoma: a clinical and pathologic study of 309 cases. *Cancer* 1971;28:1165–1177

270. Lokich JJ, Harrison JH: Renal cell carcinoma: natural history and chemotherapeutic experience. *J Urol* 1975;114:371–374

271. Robson CJ, Churchill BM, Anderson W: The results of radical nephrectomy for renal cell carcinoma. *J Urol* 1969;101:297–302

272. Hulten L, Rosencrantz M, Seeman T: Occurrence and localization of lymph node metastases in renal carcinoma: a lymphographic and histopathological investigation in connection with nephrectomy. *Scand J Urol Nephrol* 1969;3:129–133

273. Lang EK: Superselective arterial catheterization as a vehicle for delivering radioactive infarct particles to tumors. *Radiology* 1971;98:391–399

274. Almgard LE, Fernström I, Haverling M: Treatment of renal adenocarcinoma by embolic occlusion of the renal circulation. *Br J Urol* 1973;45:474–479

275. Wallace S, Chuang VP, Swanson D, Bracken B, Hersch EM: Embolization of renal carcinoma. *Radiology* 1981;138:563–570

276. Kaisary AV, Williams G, Riddle PR: The role of preoperative embolization in renal cell carcinoma. *J Urol* 1984;131:641–646

277. Sandoval Parra R, Wingartz Plata HF, Gonzalez Gonzalez HJ, et al: Renal embolization: experience in 81 cases. *World Urol Update Ser* 1983;11(3):2–7

278. Becker GJ, Holden RW, Klatte EC: Therapeutic embolization with absolute ethanol. *Semin Intervent Radiol* 1985;1:118–129

279. Cho KJ, Nichiyama RH, Shields JJ: Functional, angiographic and histologic studies in experimental renal infarction. Presented at the 27th Annual Meeting of the Association of University Radiologists, Rochester, NY, May 1979

280. Hald T, Mygind T: Control of life-threatening vesical hemorrhage by unilateral hypogastric artery muscle embolization. *J Urol* 1974;112:60–63

281. Lang EK, Deutsch JS, Goodman JR, Barnett TF, Lanasa JA Jr, Duplessis GH: Transcatheter embolization of hypogastric branch arteries in the management of intractable bladder hemorrhage. *J Urol* 1979;121:30–36

282. Bree RL, Goldstein HM, Wallace S: Transcatheter embolization of the internal iliac artery in the management of neoplasms of the pelvis. *Surg Gynecol Obstet* 1976;143:597–601

283. Miller FJ Jr, Mortel R, Mann WJ, Jahshan AE: Selective arterial embolization for control of hemorrhage in pelvic malignancy: femoral and brachial catheter approaches. *AJR* 1976;126:1028–1032

284. Athanasoulis CA, Waltman AC, Barnes AB, Herbst AL: Angiographic control of pelvic bleeding from treated carcinoma of the cervix. *Gynec Oncol* 1976;4:144–150

285. Higgins CB, Bookstein JJ, Davis GB, Galloway DC, Barr JW: Therapeutic embolization for intractable chronic bleeding. *Radiology* 1977;122:473

286. Mitchell ME, Waltman AC, Athanasoulis CA, Kerr WS Jr, Dretler SP: Control of massive prostatic bleeding with angiographic techniques. *J Urol* 1976;115:692–695

287. Feldman F, Casarella WJ, Dick HM, Hollander BA: Selective intra-arterial embolization of bone tumors: a useful adjunct in the management of selected lesions. *AJR* 1975;123:130–139

288. Hilal SK, Michelsen JW: Therapeutic percutaneous embolization for extra-axial vascular lesions of the head, neck and spine. *J Neurosurg* 1975;43:275–287

289. Dick HM, Bigliani LU, Michelsen WJ, Johnston AD, Stinchfield FE: Adjuvant arterial embolization in the treatment of benign primary bone tumors in children. *Clin Orthop* 1979;139:133–144

290. Channon GM, Williams LA: Giant-cell tumour of the ischium treated by embolisation and resection: a case report. *J Bone Joint Surg (Br)* 1982;64:164–165

291. Chuang VP, Wallace S, Swanson D, et al: Arterial occlusion in the management of pain from metastatic renal carcinoma. *Radiology* 1979;133:611–614

292. Keller FS, Rösch J, Bird CB: Percutaneous embolization of bony pelvic neoplasms with tissue adhesive. *Radiology* 1983;147:21–27

293. Rowe DM, Becker GJ, Rabe FE, et al: Osseous metastases from renal cell carcinoma: embolization and surgery for restoration of function. *Radiology* 1984;150:673–676

294. Wallace S, Granmayeh M, deSantos LA, et al: Arterial occlusion of pelvic bone tumors. *Cancer* 1979;43:322–328

295. Murphy WA, Strecker WB, Schoenecker PL: Transcatheter embolisation therapy of an ischial aneurysmal bone cyst. *J Bone Joint Surg (Br)* 1982;64:166–168

296. Chiang V, Soo C–S, Wallace S, Benjamin R: Arterial occlusion: management of giant-cell tumor and aneurysmal bone cyst. *AJR* 1981;136:1127–1130

4

Extracranial Embolotherapy with Detachable Balloons

KLEMENS H. BARTH, M.D.

Balloon embolotherapy has received most of its developmental impetus through neurovascular applications, with the pioneering work having been reported by Serbinenko in 1974.[1-6] Now detachable balloons are the preferred device for embolization where precise placement and a high margin of safety are required.

Detachable balloon embolization, as is any other catheter-guided embolization, is achieved via remote fluoroscopic control; however, unlike other techniques, it uses the bloodstream to advance the occluding device to its destination remote from the introducing catheter. Control over balloon position is maintained via a radiopaque catheter on which the balloon is mounted. Because this catheter serves the function of a "leash," it needs to be both strong enough to retain the balloon at any distance and flexible enough not to impede balloon travel through curved vessels and branch angles. A competent balloon–catheter connection is a crucial element in the delivery system, and this aspect proved to be most difficult during the development of various systems. For this and other reasons, only four balloon embolization systems have, to the author's knowledge, reached broader practical application, and only one of those[7] has been approved to date by the US Food and Drug Administration (FDA) for marketing (Mini-Balloon; Bard–Parker Division of Becton Dickinson Inc., Lincoln Park, NJ). Two systems, among them the first one introduced, have latex balloons[2,6]; the other systems have silicone balloons.[7,8]

GENERAL PRINCIPLES OF BALLOON EMBOLIZATION SYSTEMS

To embolize a balloon, a specific delivery system is required, in contrast to embolization with particles, steel coils, or ethanol, which can be pushed or injected through standard angiographic catheters. Three components are essential to deliver a balloon embolus: the balloon itself, the delivery (balloon) catheter to which the balloon is attached, and the catheter through which the balloon catheter is introduced or injected (introducer catheter)(Fig. 4–1). Some systems also include a coaxial catheter that is passed over the balloon catheter for balloon detachment.[8,9] None of the available balloons is radiopaque, although one system has a silver clip in the balloon tip to make it visible fluoroscopically.[2]

Silicone is a semipermeable membrane that preserves balloon volume when inflated with a liquid isosmolar to blood (285 mosm/liter) but which expands when filled with a hyperosmolar liquid and contracts when filled with a hyposmolar liquid.[8,10-12] Therefore, use of a hyperosmolar liquid leads to balloon overdistention and rupture, whereas use of a hyposmolar liquid causes balloon shrinkage and dislodgment. For convenience, silicone balloons are filled with isosmolar angiographic contrast material.[8,10-12] Because most ionic contrast media used for angiographic procedures have osmolalities much higher than blood (>1000 mosm/liter), the required dilution would greatly reduce visibility.[11] Before low-osmolality contrast medium became available, a popular solution was 52% iodipamide meglumine (Cholografin; Squibb) mixed 1:1 with water, which was radiopaque and only slightly hyperosmolar (430 mosm/liter).[7] Isosmolar metrizamide (Amipaque; Winthrop) (175 mg of iodine/ml), which is densely radiopaque, has been found suitable,[11] and the recently licensed ioxaglate meglumine sodium (Hexabrix; Mallinckrodt) also appears suitable for isosmolar dilution.

Ultrastructurally, latex is a coarse lattice that leaks liquid over time. Therefore, detachable latex balloons do not remain inflated very long with contrast medium[13]; the most appropriate long-term balloon filler is a hardening liquid such as medical grade silicone. Silicone is obtainable as two components, one of which is a catalyst (Ingenol; Ingenor Co., Paris), that are mixed in a 1:1 ratio for each application. To render the mixture radiopaque without interfering with the vulcanization process, tantalum powder can be added. The hardening time of the mixture (10–15 min) is monitored individually by observing the setting of a sample *in vitro* at body temperature.

It is important to realize that the silicone compound does not completely replace the nonsolidifying liquid (contrast) used for test inflation because of the dead space of the catheter and balloon. Since the dead space of the catheter is fixed, the smaller the balloon, the larger the percentage of dead space. Silicone filling is not effective if the dead space is ≥50% of the balloon volume.[13] The problem can be solved by using a double-lumen balloon catheter, but this catheter is larger and more rigid

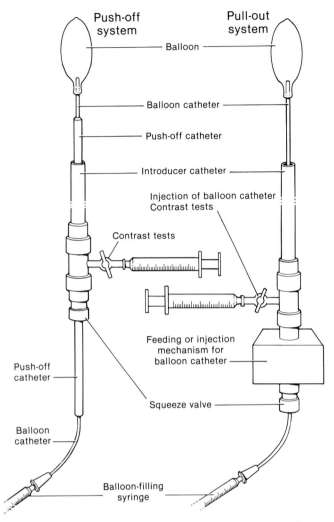

Fig. 4–1   Available detachable balloon embolization systems. Injection of the balloon is possible only with pushoff catheter (pullout detachment).

Limits in the tensile strength of the balloon determine its maximum inflated size and the vessel lumen it can occlude. For present silicone balloons filled with liquid, the expansion limit is about four times the uninflated diameter,[10] whereas it is about six times for latex balloons. The internal pressure of a balloon detached in an artery may be >200 mm Hg (lower in a vein) and represents a combination of the inflation pressure and the counterpressure of the vessel wall. Barth et al's *in vivo* experiments have shown that the chronic pressure exerted by the balloon on the vessel wall leads to intimal fibrosis (collagen deposition) and thinning of the muscle layer (Fig. 4–2).[11] Interestingly, there is little foreign body reaction in the vessel wall adjacent to a silicone balloon, in contrast to the response to other embolization agents.[11] The embolic occlusion produced by the balloon was short, with just a covering organized thrombus on both ends of the balloon (Fig. 4–2).[11] Therefore, balloon embolization can be considered to produce a vascular occlusion similar to that of surgical ligation.

As mentioned earlier, the catheter–balloon connection is an important element. Pressure cuffs and miter valves are the principal designs.[4,6–8,13] One system (Mini-Balloon) uses an interconnecting metal cannula between the balloon pressure cuff and the catheter,[10] allowing pullout detachment (described below). The miter valve of the other silicone balloon system (Hieshima) allows both pullout and pushoff detachment.[8] The latex balloon (Debrun) is designed for pushoff detachment with a coaxial catheter (Figs. 4–1 and 4–3).[2,13] The other latex balloon system, developed by Taki and coworkers and not yet available in the US, uses a twist-off detachment mechanism and a vinyl polymer for permanent filling.[6]

None of the existing balloon systems is completely safe from premature detachment, particularly when the balloon is exposed to rapid flow. This becomes an important consideration for embolization of arteriovenous fistulae (AVFs). Conversely, resistance to balloon detachment may be encountered occasionally and cannot be detected until the balloon has been inflated and detachment is attempted. Under no circumstances should the detachment force lead to overstretching of the balloon catheter.

than the usual balloon catheter.[13] The dead space problem exists for any exchange of two nonmiscible balloon fillers; it is irrelevant when using contrast medium only.

AVAILABLE BALLOON EMBOLIZATION SYSTEMS (TABLE 4–1)

Detachable Latex Balloon System (Pushoff Type)

This balloon system, developed and introduced clinically by Debrun,[2] features a radiolucent latex balloon that is available in a variety of sizes and shapes with or without a silver clip in its distal end to ease radiologic observation (Ingenor).[9,13] This balloon is hand tied by latex strings to the tip of a 2F Teflon catheter, a procedure that requires practice (Fig. 4–4A). Recently, balloon cuffs have been shaped to fit rather tightly around the 2F catheter so that tying with latex strings is required only if the risk of accidental detachment is considerable, as in AVFs. For balloon detachment, a 4.5–5F polyethylene catheter is advanced coaxially over the balloon catheter to "push" the balloon off. (Actually, this catheter is

advanced until it contacts the balloon, then held in position while the 2F catheter is pulled out.) This coaxial catheter assembly is inserted, not injected, through an 8.8F or 9F thin-walled, nontapered introducer catheter (Fig. 4–4B).

The advantage of the latex balloon system is the availability of assorted balloon sizes and shapes, allowing embolization of small aneurysms and vessels with lumens ≤14 mm. Its disadvantages are the need for considerable practice to tie the balloon correctly to the catheter, the need for a pushoff catheter, the limited shelf life of latex balloons, the need to fill the balloon with a hardening liquid (silicone) to maintain long-term occlusion, the inability to use silicone in small balloons due to the extent of the dead space, and, finally, the latex membrane itself,

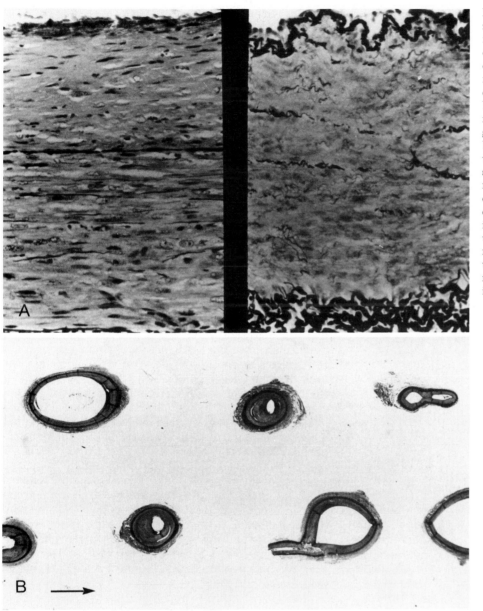

Fig. 4–2 Histologic effects of embolization balloons. A. Cross-section of intima and adjacent muscle layer of canine deep femoral artery through site of balloon embolization (left) or of normal vessel (right). Note stretching of elastic fibers and thickening of intima by collagen deposits. There is also thinning and stretching of muscle layer. No giant cells or other evidence of foreign body reaction is apparent. Van Gieson trichrome stain; × 40. B. Serial cross-sections at low power of canine deep femoral artery between proximal and distal limits of balloon occlusion (in direction of arrow). Immediately proximal and distal to balloon, intramural thrombus is present. Balloon did not match caliber of artery and overdistended it; this was done to investigate reactive changes in vessel wall as seen in part A.

which, unlike silicone rubber, is not an established medical implant material.

Detachable Silicone Balloon System (Pushoff/Pullout Type)

This system, developed by Hieshima,[8] remains an investigational device. Several balloon sizes have been developed. The balloon is connected to a 2F polyethylene catheter via a miter valve. The pushoff detachment mechanism is similar to that of Debrun's system; however, the balloon can also be detached by pullout (Fig. 4–5). Balloons are filled with blood-isosmolar angiographic contrast material. Intracranial and extracranial (particularly renal) embolizations have been described by Hieshima and coworkers. Filling with an inert polymerizing agent is being tested as a means of expanding the balloon beyond the 4:1 ratio considered safe for long-term occlu-

sion with liquid fillers. The problem of dead space again becomes a limitation for smaller balloons when a nonmiscible hardening liquid is used.

Detachable Silicone Balloon System (Pullout Type)

This is the only detachable embolization balloon system approved for intravascular use by the FDA and so will be described in some detail. It has been applied for several types of extracranial embolizations.[7,8,10–12] It is marketed under the trade name Mini-Balloon (Bard–Parker). Only two balloon sizes are available at present. The smaller balloon, with an outer diameter (OD) of about 1 mm (0.039 inch), passes through a 0.044-inch lumen introducer catheter (5F thin-walled, nontapered polyethylene catheter (Bard–Parker) or 6.5F reinforced-wall, nontapered catheter (Cook, Inc)). The larger 2-mm

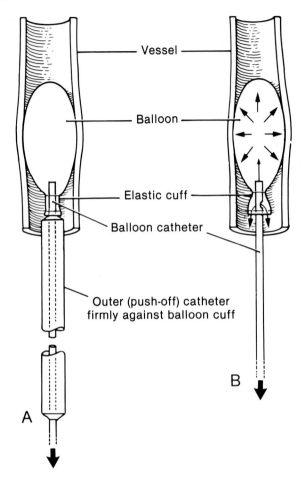

Fig. 4–3   Technique of balloon detachment.

OD (0.079-inch) balloon passes through a 0.096-inch (8.8F) thin-walled nontapered polyethylene catheter (Cook)(Fig. 4–6). The thin-walled catheters can be shaped over steam to the appropriate configuration for selective catheterization; the reinforced-wall torque catheters are preshaped.

The balloon is mounted on a 2F radiopaque polyurethane catheter. Catheter and balloon are connected via a metal cannula. The balloon has a pressure cuff over the cannula that seals upon detachment (Fig. 4–7).

The detachment mechanism is activated as the balloon pressure rises sharply when the expanding balloon encounters counterpressure from the vessel wall during filling (Fig. 4–8A). The cuff portion loosens slightly around the cannula, permitting fluid to exit through side-holes in the cannula (Fig. 4–8B). At this time, the cannula can be retracted, whereupon the excess pressure in the cuff is released momentarily, and the cuff collapses to seal the balloon (Fig. 4–8C). The polyurethane catheter is strong enough to transmit the necessary pullout force, which is best described as a quick manual tug on the catheter while filling pressure is maintained on the balloon. The detachment force can be transmitted around vascular curves; however, tight curves, such as in the carotid siphon, may present an obstacle to this detachment mechanism. Under no circumstances should the pulling force lead to stretching of the balloon catheter. If this occurs, the balloon cannot be detached safely and should be deflated and repositioned. Since successful detachment with this system requires firm engagement of the balloon in the vessel, the angiographer judges the time for detachment by observing the size and shape of the balloon in the vessel, slightly tugging on the balloon catheter to see if it can be pulled out of its position and observing the amount of filler injected, which should not exceed 0.15 ml for the 1-mm balloon and 0.6 ml for the 2-mm balloon (Figs. 4–6 and 4–7). Once these criteria are met, the detached balloon can be expected to remain inflated for an indefinite time. The maximum expanded diameter of the 1-mm balloon is 4 mm and of the 2-mm balloon up to 9 mm (Fig. 4–6). These balloons are cylindrical to maximize contact between their surface and the embolized vessel (Fig. 4–7). The balloon remains cylindrical in arteries, whereas in veins with thinner walls, such as the spermatic vein, the balloon may assume an oval shape.

Table 4–1
Comparison of Detachable Balloon Embolization Systems

Origin	Balloon Material	Balloon Filler	Detachment Mechanism	Catheter Outer Diameter (F) and Material[a]			Balloon Diameter/ Length (mm)			
				Balloon	Pushoff	Introducer	Uninflated	Volume (ml)	Inflated Maximum	Maximum Expansion
Bard	Silicone	Isosmolar iodinated contrast	Pullout	2/PU		4.9/PE	1/5	4/14	0.15	4×
						8.8/PE	2/8	8.8/17	0.60	
Ingenor (Debrun)	Latex	2-component silicone elastomer	Pushoff	1.8/Te	3.3/PE	6/PE	0.8/2	4.5/8.5	0.12	6–7×
						7/PE	1.1/2.4	6.0/10	0.4	
						8/PE	1.3/2.5	7.8/14	0.5	
							1.6/6	10/20	1.5	
						9/PE	2.3/2.2	13/12	1.3	
							2/5	14/25	3.0	
Hieshima	Silicone	Isosmolar iodinated contrast	Pushoff/ pullout	2/PE	4/PE		1.3/5	5/9	0.16	4×
							1.5/6	7/14	0.26	

[a]PU = polyurethane; Te = Teflon; PE = polyethylene.

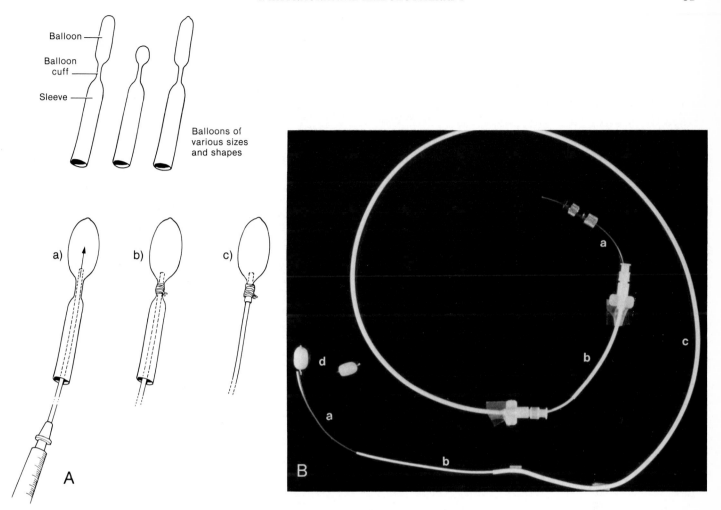

Fig. 4–4   Debrun latex balloon preparation. A. Balloons of various sizes and shapes are available. After balloon catheter has been inserted through sleeve (a), fluid injection distends balloon cuff and allows advancement of catheter into balloon. Latex tie (b) is placed under tension around balloon cuff. Sleeve (c) has been cut off. Balloon is now ready for use. B. Coaxial catheter assembly for detachable Debrun latex balloon, showing (a) catheter passed through (b) pushoff catheter, (c) introducer catheter, and (d) two detached silicone-filled balloons 12 mm in diameter.

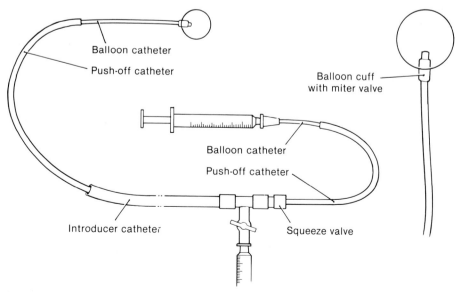

Fig. 4–5   Hieshima balloon system.

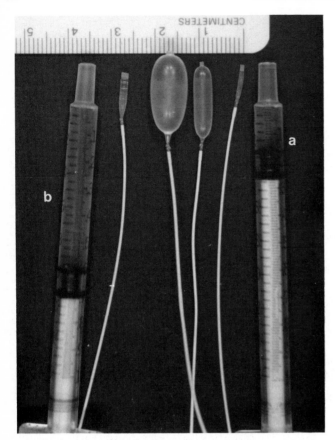

Fig. 4–6 Side-by-side comparison of inflated and uninflated diameters of 1-mm and 2-mm silicone balloons (Mini-Balloons) with filling volume indicated by 1-ml syringes: 0.15 ml for 1-mm balloon (a) and 0.6 ml for 2-mm balloon (b).

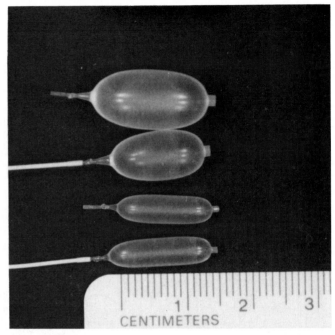

Fig. 4–7 Side-by-side comparison of inflated dimensions of 1-mm and 2-mm silicone Mini-Balloons.

If the tests described above do not wedge the balloon firmly within the vessel, the balloon cannot be safely detached. Either the next larger size must be used or the procedure must be abandoned. The angiographer should therefore carefully measure the lumen of the vessel to be occluded on a conventional cut-film angiogram with allowance for magnification (usually 10%) before the procedure is started.

Fig. 4–8 Technique of pullout Mini-Balloon detachment. A. Balloon expanding with liquid filler (arrows) within vessel lumen. Metal cannula connects balloon catheter to balloon; fluid passes through end hole of cannula into balloon. B. Having been filled adequately, balloon is subject to counterpressure from vessel wall, increasing intraluminal pressure, which allows fluid to exit through sidehole of valve cannula (arrows). This flow widens balloon cuff and allows pullout of catheter with cannula. C. Detached balloon with cuff collapsed after cannula (arrows) has been pulled out.

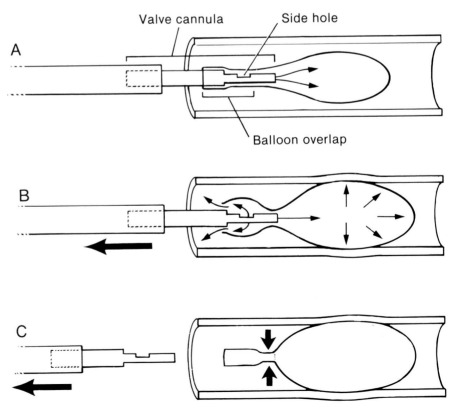

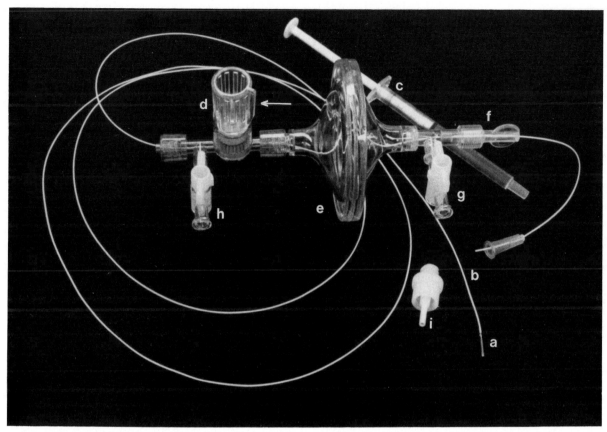

Fig. 4–9   Mini-Balloon assembly as supplied by manufacturer: (a) balloon, (b) balloon catheter threaded through coaxial valve and coiling chamber, (c) 1-ml syringe for balloon filling, (d) coaxial valve in open position (arrow), (e) coiling chamber, (f) winged squeeze valve to hold balloon catheter in place, (g) filling port, (h) injection port, (i) protective cap for balloon (balloon guide).

The balloon filler is blood-isosmolar contrast medium, as described above. Hardening silicone liquid cannot be used, since it would soften the balloon membrane and also interfere with the detachment mechanism.

The manufacturer supplies the balloon catheter threaded through an injection port in line with a coaxial valve and an injection chamber with a Tuohy–Borst valve at its end through which the end of the catheter extends (Fig. 4–9). The injection chamber has a filling port for heparinized saline. Before the balloon is used, the residual air is removed from it and the catheter by filling the balloon halfway with isosmolar contrast medium and allowing the air, which is pushed ahead of the contrast medium, to diffuse out. This diffusion process requires about 10–15 min. Thereafter, the balloon is allowed to collapse without aspiration by letting the contrast drip out of the end of the catheter. This way, collapse of the balloon is avoided. It is necessary to keep the balloon in a cylindrical shape with a residual volume for proper injection and flow direction. If the balloon is totally collapsed, it tends to fold backward during injection, impairing emptying.

After the balloon has been prepared, the catheter is coiled in the fluid-filled coiling chamber until only the balloon protrudes from the injection port. The balloon is covered with a protective plastic cap before the entire assembly is connected to the hub of the introducer catheter (Fig. 4–10). A final check of the position of the

introducer catheter is made to be certain the tip will be free in the vascular lumen. The balloon is now ready for injection into the vessel to be embolized.

Injection of the balloon is carried out after opening the coaxial valve between the injection port and the coiling chamber with a half turn (Fig. 4–9); then, 5–10 ml of heparinized saline is injected quickly, propelling the balloon catheter through the introducer catheter. The balloon may travel a considerable distance from the tip of the introducer catheter and will then need to be pulled back into the desired position. To permit the balloon catheter to be pulled back into position, the coaxial valve is opened, and the squeeze valve at the end of the coiling chamber is loosened (Fig. 4–9). If the balloon needs to be further advanced, enough of the catheter is coiled within the coiling chamber, the squeeze valve is tightened, and injection is performed as described. Flow-guided balloon advancement is facilitated by partial balloon inflation. Once the balloon is in the proper position, a test inflation is carried out, followed by contrast injection through the introducer catheter to check the occlusion. This step can be repeated as often as necessary. Before final balloon inflation, it is recommended that the balloon be evacuated completely in order to determine exactly the filling volume at the time of detachment.

After the balloon catheter has been injected, the coiling chamber can be detached from the coaxial valve for ease of handling. However, the author prefers to leave it

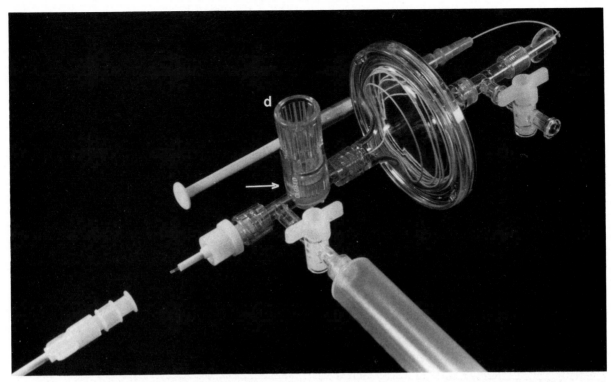

Fig. 4–10 Balloon delivery system ready to attach to introducer catheter. Note that protective cap (balloon guide) is fitted over bal-loon to ease passage through hub of introducer catheter and prevent backfolding. Note coaxial valve (d) in closed position (arrow).

attached so that he is ready to reinject the balloon at any time. Air that has leaked into the coiling chamber during balloon catheter movements can be vented by injecting flushing solution through the filling port with the detached chamber upright (Fig. 4–11).

INDICATIONS FOR BALLOON EMBOLIZATION

Because the detachable balloon provides only a short occlusion, its application to most tumor embolizations and embolization of extensive arteriovenous (AV) malformations is limited. However, it is a superior tool and an agent of choice in the occlusion of AVFs and false aneurysms of medium size and larger arteries. Other short occlusion agents such as steel coils are cheaper and simpler to use and are therefore preferred when the specific advantages of a detachable balloon are insignificant.

In order to define a rational indication for balloon embolotherapy, the following pros and cons need to be weighed. The advantages include flow directability to vessels far distal to the introducer catheter and correctability of the occlusion, increasing the precision of embolic occlusion. These advantages must be balanced against the disadvantages, including the need for nontapered catheters and introducer sheaths, 9F introducer catheters for the occlusion of vessels >4 mm in diameter, the complexity of the embolization system, and its cost.

If, for example, embolization of an AVF is required, the advantages of the balloon system outweigh those of the alternative methods. If, however, rerouting of hepatic artery blood flow is to be accomplished, e.g., for chemotherapy infusion, by occluding either the origin of the gastroduodenal artery or the left hepatic artery branch of the left gastric artery, coil occlusion is preferred as long as the catheter can be placed in the branch origin. If the vessel to be occluded cannot be selectively catheterized, flow-directable balloon embolization becomes a reasonable alternative.[14] Balloons can also be used conveniently as reliable proximal occluders after distal embolization with particles, especially since steel coils are not necessarily permanent large-vessel occluders.[15]

Once the balloon system is mastered, the radiologist is usually inclined to employ rational criteria for its use, rather than settling for technical ease with a compromise in safety and efficiency. The following are considered specific indications for balloon embolotherapy and will be discussed in detail:

1. Pulmonary AV malformations or AVFs;
2. Systemic false aneurysms and AVFs;
3. Certain systemic AV malformations;
4. Artificially created shunts;
5. Internal spermatic veins (for correction of varicocele).

Secondary applications are those already mentioned in which balloon occlusion may either be combined with use of embolic particles, such as Ivalon spheres, or with ethanol or in which balloon embolization is selected only after other methods turn out to be ineffective. Also, non-

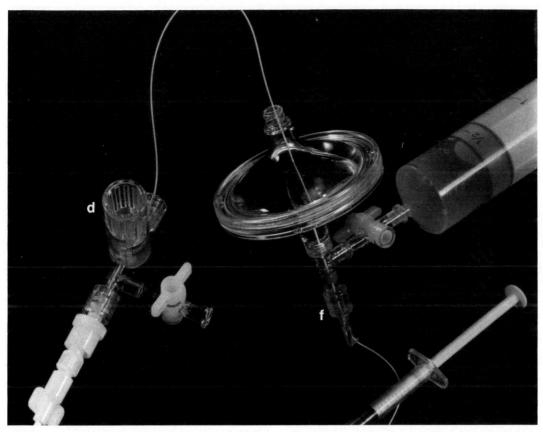

Fig. 4–11 Purging air from coiling chamber. Winged squeeze valve (f) tight around balloon catheter; coiling chamber upright to push air ahead of fluid. Thereafter, chamber is ready for reconnection with coaxial valve (d).

vascular balloon embolizations have been reported for ureters and fistulae.[15,16] Because the Mini-Balloon is generally available, the following discussion is based on the use of this system unless otherwise noted.

Embolization for Pulmonary Arteriovenous Malformations and Fistulae

GENERAL CONSIDERATIONS

As do other AV malformations, pulmonary AV malformations originate from abnormal capillary development. These lesions may be single or multiple and may enlarge with time.[17–20] Patients with multiple pulmonary AV malformations are more likely to have hereditary hemorrhagic telangiectasis (Osler–Weber–Rendu disease).[18] Pulmonary AV malformations are located predominantly in the lower lobes and near the pleural surface.[19,20] Their important anatomic features are their almost universal development from low-pressure pulmonary, rather than systemic, arteries and the frequency of a single artery to single vein connection.[18–28] The less common type consists of multiple arterial feeders to a network of small tortuous AV connections.[28] Since the symptomatology of pulmonary AV malformations is directly related to the magnitude of the right-to-left shunting, these lesions are often referred to as pulmonary AVFs.[18–20,24] Shunt-related cyanosis and fatigue caused by progressive hypoxemia are the most frequent signs. Other clinical presentations include systemic embolization and brain abscess in approximately 10% of patients and, infrequently, severe hemoptysis.

Surgical removal has been successful for solitary or even multiple fistulae as long as the extent of loss of functioning lung tissue can be tolerated. Lobectomy or segmental resections are the usual surgical procedures.[18–20] In contrast, surgical managment of patients with multiple AV malformations, in particular those with hereditary hemorrhagic telangiectasia, has limited usefulness because the natural history of this condition includes development of new pulmonary AV malformations with time.[18,21,24]

In recent years, successful transcatheter embolization of pulmonary AV malformations has been reported.[21,22] After selective catheterization of the feeding artery, an embolic device that safely occludes the fistula is inserted. Coils have been successful in some patients.[21,22,27] However, because this device, until recently, was not retrievable, vessel caliber and coil diameter must be estimated accurately before embolization. Even if this is done, there is still no assurance that a nonretrievable device like the coil will not embolize through the fistula. Therefore, the author considers detachable balloons the embolic agent of choice for pulmonary AV malformations.[23–26] Since it is frequently impossible to occlude all the AV connections in patients with Osler–Weber–Rendu disease, the strategy is to occlude the largest lesion first. Oximetry data indicating a satisfactory increase of blood oxygen in many

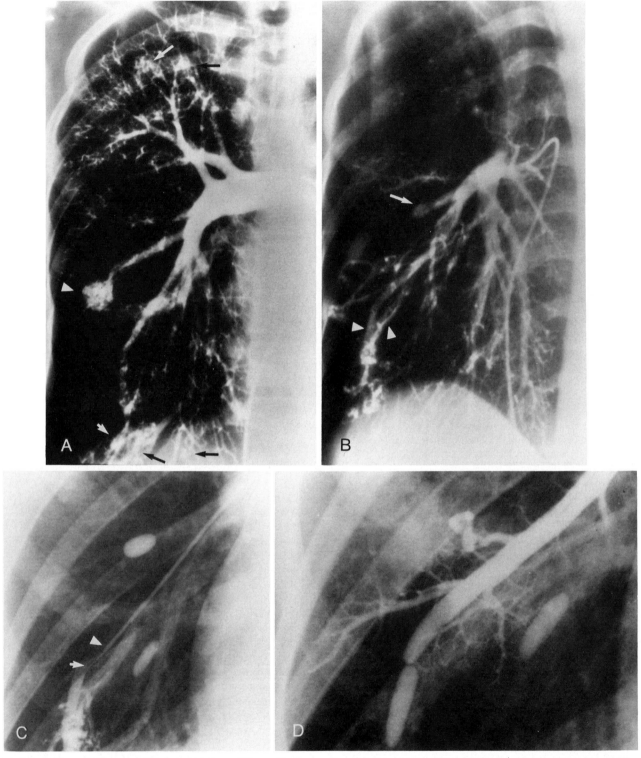

Fig. 4–12 A 26-year-old man with chronic fatigue; $PO_2 = 40$ mm Hg; hematocrit $= 59\%$. Several nodules were visible on chest radiograph. A. Right pulmonary survey arteriogram shows several small AV malformations in basilar portion of lower and upper (arrows) lobes and medium-sized malformation (arrowhead) in lower lobe. B. Selective right lower lobe pulmonary arteriogram after balloon embolization of feeder artery (arrow) to larger AV malformation with 2-mm balloon better delineates feeder arteries to smaller malformation (arrowheads). C. A 5F introducer catheter in feeding artery (arrowhead) with balloon catheter in malformation (arrow) after embolization of two adjacent lesions. D. Immediately after embolization with 1-mm balloon. E. After embolization, right lower lobe pulmonary arteriogram shows occlusion of all embolized lesions. In one session, PO_2 rose to 60 mm Hg.

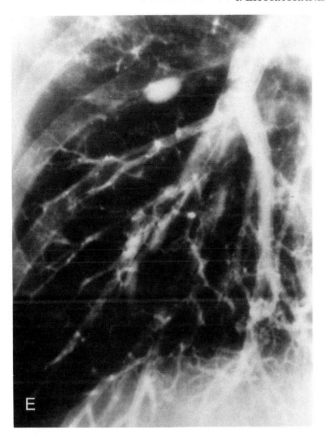

Fig. 4-12E

instances determine the end of the embolization procedure.

TECHNIQUE

Pulmonary arteriography must demonstrate the location, size, and inflow and outflow vessels of single or multiple pulmonary AV malformations. Cut-film studies are important for direct caliber measurements; however, rapid flow through the malformation frequently superimposes arterial and venous channels, masking the best point for embolic occlusion (Fig. 4–12).[29] Angled high-speed digital subtraction arteriography (DSA) (15–30 films/sec) complements cut-film arteriograms.[29] Baseline blood oximetry and pulmonary artery pressure measurements are obtained.

The caliber of the feeding artery to be embolized determines the choice of the appropriate embolization balloon(s). If the caliber of that feeding artery exceeds 9 mm (the largest Mini-Balloon), latex balloons, with sizes up to 14 mm, must be considered (Fig. 4–13). The potential use of latex balloons, an experimental device, should be specifically discussed with the referring physician, as well as with the patient, and be considered only if the radiologist is thoroughly familiar with this balloon system.

The embolization procedure is performed under full heparinization, with placement of an introducer catheter into the lobar or, if feasible, the segmental artery feeding the AV malformation (Fig. 4–12). If more than one AV malformation is to be embolized, the catheter required for the largest occlusion balloon is chosen. The femoral vein is the preferred entry site, starting with placement of a self-sealing sheath to accommodate the largest catheter. The thin-walled balloon introducer catheters, particularly the 9F size, cannot be placed directly. Therefore, negotiation of the right side of the heart and the pulmonary bifurcation with a regular angiographic catheter or a balloon-tipped catheter, followed by exchange for the balloon introducer over a guidewire, is recommended (Fig. 4–14).[26–28] Guidewire exchange is performed with the intention of placing the tip of the introducer catheter as close to the AV malformation as possible, and this requires advancing the guidewire far into the periphery for good anchoring. For the 9F catheter, guidewire anchoring may be insufficient. In this situation, the 9F catheter can be loaded over a long 5F balloon-tipped catheter, which must extend sufficiently beyond the 9F catheter to allow free negotiation through the heart and proximal pulmonary arteries.[26] The balloon tip is advanced as peripherally as possible, and the balloon is inflated to anchor the advancing introducer catheter (Fig. 4–14). Sometimes, a large-curvature (15-mm) deflector wire will help position the tip of the introducer catheter in individual segmental branches. Tightly curved deflector wires are to be avoided because of the risk of kinking or otherwise damaging the thin-walled catheter.

Once the introducer catheter is in place, definitive exploration of the embolization site is carried out, including videotape recording with freeze-framing or DSA roadmapping.[29] The latter is most useful, since it allows superimposition of the pre-embolization anatomy over the course of the embolization balloon; it also reduces substantially the amount of contrast medium required for test injections, which is particularly critical if several AV malformations are to be embolized in a single session. Oximetry and pulmonary pressure recording are repeated at this time. Meanwhile, the proper-sized embolization balloon has been prepared and is now injected to the site chosen for embolization. Sometimes, the balloon will travel through the fistula and must be retracted to the proper position; in other cases, it may stop short of the occlusion site. Then, partial inflation is applied to further flow-direct the balloon. If the balloon enters the wrong branch artery, it is partially retracted and reinjected and the above maneuvers are applied. During these manipulations, it is of the utmost importance to avoid any air accumulation in the embolization system because of the risk of systemic, in particular cerebral, embolization.

With the balloon in the intended embolization position, a test inflation is performed to demonstrate complete occlusion. Firm fit of the balloon can be tested by slight tugging on the balloon catheter. The balloon position should be adjusted until a site is found that avoids as many side branches to normal pulmonary parenchyma as possible (Fig. 4–15). If a firm fit cannot be achieved, a larger balloon needs to be selected (Fig. 4–13). However, before this decision is made, one needs to consider that the smallest caliber of the feeding artery is usually found close to its junction with the usually much larger venous portion of the AV malformation.

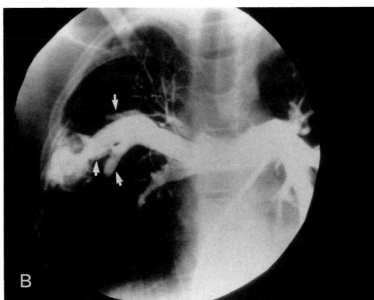

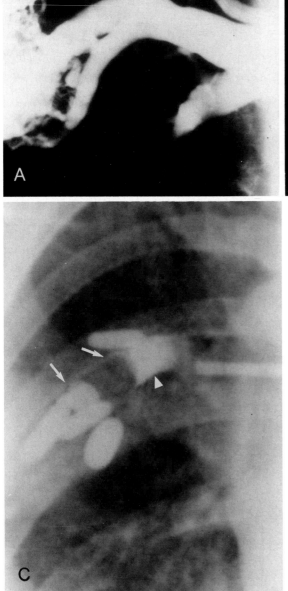

Fig. 4–13   A 9-year-old girl with cyanosis and digital clubbing; hematocrit = 59%; right pleural-based mass seen on chest radiograph. A. Right pulmonary arteriogram shows several feeder arteries to large malformation in anterior segment of right upper lobe. B. After occlusion of smaller feeder branches with 2-mm silicone balloons (arrows); largest branch remained open and necessitated placement of 12-mm latex balloon. C. In separate procedure, 12-mm latex balloon was placed in largest feeder (arrows) and filled with silicone polymer. Contrast stasis (arrowhead) indicates total occlusion of AV malformation.

Once the definitive embolization position has been found, the balloon is completely emptied as described and then filled to the required volume. Immediately before it is detached, it is observed carefully for any dislodgment while the pullout force is increased and the injection pressure on the balloon is maintained. Sometimes, the pulling force may move the artery slightly with the balloon. To differentiate this from loosening of the balloon, a test injection is made through the introducer catheter. Once the balloon is detached, a documentation angiogram is obtained, followed by repeat oximetry and pulmonary pressure recording.

Several pulmonary AV malformations can be embolized in one session, with each individual embolization being carried out as described.[26,29] The limitations are maximum contrast dose and the total amount of time required in view of operator fatigue and the ability of the patient to cooperate. A high degree of alertness is required of the operator throughout the procedure, and it may be better to resume the embolization in a subsequent

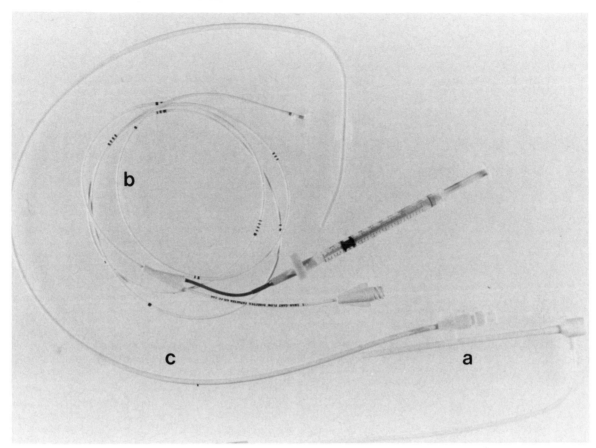

Fig. 4–14 Introducer system for pulmonary balloon embolization. (a) Percutaneous introducer sheath for femoral vein entry; (b) Swan– Ganz or Berman-type balloon catheter; (c) 5F or 8.8F nontapered introducer catheter.

session (Fig. 4–13). All these procedural details should be discussed with the patient when presenting the treatment plan.

In the author's experience with embolization of multiple pulmonary AV malformations, as many as six separate procedures have been carried out to complete the embolization and to reach the therapeutic goal, which was to raise the patient's blood oxygen saturation to 90% (a partial arterial oxygen pressure of 60 mm Hg).[24–26,29] Definitive oximetry readings should be obtained with the patient sitting or standing in room air, since changes in blood flow distribution between the upper and lower lobes must be considered.

COMPLICATIONS

A significant risk of embolotherapy of pulmonary AV malformations is inadvertent systemic embolization, for which the detachable balloon technique provides, in the author's opinion, the best possible prevention compared to particles or steel coils. Among the author's earlier patients, there was one instance in which a balloon dislodged into a pelvic artery after passing through the AVF; this was the result of poor visibility of the occlusion point because of the juxtaposition of several AV malformations in the lower lobe region. Another risk is occlusion of normal pulmonary arteries, which may lead to a pulmonary

infarction. This happened to the author in two separate procedures but was judged unavoidable due to the closeness of a normal artery branch to the most appropriate point of occlusion.[26–29] Both patients suffered transient pain and slight fever without significant morbidity.

Although the treatment of pulmonary AV malformations, particularly of multiple lesions, may present a time-consuming and demanding task for all persons involved, its successful completion is gratifying and benefits an often severely incapacitated patient whose life expectancy may thereby be increased and whose working ability may be restored.

Systemic False Aneurysms and Arteriovenous Fistulae

These spontaneous or post-traumatic lesions may occur anywhere and may be an indication for balloon embolotherapy unless surgical repair is simpler, as it is in many extremity AVFs. Balloon embolization of lesions in the abdomen and retroperitoneum, which often present technical problems, will be discussed. This is not to say the technique is not equally effective elsewhere.[30,31]

HEPATIC ARTERY EMBOLIZATION

Among lesions in the liver, post-traumatic AVFs and false aneurysms are prime targets for balloon emboliza-

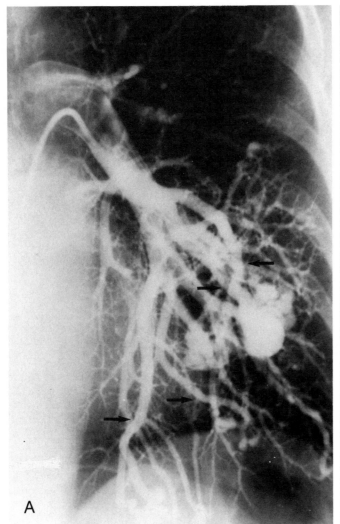
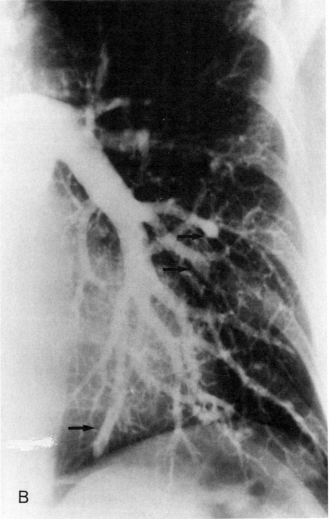

A.

B.

Fig. 4–15   Embolization of lower lobe pulmonary AV malformation. A. Several single-feeder malformations (arrows). B. Selective embol- ization with 1-mm silicone balloons (arrows) spared most of normal pulmonary artery branches.

tion. Hemobilia as a result of arteriobiliary fistula after iatrogenic trauma during operation, needle biopsy, per- cutaneous cholangiography, and biliary drainage is a well- recognized entity.[32] The fistula is usually located near the porta hepatis (Fig. 4–16). Mycotic aneurysms may neces- sitate embolization to control acute rupture,[33,34] as in other areas.[35,36] Infantile hepatic hemangioendothelioma can be a rare indication for emergency embolotherapy when large-volume transhepatic shunting leads to high- output cardiac failure. Most of these tumors regress spon- taneously if the child survives. Several emergency trans- catheter embolizations have been reported, including some using balloon embolization.[25,37,38]

The technical aspects of hepatic artery balloon embol- ization include careful angiographic mapping with exact localization of the false aneurysm or AVF to determine the most appropriate balloon size and catheterization approach. Balloons will not float as readily into false aneurysms as into AVFs for obvious reasons, so subselec- tive placement of the introducer catheter is frequently necessary (Fig. 4–16). In most instances, the 1-mm sili-

cone balloon will suffice. This will allow use of a 5F introducer catheter. Although the 5F thin-walled cathe- ter does not offer a great deal of torque, it is adequate for catheterization from the axillary or brachial artery, anal- ogous to placement of hepatic artery infusion catheters. An introducer catheter with a shallow double curve (H1H) serves best to enter the celiac axis downstream, aided by a floppy straight guidewire. A straight or 1.5-mm (0.035-inch) J guidewire is used to help the introducer catheter select the common and proper hepatic arteries. From there, the balloon can be floated toward the embol- ization site if the right hepatic artery branches are to be embolized. For left hepatic artery embolization, it is nec- essary to place the introducer catheter directly in the ori- gin of the left hepatic artery; this is best accomplished by steerable guidewires. Flow direction of the balloon may be compromised by vasospasm, which needs to be elimi- nated by a combination of slight catheter retraction and injection of a vasodilator such as 15–20 mg of papaverine. To position the balloon, repeated partial inflations, defla- tions, and reinjections may be required.

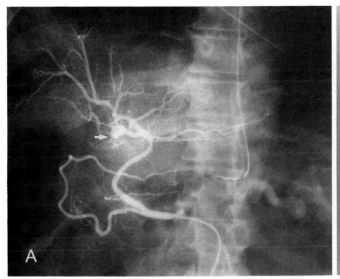
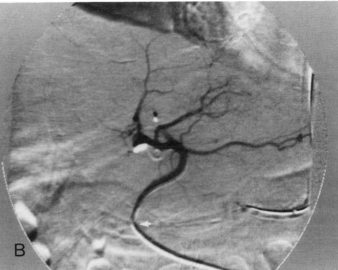

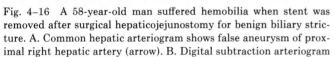

Fig. 4–16 A 58-year-old man suffered hemobilia when stent was removed after surgical hepaticojejunostomy for benign biliary stricture. A. Common hepatic arteriogram shows false aneurysm of proximal right hepatic artery (arrow). B. Digital subtraction arteriogram with balloon inflated in false aneurysm before detachment. Introducer catheter tip (arrow) in proper hepatic artery; all right hepatic artery branches distal to balloon are occluded. (Courtesy of Steven L. Kaufman, M.D., Johns Hopkins Hospital, Baltimore, MD.)

In this setting, one must be aware of the balloon folding back over its catheter (see reference 29 for pictorial display), preventing adequate inflation and emptying. This problem should be suspected any time the balloon does not drain spontaneously after partial filling. The balloon will unfold, either after the balloon catheter has been pulled back or, if this does not readily occur, after the balloon has been partially filled to give it more drag away from the retreating catheter. The latter maneuver is not advisable in low-flow situations, because the balloon may not move with the blood flow and may become impacted. If these maneuvers fail, the backfolded balloon should not be pulled into the introducer catheter, since this may shear it off. Instead, the entire assembly, including the introducer catheter, should be retracted as a unit. As soon as the balloon is in a larger vessel (common hepatic artery, celiac axis), it will spontaneously unfold. Since backfolding is most frequently encountered during maneuvering in a tight space, the need to relieve vasospasm should be appreciated.

For the transfemoral approach to the celiac axis, 6.5F torque nontapered catheters are required.

SPLENIC ARTERY EMBOLIZATION

Lesions of splenic artery branches also can be treated. The tip of the introducer catheter can be left in the proximal splenic artery and the balloon flow-directed distally.

RENAL ARTERY EMBOLIZATION

Balloon embolization of renal artery lacerations and AVFs may be one of the most common applications of small balloons.[34,39,40] Virtually any embolization tech-

nique known today has been used to treat traumatic renal hemorrhage; however, from the standpoint of tissue preservation, selective balloon embolotherapy is preferable.

Traumatic lesions include those complicating biopsy, nephrostomy, percutaneous stone extractions, anatrophic lithotomies, and nephrectomies. Most smaller branch artery lacerations obliterate spontaneously; however, interlobar or hilar branches may continue to bleed or create AVFs requiring treatment. Stump AVFs following nephrectomies may not be detected until high-output cardiac failure appears.

For balloon embolotherapy, the introducer catheter must be placed in the main renal artery or the bifurcation (Figs. 4–17 and 4–18). The balloon will, in most instances, float directly toward the lesion. Thin-walled 5F introducer catheters or torque catheters may be used as described above. The 1-mm balloon is the size usually required; infrequently, the 2-mm balloon is needed. Diagnostic arteriography in any obliquity is necessary before embolization to demonstrate the course of the artery and the position of the side branches to the lesion. For a larger AVF, it is important to know that the lesion is no larger than the largest balloon available.

Unlike low-pressure pulmonary AV malformations, flow through systemic AVFs can exert a tremendous pulling force on the balloon during inflation, resulting in spontaneous detachment and pulmonary embolization. It is important to realize that spontaneous detachment occurs before the balloon is able to reach its fully inflated size and occlude the fistula. Therefore, blood flow needs to be reduced before balloon embolization. In the author's experience, this is definitely required in AVFs larger than 3 mm. Flow reduction is accomplished by placing a nondetachable balloon catheter upstream and impeding the flow just enough to allow flow direction and determination of balloon occlusion. Alternatively, a stain-

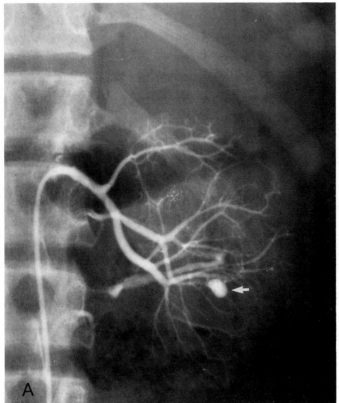

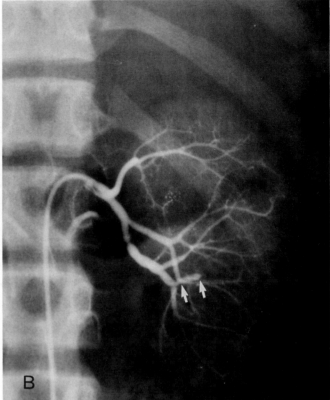

Fig. 4–17 An 11-year-old girl with chronic glomerulonephritis; intermittent hematuria occurred 11 days after needle biopsy of left kidney. A. Left renal arteriogram shows AV fistula of lower pole branch (arrow). B. After embolization of branch artery with 1-mm silicone balloon (arrows), fistula is occluded. Introducer catheter remained at renal artery bifurcation. Note spasm ring in lower pole artery.

less-steel spider can be placed first, to form a baffle for the balloon behind it.

In postnephrectomy stump AVFs (renal artery to renal vein or inferior vena cava), the arterial stump may not allow flow reduction maneuvers, so it may be impossible to treat such fistulae with a detachable balloon. Surgical ligation can be helped by leaving a nondetachable occlusion balloon in place until the surgeon is ready to place the ligature, at which time the radiologist deflates the balloon and pulls the catheter out.[41] In this way, potentially serious intraoperative bleeding can be avoided.

As previously indicated, embolization of AVFs with detachable balloons should always be carried out under full heparinization. The AVFs of interlobar or smaller branch arteries are readily embolized with the 1-mm balloon which, in most instances, will readily follow the flow and can be detached close to or in the fistula, occluding a minimum of parenchymal branches (Fig. 4–18).

RETROPERITONEAL AND PELVIC ARTERY EMBOLIZATION

In the retroperitoneum and pelvis, a balloon embolization for arterial lesions is approached first with a standard diagnostic catheterization technique, for which the 6.5F torque catheters are most suitable. In lumbar and intercostal arteries, some lesions may be closer than 1 cm to the origin of the aorta; in such cases, available balloons are too long to fit into the proximal limb. Pre-embolization arteriography should therefore include oblique views to reveal the true length of the lumbar artery, which curves posteriorly from its origin on the aorta. One may need a suitably shaped latex balloon or a shorter Hieshima silicone balloon (Table 4–1). Lesions in the more distal distribution of these arteries are reached through flow direction, which can negotiate even sharp turns (Fig. 4–19).[36]

Post-traumatic pelvic AVFs usually require flow reduction. For this purpose, crossover nondetachable balloon occlusion of the proximal internal iliac artery is preferred; however, circumstances may call for temporary crossover or ipsilateral retrograde occlusion of the common iliac artery. Alternatively, as previously discussed, a steel spider may be placed in the fistula in front of the balloon.[42]

Systemic Arteriovenous Malformations

An AV malformation can be treated only by excluding the nidus from the circulation; otherwise collateral channels will develop promptly. A particularly complex situation exists in pelvic AV malformations, where multiple feeders are the rule and numerous potential collaterals are present.[25,43] These lesions become clinically apparent through bleeding, local pain, or high-output cardiac fail-

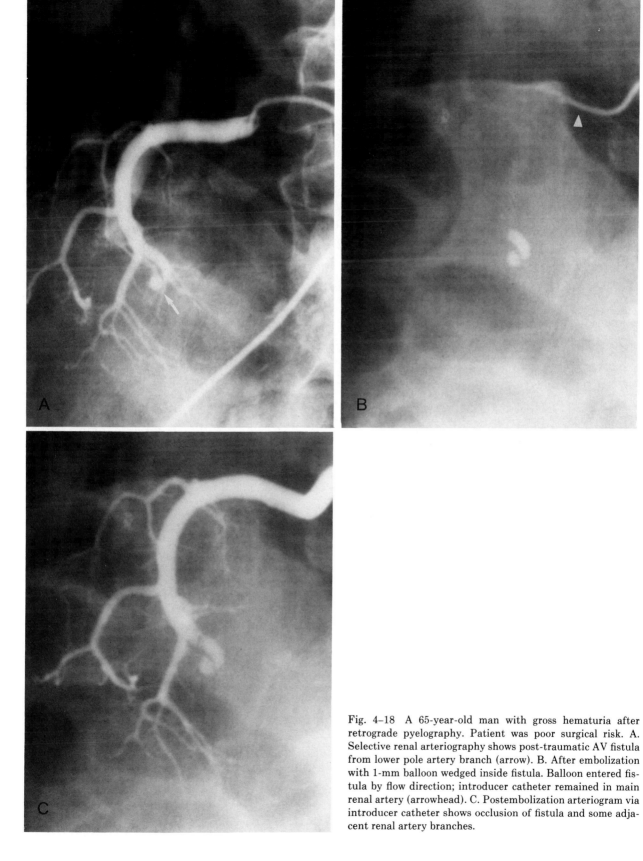

Fig. 4–18 A 65-year-old man with gross hematuria after retrograde pyelography. Patient was poor surgical risk. A. Selective renal arteriography shows post-traumatic AV fistula from lower pole artery branch (arrow). B. After embolization with 1-mm balloon wedged inside fistula. Balloon entered fistula by flow direction; introducer catheter remained in main renal artery (arrowhead). C. Postembolization arteriogram via introducer catheter shows occlusion of fistula and some adjacent renal artery branches.

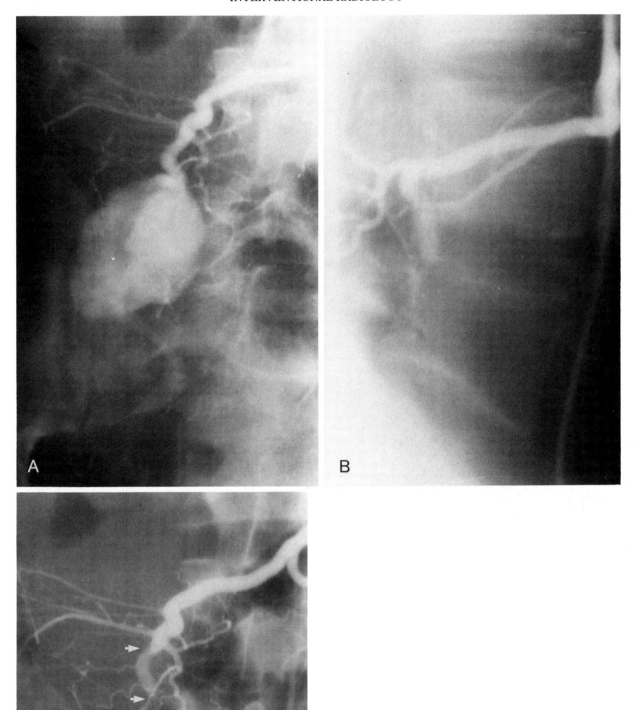

Fig. 4–19 A 27-year-old male renal allograft recipient with severe right flank pain radiating to groin with swelling of groin. There was no history of trauma. A. Selective right fourth lumbar arteriogram reveals enlargement of artery and large bleeding false aneurysm. B. Lateral view shows typical angled course of lumbar artery, with introducer catheter remaining in arterial orifice. Flow carried balloon into neck of false aneurysm, occluding it. C. Anteroposterior view shows 1-mm silicone balloon (arrows) occluding aneurysm.

ure. Embolotherapy with detachable balloons is indicated only as a palliative procedure to close large AV shunts[25]; embolizing with multiple balloons in an attempt to eradicate the lesion is futile. Before balloon embolization, the same careful diagnostic mapping is required as for other areas to determine the approach to, and the diameter of, the AVF to be occluded.

Should a balloon detach prematurely despite flow reduction measures and embolize to the lung, an attempt can be made either to rupture it by percutaneous thin-needle puncture or to retrieve it with a basket. One should consider, however, that in otherwise normal lungs even a 5-mm balloon will in all likelihood not cause symptoms if left untouched.[44]

Embolization of the Internal Spermatic Vein for Varicocele

GENERAL CONSIDERATIONS

Balloon embolization is one of several methods for non-operative occlusion of the internal spermatic vein in patients with varicocele (Chapter 6).[45-49] The clinical pre-sentation, pathology, and pathophysiology of varicocele have been described in several articles[50-52]; the present discussion is limited to the technical aspects of balloon embolotherapy. Briefly, the purpose of treatment is prevention of retrograde blood flow in the right or left internal spermatic vein and its branches, which interferes with spermatogenesis and is often associated with a clinically evident varicocele.

Left-sided varicoceles are found more frequently than bilateral or isolated right-sided varicoceles. The left internal spermatic vein always enters the left renal vein (Fig. 4–20), although duplications of the left renal vein and circumaortic rings will occasionally be encountered.[53-55] The spermatic vein is best approached by selective catheterization with a large-curve cobra catheter. The catheter tip searches the inferior aspect of the renal vein for the orifice of the left internal spermatic vein, which enters at a variable distance from the vena cava. Anatomic variations are frequent (summarized in reference 56). The closer the inferior vena cava runs to the paraspinal lumbar veins, the more likely are direct communications with those veins.[54] Two consistent branch veins of the spermatic vein, one to the renal capsule and one to the left abdominal wall, are found in the mid to lower lumbar

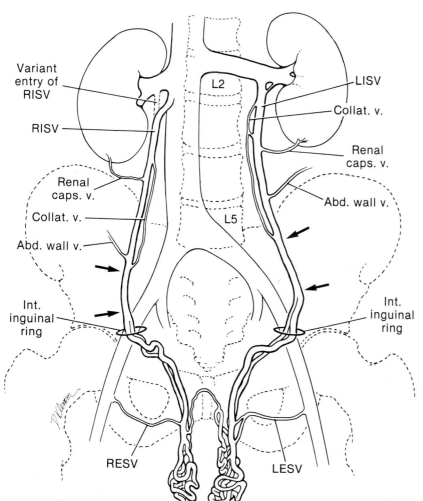

Fig. 4–20 Internal spermatic vein with insufficiency of valves on both left (LISV) and right (RISV), producing bilateral varicocele. Region between arrows on RISV and LISV is most common single-channel site for embolization with single balloon. Left (LESV) and right (RESV) external spermatic vein.

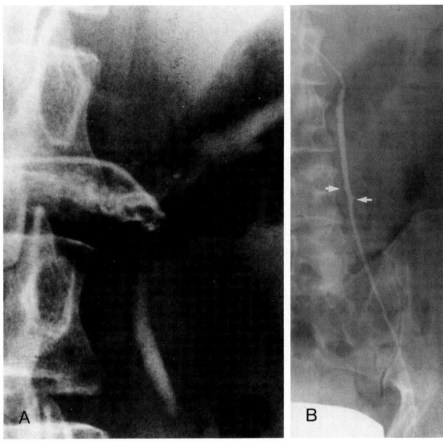

Fig. 4–21 A 31-year-old subfertile man with small varicoceles bilaterally. A. Semiselective left-sided internal spermatic venogram shows narrow orifice and reflux; there is no proximal valve. B. Selective left-sided internal spermatic venogram via 5F introducer catheter shows valveless vein with retrograde flow. Small protrusions from lumen (arrows) indicate branch and collateral venous entries, which could cause recurrence if occlusion balloon is placed proximally. Note testicular shield over symphysis. C. A 1-mm silicone balloon in intrapelvic portion of vein for definitive occlusion. D. Selective right-sided internal spermatic venogram shows reflux to level of iliac crest in single-channel vein. Occluding agent needs to be placed in each branch vein or above bifurcation (arrow) and below branch vein entry (open arrow). E. After embolization of each of two small-caliber branch veins twice with 0.2 ml of ethanol through open-end guidewire; occlusion at level of bifurcation and below branch vein entry (open arrow).

region.[54] The mid-iliac portion of the spermatic vein is the most common single-channel segment.[45,55] Above the inguinal canal, the vein usually divides into two or three branches; therefore, the preferred place for balloon embolotherapy is the single-channel segment in the mid-iliac region (Fig. 4–20).

TECHNIQUE

To gauge the venous caliber properly and to determine the anatomy, a single-film venogram is obtained, which, in a typical insufficient spermatic vein, should opacify the vein and collaterals from the left renal vein down to the inguinal area. There is no need to film or to observe fluoroscopically the spermatic vein distal to the pubic ramus.[47] The testicle is shielded by a leaded wrap throughout the procedure.

In most patients with clinically evident varicoceles, an insufficient vein 5–8 mm in diameter will have to be occluded; this requires the 2-mm balloon. The angiographer needs to study carefully all collateral channels and place the balloon distal to any communication that could allow collateral retrograde flow (Fig. 4–21).

For balloon embolotherapy, the introducer catheter must be firmly placed within the orifice of the spermatic vein, although it does not have to be introduced any further distally (Figs. 4–21 through 4–23). Since the initial diagnostic catheter is exchanged for the 8.8F introducer catheter in most instances, the guidewire will have to be advanced well into the vein to allow sufficient anchoring for the advancing introducer catheter. This introducer catheter should have a gentle (180°) curve. Frequently, despite careful maneuvering, venospasm results during the exchange. It should be allowed to resolve before balloon injection and embolization, because, in the author's experience, the only pulmonary embolization occurred after embolization of a spastic spermatic vein.[47] The best method, in the author's experience, has been slow infusion of body-temperature saline into the vein. When spasm has resolved, the embolization balloon can be injected and usually travels down to the inguinal canal. It is positioned and test inflated as described previously (Fig. 4–22). In the venous system, the balloon may

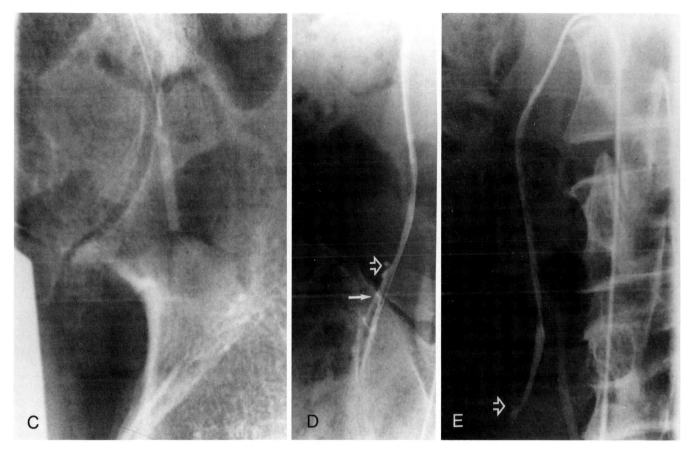

Fig. 4–21C–E

assume an oval shape due to the more compliant venous wall. Expect movement of the vein when tugging on the balloon to test firm fit. The venous occlusion site is documented on a photospot film.

The right internal spermatic vein typically enters the anterolateral aspect of the inferior vena cava caudad to the right renal vein. In about 10% of patients, however, the vein enters the right renal vein or a lower pole branch vein. Collateral veins and variations are at least as common, if not more so, on the right side than on the left.[55]

Even in patients with clinically evident right-sided varicocele, the right spermatic vein is usually smaller than the left. Therefore, a nontapered, preshaped 6.5F catheter should be used initially to enter the vein and is in many instances sufficient to carry out embolization with the 1-mm balloon. In this way, vasospasm associated with catheter exchange can be avoided. As on the left side, the preferred place for right-sided balloon embolization is in the mid-pelvic region, where most of the collaterals will have re-entered the main channel (Fig. 4–21).

Collateral veins occasionally require separate embolization and may be difficult to catheterize. Any collateral veins ≥1 or 2 mm that could bypass the balloon need to be embolized during the initial procedure in order to prevent recurrence by progressive enlargement of these channels (Figs. 4–21 through 4–23). If the balloon introducer catheter cannot enter these veins, an open-ended

guidewire with a steerable tip can be advanced into the collateral vein, which is then embolized with ≤5 ml of ethanol (Fig. 4–21). During alcohol injection, the patient will experience pain, which relents within 10–15 min; during this time, intravenous analgesics should be given. Otherwise, the embolization procedure is largely painless except during periods of vasospasm, when a dull lumbar pain may be felt. The entire embolization procedure is carried out on an outpatient basis, and the patient is allowed full physical activity after 24 hr.

Despite careful embolization technique, 5–7% of patients have recurrences, usually through collaterals that have not appeared on initial and postembolization venography.[49,57,58] Repeat venography and embolization are usually successful in these instances. Balloon embolization may not be required; ethanol or small coils may suffice to occlude these collateral channels.

Effective treatment of varicocele may not improve spermatogenesis enough to generate offspring, which is, after all, the most frequent reason for the treatment. However, for patients with fertility problems, treatment of varicocele may be the only chance for improvement, and, given the minimal invasiveness of embolotherapy, this procedure appears to present an acceptable risk. With shielding applied throughout the procedure, total radiation exposure to the testicle should not exceed 50 mrem.[58]

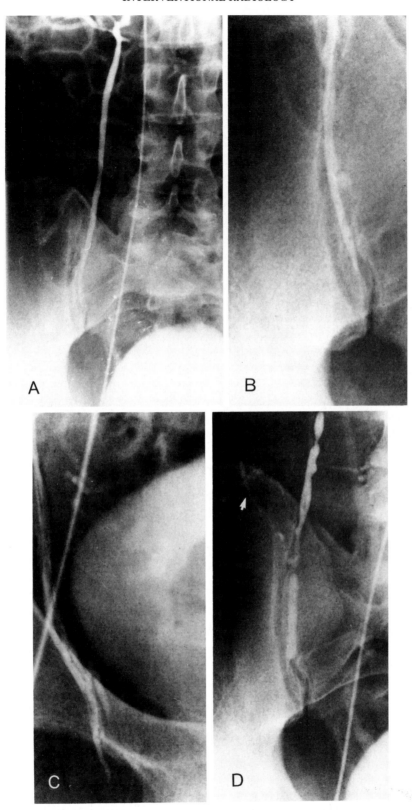

Fig. 4–22   A 26-year-old man with recurrent right-sided varicocele along with decreased sperm count after bilateral suprainguinal internal spermatic vein ligation. A. Right single channel internal spermatic vein arising from lower pole renal vein is valveless with slow retrograde flow. B. Severe spasm after insertion of open-end guidewire into distal internal spermatic vein, preventing reflux; this reaction should not be misread as effective distal ligation. C. After relief of spasm, distal filling shows suprainguinal bifurcation of vein. D. Occlusion of internal spermatic vein after embolization with 1-mm silicone balloon in typical area proximal to bifurcation and distal to renal capsular vein (arrow).

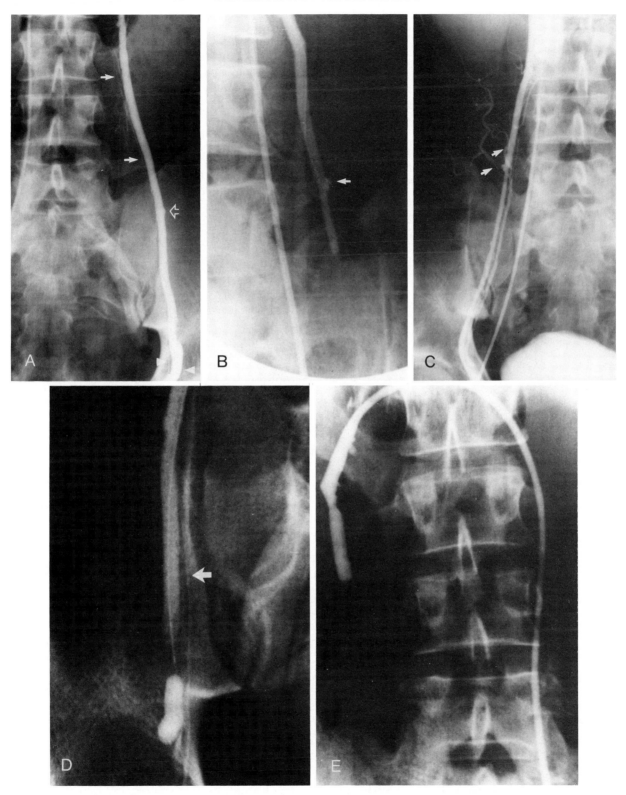

Fig. 4–23 A 28-year-old man with bilateral varicoceles and subfertility. A. Left-sided internal spermatic venogram via 8.8F introducer catheter in vein orifice shows typical valveless vein with retrograde flow. Small proximal collateral vein (arrows). Branch vein entry below iliac crest (open arrow); bifurcation above inguinal canal and distal collateral vein (arrowheads). B. Balloon distal to branch vein inflow (arrow). C. Right-sided internal spermatic venogram shows smaller caliber right-sided vein with several collateral channels and renal capsular branches (arrows). D. Balloon distally does not occlude collateral channel (arrow), which could allow recurrence. E. Proximal placement of balloon to occlude collateral inflow. This balloon alone would not have prevented retrograde flow from renal capsular veins, which is blocked by distal balloon. (Courtesy of Steven L. Kaufman, M.D., Johns Hopkins Hospital, Baltimore, MD.)

References

1. Serbinenko FA: Balloon catheterization and occlusion of major cerebral vessels. *J Neurosurg* 1974;41:125–145

2. Debrun G, Lacour P, Caron JP, et al: Inflatable and released balloon technique: experimentation in dog—application in man. *Neuroradiology* 1975;9:267–271

3. Kerber C: Balloon catheter with a calibrated leak. *Radiology* 1976;120:547–550

4. Laitinen L, Servo A: Embolization of cerebral vessels with inflatable and detachable balloons. *J Neurosurg* 1978;48:307–308

5. DiTullio MV, Rand RW, Frisch E: Detachable balloon catheter: its application in experimental arteriovenous fistula. *J Neurosurg* 1978;48:717–723

6. Taki W, Handa H, Yamagata S, et al: Embolization and superselective angiography by means of balloon catheters. *Surg Neurol* 1979;12:7–14

7. White RI Jr, Kaufman SL, Barth KH, et al: Embolotherapy with detachable silicone balloons: technique and clinical results. *Radiology* 1979;131:619–627

8. Hieshima GB, Grinnell VS, Mehringer CM: A detachable balloon for therapeutic transcatheter occlusions. *Radiology* 1981;138:227–228

9. Debrun G, Lacour P, Caron JP, et al: Detachable balloon and calibrated-leak balloon techniques in the treatment of cerebral vascular lesions. *J Neurosurg* 1978;49:635–649

10. White RI Jr, Ursic TA, Kaufman SL, et al: Therapeutic embolization with detachable balloons: physical factors influencing permanent occlusion. *Radiology* 1978;126:521–523

11. Barth KH, White RI Jr, Kaufman SL, Strandberg JD: Metrizamide, the ideal radiopaque filling material for detachable silicone balloon embolization. *Invest Radiol* 1979;14:35–40

12. Kaufman SL, Strandberg JD, Barth KH, et al: Therapeutic embolization with detachable silicone balloons: long term effects in swine. *Invest Radiol* 1979;14:156–161

13. Debrun G: Balloon catheter techniques in neuroradiology, in Athanasoulis CH, et al (eds): *Interventional Radiology*. Philadelphia, WB Saunders, 1983, pp 707–730

14. White RI Jr: Embolotherapy with detachable balloons, in Abrams HA (ed): *Interventional Techniques*. Philadelphia, WB Saunders, 1983, pp 2211–2222

15. Jhaveri HS, Gerlock AJ, Ekelund L: Failure of steel coil occlusion in a case of hypernephroma. *AJR* 1978;130:556–557

16. Gunther R, Klose K, Alken P: Transrenal ureteral occlusion with a detachable balloon. *Radiology* 1982;142:521–523

17. Pace R, Rankin RN, Finley RJ: Detachable balloon occlusion of bronchopleural fistula in dog. *Invest Radiol* 1983;18:504–506

18. Dines DE, Arms RA, Bernatz PE, Gomes MR: Pulmonary arteriovenous fistulas. *Mayo Clin Proc* 1974;49:460–465

19. Lindskog GE, Laebow A, Hausel H, Janzen A: Pulmonary arteriovenous aneurysm. *Ann Surg* 1959;132:591–610

20. Gomes MR, Bernatz PE, Dines DE: Pulmonary arteriovenous fistulas. *Ann Thorac Surg* 1969;7:582–593

21. Castañeda–Zuñiga WR, Epstein M, Zollikofer C, et al: Embolization of multiple pulmonary artery fistulas. *Radiology* 1980;134:309–310

22. Jonsson K, Hellekant C, Olsson O, Holen O: Percutaneous transcatheter occlusion of pulmonary arteriovenous malformation. *Ann Radiol* 1980;23:335–337

23. White RI Jr, Barth KH, Kaufman SL, Terry PB: Detachable silicone balloons: results of experimental study and clinical investigations in hereditary hemorrhagic telangiectasia. *Ann Radiol* 1980;23:338–340

24. Terry PB, Barth KH, Kaufman SL, White RI Jr: Balloon embolization for treatment of pulmonary arteriovenous fistulas. *N Engl J Med* 1980;302:1189–1190

25. Kaufman SL, Kumar AAJ, Roland JMA, et al: Transcatheter embolization in the management of congenital arteriovenous malformations. *Radiology* 1980;137:21–29

26. Barth KH, White RI Jr, Kaufman SL, et al: Embolotherapy of pulmonary arteriovenous malformations with detachable balloons. *Radiology* 1982;149:599–605

27. Taylor BG, Cockerill EM, Manfredi F, Klatte EC: Therapeutic embolization of the pulmonary artery in pulmonary arteriovenous fistula. *Am J Med* 1978;64:360–365

28. Knudson RP, Alden ER: Symptomatic arteriovenous malformation in infants less than 6 months of age. *Pediatrics* 1979;64:238–241

29. White RI Jr, Mitchell SE, Barth KH, et al: Angioarchitecture of pulmonary arteriovenous malformations: an important consideration before embolotherapy. *AJR* 1983;140:681–686

30. Dublin AB, Lantz BMT, Link DP: Video dilution technique evaluation of an arteriovenous fistula: monitoring detachable balloon embolization. *AJR* 1981;137:1249–1250

31. Barth KH, Kumar AJ, Kaufman SL, White RI Jr: Therapeutic embolizations in the extracranial head and neck region using a new detachable balloon system. *Fortschr Röntgenstr* 1980;133:409–415

32. Franklin RH, Bloom WF, Schoffstall RO: Angiographic embolization as the definitive treatment of posttraumatic hemobilia. *J Trauma* 1980;20:702–705

33. Porter LL, Houston MC, Kadin S: Mycotic aneurysms of the hepatic artery: treatment with arterial embolization. *Am J Med* 1979;67:695–701

34. Marshall FF, White RI Jr, Kaufman SL, Barth KH: Treatment of traumatic renal arteriovenous fistulas by detachable silicone balloon embolization. *J Urol* 1979;122:237–239

35. Renie WA, Rodeheffer RJ, Mitchell S, et al: Balloon embolization of a mycotic pulmonary artery aneurysm. *Am Rev Respir Dis* 1982;126:1107–1110

36. Stewart JR, Barth KH, Williams GM: Ruptured lumbar artery pseudoaneurysm: an unusual cause for retroperitoneal hemorrhage. *Surgery* 1983;93:592–594

37. Stanley P, Grinnell VS, Stanton RE, et al: Therapeutic embolization of infantile hepatic hemangioma with polyvinyl alcohol. *AJR* 1983;141:1047–1051

38. Burrows PE, Rosenberg HC, Chuang HS: Diffuse hepatic hemangiomas: percutaneous transcatheter embolization with detachable silicone balloons. *Radiology* 1985;156:85–88

39. Kadir S, Marshall FF, White RI Jr, et al: Therapeutic embolization of the kidney with detachable silicone balloons. *J Urol* 1983;129:11–13

40. Grinnell VS, Hieshima GB, Mehringer CM, et al: Therapeutic renal artery occlusion with a detachable balloon. *J Urol* 1981;126:223–237

41. Kadir S, Kaufman SL, Barth KH, White RI Jr: *Selected Technique in Interventional Radiology*. Philadelphia, WB Saunders, 1982

42. Grinnell VS, Flanagan KG, Mehringer MC, Hieshima GB: Occlusion of large fistulas with detachable valved balloons and the spider. *AJR* 1983;140:1259–1261

43. Palmaz JC, Newton TH, Reuter SH, Bookstein JJ: Particulate intraarterial embolization in pelvic arteriovenous malformations. *AJR* 1981;137:117–122

44. Florentine M, Wolfe RR, White RI Jr: Balloon embolization to occlude a Blalock-Taussig shunt. *J Am Coll Cardiol* 1984;3:200–202

45. Kunnen M: New technique for embolization of the internal spermatic vein: intravenous tissue adhesive. *Fortschr Röntgenstr* 1980;133:625–629

46. Formanek A, Rusnak B, Zollikoffer C, et al: Embolization of the spermatic vein for treatment of infertility: a new approach. *Radiology* 1981;139:315–321

47. White RI Jr, Kaufman SL, Barth KH, et al: Occlusion of vari-coceles with detachable balloons. *Radiology* 1981;139:327–334

48. Seyferth W, Jecht E, Zeitler E: Percutaneous sclerotherapy of varicocele. *Radiology* 1981;139:335–340

49. Barth KH, Kaufman SL, Kadir S, White RI Jr: Treatment of varicoceles by embolization with detachable balloons, in Jecht EW, Zeitler E (eds): *Varicocele and Male Infertility.* Berlin, Springer, 1982

50. MacLeod J: Further observations on the role of varicocele in human male infertility. *Fertil Steril* 1969;20:545–563

51. Klosterhalfen H, Schirren C, Wagennecht LV: Pathogenesis and therapy of varicocele. *Urologe* 1979;18:187–192

52. Cockett ATK, Takihara H, Cosentino MJ: The varicocele. *Fertil Steril* 1984;41:5–11

53. Lien HH, Kolbenstvedt A: Phlebographic appearances of the left renal and left testicular veins. *Acta Radiol [Diagn]* 1977;18:321–332

54. Riedl P: Selective phlebography and catheter sclerosation of the spermatic vein in primary varicocele. *Wien Klin Wochenschr* 1979;91(Suppl 99):3–20

55. Comhaire F, Kunnen G, Nahoum C: Radiological anatomy of the internal spermatic vein(s) in 200 retrograde venograms. *Int J Androl* 1981;4:379–387

56. Gonzalez R, Narayan N, Castañeda–Zuñiga WR, Amplatz K: Transvenous embolization of the internal spermatic vein for the treatment of varicocele scroti. *Urol Clin North Am* 1982;9:177–184

57. Kaufman SL, Kadir S, Barth KH, et al: Mechanisms of recurrent varicocele after balloon occlusion or surgical ligation of the inter-nal spermatic vein. *Radiology* 1983;147:435–440

58. Walsh PC, White RI Jr: Balloon occlusion of the internal sper-matic vein for the treatment of varicoceles. *JAMA* 1981;246:1701–1702

5

Ablation with Absolute Ethanol

GARY J. BECKER, M.D., ROBERT W. HOLDEN, M.D., HEUN Y. YUNE, M.D., AND EUGENE C. KLATTE, M.D.

The current body of knowledge concerning absolute ethanol as an embolic agent derives largely from uncontrolled clinical applications. However, laboratory work in animals by several investigators has begun to elucidate important basic information, particularly regarding the mechanisms of action.[1-11] A large body of clinical information about other embolic agents[12-17] has been applied to the development of techniques for clinical use of absolute ethanol. This chapter encompasses the indications, contraindications, methods of administration, results, and complications of the use of absolute ethanol in interventional radiology. References to animal work are included to enlighten the reader about current understanding of the mechanisms of action of this embolic agent.

RENAL EMBOLIZATION

Animal Studies

The use of particulate embolic agents, autologous clot, and coils is complicated by difficulties in handling the agents, incomplete infarction of target tissue, vascular recanalization, and inadvertent reflux that occludes nontarget vessels. These problems, which are discussed in Chapter 3 of this volume, led Ellman et al to study the potential for transcatheter therapeutic infarction of the kidney with absolute ethanol.[1] In their canine study, transcatheter injection of high concentrations of ethanol into the renal artery produced complete renal infarction. This dramatic result was attributed to the protein-denaturing property of ethanol administered in high concentration and to vascular thrombosis attributable to endothelial damage. Low concentrations (10%) did not damage the kidney, and reflux of ethanol into the aorta in concentrations as high as 10% produced no damage.

In a study of therapeutic renal infarction in eight rabbits and one pig, Ekelund et al found absolute ethanol easy to administer, reliable in producing complete renal infarction with renal artery thrombosis, and entirely safe despite a small amount of reflux into the aorta that may occur with slow renal artery injection. Indeed, they injected 2 ml of absolute ethanol directly into the abdominal aorta in one animal and found no injury.[2] For canine renal artery embolization, Buchta et al infused 0.2 ml/kg of absolute ethanol at rates of 1–2 ml/sec. Angiograms showed complete vascular occlusion.[3] Light and electron microscopic studies showed glomerular necrosis, a proteinaceous precipitate in Bowman's capsules, and vascular congestion without thrombosis, changes that were thought to represent the effect of direct toxicity to the cells rather than thrombosis-induced hypoxia. The 1 ml/ sec injection rate produced necrosis in approximately 50% of the glomeruli, whereas the 2 ml/sec injection produced necrosis in all glomeruli.

Recently, Ellman et al studied more thoroughly the light and electron microscopic changes in the kidney as a function of the rate of injection of absolute ethanol.[11] In this series of elegant experiments, the authors made a number of pertinent negative and positive findings, of which the following are most important:

1. Renal artery spasm, which had been thought important in producing vascular occlusion after ethanol injection, was not demonstrable radiographically when animals were given a metrizamide–ethanol mixture.
2. Renal infarction can be produced without vascular thrombosis in heparinized kidneys made bloodless with an occlusion balloon inflated and saline infused for 3 min before ethanol administration. Vasculitis with marked pruning is found angiographically, while parenchymal necrosis and vascular injury with endothelial sloughing are demonstrable histologically.
3. With slow (<0.5 ml/sec) ethanol injection, there is a high likelihood of acute major vascular occlusion, because the ethanol interacts with blood components, particularly red cells, creating denatured protein debris that embolizes within the renal vasculature. Extensive parenchymal necrosis is also observed.
4. Rapid (> 0.5 ml/sec) ethanol infusion produces angiographic evidence of vasculitis without vascular occlusion, as well as histologic evidence of severe endothelial injury, and extensive parenchymal necrosis. Vascular occlusion occurs late and is a secondary phenomenon.

Human Experience

RENAL TUMORS

Published Reports

Transcatheter renal devitalization using particulate emboli, steel coils, and other agents for renal cell carcinoma has been practiced widely. Although probably not effective as primary therapy, it has proved a useful adjunct to operation and an excellent means of palliation in cases of inoperable advanced and metastatic disease.[18–22] However, when particulate agents or steel coils are used, there may be incomplete infarction of the kidney,[22] unintentional embolization of nontarget organs,[23–27] and difficulty in handling and administering the agent.[26] Greenfield et al were the first to describe prevention of reflux of embolic materials and prevention of unintentional embolization by using a balloon occlusion catheter.[28] This technique, originally used with particulate embolic agents, has proved useful for embolization with absolute ethanol.

Klatte first reported clinical use of absolute ethanol for transcatheter renal artery occlusion in renal cell carcinoma in 1980. Subsequently, Rosenkrantz et al reported three patients who underwent prenephrectomy embolization with absolute ethanol.[29] Following the lead of Wallace and colleagues, Rosenkrantz et al left at least a 2-day interval between the diagnostic angiogram and the embolization in an effort to minimize the risk of renal failure. They used epidural anesthesia and an ethanol dose of 0.2 ml/kg of body weight, a dose that did not produce systemic toxicity in animal studies. Ethanol injection rates approximated rates of contrast injection which did not produce reflux from the renal artery into the aorta at angiography. As others did before them, Wallace and colleagues delayed nephrectomy for 10 days in an effort to maximize the potential immune response.[22] (Importantly, there are insufficient data to prove the enhanced immune response hypothesis, as discussed below.) Each embolization procedure resulted in a relatively bloodless nephrectomy. Angiographic and pathologic findings in all cases were similar to those of early animal studies: complete renal necrosis and tumor necrosis, with no evidence of thrombosis in the renal arteries. This finding is to be expected with relatively high (>0.5 ml/sec) injection rates of ethanol according to the work of Ellman et al. The highest blood ethanol level attained in any of the patients was 0.07% by volume, well below legal intoxication levels. Patients experienced a postembolization syndrome similar to that which follows renal artery occlusion with other agents,[22] with nausea, vomiting, pain, and fever that generally lasted 1–5 days. Narcotic analgesia, antipyretics, antiemetics, and intravenous fluids were often indicated. It was this pain that led Rosenkrantz et al to give their patients epidural anesthesia for 36–72 hr after ethanol transcatheter embolization or until patients were able to tolerate oral analgesics with minimal symptoms.

Gas was found in the tumors by computed tomography (CT) after embolization. Although this finding may appear alarming, seeming to indicate infection, Bernardino et al have attributed it to tumor necrosis.[30] Furthermore, the experimental findings of Carroll and Walter indicate that some of the gas might actually be introduced during the embolization procedure.[31]

Ellman et al reported successful renal ablation with absolute ethanol in six patients, two preoperatively and four palliatively, with good results and only mild postembolization syndromes.[32]

Rabe et al infarcted 15 renal cell carcinomas and one angiomyolipoma with absolute ethanol.[33] Embolizations were performed for palliation of symptoms in metastatic disease (10 patients, 9 of whom improved), preoperatively to reduce blood loss during radical nephrectomy (three patients, all of whom were alive and well without further evidence of disease 1–26 months postoperatively), or as primary therapy in two patients. One of these two had earlier undergone a right nephrectomy for renal cell carcinoma, so the carcinoma of the left lower pole necessitated a limited approach, which culminated in a selective lower pole embolization with absolute ethanol. The patient was alive and well 4 months after embolization. The second patient in whom embolization was the primary treatment was a young woman who presented with a large retroperitoneal hemorrhage due to rupture of an aneurysm in a left lower pole angiomyolipoma. After surgical evacuation of the hematoma and a second severe hemorrhage, she underwent transcatheter embolization of the tumor. The patient returned 3 weeks later with a large perinephric abscess, the only complication of the series. She had not been given antibiotics before embolization, had been receiving corticosteroids for an unrelated condition, and had undergone the aforementioned operation. Any or all of these factors could have contributed to the formation of the abscess. Although there is no conclusive evidence of the need for antibiotic prophylaxis, Rabe et al recommend that broad-spectrum antibiotics be administered to all patients beginning the night before embolization and continuing for 5 days afterward.

Injection of ethanol through a balloon occlusion catheter positioned in the midportion of the main renal artery, now universally accepted, is the technique that was used by Rabe et al. The balloon was inflated immediately before ethanol injection, remained inflated for 2 min, and was deflated during a 10-min waiting period, after which the catheter was aspirated to remove residual ethanol and then cleared with saline. A repeat angiogram was performed. Although the endpoint in each case in this series was total occlusion of the main renal artery, the reader is reminded that the aforementioned study of Ellman et al indicates that total renal infarction can be achieved without angiographic evidence of thrombus in the main or interlobar renal arteries, particularly with slow injection rates. Rabe et al cited several potential benefits of balloon occlusion: interruption of renal blood flow, thus prolonging the contact of the ethanol with the endothelium; prevention of unintended reflux into the aorta; and effective infarction achieved by injection of ethanol into the main renal artery. The latter obviates the segmental renal artery injections frequently required with particulate embolic agents in cases requiring total

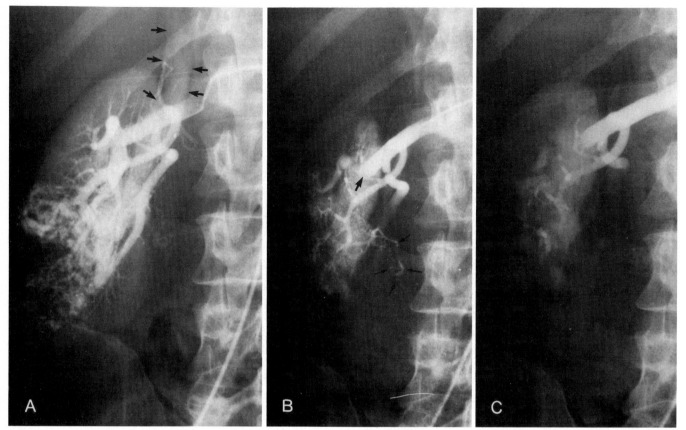

Fig. 5–1 Patient with metastatic right renal cell carcinoma and flank pain. A. Selective right renal arteriogram; in addition to the neoplasm, early opacification of right renal vein and inferior vena cava (arrows) provides evidence of rapid shunting through tumor bed. B. Selective right renal arteriogram after 10 ml of absolute ethanol shows occlusion of main renal artery (large arrow) and min- imal residual tumor vascularity (small arrows). C. After another 5 ml of ethanol has been injected, there is no residual tumor vascularity. Flank pain resolved after embolization. This patient also had a metastasis in the right proximal humerus, which was managed with transcatheter Ivalon and surgical fixation.

renal infarction and so reduces the procedure time. Patients treated before the advent of the balloon occlu- sion method commonly required a subsequent emboliza- tion procedure, the need for which was determined by either ^{99m}Tc red blood cell dynamic and static imaging of renal blood flow or by contrast-enhanced CT scanning. Figures 5–1 and 5–2 are examples of renal cell carcinoma treated by transcatheter injection of absolute ethanol.

The importance of balloon occlusion became certain when Cox et al reported two cases of left colon infarction following renal embolization with ethanol using conven- tional catheters.[34] The authors postulated that any ethanol that refluxed into the aorta during injection lay- ered because of the differences in density and viscosity of ethanol and blood and that laminar flow in the aorta pre- vented dilution of the layered ethanol by blood. Conse- quently, the concentration of ethanol in the blood enter- ing the inferior mesenteric artery must have been considerably higher than would have been expected fol- lowing a midstream aortic injection (such as that used in the animal study of Ekelund et al).[2] Clearly, one cannot simply use a standard angiographic catheter without an occlusion balloon, determine the rate of flow of contrast medium that does not produce fluoroscopic evidence of

reflux, and then attempt to reproduce that injection rate for safe transcatheter renal ablation with ethanol. Bal- loon occlusion catheters must be used.

Recently, several additional clinical series have been published.[35–38] Ekelund et al reported 20 patients with renal cell carcinoma; 14 with locally advanced disease or distant metastases underwent embolization with ethanol for palliation of pain or hematuria, and six underwent postembolization nephrectomy.[35] Those authors found that intraprocedural pain was diminished when lidocaine was administered through the catheter before the ethanol. This has been true in the present authors' expe- rience as well. Ekelund's group also found the postem- bolization syndrome to be milder with ethanol ablation than with other methods of embolization. Although some other investigators also believe this to be true, the expe- rience has not been common to all series. Ekelund et al found gas in the kidney and tumor on CT to be common after embolization and suggested that it probably arose from carbon dioxide from anerobic metabolism or the release of oxygen from oxyhemoglobin.

To investigate the hypothesis that *in vivo* necrosis enhances the patient's immune response to the tumor, the authors evaluated the natural killer (NK) cell activity

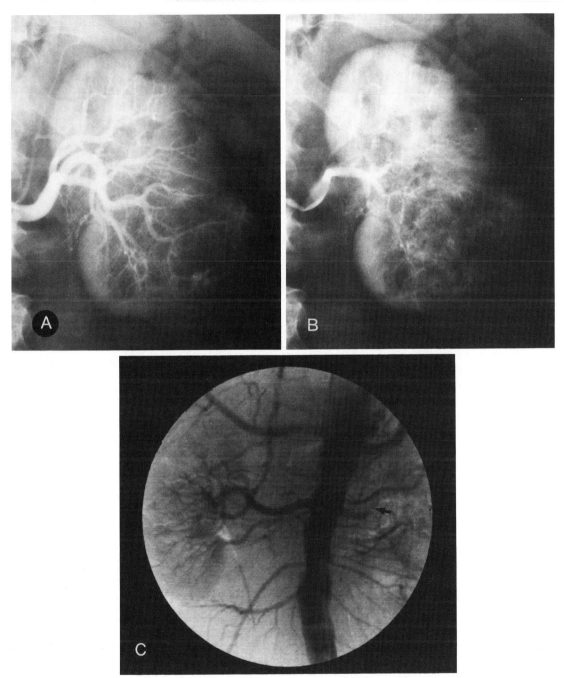

Fig. 5–2 A 57-year-old man with left renal cell carcinoma. Early (A) and late (B) arterial phases of selective left renal arteriogram reveal moderately vascular left lower pole neoplasm. C. Intra-arterial digital subtraction angiography after transcatheter ethanol embolotherapy reveals occluded stump of left renal artery (arrow).

of circulating monocytes in seven of their patients before and after embolization. All patients had low baseline NK activity. After embolotherapy, NK activity increased in four patients, decreased in two, and was unchanged in one. Although the mean cytotoxicity increased, the increase was not statistically significant. Thus, these investigators found no support for the immunity enhancement hypothesis.

Klimberg et al reported 34 patients who underwent renal ablation, 25 for renal cell carcinoma, with a balloon occlusion catheter and an average absolute ethanol dose of 15 ml.[36] Of these, 21 underwent transabdominal radical nephrectomy several hours to 57 days after renal ablation. At operation, tumor was confined to the renal capsule in six patients (stage I); had penetrated into perinephric fat but not beyond Gerota's fascia in four (stage II); involved the renal vein, vena cava, or regional nodes in nine (stage III); and had metastasized in two (stage IV). The mean tumor mass was 830 g and the median blood loss was 725 ml. The authors were convinced that dissection had been greatly facilitated, particularly in the large vascular tumors, but this contrasts with two recent reports in which the authors question the value of preoperative angioinfarction for renal cell carcinoma.[37,38] Thus, MacErlean et al believe that the usefulness of preoperative angioinfarction for renal carcinoma is limited to cases involving large hypervascular tumors.[37] Also, in the series of Teasdale et al, 28 patients underwent transcatheter renal embolization, 26 as prenephrectomy procedures, and the authors question the value of embolization largely because histologic examination did not demonstrate complete infarction of the tumor in 24 of the embolized kidneys, in 8 of which it appeared that the tumor had completely escaped infarction.[38] However, these embolizations had been performed using gelatin sponge, stainless-steel coils, or both. Importantly, in the series of both Ekelund et al and Klimberg et al, extensive tumor necrosis was found at histopathologic examination after transcatheter absolute ethanol renal ablation.[35,36] In both series, balloon occlusion catheters were used. Klimberg et al also found the postembolization syndrome to be milder with the ethanol method than with other agents and the immediate pain of renal infarction to be diminished with pre-embolization transcatheter injection of 2 ml of lidocaine. They concluded that ethanol is the embolic agent of choice in renal cell carcinoma, not only for these reasons, but also because it is inexpensive, readily available in sterile form, greatly simplifies angioinfarction, and decreases the procedure time.

Mebust et al, in their experience with 46 patients who underwent transcatheter angioinfarction for renal cell carcinoma, concluded that no reduction in operative blood loss or operating time could be documented in patients who underwent preoperative embolization.[39] However, only five of their patients had transcatheter ethanol angioinfarction, the other procedures being done with gelatin sponge or Gianturco coils. Two of their patients suffered left colon infarction after embolotherapy, but balloon occlusion was not used, and it would appear that reflux into the aorta was involved, as in the previously described cases.

Recently, Earthman et al used subselective ethanol embolotherapy to treat two patients with a total of three hemorrhaging angiomyolipomas. They also reviewed the world literature and concluded that the method is one of the best for achieving safe, permanent, and complete ablation.[40]

Technical Guidelines

The following guidelines, derived from the collective experience of many investigators including the present authors,[41,42] should aid angiographers who use absolute ethanol embolotherapy for renal tumors.

The indications for transcatheter absolute ethanol devitalization of renal tumors are:

1. Immediate preoperative devascularization of the tumor to facilitate surgical resection. Since available data do not strongly support the enhanced immune response hypothesis, there is no need to delay the operation for 10–14 days after embolization; rather, a period of 1–6 hr is recommended, since the shorter delay decreases the duration of symptoms of the postembolization syndrome. Case selection need not be limited to patients with renal cell carcinoma; palliation and preoperative devascularization may be useful also in benign lesions such as angiomyolipoma;
2. Palliation of hematuria, fever, and other tumor-related problems such as secondary polycythemia;
3. Primary therapy in selected cases, such as subselective tumor embolization in a solitary kidney.

Pre-embolization broad-spectrum antibiotics are used by some radiologists to prevent abscess formation in the devitalized renal and tumor tissue. Those who use them tend to continue administration for approximately 5 days after the procedure. Most interventionalists agree that antibiotics should be used in patients with ureteronephrolithiasis or urinary tract infection.

Most investigators believe it is wise to delay the embolization procedure for at least 2 days after diagnostic angiography to minimize the risk of renal failure.

Pre-embolization parenteral analgesia is essential. Although epidural anesthesia may be used, the shortened postembolization syndrome attending the author's recommendations should reduce the need for it.

The technique is as follows:

1. The standard transfemoral approach should be used to position a balloon occlusion catheter in the midportion of the main renal artery beyond the origins of the inferior adrenal and gonadal arteries. (See below under "Adrenal Ablation" for an explanation of the potential ill effects of transcatheter adrenal ablation with ethanol.) To reiterate, one should avoid using a diagnostic angiographic catheter without an occlusion balloon and simply estimating the proper ethanol injection rate by fluoroscopic monitoring of an injection of contrast medium; such estimation can cause reflux of ethanol into the aorta and inferior mesenteric artery, with left colon infarction.
2. Parenteral analgesics should be used during the procedure, because the pain of renal infarction is often severe. Morphine is probably the drug of choice. In the authors' experience, as well as in that of others, 3–5 ml of 2% lidocaine given through the catheter after inflation of the occlusion balloon and before ethanol administration also help reduce pain.
3. The occlusion balloon should be inflated immediately before ethanol injection and remain inflated during and for 2 min after the injection in order to increase the endothelial contact time by eliminating or markedly reducing renal blood flow. This maneuver also prevents reflux of ethanol into the aorta. Furthermore, balloon occlusion provides more effective total renal necrosis with a main renal artery injection, thereby eliminating the need for segmental injections and dramatically reducing the procedure time.
4. As much as 0.2 ml of absolute ethanol (95% ethyl alcohol)/kg of body weight may be administered on the first (and often only) injection. Injection rates from

<0.5 ml/sec to 2.0 ml/sec can be justified by available evidence, and it is likely that either of these extremes will provide the desired extensive tumor necrosis, albeit by different mechanisms.[11] These doses and rates produce total renal necrosis without creating toxic ethanol levels in either animals or humans. Importantly, the authors have used as much as 0.4 ml/kg in thromboembolotherapy for gastroesophageal varices in average-sized adults without creating signs of systemic toxicity. They also frequently exceed 0.2 ml/kg in patients undergoing renal ablation with ethanol when a second injection is required to complete the embolization. The authors have not measured the ethanol levels in these patients.

5. The balloon is deflated after 2 min, and the catheter is left undisturbed for another 10 min. The catheter is then aspirated to removed residual ethanol and any particulate debris and flushed with heparinized saline.

6. A repeat angiogram is obtained. In the past, the authors believed that total renal artery occlusion was the only desirable endpoint, but they now know that this angiographic picture is most likely to result from very slow ethanol injection rates (<0.5 ml/sec), whereas more rapid injections (≤2 ml/sec) are more likely to result in an immediate postembolization angiographic pattern of severely pruned intrarenal vessels, stasis of contrast medium in the pruned renal artery branches, absence of the nephrographic picture obtained at diagnostic angiography, and no evidence of contrast washout.[11] It is likely that long-term follow-up of patients with the latter angiographic appearance will usually show renal artery occlusion. In any event, both of these angiographic pictures indicate that the desired result probably has been achieved. If the maximum ethanol dose has not been administered on the first attempt and the desired result has not been obtained, then the procedure may be repeated.

On follow-up CT, ultrasound, or plain film examination, gas in the infarcted kidney and tumor is to be expected. It probably is the result of tissue necrosis, air injected during the embolization procedure, or postembolization accumulation of carbon dioxide from anaerobic tissue metabolism or of oxygen from oxyhemoglobin dissociation. It should not be misconstrued as a sign of abscess. If, however, increasing gas, or gas associated with a soft tissue mass, is found, particularly in association with continued pain, tenderness, and fever, one should consider the possibility of a renal or perinephric abscess.

In the follow-up of patients not undergoing nephrectomy, continuation or recurrence of the symptoms for which the embolization was originally performed may herald the need for repeat embolization. An increase in tumor size may indicate the same. In these instances, verification of continued blood flow to the tumor may be accomplished with either a contrast-enhanced CT scan or ^{99m}Tc red blood cell dynamic and static images of renal blood flow.

Other possible complications include transient elevation of both systolic and diastolic blood pressure for 2–4 hr after embolization, temporary or irreversible renal failure, and pulmonary, or even systemic, embolization of nontarget tissues with high concentrations of ethanol.

HYPERTENSION AND OTHER COMPLICATIONS OF END-STAGE RENAL DISEASE

Nanni et al reported five patients who underwent renal ablation with ethanol for uncontrolled hypertension.[43] Although the present authors do not consider renal ablation for just any case of uncontrolled hypertension, one must remember that 80% of patients with end-stage renal failure develop systemic hypertension and that those who do not respond to antihypertensive drugs or dialysis typically have elevated renal vein renin concentrations.[44] Surgical nephrectomy has been used, but given the current effectiveness of transcatheter "medical nephrectomy" with absolute ethanol, one must consider the newer technique seriously. Before embolization, Nanni et al demonstrated elevated renal vein renin concentrations in four of their patients. Using a technique similar to the one described above, they injected smaller quantities of ethanol. Of the two patients with functioning renal allografts at the time of embolization, one eventually developed a second acute rejection, the only complication in the small series. No hypothesis was offered to explain this occurrence. In each of the five embolized patients, the result was normotension on either no drugs or on reduced doses. Since the original publication, this series has expanded to nine patients.

Recently, Denny et al reported a patient with severe hypertension despite a multiple-drug antihypertensive regimen and renin lateralizing to the left kidney who had a completely occluded left renal artery and only collateral flow to the left kidney at angiography.[45] After recanalization using a curved catheter and a straight guidewire, percutaneous transluminal angioplasty was performed. When this procedure failed to control the patient's hypertension, the poorly functioning kidney was embolized with ethanol. The result was normotension on a two-drug regimen. A renal scan 6 months later showed no flow to the left kidney.

Keller et al recently reported their experience with renal ablation in 18 kidneys of 10 patients with end-stage renal disease.[46] Embolic material varied from isobutyl-2-cyanoacrylate to sodium tetradecyl sulfate-soaked gelatin sponge pledgets to Gianturco spring coils to ethanol. Since 1978, ethanol has been used in all renal ablations (7 patients, 13 renal ablations). Indications included nephrotic syndrome with massive protein loss (7 patients, 13 kidneys), poorly controlled post-transplantation, hypertension in the absence of transplant renal artery stenosis (2 patients, 3 kidneys), and diabetic nephropathy with persistent urine leak from ureterocutaneous fistulae following pelvic irradiation (1 patient, 2 kidneys). Desired clinical results were achieved in all cases.

The proper indications and potential complications of this treatment method need to be more fully elucidated. For the present, suffice it to say that some patients with complications of end-stage renal disease appear to be good candidates for renal ablation with transcatheter ethanol.

PERCUTANEOUS TRANSHEPATIC SCLEROSIS OF ESOPHAGEAL VARICES

Published Reports

Patients with bleeding esophageal varices due to cirrhosis continue to frustrate gastroenterologists, surgeons, and interventional radiologists. The involvement of interventional radiology stems from the availability of the transhepatic approach for catheterization of the portal vein, with selective catheterization and obliteration of the coronary (left gastric) and short gastric veins that are tributary to the varices.[47–52] Widrich et al, who used primarily autologous clot, balloon occlusion, and gelatin sponge soaked in sodium tetradecyl sulfate, helped to pioneer this temporizing treatment.[51] Many of their important experiences and observations are applicable to transcatheter coronary vein sclerosis with absolute ethanol. Therefore, some of their concepts are included below the recommended technique.

The aforementioned problems with particulate embolic agents led to investigation with ethanol. Ethanol provides the following additional advantages: easy handling, shortened procedure time, and apparent permanence as a vaso-occlusive agent. It is also inexpensive and readily available in sterile containers.

The first report of a series was by Yune et al and encompassed 12 cirrhotic patients.[53] This series has now been expanded to 50 patients,[54] 13 of whom were Child class B and 37 class C.[55] The etiologies of the cirrhosis were alcoholic in 22, postnecrotic in nine, primary biliary in two, and unknown in two. All patients had endoscopic confirmation of esophageal varices within the 24 hr preceding treatment, with documentation of active or recent bleeding. The latter was suggested by the presence of fresh blood clot on the surface of prominent varices. All had varices treated by transhepatic selective catheterization and embolization with absolute ethanol via a balloon occlusion catheter whenever possible. Gelatin sponge pledgets and stainless-steel Gianturco coils were used adjunctively in several cases. Technical failure due to one or more of the following was encountered in 13 instances: severe ascites, small rigid liver, cavernous transformation of the main portal vein, and severe coagulopathy. Of these failures, 12 were in patients in Child class C. Of the 37 patients initially treated successfully, 13 had recurrent hemorrhage, and nine of these were Child class C. Rebleeding, which was fatal in five of the nine patients, was due to recanalization of previously thrombosed veins in two. Nine patients died of other medical conditions despite successful variceal obliteration with ethanol. Of the 24 patients (48%) who have survived 6–36 months after the initial procedure with or without recurrent hemorrhage, only one was an initial technical failure. The authors concluded that patients in Child class B are better candidates than those in class C for this form of therapy. In addition, they concluded that class C patients with extensive ascites and severely contracted and rigid livers pose a difficult technical challenge, which is overcome to the point of control of bleeding in only one-third of cases. Most of the long-term survivors had lessening of signs and symptoms.

Transient pain upon ethanol injection was experienced by all patients. Death due to sepsis occurred in two patients with adult respiratory distress syndrome. One patient died 3 days after the procedure of small bowel infarction, the cause of which was not determined. Portal vein thrombosis with cavernous transformation developed in three patients. These patients, who experienced recurrent hemorrhage as early as 3 weeks and as late as 2½ years after initial thrombotherapy with ethanol, were treated with transendoscopic sclerotherapy or conservative medical management.

In the initial series report, Yune et al stated that ethanol can coagulate blood cells and plasma and thus is able to occlude small branch vessels. In addition, they assumed that there is instantaneous physical injury to the vascular endothelium upon contact with ethanol that accounts for the permanent occlusion.

Fifteen patients (13 in Child class C and 2 in class B) reported by Keller et al had acute hemorrhage from gastroesophageal varices that was managed by transhepatic sclerosis with absolute ethanol.[56] All were uncontrolled by Sengstaken–Blakemore tube, intravenous vasopressin, or both, and all underwent pre-embolization endoscopy, to document variceal bleeding, as well as arterial portography, to document the patency of the portal venous system. Although initial control and angiographic success were achieved in 13, two died within 48 hr from unrelated causes. All experienced chest pain at the time of embolization and an average initial rise in portal venous pressure of 10.6 mm Hg. Of the 11 with initial control who survived, 7 rebled 1 week to 13 months after embolization. Of the four who did not rebleed, two died 4 weeks and 6 months after embolization. Only two were alive (at 14 and 16 months) after embolization without evidence of rebleeding. The authors expressed their dislike for the radiolucency of ethanol and the seemingly long procedure times. They also reported a 20% frequency of portal vein thrombosis, which may have resulted from unintended reflux of ethanol into the portal vein or from the catheterization procedure itself. The problem of radiolucency is readily handled by mixing the ethanol with nonionic contrast media, which the present authors have done in a few cases. Unfortunately, these media are expensive. The ionic media cannot readily be mixed with absolute ethanol, because this often produces a precipitate that can occlude the catheter. In the present authors' experience, the problems of reflux and of procedure time are best handled by using balloon occlusion catheters. More recently, other investigators have begun to use them and have noted a decrease in the volume of ethanol needed to produce complete coronary venous occlusion.

In Uflacker's series of 11 patients with variceal bleeding treated with transhepatic ethanol, five had alcoholic cirrhosis, five had postnecrotic cirrhosis, and one had portal hypertension and varices of unknown cause.[57] Six were treated with ethanol alone; three with ethanol and gelatin sponge; and two with ethanol, gelatin sponge, and coils. Two patients died of recurrent hemorrhage and two died without rebleeding. The remaining seven had had no rebleeding 13–19 months after embolization. The hypothesis that distal embolic occlusion of the varices occurs with ethanol thrombotherapy could not be substantiated in those who died. Since this initial report, Uflacker has treated six more patients. Of three who rebled, two had angiographically documented portal or splenic vein thrombosis, adding to the experience of Keller and his colleagues and to our experience. All three died. The three patients who survived without rebleeding had endoscopic re-examination that showed a decrease in the size and number of varices. Of potential importance regarding Uflacker's frequency of portal vein thrombosis is the fact that he reports inserting a catheter as far as possible into the coronary vein in each instance in order to avoid reflux of ethanol into the portal vein. He did not use balloon occlusion catheters.

Using transhepatic cineportography, Sano and Kuroda demonstrated macrofistulous portopulmonary venous anastomoses in 10 of 40 cirrhotic patients with esophageal varices.[58] In most instances, the communication between the gastroesopheageal and pulmonary veins was easily identified at the level of the seventh thoracic vertebra, with drainage into the left atrium by way of the left lower lobe pulmonary veins. Portopulmonary anastomoses also occurred on the right. A serious implication of this finding is that particulate embolic materials used to obliterate varices may enter the systemic circulation. To avoid this complication, Sano and Kuroda recommend one further diagnostic study to aid in case selection: they used contrast-enhanced left atrial echocardiography, in which the fistulous communications were easily demonstrated by the real-time sonographic appearance of microbubbles in the left atrium after transcatheter injection of saline into the portal or splenic vein. Imaging of these microbubbles, cineportography, or both should help interventional angiographers identify patients unsuitable for embolization with particulate agents. The authors believe that ethanol thrombotherapy in patients with macrofistulous portopulmonary venous anastomoses may not be as fraught with the problems of systemic embolization because of the dilution that follows injection of absolute ethanol. However, it has not been proved that the concentration of ethanol reaching the left atrium and systemic circulation in these patients is harmless.

Widrich et al described collateral pathways of the left gastric vein in portal hypertension.[59] In their study of 347 portal venograms, the authors identified portopulmonary anastomoses in a small percentage of patients and believed that had cineportography been performed on all patients, the recognized frequency of this finding would have been much higher. They also reported a high frequency of multiple coronary veins with intercommunication and other tributaries to gastroesophageal varices, all of which, the authors emphasize, need to be properly mapped with splenic venography if thromboembolotherapy is planned.

Technical Guidelines

The following recommendations for transcatheter ethanol embolotherapy in gastroesophageal varices have been listed in two previous publications.[41,42] They derive from the present authors' experience and that of other investigators.

1. Before considering embolization, the interventional radiologist must consult with the gastroenterologist and vascular surgeon. Referring practices for such cases vary from one community to another. Alternative treatment modalities, including distal splenorenal shunt[60–62] and transendoscopic variceal sclerosis with 5% sodium morrhuate, must be considered.[63]

2. Verification of the patency of the portal vein is necessary before attempting the percutaneous transhepatic approach. Keller et al used arterial portography[56]; the present authors advocate the use of real-time ultrasound to determine the patency of the portal vein and its intrahepatic radicles. They also obtain a depth measurement with the transducer positioned at the desired entry site. This simple procedure is extremely helpful in gaining access to the portal vein and in minimizing the number of passes with the sheathed needle. Portal vein thrombosis and cavernous transformation of the portal vein can be detected by ultrasound.[64,65]

3. Intravenous or intramuscular analgesia and local anesthesia should be used.

4. A 5-mm skin incision that exposes subcutaneous fat is needed. The optimal location of the incision is generally on the right side of the chest wall between two of the lowest ribs laterally or anterolaterally. An anterior approach should be avoided in order to reduce irradiation of the examiner's hands. Fluoroscopic control should be used to avoid puncturing the pleura; real-time ultrasonography should have already aided the angiographer in avoiding the gallbladder and the hepatic flexure of the colon.

5. A sheathed 19- or 18-gauge needle is used to enter the liver and portal vein. One should use a sheath made of stiff material; thin-walled polyethylene sheaths are inadequate, as they tend to kink or "accordion" in cirrhotic livers. A large amount of ascites can prevent successful entry into the liver and portal vein, particularly if the liver is hard; for this reason, some angiographers consider tense ascites a contraindication to transhepatic variceal obliteration. The needle puncture should be made during midexhalation, as should the initial sonogram for portal vein location, because if the patient is asked to hold his breath in deep inhalation or exhalation during needle puncture, but then necessarily breathes quietly throughout the remainder of the procedure, one often finds that the skin entry point is remote from the liver entry point, sometimes as much as 5–10 cm cephalocaudal, so that the entire procedure is hampered by the uneven catheter tract to the portal vein.

Once the sheath and guidewire are in the vein, the sheath is advanced along the guidewire to gain optimal position in the portal venous system. The guidewire may then be advanced into the splenic vein, and the sheath may be replaced with an angiographic catheter. The authors usually attempt to use a C-1 catheter (7.0F Cordis with occlusion balloon), because subselection of the coronary vein will be necessary and balloon occlusion will be desired. If this C-1 or a 6.5F or 7F Cook catheter cannot be advanced

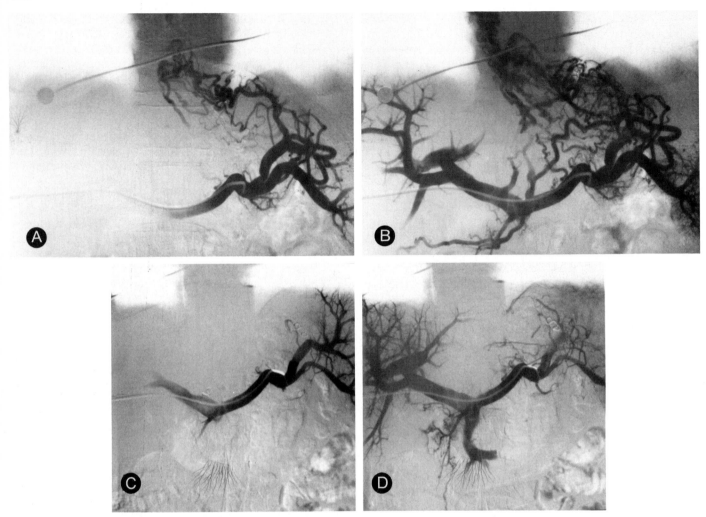

Fig. 5–3 A 53-year-old alcoholic man with cirrhosis and bleeding esophageal varices. Early (A) and late (B) phases of percutaneous transhepatic portal venogram reveal large esophageal varices. Note: one does not ordinarily identify a bleeding site on these studies. After subselective catheterization of the coronary and short gastric veins and obliterative therapy with absolute ethanol and Gianturco coils, early (C) and late (D) phases of transhepatic portal venogram show no evidence of varices.

all the way into the splenic vein because of ascites or resistance in the liver, the authors frequently use an exchange wire and a straight Teflon catheter with a tapered tip. The latter can usually be advanced into the portal vein and will follow a guidewire into the splenic vein. This catheter dilates the liver parenchyma and thereby facilitates subsequent selective catheterization. On occasion, use of a sheath is desirable or necessary to bridge the distance between the parietal peritoneum and the portal vein. This space contains a variable amount of ascites and, typically, rather firm liver substance, with much resistance. Once the sheath enters the portal vein, all subsequent selective catheter manipulations are relatively easy. Care should be taken in selecting a sheath with sufficient length to enter the portal vein. However, if the sheath is too short but a guidewire remains in place throughout all exchanges, access to the portal system will not be lost, and a catheter can be re-introduced.

6. After the portal venous pressure has been measured, a portal venogram should be performed. The authors most frequently inject contrast medium at 12 ml/sec for a total volume of 36 ml of a 76% mixture of meglumine diatrizoate and sodium diatrizoate or iohexol (350 mg iodine/ml) and use an angiographic film sequence of two films/sec for 3 sec, one film/sec for 3 sec, and one film every 2 sec for 6 sec. Once the portal venous anatomy is understood, the proper embolization procedure can be planned.

7. Selective coronary venography should be performed to identify the varices, intercommunications with other variceal tributaries, portopulmonary venous anastomoses (one must film over the lung fields for this, preferably with cineportography), and portosystemic shunts.

8. After balloon occlusion, 10–12 ml of absolute ethanol are injected into the coronary vein at a rate of approximately 2 ml/sec. After a 10-min waiting period, a repeat venogram is performed to search for continued flow into the varices. If there is flow, the procedure is repeated. If balloon occlusion is not possible, the angiographer may consider using particu-

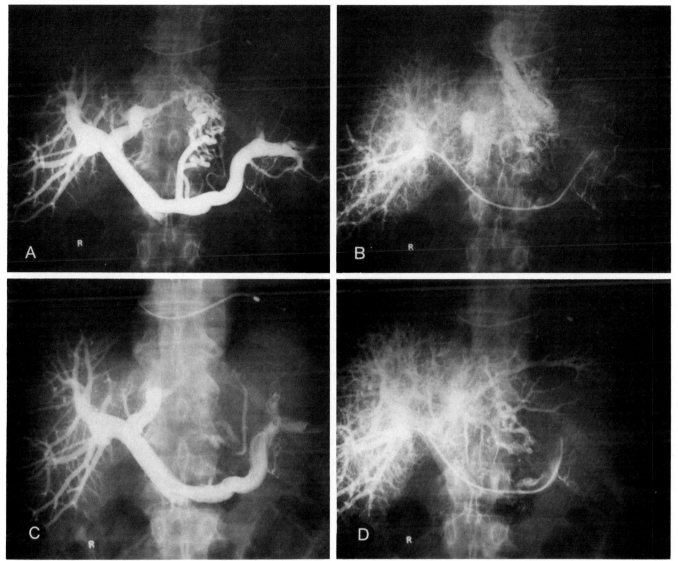

Fig. 5–4 A 68-year-old man with alcoholic cirrhosis and bleeding esophageal varices. Mid (A) and late (B) phases of transhepatic portal venogram reveal esophageal varices. After subselective catheterization of all identifiable tributaries and obliterative therapy with absolute ethanol, mid (C) and late (D) phases of repeat portal venogram show no evidence of esophageal varices. Several small varices not in direct communication with portal or splenic vein are seen in D.

late emboli to retard blood flow prior to ethanol administration. Gelfoam or sodium tetradecyl sulfate-soaked Gelfoam pledgets may be used for this purpose.

9. After coronary vein occlusion, a repeat portal venogram should be performed to document the occlusion and to search for other pathways to the varices that become visible after the initial procedure. If no accessible pathways are found, the procedure is complete. The portal venous pressure is measured again; it is usually higher than before the embolization.

10. As the catheter is removed from the liver, Gelfoam pledgets are placed in the catheter tract. The catheter is removed when blood return is minimal or absent.

11. Potential complications include infection, pleural effusion, pneumothorax, arteriovenous fistula, renal failure, hemorrhage, subcapsular hematoma, and portal vein–splenic vein thrombosis with or without recurrent hemorrhage. The latter may occur at higher frequency with ethanol thromboembolotherapy, but it is likely that this problem can be minimized by using balloon-occlusion catheters. To minimize the risk of infection, caps, gowns, masks, and gloves are used for these procedures.

Figures 5–3 and 5–4 are examples of patients with cirrhosis and esophageal varices managed by transcatheter ethanol thromboembolotherapy.

Each of the remaining interventional applications of absolute ethanol is either entirely experimental or has been used only on a limited basis clinically.

HEPATIC ARTERIAL EMBOLIZATION

Hepatic arterial embolization has been used extensively for palliation in patients with liver neoplasms.[66–70] Interest in this method has evolved because of evidence that hepatic neoplasms are supplied principally by the hepatic arterial circulation rather than by the portal venous circulation.[71–72] In the hope of deriving the same advantages of absolute ethanol over the particulate embolic agents and steel coils described earlier in this chapter, investigators have begun to study the potential application of this agent in hepatic neoplasms.

Animal Studies

Stridbeck et al reported on segmental hepatic arterial ethanol administration in pigs.[7] Using 4–5 ml of ethanol manually injected at approximately 0.5 ml/sec, they produced angiographically demonstrable acute segmental hepatic arterial occlusion in all of their eight animals. Liver enzyme concentrations rose transiently to moderately high levels. Follow-up angiography at various times up to 3 months after embolization disclosed occlusions in all animals and common hepatic-artery occlusions in half. All animals had reconstitution of intrahepatic arterial branches by way of intrahepatic collaterals; some also had prominent extrahepatic collaterals. They were killed at various times after embolization, and the gross evidence of liver infarction was seen to be inversely related to the length of the observation (survival) period. Only four animals underwent microscopic examination. In the earliest specimen (4 days after embolization), there was midzonal necrosis similar to that seen with hepatotoxic agents, inflammation, edema, and bile duct proliferation. Necrosis was found in the walls of hepatic artery branches, which were also occluded by fresh thrombi. In longer survivors, the areas of necrosis were less extensive and were demarcated by granulation tissue. The thrombi were more organized, and there was more bile duct proliferation. For unknown reasons, no macroscopic or microscopic abnormalities were found in the animal killed 3 months after embolization. The authors concluded that ethanol produces effective and permanent occlusion of injected vessels in the liver, but that the occluding effect is counteracted by the development of collaterals.

O'Riordan et al studied proper hepatic arterial administration of ethanol in dogs in doses ranging from 0.3 ml/kg to 1.0 ml/kg (4.5–20 ml total).[9] Doses were given through a standard angiographic catheter over a 20-sec period. All animals had significant pain requiring analgesia within 24 hr. One animal died of pancreatitis, presumably secondary to reflux of ethanol into the pancreaticoduodenal arterial supply during the procedure. Although this study also showed effective occlusion of target hepatic vessels, collaterals did develop. Only one animal had recanalization of a major vessel. Dogs experienced leukocytosis, serum enzyme elevation (alanine aminotransferase and alkaline phosphatase), and hyperbilirubinemia (which occurred in only two dogs). At microscopic examination, vessel intimas were split, thrombi were present, hemorrhage and coagulative necrosis were found in the involved parenchyma, and inflammatory infiltrate with polymorphonuclear leukocytes was identifiable throughout the liver. In animals killed at 4 weeks, the pathologic changes had regressed, but there was marked perisinusoidal fibrosis. The authors emphasized that arteriograms taken 15 min after embolization with absolute ethanol do not indicate the true extent of infarction, since the changes tend to progress over at least 1 week, as demonstrated by angiography, leukocyte count, liver enzyme alterations, and histopathologic analysis.

In a study of six adult rhesus monkeys, Doppman and Girton tested the hypothesis that absolute ethanol is an ideal transarterial embolic agent for liver lesions because portal venous flow should protect normal hepatocytes by dilution.[8] Although they found that injury to hepatocytes was minimal, they also discovered that absolute ethanol perfuses the peribiliary plexus (the plexus of vessels surrounding the bile ducts in the portal tracts[73,74]) and produces scarring of the bile ducts, resulting in a cholangiographic pattern similar to that of sclerosing cholangitis. The authors recommend that continued careful investigation into the role and effects of ethanol in hepatic embolization be undertaken before clinical trials of this treatment are contemplated.

Ekelund et al examined the blood supply of experimental liver tumors in rats after intra-arterial embolization with Gelfoam powder in some animals and ethanol in others.[10] They studied the remaining vascular supply in these experimental and in other control animals by postmortem Microfil perfusion. Filling of tumor lakes from the portal venous supply was seen in only 20% of control animals but in 50% of the animals embolized with Gelfoam and in 85% of those embolized with ethanol. The authors explain that histologic studies have shown tumor lakes to be abnormally dilated blood vessels. Their study with Microfil showed that tumor lakes can be filled from either arterial or portal venous routes. They further remind us that there are numerous routes of arterioportal communication within the liver,[75,76] including direct arterioportal connections in the sinusoids, as well as the vasa vasorum of the portal vein and the peribiliary arterial plexus, all of which may provide supply in the event of arterial occlusion. Other investigators have not overlooked the potential importance of the portal-venous supply to the tumor.[77–79] Ekelund et al postulate that transcatheter arterial occlusion combined with intraportally administered chemotherapeutic agents may prove more effective in the treatment of hepatic neoplasms than an entirely arterial approach. Of importance with respect to studies involving transarterial ethanol hepatic embolization is the fact that one can expect to witness increased portal venous supply to regions treated with arterial occlusion therapy.

Human Experience

Of 325 patients who underwent transarterial therapy for hepatic neoplasms, Wallace and his colleagues treated 20 with 1–5 ml of absolute ethanol alone or in combination with Ivalon (5 ml of absolute ethanol with 100 mg of

Ivalon, 150-μm particles).[80,81] Injections were not made in wedged positions, nor was balloon occlusion used. Their longest follow-up has been 2 years without evidence of biliary obstruction, but the biliary tract has not been imaged for evidence of sclerosing cholangitis.[82] These investigators have been able to demonstrate the development of arterial collaterals on follow-up angiography that have been significant enough to necessitate sequential hepatic artery embolizations. Wallace and colleagues have summarized both their assessment of current animal data and their own clinical experience by stating that the optimal indications for the use of ethanol in hepatic artery embolization have yet to be established.

TRANSCATHETER SPLENIC EMBOLIZATION

Animal Studies

Mineau et al reported a study of artery embolization with absolute ethanol in swine and dogs.[6] Importantly, three of the five pigs treated in this study developed gastric perforation without evidence of peritonitis. The work of Spigos and his colleagues outlines the need for controlled segmental splenic infarction, and Mineau et al were mindful of this in their animal work. There were 11 successful splenic infarctions in 14 attempts, and two of those successes involved flow-directed balloon catheters to guide segmental infarction. Although these results are promising, the gastric perforations are of great concern, and the technique must still be viewed as experimental.

Human Experience

Many of the indications, techniques, and complications of splenic artery occlusion in place of surgical splenec-tomy have been described.[83–86] The many indications include thrombocytopenia, other signs of hypersplenism, and hemorrhage due to trauma. Spigos et al described partial splenic embolization for hypersplenism as a means of treating the patient while preserving splenic function.[87] All human series have involved particulate embolic material, stainless-steel coils, or both. Risks and complications include pain, fever, leukocytosis, abscess formation (low incidence), left pleural effusion (in approximately half the patients), transient hyperkalemia, transient hyperamylasemia, and splenic rupture. Another potential complication is overt pancreatitis or pancreatic infarction. Because these techniques are complex, often requiring a staged approach for completion, the reader is advised to consult the references before attempting treatment in any given case. To the authors' knowledge, ethanol has not been used clinically to produce a transcatheter splenectomy.

ADRENAL ABLATION

Doppman and Girton investigated unilateral adrenal ablation in rhesus monkeys by direct injection of absolute ethanol into the adrenal veins as a means to ablate functioning neoplasms and hyperplasia.[5] The investigators found that the injections resulted in severe hypertensive crises due to torrential catecholamine release. Postmortem histologic studies showed residual viable glandular tissue. Because of this residual viable tissue and the severe hypertensive episodes, the authors concluded that the technique was both dangerous and ineffective. Some of the animals premedicated with sympathetic blocking agents exhibited less severe or absent hypertensive responses. It should be noted that although the investigators wedged the catheters into the veins before injection, balloon occlusion was not used. Balloon occlusion might have helped induce more effective organ ablation. Recently, Fink et al reported that transcatheter injec-tion of 0.4 ml of ethanol into the adrenal artery in each of three rhesus monkeys resulted in a mean increase of 60 mm Hg in systolic pressure and 50 mm Hg in diastolic pressure within 2 min after injection.[88] The injections also caused cardiac arrhythmias, and the authors postulated that all of the ill effects were due to catecholamine release upon embolization. In the same study, inferior phrenic artery embolization with Gelfoam powder produced only mild (6 mm Hg systolic, 10 mm Hg diastolic) increases in blood pressure in an additional three monkeys. The authors are aware of no studies involving ethanol adrenal ablation in humans. Although these methods may eventually prove useful, the current experimental evidence is not promising. Injection of absolute ethanol into any vessel for adrenal ablation must be regarded as dangerous.

BRONCHIAL ARTERY EMBOLIZATION

Naar et al used absolute ethanol embolization of a bronchial artery to control severe hemoptysis in a patient with a small bronchial artery orifice and a catheter too tenuously positioned at the orifice to allow particulate embolization.[87] Other authors have reported embolization for hemoptysis using other agents.[90,91] Absolute ethanol is considered to be vaso-occlusive at the level of minute vessels, as is isobutyl-2-cyanoacrylate. One month after the report of Naar et al, Grenier et al reported using the latter agent to embolize the bronchial arteries in 14 patients.[92] Bookstein criticized the use of capillary occlusive agents for bronchial artery embolization, citing the theoretically greater tendency of such agents to produce injury to bronchial, mediastinal, and spinal structures.[93] Subsequently, Ivanick et al reported infarction of the left mainstem bronchus as a complication of bronchial artery embolization with ethanol.[94] The present authors agree with Bookstein and therefore strongly discourage the use of ethanol for bronchial artery embolization.

ARTERIAL EMBOLIZATION FOR GASTROINTESTINAL BLEEDING

In keeping with the above-mentioned complications and risks, as well as concern about the capillary occlusive potential of ethanol, the authors strongly discourage its use for bleeding Mallory–Weiss tears, gastric or duodenal ulcers, or bleeding small bowel or colon lesions. They are not aware of any reports of these uses of ethanol in humans.

CONTROL OF BLOOD LOSS FROM NONVISCERAL SOURCES

McLean et al reported successful use of ethanol to manage bleeding from an internal mammary artery.[95] The hemorrhage was from a chest wall ulcer due to carcinoma of the breast. The authors emphasized that the internal mammary artery was functioning as an end vessel in this instance, and that no clinically apparent necrosis followed embolization. It is important to note that because of the potential for necrosis in the distribution of the feeding vessel, applications of the type described by McLean and his colleagues are limited.

TREATMENT OF ARTERIOVENOUS MALFORMATIONS AND VASCULAR TUMORS OF THE EXTREMITIES

Arteriovenous malformations are difficult to manage, and surgical ligation of feeding arteries is fraught with the long-term problems of reconstitution of the lesion by smaller vessels, which are more difficult to manage. Because of these problems, good transcatheter embolization techniques using particulate materials have evolved, as discussed in Chapter 3.[96–98] Use of transcatheter absolute ethanol in the treatment of these lesions is contraindicated in certain instances. As has been stated above, the potential for complete capillary obliteration and tissue necrosis with absolute ethanol is significant. In one patient whose only other option was hemipelvectomy, the technique was used to embolize a vascular sarcoma of the pelvis. Inadvertent total occlusion of the superior gluteal artery, probably at the capillary level, resulted in marked tissue necrosis, with external breakdown together with necrosis of the sciatic nerve. Another lesion that might cause similar problems is a vascular renal cell carcinoma metastasis to an extremity; in one such case, a patient sloughed a small patch of skin from the lower leg after ethanol embolotherapy for a metastasis in the proximal tibia.[99]

Some investigators feel that superselective catheter position allows embolization of renal cell carcinoma osseous metastases with absolute ethanol or other capillary occlusive agents. Indeed, at the authors' institution this procedure has repeatedly been performed successfully and safely in lesions involving the vertebrae. However, they have recently witnessed a case of postembolization sympathectomy in a woman whose distal femur renal cell carcinoma metastasis was superselectively embolized with ethanol. Fortunately, this complication resolved within 3 weeks.

Although some lesions of this type may be amenable to transcatheter vaso-occlusion with absolute ethanol, the angiographer must be careful not to occlude end vessels supplying the capillary beds of muscle, skin, and other nontarget tissues. There are other agents available that cause sufficient small vessel occlusion to devascularize such lesions without inducing complete tissue necrosis in nontarget areas.

INTERVENTIONAL THERAPY OF NEUROVASCULAR LESIONS

Transcatheter ablation of neurovascular lesions with absolute ethanol in humans must be viewed as entirely experimental. Pevsner et al recently reported their experience with selective alcohol injection into the middle cerebral artery in six rhesus monkeys using a flexible version of the Pevsner Mini-Balloon catheter coaxially positioned through a 5F catheter.[4] Thrombus was identified in a short segment of vessel beyond the catheter tip but not in the more distal branches. Although the initial results appear promising, the technique is not ready for human application.

NONANGIOGRAPHIC USES OF ETHANOL IN INTERVENTIONAL RADIOLOGY

Ablation of Renal Cysts

Bean reported transcatheter ablation at the time of ultrasound-guided diagnostic aspiration of 34 benign renal cysts in 29 patients.[100] Knowing that most renal cysts are benign and that only a few cause hypertension or pyelocaliectasis, he still argued in favor of this form of therapy. Bean ablates the cysts with ethanol at the time of diagnostic aspiration, because, in his experience, the incidence of complications from treatment is no higher than that of diagnositic aspiration alone. Hence, he stated, one can treat the cysts in order to prevent complications. Bean recommends placement of a small pigtail catheter in the cyst before ethanol injection to prevent extracystic injections of ethanol, which can occur if the injection is made through a sharp needle. Bean also emphasized the need for injection of contrast medium into the cyst before the therapeutic procedure in order to ensure intracystic location. Confusion can arise otherwise, since there is a morphologic similarity between benign cysts and diverticula. After the injection, ethanol inactivates the secreting cells rapidly (within 3 min). Ethanol is withdrawn through the pigtail catheter, which is removed. No leakage of ethanol occurred in Bean's series, and only about one-eighth of the volume of the cyst had to be injected to inactivate epithelial cells. Only one cyst recurred.

Parathyroid Tumor Ablation

Solbiati et al recently reported 12 uremic patients with secondary hyperparathyroidism, in whom 13 parathyroid tumors were detected by sonography and confirmed by fine needle aspiration biopsy.[101] These patients were treated by percutaneous injection of absolute ethanol into the tumors under ultrasound guidance for a variety of indications, including recurrence after previous subtotal resection, high surgical risk, and refusal of operation. In the large glands, volume decreased after ablative therapy; in most cases of single hyperplastic glands, therapeutic clinical and biochemical effects were obtained. Maximum volume reductions were noted by sonography at 6 months following treatment.

Three treatments were unsuccessful. In two of these the injected alcohol diffused anterior to the gland, and in one the lesion had partially calcified walls, which prevented adequate intraglandular injection. Complications included 24 hr of dysphonia in one patient after fine needle aspiration biopsy and a small hematoma in one gland after injection with ethanol. The latter sometimes occurs with needle biopsy alone. After considering the structural, clinical, and biochemical results of their series, Solbiati et al concluded that percutaneous ethanol ablation of enlarged parathyroid glands can be used in certain cases of secondary hyperparathyroidism and that it can improve responsiveness to medical therapy and delay the need for operation.

SUMMARY

Transcatheter absolute ethanol embolization is indicated in many instances of primary renal tumor, in some instances of complicated end-stage renal disease, in the management of gastroesophageal varices, and in a few other instances. In most cases of arteriovenous malformation and vascular metastasis to an extremity, ethanol-mediated ablation is contraindicated. In these instances, extensive capillary damage can result in widespread myonecrosis and necrosis of other nontarget tissues. The techniques are exciting but fraught with real and potential complications. The interventional radiologist should be familiar with all aspects of absolute ethanol embolization prior to attempting it in any case.

References

1. Ellman BA, Green EC, Elgenbrodt E, Garriott JC, Curry TS: Renal infarction with absolute ethanol. *Invest Radiol* 1980;15:318–322
2. Ekelund J, Jonsson N, Treugut H: Transcatheter obliteration of the renal artery by ethanol injection: experimental results. *CardioVasc Intervent Radiol* 1981;4:1–7
3. Buchta K, Sands J, Rosenkrantz J, Roch WD: Early mechanism of action of arterially infused alcohol U.S.P. in renal devitalization. *Radiology* 1982;145:45–48
4. Pevsner PH, Klara P, Doppman J, George E, Girton M: Ethyl alcohol: experimental agent for interventional therapy of neurovascular lesions. *AJNR* 1983;4:388–390
5. Doppman JL, Girton M: Adrenal ablation by retrograde venous ethanol injection: an ineffective and dangerous procedure. *Radiology* 1984;150:667–678
6. Mineau DE, Miller FJ Jr, Lee RG, Nakashima EN, Nelson JA: Experimental transcatheter splenectomy using absolute ethanol. *Radiology* 1982;142:355–359
7. Stridbeck H, Ekelund L, Jonsson N: Segmental hepatic arterial occlusion with absolute ethanol in domestic swine. *Acta Radiol* [*Diagn*] 1984;25:331–335
8. Doppman JL, Girton ME: Bile duct scarring following ethanol embolization of the hepatic artery: an experimental study in monkeys. *Radiology* 1984;152:621–626
9. O'Riordan D, McAllister H, Sheahan BJ, MacErlean DP: Hepatic infarction with absolute ethanol. *Radiology* 1984;152:627–630
10. Ekelund L, Lin G, Jeppsson B: Blood supply of experimental liver tumors after intraarterial embolization with Gelfoam powder and absolute ethanol. *CardioVasc Intervent Radiol* 1984;7:234–239
11. Ellman BA, Parkhill BJ, Marcus PB, Curry TS, Peters PC: Renal ablation with absolute ethanol: mechanism of action. *Invest Radiol* 1984;19:416–423
12. Harley JD, Killien FC, Peck AG: Massive hemoptysis controlled by transcatheter embolization of the bronchial arteries. *AJR* 1977;128:302–304
13. Gianturco G, Anderson JH, Wallace S: Mechanical device for arterial occlusion. *AJR* 1975;124:428–435
14. Reuter SR, Chuang VP, Bree RL: Selective arterial embolization for control of massive upper gastrointestinal bleeding. *AJR* 1975;125:119–126
15. Gomes AS, Rysavy JA, Spadaccini CA, Probst P, D'Souza V, Amplatz K: The use of the bristle brush for transcatheter embolization. *Radiology* 1978;129:345–350
16. Tadavarthy SM, Moller JHJ, Amplatz K: Polyvinyl alcohol (Ivalon)—a new embolic material. *AJR* 1975;125:609–616
17. White RI, Kaufman SL, Barth KH, Kadir S, Smyth JW, Walsh PC: Occlusion of varicoceles with detachable balloons. *Radiology* 1981;139:335–340
18. Lalli AF, Peterson N, Bookstein JJ: Roentgen-guided infarctions of kidneys and lungs: a potential therapeutic technic. *Radiology* 1969;93:434–435
19. Lang EK: Superselective arterial catheterization as a vehicle for delivering radioactive infarct particles to tumors. *Radiology* 1971;98:391–399
20. Almgard LE, Fernström I, Haverling M, et al: Treatment of renal adenocarcinoma by embolic occlusion of the renal circulation. *Br J Urol* 1973;45:474–479
21. Lang EK, Sullivan J, de Kernion JB: Work in progress: trans-

catheter embolization of renal cell carcinoma with radioactive infarct particles. *Radiology* 1983;147:413–418

22. Wallace S, Chuang VP, Swanson D, et al: Embolization of renal carcinoma: experience with 100 patients. *Radiology* 1981;138:563–570

23. Woodside J, Schwarz H, Gergreen P: Peripheral embolization complicating bilateral renal infarction with Gelfoam. *AJR* 1976;126:1033

24. Chuang VP: Nonoperative retrieval of Gianturco coils from the abdominal aorta. *AJR* 1979;132:996–999

25. Mukamel E, Hadar H, Nissenkorn I, Servadio C: Widespread dissemination of Gelfoam particles following occlusion of renal circulation. *Urology* 1979;14:194

26. Mazer MJ, Baltaxe HA, Wolf GL: Therapeutic embolization of the renal artery with Gianturco coils: limitations and technical pitfalls. *Radiology* 1981;138:37–46

27. Kuntslinger F, Brunelle F, Chaumont P, Doyon D: Vascular occlusive agents. *AJR* 1975;136:151–156

28. Greenfield AJ, Athanasoulis CA, Waltman AC, LeMoure ER: Transcatheter embolization: prevention of embolic reflux using balloon catheters. *AJR* 1978;138:651

29. Rosenkrantz H, Sands JP, Buchta KS, Healy JF, Kmet JP, Gerber F: Renal devitalization using 95 per cent ethyl alcohol. *J Urol* 1982;127:873–875

30. Bernardino ME, Chuang VP, Wallace S, Thomas JL, Soo CS: Therapeutically infarcted tumors: CT findings. *AJR* 1981;136:527–532

31. Carroll BA, Walter JF: Gas in embolized tumors: an alternative hypothesis for its origin. *Radiology* 1983;147:441–444

32. Ellman BA, Parkhill BJ, Curry TS III, Marcus PB, Peters PC: Ablation of renal tumors with absolute ethanol: a new technique. *Radiology* 1981;141:619–626

33. Rabe FE, Yune HY, Richmond BD, Klatte EC: Renal tumor infarction with absolute ethanol. *AJR* 1982;139:1139–1144

34. Cox GG, Lee KR, Price HI, Gunter K, Noble MJ, Mebust WK: Colonic infarction following ethanol embolization of renal cell carcinoma. *Radiology* 1982;145:343–345

35. Eklund L, Ek A, Forsberg L, et al: Occlusion of renal arterial tumor supply with absolute ethanol: experience with 20 cases. *Acta Radiol [Diagn]* 1984;25:195–201

36. Klimberg I, Hunter P, Hawkins IF, Drylie DM, Wajsman Z: Preoperative angioinfarction of localized renal cell carcinoma using absolute ethanol. *J Urol* 1985;133:21–24

37. MacErlean DP, Owens AP, Bryan PJ: Hypernephroma embolization: is it worthwhile? *Clin Radiol* 1980;31:297

38. Teasdale C, Kirk D, Jeans WD, Penry JB, Tribe CT, Slade N: Arterial embolization in renal carcinoma: a useful procedure? *Br J Urol* 1982;54:616–621

39. Mebust WK, Weigel JW, Lee KR, Cox GG, Jewell WR, Krishnan EC: Renal cell carcinoma—angioinfarction. *J Urol* 1984;131:231–234

40. Earthman WJ, Mazer MJ, Winfield AC: Angiomyolipomas in tuberous sclerosis: subselective embolotherapy with alcohol, with long-term follow-up study. *Radiology* 1986;160:437–441

41. Becker GJ, Holden RW, Klatte EC: Absolute ethanol in interventional radiology. *Rev Interam Radiol* 1984;9:31–39

42. Becker GJ, Holden RW, Klatte EC: Therapeutic embolization with absolute ethanol. *Semin Intervent Radiol* 1984;1:118–129

43. Nanni GS, Hawkins IF Jr, Orak JK: Control of hypertension by ethanol renal ablation. *Radiology* 1983;148:51–54

44. Vertes V, Cangiano JL, Berman LB, Gould A: Hypertension in end stage renal disease. *N Engl J Med* 1968;280:978–981

45. Denny DF, Perlmutt LM, Bettmann MA: Percutaneous recanalization of an occluded renal artery and delayed ethanol ablation of the kidney resulting in control of hypertension. *Radiology* 1984;151:381–382

46. Keller FS, Coyle M, Rosch J, Dotter CT: Percutaneous renal ablation in patients with end stage renal disease: alternative to surgical nephrectomy. *Radiology* 1986;159:447–451

47. Lunderquist A, Vang J: Transhepatic catheterization and obliteration of the coronary vein in patients with portal hypertension and esophageal varices. *N Engl J Med* 1974;291:646–649

48. Scott J, Dick R, Long RG, Sherlock S: Percutaneous transhepatic obliteration of gastroesophageal varices. *Lancet* 1976;2:53–55

49. Pereiras R, Viamonte M Jr, Russell E, LePage J, White P, Hutson D: New techniques for interruption of gastroesophageal venous bloodflow. *Radiology* 1977;124:313–323

50. Viamonte M Jr, Pereiras R, Russell E, LePage J, Hutson D: Transhepatic obliteration of gastroesophageal varices: results in acute and nonacute bleeders. *AJR* 1977;129:237–241

51. Widrich WC, Robbins AH, Nabseth DC, Johnson WC, Goldstein SA: Pitfalls of transhepatic portal venography and therapeutic coronary vein occlusion. *AJR* 1978;131:637–643

52. Pereiras R, Schiff E, Barkin J, Hutson D: The role of interventional radiology in disease of the hepatobiliary system and the pancreas. *Radiol Clin North Am* 1979;17:555–605

53. Yune HY, Klatte EC, Richmond BD, Rabe FE: Absolute ethanol in thrombotherapy of bleeding esophageal varices. *AJR* 1982;138:1137–1141

54. Yune HY, O'Conner KW, Klatte EC, Olson EW, Becker GJ, Strickler SA: Ethanol thrombotherapy of esophageal varices: further experience. *AJR* 1985;144:1049–1053

55. Child CG III: *Hepatic Circulation and Portal Hypertension.* Philadelphia, WB Saunders, 1954

56. Keller FS, Rosch J, Dotter CT: Transhepatic obliteration of gastroesophageal varices with absolute ethanol. *Radiology* 1983;146:615–619

57. Uflacker R: Percutaneous transhepatic obliteration of gastroesophageal varices using absolute alcohol. *Radiology* 1983;146:621–625

58. Sano A, Kuroda Y: Cine-portographic characteristics of portopulmonary venous anastomosis in portal hypertension. Presented at the 83rd Annual Meeting of the American Roentgen Ray Society, Atlanta, GA, 1983

59. Widrich WC, Srinivasan M, Semine MC, Robbins AH: Collateral pathways of the left gastric vein in portal hypertension. *AJR* 1984;142:375–382

60. Galambos JT, Warren WD: Surgery for portal hypertension. *Clin Gastroenterol* 1979;8:525–541

61. Adson MA, van Heerden JA, Ilstrup DM: The distal splenorenal shunt. *Arch Surg* 1984;119:609–614

62. Langer B, Rotstein LE, Stone RM, et al: A prospective randomized trial of the selective distal splenorenal shunt. *Surg Gynecol Obstet* 1980;150:45–48

63. Allison JG: The role of injection sclerotherapy in the emergency and definitive management of bleeding esophageal varices. *JAMA* 1983;249:1484–1487

64. Merritt CRB: Ultrasonographic demonstration of portal vein thrombosis. *Radiology* 1979;133:425–427

65. Kauzlaric D, Petrovic M, Barmeir E: Sonography of cavernous transformation of the portal vein. *AJR* 1984;142:383–384

66. Clouse ME, Lee R, Duszlak E, et al: Peripheral hepatic artery embolization for primary and secondary hepatic neoplasms. *Radiology* 1983;147:407–413

67. Lunderquist A, Ericsson M, Nobin A, Sanden G: Gelfoam powder embolization of the hepatic artery in liver metastases of carcinoid tumors. *Radiologe* 1982;22:65–73

68. Nakamura H, Tanaka T, Hori S, et al: Transcatheter embolization of hepatocellular carcinoma: assessment of efficacy in cases of resection following embolization. *Radiology* 1983;147:401–409

69. Wallace S, Chuang VP: The radiologic diagnosis and management of hepatic metastases. *Radiologe* 1982;22:56–66

70. Soo C–S, Chuang VP, Wallace S, Charnsangavej C, Carradsco H: Treatment of hepatic neoplasm through extrahepatic collaterals. *Radiology* 1983;147:45–48

71. Breedis C, Young G: The blood supply of neoplasms in the liver. *Am J Pathol* 1954;30:969–981

72. Lien WM, Ackerman NB: The blood supply of experimental liver metastases: a microcirculatory study of the normal and tumor vessels of the liver with the use of perfused silicone rubber. *Surgery* 1970;68:334–337

73. Grisham JW, Nopanitaya W: Scanning electron microscopy of casts of hepatic microvessels: review of methods and results, in Lautt WW (ed): *Hepatic Circulation in Health and Disease.* New York, Raven Press, 1981, pp 87–95

74. Ohtani O: The peribiliary portal system in the rabbit liver. *Arch Histol Jpn* 1979;42:153–159

75. Cho KJ, Lunderquist A: Experimental hepatic artery embolization with Gelfoam powder. *Invest Radiol* 1983;18:189–193

76. Bookstein JJ, Cho KJ, Davis GB, Dail D: Arterioportal communications: observations and hypotheses concerning transsinusoidal and transvasal types. *Radiology* 1982;142:581–590

77. Honjo I, Matsumura H: Vascular distribution of hepatic tumors: experimental study. *Rev Int Hepatol* 1965;15:681–690

78. Honjo I, Suzuki T, Ozawa K, Takasan H, Kitamura O, Ishikawa T: Ligation of a branch of the portal vein for carcinoma of the liver. *Am J Surg* 1975;130:296–302

79. Nilsson LAV, Zettergren L: Effect of hepatic artery ligation on induced primary liver carcinoma in rats: preliminary report. *Acta Pathol Microbiol Scand* 1967;71:187–193

80. Chuang VP, Wallace S, Soo C–S, Charnsangavej C, Bowers T: Therapeutic Ivalon embolization of hepatic tumors. *AJR* 1982;138:289–294

81. Carrasco CH, Chuang VP, Wallace S: Apudomas metastatic to the liver: treatment by hepatic artery embolization. *Radiology* 1983;149:79–83

82. Wallace S, Charnsangavej C, Carrasco CH, Bechtel W: Ethanol for hepatic artery embolization. *Radiology* 1984;152:821–822

83. Castañeda–Zuñiga WR, Hammerschmidt DE, Sanchez R, Amplatz K: Nonsurgical splenectomy. *AJR* 1977;129:805–811

84. Wholey MH, Chamorro HA, Rao G, Chapman W: Splenic infarction and spontaneous rupture of the spleen after therapeutic embolization. *Cardiovasc Radiol* 1978;1:249–253

85. Witte CL, Ovitt TW, Van Wyck DB, Witte MH, O'Mara RE, Woolfenden JM: Ischemic therapy in thrombocytopenia from hypersplenism. *Arch Surg* 1976;111:1115–1121

86. Yoshioka H, Kuroda C, Hori S, et al: Splenic embolization for hypersplenism using steel coils. *AJR* 1985;144:1269–1274

87. Spigos DG, Honasson O, Mozes M, Capek V: Partial splenic embolization in the treatment of hypersplenism. *AJR* 1979;132:777–782

88. Fink IJ, Girton M, Doppman JL: Absolute ethanol injection of the adrenal artery: hypertensive reaction. *Radiology* 1985;154:357–358

89. Naar CA, Soong J, Clore F, Hawkins IF Jr: Control of massive hemoptysis by bronchial artery embolization with absolute ethanol. *AJR* 1983;140:271–272

90. Wholey MH, Chamorro HA, Rao G, Ford WB, Miller WH: Bronchial artery embolization for massive hemoptysis. *JAMA* 1976;236:2501–2504

91. Uflacker R, Kaemmerer A, Neves C, Picon P: Management of massive hemoptysis by bronchial artery embolization. *Radiology* 1983;146:627–634

92. Grenier P, Cornud F, Lacombe P, Via UF, Nahum H: Bronchial artery occlusion for severe hemoptysis: use of isobutyl-2-cyanoacrylate. *AJR* 1983;140:467–471

93. Bookstein J: Editorial comment. *AJR* 1983;140:471

94. Ivanick MJ, Thorwarth W, Donohue J, Mandell V, Delany D, Jaques PF: Infarction of the left main-stem bronchus: a complication of bronchial artery embolization. *AJR* 1983;141:535–537

95. McLean GK, Mackie JA, Hartz WH, Freiman DB: Percutaneous alcohol injection for control of internal mammary artery bleeding. *AJR* 1983;141:181–182

96. Gomes AS, Mali WP, Oppenheim WL: Embolization therapy in the management of congenital arteriovenous malformations. *Radiology* 1982;144:41–49

97. Stanley RJ, Cubillo E: Nonsurgical treatment of arteriovenous malformations of the trunk and limb by transcatheter arterial embolization. *Radiology* 1975;115:609–612

98. Kaufman SL, Kumar AAJ, Roland JA, et al: Transcatheter embolization in the management of congenital arteriovenous malformations. *Radiology* 1980;137:21–29

99. Rowe DM, Becker GJ, Rabe FE, et al: Osseous metastases from renal cell carcinoma: embolization and surgery for restoration of function. *Radiology* 1984;150:673–676

100. Bean WJ: Renal cysts: treatment with alcohol. *Radiology* 1981;138:329–331

101. Solbiati L, Giangrande A, De Pra L, Bellotti E, Cantu P, Ravetto C: Percutaneous ethanol injection of parathyroid tumors under US guidance: treatment for secondary hyperparathyroidism. *Radiology* 1985;155:607–610

6

Embolization of the Internal Spermatic Vein with Mechanical Devices for the Treatment of Varicocele

WILFRIDO R. CASTAÑEDA-ZUÑIGA, M.D., M.Sc., CESAR ERCOLE, M.D., CAROL C. COLEMAN, M.D., GUNNAR LUND, M.D., DAVID W. HUNTER, M.D., TONY P. SMITH, M.D., MICHAEL D. DARCY, M.D., ANDREW H. CRAGG, M.D., FLAVIO CASTAÑEDA, M.D., AND KURT AMPLATZ, M.D.

The term "varicocele" originally designated a visible enlargement of the veins of the pampiniform plexus, nearly always on the left. The relation between the condition and male subfertility was suspected as early as 1929 and was confirmed by the frequent improvement in semen quality after operative correction of this condition.

In the past several years, studies with Doppler ultrasonography, thermography, radionuclide scanning, and venography have shown that classical varicoceles result from absent or inadequate valves in the internal spermatic veins. Such studies also have proved that valvar inadequacy can be present without being clinically apparent, a condition known as subclinical varicocele (reviewed in reference 1). Although subclinical varicocele is most often encountered on the right side in patients with obvious varicocele on the left, it can also be bilateral. Its lack of signs and symptoms does not mean that it can be ignored in the evaluation of the subfertile man, because the size of the varicocele does not correlate with the extent of testicular and epididymal dysfunction associated with it.[2,3]

WHICH VARICOCELES SHOULD BE CORRECTED?

For the purposes of this discussion, two kinds of varicoceles can be distinguished: those large enough to be a nuisance to the patient and those in men complaining of subfertility.

Annoying Varicoceles

If a varicocele is large enough to interfere with the patient's activities, it may be ablated. Although this can be achieved by a traditional Ivanissevitch operation, this approach usually requires general anesthesia and fails in many cases because not all of the contributing vessels are ligated.

It must be mentioned that an evident varicocele appearing for the first time in a middle-aged or older man often indicates tumor invasion of the veins upstream.

Varicocele Associated with Subfertility

The past few years have seen an enormous increase in the sophistication of understanding of male subfertility (reviewed in reference 4). Unfortunately, this development has not been accompanied by an equal increase in the ability to correct the problems that have been identified.

One problem that can be corrected is varicocele. Increasingly, venous embolization is the method of choice, because it can be carried out, together with venography to identify the unusual venous anatomy so common in these patients,[5] as an outpatient procedure using only local anesthesia.[6] In nearly all patients, a significant improvement in sperm count and motility index follows.[6]

SPERMATIC VENOGRAPHY AND EMBOLIZATION

Therapeutic embolization is indicated in men with clinical or subclinical varicoceles who have been infertile for at least 2 years and who have oligoasthenospermia and no other apparent cause of infertility. A coagulation profile should be obtained 1 or 2 days before admission.

For outpatient venography and embolization, the patient is admitted early in the morning, and the radiologist discusses the procedure with the patient. The procedure itself can be performed via the femoral vein, but an approach via the right internal jugular vein generally makes catheterization of the internal spermatic veins easier.[7] Local anesthesia suffices.

Method of Venography

Two approaches to spermatic vein catheterization and embolization have been used in the authors' institution: femoral and jugular. The standard femoral approach is adequate for routine venography, although it is difficult to advance a catheter deep into either the right or the left spermatic vein if embolization is to be attempted. It is, however, adequate for the injection of sclerosing agents. A jugular approach facilitates deep catheterization of both spermatics; thus the authors use this technique whenever embolization is planned.

FEMORAL APPROACH

The femoral vein is punctured using the Seldinger technique, and a gently curved 7F or 8F modified headhunter no. 1 or cobra catheter is advanced over a guidewire into the inferior vena cava. Under fluoroscopic control, the left renal vein is selectively catheterized and its inferior surface probed until the left spermatic vein is engaged; usually the orifice is 2–3 cm from the junction of the renal vein and vena cava. In a high percentage of cases, the spermatic vein has a common origin with lumbar veins that arise from the inferior surface of the renal vein, just to the left of the lumbar vertebral bodies. In a small number of cases, the left spermatic vein arises from intrarenal venous branches or from elsewhere in the vena cava.

Once the orifice of the left spermatic vein has been engaged, a test injection is made to determine the competence of the valves (Fig. 6–1A,B). If they are incompetent, a wire is advanced deep into the spermatic vein, and the catheter is passed over the wire. It is frequently difficult to advance the catheter, since it tends to buckle as it enters the renal vein, pulling the wire out of the spermatic vein. Exchange of the rigid torque control catheter for a soft 5F polyethylene catheter may facilitate this manuever. Both venograms and embolization procedures can be carried out once deep catheterization of the vein has been accomplished. Usually, venography will demonstrate a common collateral channel at the level of the iliac crest communicating with lumbar veins (Fig. 6–2).

The right spermatic vein is difficult to catheterize from the femoral approach. A 7F sidewinder II catheter is used to probe the anterolateral surface of the inferior vena cava, just caudal to the orifice of the right renal vein. When the catheter tip engages the orifice of the right spermatic vein it is pulled down into the vein (Fig. 6–3). The right spermatic vein enters the right renal vein in 10% of cases. In this situation, the sidewinder can be used to probe the inferior surface of the right renal vein.

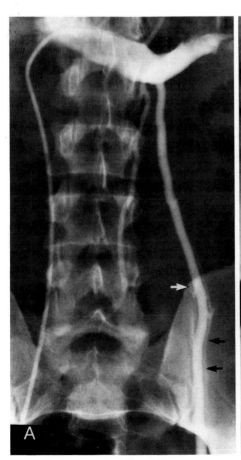
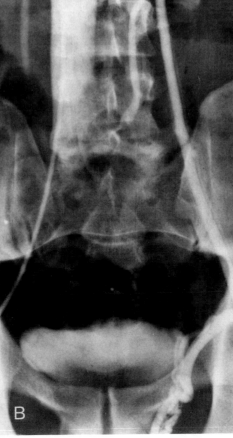

Fig. 6–1 A,B. Left renal venogram; incompetence of venous valves in left spermatic veins with marked reflux of contrast medium to level of the testicle. Small accessory channels are seen alongside large left spermatic vein (arrows).

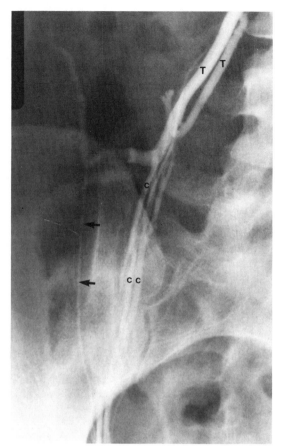

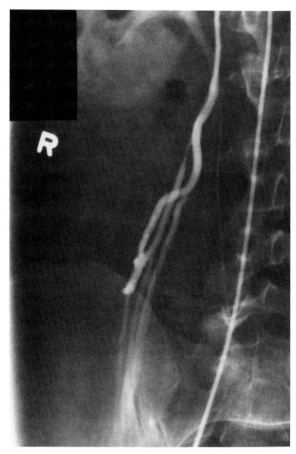

Fig. 6–2 Right spermatic venogram; multiple venous channels within pelvis (c) with two large common trunks (T) in most proximal segment. Collaterals to retroperitoneal veins are present (arrows).

Fig. 6–3 Multiple large communicating veins joining to form a common trunk before entering the inferior vena cava. Large or multiple veins such as these contain enough blood moving fast enough to cool hot contrast medium below temperature needed to damage vessel wall.

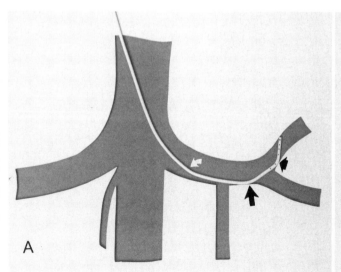

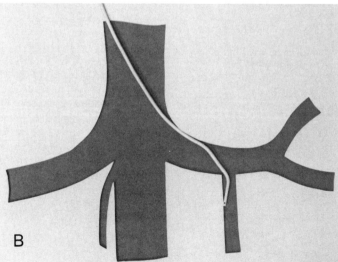

Fig. 6–4 A. Left catheter is shaped so that it will easily enter left renal vein. Primary (arrowhead) and secondary (arrow) curves are unaltered. Tertiary curve (curved arrow) has been reversed. B. When rotated 180° long tertiary curve holds the tip firmly against inferior wall of the vein, entering easily into the spermatic vein. (Reproduced from Hunter DW, Castañeda–Zuñiga WR, Coleman CC, et al: Spermatic vein embolization with hot contrast medium or detachable balloons. *Semin Intervent Radiol* 1984;1(2):163–169.)

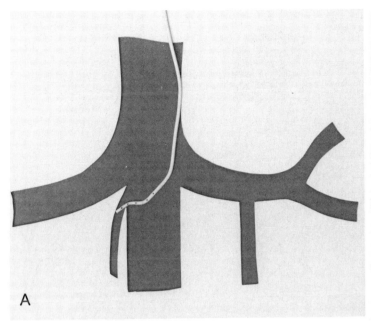

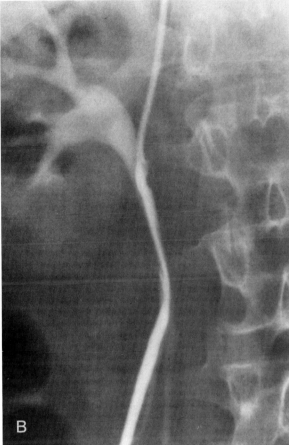

Fig. 6–5 Catheterization of right side. A. Right-sided catheter tip points inferiorly. No other changes are made to convert a left catheter into a right. B. Right spermatic vein most commonly originates from inferior vena cava anterior and inferior to right renal vein at a steep downward angle.

JUGULAR TECHNIQUE

Because deep catheterization of both spermatic veins is difficult using the femoral route, the authors have developed a transjugular approach that greatly facilitates catheterization and embolization.[7] The patient's head is turned 45° to the left, and the carotid artery 5–6 cm above the level of the clavicle is palpated. Local anesthesia is administered just lateral to this point, and a 19-gauge needle is directed to a point approximately 5 cm lateral to the sternoclavicular joint. (A 19-gauge needle is used to minimize trauma during localization of the vein.) Once venous blood has been aspirated, the needle is withdrawn, and a larger needle is inserted in the same direction. Puncture of the vein is aided by having the patient perform a Valsalva maneuver.

Catheterization can usually be accomplished with a modified headhunter catheter for the left spermatic vein (Fig. 6–4A,B) and a modified cobra catheter for the right (Fig. 6–5A,B). Deep catheterization of both veins is easily accomplished by advancing the catheter over a wire once the spermatic vein has been entered.

Venograms are obtained by the manual injection of 20–30 ml of contrast medium. Four to six exposures are generally made in order to demonstrate the proximal and distal segments of the spermatic vein. Alternatively, digital subtraction studies may be obtained. It is particularly

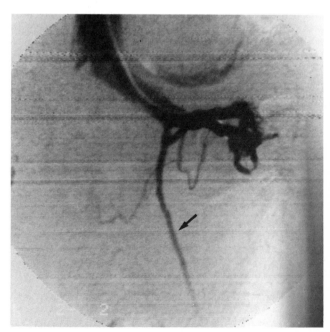

Fig. 6–6 Digital subtraction studies provide excellent detail with minute doses of dilute (20%) contrast medium injected into the left renal vein; reflux into spermatic vein (arrow).

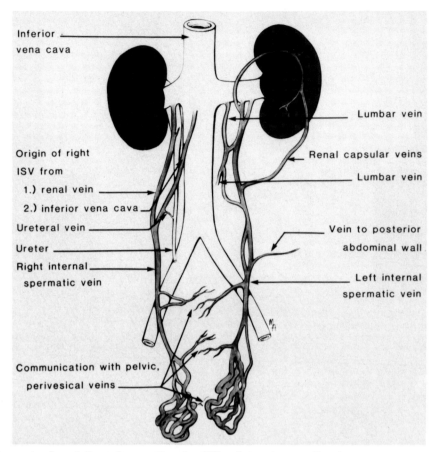

Fig. 6–7   Diagram showing anatomic variations of spermatic veins. ISV = Internal spermatic vein.

important to demonstrate all collaterals present, because occlusion of all of them is needed in order to prevent recurrence. Digital subtraction angiography provides a useful technique to demonstrate the anatomy while using limited amounts of contrast medium (Fig. 6–6).

Anatomic variations in the spermatic system are common (Fig. 6–7). Anastomoses of the internal spermatic veins with other retroperitoneal veins (capsular, periureteral (Fig. 6–8), internal iliac (Fig. 6–9), and femoral (Figs. 6–10 and 6–11)) are frequently seen.[8,9] Such collateral anastomoses make the precise placement of occluding devices imperative.

TREATMENT

Surgery

The traditional treatment of varicocele has been high ligation of the left internal spermatic vein at the level of the internal inguinal ring. Although the technique has recently been performed under local anesthesia,[10] thus increasing its appeal, it still has a failure rate of 5% caused by incomplete ligation of all branches of the spermatic vein.[11]

Nonsurgical Spermatic Vein Occlusion

COILS, SPIDERS, IVALON

Transcatheter embolization of the spermatic veins can be carried out at the time of venography. Stainless-steel coils, compressed Ivalon plugs, and detachable spiders[1,12,13] can be passed through a thin-walled, 9F polyethylene catheter. If coils are used, their diameter should be slightly larger than that of the spermatic vein and their ends should be modified to prevent dislodgment (Fig. 6–12).[14] The introduction of a spider in a proximal portion of the vein reduces the possibility of coil or Ivalon plug embolization (Fig. 6–13). A spider combined with an Ivalon plug (spiderlon) can be used for a one-step embolization (Fig. 6–14). Because duplication and collateralization of the internal spermatic vein system are common (Fig. 6–15), embolic devices are usually placed at the level of the pelvis and also as near as possible to the level of the renal vein (Fig. 6–16).

The advantage of this technique is that precise occlusion of the spermatic vein relative to collateral vessels is

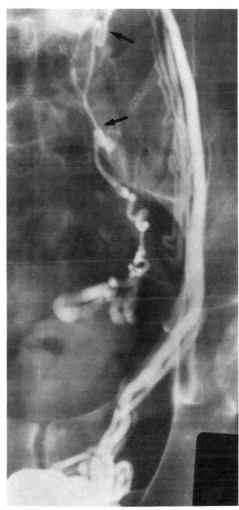

Fig. 6–8   Left spermatic venogram; one large venous channel with multiple accessory channels; note also collaterals to retroperitoneal venous channels (arrows).

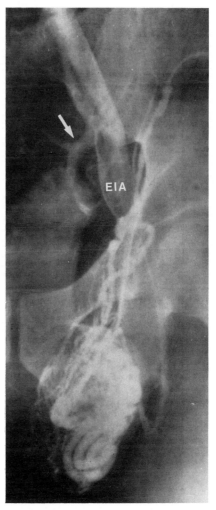

Fig. 6–9   Incompetent left spermatic vein; observe collaterals to hypogastric artery (white arrow). EIA = External iliac artery.

achieved. The disadvantages are those associated with placement of a foreign body and the attendant risk of embolization. It is also often difficult to pass embolic devices when the spermatic vein has been catheterized by the femoral route. For this reason, the authors recommend a jugular approach when embolization with particulate material or mechanical devices is attempted.

TISSUE GLUE

Cyanoacrylate-based tissue glue has been used to occlude the spermatic veins.[15] Isobutyl-2-cyanoacrylate is a rapidly polymerizing agent that hardens immediately on contact with an ionic solution such as blood. The glue is injected through a 3F catheter placed coaxially through a 7F or 8F catheter. The advantage of tissue glue is that an immediate selective vessel occlusion is obtained. In addition, it may be easier to introduce from a femoral route than are other embolic agents. Unfortunately, there are numerous drawbacks associated with the technique.

The catheter system must be flushed with a nonionic solution such as glucose to prevent polymerization of the glue in the catheter. If the agent is flushed too rapidly, it may reflux and embolize the renal vein or lung. Considerable experimental skill should be obtained in the laboratory before this agent is used clinically.

SCLEROTHERAPY

The first transvenous occlusion of the spermatic vein was accomplished by injection of a sclerosing agent directly into the vein.[16] Since that time, numerous reports have been made of the efficacy of this technique.[17–20] The most popular sclerosing agent is Varicosid 5%, the salt of a fatty acid of cod liver oil.[20] Other agents include 80% iothalamate sodium and 3% ethoxysclerol.[18]

Approximately 3 ml of a sclerosing agent is introduced into the distal third of the spermatic vein, left in place for 5–15 min, and then aspirated. The patient is instructed to perform a Valsalva maneuver during injection of the

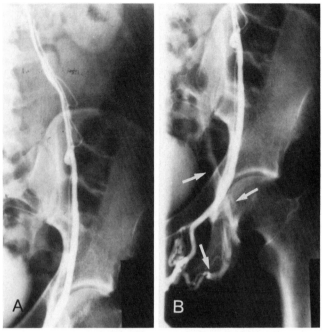

Fig. 6–10 A. Left spermatic venogram; incompetence of venous valves with reflux of contrast medium down to the testicle. B. Collaterals are seen below level of inguinal ligament to common femoral vein (arrows).

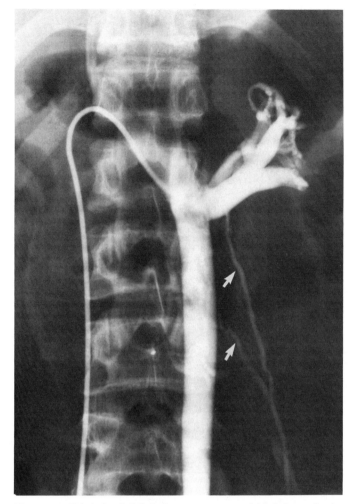

Fig. 6–11 Persistent left inferior vena cava to which left renal vein is connected. Two left spermatic veins are seen, one arising from left renal vein and one from left inferior vena cava (arrows).

sclerosant to facilitate its passage down the spermatic vein. Venography is repeated 15–30 min after the procedure, and, if necessary, sclerosing is repeated.

The advantages of sclerotherapy include ease of delivery and ability to occlude collateral vessels that may be the cause of persistent or recurrent varicocele (Fig. 6–17). Disadvantages include possible reflux of the agent into the renal vein and testicular thrombophlebitis when the sclerosing agent is allowed to fill the pampiniform plexus.[17,18,20]

DETACHABLE BALLOONS

Selective occlusion of the spermatic vein has also been achieved with detachable balloons.[21] Depending on the size of the spermatic vein, 1- or 2-mm Mini-Balloons are passed through an untapered 9F polyethylene catheter placed in the spermatic vein. The balloons are inflated with a 50/50 mixture of contrast medium and sterile water, and a test injection is made through the introducing catheter to determine if the balloons are optimally placed in relation to any collateral vessels. When detached, the balloons are supposed to remain inflated for 30 days or longer.

The advantages of detachable balloons are the same as with other mechanical occluding agents, primarily selective occlusion of the spermatic vein relative to collaterals. An additional advantage not shared by other embolic agents is the ability to determine the optimal balloon position by a test inflation prior to detachment. Disadvantages of detachable balloons include their high cost and the possibility of their embolization to the lung if too small a balloon is selected or if the balloon is placed while the vein is in spasm.[21]

THERMAL VESSEL OCCLUSION

The authors have recently developed a new, as yet experimental, technique, transcatheter thermal vessel occlusion, that may obviate many of the disadvantages of present techniques.[22–24] The injection of 3–6 ml of boiling contrast medium into canine spermatic veins produces complete long-term occlusion without evidence of collateralization or systemic effects. Contrast media are inexpensive and readily available and can be injected through small catheters. A femoral rather than a jugular approach can be used, since deep catheterization of the spermatic vein is not necessary. Hot contrast medium produces thermal sclerosis of both the spermatic vein and its collaterals, which may decrease the rate of varicocele recurrence associated with mechanical occluding devices provided the anatomy is suitable (Fig. 6–13). In addition, hot

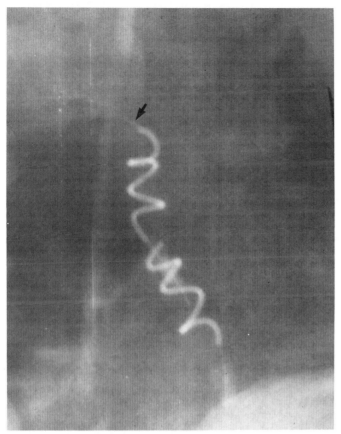

Fig. 6–12   Spot film showing position of two coilons within left spermatic vein in patient with infertility due to large left-sided varicocele. Observe that proximal end of most proximal coilon has been modified (arrow) for better fixation within venous wall to prevent migration.

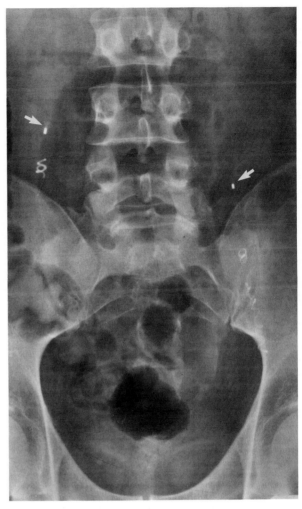

Fig. 6–13   Bilateral spermatic vein embolization in patient with infertility and bilateral varicoceles. Spider has been placed on left side proximal to a GWC spring embolus to prevent migration (arrow). Spider has been placed on right side proximal to spring coil (arrow).

contrast may be superior to sclerosing agents because it is rapidly converted to a nontoxic substance by cooling. Clinical trials are under way.

Postembolization Management

Repeat venograms are obtained 10–30 min after the procedure. After removal of the catheter, light pressure is maintained over the neck or groin for 5 min, and the patient is then monitored for 2–4 hr before discharge.

Follow-up angiography is generally not needed. Varicocele regression can be monitored clinically at the time that spermiograms are checked; usually every 3 months for 1 year.

RESULTS

Catheterization of the spermatic veins is difficult in many cases, perhaps due to anatomic abnormalities so often associated with varicocele. In 3%–40% of patients, the spermatic vein cannot be embolized[7,17,18,20]; therefore, both nonsurgical occlusion and traditional operative interruption of the spermatic vein have a place. The importance of right spermatic vein incompetence has recently been stressed.[1,7] If treated surgically, bilateral spermatic vein ligation would, of course, require two separate incisions.

The fact that interruption of the spermatic veins causes regression of varicoceles and improvement in semen characteristics in a significant number of patients is well documented.[1,6,7] Semen quality is improved in 55%–85%, and impregnation has been reported in 25%–55% for those treated.[1,6,7,25] Results with both surgical and nonsurgical techniques appear similar, although long-term follow-up of patients treated nonsurgically is not yet available. Whether transcatheter spermatic vein occlusion is more effective than operation in preventing

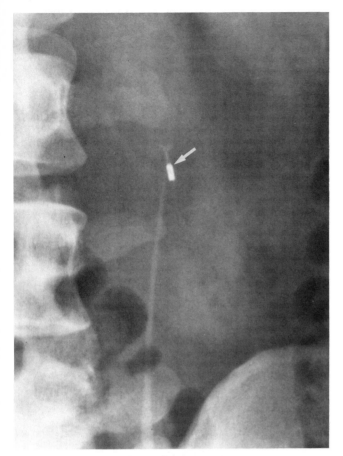

Fig. 6–14   Spiderlon in left spermatic vein.

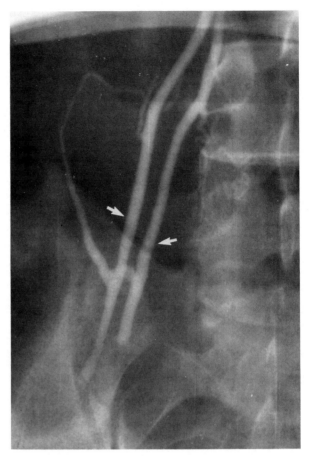

Fig. 6–15   Right spermatic venogram reveals incompetent venous valves and dual venous trunk (arrows).

varicocele recurrence is also not yet known. Theoretical' the ability to place embolic devices selectively shoud eliminate the surgical problem of incomplete ligation of the spermatic vein and its collaterals. In addition, by also causing thrombosis of existing collaterals, sclerotherapy may decrease the rate of varicocele recurrence.

Complications associated with transcatheter spermatic vein occlusion are infrequent and usually self-limiting. The most significant complication is embolization of a mechanical occluding device to the lung. Other, less serious, complications include testicular phlebitis, spermatic vein perforation, and hematoma at the puncture site.

References

1. Gonzalez R, Narayan P, Castañeda–Zuñiga WR, Amplatz K: Transvenous embolization of the internal spermatic veins for the treatment of varicocele scroti. *Urol Clin North Am* 1982;9:177–184

2. Verrstoppen GR, Steeno OP: Varicocele and the pathogenesis of the associated subfertility: a review of the various theories. 1: Varicocelogenesis. *Andrologia* 1977;9:133–140

3. Coolsaet BRRA: The varicocele syndrome: venography determining the optimal level for surgical management. *J Urol* 1980;124:833–841

4. Ross LS: Diagnosis and treatment of infertile men: a clinical perspective. *J Urol* 1983;130:847–859

5. Narayan P, Amplatz K, Gonzalez R: Varicocele and male subfertility. *Fertil Steril* 1981;36:92–96

6. Castñeda–Zuñiga WR, Gonzalez R, Amplatz K: Spermatic vein embolization in the treatment of infertility, in Kaye KW (ed): *Outpatient Urologic Surgery*. Philadephia, Lea and Febiger, 1985, pp 165–172

7. Formanek A, Rusnak B, Zollikoffer C, et al: Embolization of the spermatic vein for treatment of infertility: a new approach. *Radiology* 1981;139:315–321

8. Comhaire F, Kunnen M: Selective retrograde venography of the internal spermatic vein: a conclusive approach to diagnosis of varicocele. *Andrologia* 1976;8:11–24

9. Johnsen SG, Agger P: Quantitative evaluation of testicular biopsies before and after operation for varicocele. *Fertil Steril* 1978;29:58–63

10. Ross LS, Lipson S, Dritz S: Surgical treatment of varicocele. *Urology* 1982;19:179–180

11. Palomo A: Radical cure of varicocele by a new technique: preliminary report. *J Urol* 1979;61:604

12. Thelen M, Weibback L, Franken T: Die Behandlung der idiopathischen Varikozele durch transfemorale Spiralokklusion der vena testicularis sinistra. *RöFo* 1979;131:24–29

13. Zollikofer C, Castañeda–Zuñiga WR, Galliani C, et al: Therapeutic blockage of arteries using compressed Ivalon. *Radiology* 1980;136:635–640

14. Castañeda–Zuñiga WR, Tadavarthy SM, Gonzalez R, Rysavy J, Amplatz K: Single barbed stainless steel coils for venous occlusion: a simple but useful modification. *Invest Radiol* 1982;17:186–188

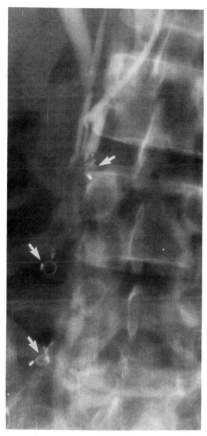

Fig. 6–16 Both venous channels have been obliterated with GWC spring embolus (arrows). The postembolization venogram reveals complete thrombosis of both channels.

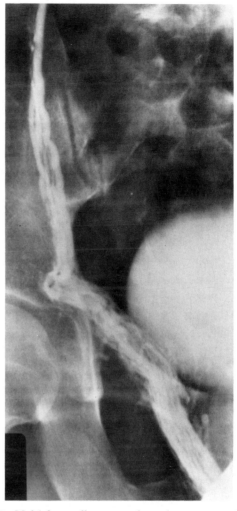

Fig. 6–17 Multiple small venous channels are seen within the inguinal canal extending into the pelvis and finally forming a common trunk at the level of the iliac crest.

15. Kunnen M: Traitment des varicoceles par embolization a l'iso-butyl-2-cyano-acrylate. *Ann Radiol* 1981;24:406–409

16. Lima SS, Castro MP, Costa OF: A new method for the treatment of varicocele. *Andrologia* 1978;10:103–106

17. Riedel P, Lunglmayr G, Stackl W: A new method of transfemoral testicular vein obliteration for varicocele using a balloon catheter. *Radiology* 1981;139:323–325

18. Iaccarino V: A nonsurgical treatment of varicocele: transcatheter sclerotherapy of gonadal veins. *Ann Radiol* 1980;23:369–370

19. Zeitler E, Jecht E, Richter EI, Seyferth W: Selective sclerotherapy of the internal spermatic vein in patients with varicocele. *Ann Radiol* 1980;23:371–373

20. Seyferth W, Jecht E, Zeitler E: Percutaneous sclerotherapy of varicocele. *Radiology* 1981;139:335–340

21. White RI Jr, Kaufman SL, Barth KH, Kadir S, Smyth JW, Walsh PC: Occlusion of varicoceles with detachable balloons. *Radiology* 1981;139:327–334

22. Cragg AH, Galliani CA, Rysavy JA, Castañeda–Zuñiga WR, Amplatz K: Endovascular diathermic vessel occlusion. *Radiology* 1982;144:303–308

23. Rholl KS, Rysavy JA, Vlodaver Z, et al: Transcatheter thermal venous occlusion: a new technique. *Radiology* 1982;145:333–337

24. Rholl KS, Rysavy JA, Vlodaver Z, et al: Spermatic vein obliteration using hot contrast medium. *Radiology* 1983;148:85–87

25. Greenberg SH: Varicocele and male fertility. *Fertil Steril* 1977;28:699–706

7

Nonsurgical Cure of Varicocele by Transcatheter Embolization of the Internal Spermatic Vein(s) with a Tissue Adhesive (Bucrylate)

MARC KUNNEN M.D., Ph.D., AND FRANK COMHAIRE, M.D., Ph.D.

Varicocele is the most common detectable cause of male infertility. It is caused by a disturbance of the efflux of venous blood from the testicle(s) due to inversion of blood flow in the internal spermatic vein(s). Impairment of testicular and epididymal function probably results from countercurrent exchange of noradrenaline from the refluxing venous blood into the testicular arterial blood, at the level of the pampiniform plexus. The latter causes chronic vasoconstriction of the intratesticular arterioles and decreased tissue perfusion with degeneration of the Sertoli cells and, finally, decreased production of spermatozoa.[1]

Varicoceles may cause local discomfort and are associated with prostatovesiculitis as well as sexual inadequacy. Although Ahlberg et al[2] showed in 1966 that varicoceles could be detected by retrograde phlebography, this technique was rarely used, whereas many investigators performed ascending phlebography during varicocelectomy.[3,4]

In 1976, the authors described a method for selective venography of the internal spermatic vein(s),[5,6] which was claimed to be safe and suitable for routine use. At present, this method is in practice throughout the world.

In 1979, Kunnen developed a new method for nonsurgical cure of varicocele disease, namely, transcatheter embolization with the tissue adhesive isobutyl-2-cyanoacrylate (IBCA, Bucrylate from Ethicon/Somerville).[7-10] To date, more than 400 patients have been treated with this technique. The procedure will be described and the results presented.

GENERAL INFORMATION

Diagnostic Venography

The catheterization is performed from the right groin under local anesthesia and according to a strict protocol, using coaxial catheters exclusively. Diagnostic venography should always precede the therapeutic procedure.

One starts with the cobra catheter, which is the outer part of the Kunnen Left Spermatic Set (No. 2247, Meadox-Surgimed, Denmark)(Fig. 7–3A). At first, the right renal and internal spermatic veins are examined. The right renal vein is catheterized, probing the segmentary veins with a J-tipped 0.038-inch guidewire with a movable core (Fig. 7–2A). The venogram has to show the segmentary veins clearly. Connecting collaterals to the spermatic vein or a direct connection between the renal and the spermatic vein (Fig. 7–6 and 7A) have to be searched for. If these are not found, and if the outlet of the right internal spermatic vein is not easily catheterized from the inferior caval vein, or if it shows a competent valve, the right-sided venography is regarded as negative.

Even if the right-sided venography is positive—which occurs in 32% of the authors' patients presenting with a left varicocele—one has to proceed with the left-sided diagnostic venography using the same cobra-shaped catheter.

The catheter is pushed into the segmentary renal veins, probing them with with the J-tip of the 0.038-inch guidewire. The venogram has to show the segmentary veins together with the presence (Fig. 7–5A) or absence of perirenal collaterals (Fig. 7–1A), as well as the competence of (Fig. 7–14A) or insufficiency (Fig. 7–1A) of the valve at the outlet of the left internal vein.

If the left venography is positive; *i.e.*, if retrograde opacification of the left spermatic vein is seen, this vein should be catheterized coaxially, opacified superselectively, and embolized with IBCA. The occlusion should be monitored by means of a control selective venogram.

If the right-sided venography is positive, the cobra catheter is exchanged for a hooked catheter—outer part of the Kunnen Right Spermatic Set (No. 2248, Meadox-Surgimed, Denmark)(Fig. 7–3B)—for easier coaxial catheterization of the right internal spermatic vein. Superselective venography of the right internal spermatic vein, followed by embolization with IBCA and control selective venography to monitor the occlusion, are the final steps of the procedure.

It should be noted that diagnostic venographies must be carried out carefully in order to demonstrate not only retrograde filling of the internal spermatic vein(s), but also all accompanying, connecting, or collateral veins. Superselective venography by means of the small, straight coaxial catheter yields more precise information on the most suitable site for embolization.

Also, if one fails to achieve a clearly filled venogram of the right renal vein when using the cobra catheter, the examination should be interrupted on this side; the procedure is continued on the left side, and finally the right

venography is repeated using the hooked catheter. This, however, rarely occurs.

Superselective Coaxial Catheterization and Embolization

The outer cobra-shaped catheter (for the left side; Fig. 7–1) or the hooked catheter (for the right side; Fig. 7–2) is placed in the outlet of the internal spermatic vein. The thin inner catheter, fitted with the small (0.025-inch) guidewire included in the left spermatic set, is pushed through the outer catheter to enter the spermatic vein. The catheters are moistened with 5% glucose through a T-adapter (Fig. 7–3).

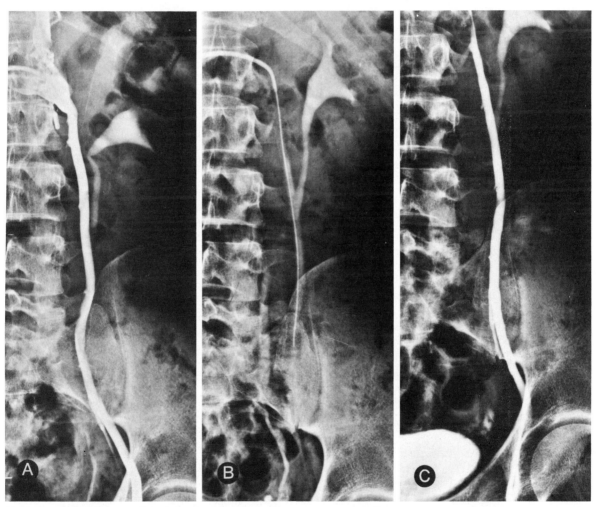

Fig. 7–1 Typical embolization procedure in left internal spermatic vein with the left spermatic set. A. Selective venogram with cobra catheter in the outlet. The vessel presents a bifurcation at the level of the sacroiliac joint. B. The thin inner catheter fitted with 0.025-inch guidewire is pushed through outer catheter into spermatic vein. C. Superselective venography through thin catheter clearly shows anatomic details, especially bifurcation and competent valves of connecting vessels. The exact site for embolization is selected just superior to the bifurcation. D. Tip of thin catheter is moved to embolization site, guidewire is removed, and exact location is monitored by injecting small quantities of 60% Isopaque. Tilting table is moved so as to stop circulation in spermatic vein completely. E. Tissue adhesive is injected, inner catheter is immediately withdrawn, and outer catheter is pulled backward into vena cava. Blood is aspirated to assure absence of adhesive in cobra catheter. The embolus is clearly visible at the level of the left sacroiliac joint. F. Ten minutes later, control venogram is performed with the cobra catheter; renal vein injection during Valsalva maneuver shows incomplete filling of spermatic vein. G. Selective spermatic venogram during Valsalva maneuver confirms complete occlusion.

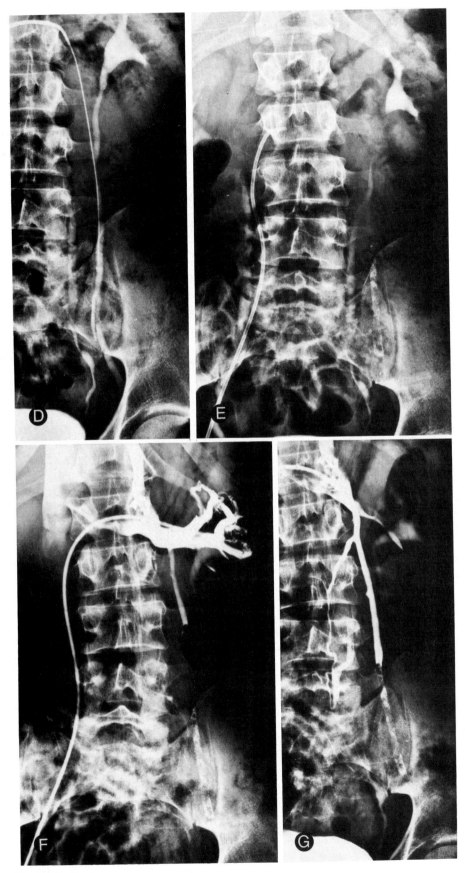

Fig. 7–1 D–G

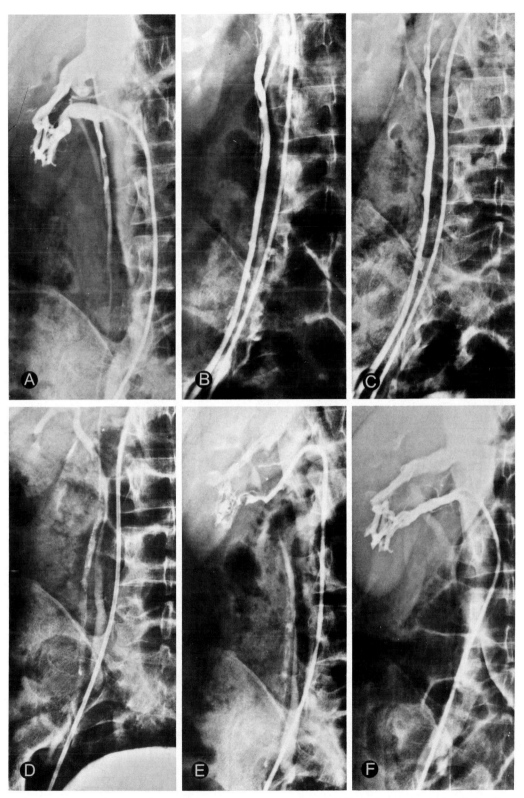

Fig. 7–2 Typical embolization procedure in right internal spermatic vein with the right spermatic set. A. Diagnostic venography with injection into caudal segment of right renal vein using cobra catheter. Right internal spermatic vein is connected directly with renal vein and displays pathologic reflux. B. After examination (and possibly embolization) of the left side with the cobra catheter, the hooked catheter is introduced into outlet of right spermatic vein, and selective venography is performed. C. Thin catheter is introduced into spermatic vein through outer hooked catheter. Superselective venography reveals valves of connecting vessels and bifurcation at the level of the sacroiliac joint. D. X-ray picture taken during injection of embolus above the bifurcation. E. Control renal venogram 10 min after embolization shows no more reflux. F. Control renal venogram 15 months after embolization shows integrity of renal veins and absence of reflux. The embolus is no longer visible.

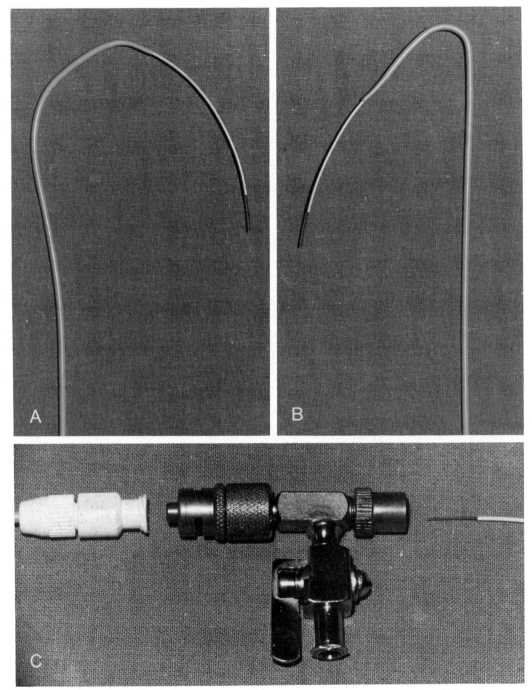

Fig. 7–3   Catheter and guidewire assembly. A. Thin inner catheter fitted with small guidewire is pushed through cobra catheter. B. Thin inner catheter fitted with small guidewire is pushed through hooked catheter. C. T-adapter (Cook sidearm design, catalog number SOWS-PCF-MLL-RA-TO) for moistening catheters with 5% glucose.

Under fluoroscopic control, the tip of the catheter is brought to the exact site selected for embolization. This site should be inferior to the lowest anastomosis between the spermatic vein and the (peri)renal venous plexus and preferably superior to any bifurcations (Fig. 7–1C). The catheter moves more easily when the patient coughs. The guidewire is removed, and the exact location of the catheter is determined by injecting a small quantity of Isopaque 60% (sodium, calcium, and magnesium metri-zoate; 350 mg iodine/ml). The patient is examined on a remote-controlled tilting table, which is brought into a nearly horizontal position (2°–10°) in order to stop the circulation in the internal spermatic vein completely. The latter is controlled by injecting a small bolus of contrast medium (Fig. 7–1D). This procedure is extremely important because it excludes accidental thrombosis of the renal vein as well as injection into the pampiniform plexus.

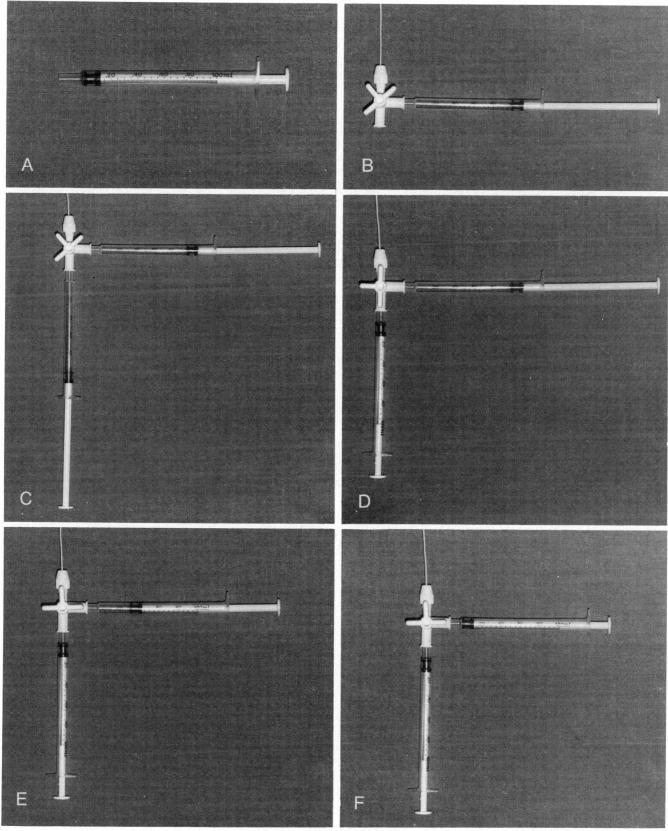

Fig. 7–4   Tuberculin syringes and 3-way stopcock on small straight embolization catheter. The manipulation is described in the text.

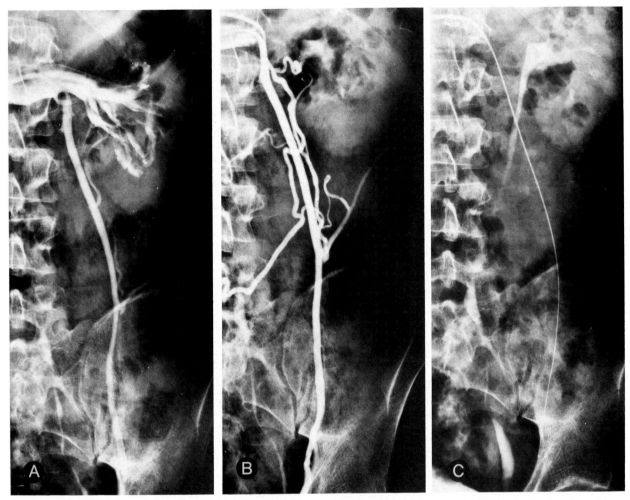

Fig. 7–5 Typical embolization at the level of the lowest anastomosis between perirenal plexus and left spermatic vein. A. Reflux in left spermatic vein during injection of contrast medium into renal vein. Some connecting vessels are visible. B. Selective spermatic venogram shows these vessels better. C. The small catheter fitted with the guidewire is introduced into spermatic vein. D. Superselective injection of small amount of contrast medium at site of lowest anastomosis shows the different branches and also the caudal lateral accompanying vein, which were not clearly seen on selective venograms. E. As some dye is still moving up through the tortuous cranial collateral, remote-controlled table has to be tilted a few more degrees upward, in order to stop blood circulation in spermatic venous system completely. F. Embolus enters all vessels, but only for a few centimeters. G. No blood could be aspirated from cobra catheter when pulled back in vena cava because caval wall adhered to tip of catheter. Catheter is therefore brought into left iliac vein, and blood is aspirated. Catheter may be used for control venograms. H. Control renal venogram during Valsalva maneuver 10 min after embolization; slight filling of spermatic vein. I. Selective control venogram shows total occlusion of spermatic venous system at the embolus.

A tuberculin syringe is filled with 1 ml of 10% glucose and connected to the plastic 3-way stopcock of the embolization catheter, which is filled with 5% glucose (Fig. 7–4A,B). The glucose solution slows down the polymerization of the tissue adhesive. Into a second syringe, the following substances are aspirated in sequence and without mixing: 0.1 ml of 60% Isopaque, 0.4–0.6 ml of IBCA, and another 0.1 ml of 60% Isopaque. One should never use more than 1 ampule (0.6 ml) of IBCA. The contrast medium is used not only to delineate the nonopaque bolus of IBCA on the TV monitor and the X-ray films, but also to initiate the polymerization; once the IBCA is in contact with the Isopaque, one must proceed quickly. The second syringe is connected to the stopcock (Fig. 7–4C), and its contents are injected into the embolization catheter (Fig. 7–4D) and pushed into the spermatic vein with the contents of the first syringe; i.e., 0.7 ml of 10% glucose from the first syringe is injected in order to push the embolus completely into the spermatic vein (Fig. 7–4E). The coaxial embolization catheter is immediately pulled back 2–3 cm, and the remaining 0.3 ml of 10% glucose from the first syringe is injected to remove all IBCA from this catheter (Fig. 7–4F).

The inner catheter is withdrawn from the outer one, which is pulled back into the vena cava, where blood is aspirated (Fig. 7–1E). If it is not possible to aspirate blood, the caval wall may adhere to the tip of the catheter; this can be avoided by placing the tip of the catheter in the left common iliac vein.

Whenever aspiration of blood remains impossible,

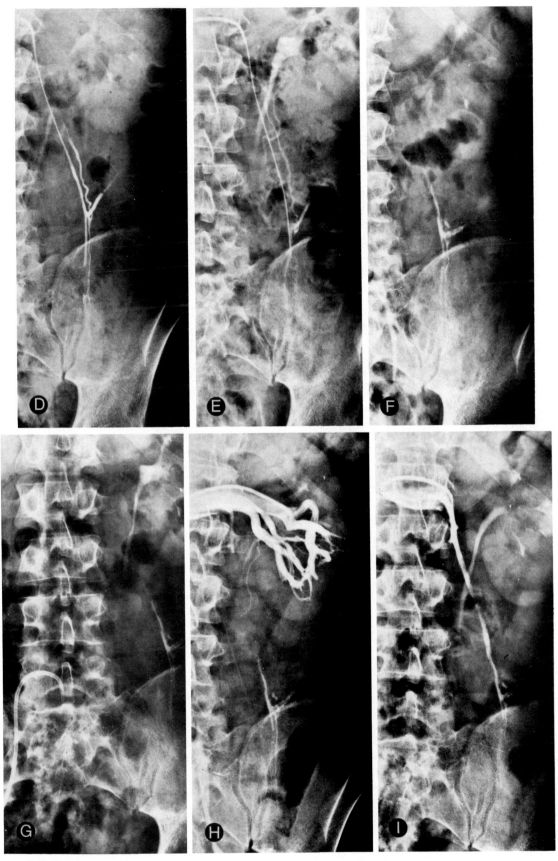

Fig. 7–5 D–I

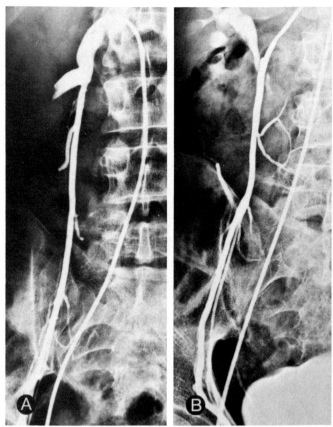
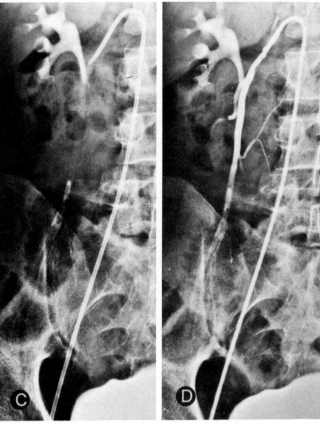

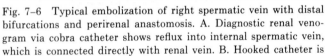

Fig. 7–6 Typical embolization of right spermatic vein with distal bifurcations and perirenal anastomosis. A. Diagnostic renal venogram via cobra catheter shows reflux into internal spermatic vein, which is connected directly with renal vein. B. Hooked catheter is introduced into spermatic vein; top of thin catheter is located at the junction of the perirenal anastomosis with bifurcated distal branches. C. IBCA embolus opacified with Isopaque. D. Selective control venogram demonstrating total occlusion.

occlusion of the outer catheter by a residue of IBCA should be suspected, and the outer catheter should be withdrawn and replaced by a new outer catheter. (In these rare cases, one can cut the external part of the catheter obliquely, introduce an 8F sheath over it, and withdraw and replace the catheter by the new one fitted with the 0.038-inch guidewire).

As soon as the tissue adhesive comes in contact with blood, it polymerizes to form a permanent occlusion. The embolus is seen on the X-ray pictures (Figs. 7–1E–G and 7–2D,E). A control venogram is performed about 10 min later through the outer catheter. First, the renal vein is injected without a Valsalva maneuver in order to check its integrity. The renal vein is then injected during a Valsalva maneuver (Figs. 7–1F and 7–2E), and finally the thrombosed spermatic vein is selectively opacified (Fig. 7–1G) to confirm the absence of residual reflux.

During the whole procedure, 5% glucose is used as a moistening and rinsing solution. Physiologic saline is absolutely *contraindicated*, because it will cause premature polymerization of the IBCA.

Never try to perform more than one embolization through the same inner catheter! However, the outer catheter can be used for a second or, rarely, a third embolization.

Examples of the Technique

In Figure 7–5, another example of a typical left spermatic venous embolization is shown. The embolus is placed at the level of the lowest anastomosis between the perirenal plexus and the spermatic vein (also called the renospermatic bypass). The liquid embolus enters the different connecting vessels and occludes them all in one procedure (Fig. 7–5F); this is one of the great advantages of the authors' technique over the methods in which detachable balloons or coils are used. On the other hand the embolus will never move further than a few centimeters, as IBCA polymerizes rapidly when it is in contact with blood. Hence, there is no danger of damaging surrounding tissues, unlike the situation when large amounts of sclerosing agents are used (sclerotherapy).

In Figure 7–6, an embolization is shown in a patient with bifurcations of the caudal part of the right internal spermatic vein together with an anastomosis with the perirenal plexus. The IBCA embolus is located at the junction of these vessels, near the level of the right sacroiliac joint. Figure 7–7 demonstrates how several distal branches are occluded with a single embolus, which is injected at the site of their distal connections.

If the spermatic vein has high bifurcations but no

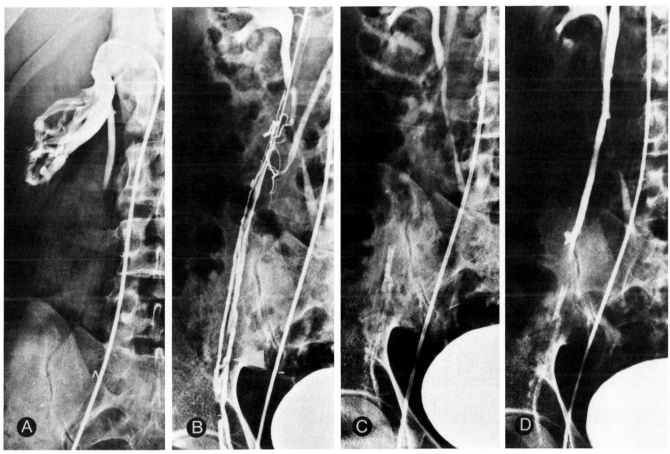

Fig. 7–7 Embolization of right spermatic vein with bifurcated vessels in distal segments. A. Diagnostic renal venogram via cobra catheter shows slight reflux in internal spermatic vein, which is connected directly to renal vein. B. Via hooked outer catheter lying in outlet of spermatic vein, thin catheter is brought into the medial bifurcated vessel at the level of distal connection with the lateral one (arrowhead). C. Embolus is located in both vessels. D. Control selective venogram reveals total occlusion and anastomosis with perirenal plexus superior to the embolus.

renospermatic bypass, one can embolize the superior part of the vein. One must completely stop the spermatic circulation as usual by tilting the table and monitoring the circulation with small contrast injections. If, on the contrary, there is an anastomosis with the perirenal plexus, as suggested by the presence of a lateral valve (Fig. 7–8), embolization of the cranial segment is to be avoided. In this case, the embolization catheter did enter the small medial branch of the bifurcation. One can embolize via the small vessel, as shown here, and expect occlusion of the whole system by one embolus if contrast injections have revealed runoff through the connections. If there is no evident runoff, or if the catheter lies for more than 10 cm in such a thin accompanying vein, the authors advise against using this procedure, because the catheter may be trapped in the embolus.

Large veins are also easily occluded, usually with one single embolization. A slightly different technique is used, in that the embolus is pushed into the vessel with the entire 1-ml volume of 10% glucose in order to concentrate all the IBCA in one single spot. Figure 7–9 shows embolization of a left spermatic vein 9 mm in diameter just above its distal bifurcation. Figure 7–10 shows the

occlusion of an 8-mm thick vessel at the level of the lowest renospermatic bypass and of the connections with medial–caudal and lateral–superior accompanying veins.

Procedures in More Complex Anatomic Conditions

PERIRENAL ANASTOMOSIS CONNECTED TO BIFURCATED DISTAL PART OF SPERMATIC VEIN

In the cases shown in Figures 7–11 and 7–12, the lateral branch of a bifurcated distal part of the spermatic vein is connected to the lowest perirenal anastomosis on a slightly lower level than the bifurcation. The embolization catheter must be placed in the lateral branch, and the embolus should be injected at the site of the perirenal anastomosis. Usually, the embolus will ascend into the bifurcation after the first part begins polymerizing in the lateral vessel, and it will occlude all the branches and anastomoses. In the majority of cases, this can be

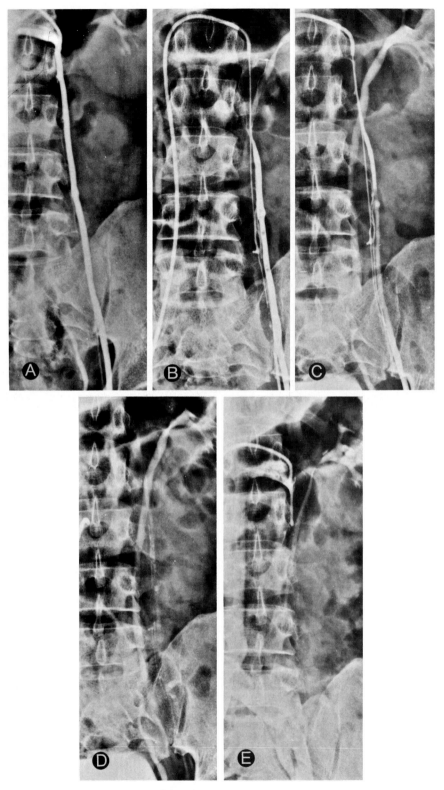

Fig. 7–8   Embolization via small branch of bifurcation situated in the cranial segment with distal connections. A. Selective injection of insufficient spermatic vein with small medial accompanying vein. B. Upon coaxial catheterization, small catheter enters medial vein and reveals bifurcation in cranial segment. Connections to principal vein are shown by superselective venography, which reveals a lateral valve at the level of L4, suggesting the presence of a renospermatic bypass. C. During further injection of contrast medium, definite runoff is shown and another distal accompanying vessel revealed. After the vessels have been cleared with 5% glucose, IBCA is injected, pushed by 1 ml of 10% glucose. D. Embolus is clearly visible in the two small branches and in principal vessel. E. Control venogram shows complete occlusion with superior limit at level of L2/3.

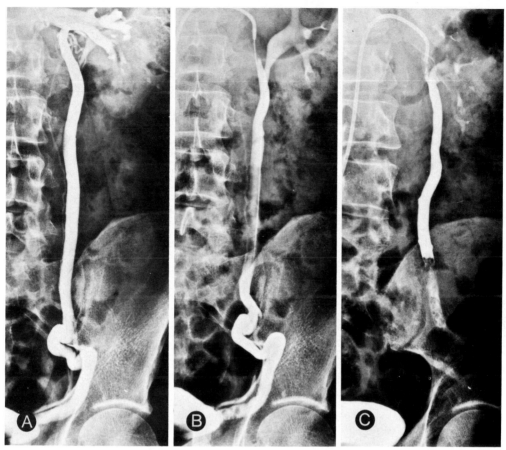

Fig. 7–9 Embolization of large (9-mm) left spermatic vein. A. Renal venography reveals massive reflux through spermatic vein, which presents distal bifurcation as well as small medial accompanying vein. B. Tip of coaxial catheter is just above bifurcation. Small medial accompanying vein is found to be connected to principal sper-matic vein immediately above bifurcation; it presents retrograde fill-ing. Embolus is concentrated on this spot (see text). C. Control selec-tive venogram shows total occlusion. Embolus is clearly seen; it is large and rather short. Accompanying vein is blocked at its junction.

achieved by means of the straight guidewire of the sper-matic set. If this procedure is unsuccessful, one should exchange the wire for a steerable J-wire manufactured for coronary angioplasty (Fig. 7–13), which is useful in nego-tiating eccentric connections and in passing minute branches. The direction of the flexible J-tip can be changed by rotating the bent end of the guidewire around its axis. As shown in Figure 7–12, one can even reach the perirenal anastomosis itself.

If one were to occlude only the medial vein, the vari-cocele would persist as a result of the bypassing anasto-mosis and the lateral branch. The latter would now be unreachable for nonsurgical cure! If, after embolization of the lateral vein, the medial one would not be occluded, one has only to inject a second embolus. This will always be the case if the distance between the bifurcation and the renospermatic bypass is great (Fig. 7–14).

The authors stress that one should always first embol-ize the more distal connections and be aware of the fact that it is easy to put a second embolus higher up when necessary, whereas once a particular vessel is embolized, it is impossible to reach the more distal parts.

Perirenal anastomoses can never be coaxially cathet-erized in the caudal direction but only in the cranial direction from the spermatic vein.

REFLUX THROUGH BYPASSING COLLATERAL IN CASES WITH COMPETENT OUTLET VALVES

In a relatively large proportion of patients with a vari-cocele (in the authors' series, more than 25%), renal venography reveals one or even several competent valves in the cranial part of the internal spermatic vein. How-ever, reflux occurs through one or more bypassing reno-spermatic anastomoses. It is clear that these patients can be treated nonsurgically only if the spermatic vein is occluded distal to these renospermatic bypasses. The cor-rect site for embolization can be reached only after cath-eterization through the competent valves. With the authors' coaxial technique, they generally succeed in passing these valves, which is another advantage of this procedure. Usually, they place the appropriate catheter in, or just above, the competent outlet valve and pass the valve with the guidewire reaching slightly out of the thin catheter, just as in cases without outlet valves. The trick consists of bringing the patient to a Trendelenburg posi-tion, which opens the valves as blood effluxes. If this pro-cedure fails, the patient is asked to cough or to perform a Valsalva maneuver. Once the ideal site for embolization is reached, i.e., the distal part of the spermatic vein, they proceed as described above. The completeness of the

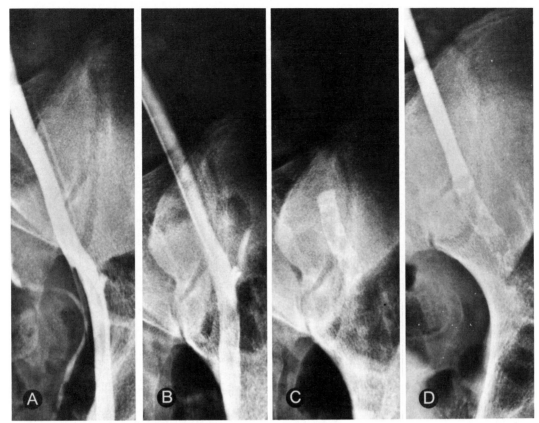

Fig. 7–10 Embolization of large (8-mm) left spermatic vein at level of its lowest anastomosis with perirenal plexus and of connection with medial–caudal and lateral–superior accompanying veins. A. Selective venography shows medial–caudal and lateral–superior accompanying veins connected to principal spermatic vein at level of sacroiliac joint. (Projection may differ as function of the position of the patient—erect or horizontal—and performance of Valsalva maneuver.) Slight filling of renal anastomosis. B. Embolization catheter is placed distal to connection of this lowest anastomosis, which is clearly visible now. C. Large and rather short "concentrated" embolus. D. Selective control venogram demonstrates total occlusion of all vessels.

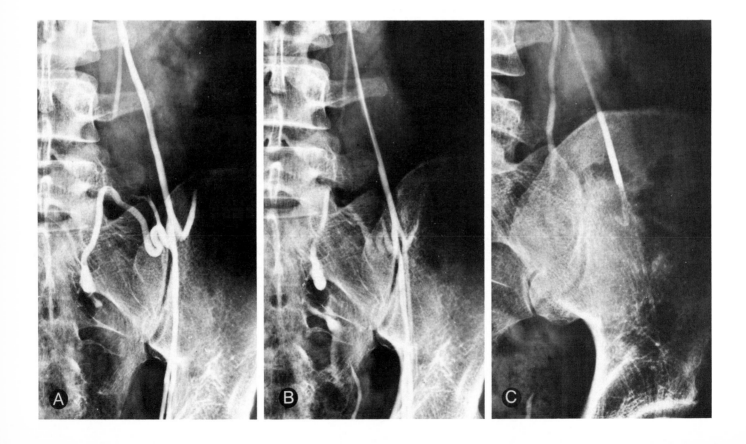

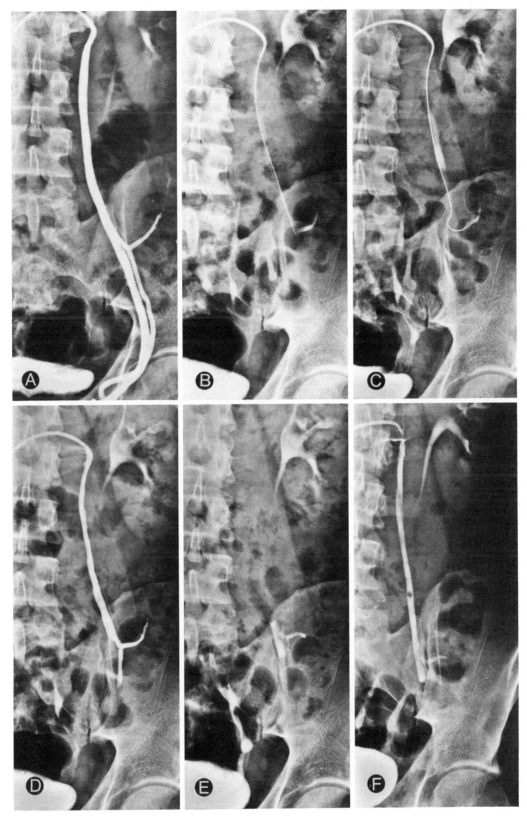

Fig. 7–12 (above) Use of steerable J-guidewire to reach perirenal anastomosis connected to lateral branch of bifurcated spermatic vein. A. Selective venography in insufficient spermatic vein which is bifurcated and shows renospermatic bypass connected to its lateral branch that ends below level of bifurcation. B. Coaxial catheterization. C. The J-wire is pushed into anastomosis. D. Coaxial catheter is pushed into anastomosis. E. Embolus fills part of branches, including bypass. F. Control selective venogram shows complete occlusion.

←

Fig. 7–11 (previous page) Embolization of bifurcated left spermatic vein with a perirenal anastomosis connected to lateral branch. A. Selective spermatic venography shows medial collateral and renospermatic bypass. A bifurcation can be suspected. B. Coaxial catheterization of lateral limb of bifurcation shows lateral branch, which is connected with renospermatic bypass. Embolization is performed at the level of this connection. C. Control venogram shows embolus in the different vessels; occlusion is complete.

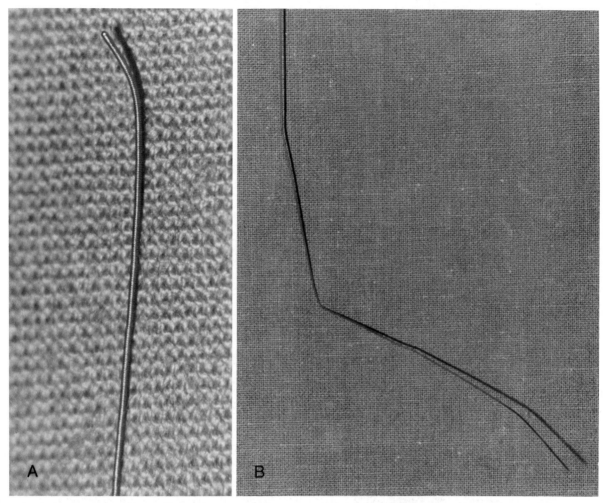

Fig. 7–13   Steerable J-guidewire designed for coronary angioplasty. A. Direction of flexible J-tip can be steered by rotating bent end (B) of guidewire around its axis.

occlusion is checked by a control renal venogram, which should demonstrate lack of filling or the opacification of only the cranial part of the collaterals without further reflux.

In Figure 7–15, an example of this situation is demonstrated. The competent valves are clearly seen. They are bypassed by several short collaterals (Fig. 7–15B) and by long renospermatic anastomoses (Fig. 7–15B,C and, especially, E). The tip of the catheter is placed at the level of the sacroiliac joint, where the lower part of the embolus is injected (Fig. 7–15F). The embolus also fills the distal part of the renospermatic bypass. Upon control venography with injection of the renal vein, the collaterals are no longer filled (Fig. 7–15G). Moreover, the outlet valve remains competent (Fig. 7–15H).

In the case shown in Figure 7–16, the competent outlet valve is further bypassed by a hooked medial collateral vessel. This collateral is used for selective venography before (Fig. 7–16C) and again after the embolization (Fig. 7–16F), whereas the competent valve is passed coaxially (Fig. 7–16D,E) to achieve the embolization. Also shown is the right side of the same patient (Figs. 7–16G–J). The right spermatic vein shows a typical outlet in the vena cava but, in addition, a direct communication with the right renal vein (Fig. 7–16G). The latter remained open

(Fig. 7–16J) after embolization through the thin catheter, which was brought to the site via a cobra catheter passing through a small lateral accompanying vein (see arrow in Fig. 7–16H). Control venography performed from the vena cava demonstrated total occclusion of the spermatic vein at the site selected for embolization (Fig. 7–16I).

In some cases, such as that illustrated in Figure 7–17, the upper part of the spermatic vein is very narrow. Nevertheless, it can be catheterized coaxially to permit embolization in the distal part of the spermatic system. In Figure 7–14, an association of a competent outlet valve and bypassing renospermatic bypasses is illustrated. Treatment consisted of two applications of IBCA for anatomic reasons.

An example is presented of the few cases with competent outlet valves and bypassing collaterals in which the coaxial catheter could not be passed through the valve via a cobra catheter because the spermatic vein was situated too medially. By using a 7F catheter with a curve of 180° (F-curve; Fig. 7–18), the authors succeeded in catheterizing and embolizing this spermatic vein also (Fig. 7–19).

It should be admitted that, despite all of these procedures, the authors do not succeed in passing competent valves in a few cases. These are the only technical failures of this technique.

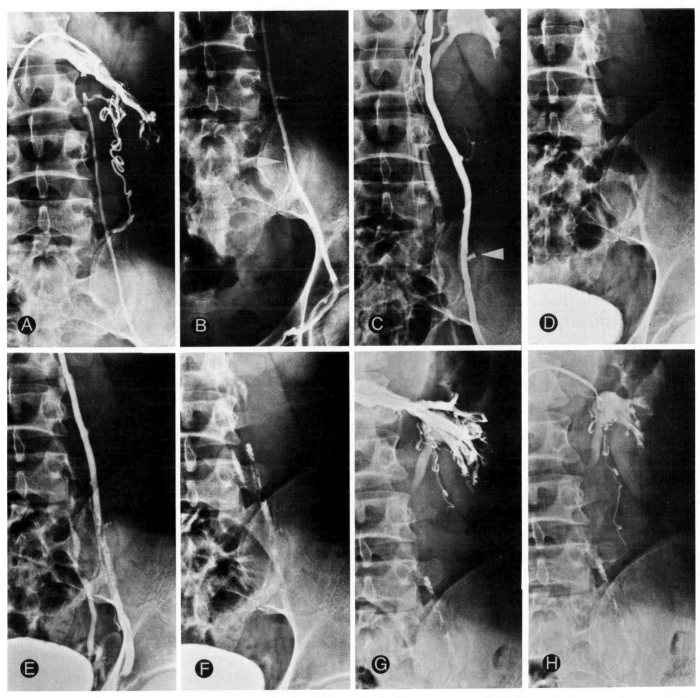

Fig. 7–14 Association of competent outlet valve with bypassing perirenal collaterals, compelling application of two emboli for anatomic reasons. A,B. Diagnostic renal venography shows competent spermatic outlet valve together with bypassing anastomosis. There is a distal bifurcation and a small medial branch (arrowhead in B). C. Superselective venography reveals connection of a low anastomosis at level of sacroiliac joint (arrowhead). D. First embolus is placed at level of lower anastomosis. E. Superselective control venography shows that medial bifurcated branch is not occluded. F. Use is made of a new 3F straight catheter, while cobra catheter is reused. Second embolus is placed at site of bifurcation (compare D). G,H. Control venography after complete embolization. Only one collateral is filled; the contrast medium is blocked at connection with spermatic vein.

TREATMENT OF PERSISTENT VARICOCELES

Most varicoceles that persist after either surgical or nonsurgical treatment can be cured by coaxial embolization with IBCA.

Persistence after Surgery

According to Weissback et al, the failure rate after surgical treatment of varicocele ranges from 0.2%–25%.[11]

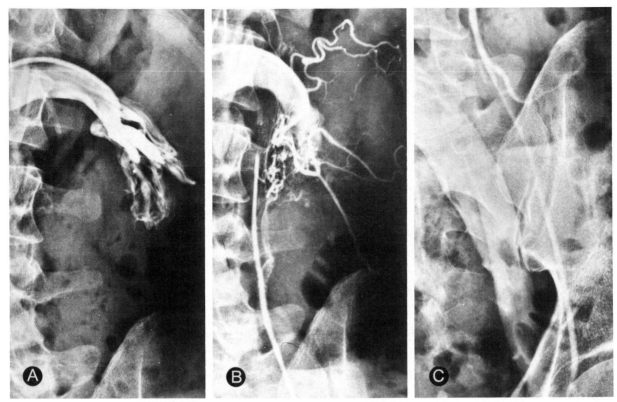

Fig. 7–15   Embolization in a typical case with a competent valve at spermatic venous outlet but reflux through bypassing collaterals. A. Diagnostic renal venography, early phase. Contrast enters internal spermatic vein for 2 cm and is then stopped by competent valve. B. Two seconds later, distal, insufficient part of spermatic vein is filled via several short and tortuous collaterals. Long renospermatic bypass is also filled. C. Two more seconds later, contrast medium in one of these anastomoses reaches spermatic vein at the level of L4/5. D. Tip of cobra catheter is placed above competent valve. E. Competent valve is passed by coaxial catheter fitted with 0.025-inch guidewire. Superselective venography reveals a second renospermatic anastomosis, which is situated more caudally and is connected to spermatic vein halfway to the level of sacroiliac joint. This site must be included in the occlusion. F. Embolus is clearly visible; its lower limit occludes distal anastomosis and its upper part occludes cranial one. G. Control renal venogram shows that anastomoses no longer fill because they are occluded more distally. H. Selective spermatic venography shows competent valve, which has not been damaged by procedure.

The persistence of varicoceles after ligation has stimulated the authors to examine such cases by selective venography and to treat them by embolization. In general, these patients had been operated on by a low ligation, and therefore the vessels could be catheterized and embolized according to the authors' standard procedure. It usually proved to be the case that one or more contributing vessels had not been ligated, and it was not uncommon to find no ligation at all. One patient presented with persistent bilateral varicoceles after bilateral surgery. He had competent outlet valves on both sides and bypassing perirenal anastomoses. His disease was cured by bilateral embolization.

Persistence after Coil Embolization

This problem commonly results from embolization performed in the cranial segment of the spermatic vein, leaving the accompanying veins or renospermatic anastomoses open. Moreover, coil-treated vessels may also remain open or become partly patent later.

The presence of coils may render distal coaxial catheterization of the spermatic vein and correct embolization with IBCA impossible. All these factors were noticed in a patient presenting with primary infertility due to persistent bilateral varicoceles. Two years previously, this patient had undergone operation on the left side. Because surgery was unsuccessful, he was subsequently treated on the same side by coil embolization at the level of L4. Because he was not doing any better afterward, two additional coils were placed at the level of L3 in a further session. At the same time, an embolization with two coils was performed in the caval outlet of the right spermatic vein. All of this treatment remained ineffective, and the patient was referred to the authors for further treatment.

Upon right-sided renal venography, an insufficient branch of the right spermatic vein was detected, which connected to the superior of the two renal veins. Furthermore, selective venography showed a bifurcation of the distal spermatic vein. The coaxial catheter was pushed more caudally until its tip was situated at the level of the sacroiliac joint. By means of superselective venography a renospermatic bypass was revealed. The arrest of blood flow was monitored by injecting a small amount of contrast medium which filled the different branches over a few centimeters. An embolus of IBCA was injected according to the authors' standard procedure. Upon control renal venography, no further reflux in the spermatic system on the right side was found. The embolus reached from the sacroiliac joint almost as high as the coils. Left

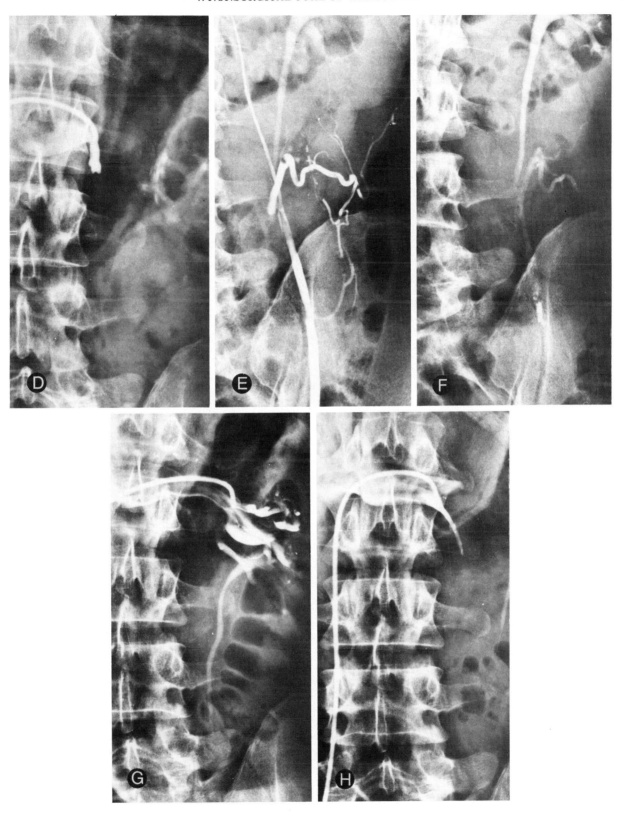

Fig. 7–15 D–H

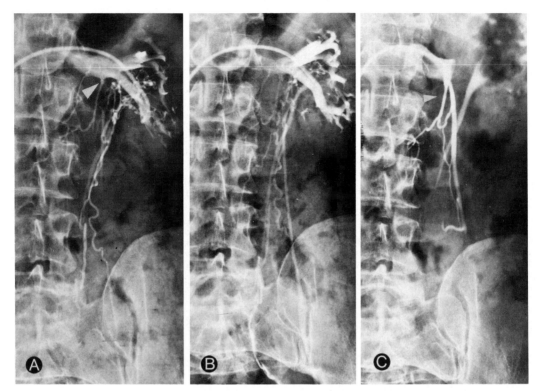

Fig. 7–16 This patient presented with bilateral varicoceles with a competent valve and bypassing collaterals on the left side and an outlet to the vena cava as well as a direct connection to the renal vein on the right side. Bilateral embolization is performed with the left spermatic set (cobra catheter). On left, catheter was introduced through the competent valve; on right, catheter was introduced via renal vein and a small lateral collateral. A. Diagnostic left renal venography, early phase. Competent outlet valve (arrowhead) is bypassed by hooked medial collateral and by several short tortuous and one long renospermatic bypasses. There is opacification of a small upper and a larger lower segment of principal spermatic vein. B. Same injection as in A, 1 sec later. Outlet valve is more clearly visible. Principal vein is almost completely opacified; only upper 2 cm are not visible. C. When medial hooked bypass is injected (arrowhead), upper part of principal vein and the renal vein are opacified. Accompanying veins are disclosed. D. Coaxial catheter is pushed through competent outlet valve. E. Superselective venogram reveals additional branches and distal bifurcation. All vessels are connected at level of iliac crest. F. Control venogram through medial hooked anastomosis reveals total occlusion after embolization at level of iliac crest. G. Right renal diagnostic angiography via cobra catheter. Right spermatic vein has two outlets, one in vena cava and one in renal vein; the communication stands out clearly. H. Superselective catheterization performed with left spermatic set passing from renal vein through a small lateral accompanying vein (upper arrowhead). Embolization must be performed at site of cranial bifurcation (lower arrowhead). I. Control venogram with cobra catheter in caval outlet of right spermatic vein. Total occlusion is achieved at level of bifurcation. J. Control venogram with cobra catheter in renal outlet of right spermatic vein. As planned, these vessels are free of embolus.

venography revealed a huge renospermatic anastomosis bypassing to the insufficient caudal part of the spermatic vein and shunting the coils (Fig. 7–20). Moreover, the superior coils seemed to be unable to withstand the blood flow, whereas the inferior one was located in the lateral, smaller branch of a bifurcation (Figs. 7–20A–D). Unfortunately, the superior coils prevented passage of the tip of the coaxial guidewire, and *a fortiori*, IBCA embolization of the distal spermatic vein was impossible. For this reason, the patient was operated on through a suprainguinal incision on the left side. Three months later, he impregnated his wife.

Persistence after IBCA Embolization

FALSE PERSISTENCE

In the authors' first series of patients, they commonly embolized only the left side, rarely the right side. As a matter of fact, they experienced difficulties in catheterizing the right spermatic vein coaxially with the cobra catheter, because its tip struck the vessel wall at too steep an angle. As a result, they observed four patients with bilateral varicoceles who were embolized only in the left spermatic vein and presented with clinical persistence of left-sided varicocele. Upon control venography, the occlusion was found to be complete on the left side and absolutely unchanged (Fig. 7–21). In all these cases, however, intrascrotal connections filled the left-sided varicocele from the right spermatic vein. Embolization of the right spermatic vein cured these patients.

The same situation can be found after left-sided surgical ligation.

TRUE PERSISTENCE

Of the 435 patients the authors have embolized to date, clinical persistence was observed in only seven (less than

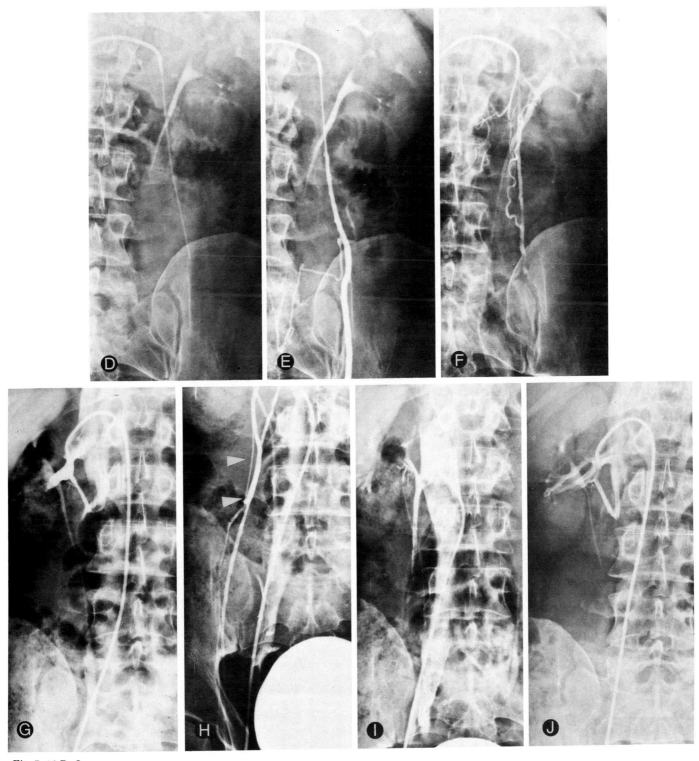

Fig. 7–16 D–J

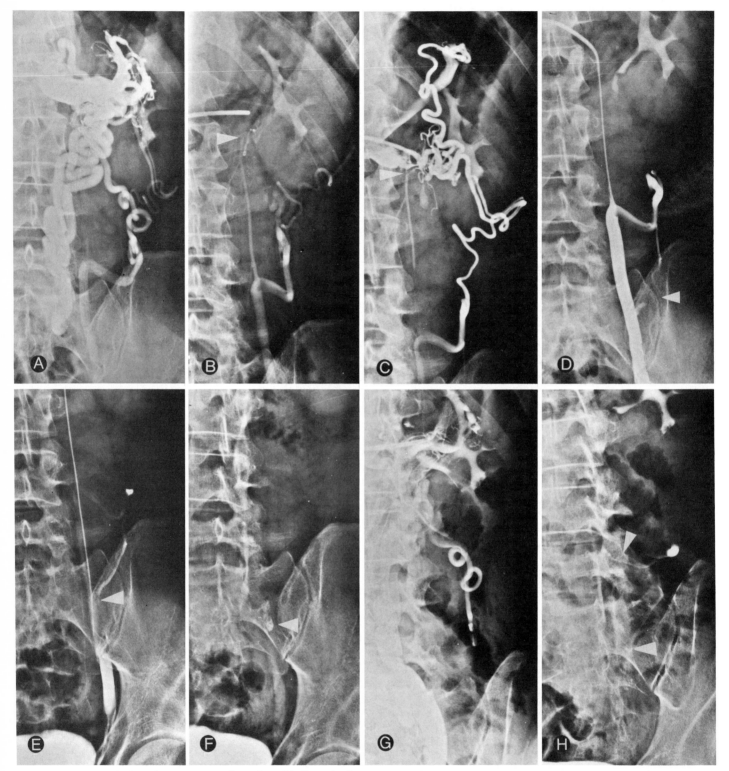

Fig. 7–17 Association of competent outlet valve with hypoplastic cranial segment of spermatic vein and renospermatic anastomoses. A. Diagnostic renal venography. Voluminous periureteral varices are of no importance for the varicocele, since they do not drain into pampiniform plexus. Note presence of tortuous lateral perirenal anastomosis bypassing to thick distal segment of spermatic vein. B. Hypoplastic upper part of spermatic vein opacifies antegrade; competent valve is indicated by the arrowhead. C. Selective injection of perirenal plexus clearly shows anastomosis but also reveals small anastomosis ending just below competent valve (arrowhead). D. Hypoplastic upper part of spermatic vein is passed coaxially. Superselective venography reveals an additional anastomosis ending at level of sacroiliac joint (arrowhead). E. Small injection shows tip of embolization catheter situated distal to lowest anastomosis (arrowhead). F. Lower limit of embolus (arrowhead) is distal to outlet of lower anastomosis. G. Control venography, injecting perirenal plexus (compare C). H. Anastomoses fill very slowly and are all occluded at their connection with spermatic vein (arrowheads).

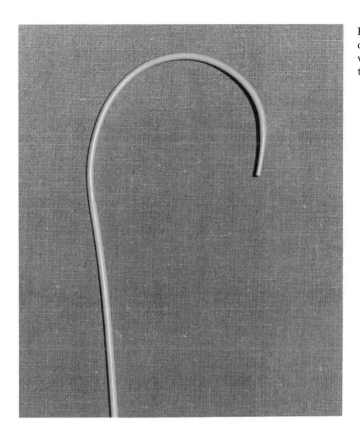

Fig. 7–18 A 7F catheter with F-curve of 180° (Meadox–Surgimed, catalog no. 4465F070) used for coaxial catheterization of competent valves in cases where outlet of left spermatic vein is situated close to the vena cava.

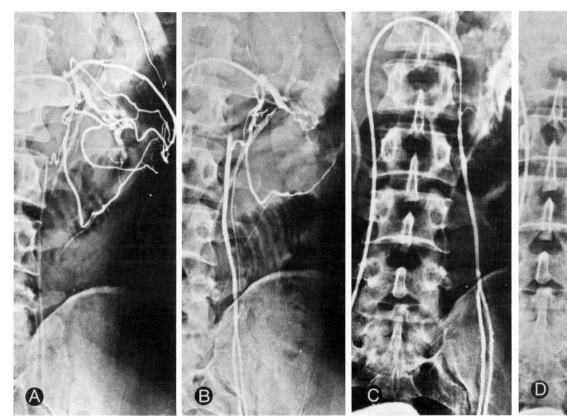

Fig. 7–19 Coaxial catheterization and embolization using F-curve instead of cobra catheter in patient with competent outlet valve and medially situated left spermatic vein. A. Diagnostic venography, early phase. Perirenal anastomoses bypass to distal part of spermatic vein, which is insufficient. B. A few seconds later, distal bifurcation and cranial lateral accompanying branch are revealed. The competent outlet valve could not be passed because distance from vena cava cannot be properly put ("streamlined") in outlet valve. At each attempt to pass valve with coaxial catheter, cobra recoiled. With F-curved catheter, 3F straight catheter, and 0.025-inch wire of the left spermatic set, competent valve is passed rather easily. C. Superselective venography via F-curve and coaxial catheter. Embolization is performed at junction of all branches (iliac crest). D. Control venography via F-curve catheter shows total occlusion of spermatic venous system at level of L4/5.

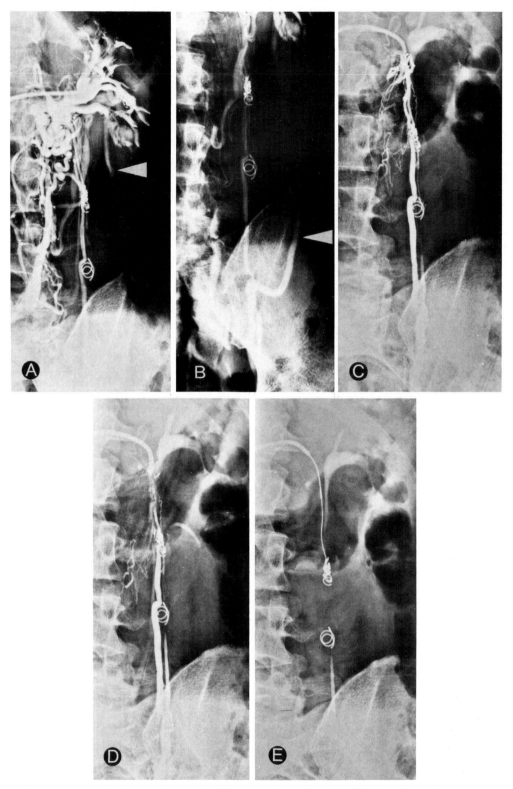

Fig. 7-20 Postoperative persistence of varicocele after surgical ligation and two sessions of coil embolization. A,B. Diagnostic renal
venography reveals huge renospermatic anastomosis (arrowheads)
that bypasses to the insufficient caudal part of spermatic vein and
shunts the coils. C,D. Superior coils (2 or 3 at level of L3) are unable
to withstand the bloodstream. Inferior coil (L4) is placed in a lateral,
smaller branch of bifurcation, leaving major medial branch open. E.
Superior coils block passage of coaxial catheter.

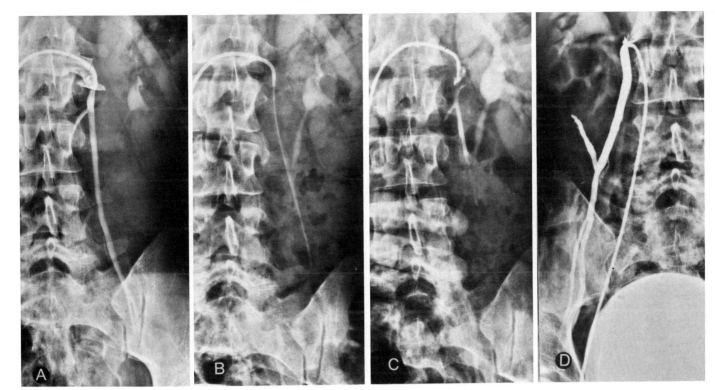

Fig. 7–21 In this patient, clinical persistence of left-sided varicocele after left-sided embolization is due to insufficiency of right spermatic vein together with intrascrotal collaterals. A. Diagnostic left venography shows distal bifurcations. B. Tip of coaxial catheter at site of superior bifurcation. C. Control venography after embolization shows complete occlusion at level of L3. D. Diagnostic right-sided venogram via cobra catheter clearly reveals reflux through bifurcated right spermatic vein, as well as presence of perirenal anastomosis. Right spermatic vein was not treated during the first session (see text). E. Control left venography 4 months later because of clinical persistence shows that occlusion is unchanged (arrowhead indicates spermatic occlusion lying upon ureter). Lumbar ascending vein is opacified. F–H. Right-sided venography with hooked catheter confirms the finding of D and shows right-sided varicocele with intrascrotal connections that fill left pampiniform plexus. Normally, the testicles are X-ray shielded with 1 mm lead and varicoceles are not depicted. I. Upon coaxial superselective venography, all branches are found to be connected at level of iliac crest. J. Embolization is performed at this level. K. Right venography shows complete occlusion.

2%), in whom a residual reflux was detected on the side embolized. In six, the embolized vessel was still occluded, but other insufficient vessels were found that had not been detected at the initial venography. These patients were treated by repeat embolization. Because four of these cases occurred in the first 76 patients treated, as against only two in the subsequent 359 cases, the authors concluded that systemic superselective venography has dramatically improved the results.

The authors registered only one patient with true persistence where the embolized vessel was found to be patent upon control venography. Repeat embolization of the same vessel cured the patient. Thus, persistence after IBCA embolization is rare and "recanalization" of the embolized vessel seems to be exceptional.

Complications and Technical Results

Usually, the patients express no complaints during or after the embolization procedure. Examination and treatment are performed under local anesthesia and on an outpatient basis. The obliteration using IBCA can be localized very selectively, and its site is always checked by superselective venography. By using coaxial catheters and stopping the blood circulation in the spermatic venous system, it is ascertained that the drug cannot reach the general circulation and that contact with the testis will not occur. Pain, thrombophlebitis, or hydrocele never occurred in the authors' patients.

Only two complications have occurred. In one man, the third case treated, the coaxial catheter was not pulled back immediately, and after a few minutes, it was found to be trapped in the embolus. In a 12-year-old boy who had already been operated on without success on the left side, the authors first embolized the persistent varicocele. Because reflux through the right spermatic vein was also detected, this side was embolized also. The right spermatic venous system consisted of at least four small, interconnected branches. The coaxial catheter was placed distally, partly wedged in one of the branches. During the injection of contrast medium, there was no clear runoff. Immediately after injection of the embolus, the catheter could not be removed because it was trapped in the embolus. At present, the authors consider such wedging with poor evacuation to be a contraindication to the injection of IBCA, and a better site for embolization must be selected. Both patients were immediately operated on and recovered uneventfully.

The high accuracy of this method is emphasized by the results achieved in the last 18-month period, during

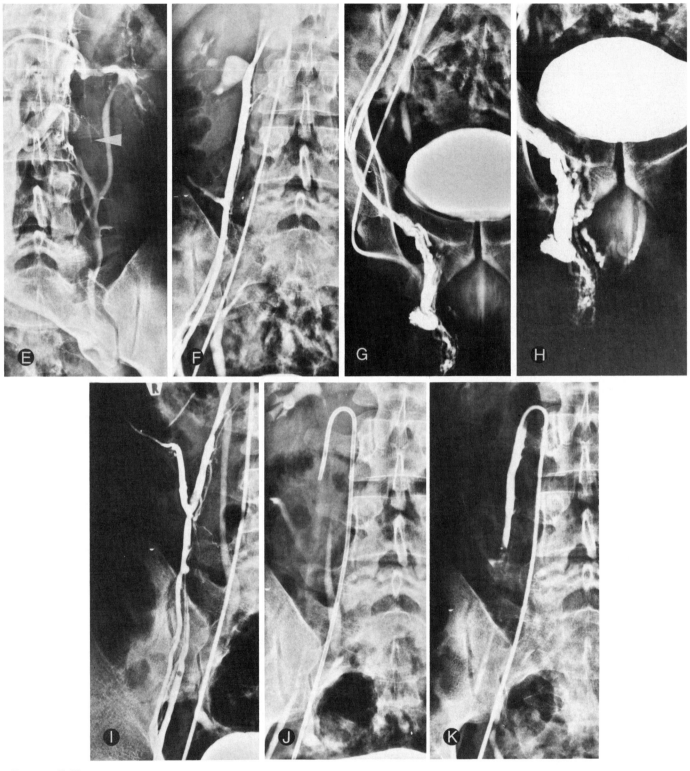

Fig. 7–21 E–K

which 140 patients were treated. Six of these had normal selective venograms. Of the 134 patients with abnormal venograms, six of whom had been operated on without success, only five patients (3.7%) could not be cured by embolization. All five had a left renospermatic bypass and a competent spermatic outlet valve that could not be passed by the coaxial catheter. Such a valve was found in

35% of the cases with left-sided varicoceles and could be passed in 90% of these. Thirty-two per cent of the patients presented with bilateral varicoceles, but only one patient had a unilateral right varicocele. All 43 right-sided varicoceles could be embolized. Eight of these patients had a renospermatic bypass together with a competent outlet valve.

EFFECT OF VARICOCELE TREATMENT ON SEMEN AND PREGNANCIES

Treatment of varicocele aims at repair of testicular function, namely recovery of fertility and normalization of androgen production. The latter was indeed observed in most of the men consulting the authors for sexual inadequacy and who presented with subnormal plasma testosterone concentration.[12] Slightly more than half of the couples who consulted for varicocele-associated infertility achieved pregnancy. The probability of success was 4% per cycle (Fig. 7–22). This is significantly better than the expected treatment-independent pregnancy rate, which is estimated to be no more than 1.5% per cycle. The causal relation between varicocele treatment and the occurrence of pregnancies is further substantiated by the observation that no significant improvement of semen quality occurred in men who were unsuccessful in impregnating their wives, whereas those who were successful did present a significant improvement.

The success rate of varicocele treatment was 60%–80% in men with normal testicular volume, below-average serum follicle-stimulating hormone (FSH) concentra-

tions, and moderate impairment of spermatogenesis. The success rate was moderate (20%–50%) in men combining varicocele with other pathology that may influence fertility and in patients with below-normal testicular volume and/or above-average mean serum FSH concentrations. The probability of conception was <20% if serum FSH concentration was grossly elevated, if testicular volume was severely reduced, if the man had circulating sperm antibodies, or if he had azoospermia (absence of spermatozoa in his ejaculate). The latter patients stand such poor chances of success that treatment probably should not be offered to them.[13]

References

1. Comhaire F, Simons M, Kunnen M, Vermeulen L: Testicular arterial perfusion in varicocele: the role of rapid sequence scintigraphy with technetium in varicocele evaluation. *J Urol* 1983;130:923

2. Ahlberg NE, Bartley O, Chidekel N, Fritjofson A: Phlebography in varicocele scroti. *Acta Radiol[Diagn]* 1966;4:517

3. Brown JS, Dubin L, Hotchkiss RS: The varicocele as related to fertility. *Fertil Steril* 1967;18:46

4. Hiel JT, Green NA: Varicocele: a review of radiological and anatomical features in relation to surgical treatment. *Br J Surg* 1977;64:747

5. Comhaire F, Kunnen M: Selective retrograde venography of the internal spermatic vein: a conclusive approach to the diagnosis of varicocele. *Andrologia* 1976;8:11

6. Comhaire F, Kunnen M: The value of scrotal thermography as compared with selective retrograde venography of the internal spermatic vein for the diagnosis of "subclinical" varicocele. *Fertil Steril* 1976;27:694

7. Kunnen M: Neue technik zur Embolisation der Vena spermatica interna: intravenöser Gewebekleber. *Fortschr Röntgenstr* 1980;133:625

8. Kunnen M: Traitement des varicocèles par embolisation à l'isobutyl-2-cyanoacrylate. *Ann Radiol* 1981;64:406

9. Kunnen M: Nonsurgical cure of varicocele by transcatheter embolization of the internal spermatic vein with bucrylate, in Zeitler E, Jecht E: *Varicocele and Male Infertility (Recent Advances in Diagnostic and Therapy).* Berlin, Springer–Verlag, 1982, p 153

10. Kunnen M, Comhaire F: Transcatheter embolization of the internal spermatic vein(s) with Bucrylate: further improvments. *Ann Radiol* 1984;27:303

11. Weissbach L, Thelen M, Adolphs HD: Treatment of idiopathic varicoceles by transfemoral testicular vein occlusion. *J Urol* 1981;126:354–

12. Comhaire F, Vermeulen A: Plasma testosterone in patients with varicocele and sexual inadequacy. *J Clin Endocrinol Metab* 1975;40:824

13. Comhaire F, Kunnen M: Factors affecting the fertility outcome after treatment of subfertile men with varicocele by transcatheter embolization with Bucrylate. *Fertil Steril* 1985; 43:781

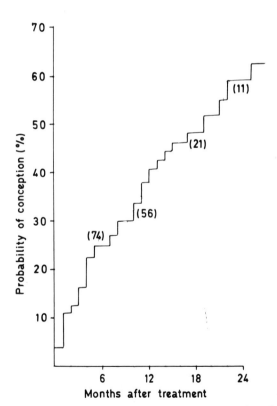

Fig. 7–22 Cumulative probability of pregnancy related to the time elapsed after treatment in a group of 100 couples with varicocele-associated infertility. The numbers in parentheses indicate the number of couples under follow-up at 6, 12, 18, and 24 months.

8

Ferromagnetic Microembolization for Treatment of Hepatocellular Carcinoma

MASAO SAKO, M.D.

Transcatheter arterial embolization is one of the most reliable adjuncts for the treatment of well-localized neoplasms. Various occlusive agents have been used, most of which primarily obliterate major feeding arteries rather than small peripheral vessels. As a result, collateral circulation to the distal vascular bed subsequently develops, thus reducing the therapeutic effects of the embolization.

For optimal tumor infarction, occlusive agents must be small enough to reach the precapillary vascular bed of the tumor but too large to stray into the venous vascular bed through tumoral arteriovenous communications. To serve this purpose, the ferromagnetic effect has been investigated to try to entrap small iron particles within the target vessels.[1-4]

REAGENTS AND EQUIPMENT

Ferropolysaccharide

Ferropolysaccharide (FPS) is a dark gray, viscous, aqueous suspension of iron microspheres (Fig. 8–1). The particles are pure (99.99%) iron, 10–30 μm in diameter, with numerous micropores (Iron Metal Sponge; Wako Pure Chemical Industries, Ltd). The polysaccharide solution consists of 14% dextran 40, and 2% sodium carboxymethyl cellulose in saline. Dextran 40 is a popular plasma expander that can be excreted by the kidneys (mol wt: 40,000). Sodium carboxymethyl cellulose, a nontoxic polysaccharide (mol wt: 60,000–80,000), is widely used as a protective colloid for food, cosmetics, and medicines and is added to increase the dispersion of the iron particles. The pH of the solution is 5.1. For storage, 20 ml of the polysaccharide solution and 1 g of the iron sponge are sterilized in glass ampules by autoclaving. Before use, 1 g of the iron sponge is suspended homogeneously in 10 ml of polysaccharide solution by thorough shaking for a few minutes in a sterile test tube.

Microembolization with FPS works by macroaggregation of the iron particles: when exposed to a strong magnetic field, they become magnetized and subsequently exert a magnetic force on each other, forming larger conglomerates of particles, which grow by aggregating with fibrin in the blood until occlusion occurs.[4] The high molecular weight polysaccharide solution lowers the velocity of blood flow, allowing the viscous medium to adhere to some degree to the vascular intima, where the iron particles can be held while they aggregate progressively in the magnetic field. The iron particles can be demonstrated within the vessels by computed tomography (CT) examinations as a high-density striated pattern. The autopsy specimen of a patient who died from hepatic failure due to severe cirrhosis 1 year after treatment showed that small vessels around the lesion were still filled with aggregated iron particles, indicating long-term or permanent vascular occlusion.[4]

If excessive doses of FPS are injected, the aggregated iron particles will occlude, at the proximal subsegmental or segmental level, the arteries feeding not only neoplastic tissue, but also normal liver tissue. However, liver infarction does not necessarily occur, as demonstrated by CT examination, if portal blood flow was normal before embolization.

The Magnetic Device

Early experimental studies have shown the optimal magnetic intensity for microembolization with FPS to be about 300 gauss; a magnetic intensity of >500 gauss causes occlusion of vessels >400 μm in diameter (Fig. 8–2).[5]

A box-shaped, 10 × 10 × 5 cm, rare earth–cobalt magnet (Toshiba Corporation) is used. It can be placed over any part of the body surface by using an antimagnetic holder attached to the angiographic table (Fig. 8–3). The magnetic field intensity curves at various distances (Fig. 8–4) indicate that 300 gauss can be exerted at a depth of 10 cm.

Care should be taken to prevent a magnetic effect on the fluoroscopic units, because use of a strong magnet close to an image intensifier temporarily or permanently distorts the image. To prevent this, before the magnet is activated, the patient is moved at least 1 m away from the image intensifier. This has the disadvantage that fluoroscopic observation is not available during FPS injection. An antimagnetic fluoroscopic unit is now available commercially for observation during the injection.

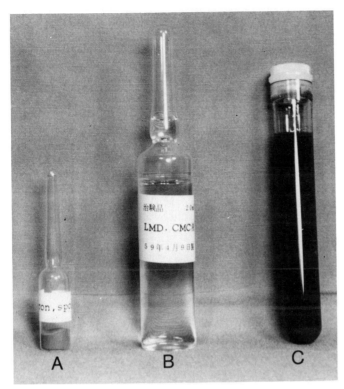

Fig. 8–1 Ferropolysaccharide: iron sponge microspheres (30–50 μm) (A) and viscous polysaccharide solution (B) were each enclosed in glass ampules and sterilized. Prior to use, 1 g of the particles was homogeneously suspended in 10 ml of polysaccharide solution by thorough shaking for a few minutes in a sterilized test tube (C).

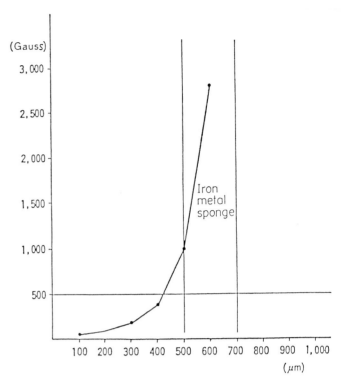

Fig. 8-2 Relation between magnet intensity and size of vessel occluded.

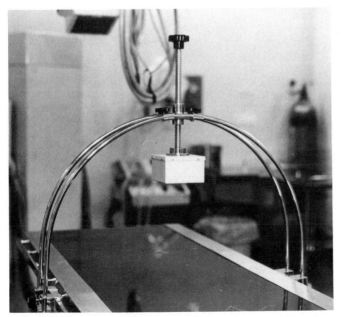

Fig. 8–3 The magnetic device: a box-shaped, rare earth–cobalt magnet (3000 gauss) can be placed on any part of the body surface by using an antimagnetic steel holder attached to the angiographic table.

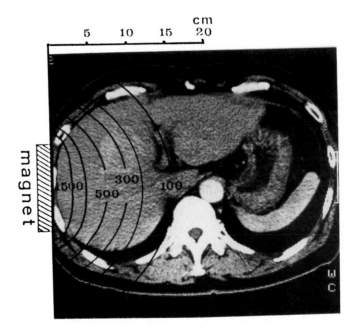

Fig. 8–4 The magnetic field strength curves at various distances. Before embolization, the strength curves were projected on the CT image of a patient to obtain optimal positioning of the magnet.

CLINICAL APPLICATIONS OF FERROMAGNETIC MICROEMBOLIZATION TO PATIENTS WITH HEPATOCELLULAR CARCINOMA

Technique

Forty-five ferromagnetic microembolization (FME) procedures have been performed in 25 men and 5 women aged 37–81 years with unresectable hepatocellular carcinoma. In 15 patients, embolization was repeated as many as 4 times (mean total: 2.5 treatments). The diagnosis was established by biopsy, autopsy, or clinical examination such as angiography and α-fetoprotein assay.

Before the embolization, preliminary celiac and superior mesenteric arteriography is carried out to identify the feeding arteries as well as to evaluate the extent of the tumor and the presence or absence of portal vein involvement. If the portal trunk or the right or left main branch of the portal vein is occluded, embolization is contraindicated. If portal vein patency is demonstrated, superselective catheterization is done with a soft, long (3–10-cm), tapered 6.5F catheter (inner diameter: 1.4 mm). If the tumor is located in the right lobe of the liver, the catheter tip is advanced beyond the origin of the cystic artery to avoid gallbladder infarction; for lesions in the left lobe of the liver, the catheter tip is introduced into the left hepatic artery.

After selective catheterization has been achieved, the patient is moved away from the angiographic table to avoid damage to the image intensifier by the magnet. The magnet is then positioned and activated over the area of interest, and FPS is injected slowly through the catheter. After completion of the injection, the catheter is rinsed with 2–3 ml of saline, and the magnet is left in place for 10 min.

The dose of FPS depends on the size and vascularity of the tumors; 1–2 ml is routinely injected initially, and the need for additional injections is determined by fluoroscopic evaluation of hepatic blood flow or by repeat angiography. Usually, tumors of 5–6 cm in diameter require 3–4 ml of FPS. When necessary, FME was repeated in a subsequent session in the same manner.

Evaluation of Therapeutic Effect

The therapeutic effect of embolization of hepatic tumors is generally evaluated by tumor markers, ultrasonography, CT, and angiography. However, determination of tumor extent, including size, presence of small (<1 cm) metastatic nodules, recanalization, and development of collateral circulation, can be done accurately only by angiography.

Angiograms are studied for tumor type (solitary, sharply defined lesion; multinodular (more than two sharply defined lesions), infiltration (ill-defined lesions), and mixed), extent (number of feeding vessels, rated T1 to T4), vascularity (+ to +++), size of tumor stain (width × length), portal vein involvement (of main branch of the right or left lobe (P3), of a first-order branch (P2), of a second-order branch (P1), or of a third-order or more peripheral branch (P0)), and presence of intrahepatic metastases (d) (Fig. 8–5). For example, an ill-defined lesion with two feeding vessels, considerable vascularity, involvement of a main branch of the portal vein, and intrahepatic metastases would be classified as infiltrative T2, ++, P3, d, and the extent of the tumor stain in centimeters would be specified.

Regression of the primary tumor is evaluated by comparing tumor stain before and after embolization. The degree of tumor regression is divided into three categories: "good," when there is complete disappearance or >50% decrease in tumor size, "moderate" (between 25% and 50% regression), and "poor" (<25% regression).

RESULTS

Primary Tumor Regression

A good result was noted in 13 cases, including 9 in which there was complete disappearance of the tumor stain (Fig. 8–6A,B). Moderate results were seen in 5 patients and poor results in 7 (Table 8–1).

The relation between primary tumor regression and angiographic findings is shown in Table 8–2. In the patients with good and moderate results (77%–80% of the cases), tumors were localized within a segment (T1), and 60%–100% had portal vein involvement limited to third-order branches (P0). The tumors in these groups were for

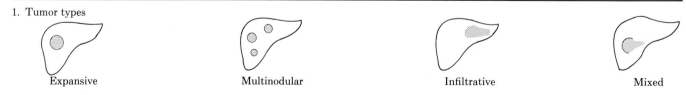

1. Tumor types

    Expansive   Multinodular   Infiltrative   Mixed

2. Tumor extent: T1~T4 (no. of involved segment)
3. Tumor vascularity: (+)~(+++)
4. Tumor stain: size (width × length cm)
5. Portal involvement: P0~P3 (main trunk)
6. Intrahepatic metastases: d

Fig. 8–5 Angiographic classification of hepatocellular carcinoma as tumor factors.

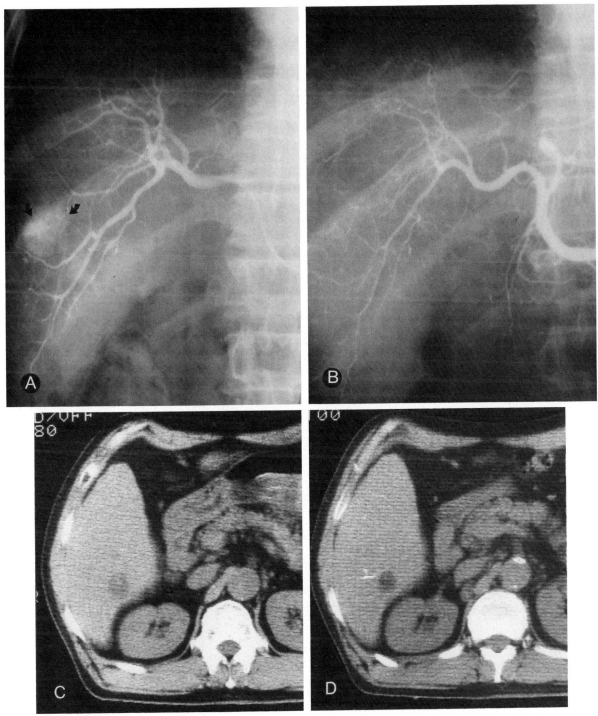

Fig. 8–6   A 54-year-old man with hepatoma in posterior segment of right lobe. A. Angiographic tumor characteristics: large vascular mass in right lobe of the liver with dense tumor stain (arrows). Ferromagnetic microembolization with 3 ml of FPS. B. Follow-up angiography performed 10 months after embolization shows no tumor stain (*i.e.,* primary tumor regression "marked"). C. CT scan before embolization shows sharply defined, round, low-density area at posterior segment of right lobe. D. CT scan 10 months after procedure shows diminution in both density and size of mass. Aggregated iron particles are visible as high-density striated pattern (arrow) without any abnormal density on the normal parenchyma to indicate infarction. Unfortunately, patient died of rupture of esophageal varices 45 months after embolization.

Table 8-1 Angiographic Comparison of Tumor Size Before and After Ferromagnetic Microembalization

Degrees of Tumor Diminution	No. of Cases	Angiographic Evaluation of Primary Effect
Disappearance	9 (36%)	Marked
More than 50%	4 (16%)	Marked
25%–50%	5 (20%)	Moderate
Less than 25%	7 (28%)	Poor

[a]Angiography performed 2–5 months after ferromagnetic microembolization.

Table 8-2 Relation between Primary Effect and Tumor factors

Tumor Factors	Primary Effect (%)		
	Marked Group (13)	Moderate Group (5)	Poor Group (7)
Extent			
T1	77	80	29
T2	15	20	57
T3	8		14
Portal involvement			
P0	100	60	29
P1		40	29
P2			42
Tumor types			
Expansive	39	60	29
Multinodular	38	40	
Infiltrative			29
Mixed	23		42

the most part sharply demarcated, either solitary or multiple. In contrast, the group with poor results had tumors that were >T2 in 71% of cases, with portal vein involvement of >P1 in 71%. The degree of vascularity had no relation to the frequency of primary tumor regression. Intrahepatic metastases were present in 14 cases, and in

10 disappearance or marked diminution in number and size occurred (Fig. 8–7).

Development of collateral bypassing circulation was observed in only three patients, one with infiltrative and two with mixed-type hepatomas, in whom the extrahepatic collaterals developed from duodenal, omental, and subphrenic arteries. In these cases, the results were poor (Fig. 8–8).

It is difficult to compare the frequency of recanalization with the results of other vaso-occlusive agents, because FME is used with the intention of occluding peripheral intraparenchymal tumor vessels. In fact, 44% of the patients had occlusion only of the tumor vasculature. The remaining 14 patients showed occlusion of subsegmental or segmental arteries, probably because of injection of excessive amounts of FPS. Of these 14 cases, 8 showed recanalization.

Cumulative Survival Rates

The cumulative survival rate calculated by the Kaplan–Mayer method was 65.4% at 1 year and 52% in 2 years. In 18 patients with tumors <5 cm in diameter, the survival rate was 82.5% at 1 year and 68.5% at 2 years (Fig. 8–9).

Primary tumor regression correlated well with the survival rates (Fig. 8–10). The 1-year survival rate in patients with good and moderate results was 77%–80%, and five patients survived for >2 years. In these cases, the tumors were T1, P0, and either solitary or multinodular. In contrast, the 1-year survival rate for the poor results group was only 33%.

Six patients died within 1 year, two of them due to rupture of esophageal varices. In the remaining four, the tumor characteristics were: T2, P0, multinodular; T2, P2, solitary; T2, P1, infiltrative; and T3, P2, mixed. Primary tumor regression was poor in three and moderate in one.

Tumor vascularity and intrahepatic metastases did not correlate with the 1- and 2-year survival rates.

POSTEMBOLIZATION SYMPTOMS AND SEROLOGIC DATA

The most common postembolization symptoms were abdominal pain of various intensities and abdominal distension. Pain usually subsides within 24–48 hr with the administration of sedatives and analgesics. Fever (37.5–39° C) was noted in 95% of the patients and lasted for 3–

7 days. The patients with fever >38° C were usually given steroids and antipyretics. Serum liver enzymes, total bilirubin, and albumin all increased transiently. However, all the concentrations returned to the preembolization levels within 1–2 weeks (Fig. 8–11).

DISCUSSION

Hepatocellular carcinoma is one of the most common tumors in Japan. Unfortunately, it is often unresectable because of advanced cirrhosis. In such cases, hepatic embolization, usually with Gelfoam, has been widely used, with 1- and 2-year survival rates of 44% and 29%, respectively.[6] With FME, better survival rates are obtained: 65% at 1 year and 52% at 2 years. This improved survival has several causes, including microembolization of tumor vessels, with histologically proven widespread tumor necrosis (Fig. 8–12); long-acting or per-

manent occlusion; rare collateral formation; no reflux of particles; reliable effects on small (<5 mm) lesions; and ease of repeat embolization.

Collateral formation has been reported in 65%–80% of cases after embolization with Gelfoam due to primary occlusion of major feeding arteries. This makes repeat embolization difficult, yet this procedure is considered essential to improve survival rates in patients with hepatocellular carcinoma. In contrast, FME has prevented the development of collaterals from both intrahepatic and

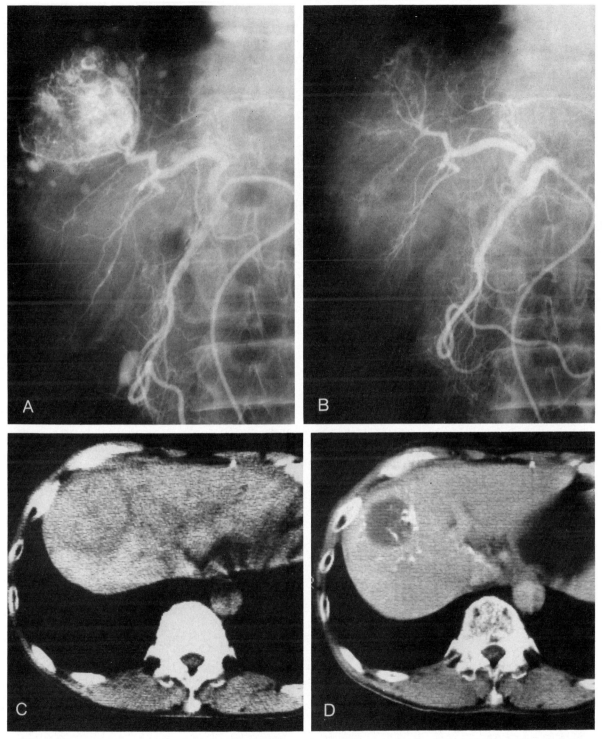

Fig. 8–7 A 62-year-old man with hepatoma. A. Preliminary angiography reveals hepatoma in anterior segment of right lobe. Angiographic tumor characteristics: expansive, T1, + + + vascularity, 6 × 6-cm stain, P1, and multiple 3–20-mm intrahepatic metastases. Embolization with 5 ml of FPS. B. Follow-up angiography 2 months after embolization shows almost complete disappearance of tumor vessels, stain, and minute (<5-mm) intrahepatic metastases, while normal hepatic arteries, which had been distributed along the lesion, remain encircled. C. CT scan before embolization shows round mass in right lobe. D. Scan made 3 months after embolization reveals markedly diminished density and size of mass, indicating widespread necrosis. Scattered, aggregated iron particles noted around and within the lesion. Patient lived for 34 months.

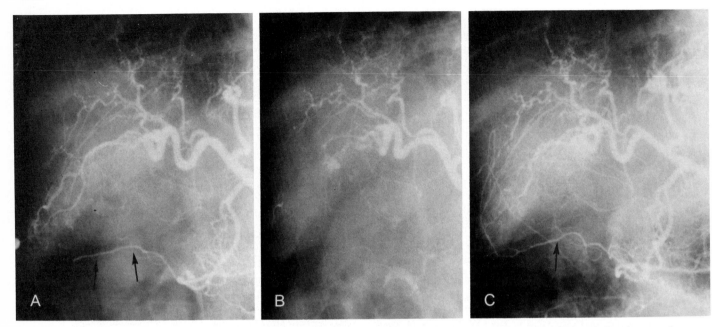

Fig. 8–8 A 65-year old man. A. Preliminary angiograms reveal hepatoma with ill-defined margin in posterior segment of right lobe.
Extrahepatic collaterals from both omental and duodenal branches
are noted. Superior mesenteric arteriography revealed occlusion of
the first-order portal branch. Thus, tumor factors are: infiltrative,
T1, + + + vascularity, 3 × 8-cm stain, P2. Embolization with 5 ml
of FPS. B. Angiograms immediately after embolization reveal complete disappearance of tumor vessels and stain. C. Angiograms 3
months later show development of extrahepatic collaterals and recanalization of posterior segmental artery to feed the tumor, which has
grown slightly. Embolization with FPS was repeated. Patient lived 7
months after repeat embolization.

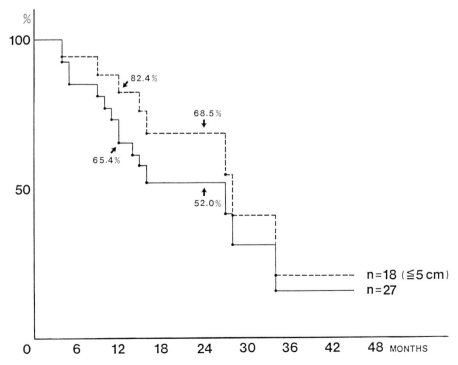

Fig. 8–9 Cumulative survival rate.

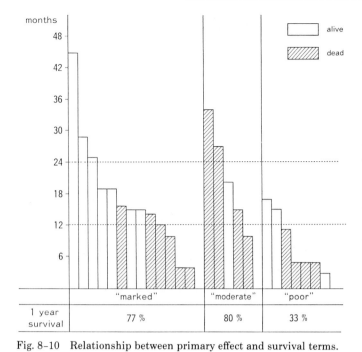

Fig. 8–10 Relationship between primary effect and survival terms.

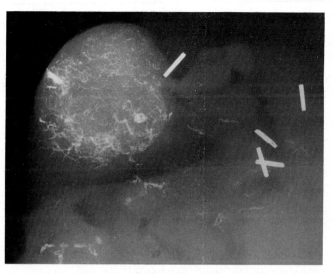

Fig. 8–12 Low-kilovolt soft-tissue examination of specimen resected after ferromagnetic microembolization; note widespread occlusion of tumor vessels with aggregated iron particles. Histologic examination confirmed necrosis throughout the lesion.

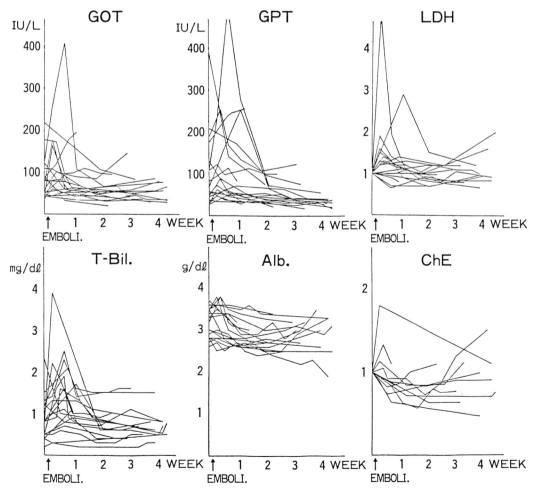

Fig. 8–11 Serologic data after ferromagnetic microembolization. GOT, glutamic oxaloacetic transaminase; GPT, glutamic pyruvic transaminase; LDS, lactate dehydrogenase; T-Bil, total bilirublin; Alb, albumin.

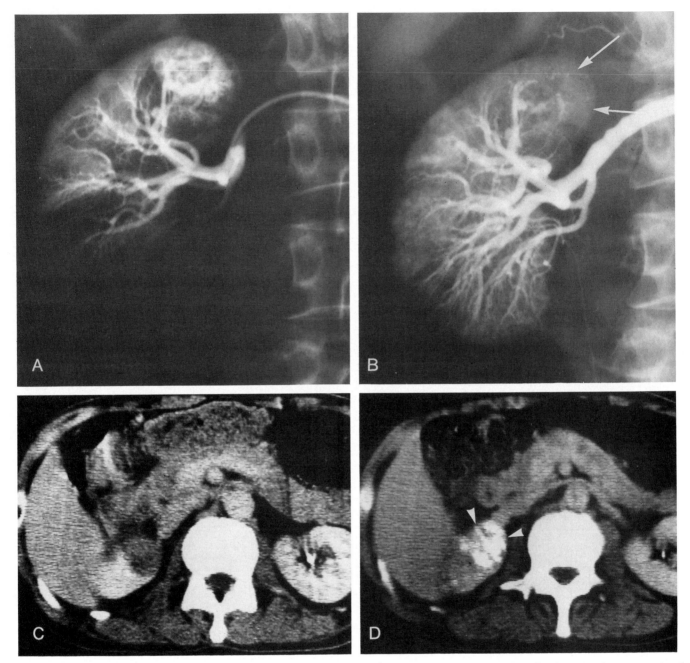

Fig. 8-13 A 51-year-old man with renal cell carcinoma. A. Preliminary angiography reveals tumor in ventral segment of right kidney. B. Angiograms immediately after embolization with 6 ml of FPS show almost complete disappearance of tumor vessels. C. Pre-embolization CT scan demonstrates low-density mass in upper pole of right kidney. D. Plain CT film obtained 10 days later shows aggregated iron particles as scattered high-density areas corresponding to the lesion. Histologic examination confirmed widespread necrosis.

extrahepatic pathways in 88% of patients. An additional procedure was easily performed when required, since major feeding arteries were commonly (76%) patent.

It is well known that distal embolization with small particles is more effective against tumors than is occlusion of proximal vessels with other types of agents. However, small particles are more prone to reflux into proximal arteries, causing undesirable infarction of the gallbladder or pancreas, even if the injection is made at a peripheral level. An FPS embolization utilizing 30–50-μm particles provides sufficient microembolization, with

reflux of particles being prevented by the use of external magnetic control.

One of the disadvantages of FME is the need for a superselective catheterization to avoid gallbladder infarction. If catheterization of target vessels is not successful due to anatomic variations or to arteriosclerosis, FME must be forgone in favor of Gelfoam embolization. To extend the indications of this procedure, new devices or techniques to permit superselective catheterization will be required.

In addition to its use for hepatic embolization, FME

has been applied to eight patients with renal cell carcinoma (Fig. 8–13) and one patient with advanced lung cancer, resulting in excellent tumor infarction. No severe complications or abnormal serologic data due to FME were observed.[8,9]

In summary, FME provides widespread microembolization of tumors with reliable, excellent therapeutic effect and without any undesirable reactions by the normal organs. In general, the therapeutic effect of FME on hepatocellular carcinoma depends on tumor characteristics: tumors of the mixed and infiltrative types are less susceptible than those of the sharply localized type.[10,11] In addition, the therapeutic effects are less prominent in the presence of portal vein involvement. To overcome this limitation, chemoembolotherapy is being tested.[12] In addition, induction heating (hyperthermia) of the magnetic particles placed in the target lesion can be used for selective heating of the lesions.[13] This induction heating is still in the experimentation stage, but recent results look promising for use in clinical practice.

In conclusion, the author considers FME to be one of the most reliable potential methods for extending the capability of interventional radiology in oncologic patients.

References

1. Mosso JA, Rand WR: Ferromagnetic silicone vascular occlusion: a technique for selective infarction of tumors and organs. *Ann Surg* 1973;178:663
2. Albrechtsson U, Hansson GA, Olin T: Vascular occlusion with a ferromagnetic particles suspension: an experimental investigation in rabbits. *Acta Radiol [Diagn]* 1977;18:279
3. Barry JW, Bookstein JJ, Alksne JF: Ferromagnetic embolization: experimental evaluation. *Radiology* 1981;138:341
4. Sako M, Yokogawa S, Sakamoto K, et al: Transcatheter microembolization with ferropolysaccharide: a new approach to ferromagnetic embolization of tumors (preliminary report). *Invest Radiol* 1982;17:573
5. Sako M, Ohtsuki S, Arai M, et al: Cancer therapy by ferromagnetic microembolization: studies on a new electromagnetic device. *J Jpn Soc Cancer Ther* 1983;18:92
6. Yamada R, Sato M, Kawabata M, et al: Hepatic artery embolization in 120 patients with unresectable hepatoma. *Radiology* 1983;148:397
7. Yuri H, Sako M: Ferromagnetic microembolization in the treatment of metastatic tumors of the liver. *J Jpn Soc Cancer Ther* 1984;19:50
8. Hirota S, Sako M: Experimental and clinical study of ferromagnetic microembolization for a treatment of malignant tumors. *J Jpn Soc Cancer Ther* 1982;17:1936
9. Morita M, Sako M: Experimental and clinical studies on embolotherapy of lung cancer. *J Jpn Soc Cancer Ther* 1985;20:71
10. Sato M: Experimental and clinical studies on the hepatic artery embolization for treatment of hepatoma. *Nippon Acta Radiol* 1983;43:977
11. Nakashima T: Vascular changes and hemodynamics in hepatocellular carcinoma, in Okuda K, Peter R (eds): *Hepatocellular Carcinoma.* New York, John Wiley & Sons, 1976, p 169
12. Sako M, Shimizu T, Hirota S, et al: Intraarterial infusion therapy with polysaccharide solution as a carrier of anticancer drugs. *Nippon Acta Radiol* 1985;45:26
13. Sako M, Morita M, Ohtsuki S, et al: Studies on selective embolohyperthermic therapy of tumors by using ferromagnetic particles. *J Jpn Soc Cancer Ther* 1984;19:2168

9

Vasoactive Drugs and Embolotherapy in the Management of Gastrointestinal Bleeding

JOHN F. CARDELLA, M.D., S. MURTHY TADAVARTHY, M.D., FLAVIO CASTAÑEDA, M.D., CAROL C. COLEMAN, M.D., GUNNAR LUND, M.D., TONY P. SMITH, M.D., MICHAEL D. DARCY, M.D., DAVID W. HUNTER, M.D., ANDREW H. CRAGG, M.D., AND WILFRIDO R. CASTAÑEDA-ZUÑIGA, M.D., M.Sc.

No aspect of angiographic and interventional radiology can be at once so frustrating and so gratifying as the diagnosis and therapy of gastrointestinal bleeding. This chapter considers the use of vasoactive drugs and embolotherapy for this purpose. The preceding chapters review embolotherapy in more detail.

The literature has an abundance of estimates of how briskly a patient must bleed for it to be detectable angiographically, ranging from 0.5–3.0 ml/min (1.5–9 units/24 hr).[1-4] The authors' experience has shown that bleeding of 1.5–2.0 ml/min (4–6 units/24 hr) is usually detectable, whereas less rapid bleeding is difficult to detect. The other component of detectability is constancy, *i.e.*, the patient must be bleeding during the angiographic run.

NONINVASIVE DIAGNOSTIC EVALUATION

Radionuclide studies using tagged red blood cells have enhanced the ability to detect and document gastrointestinal (GI) bleeding with an image.[5-17] However, although these studies are useful for confirmation of slow oozing and widely spaced intermittent episodes by virtue of their high sensitivity, they contribute little information about etiology because of their poor specificity. Nevertheless, if properly performed with carefully timed scans, the site of bleeding can be placed at least in the proper quadrant of the abdomen and frequently in the stomach, small bowel, or colon (Fig. 9–1), and this information can guide the angiographer in the search for the actual site of extravasation.

OVERVIEW OF PHARMACOTHERAPY

Once a bleeding site has been identified, recent progress in occlusive therapy allows the angiographer to step from diagnostician to therapist.[18-28] Transcatheter treatment for GI bleeding includes pharmacologic agents and embolic materials. The mainstay of pharmacologic control is vasopressin (Pitressin). Epinephrine, which was used in early trials, is seldom used now.

Vasopressin can be administered intravenously without diagnostic arteriography or empirically when no bleeding site is located to produce a systemic vasoconstrictive effect to slow or arrest bleeding. Doses are 1000–2000 units/hr, with administration being continued for 48 hr if the patient shows decreased melena-hematemesis, decreasing blood transfusion requirements, and stabilized hemodynamics. If 48 hr of intravenous vasopressin produces no slowing in the rate of GI blood loss, the drug should be discontinued, because further administration is unlikely to be successful.

Intra-arterial vasopressin can be used effectively immediately after arteriogrqaphy when a bleeding site is identified.[26-31] Although ideally the drug is delivered selectively into the bleeding branch, when selective catheterization is not possible, delivery into the superior or inferior mesenteric artery is adequate. The danger in nonselective delivery is, of course, constrictive bowel ischemia.[32,33] The currently recommended intra-arterial dose is 0.2 unit/min initially. If, after 20–30 min of infusion, repeat arteriography shows no vasoconstrictive effect, the dose should be doubled to 0.4 unit/min. Higher doses are seldom required. Intra-arterial infusion is continued until angiographic evidence of vasoconstriction is seen or until bleeding stops. Patients then leave the procedure room with the arterial catheter in place and the infusion running by means of a pump (Harvard pump) capable of generating suprasystemic pressure. Generally, patients undergo follow-up angiography 12–24 hr after the infusion was started. At that time, if bleeding has been arrested clinically and angiographically, the vasoconstrictor is slowly withdrawn by reducing the dose every 6–8 hr over a 12–24-hr period. When the vasoconstrictor infusion has been discontinued, the catheter is left in place and kept open with an infusion of 5% dextrose or lactated Ringer's solution so that one will be prepared in the event bleeding necessitates restarting the infusion. If all goes well and bleeding remains arrested, the catheter is removed at a convenient time. Success rates for intra-arterial vasopressin infusions are between 65% and 85%, depending on the size of the bleeding vessel.[31-33] Most investigators contend that intra-arterial vasopressin is more effective than intravenous systemic therapy, even with the lower doses allowed by selective delivery.

Epinephrine was also given intra-arterially for pharmacotherapy of GI bleeding in the early experience.[32,33] Its alpha-agonist properties caused vasoconstriction of the splanchnic bed, but its beta-agonist properties caused chronotropic cardiac effects, which were a problem in some patients during long-term infusion. The reported dosages for epinephrine are:

1 mg/kg/min infused into the celiac trunk in dogs[32];

8–16 mg/min for the left gastric, gastroduodenal, or inferior mesenteric arteries in humans;

20–30 mg/min for the celiac or superior mesenteric arteries of humans.[33]

Because of the cardiac effects of epinephrine, it has been supplanted by vasopressin in most medical centers.

OVERVIEW OF EMBOLOTHERAPY

Alternatively, GI bleeding can be arrested by embolotherapy with various temporary or permanent materials. Bleeding from transient lesions—such as ulcers, erosions, diverticula, spontaneous leaks, and traumatic tears—requires embolization with temporary materials to get the patient through the acute episode and then to permit vessel recanalization so that organ function loss in minimized. On the other hand, bleeding resulting from tumors, arteriovenous malformations (AVMs), large areas of angiodysplasia, and varices that will not heal spontaneously requires permanent embolization, both to control the immediate bleeding problems and as definitive therapy for the underlying pathologic process.

Temporary embolic agents include Gelfoam in powder and pieces[18-20] and autologous blood clot.[24,25,34,35] Gelfoam is prepared as a suspension in dilute contrast medium to facilitate viewing as the particles are deposited. The particle size is chosen on the basis of the pathology of the lesion and the size of the vessels requiring embolization; the general principle is to deposit the smallest particles that arrest bleeding and to deposit them as far peripherally as possible. The authors typically "backpack" a vessel with larger particles as the catheter is withdrawn.

Autologous blood clot is an agent mainly of historical interest[24,25]; particle (clot) size is difficult to control, the clots tend to sludge in the catheter because of their gelatinous nature, and deranged coagulation status in the patient makes clot induction difficult in some cases.

Permanent embolic agents are more numerous and include polyvinyl alcohol (Ivalon), coils, balloons, polymers and glues, alcohol, and hot contrast medium. The first two are characteristically used for bleeding in the GI tract; the last four are not used because the far distal occlusion they produce may induce wall ischemia.[36] Ivalon is prepared in a slurry with 2:2:1 contrast medium, albumin, and high molecular weight dextran (e.g., 20 ml of contrast, 20 ml of albumin, 10 ml of dextran).[37] Enough Ivalon particles are then added to make a slurry that will pass through the catheter without occluding it. The small size of the Ivalon powder (0.5-mm diameter) provides good end-organ embolization; injection of powder can be followed by Ivalon particles 1.0–2.0 mm in diameter for occlusion of small feeding branches. For bleeding resulting from a large AVM or tumor that has caused hypertrophy of the feeding artery(ies), the authors have used Ivalon powder followed by 3-, 5-, or 8-mm GWC coils, a combination that gives excellent permanent embolization.

Whether temporary or permanent embolotherapy is chosen, a postembolization angiogram must be obtained to document arrest of bleeding, because clinical signs are not accurate. The colon, in particular, can continue to clear melanotic stool long after active bleeding has been stopped. Theoretically, the catheter could be left in place after embolization, as with infusions of vasopressin, but the authors do not do this routinely because of the thrombogenicity of that foreign body and the need for intensive care unit (ICU) monitoring of a patient with an arterial catheter in place.

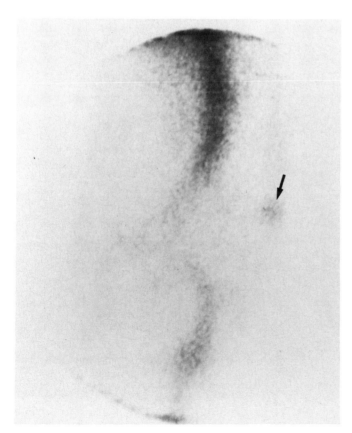

Fig. 9–1 Nuclear medicine scan with tagged red blood cells shows accumulation of radionuclide activity in left flank (arrow).

INDICATIONS FOR INTERVENTION

Gastrointestinal bleeding can be caused by a wide variety of lesions that may be located anywhere from the esophagus to the anus. The next section of this chapter discusses specific bleeding entities from a pathophysiologic and therapeutic approach.

Mallory–Weiss Esophageal Tears

Spontaneous rupture of the esophagus is uncommon and most often is caused by severe coughing or vomiting, particularly in alcoholic patients; presumably, an existing weakness in the esophageal wall ruptures under the increased intraesophageal pressure. Typically, the lower third of the esophagus ruptures longitudinally along its posterolateral wall. The symptoms include sudden onset of excruciating epigastric and left-sided chest pain radiating to the back. Pneumothorax or hydropneumothorax, particularly on the left side, and pneumomediastinum are worrisome radiographic findings in a patient with the symptoms described. Frequently, the patients present in shock of sudden onset. Many patients have profound hematemesis.

The arterial blood supply of the esophagus is complex. The primary supply of the cervical portion is from the terminal branches of the inferior thyroid artery, which gives rise to multiple ascending and descending esophageal branches. The inferior thyroidal arteries, in turn, originate from the left and right subclavian arteries. There is considerable variability in the arterial supply to the esophagus, with accessory cervical esophageal arteries originating from the subclavian, carotid, and vertebral arteries as well as from the ascending pharyngeal and caudal cervical trunk.

The thoracic segment of the esophagus receives arterial blood from the bronchial arteries, the aorta, and the right intercostal arteries. Bronchial artery patterns are variable, but the most common pattern is two left and one right bronchial arteries (about 50% of individuals). Other variations include one right and one left (25% of the population), two right and two left (15% of the population), and one left and two right bronchial arteries (8% of the population). A few instances of three right and three left bronchial arteries have been described.

There are two direct aortic branches to the esophagus, which are unpaired. The superiormost branch is 3–4 cm long and usually arises from the aorta at the T6 or T7 level. The inferior aortic branch is longer, measuring 6–7 cm, and arises at the T7 to T8 level.

The abdominal portion of the esophagus receives its blood supply from branches of the left gastric, short gastrics, and left inferior phrenic arteries. The complex arterial supply to the esophagus and its segmental nature make selective arterial embolization of the esophagus possible, particularly in cases of refractory bleeding from Mallory–Weiss tears.

The angiographic evaluation of a Mallory–Weiss tear requires a methodical search for esophageal branches, first in the brachiocephalic vessels, then progressively down the thoracic aorta, and finally into the celiac axis to locate any arterial bleeding in the distal esophagus (Fig. 9–2).

Variable success has been achieved with embolization of esophageal bleeding from Mallory–Weiss tears.[38–40] Because of the multiple sources of arterial bleeding, successful embolization of bleeding lesions may be difficult if collateral pathways can deliver blood to the bleeding site. If a definite site of bleeding can be identified angiographically (Fig. 9–2), the feeding artery should be embolized with Gelfoam plugs to control these vessels while the torn tissues heal and then allow recanalization of the vessels to maintain esophageal viability.

Large Mallory–Weiss tears that involve multiple arterial sites of bleeding are difficult to embolize, and these patients are probably better managed by operation. Preoperative occlusion of bleeding sites makes surgery less difficult.

Successful use of intra-arterial vasopression for Mallory–Weiss tears has not been reported.

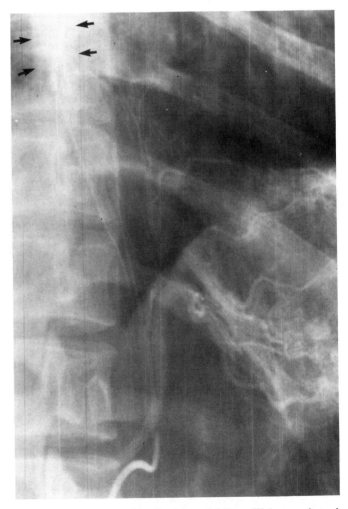

Fig. 9–2 Patient with bleeding from Mallory–Weiss esophageal tear; selective injection into left inferior phrenic artery shows extravasation of contrast medium from lower esophagus (arrows).

Bleeding Esophageal Varices

Esophageal varices develop by one of two mechanisms. Varices in the lower portion develop in response to high resistance to blood flow through the liver parenchyma and may have presinusoidal or postsinusoidal causes. In each case, passage of blood from the portal venous system to the systemic venous system is impeded. As the disease worsens, the portal hypertension causes retrograde flow through the portal venous system, with reversal of blood flow through the splenic, mesenteric, and coronary veins, causing tremendous collateralization and dilatation of the esophageal venous plexus and allowing portal venous blood to reach the systemic venous system via the azygous-hemiazygous system and the superior vena cava (Figs. 9–3 and 9–4). The other type, "downhill" esophageal varices, can develop, predominently in the upper esophagus, in response to superior vena caval obstruction. In this case, the blood flow in the esophageal venous plexus is reversed, and portal venous blood flow is in the normal direction, allowing communication with the inferior vena cava.[41,42]

Historically, the diagnosis of esophageal varices has been made with an upper GI series and a barium eso-phagogram or esophageal endoscopy. Techniques for endoscopic sclerosis of esophageal varices with absolute ethanol or isobutyl-2-cyanoacrylate polymers are well accepted.[43] Sclerosis has been used primarily for prophylaxis, because the technique is technically more difficult and less successful in cases of bleeding esophageal varices, particularly those in which bleeding is brisk.[44–47] Intravariceal vasopressin injection was abandoned because of its ineffectiveness, but intravenous systemic vasopressin will arrest bleeding in some cases in combination with the Sengstaken balloon. This result would obviate transhepatic portal venography.[44]

Transcatheter embolization of bleeding esophageal varices is performed using a transhepatic portal vein approach from the right midaxillary line, as first described by Wiechal in 1964.[48] Lunderquist introduced the transhepatic portal vein catheterization technique to the United States in 1974.[48] More recently, Widrich and others have performed more than 300 transhepatic portal venograms at the Boston Veterans Administration Medical Center.[49] The technique has been modified and improved in recent times.[41,43,50–54] Basically, a portal vein branch in the liver parenchyma is entered with the aid of a skinny (22-gauge) needle in a fashion similar to that

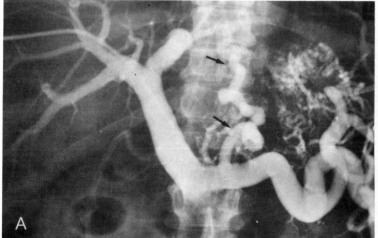

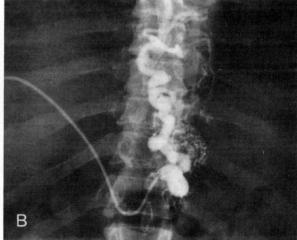

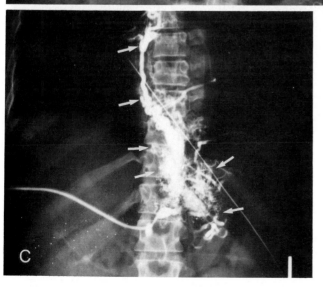

Fig. 9–3 Forty-year-old man with alcoholic cirrhosis and esophageal varices who had several bleeding episodes. A. Percutaneous transhepatic portal venogram shows large coronary vein (arrows). B. Selective coronary venogram shows large coronary vein with flow toward lower esophageal venous plexus. C. Selective injection into coronary vein reveals extensive esophageal and gastric varices (arrows). (Reproduced from Becker GJ, Holden RW, Klatte EC: On therapeutic embolization with absolute ethanol. *Semin Intervent Radiol* 1984;1:118–129 with permission from Thieme-Stratton.)

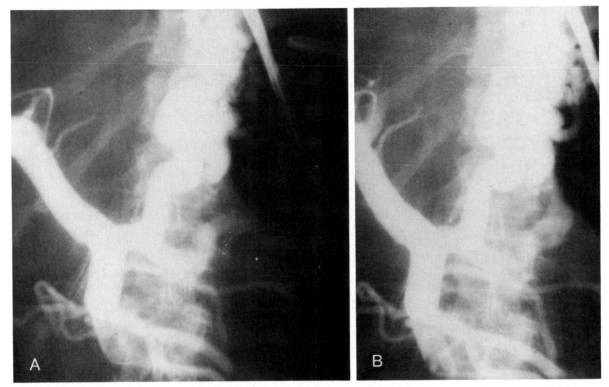

Fig. 9–4 A, B. Transhepatic portal venogram shows markedly dilated coronary vein with large esophageal varix connecting directly to azygous vein. (Courtesy of E. Russell, M.D., University of Miami.)

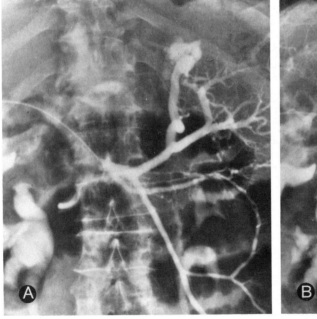 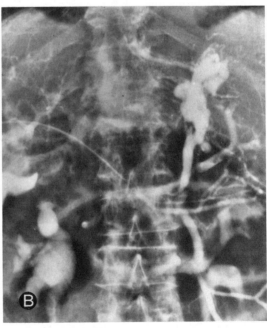

Fig. 9–5 Patient with alcoholic cirrhosis and bleeding esophageal varices. A, B. Transhepatic portal venography performed with tip of catheter within splenic vein shows huge varices arising from short gastric veins.

used for percutaneous transhepatic cholangiography. Gentle aspiration of the needle is performed until blood is obtained. Small test injections are then given to distinguish portal radicles from hepatic veins and hepatic artery branches. Once the correct vessel has been entered, a guidewire is introduced and a steerable catheter is passed into the portal vein (Fig. 9–5A). Under fluoroscopy, the guidewire and catheter are manipulated into the splenic vein, and an angiogram is performed to demonstrate the dilated, varicose venous channels (Fig. 9–5B). Subsequently, the catheter is passed into the coronary vein and then into the different varices as far

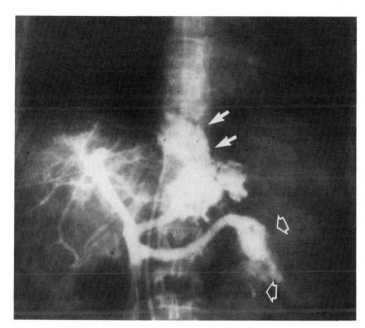

Fig. 9–6   Transhepatic portal venogram shows spontaneous spleno-renal shunt (open arrow). Huge gastroesophageal varices arise from coronary vein (large arrows). (Courtesy of E. Russell, M.D., University of Miami.)

Fig. 9–7   Patient with cirrhosis and bleeding esophageal varices. A. Complete thrombosis of coronary vein after embolization with Gelfoam; large black arrows point to left gastric vein and small open arrow points to distal stump. There is now opacification of a smaller short gastric vein supplying additional gastric varices (small white arrows). Note increased flow across splenorenal shunt (large open arrow). B. Bleeding recurred 5 years postembolization; injection into splenic vein shows enlargement of gastric varices arising from short gastric vein (arrow) and spontaneous splenorenal shunt (s). C. After occlusion of short gastric veins, repeat splenic venogram shows additional varices arising from most proximal part of splenic vein (arrows). D. Repeat portal venogram shows obliteration of all short gastric and coronary vein feeders with patent splenorenal shunt (s). Patient is alive 7 years after embolization. (Courtesy of E. Russell, M.D.)

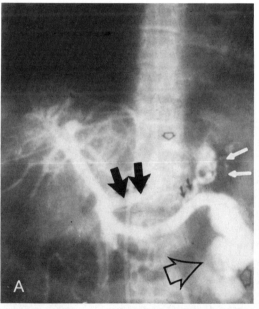

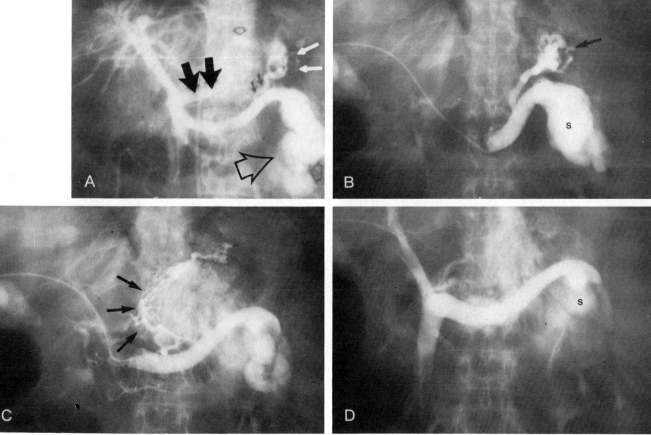

peripherally as possible to demonstrate anatomy, size of venous channels, and associated anomalies (Fig. 9–6A,B).

Various embolic materials have been used to obliterate varices.[49–54] Lunderquist and his coworkers have used a coaxial catheter system for embolization, with isobutyl-2-cyanoacrylate (Bucrylate) being injected through the smaller catheter. The polymer is immediately flushed from the catheter with isotonic glucose solution and the coaxial system is immediatey withdrawn 1–2 cm to prevent its adherence to the vessel wall.[43] If Bucrylate or other suitable polymers are not available, other embolic materials such as Gelfoam/Sotradecol (Fig. 9–7),[51,53] ethanol (Fig. 9–8), and GWC steel coils[49] can be used to obliterate the large feeding veins.

The present authors have used a combined technique for embolization of esophageal varices in which a catheter is passed as far peripherally into the varix as possible. Gelfoam soaked in Sotradecol is then injected to obliter-ate and sclerose the venous channels. Following this, GWC coils are introduced to obliterate the large varicose channel proximally (Fig. 9–9A,B). This combined approach has arrested active bleeding, and the rebleeding rate has been low, certainly similar to that following decompressive portal-to-systemic surgical shunts and other embolic techniques. All visible varices should be embolized (Fig. 9–7) after which angiography is performed to demonstrate the complete obliteration of all the varicosities (Fig. 9–8).

Two other approaches to varices are available. An umbilical vein approach through a surgical cutdown has been advocated[55] for entering the portal system by passing through the connection of the umbilical vein with the left portal vein (Fig. 9–10). Another approach is a transjugular route.[56] The hepatic veins are catheterized selectively, and the portal system is entered using a sharp needle passed through the guiding catheter and advanced

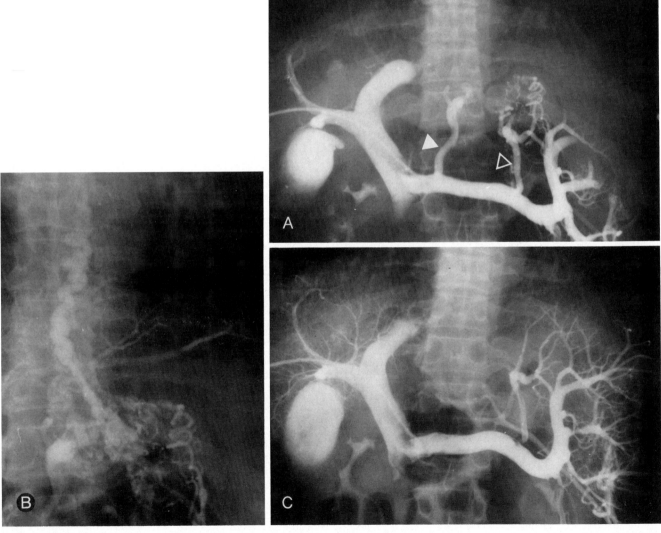

Fig. 9–8 Patient with cirrhosis and esophageal varices with endo-scopically documented variceal bleeding. A. Percutanous transhe-patic portal venogram shows large coronary vein (white arrowhead) and short gastric vein (open arrowhead). B. Selective coronary ven-ogram shows esophageal varices and intercommunication with short gastric veins. C. Portal venogram after embolization with ethanol shows obliteration of coronary vein, short gastric veins, and esopha-geal varices. (Reproduced from Becker GJ, Holden RW, Klatte EC: On therapeutic embolization with absolute ethanol. *Semin Intervent Radiol* 1984;1:118–129 with permission from Thieme-Stratton.)

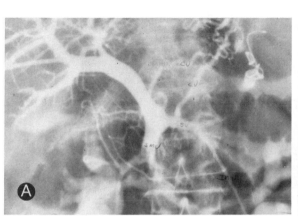

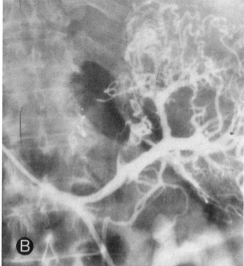

Fig. 9–9 Portal venogram after embolization of short gastric veins with GWC spring embolus shows complete thrombosis of these vessels, but additional varices are seen arising from coronary veins. B.

Repeat portal venography after embolization of all the short gastric and coronary vein varices shows no further opacification of varices.

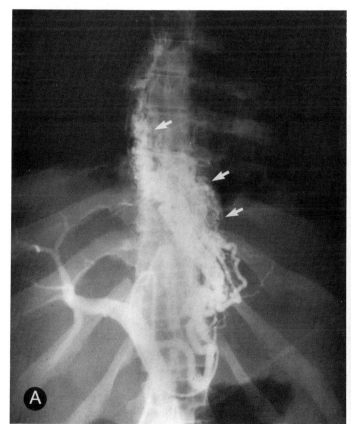

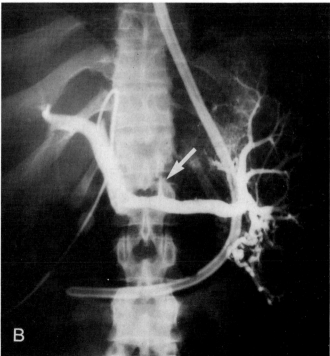

Fig. 9–10 Transumbilical catheterization of portal vein. A. Through transumbilical approach, portal vein has been catheterized; tip of catheter is placed in coronary vein. Observe huge gastroesophageal varices (arrows). B. After embolization of coronary vein with Gelfoam plugs, observe complete thrombosis of esophageal varices (arrow). (Courtesy of Dimitri Spigos, M.D., University of Illinois.)

blindly. Once the needle's position within the portal vein has been confirmed by injection of contrast medium, a guidewire is passed through the needle into the vein, and the needle and guiding catheter are replaced by an angiographic catheter that is passed over the guidewire. Catheterization and embolization of the varices are then performed. With embolization, Widrich and others report effective control of esophageal variceal bleeding at 1 month in 60% of 86 patients.[49] Complications of transhepatic portal vein embolization therapy include intraabdominal bleeding from the transhepatic puncture, particularly in patients with coagulopathy secondary to the liver disease and with diminished platelet number or poor platelet function. The transvenous or transumbilical routes are better approaches in these patients, since they avoid extrahepatic extravasation. Intrapleural bleeding and hemothorax have been reported when the lateral costophrenic angle has been crossed during the transhepatic approach. By careful fluoroscopy monitoring during deep inhalation and exhalation by the patient, this complication should be avoided. Portal vein thrombosis has been described related both to manipulation within the portal vein and as a response to a backflow of embolic material, such as particles (Gelfoam, Ivalon), polymers, or alcohol. This complication should be uncommon if occlusion balloon techniques are used for fluid embolic materials and with judicious deposition of particles and coils. To avoid complications such as intraperitoneal or intrapleural bleeding, the authors have been reluctant to undertake transhepatic portal venography in patients with a platelet count <50,000/ml or in patients with prothrombin times or partial thromboplastin times >1.5 of control values. These contraindications become relative in the presence of exsanguinating esophageal bleeding, when the procedure is undertaken to save the patient's life. To help decrease bleeding from the puncture tract, a plug of Gelfoam can be inserted at the conclusion of the procedure.

Gastritis

Gastritis has two basic causes: drug- or alcohol-induced injury and idiopathic factors. Stress ulceration will be discussed under "Gastric Peptic Ulcer." In the diagnostic study of a patient presumed to have gastrointestinal bleeding from gastritis, a single focus of extravasation into the stomach is unlikely to be identified; instead, multiple sites of extravasation may be seen in the lumen of the stomach, which is diffusely hyperemic (Fig. 9–11).

The evaluation of these patients should include a selective left gastric artery injection if possible, because this study will often identify extravasation into the lumen and provide a more interpretable study inasmuch as there is no superimposition of splenic and pancreatic branches, as occurs with a celiac trunk injection. Depending on the size of the patient and the aorta, selective left gastric artery catheterization can be most easily performed using a left gastric, sidewinder-1, or sidewinder-2 type of catheter in which the distal tip has been turned upward with steam. Once the sidewinder is engaged in the celiac trunk, it is pulled down slowly, with small contrast injections, until it is nearly straightened, at which point the tip will be directed superiorly and in most cases will engage the

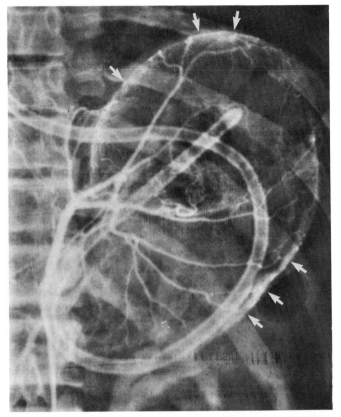

Fig. 9–11 Selective left gastric arteriogram in patient with diffuse mucosal bleeding in erosive gastritis demonstrated by endoscopy. Note diffuse mucosal stain (arrows) suggestive of mucosal extravasation of contrast medium.

left gastric artery selectively. When gastroscopy has identified ooze or bleeding from gastritis in the distal part of the stomach, it may be necessary to perform a selective gastroduodenal artery injection with filling of the gastroepiploic arcade along the greater curvature of the stomach. Selective catheterization of the gastroduodenal artery is more difficult, especially when the vessel arises far to the right of a long common hepatic artery.

Once an area of extravasation has been identified along with the confirmatory hyperemic changes of gastritis, intra-arterial vasopressin should be given for the control of diffuse bleeding. In general, the bleeding from gastritis is from small (arteriolar-size) vessels, and vasoconstriction is adequate to control it. The standard infusion rate and doses outlined earlier are adequate for control in most cases, although the authors recommend extending the infusion time to 24–36 hr after a response has been achieved before starting to decrease the dose, because otherwise rebleeding is more likely.[34,36,57,58] Selective infusion of vasopressin into the left gastric artery controls bleeding from gastritis in slightly more than 80% of cases[57]; in this report, approximately 16% of patients had recurrent bleeding and were judged to be suitable candidates for a repeat vasopression infusion. Only in extremely refractory cases of gastritis bleeding, bleeding from a large hyperemic vessel, or severe coagulation abnormalities should particulate embolization for gastritis be necessary.[59,60]

Gastric Peptic Ulcer

Gastric peptic ulcers occur by three mechanisms: (1) idiopathic; (2) in association with hypergastrinemia (Zollinger–Ellison syndrome); and (3) stress, particularly postoperatively or in burns. Regardless of the etiology of the ulceration, gastrointestinal bleeding is caused by erosion into a small artery. The angiographic evaluation of the hemorrhage is generally performed by selective injections of the left gastric artery, the gastroduodenal artery, or the superior pancreaticoduodenal arteries. In contradistinction to the arteriographic picture of gastritis, the angiographic appearance of a bleeding ulcer is one in which stomach vascularity is normal, and the bleeding is usually confined to one or two locations rather than being diffuse (Fig. 9–12). Occasionally, with erosions into large branch arteries, extravasation of contrast medium from the vessel can be identified.

After identification of a bleeding site, the angiographic catheter is left in place for intra-arterial vasopressin infusion. In most cases in which the bleeding originates from a small branch vessel, this treatment controls the hemorrhage. However, when the ulcer crater erodes into a larger vessel, such as the gastroduodenal or left gastric artery, vasopressin usually fails (Fig. 9–13A).[21,60] Particulate embolization of the bleeding vessel is frequently required (Fig. 9–13B).[21,60–63]

The philosophy of management of patients with gastric ulcer bleeding is evolving, especially with the advent of histamine antagonists (cimetidine) and antacid therapy.[64] In addition, gastroscopy enables peroral coagulation of bleeding points with electrocautery. Endoscopic management of GI bleeding, as well as transcatheter embolization and pharmocotherapy, has significantly reduced the frequency of surgery for bleeding ulcer disease.

Vasopressin infusion into the left gastric, gastroduodenal, or pancreaticoduodenal arteries has resulted in almost no complications.[29,32,54] Similarly, particulate embolization of these same vessels has not caused infarction of the stomach.[65,66] The particulate material chosen for embolization should be a temporary one such as Gelfoam.[67,68] The luxurious four-quadrant blood supply of the stomach provides such excellent collateral flow that, even in the stomach that has been operated on, embolization has been almost complication free. Indeed, the dual blood supply to some areas makes control of bleeding difficult by either vasoconstrictor infusion or selective embolotherapy (Fig. 9–13C, D). Nonetheless, embolization should be approached cautiously in patients with previous gastric surgery; the extent of the surgical interruption of the vascular bed is unknown, and embolization of an additional vessel can cause gastric infarction.[65,66]

Malignant Gastric Ulcers

Malignant gastric neoplasms are a well-recognized cause of bleeding. Frequently, the site is identifiable angiographically as extravasation into the lumen of the stomach (Fig. 9–14) as well as by neovascularity within the tumor itself. The general principle of placing a catheter superselectively as near the lesion as possible also applies to malignant tumors. The selective infusion of tumors with drugs such as epinephrine or vasopressin has not been successful, as the abnormal tumor vessels appear unresponsive to these agents.

Goldstein et al reported their experience with embolization of bleeding gastrointestinal tumors.[20] The preferred method of dealing with tumors in the stomach and duodenum has been embolization with permanent agents, particularly Ivalon, when superselective catheterization can be performed; not only has this been helpful in stopping the hemorrhage, but it has caused considerable tumor shrinkage prior to resection. When the tumor is larger and more diffuse and superselective embolization is not possible, subselective embolization with a temporary particulate material such as Gelfoam can be used to control the acute hemorrage and allow time for the patient to be stabilized and to achieve a better condition for surgical resection.[20,69]

Duodenal Peptic Ulcer Disease

Bleeding originating in the region of the pylorus or duodenum has been managed both by vasopressin infusion and by embolization, as well as by a combination of the two (Fig. 9–15). Vasopressin's success rate for control of bleeding in the duodenum has been only 35%–45%.[60,61,64] Of those patients who underwent embolization after vasopressin failure, the procedure has been successful in 65%–70%.[60,61,64,69,70] The success rate and expected outcome of vasopressin or embolization for duodenal ulcer bleeding can be predicted from the size of the vessel supplying the bleeder. A small tertiary branch of the gastroduodenal artery should respond to vasopressin, whereas more proximal large feeders from the gastroduodenal artery will require particulate embolization (Fig. 9–16).

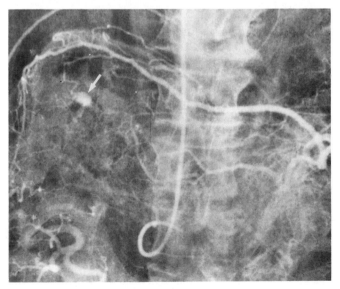

Fig. 9–12 Stress ulceration demonstrated by a common hepatic artery injection (arrow) in patient with massive bleeding after major surgery for multiple trauma.

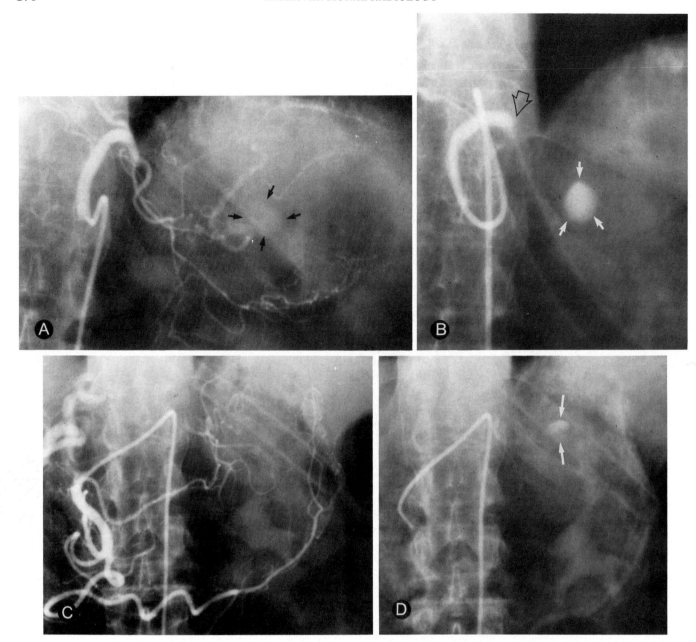

Fig. 9–13   Fifty-year-old man bleeding from ulcer in gastric fundus. A. Selective left gastric arteriogram after infusion of vasopressin shows continued extravasation of contrast medium, which collects within ulcer crater (arrows). Observe marked decrease in caliber of left gastric artery branches due to the vasopressor effect. B. Selective left gastric arteriogram after embolization with Gelfoam plugs; note stump of left gastric artery (open arrow) and collection of contrast medium at level of ulcer crater (small arrows). C. Because of persistent bleeding, arteriography was repeated. Selective gastroduodenal arteriogram shows good opacification of right gastric and gastroepiploic arteries, with extravasation of contrast medium in area of ulcer crater in gastric fundus in late phase (D) (arrows).

The diagnosis is established by a combination of gastroscopy to identify potential ulcer bleeding sites and, if possible, by superselective arteriography into the gastroduodenal artery.

Postsurgical Anastomotic Bleeding

The basic principle of hemorrhage control at surgical anastomoses in the GI tract is selective injection of the appropriate vessel supplying the segment of bowel used in the anastomosis.[71,72] In cases of esophagogastrostomy, it is important to study the blood supply of the native upper esophagus and stomach used to create the anastomosis. In gastrojejunostomy anastomoses, it is important to study the blood supply of the remaining stomach and jejunum. The jejunum is supplied by the superior jejunal branches of the superior mesenteric artery. Gastroenterostomies are studied primarily by superior mesenteric arteriography. In these situations (Fig. 9–17) it is frequently necessary to perform superselective catheterization into second- and third-order branches of the superior mesenteric artery, not only to identify the bleeding site

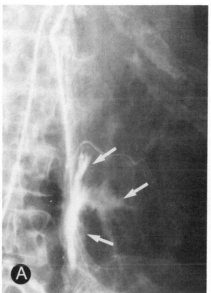
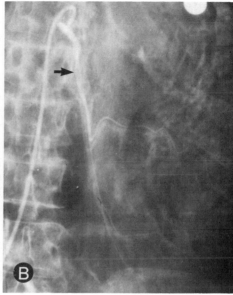

Fig. 9–14 Fifty-two-year-old patient with lymphocytic leukemia presenting with gastrointestinal bleeding from diffuse erosive gastritis during chemotherapy. A. Selective left gastric arteriogram shows extensive extravasation of contrast medium (arrows) from branch of left gastric artery. B. Postembolization with 2 × 2-mm Gelfoam plugs; observe selective occlusion of branches in area of previous extravasation. Filling defects within proximal left gastric artery (arrow) represent Gelfoam plugs.

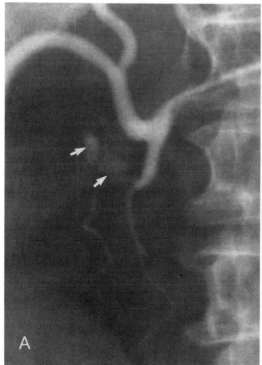
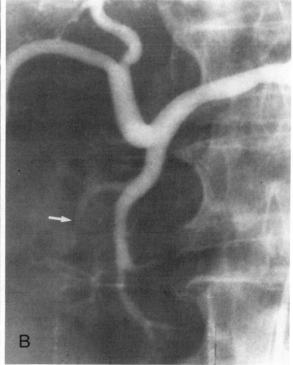

Fig. 9–15 Sixty-two-year-old man with metastatic renal cell carcinoma presenting with severe gastrointestinal bleeding from malignant ulcer in second portion of duodenum. A. Selective gastroduodenal arteriogram shows extravasation from a pancreatoduodenal arterial branch (arrows). B. Common hepatic arteriogram after selective embolization of bleeding vessel shows thrombosis of this artery with no evidence of extravasation (arrow).

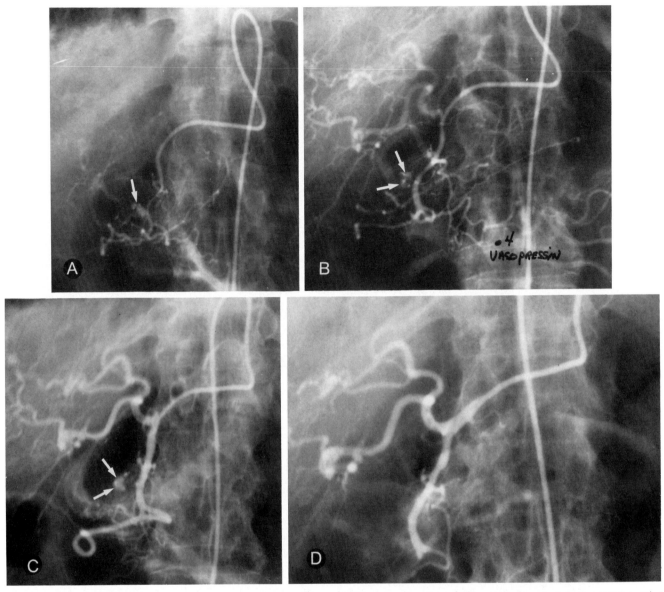

Fig. 9–16   Patient with bleeding from duodenal ulcer. A. Selective infusion of vasopressin into gastroduodenal artery (0.2 unit/min) fails to halt bleeding (arrow). B. Repeat gastroduodenal arteriogram after infusion of 0.4 unit of vasopressin per minute shows continued extravasation of contrast medium (arrows). C. Repeat gastroduodenal arteriogram after 2 1/2 hr of vasopressin infusion at 0.6 unit/min shows continued extravasation (arrows). D. Repeat gastroduodenal arteriogram after embolization with Gelfoam shows adequate control of bleeding.

without superimposition of other vessels, but also to attempt vasopressin infusion (Fig. 9–12). Ileocolostomies and colocolostomies require study of the appropriate superior mesenteric arterial branches, branches of the inferior mesenteric artery, or both.

The primary means of bleeding control postoperatively is vasopressin infusion, which provides good short-term cessation of bleeding and allows time for healing so that bleeding does not recur.[71]

Because GI resective surgery and bowel anastomoses frequently involve the ligation of several collateral vessels, permanent embolization is to be avoided if at all possible because of the risk of bowel infarction, particularly after previous partial gastrectomies. Also, in cases involving resection of long segments of small bowel, many potential collateral pathways are eliminated, so again,

embolization in the small bowel is to be avoided. A similar principle applies to patients with previous colonic resections.

Bleeding in Meckel's Diverticulum

The classic picture of small bowel bleeding occurs in the young patient with a Meckel's diverticulum. The presence of Meckel's diverticulum can be established with high sensitivity and high specificity by radionuclide scanning using ^{99m}Tc-pertechnetate preparations,[12,14–16,73,74] which are avidly taken up and secreted by gastric mucosa, with which the diverticulum typically is lined (Fig. 9–18A). In the proper setting of GI bleeding in a young patient, in whom endoscopy is negative and who has a positive radionuclide Meckel's scan, superior

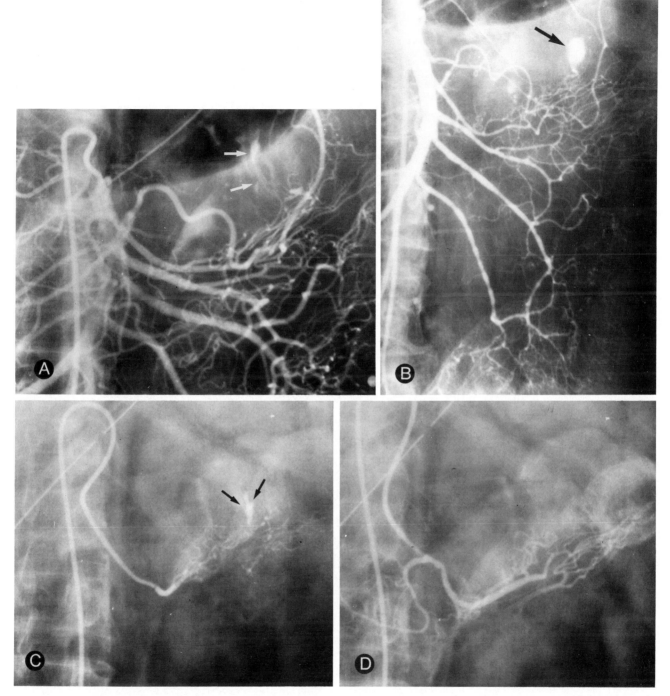

Fig. 9–17   Gastrointestinal bleeding after Billroth I anastomosis in patient who had ingested acid. A. Selective superior mesenteric arteriogram shows extravasation of contrast medium from proximal jejunal branch (arrows). B. Repeat superior mesenteric arteriogram after infusion of 0.4 unit of vasopressin per minute into superior mesenteric artery shows continued extravasation of contrast medium from jejunal branch (arrow). C. Selective catheterization of jejunal branch shows persistence of bleeding after selective infusion of 0.4 unit of vasopressin per minute (arrows). D. Repeat jejunal branch arteriogram after embolization with Gelfoam shows complete occlusion of bleeding artery with no further extravasation.

mesenteric arteriography can be undertaken to identify the bleeding site. If a bleeding site is identified, superselective catheterization of the superior mesenteric artery branch supplying the region can be attempted for vasopressin infusion.[75] If superselective catheterization is difficult or impossible, infusion into the superior mesenteric artery itself is effective in stopping Meckel's diverticular bleeding, although understandably less so than direct superselective infusion.

Diverticular Disease in the Small Bowel

Occasionally, adult patients with diverticular disease in the small bowel also demonstrate gastrointestinal hem-

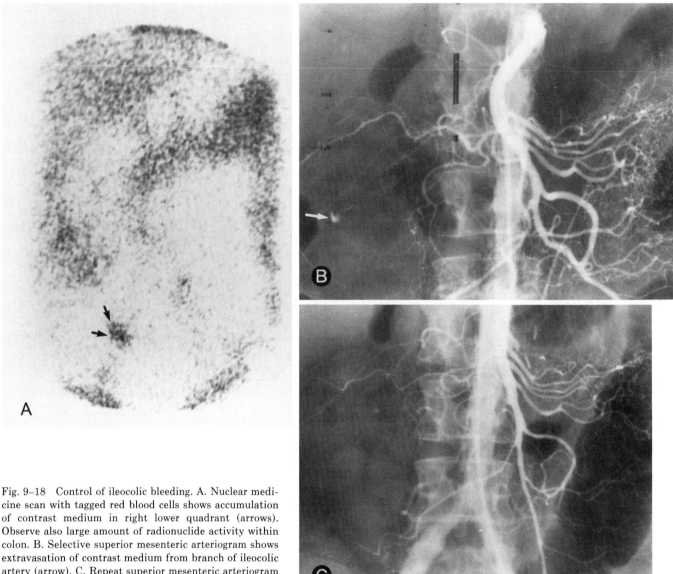

Fig. 9–18 Control of ileocolic bleeding. A. Nuclear medicine scan with tagged red blood cells shows accumulation of contrast medium in right lower quadrant (arrows). Observe also large amount of radionuclide activity within colon. B. Selective superior mesenteric arteriogram shows extravasation of contrast medium from branch of ileocolic artery (arrow). C. Repeat superior mesenteric arteriogram after infusion of vasopressin shows adequate control of bleeding with no extravasation of contrast medium.

orrhage beyond the ligament of Treitz, particularly when the diverticulum is large and has been colonized by enteric organisms.[75,76] In such cases, the bleeding is of an oozing nature and is frequently difficult to identify angiographically, especially as it often is intermittent. Radionuclide scanning with [99mTc]-labeled red blood cells may help confirm and, to a lesser extent, locate the region of bleeding (Fig. 9–18A). Again, vasopressin infusion as superselectively as possible is the mainstay of therapy (Fig. 9–18B, C). Antibiotics in high enteral doses should also be given to attempt to sterilize the diverticulum. Vasopressin infusion for bleeding small bowel diverticula is a temporary measure, and operation is the preferred definitive therapy.

Small Bowel Ulcerations

For the most part, ulcerations in the small bowel are ischemic, most commonly from emboli. The angiographic series may show an abruptly truncated superior mesenteric artery branch with a small embolus within the vessel, although it is rare to demonstrate the blockage. Other arteriographic signs of ischemic lesions include an intense blush of the bowel wall in the region. The mechanism by which bleeding occurs is thought to be sloughing of the bowel mucosa and erosion into small arterioles in the submucosal layers of the bowel wall. The use of vasopressin in the management of these patients may at first seem paradoxical, but bear in mind that the vessels that respond to this hormone are the medium-sized arterioles, i.e., those vessels containing smooth muscle fibers. Again, vasopressin administration is a temporizing measure and should be used only to permit stabilization of the patient in preparation for a definitive operation.

It has been helpful to leave the catheter in the superior mesenteric vessels when the patient is sent to surgery so that intraoperative injections of methylene blue can be given to assist the surgeon in locating the ulcerated,

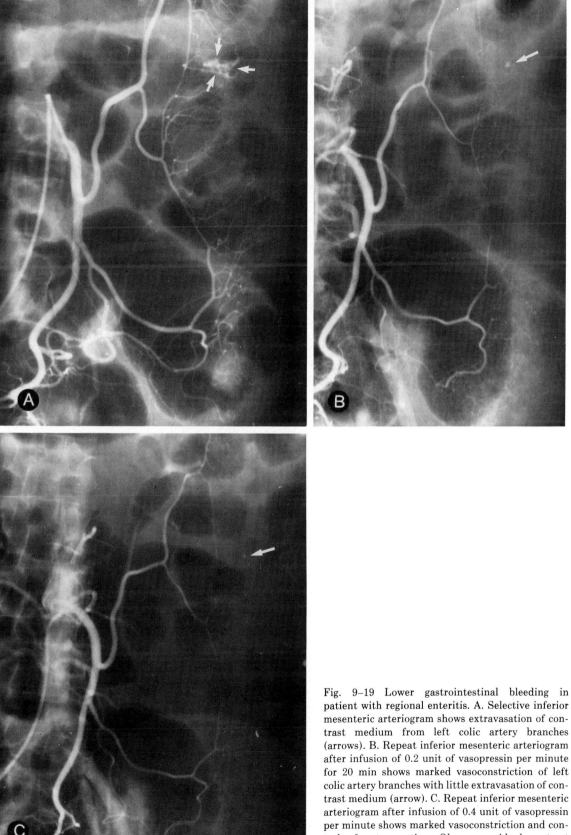

Fig. 9–19 Lower gastrointestinal bleeding in patient with regional enteritis. A. Selective inferior mesenteric arteriogram shows extravasation of contrast medium from left colic artery branches (arrows). B. Repeat inferior mesenteric arteriogram after infusion of 0.2 unit of vasopressin per minute for 20 min shows marked vasoconstriction of left colic artery branches with little extravasation of contrast medium (arrow). C. Repeat inferior mesenteric arteriogram after infusion of 0.4 unit of vasopressin per minute shows marked vasoconstriction and control of extravasation. Observe residual contrast medium in ulcer (arrow).

bleeding segment of the small bowel.[77,78] In this way, the extent of small bowel resection is minimized, reducing postoperative morbidity and avoiding the inconvenience to the patient of short bowel syndrome.

Tumors of the Small Bowel

Generally, small bowel tumors bleed intermittently, and because these patients are frequently studied electively between bleeding episodes, it is unusual to identify the actual site of extravasation or bleeding.[75,79,80] Tumor neovascularity itself may be seen within the small bowel. In cases of multiple small bowel tumors, the angiographic evaluation is particularly frustrating, inasmuch as any of these tumors could be the bleeding site and, in all likelihood, bleeding will be in abeyance at the time of the study.

Leiomyomas and leiomyosarcomas in the small bowel display a typical angiographic appearance, with hypervascularity and irregular corkscrew tumor vessels.[79] Intra-arterial vasopressin therapy is, again, primarily a temporizing measure while the patient is prepared for surgery. Definitive particulate embolization of these tumors is both technically difficult, because of the superselective catheterization techniques required, and fraught with complications, particularly small bowel infarction, and thus it should be undertaken reluctantly.[79,81]

A small bowel carcinoid is identifiable arteriographically by the fibroblastic reaction in the mesenteric root, which causes retraction, displacement, and occlusion of multiple superior mesenteric artery branches.[82] Vasopressin infusion is, again, a temporizing measure until definitive operation can be done when the patient is in stable condition.

Birns and coworkers reported a case of intramural small bowel hematoma presenting with severe upper GI bleeding.[83] Crawford et al reported locating a jejunoileal arteriovenous malformation using segmental bowel staining.[84]

Granulomatous Disease of the Small Bowel (Inflammatory Bowel Disease)

Angiographically, the bowel wall involved by Crohn's disease reveals hyperemia with arteriovenous shunting and, frequently, intense venous opacification during midarterial films. The bleeding associated with inflammatory bowel disease is generally diffuse, similar to that seen with gastritis; rarely is a focal site of extravasation identified (Fig. 9–19A).[85,86] Gastrointestinal bleeding can be controlled acutely with intra-arterial vasopressin infusion (Fig. 9–19B), but the definitive therapy is surgical, particularly in Crohn's disease severe enough to cause stenosis in the terminal ileum or other segments of small bowel. Vasopressin may actually be contraindicated in these situations because of the risk of infarcting segments of bowel whose blood supply is already severely compromised by granulomatous infiltration of the wall.

Cecal Ulceration in Immunosuppressed Patients

Immunosuppressed patients can present with severe GI bleeding secondary either to steroid administration or to overwhelming cytomegalovirus infection that can cause miliary ulcerations in the GI tract. Frequently, the latter presents as localized cecal ulcerations that respond transiently to vasopressin infusion via the superior mesenteric artery but resume bleeding as soon as the vasoconstrictor is discontinued.[81] Stopping the immunosuppressors and operation are the main avenues of therapy.[87]

Arteriovenous Malformations in the Colon

Arteriovenous malformations in the colon are congenital abnormalities, anatomically different from the acquired angiodysplastic lesions in aortic stenosis. The angiographic characteristics of both angiodysplasis and AVMs include early filling of draining veins, slow emptying of tortuous intramural venous channels, and dilatation of the feeding arteries (Fig. 9–20). Less commonly seen are a local stain within the colonic wall, a true vascular tuft of tangled vessels, and prolonged venous opacification (Fig. 9–21).[88–90] True congenital AVMs are most commonly encountered in the rectum and sigmoid colon.[91] Both angiodysplasia and AVMs of the colon tend to bleed intermittently (Fig. 9–22); therefore, arteriographic diagnosis is difficult, and false-negative results are frequently obtained. Identification of the nonbleeding lesions with barium enema studies and, more commonly, by colonoscopy are important prior to angiography, especially in the patient with documented slow or intermittent colonic blood loss.[92] The abnormal vessels in both of

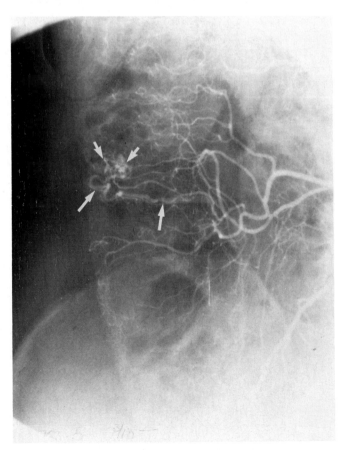

Fig. 9–20 Abnormal cluster of vessels in cecal area, with early venous opacification (arrows).

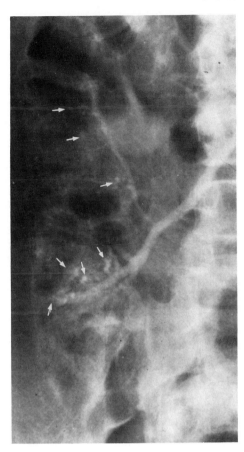

Fig. 9–21 A 56-year-old man with repeated episodes of lower gastrointestinal bleeding. Selective superior mesenteric arteriogram reveals a localized area of dense vascular stain (small arrows) and early venous opacification.

these entities preclude success with intra-arterial vasopressin. The lesions can be managed by embolization either with Gelfoam, if temporary embolization is required, or with Ivalon particles, when permanent embolization is indicated (Fig. 9–22B, C).[26,93]

Grossly visible AVMs do not present a difficult surgical problem and can be resected easily. On the other hand, small angiodysplastic lesions are nearly invisible intraoperatively, and empiric colon resection frequently is necessary when bleeding is a problem. The specimen must be sent for high-resolution magnification angiography, if possible using a small focal spot unit. In addition, the predominant feeding arteries of the colon should be injected with a silicone preparation when the specimen is sectioned by the pathologist in the hope of locating AVMs.

Diverticulitis of the Colon

Diverticulosis is the most common cause of bleeding in the large intestine and generally occurs in patients older than 60 years.[94] Although diverticula are more common in the left side of the colon, bleeding from diverticula occurs three times more often from the right side. The primary origin of diverticular bleeding is thought to be erosion into a peridiverticular artery by fecal material or bacterial overgrowth. The only definite angiographic criterion for diverticular bleeding is extravasation into the precise diverticular site (Fig. 9–23A). Intra-arterial vasopressin is reportedly the more successful way to control diverticular bleeding (Fig. 9–23B).[93,94] Those cases in which vasopressin infusion fails are thought to be the result of the age of the patient and the atherosclerotic changes in the vessels involved. In this situation, the arterioles may not be capable of constricting in response to the infusion of vasopressin.

Inflammatory Bowel Disease (Granulomatous and Ulcerative Colitis)

Boijsen and Reuter have shown that in granulomatous enterocolitis, the arteries and veins fill more rapidly than in the surrounding normal bowel, with increased vascularity, and that there is a slight dilatation of the feeding arteries, with dilatation and tortuosity of the draining veins.[85] Those authors also showed that during the capillary phase of the arteriogram, thickened, edematous bowel wall can be detected in the presence of active ulcerative or granulomatous colitis.

The bleeding from inflammatory bowel disease of the colon, whether it be granulomatous or ulcerative, is generally diffuse oozing from the involved segment.[27,28] Correspondingly, the bleeding from inflammatory bowel disease is perhaps amenable to vasopressin infusion but certainly is not an appropriate indication for embolization. Again, the bleeding is intermittent and oozing, and frequently no evidence of the bleeding site will be visible on arteriography. Several publications discuss in detail the angiographic findings in both ulcerative and granulomatous colitis and the differentiation of the two.[27,28,85]

Tumors of the Colon

More than 75% of all polyps and cancers in the colon occur in the tissue served by the inferior mesenteric artery.[95–97] Several reports have suggested a role for arteriography in the diagnosis of carcinoma of the colon, but more recently, these techniques have been abandoned as insufficiently sensitive and certainly not cost effective in screening for this common cancer.[85,98–100] When changes are visible, the angiographic appearance is one of tortuous vessels that are randomly distributed, have irregular walls, and taper more rapidly than adjacent normal vessels. Many colon carcinomas accumulate contrast medium with some puddling in the capillary and early venous phase, and many also demonstrate premature venous filling.[101]

The role of vasopressin infusion for bleeding carcinomas has not been established, but this method is generally ineffective because of the nonresponsiveness of the tumor vessels. Particulate embolization with permanent agents such as Ivalon is a theoretical, although not widely accepted, method of dealing with the bleeding carcinoma of the colon. However, embolization for tumor control is difficult in the inferior mesenteric arterial circulation because of the frequent inability to pass catheters superselectively into this vessel. In addition, operation remains the definitive treatment for the disease because problems of obstruction, tumor bulk, and detection of metastases

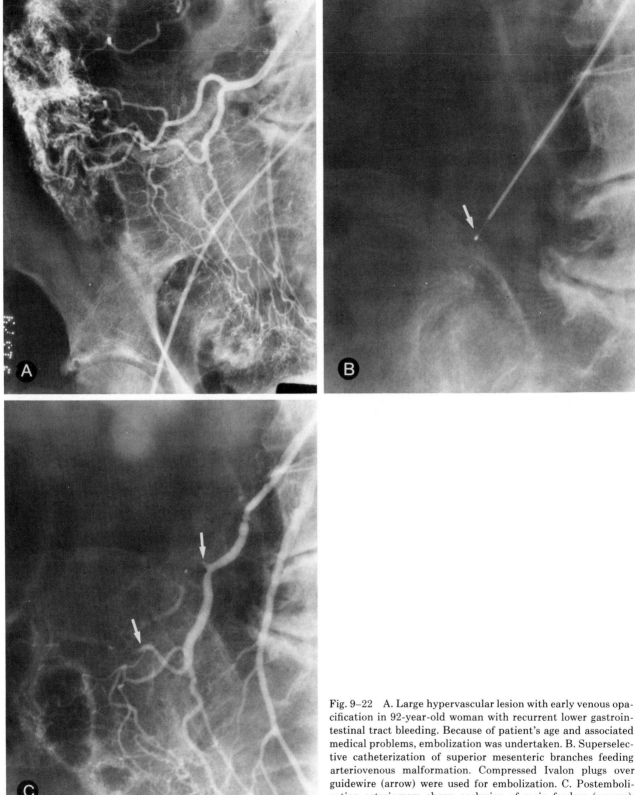

Fig. 9–22   A. Large hypervascular lesion with early venous opacification in 92-year-old woman with recurrent lower gastrointestinal tract bleeding. Because of patient's age and associated
medical problems, embolization was undertaken. B. Superselective catheterization of superior mesenteric branches feeding
arteriovenous malformation. Compressed Ivalon plugs over
guidewire (arrow) were used for embolization. C. Postembolization arteriogram shows occlusion of main feeders (arrows);
lesion is significantly devascularized.

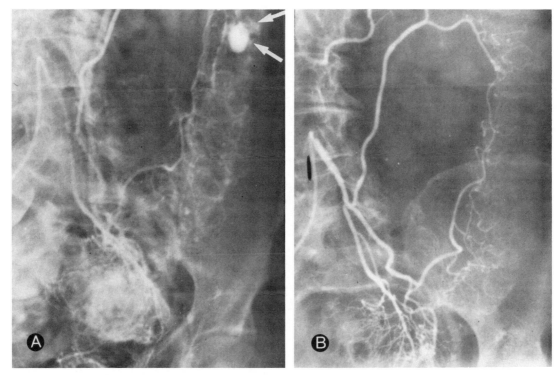

Fig. 9–23 Seventy-six-year-old woman with bright red hemorrhage through rectum. A. Selective inferior mesenteric arteriogram shows extensive extravasation of contrast medium from diverticulum in descending colon (arrows). B. Repeat inferior mesenteric arteriogram after vasopressin infusion for 24 hr shows thrombosis of bleeding vessel with no further extravasation of contrast medium.

cannot be managed percutaneously at this time. The primary tumors in the colon that contribute to lower GI bleeding are villous adenomas, adenocarcinomas, and, less frequently, carcinoids in the region of the cecum.

COMPLICATIONS

The complications of percutaneous management of gastrointestinal bleeding can be divided into three categories. The first are problems related to the catheter, which, with modern equipment and technology, should be uncommon. Thrombosis at the arterial puncture site probably occurs most frequently (about 0.1% of the studies performed in the United States[102,103]).

With long-term vasopressin infusion, the catheter is frequently left in place for several days, during which time it accumulates a fibrin sheath. However, this sheath appears to be well tolerated by the patient if care is exercised during catheter removal. The present authors remove the catheter in the following way. First, peripheral pulses in the leg are checked. Then the physician's assistant applies gentle continuous suction to a large syringe attached to the catheter as it is slowly withdrawn. The artery is compressed below the puncture site, and the catheter is removed under continuous suction. After the catheter leaves the artery, the vessel is allowed to bleed for several seconds to expel any thrombus or fibrin sheath that has been stripped off the catheter at the puncture site. After several seconds of bleeding, the vessel is controlled from above and the artery compressed in the standard fashion. Using this pull-out technique, the authors have had no distal embolization from long-term indwelling catheters.

The second category of complications is those attributable to vasopressin. Most patients complain initially of some abdominal cramping, which is thought to be related to the direct effect of the hormone on the smooth muscle of the gut, with increased peristalsis. This cramping persists for as long as 1/2 hr and is unlikely to recur. The physicians performing this study and the staff caring for the patient should be alert for abrupt changes in the patient's comfort level, with complaints of severe localized pain. This frequently indicates a shift in catheter position to a more superselective location, such that the vasopressin is being delivered into a smaller blood vessel, producing intense vasospasm and local ischemia. Third, although the intra-arterial vasopressin dose is low in comparison to the systemic dose, during long-term infusion the antidiuretic effect appears, usually after 6–8 hr. Therefore, the patient's urinary output and electrolyte status must be monitored and a diuretic and electrolyte replacement started if appropriate. Lastly, some patients experience serious peripheral vasoconstriction, which is believed to be an idiosyncratic reaction to vasopressin. The extremities can become mottled and painful to the point of necessitating discontinuation of the drug. At the recommended local doses, reduction in cardiac output should not be a problem, but this is almost certainly dependent on the individual patient's cardiac status.

The third category of complications involves improper deposition of embolic material. Generally, once embolic particles or devices are released from the catheter, they cannot be retrieved, so it is incumbent upon the physician performing the procedure to be absolutely meticulous in positioning the catheter tip so that the embolic material is deposited as close to the bleeding site as possible and so that there is no backflow of material into blood vessels supplying normal tissue. The complications resulting from embolic particulate matter include end-organ necrosis and reflux of embolic material. As mentioned earlier in this chapter, embolic reflux should be avoidable with the use of occlusion balloon techniques, especially when fluid embolic material, such as absolute alcohol or cyanoacrylate, is used.

After embolizations, particularly extensive ones, the patients may have fever as high as 102° F. Local areas of ischemic pain and pain from necrotic tissue may also be experienced.

PERIPROCEDURAL CARE

Patient Preparation

Close cooperation between the interventional radiologist and the referring clinician is mandatory in the management of these patients. Adequate preangiographic workup is also necessary to facilitate a tailored examination in which selected high-suspicion areas within the GI tract can be examined. "Search and destroy" arteriographic procedures are to be avoided, because they require large contrast volumes and are frequently nonrewarding diagnostically. Collection of all available data, including barium GI studies and radionuclide bleeding studies, should be the responsibility of the interventional radiologist before diagnostic or therapeutic angiography.

Patients should be in as good a coagulation status as possible, which is usually not a problem in cases of GI bleeding. Exceptions are the patient with bleeding esophageal varices secondary to cirrhosis, patients receiving chemotherapy, and recipients of bone marrow transplants, in whom coagulation studies are likely to be significantly abnormal. If the hemorrhage is not life-threatening, the authors prefer to correct the coagulation factors with fresh-frozen plasma, cryoprecipitate, vitamin K, and platelet transfusions as appropriate. An additional consideration is the frequent coagulation abnormality in patients who have received several transfusions before angiography. Although these patients may have coagulation studies within the normal range, they frequently bleed extensively at the time of catheter removal.

It is imperative that the interventional radiologist discuss the diagnosis and treatment plan with the patient. At the authors' institution, the patient's permission is obtained for both diagnostic angiography and therapeutic embolization as indicated before preprocedure drugs are given.

Sedative medication that will transiently lower blood pressure is to be avoided in the preangiographic period, because a decrease in blood pressure in response to narcotic medications can transiently stop or slow the bleeding and add to the frustration of the examination. The GI bleeding evaluation, particularly if embolization is being considered, is performed in the operating room of a special angiographic suite. This gives the radiologist ready access to anesthesia and patient monitoring services.

Postprocedure Care

If the patients are receiving a vasopressin infusion, they will of necessity return from the procedure room with an arterial catheter in place. This is best monitored in an ICU setting in which the patient has a primary, one-to-one nurse. Frequent catheter checks and groin observation for hematoma are essential. The authors deliver 0.2–0.4 unit of vasopressin per minute using an autosyringe or Harvard pump mechanism, both of which are capable of generating suprasystemic pressures and the delivery rate of which can be precisely controlled. Generally, with a 6F or 7F catheter, flow rates of 50–75 ml/hr are required to keep the catheter open, and the concentration of vasopressin is formulated by the pharmacy to fulfill this requirement.

The typical GI bleeding case is referred to the authors late in the afternoon or in the early evening. Assuming the bleeding site is identified and vasopressin is begun, an angiogram is performed after 20–30 min of infusion. If bleeding is still identified, the dose is doubled to 0.4 unit/min. In another 20–30 min, angiography is repeated to see if bleeding has been controlled, and the patient is sent to the ICU with the infusion running. Generally, the patient is returned for the first follow-up angiogram 12–24 hr after the infusion was started. If bleeding has subsided clinically and angiographically, the infusion is continued at the same rate for another 12 hr and then slowly reduced, as described earlier. If bleeding does not resume, the vasopressin infusion is stopped and the patient is sent to the ward with 5% dextrose or lactated Ringer's solution infusing through the catheter. If there are no clinical signs of bleeding over the next 8–12 hr the catheter is removed.

References

1. Baum S, Nusbaum M, Blakemore A, Finkelstein K: The preoperative radiographic demonstration of intra-abdominal bleeding from undetermined sites by percutaneous selective celiac and superior mesenteric arteriography. *Surgery* 1965;58:797
2. Margulis AR, Heinbecker P, Bernard HR: Operative mesenteric arteriography in the search for the site of bleeding in unexplained gastrointestinal hemorrhage. *Surgery* 1960;48:534
3. Nusbaum M, Baum S: Radiographic demonstration of unknown sites of GI bleeding. *Surg Forum* 1963;14:374
4. Rahn NH III, Tishler JMA, Han SY, Russinovich NAE: Diagnostic and interventional angiography in acute gastrointestinal hemorrhage. *Radiology* 1982;143:361
5. Kalff V, Kelly MJ, Dudley F, et al: Management of acute intermittent gastrointestinal bleeding. *Radiology* 1984;152:270
6. Smith RK, Arterburn JG: Advantages of delayed imaging and

radiographic correlation in scintigraphic localization of gastrointestinal bleeding. *Radiology* 1981;136:707

7. Smith RK, Arterburn JG: Detection and localization of gastrointestinal bleeding using Tc-99m-pyrophosphate in vivo labeled red blood cells. *Radiology* 1980;136:287

8. Bunker SR, Brown JM, McAuley RJ, et al: Detection of gastrointestinal bleeding sites: use of in vitro technetium Tc 99m-labeled RBC's. *Radiology* 1982;145:286

9. Winzelberg GG, McKusnick KA, Froelich JW, et al: Detection of gastrointestinal bleeding with 99m-Tc-labeled red blood cells. *Radiology* 1982;142:139

10. Alavi A: Detection of gastrointestinal bleeding with 99m-Tc-sulfur colloid. *Radiology* 1982;12:126

11. Som P, Oster ZH, Atkins HL, et al: Detection of gastrointestinal blood loss with 99m-Tc-labeled, heat-treated red blood cells. *Radiology* 1981;138:207

12. Markisz JA, Front D, Royal HD, et al: Evaluation of Tc-99m labeled red blood cell scintigraphy for the detection and localization of gastrointestinal bleeding sites. *Radiology* 1983;147:316

13. Winn M, Weissmann HS, Sprayregen S, et al: Radionuclide detection of lower gastrointestinal bleeding sites. *Radiology* 1984;151:835

14. Alavi A: Radionuclide localization of gastrointestinal hemorrhage. *Radiology* 1982;142:801

15. Miskowiak J, Nielsen SL, Munck O: Scintigraphic diagnosis of gastrointestinal bleeding with 99m-Tc-labeled blood-pool agents. *Radiology* 1981;141:499

16. Bunker SR, Lull RJ, Tanasescu DE, et al: Scintigraphy of gastrointestinal hemorrhage: superiority of 99m-Tc red blood cells over 99m-Tc sulfur colloid. *Radiology* 1984;143:543

17. Ferrant A, Dehasque N, Leners N, et al: Scintigraphy with In-111-labeled red cells in intermittent gastrointestinal bleeding. *Radiology* 1981;139:270

18. Rosch J, Antonovic R, Dotter CT: Current angiographic approach to diagnosis and therapy of acute gastrointestinal bleeding. *Fortschr Röntgenstr* 1976;125:301–310

19. Goldman ML, Land WC, Bradley EL III, Anderson J: Transcatheter therapeutic embolization in the management of massive upper gastrointestinal bleeding. *Radiology* 1976;120:513

20. Goldstein HM, Medellin H, Ben-Menachem Y, Wallace S: Transcatheter arterial embolization in the management of bleeding in the cancer patient. *Radiology* 1975;115:603

21. Rosch J, Dotter CT, Brown MJ: Selective arterial embolization. *Radiology* 1972;102:303

22. Ring EJ, Oleaga JA, Freiman D, Husted JW, Waltman AC, Baum S: Pitfalls in the angiographic management of hemorrhage: hemodynamic considerations. *AJR* 1977;129:1007

23. Higgins CB, Bookstein JJ, Davis GB, Galloway DC, Barr JW: Therapeutic embolization for intractable chronic bleeding. *Radiology* 1977;122:473

24. Reuter SR, Chuang VP, Bell RL: Selective arterial embolization for control of massive upper gastrointestinal bleeding. *AJR* 1975;125:119

25. Reuter SR, Chuang VP: Control of abdominal bleeding with autologous embolized material. *Radiology* 1974;14:86

26. Kaufman SL, Kumar AAJ, Harrington DP, et al: Transcatheter embolization in the management of congenital arteriovenous malformations. *Radiology* 1980;137:21

27. Lunderquist A: Angiography and ulcerative colitis. *AJR* 1967;99:18

28. Tsuchiaya M, Miura S, Asakura H, et al: Angiographic evaluation of vascular changes in ulcerative colitis. *Angiology* 1980;31:147

29. Clark RA, Colley DP, Eggers FM: Acute arterial gastrointestinal hemorrhage: efficacy of transcatheter control. *Radiology* 1981;136:1185

30. Jander HP, Russinovich NAE: Transcatheter Gelfoam embolization in abdominal, retroperitoneal, and pelvic hemorrhage. *Radiology* 1980;136:337

31. Feldman L, Greenfield AJ, Waltman AC et al: Transcatheter vessel occlusion: angiographic results versus clinical success. *Radiology* 1983;147:1

32. Baum S, Nusbaum M: The control of gastrointestinal hemorrhage by selective mesenteric arterial infusion of vasopressin. *Radiology* 1971;98:497

33. Nusbaum M, Baum S, Blakemore WS, Tumen H: Clinical experience with selective intra-arterial infusion of vasopressin in the control of gastrointestinal bleeding from arterial sources. *Am J Surg* 1972;123:165

34. Baum S, Athanasoulis CA, Waltman AC, Ring EJ: Angiographic diagnosis and control. *Adv Surg* 1973;7:49

35. Bookstein JJ, Chlosta EM, Foley D, Walter JF: Transcatheter hemostasis of gastrointestinal bleeding using modified autogenous clot. *Radiology* 1974;113:227

36. White RI, Harrington DP, Novak G, Miller FJ, Giargiana FA, Sheff RN: Pharmacologic control of hemorrhagic gastritis: clinical and experimental results. *Radiology* 1974:111:549

37. Herrera M, Castañeda WR, Kotula F, Rysavy J, Rusnak B, Amplatz K: Ivalon shavings, a new embolic agent: technical considerations. *Radiology* 1982;144:683

38. Carsen GM, Casarella WJ, Spiegel RM: Transcatheter embolization for treatment of Mallory–Weiss tears of the esophagogastric junction. *Radiology* 1978;128:309

39. Fisher RG, Schwartz JT, Graham DY: Angiotherapy with Mallory–Weiss tear. *Radiology* 1980;134:679

40. Eisenberg H, Steer ML: The nonoperative treatment of massive pyloroduodenal hemorrhage by retracted autologous clot embolization. *Surgery* 1976;79:414

41. Lunderquist A, Hoevels J, Owman T: Transhepatic portal venography, in Abrams HL (ed): *Abrams' Angiography: Vascular and Interventional Radiology,* Ed 3. Boston, Little, Brown, and Company, 1983, p 1505

42. Fleig WE, Stange EF, Ditschuneit H: Upper gastrointestinal hemorrhage from downhill esophageal varices. *Radiology* 1982;144:699

43. Lunderquist A, Borjesson B, Owman T, Bengmark S: Isobutyl II cyanocrylate (Bucrylate) in obliteration of gastric coronary vein in esophageal varices. *AJR* 1978;130:1

44. Hanna SS, Warren WD, Galambos JT: Bleeding varices: emergency management. *Radiology* 1981;140:583

45. Hanna SS, Warren WD, Galambos JT: Bleeding varices: elective management. *Radiology* 1981;140:585

46. Agha FP: Esophagus after endoscopic injection sclerotherapy: acute and chronic changes. *Radiology* 1984;153:37

47. Tihansky DP, Reilly JJ, Schade RR, Van Thiel DH: Esophagus after injection sclerotherapy of varices: immediate postoperative changes. *Radiology* 1984;153:43

48. Wiechal KL: Tekniken vid perkutan transhepatisk portapunktion (PTP). *Nord Med* 1971;86:912

49. Widrich WC: Embolization therapy of esophageal varices. Presented at the Eighth Annual Course on Diagnostic and Therapeutic Angiography and Interventional Radiology, Society of Cardiovascular Radiology, San Francisco, February 1983

50. Widrich WC, Robbins AH, Nabseth DC, Johnson WC, Goldstein SA: Pitfalls of transhepatic portal venography and therapeutic coronary vein occlusion. *AJR* 1978;131:637

51. Pereiras R, Viamonte M Jr, Russel E, LaPage J, White P, Hutson D: New technique for interruption of gastroesophageal venous blood flow. *Radiology* 1977;124:313

52. Mendez G Jr, Russell E: Gastrointestinal varices: percutaneous transhepatic therapeutic embolization in 54 patients. *Radiology* 1980;135:1045

53. Funaro AH, Ring EJ, Freiman DB, Oleaga JA, Gordon RL: Transhepatic obliteration of esophageal varices using the stainless steel coil. *AJR* 1979;133:1123

54. Viamonte M Jr, Pereiras R, Russel R, LaPage J, Hutson D: Transhepatic obliteration of gastro-esophageal varices: results in acute and nonacute bleeders. *AJR* 1977;129:237

55. Spigos DG, Tauber JW, Tau WS, Mulligan BD, Espinoza GL: Umbilical venous cannulation: a new approach for embolization of esophageal varices. *Radiology* 1983;146:53

56. Goldman ML, Fajman W, Galambos J: Transjugular obliteration of the gastric coronary vein. *Radiology* 1976;118:453

57. Athanasoulis CA, Baum S, Waltman AC, Ring EJ, Imbembo A, Vander Salm TJ: Control of acute gastric mucosal hemorrhage: intra-arterial infusion of posterior pituitary extract. *N Engl J Med* 1974;290:597

58. Rosch J, Dotter CT, Antonovic R: Selective vasoconstrictor infusion in the management of arterio-capillary gastrointestinal hemorrhage. *AJR* 1972;116:279

59. Rosch J, Keller FS, Kozak B, Niles N, Dotter CT: Gelfoam powder embolization of the left gastric artery in treatment of massive small-vessel gastric bleeding. *Radiology* 1984;151:365

60. Reuter ST, Chuang VP, Bree RL: Selective arterial embolization for control of massive upper gastrointestinal bleeding. *AJR* 1975;125:119

61. Katzen BT, McSweeney J: Therapeutic transluminal arterial embolization for bleeding in the upper part of the gastrointestinal tract. *Surg Gynecol Obstet* 1975;141:523

62. White RI Jr, Giargiana FA Jr, Bell W: Bleeding duodenal ulcer control: selective arterial embolization with autologous blood clot. *JAMA* 1974;229:546

63. Bookstein JJ, Chlosta EM, Foley D, et al: The transcatheter hemostasis of gastrointestinal bleeding using modified autologous clot. *Radiology* 1974;113:277

64. Collen MJ, Hanan MR, Maher JA, et al: Cimetidine vs. placebo in duodenal ulcer therapy. *Radiology* 1981;139:524

65. Bradley EL, Goldman M: Gastric infarction after therapeutic embolization. *Surgery* 1976;79:421

66. Prochaska JM, Flye MW, Johnsrude IS: Left gastric artery embolization for central gastric bleeding: a complication. *Radiology* 1973;107:521

67. Castañeda–Zuñiga WR, Jauregui H, Rysavy J, Amplatz K: Selective transcatheter embolization of the upper gastrointestinal tract: an experimental study. *Radiology* 1978;127:81

68. Gold RE, Grace M: Gelfoam embolization of the left gastric artery for bleeding ulcer. *Radiology* 1975;116:575

69. Waltman AC, Greenfield AJ, Novelline RA, Athanasoulis CA: Pyloroduodenal bleeding and intra-arterial vasopressin: clinical results. *AJR* 1979;133:643

70. Athanasoulis CA: Therapeutic applications of angiography. *N Engl J Med* 1980;302:1117 and 1174

71. Athanasoulis CA, Waltman AC, Ring EJ, Smith JC, Baum S: Angiographic management of postoperative bleeding. *Radiology* 1974;113:37

72. Rosenbaum A, Siegelman S, Sprayregen S: The bleeding marginal ulcer: catheterization, diagnosis and therapy. *AJR* 1975;125:812

73. Sfakianakis GN, Conway JJ: Detection of ectopic gastric mucosa in Meckel's diverticulum and in other aberrations by scintigraphy: indications and methods—a 10 year experience. *Radiology* 1982;143:299

74. Gordon I: Gastro-intestinal hemorrhage unrelated to gastric mucosa diagnosed on 99m-Tc pertechnetate scans. *Radiology* 1980;136:821

75. Briley CA Jr, Jackson DC, Johnsrude IS, Mills SR: Acute gastrointestinal hemorrhage of small-bowel origin. *Radiology* 1980;136:317

76. Spiegel RM, Schultz RW, Casarella WJ, Wolff M: Massive hemorrhage from jejunal diverticula. *Radiology* 1982;143:367

77. Fazio VW, Zelas P, Weakley FL: Intraoperative angiography and the localization of bleeding from the small intestine. *Radiology* 1980;139:524

78. Athanasoulis CA, Moncure AC, Greenfield AJ, et al: Intraoperative localization of small bowel bleeding sites with combined use of angiographic methods and methylene blue injection. *Surgery* 1980;87:77

79. Uflacker R, Amaral NM, Lima S, et al: Angiography in primary myomas of the alimentary tract. *Radiology* 1981;139:361

80. Zornoza J, Dodd GD Jr: Lymphoma of the gastrointestinal tract. *Semin Roentgenol* 1980;15:272

81. Palmaz JC, Walter JF, Cho KJ: Therapeutic embolization of the small-bowel arteries. *Radiology* 1984;152:377

82. Song-Nian L, Wan-Zhong Z, Xie Jing-Xia, et al: Gastrointestinal tract carcinoid: radiologic and pathologic morphology. *Chin Med J* 1982;95:136

83. Birns MT, Katon RM, Keller F: Intramural hematoma of small intestine presenting with major upper gastrointestinal hemorrhage: case report and review of literature. *Radiology* 1980;134:816

84. Crawford ES, Roehm JOF Jr, McGavren MH: Jejunoileal arteriovenous malformation: localization for resection by segmental bowel staining techniques. *Radiology* 1980;137:880

85. Boijsen E, Reuter SR: Mesenteric arteriography in the evaluation of inflammatory and neoplastic disease of the intestine. *Radiology* 1966;87:1028

86. Brahme F: Mesenteric angiography in regional enterocolitis. *Radiology* 1966;87:1037

87. Castañeda–Zuñiga WR, Javregui J, Garera Reyes R, Amplatz K: Bleeding from cecal ulcers in renal transplant patients. *Rev Interam Radiol* 1978;3:27

88. Boley SJ, Sprayregen S, Sammartanor J, Adams A, Kleinhaus S: The patho-physiologic basis for the angiographic signs of vascular ectasias of the colon. *Radiology* 1977;125:615

89. Nyman U, Boijsen E, Lindstrom C, et al: Angiography in angiomatous lesions of the gastrointestinal tract. *Radiology* 1981;138:521

90. Lewis HJE, Gledhill T, Gilmour HM, et al: Arteriovenous malformation of intestine. *Radiology* 1980;135:264

91. Talman EA, Dixon DS, Gutierrez FE: Role of arteriography in rectal hemorrhage due to arteriovenous malformations and diverticulosis. *Radiology* 1980;134:816

92. Max MH, Richardson JD, Flint LM Jr, et al: Colonoscopic diagnosis of angiodysplasias of the gastointestinal tract. *Radiology* 1981;140:855

93. Walker WJ, Goldin AR, Shaff MI, Allibone GW: Per catheter control of hemorrhage from the superior and inferior mesenteric arteries. *Clin Radiol* 1980;31:71

94. Shaff ME, Becker H: Diagnosis and control of diverticular bleeding by arteriography and vasopressin infusion. *S Afr Med J* 1979;56:72

95. Maglinte DDT, Keller KJ, Miller RE, Chernish SM: Colon and rectal carcinoma: spatial distribution and detection. *Radiology* 1983;147:669

96. Johnson CD, Carlson JC, Taylor WF, et al: Barium enemas of carcinoma of the colon: sensitivity of double- and single-contrast studies. *Radiology* 1983;140:1143

97. Thoemi RF, Petras AF: Detection of rectal and rectosigmoid lesions by double-contrast barium enema examination and sigmoidoscopy: accuracy of technique and efficacy of standard overhead views. *Radiology* 1982;142:59

98. Halpern N: Selective inferior mesenteric arteriography. *Vasc Dis* 1964;1:294

99. Strom BG, Winberg T: Percutaneous selective arteriography of the inferior mesenteric artery. *Acta Radiol (Stockh)* 1962;57:401

100. Wholey NH, Bron KM, Haller JB: Selective angiography of the colon. *Surg Clin North Am* 1965;45:1283

101. Stromb G, Winberg T: Percutaneous selective arteriography of the inferior mesenteric artery. *Acta Radiol (Stockh)* 1962;57:401

102. Hessel SJ, Adams DF, Abrams HL: Complications of angiography. *Radiology* 1981;138:273

103. Jacobson B, Curtin H, Rubenson A, et al: Complications of angiography in children and means of prevention. *Radiology* 1981;138:273

10

Site and Etiology of Hemobilia

IVAN VUJIC, M.D.

In 50% of cases of hemobilia, bleeding originates from the liver parenchyma, whereas the biliary ducts and the gallbladder are the source in approximately 45% of the cases. Hemobilia due to pancreatic disease is rare (see following chapter).

CAUSES

Trauma is by far the most common cause of hemobilia, accounting for 50% of the cases (Fig. 10–1). Approximately one-third are iatrogenic. With the many traffic accidents and the recent introduction of invasive percutaneous radiographic procedures, one should expect to see an increasing percentage of cases of hemobilia of traumatic origin.[1]

Although hemobilia is present in only 2.5% of cases of accidental liver trauma,[2] the incidence following diagnostic biopsy is 3%–7%[3] and that following percutaneous transhepatic cholangiography (Fig. 10–2) with an 18-gauge needle is 4%.[4] An incidence of 14% after percutaneous transhepatic biliary drainage was reported by Monden et al.[5] Similarly, late angiography in 83 patients who had undergone percutaneous transhepatic biliary drainage revealed a substantial number of vascular com-

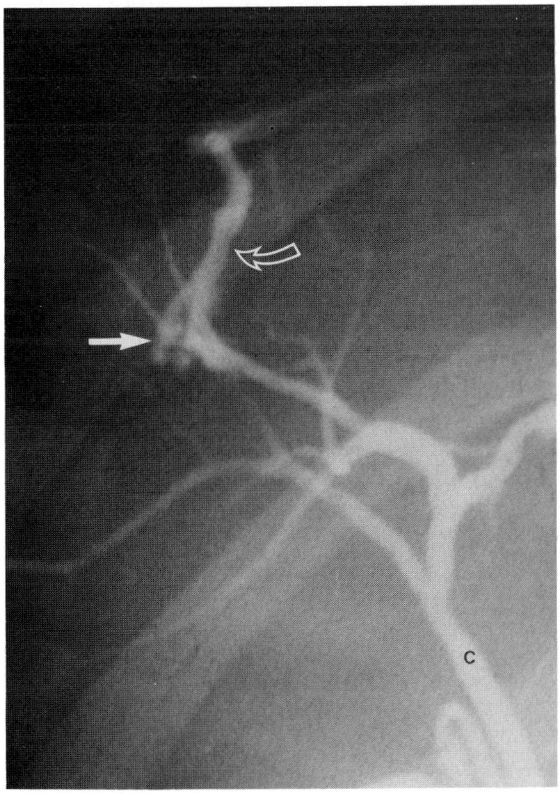

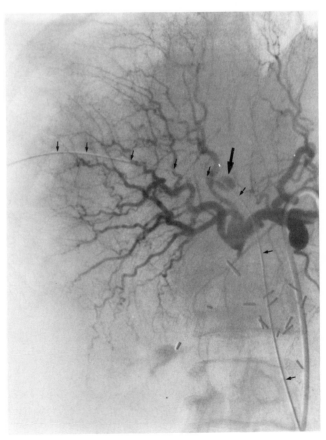

Fig. 10–1 Endoscopic retrograde cholangiogram with bile ducts injected via catheter positioned in common bile ducts (c) opacifies fistula (white arrow) and segmental branch of right hepatic vein (open arrow).

Fig. 10–2 Common hepatic arteriography reveals false aneurysm arising from right hepatic artery (large arrow) in patient following percutaneous biliary drainage. Small arrows show position of drainage catheter.

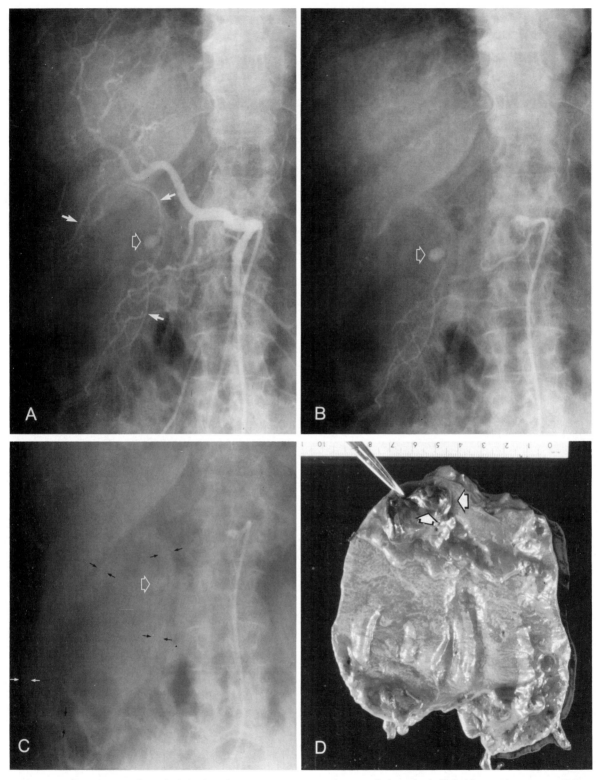

Fig. 10–3 Early arterial phase of hepatic injection demonstrates branches of cystic artery (white arrows) outlining gallbladder and pool of contrast medium (open arrow) in region of gallbladder neck. B. Late arterial phase shows persistent collection of contrast medium (open arrow) within dilated gallbladder. C. Venous phase demonstrating a thickened and irregular gallbladder wall (small arrows). Collection of contrast medium persists (open arrow). D. Approxi- mately 1 cm below the gallbladder neck, note partially organized thrombus (arrows) adherent to area of ulceration, corresponding to angiographically demonstrated bleeding site. (Reproduced from Ryvecher MY, Schatz SL, Deutch AM, Cohen HR: Angiographic demonstration of bleeding into the gallbladder. *Radiology* 1980;136:326.)

plications, with four patients presenting with severe hemobilia due to a pseudoaneurysm adjacent to the drainage catheter.[6] More recently, sporadic cases of hemobilia following endobiliary prosthesis placement and the use of an infusion pump for intra-arterial delivery of chemotherapy have been described.[1] Hemobilia is usually of no clinical significance and subsides spontaneously, although occasionally significant bleeding follows diagnostic percutaneous procedures.[7]

Another form of iatrogenic hemobilia is caused by cholecystectomy and surgical manipulations in the biliary tree.[8] The extraction of stones in conjunction with the exploration of biliary ducts can result in bleeding secondary to mucosal laceration by the instruments. Occasionally, bleeding can be due to a pseudoaneurysm following surgical exploration.[1]

Gallstones and stones in the common bile duct are associated with hemobilia in 25% and 37% of cases, respectively.[9] In most of these cases, the bleeding is caused by mucosal irritation during stone passage. This type of bleeding is minor and ceases spontaneously. Pressure necrosis of the wall, however, allows the stone to migrate to adjacent hollow structures and can cause severe hemobilia if vascular erosion occurs (Fig. 10–3).[10]

Hemobilia can also be caused by inflammatory lesions, the most common of which has been coexisting gallstones and cholecystocholangitis.[1,8,11] On the other hand, in the Far East, "tropical hemobilia" caused by *Ascaris* is by far the most common form.[12]

Extensive necrosis of the liver due to drug-induced hepatitis[13] and halothane anesthesia[14] has been blamed for severe hemobilia. Similarly, on very rare occasions, hemobilia has been associated with abscess (Fig. 10–4),[15] hydatid cyst,[16] and amebic infection.[17]

Primary or metastatic malignancy of the liver, gallbladder, or bile ducts may result in severe hemobilia. Single adenomatous polyps, diffuse biliary papillomatosis, aberrant pancreatic tissue in the wall of the gallbladder,[10] and other benign tumors[18–22] have been occasional sources of profuse hemorrhage. Coagulopathy is a rare cause.[1]

Only 7% of cases of hemobilia are caused by vascular abnormalities.[10] The passage of blood into the biliary tree is the result arteriobiliary (Fig. 10–5A,B) or, rarely, of venobiliary fistulae (Fig. 10–6). An arteriobiliary fistula is usually the consequence of penetrating trauma but may result from spontaneous rupture of hematomas, necrotic liver tissue (Fig. 10–4), or aneurysms into the bile ducts (Figs. 10–5 and 10–6). Venobiliary fistulae may occur

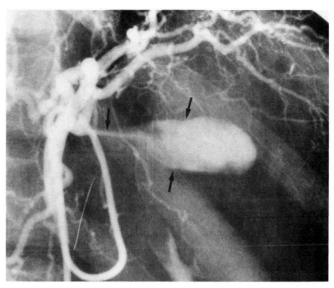

Fig. 10–4 Patient with bacterial liver abscess presenting with severe gastrointestinal bleeding. Selective left hepatic arteriography reveals extensive extravasation of contrast medium (arrows) in area of hepatic abscess.

between the portal or hepatic vein and the biliary radicles and may be associated with hemobilia (Fig. 10–7).[23,24] Aneurysms or pseudoaneurysms involving the hepatic artery have a great tendency to rupture, and if this happens, free communication with the biliary tree is not uncommon.[25] Hemobilia due to ruptured gastroduodenal and cystic arteries has been recorded in a number of patients.[26]

Arteriovenous fistulae are often present in association with hemobilia. The most common fistula is one between the hepatic artery and the portal vein.[27] If the fistula is large, it may lead to severe portal hypertension.[28,29]

Portal hypertension may cause hemobilia, most often when large varices along the biliary ducts or gallbladder wall rupture. Varices of this type have been reported accompanying severe portal hypertension due to a primary hepatic malignancy invading the portal system or to cirrhosis.[30,31] The varices can enlarge, compress nearby tissues, and subsequently cause obstructive jaundice. It is essential to realize that these patients are prone to bleed spontaneously or following any invasive radiologic or surgical procedure.[32]

CLINICAL PRESENTATION AND DIAGNOSIS

Hemobilia remains difficult to diagnose even with the newer imaging modalities. The combination of gastrointestinal bleeding and biliary colic resembling gallstone disease should raise the suspicion of hemobilia. A classic triad of gastrointestinal bleeding, biliary colic, and obstructive jaundice is present in about one-third of patients.[27] Gastrointestinal bleeding occurs as melena or hematemesis. Additional symptoms include anemia in 70% of cases, fever, a palpable mass in the right upper quadrant, and dull pain (Fig. 10–3).[10] Shock due to significant blood loss is not uncommon. When blood seeps into the duodenum slowly, the cardinal symptoms are not present, and the only manifestation may be chronic anemia. Another important feature is the time lag between the initial injury and the evidence of subtle bleeding and recurrence of hemorrhage, which may be present for weeks, months, or years.

The diagnosis of hemobilia is difficult unless the condition is suspected. Percutaneous transhepatic cholangiography (Fig. 10–1) or endoscopic retrograde cholangio-

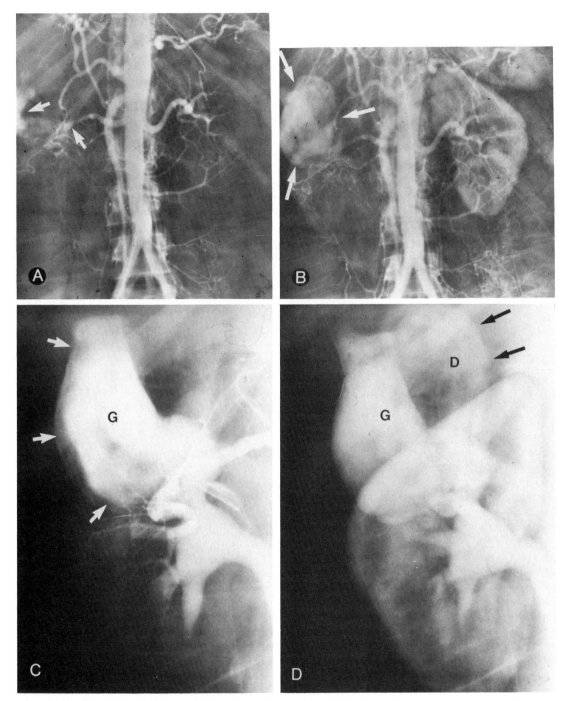

Fig. 10-5 A,B. Patient with massive upper gastrointestinal bleeding. Abdominal aortogram reveals massive extravasation from the right renal artery (A, arrows) with a localized collection in the right upper quadrant (B, arrows). C. Selective right renal arteriogram shows massive extravasation of contrast medium into the gallbladder (arrows). D. Late phase of arteriogram reveals passage of contrast medium from the gallbladder (G) into the duodenum (D) (arrows). Surgery demonstrated the presence of a communication between the gallbladder and a patch that was performed to correct severe fibromuscular dysplasia of the renal artery 10 years previously.

Fig. 10-7 Wedge hepatic venogram in patient with severe hemobilia following blunt abdominal trauma shows opacification of biliary radicles from hepatic veins (arrow).

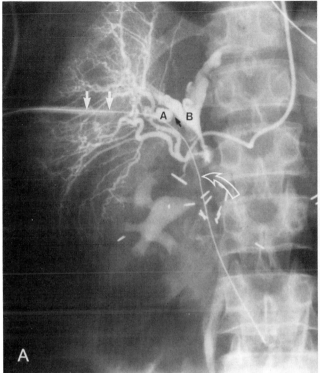

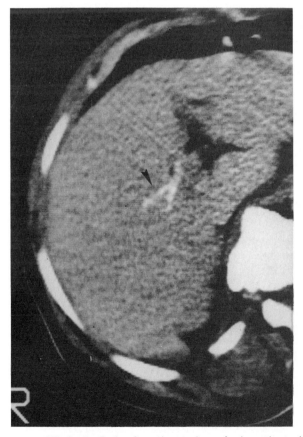

Fig. 10-6 False aneurysm. A. Selective right hepatic arteriogram confirms to better advantage the presence of a false aneurysm (A). Note also opacification of biliary radicle (B) from false aneurysm (black arrow), after partial pull-back of tamponading drainage cath-eter (white arrows) over a guidewire (curved white arrow). Same patient as in Figure 10-2. B. Repeat right hepatic arteriogram after embolization reveals occlusion of hepatic artery branch feeding false aneurysm (arrow).

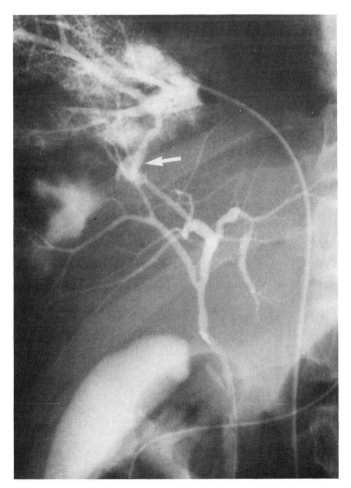

Fig. 10-8 CT obtained after hepatic arteriography in patient with known hemobilia shows dense opacification of biliary radicles (arrowhead).

pancreatography may show filling defects, but they are not pathognomonic for hemobilia. Ultrasonic examination may identify a hypoechogenic hematoma within the liver[23] or a dense echogenic intraluminal mass within the gallbladder without acoustic shadowing.[33,34]

A preliminary report suggests that computed tomography (CT) can reveal the presence of blood clots in the gallbladder[35] and therefore may serve as the initial screening procedure if hemobilia is suspected. The normal gallbladder density measures from 0–20 Hounsfield units (HU). In experimental work on monkeys, it was shown that hemobilia homogeneously or nonhomogeneously increases the attenuation coefficient of bile to > 50–60 HU (Fig. 10–8). Follow-up CT scans show a gradual increase in the attenuation coefficient of retracted blood clots over time, a feature that makes CT an attractive screening modality. On endoscopy and angiography one can miss the diagnosis because of the intermittent character of the bleeding episodes. An additional important advantage of CT is its ability to identify cholelithiasis, milk of calcium, tumors, and liver trauma as possible causes of hemobilia.

The observation of a dense accumulation of contrast medium in the biliary tree after selective hepatic angiography (Figs. 10–6A and 10–7) is another finding that suggests hemobilia.[36] However, this finding should be interpreted cautiously, because use of cholecystographic agents, vicarious excretion of urographic water-soluble contrast media, and reflux of orally administered contrast medium through the papilla of Vater due to a malfunctioning sphincter all may increase the attenuation value of bile.[35] Strax et al demonstrated that the usual increase in the density of bile follows the use of contrast medium with >37 g of iodine.[37] Therefore, the identification of contrast medium in the biliary system after angiographic examination occurs normally by itself and should be diagnostic of hemobilia only if it is associated with endoscopic proof.

A definitive diagnosis of hemobilia is made by direct observation of blood coming through the ampulla of Vater. Unfortunately, because of the intermittent character of the bleeding, endoscopic diagnosis is made in only approximately 50% of patients.[27,38] Because the principal reason for failure in diagnosis is this intermit-

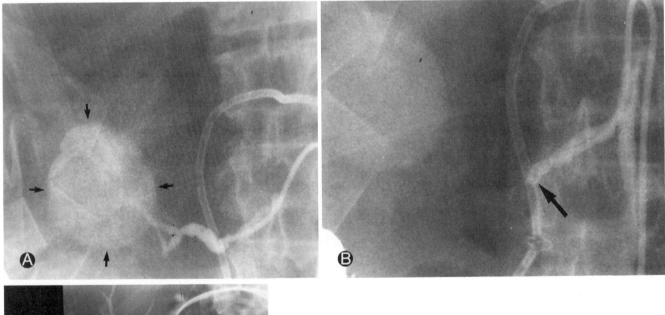

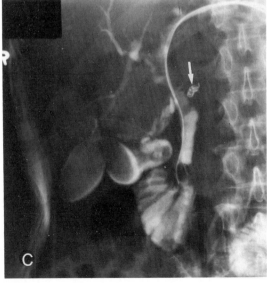

Fig. 10–9 Patient with severe bleeding after partial hepatic resection. A. Selective common hepatic arteriogram shows extravasation into large false aneurysm (arrows). B. Angiogram after embolization with GWC coils shows complete occlusion of hepatic artery branches supplying false aneurysm (arrow). C. Cholangiogram through drainage catheter shows large amount of blood clots in bile ducts and gallbladder. Arrow points to coils in hepatic artery.

tent type of bleeding, extended endoscopic observation of the papilla is recommended.[39] With minor bleeding, a hemoglobin-positive duodenal content, in the presence of otherwise normal endoscopic findings, may be the only positive test.

The most rewarding evaluation is obtained by selective celiomesenteric angiography. The angiographic feature most frequently associated with hemobilia originating in the liver and bile ducts is a pseudoaneurysm (Figs. 10–2, 10–4, and 10–6A). Hepatic artery–portal vein fistulae are also common, whereas communication between the hepatic artery and the hepatic veins is rare. Only a few cases of direct venobiliary fistulae have been reported (Fig. 10–7).[24] In spite of the proximity of the hepatic artery, portal vein, and bile ducts, extravasation of contrast medium into the biliary tree is seen in only 25% of patients.

TREATMENT

Significant hemobilia seldom ceases spontaneously and thus usually necessitates surgical or, more recently, angiographic intervention. Surgical treatment consists of either liver suturing or partial hepatic resection for peripheral lesions and ligation of the hepatic artery for more central injuries. Early recognition and prompt intervention seem to be the reasons for the gradual decrease in the mortality rate.[1] Cholecystectomy is the procedure of choice for every case in which the gallbladder is a source of bleeding (Fig. 10–3).

In recent years, since Walter et al described a case of hemobilia controlled by angiographic techniques, there has been wide acceptance of this method as the first choice for the treatment of relatively stable patients.[40] Vaughan et al, in a reveiw of 34 published cases, found that vascular embolization controlled hemobilia in every case.[38] In most cases, Gelfoam particles were successful (Fig. 10–6B), although for larger hepatoportal or hepatobiliary fistulae, the use of GWC spring coils or detachable balloons is indicated (Fig. 10–9).[41–43] The primary goal of embolic therapy should be to reduce the pulsatile blood pressure distal to the artificial occlusion rather than to devascularize the hepatic parenchyma. Peripheral placement of the catheter in the vessel feeding the abnormality and embolization with absorbable particulate material seems to be most effective. Central embolization of the main hepatic artery or one of its principal branches is indicated whenever a peripheral branch cannot be catheterized or if the patient's deteriorating condition mandates prompt intervention. Spring coils or detachable balloon catheters can be used for these occlusions. Infarctions and necrosis of liver parenchyma usually do not occur with central embolization because of enormous potential for collateral circulation distal to the site of interruption of the blood flow.

The low rate of complications of embolic therapy in the liver is the result of the dual hepatic vascular supply. The portal vein contributes 75%–80% of the oyxgen and metabolic needs, so prior to any interventional occlusive therapy, one should cautiously evaluate the portal anatomy and hemodynamics and avoid embolization procedures in patients with severely compromised portal flow. Minor

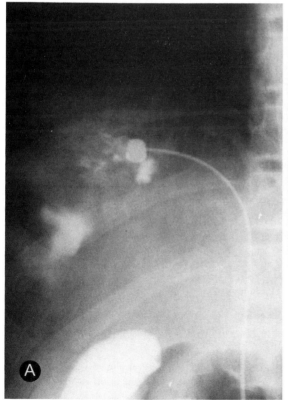

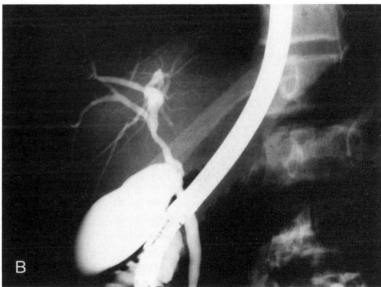

Fig. 10–10 Venobiliary fistula. A. Balloon in wedge position to occlude fistula. Same patient as in Figure 10–6. B. Endoscopic retrograde cholangiogram 3 1/2 weeks later. Normal biliary pattern. (Reproduced from Struyven J, Cremer M, Pirson P, Jennty P, Jeanmart Y: Posttraumatic bilhemia: diagnosis and catheter therapy. *AJR* 1982;138:746–747.)

liver damage manifested as a transient elevation of serum liver enzyme concentrations is present in approximately 20% of patients. Major complications are rare and associated with obstructive jaundice.[6] It is believed that decreased portal perfusion of the liver is associated with obstruction of bile ducts. As a result of this hemodynamic change, the liver parenchyma becomes more and more dependent on the arterial blood flow and consequently very sensitive to the ischemic conditions created by embolization of hepatic arteries.[44]

Venobiliary fistulae with clinical evidence of bilemia may be treated by temporary occlusion of the venous end of the fistula with a balloon catheter (Fig. 10–10A,B). This results in thrombosis and permanent occlusion of the abnormal channel.[24]

References

1. Sanblom P, Saegesser F, Mirkovitch V: Hepatic hemobilia: hemorrhage from the intrahepatic biliary tract: a review. *World J Surg* 1984;8:41

2. Fekete F, Guillet R, Giuli R, Goyer S: Hemobilies traumatiques. *Ann Chir* 1969;23:1199

3. Raines DR, VanHeertum RL, Johnson LF: Intrahepatic hematoma: a complication of percutaneous liver biopsy. *Gastroenterology* 1979;67:284

4. Cahow CE, Burell M, Greco R: Hemobilia following percutaneous cholangiography. *Ann Surg* 1977;185:235

5. Monden M, Okamura J, Kobayashi N, et al: Hemobilia after percutaneous transhepatic biliary drainage. *Arch Surg* 1980;115:161

6. Hoevees J, Nilsson U: Intrahepatic vascular lesions following nonsurgical percutaneous transhepatic bile duct intubation. *Gastrointest Radiol* 1980;5:127

7. Merion de Villasante JRE, Alvarez–Rodriquez J, Hernandez–Ortiz J: Management of post-biopsy hemobilia with selective arterial embolization. *AJR* 1977;128:668

8. Larmi TK: Hemobilia associated with cholecystitis, post cholecystectomy conditions and trauma. *Ann Surg* 1966;163:373

9. Gad P: Okkult blodning ved galdesten. *Nord Med* 1962;68:1069

10. Ryvicker MY, Schatz SL, Deutch AM, Cohen HR: Angiographic demonstration of bleeding into the gallbladder. *Radiology* 1980;136:326

11. Salem R, Boesby S, Bowley N, Blumgart LH: Haemobilia and haemoperitoneum. *J R Coll Surg Edinb* 1984;29:262

12. Chen S: On the etiology, pathogenesis, diagnosis and treatment of massive hemorrhage from the intrahepatic bile duct (abstract). In *Proceedings of the VIII National Congress of Surgery*, Peking, 1963, p 28

13. Lichtman SS: Gastrointestinal bleeding in disease of the liver and biliary tract. *Am J Dig Dis* 1936;3:439

14. Makela V, Landesmaki M: Hemobilia associated with hepatic necrosis after halothane anesthesia: a case report. *Ann Chir Gynecol Tenn* 1969;58:183

15. Karam JH, Jacobs T: Hemobilia: report of a case of massive gastrointestinal bleeding originating from a hepatic abscess. *Ann Intern Med* 1961;54:319

16. Goulston E: Massive hemobilia from an hydatid cyst of the liver. *Aust NZ J Surg* 1963;105:662

17. Forestier M: Un cas d'hemobilie aprés un absces amibien du foie. *Mem Acad Chir* 1963;34:83

18. Fisher ER, Creed DL: Clot formation in common duct: unusual manifestation of primary hepatic carcinoma. *Arch Surg* 1956;73:261

19. Rudstom P: Hemobilia in malignant tumours of the liver. *Acta Chir Scand* 1951;101:243

20. Bismuth H, Hernandez C, Hepp J: Les hemobilies d'origine vestibulaire. *Ann Chir* 1976;30:376

21. Hudson PB, Johnson PP: Hemorrhage from gallbladder. *N Engl J Med* 1946;234:438

22. Goldner F: Hemobilia secondary to metastatic liver disease. *Gastroenterology* 1979;76:595

23. Curet P, Baumer R, Roche A, Grellet Y, Mercadier M: Hepatic hemobilia of traumatic or iatrogenic origin: recent advances in diagnosis and therapy. Review of the literature from 1976 to 1981. *World J Surg* 1984;8:2

24. Struyven J, Cremer M, Pirson P, Jeanty P, Jeanmart Y: Post-traumatic bilhemia: diagnosis and catheter therapy. *AJR* 1982;138:746

25. Guida PM, Moore SW: Aneurysm of the hepatic artery: report of five cases with a brief review of the previously reported cases. *Surgery* 1966;60:299

26. Warmath MA, Usselman JA: Hemobilia developing from aneurysm of the left gastric artery. *Gastrointest Radiol* 1980;5:21

27. Foley WJ, Turcotte JG, Hoshins PA, Brant RL, Ause RG: Intrahepatic arteriovenous fistulae between the hepatic artery and portal vein. *Ann Surg* 1971;174:849

28. Cleveland RJ, Jackson BM, Newman PH, Nelson R: Traumatic intrahepatic artery–portal vein fistula with associated hemobilia. *Ann Surg* 1970;171:451

29. Markgraf WH: Traumatic hemobilia associated with hepatoportal biliary fistula. *Arch Surg* 1960;81:860

30. Barzilia R, Kleckner MS Jr: Hemocholecyst following ruptured aneurysm of portal vein. *Arch Surg* 1956;72:725

31. Martelli CF: Contributo allo studio delle emorragie colecistiche. *Arch Osp Mare* 1958;10:259

32. Meredith HC, Vujic I, Schabel SI, O'Brien PH: Obstructive jaundice caused by cavernous transformation of portal vein. *Br J Radiol* 1978;51:1011

33. Ruiz R, Teyssou H, Tessier JP: Apport de l'echographie dans le diagnostic des hemobilies: a propos d'un cas aprés ponction biopsie hepatique transparietale. *Ann Radiol* 1980;22:52

34. Grant EG, Smirniotopoulos JG: Intraluminal gallbladder hematoma: sonographic evidence of hemobilia. *J Clin Ultrasound* 1983;11:507

35. Krudy AG, Doppman JL, Bissonette MB, Girton M: Hemobilia: computed tomographic diagnosis. *Radiology* 1983;148:785

36. Vujic I, Stanley JH, Tyminski L, Cunningham JT, Adams K: Computed tomographic demonstration of hemobilia. *J Comput Assist Tomogr* 1983;7:219

37. Strax R, Toombs BD, Kam J, Rauschkolb EN, Patel S, Sandler CM: Gallbladder enhancement following angiography: a normal CT finding. *J Comput Assist Tomogr* 1982;6:766

38. Vaughan R, Rosch J, Keller FS, Antonovic R: Treatment of hemobilia by transcatheter vascular occlusion. *Eur J Radiol* 1984;4:183

39. Lehman GA, Bash D: Endoscopic observations of hemobilia. *Gastrointest Endosc* 1979;25:110

40. Walter JF, Paaso BT, Cannon BW: Successful transcatheter embolic control of massive hematobilia secondary to liver biopsy. *AJR* 1976;127:847

41. Clark RA, Frey RT, Colley DP, Eiseman WS: Transcatheter embolization of hepatic arteriovenous fistula for control of hemobilia. *Gastrointest Radiol* 1981;6:353

42. Tegtmeyer CJ, Besirdjian DR, Fergerson WW, Hess CE: Transcatheter embolic control of iatrogenic hemobilia. *Cardiovasc Intervent Radiol* 1981;4:88

43. Dunnick NR, Doppman JL, Brereton HD: Balloon occlusion of segmental hepatic arteries: control of biopsy induced hemobilia. *JAMA* 1977;238:2524

44. Doppman JL, Girton M, Vermess M: The risk of hepatic artery embolization in the presence of obstructive jaundice. *Radiology* 1982;143:37

11

Bleeding as a Complication of Pancreatic Disease

IVAN VUJIC, M.D.

Bleeding in association with pancreatic disease is not uncommon, but most of these patients bleed from peptic ulcer disease, hemorrhagic gastritis, or, rarely, Mallory–Weiss syndrome.[1] Far fewer bleed from the direct sequelae of pancreatic disease. Such bleeding is caused either by direct erosion of pancreatic or peripancreatic vessels or by thrombosis, usually involving portal vein tributaries.

MECHANISMS OF BLEEDING

Erosion of vascular structures is caused by the proteolytic activity of pancreatic enzymes, which are released during subacute or recurrent chronic pancreatitis after severe trauma. The result is acute pancreatitis, often leading to formation of a pseudoaneurysm, which has been reported by White et al in 10% of cases of pancreatitis.[2] The process is usually also associated with formation of pancreatic pseudocysts. Once formed, the pseudoaneurysm has a tendency to enlarge[3] and ultimately ruptures into the gastrointestinal tract, the abdominal cavity, or, rarely, the pancreatic ductal system. In some cases, the hemorrhage will be confined to the pseudocyst cavity; but on rare occasions, the pseudocyst erodes the large vessels such as the aorta[4] and portal vein.[5,6] The vessels most commonly involved are, in descending order of frequency, the splenic (Fig. 11–1), gastroduodenal, and pancreaticoduodenal arteries, although virtually every peripancreatic vessel may be involved (Fig. 11–2).[7] This type of hemorrhage is severe and, until recently, had a high mortality rate,[8,9] principally because of inadequate preoperative workup and too conservative treatment.

Hemorrhage may take place prior to, during, or after operation (Fig. 11–3). Frey[10] and Sankaran and Walt[11] reported severe preoperative and postoperative bleeding in 7.6%–9.8%, 6.0%–7.6%, and 7.6%–10% of patients with pancreatic pseudocysts. Similarly, Nielsen reported an 18% postoperative incidence of bleeding following internal drainage of pancreatic pseudocysts.[12] Recently, with more liberal use of angiography and earlier and more aggressive operation, the mortality rate has been reduced considerably.[8]

Although encasement of major arteries is frequently seen in disease of the pancreas, thrombosis of these arteries is not a prominent feature. Occasionally, smaller arteries may thrombose in the course of fatty necrosis in hemorrhagic pancreatitis, leading to bowel infarction.[13,14] On the other hand, thrombotic processes frequently involve the peripancreatic tributaries of the portal vein.

Splenic vein thrombosis is by far the most common, being reported in 8.5%–45% of patients with pancreatitis.[15–18]

The next most common causes of bleeding are tumors of the pancreas, usually carcinomas but occasionally islet cell tumors and cystadenomas.[19] The iatrogenic causes include thrombosis following splenectomy,[20] distal splenorenal shunt,[21] and umbilical vein catheterization.[22] The result of splenic vein thrombosis is gastric varices, which usually develop from the abundant collateral flow through the short gastric veins, which drain into the right and left gastric veins and finally the portal vein (Fig. 11–4). Another major collateral pathway consists of the left gastroepiploic vein, which drains through the omentum

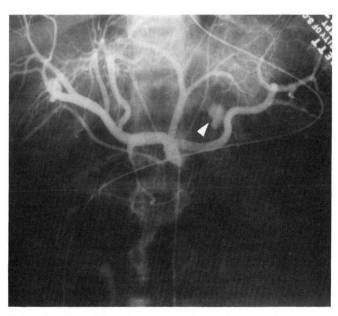

Fig. 11–1 Post-traumatic pancreatitis with pseudoaneurysm (arrowhead) originating in region of small pancreatic branches of splenic artery.

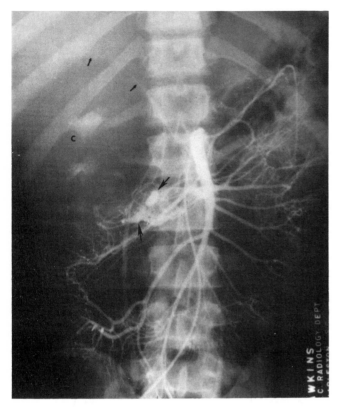

Fig. 11–2   Enlarging hemorrhagic cyst (C) with two pseudoaneurysms originating from small colic branches (large arrows). Note displacement of vessels by enlarging hemorrhagic pseudocysts in head of pancreas (small arrows).

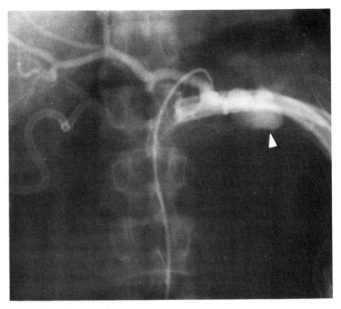

Fig. 11–3   Active bleeding from stump of splenic artery (arrowhead) into pseudocyst and abdominal cavity following splenectomy and distal pancreatotomy.

into the right gastroepiploic and superior mesenteric to the portal vein (Fig. 11–5). Occasionally, however, the left gastroepiploic vein drains through the omental branches of the left colic vein into the inferior mesenteric vein, resulting in colonic varices[23] that are highly suggestive of

splenic vein thrombosis, although in a review of the cases reported in the English language literature, Moosa and Gadd noticed that esophageal varices were present in almost 50% of cases.[19] Such varices develop when the short gastric veins are inadequate to decompress left-sided portal hypertension,[19] which is likely when the coronary vein drains into the splenic rather than the portal vein, an anatomic arrangement present in 70% of persons.[18,24]

Thrombosis involving the portal and superior mesenteric veins is rare and is associated with either a septic stage of severe necrotizing pancreatitis or with carcinoma of the pancreatic head causing pancreatitis.[13,19,25]

CLINICAL PRESENTATION AND DIAGNOSIS

Early recognition of bleeding in patients with known pancreatitis is essential for appropriate successful man-

agement. The chief presenting complaints are gastrointestinal bleeding in half the patients and vague recurrent

Fig. 11–4   Left-sided portal hypertension caused by splenic vein (SV) thrombosis (arrow) due to chronic pancreatitis. Collateral hepatopetal flow through gastric varices, coronary vein (CV) and additional vein paralleling the coronary vein serves as predominant route for decompression. PV = portal vein.

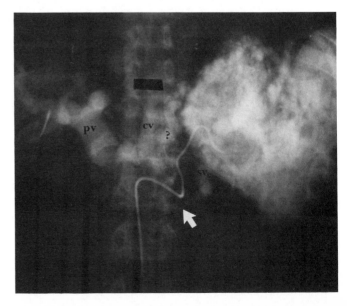

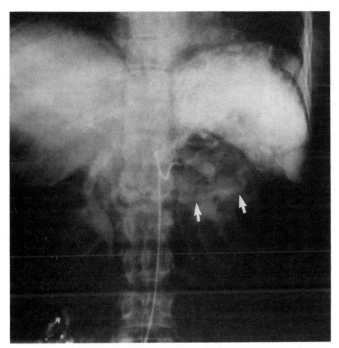

Fig. 11–5 Splenic vein thrombosis at level of splenic hilum with collateral circulation predominantly through the gastroepiploic veins (arrows).

abdominal pain in one-fourth. Splenomegaly is present in approximately one-third of patients. The combination of a palpable abdominal mass, particularly if it is pulsatile, an audible bruit in the vicinity of the mass, abdominal pain, and clinical evidence of bleeding into the gastrointestinal tract or abdominal cavity in association with hyperamylasemia should alert the clinician.

Endoscopy may rule out bleeding from peptic ulcer disease, gastritis, Mallory–Weiss tears, and varices and occasionally may permit diagnosis of pancreatic hemobilia.[26] On rare occasions, it will reveal the site of the erosion of the pseudocyst directly into the gastrointestinal tract.

Ultrasonic patterns associated with a bleeding pancreatic pseudocyst consist of rapid enlargement of a cystic mass and a sudden change in the echogenicity of the inner structures of the cystic space (Fig. 11–6).[27] Recent work suggests that an acute hemorrhagic pancreatic fluid collection presents as a well-defined mass with homogeneous echogenicity. Remote hemorrhagic collections of more than several weeks' duration present as simple appearing cysts. Hemorrhagic collections studied 1 week after a bleeding episode appear as a cystic mass containing solid tissue or septa.[28] It should be remembered, however, that occasionally the distinction between pseudoaneurysm and pseudocyst is impossible.[29]

Computed tomography (CT) is an excellent way to

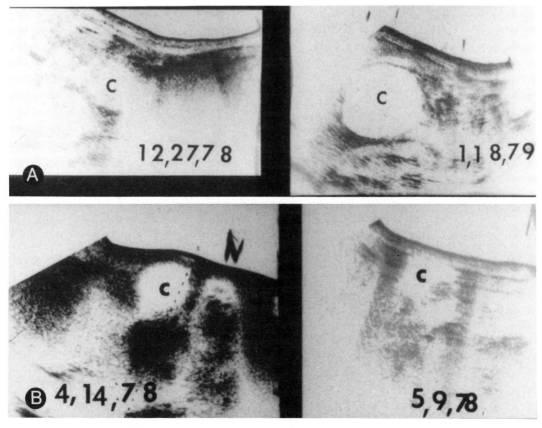

Fig. 11–6 Hemorrhagic pseudocysts. A. Bleeding manifested by the rapid enlargement of the pseudocyst over a period of 3 weeks; compare with Figure 11–2. B. Small pseudoaneurysm in region of tail of the pancreas bleeding into pseudocyst. Mild to moderate enlargement of cavity with change in internal echogenicity indicating bleeding.

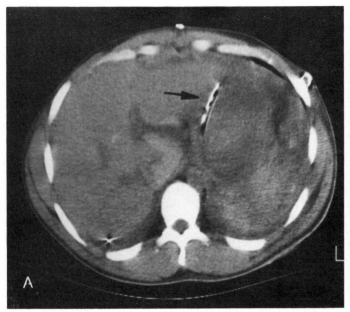

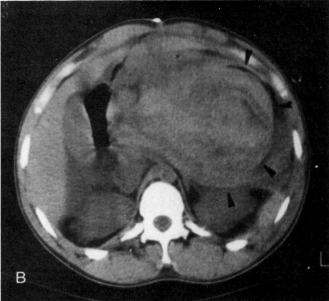

Fig. 11–7 Sudden drop in hematocrit in patient with known pancreatic disease and retrograde cystic mass. A. Acute formation of pseudocyst displacing stomach anteriorly and medially (arrow).

B. Lower level, high-density number within the pseudocyst (arrowheads), indicative of extensive bleeding.

demonstrate an acute hemorrhage in or around the pancreas. The finding of increased density numbers (>30 Hounsfield units) is diagnostic of acute bleeding (Fig. 11–7).[30] Occasionally, CT will identify the aneurysm within the pseudocyst.[31] In addition, CT is the appropriate modality for identification of abnormalities following pancreatic trauma.[32]

Angiography is the procedure of choice for identification of the site and source of bleeding. Its widespread and prompt use in the past decade has led to earlier and more accurate diagnosis, which resulted in more aggressive surgical treatment and a considerable decrease in the mortality rate.[7] Thus, the angiographic distinction of acute bleeding due to peptic ulcer disease, hemorrhagic gastritis, or the Mallory–Weiss syndrome from bleeding due to pancreatitis and its sequelae has had a tremendous impact on clinical management. Angiography is indispensable in the evaluation of the portal system, which should be part of a standard evaluation of bleeding patients with pancreatic disease. Identification of splenic vein thrombosis as the sole abnormality or confirmation of associated generalized portal hypertension due to liver

disease is important, because the surgical treatment of these two entities is completely different.

The source and site of bleeding are usually diagnosed by identification of the erosive arterial changes or pseudoaneurysm formation. If the pseudoaneurysm is huge, angiography usually confirms its nature and distinguishes it from the pseudocyst. Occasionally, however, the angiogram identifies multiple small pseudoaneurysms that cannot be diagnosed by any other means.[33] These abnormalities are usually associated with encasement of the intrapancreatic arteries and, occasionally, with active bleeding (Fig. 11–8).[34] Rarely, frank extravasation of contrast medium from the pseudoaneurysm is seen. This occurs more frequently when the pseudoaneurysm ruptures into the abdominal cavity into or around the pancreatic bed. The next most common rupture is into the gastrointestinal tract, usually the duodenum.[11] Extravasation into the pseudocyst with drainage via the pancreatic ductal system is rare.[35] In a few cases, bleeding into the pancreatic duct has been demonstrated by angiography (Fig. 11–9).[36–38]

MANAGEMENT

As a rule, bleeding complications of pancreatic disease require prompt diagnosis and an aggressive surgical approach. Preoperative angiography is one of the most important steps in patient management.

Once the source of bleeding has been identified, surgical celiotomy is indicated. The operative technique remains somewhat controversial, although recent data suggest that arterial ligation or intracystic suture ligation in conjunction with drainage procedures, splenectomy,

and gastrectomy, rather than partial or total pancreatectomy, is effective. In patients with ductal pancreatic bleeding or who bleed as a result of pancreatitis triggered by a mass lesion in the head of the pancreas, partial or total pancreatectomy is required for definitive control of bleeding.[7]

There are several situations, however, in which angiographic management of hemorrhage is appropriate. First, in unstable patients with a severely bleeding pseudoaneu-

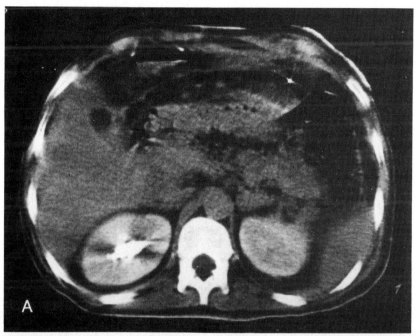

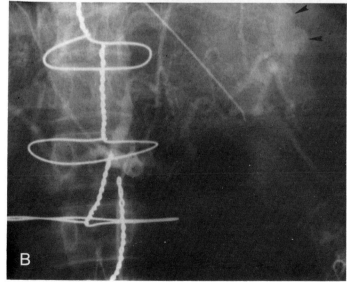

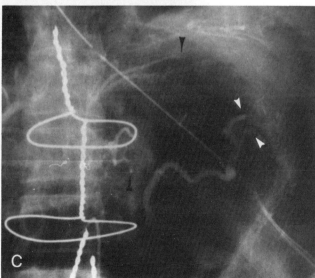

Fig. 11-8 Phlegmon. A. CT scan; pancreas and peripancreatic tissues are not recognizable. B. Celiac angiogram demonstrates severe encasement of splenic and left gastric arteries and area of extrava-sation in left upper quadrant (black arrowheads). C. Hemostasis was established by limited embolization of branches of splenic and left gastric arteries (white arrowheads).

Fig. 11–9 Left gastic angiogram after Billroth gastrectomy reveals extensive extravasation from stump of left gastric artery (lg) into a pancreatic pseudocyst and drainage via pancreatic duct into duodenum (arrowhead).

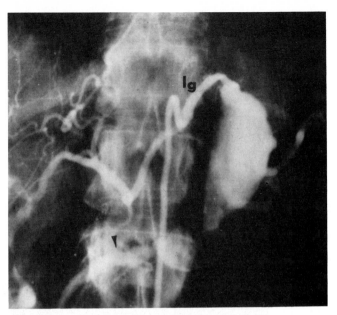

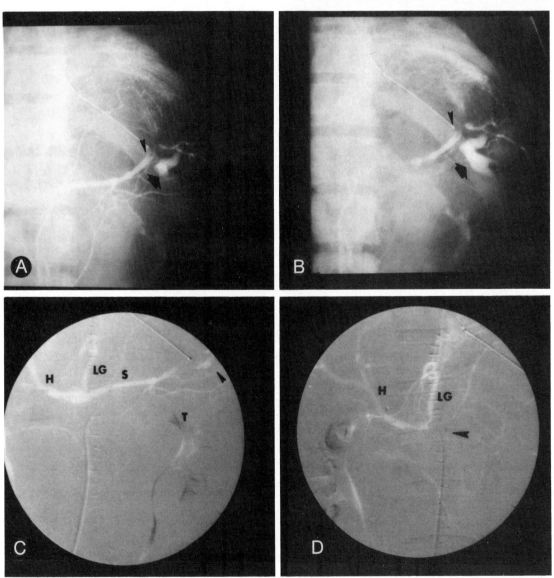

Fig. 11–10 Trauma case. A,B. Injury to distal pancreas and distal portion of splenic artery (small arrowhead) with active extravasation in the same area (large arrow). C. Digital subtraction angiography also demonstrates bleeding from distal portion of splenic artery (arrowhead). D. An occlusion balloon has been placed in origin of splenic artery for temporary control of bleeding, which was followed by definitive surgical procedure. H = hepatic artery; LG = left gastric artery; S = splenic artery; T = upper pole of left kidney.

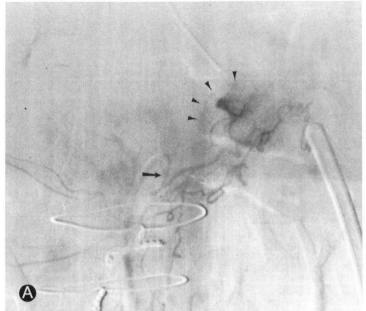
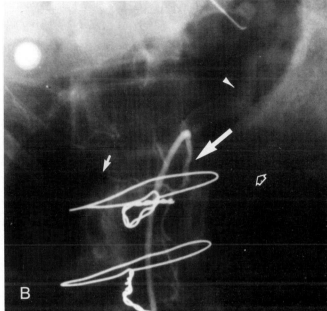

Fig. 11–11 Bleeding pseudoaneurysm. A. Dorsal pancreatic angiogram (arrow) reveals stretching of vessels in region of pancreatic head. Transverse pancreatic artery and other pancreatic branches in region of body and tail of pancreas are of increased caliber, with a pseudoaneurysm in region of tail (arrowheads). Note increased densities surrounding pseudoaneurysm, indicating extravasation into cystic space. B. Angiogram after embolization reveals patency of proximal dorsal pancreatic artery (large arrow) and at least one patent branch (small arrow) supplying pancreatic head. Main branches supplying body and tail of pancreas are occluded with Gelfoam particles. Small amount of residual extravasated contrast is identifiable in the course of the transverse pancreatic artery (arrowhead).

rysm, temporary hemostasis can be obtained by occlusion with mechanical devices (Fig. 11–10).[7,37] Occlusion balloon catheters, detachable balloons, and GWC coils are ideal for the occlusion of large arteries. However, because the bleeding vessel may be supplied by collateral pathways, which form rapidly after embolotherapy, a definitive operation should be done as soon as possible after angiographic occlusion and restoration of blood volume.

Second, if the patient bleeds from a small pseudoaneurysm involving the intrapancreatic branches, embolization with Gelfoam particles may control a bleeding episode and obviate operation (Fig. 11–11).[39–41] These small pseudoaneurysms have extremely fragile walls that are prone to rupture during the delivery of particulate embolic material, so use of the minimum volume of carrier fluid and minimal injection pressure during delivery of the emboli are appropriate (Fig. 11–12).[39]

Third, angiographic management may be indicated in patients with obvious bleeding in or around the pancreas and convincing findings on ultrasound and CT examinations who have unimpressive findings on angiography. This happens mostly in cases of encasement of small arterial branches and pseudoaneurysms. Occasionally, bleeding is demonstrated, but its source is not identified. In such cases, limited embolization of branches of the splenic and left gastric arteries with Gelfoam particles immediately stops the bleeding (Fig. 11–13). A semipermanent resorbable material rather than a permanent material is recommended in these patients, because the resorbable material occludes the vessels over a crucial period of several weeks, allowing conservative treatment of the underlying disease, yet permits restoration of flow to the diseased region as the clinical condition improves.

Finally, the angiographer may assist the surgeon in the preoperative management of patients with left-sided portal hypertension due to splenic vein thrombosis. A simple splenectomy cures this condition, but the operation is not easy because considerable venous engorgement and inflammatory reaction due to pancreatitis extend the operating time, and the procedure is often complicated by extensive bleeding during dissection of the numerous adhesions. In such cases, the relatively easy placement of an occlusion balloon catheter in the splenic artery and its inflation during the crucial stage of the operative procedures reduce the need for blood transfusion (Fig. 11–14). In addition, the catheter can be left in place with the balloon deflated for 24–48 hr postoperatively to permit control of bleeding by inflation of the balloon. Leaving the balloon catheter in place seems particularly justifiable in those patients in whom partial or total pancreatectomy or internal pseudocyst-drainage procedures are done in addition to splenectomy.[42] Published data suggest that the mortality rate from hemorrhage following surgical ligation of a bleeding vessel or pancreatic resection is almost twice that in patients with spontaneous hemorrhage due to pancreatic disease. Therefore, angiographic workup and management of postoperative bleeding in patients with pancreatic disease seems to be justified in every patient who is hemodynamically stable. Even in those patients who are hypotensive, a quick insertion of an occlusive balloon into the bleeding vessel may considerably reduce both morbidity and mortality.

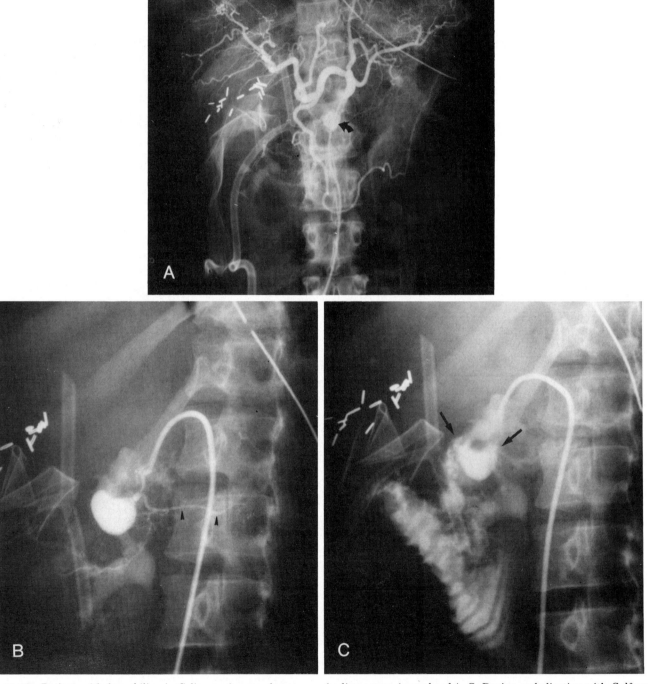

Fig. 11–12   Patient with hemobilia. A. Celiac angiogram demonstrates large pseudoaneurysm in region of pancreas (arrow). B. Subselective angiogram demonstrates dorsal pancreatic artery to be the feeding artery (arrowheads). C. During embolization with Gelfoam particles, pseudoaneurysm ruptured, with extravasation of contrast medium (arrows) into common bile duct and duodenum.

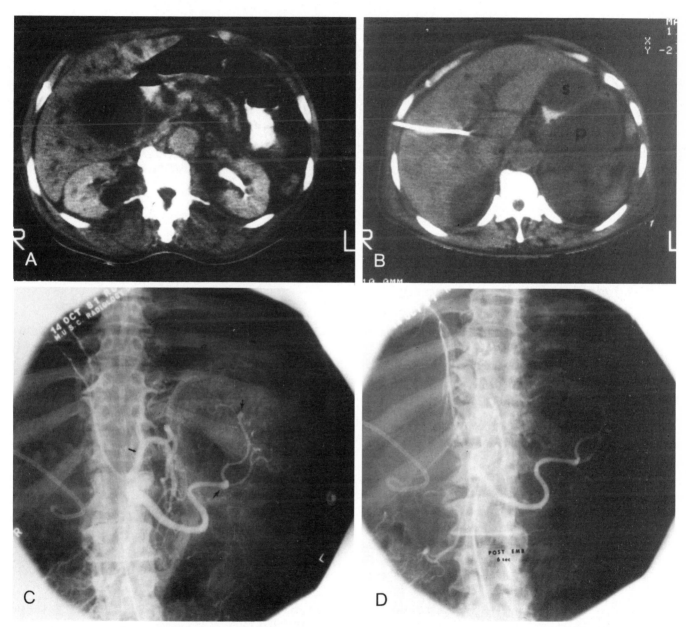

Fig. 11–13 Appearance of bleeding during percutaneous drainage. A. CT scan demonstrates dilated biliary ducts, gallbladder, and main pancreatic duct. B. After successful percutaneous external drainage of biliary tree, there was a drop in hematocrit associated with sudden appearance of pancreatic pseudocyst in retrogastric area. S = stomach; P = pancreatic pseudocyst. C. Angiogram done because of clinical evidence of continued bleeding demonstrates encasement of left gastric (small arrow) and splenic arteries with small pseudoaneurysms identified in distribution of the splenic artery (large black arrows). Note common trunk of left hepatic and left gastric arteries. D. After embolization with small particles of Gelfoam, smaller branches of splenic and left gastric arteries do not opacify.

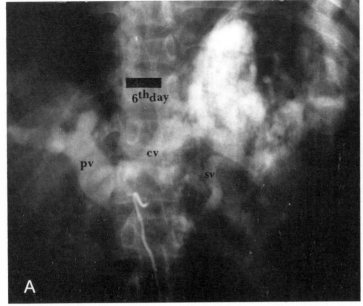

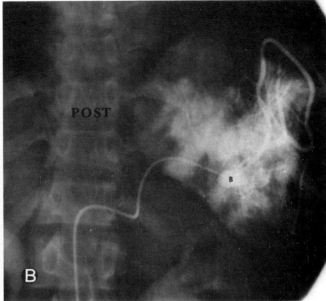

Fig. 11–14 Left-sided portal hypertension after embolization of spleen with Gelfoam particles in patient in Figure 11–4. A. Despite extensive embolization, flow to spleen is preserved. Thrombosis of splenic vein (SV) is demonstrated, with collateral circulation through gastric varices into portal vein (PV) through the dilated coronary vein (CV). B. To decrease flow to the spleen and varices, balloon catheter was placed in splenic hilum and inflated. Inflated balloon completely blocks circulation in splenic bed. Patient was immediately sent to the operating room for surgical splenectomy.

References

1. Gadacz TR, Trunkey D, Kieffer RF Jr: Visceral vessel erosion associated with pancreatitis. *Arch Surg* 1978;113:1438

2. White AF, Baum S, Buranasiri S: Aneurysm secondary to pancreatitis. *AJR* 1976;127:393

3. Boisen E, Tylen U: Vascular changes in chronic pancreatitis. *Acta Radiol[Diagn]* 1972;12:35

4. Sindelar WF, Mason GR: Aortocystoduodenal fistula: rare complication of pancreatic pseudocyst. *Arch Surg* 1979;114:953

5. Zeller M, Hetz HH: Rupture of pancreatic pseudocyst into the portal vein. *JAMA* 1966;196:869

6. Takayama T, Kato K, Katada N, et al: Radiological demonstration of spontaneous rupture of a pancreatic pseudocyst into the portal system. *Am J Gastroenterol* 1982;76:55

7. Stabile BE, Wilson SE, Debas HT: Reduced mortality from bleeding pseudocysts and pseudoaneurysms caused by pancreatitis. *Arch Surg* 1983;118:45

8. Cogbill CL: Hemorrhage in pancreatic pseudocysts: review of literature and report of two cases. *Ann Surg* 1968;167:112

9. Stanley JC, Frey CF, Miller TA, et al: Major arterial hemorrhage: complication of pancreatic pseudocysts and chronic pancreatitis. *Arch Surg* 1976;111:435

10. Frey CF: Pancreatic pseudocyst: operative strategy. *Ann Surg* 1978;188:652

11. Sankaran S, Walt AJ: The natural and unnatural history of pancreatic pseudocysts. *Br J Surg* 1975;62:37

12. Nielsen OS: Bleeding after pancreatic cystogastrostomy. *Acta Chir Scand* 1979;145:247

13. Collins JJ, Peterson LY, Wilson RE: Small interstitial infarction as a complication of pancreatitis. *Ann Surg* 1968;167:433

14. Hunt DR, Mildenhall P: Etiology of strictures of the colon associated with pancreatitis. *Am J Dig Dis* 1975;20:941

15. Leger L, Lenroit J, Lamaigre G: Hypertension portale segmentaire des pancreatities: aspects angiographiques. *J Chir (Paris)* 1968;95:599

16. Rignault D, Mine J, Moire D: Splenoportographic changes in chronic pancreatitis. *Surgery* 1968;63:571

17. LeMaitre G, L'Hermine C, Maillard JP, Toison FL: Hypertension portale segmentaire des pancreatities: aspects angiographiques. *Lille Med* 1971;16:928

18. Little AG, Moossa AR: Gastrointestinal hemorrhage from left sided portal hypertension. *Am J Surg* 1981;141:153

19. Moossa AR, Gadd MA: Isolated splenic vein thrombosis. *World J Surg* 1985;9:284

20. Zannini G, Musciariello S, Pagano G, et al: Prehepatic portal hypertension: experience with eighty-eight cases. *Int Surg* 1982;67:311

21. Nordlinger BM, Fulenwider JT, Millikan WJ, Warren WD: Splenic artery ligation in distal splenorenal shunt. *Am J Surg* 1978;136:561

22. Vos LJM, Potocky V, Broker FHL, et al: Splenic vein thrombosis with esophageal varices: a late complication of umbilical vein catheterization. *Ann Surg* 1974;180:52

23. Burbige EJ, Tarder G, Carson S, et al: Colonic varices: a complication of pancreatitis with splenic vein thrombosis. *Am J Dig Dis* 1978;23:752

24. Stone RT, Wilson SE, Passaro E Jr: Gastric portal hypertension. *Am J Surg* 1978;136:73

25. Case records of Massachusetts General Hospital. *N Engl J Med* 1945;233:443

26. Brintall BB, Laidlaw WW, Papp JP: Hemobilia: pancreatic pseudocyst hemorrhage demonstrated by endoscopy and arteriography. *Am J Dig Dis* 1974;19:186

27. Vujic I, Seymour EQ, Meredith HC: Vascular complications associated with sonographically demonstrated cystic epigastric lesions: an important indication for angiography. *Cardiovasc Intervent Radiol* 1980;3:75

28. Hashimoto BE, Laing FC, Jeffrey RB Jr, Federle MP: Hemorrhagic pancreatic fluid collections examined by ultrasound. *Radiology* 1984;150:803

29. Jhaveri HS, Gerlock AJ Jr, Smith CW, Goncharenko V: Value of

arteriography in the evaluation of a sonolucent pancreatic mass. *Cardiovasc Intervent Radiol* 1979;2:55

30. Isikoff MB, Hill MC, Silverstein W, Barkin J: The clinical significance of acute pancreatic hemorrhage. *AJR* 1981;136:679

31. Borlaza GS, Kuhns LR, Seigel R, Posderac R, Eckhauser F: Computed tomographic and angiographic demonstration of gastroduodenal artery pseudoaneurysm in a pancreatic pseudocyst. *J Comput Assist Tomogr* 1979;3:612

32. Jeffrey RB Jr, Federle MP, Crass RA: Computed tomography of pancreatic trauma. *Radiology* 1983;147:491

33. Harris RD, Anderson JE, Coel MN: Aneurysms of small pancreatic arteries: a cause of upper abdominal pain and intestinal bleeding. *Radiology* 1975;115:17

34. Vujic I, Anderson BL, Stanley JH, Gobien RP: Pancreatic and peripancreatic vessels: embolization for control of bleeding in pancreatitits. *Radiology* 1984;150:51

35. Bivins BA, Sachatello CR, Chuang VP, Brody P: Hemosuccus pancreaticus (hemiductal pancreatitis). *Arch Surg* 1978;113:751

36. Koehler PR, Nelson JR, Berenson MM: Massive extra-enteric gastrointestinal bleeding: angiographic diagnosis. *Radiology* 1976;119:41

37. Walter YE, Chuang VP, Bookstein JJ, et al: Arteriography of massive hemorrhage secondary to pancreatic disease. *Radiology* 1977;124:337

38. Vujic I, Jones WN, Bradham GB, Meredith HC: Angiographic demonstration of gastrointestinal bleeding through the pancreatic duct. *Gastrointest Radiol* 1980;5:43

39. Lina JR, Jaques P, Mandell V: Aneurysm rupture secondary to transcatheter embolization. *AJR* 1979;132:553

40. Vujic I, Anderson MC, Meredith HC, Cullom JW: Successful embolization of dorsal pancreatic artery to control massive upper gastrointestinal bleeding. *Am Surg* 1980;46:184

41. Knight RW, Kadir S, White RI Jr: Embolization of bleeding transverse pancreatic artery. *Cardiovasc Intervent Radiol* 1982;5:37

42. Vujic I: Preoperative angiographic occlusion of splenic artery. *AJR*, In Press.

12

Mechanism of Transluminal Angioplasty

CHRISTOPH L. ZOLLIKOFER, M.D., ANDREW H. CRAGG, M.D., DAVID W. HUNTER, M.D.,
WILFRIDO R. CASTAÑEDA–ZUÑIGA, M.D., M.Sc., AND KURT AMPLATZ, M.D.

Percutaneous transluminal angioplasty (PTA) was introduced by Dotter and Judkins in 1964.[1,2] After a rather slow start, it has gained wide acceptance during the past 10 years for the treatment of both atherosclerotic and nonatherosclerotic vascular disease, even though its mechanism has not been well understood until recently. This review presents the authors' experimental work on human cadavers and living animals to explain the morphologic changes seen after angioplasty. The changes in arachidonic acid metabolism induced by the dilation of arterial segments are also described. A special section deals with the theoretical consequences of drug administration for the prevention of stenosis recurrence and of thrombosis. Finally, the physical properties of balloon catheters are discussed, and the effects of compliance and bursting characteristics of the various balloon materials on the results are stressed. It is of practical value, particularly for the beginner in this field, to become familiar with the advantages and disadvantages of the different types of balloon dilation catheters.

HISTORICAL DEVELOPMENT OF TRANSLUMINAL ANGIOPLASTY

Early Equipment

On January 16, 1964, the first PTA, of a popliteal artery, was performed in an elderly woman with gangrene, and by November of that year, Dotter and Judkins could describe their experience with the new technique in 11 patients.[2] Over the next few years, Dotter and Judkins further documented the value of their nonsurgical technique.[3–6] The dilation system they used consisted of coaxial Teflon dilators, which were introduced over a guidewire after antegrade puncture of the femoral artery (Fig. 12–1). The technique was subsequently modified by Staple and Van Andel.[7,8] The latter investigator designed a series of tapered catheters of increasing size that are introduced one after another, a system with the theoretical advantage of avoiding the "snowplow effect" of the relatively blunt Dotter system. With the gradually tapered dilators, more radial than axial or longitudinal force was applied to the atheromatous vessel wall (Fig. 12–2).

In spite of the reported success in Europe,[9–15] particularly from the groups headed by Andreas Grüntzig[12] and Eberhart Zeitler,[13] minimal acceptance was given the new method in the United States. Furthermore, the Dotter procedure was limited to the femoral and popliteal arteries because larger diameter dilators were needed for the iliac arteries. Latex balloons proved unsatisfactory because of the large compliance and stretching deformity of the latex.[20,21] Then, in 1973, Porstmann described a "caged" or "corset" balloon catheter (Fig. 12–3), further modified by Dotter et al, which could be used in iliac arteries.[22] The corset or cage formed by the struts of Teflon prevented undesirable deformity of the latex balloon. However, because of fear of excessive damage to the vessel wall and because of its higher thrombogenicity, the caged balloon catheter was never widely accepted. It was not until Andreas Grüntzig reported successful transluminal angioplasty in peripheral as well as renal and coronary arteries using a new double-lumen polyvinyl chloride (PVC) balloon catheter that transluminal angioplasty finally became popular in the United States.[23–25]

Grüntzig Balloon Catheter

After his original report of a single-lumen balloon catheter,[21] Grüntzig introduced a double-lumen, single end hole balloon catheter in 1976.[23] Over an inner catheter, a PVC coaxial catheter was mounted that had an inflatable distal balloon (Fig. 12–4). This balloon could be filled via a side channel at the proximal end of the catheter, which connected to a longitudinal groove cut along the outer surface of the inner catheter. With this new design, pressures of 3–5 atm could be applied to the stenosis with balloons as large as 10 mm in diameter. This permitted dilation of iliac artery stenoses using a catheter with a maximum outer diameter of 3.0 mm. Also, with a balloon, radial rather than axial forces were applied to the atherosclerotic lesions, thereby minimizing the risk of embolization.[21]

Thanks to the ingenious Grüntzig balloon catheter, angioplasty, or the Dotter procedure, was rediscovered in the United States and spread rapidly. Continued modifications and improvements, especially in the compliance of the balloons, made it possible to treat increasingly difficult cases. Also, strictures and stenoses outside the vas-

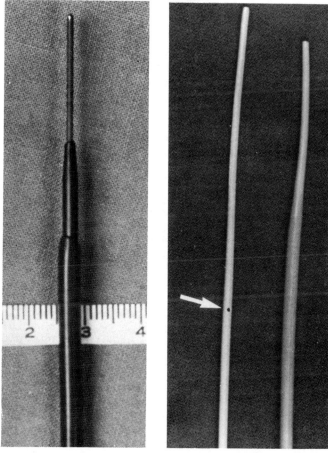

Fig. 12–1 (above left) Dotter coaxial Teflon catheter system with 1.12-mm guidewire and 8F inner and 12F outer catheter.

Fig. 12–2 (above right) Van Andel catheters with long tapered tips. Proximal sidehole (arrow) was added later by E. Zeitler for injection of contrast medium.

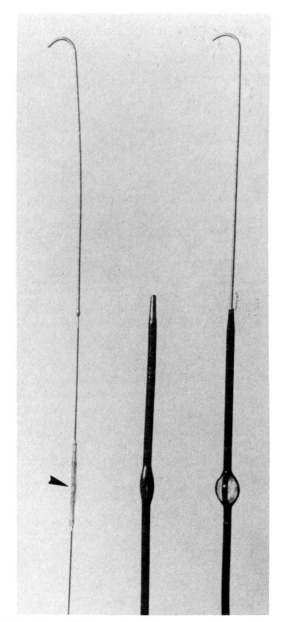

Fig. 12–3 "Corset" balloon, after Porstmann. Latex balloon (arrowhead) mounted on guidewire is inflated within Teflon catheter with three longitudinal struts. The Teflon catheter prevents overstretching of balloon.

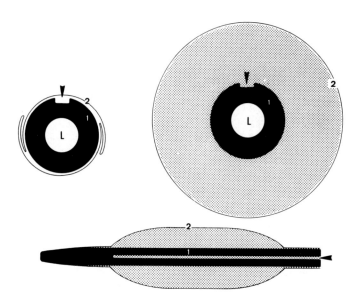

Fig. 12–4 Diagram of the Grüntzig balloon dilatation catheter in cross- and longitudinal sections. 1 = inner catheter with side channel (arrowhead); L = lumen of the inner catheter; 2 = balloon and coaxial outer catheter made of PVC. In the deflated state, balloon folds around inner catheter in umbrella-like fashion (top left). Top right and bottom: balloon inflated. (After A. Grüntzig, 1977.)

cular system, such as those in the gastrointestinal and genitourinary tracts, could be treated successfully.

By 1981, about 100,000 Grüntzig balloon catheters were being sold yearly in the United States.[26] A study by Doubilet and Abrams pointed out that, as a consequence of the use of PTA in the treatment of iliac and femoral lesions, more than 300 patients' lives and $100,000,000 in health expenses could be saved annually in the U.S.[27] The numbers for coronary artery disease are even more impressive: according to Hall and Grüntzig, 15%–20% of patients requiring coronary bypass surgery are candidates for PTA,[28] with annual savings in health expenses of $170,000,000.[29]

THEORIES OF THE MECHANISM OF TRANSLUMINAL ANGIOPLASTY

Original Theories Offered by Dotter and Other Pioneers of Transluminal Angioplasty

According to Dotter,[5,6,20,30,31] the principal mechanism of angioplasty is compression and remodeling of the atheromatous plaque. In other words, it was believed that the dilating catheter or balloon causes a cold flow that remodels the atheromatous material, much as if a balloon were being inflated in soft cheese. By this inelastic compression–remodeling of the atheromatous core—possibly with release of fluid contents—a stable autogenous tube would be formed, with maximum preservation of the existing vessel lining (Fig. 12–5).[20,30,31] This theory was largely accepted by the two other pioneers of transluminal angioplasty, Grüntzig[12,21] and Zeitler.[13] Grüntzig also mentioned a role for stretching of the media, with an increase in the outer arterial diameter, which was suggested by the work of Jester et al.[32]

Challenging the Old Theory

With the more frequent use of PTA, it became clear that the original theory was not tenable. Atheromatous plaques, being semiliquid or solid without true empty spaces, are virtually incompressible unless liquid is extruded. Therefore, if the balloon causes cold flow inside a relatively rigid tube, the plaque, like soft cheese, should spread, i.e., the stenosis should elongate (Fig. 12–6). However, this effect has almost never been seen during balloon dilatation, although with Dotter's original coaxial dilator system, some pushing of lesion material (snowplow effect) can occur.[8,13] Furthermore, fibrotic or calcified lesions also can be dilated by balloon angioplasty, yet in these lesions, remodeling by cold flow can be excluded. Significant extrusion of liquid is highly unlikely in such cases, which eliminates significant compression of the plaque as a mechanism. In addition, the radiolucent lines

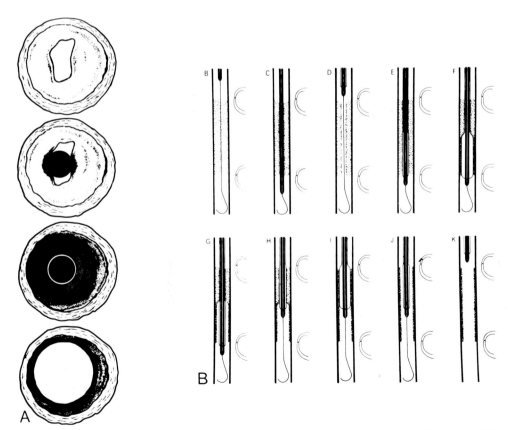

Fig. 12–5 Original theory of the mechanism of angioplasty as described by Dotter (A) and Grüntzig (B). Widening of lumen (A) or recanalization of atherosclerotic obstruction (B) occurs with no evidence of increase in caliber of artery or change in length of lesion.

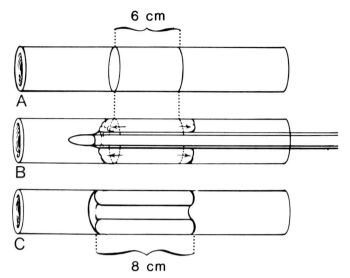

6 cm

A

B

C

8 cm

Fig. 12–6 Diagram of a 6 cm long localized obstruction (A), through which a 12F Dotter dilator is introduced (B). If no material is removed or compressed, atheroma will have to be redistributed proximally and distally to make room for dilator. The calculated volume of cylinder that has been displaced would lead to elongation of atheromatous lesion to 8 cm (C). (Reproduced from Castañeda–Zuñiga WR, Amplatz K, Laerum F, et al: Mechanics of angioplasty: an experimental approach. *Radiographics* 1981;1: 1–14.)

so frequently seen in arteriograms after successful angioplasty could not be explained on the basis of the original theory. There was a clear need for experimental data on which to base a better theory, but before 1979, there were few experimental data on the mechanism of angioplasty,[24,32–36] and all of these papers, with the exception of that by Leu and Grüntzig,[36] described experiments with coaxial dilators.

Four papers presented at the American Heart Association's 1978 annual meeting dealt with histologic changes after balloon angioplasty of coronary arteries.[37–40] However, the results were contradictory. Whereas Jester et al described extensive dissections and tears in the intima with stretching of the media during successful angioplasty,[32] Baughman et al[37] and Freudenberg et al[38] called dissection and rupture of the intima a complication. In other words, successful dilatation of an atherosclerotic stenosis was thought to be possible while leaving the intima intact and without stretching of the media and adventitia.

These contradictory findings and conclusions, together with the physical fact that solid or semisolid substances are noncompressible in the absence of extrusion of liquids, prompted the present authors to begin an extensive experimental study of the mechanism of angioplasty in 1978. Their research was conducted in three principal directions: the morphologic changes that follow PTA, the changes in vessel wall metabolism after PTA, and the physical properties of the balloon catheters and their influence on PTA results.

Experimental Data

INTRODUCTORY REMARKS ON BLOOD VESSEL ANATOMY AND PHYSIOLOGY

Anatomy of the Arterial Wall

The arterial wall consists of three layers, the tunica intima, the tunica media, and the tunica adventitia. This three-layer design is found in all mammalian arteries (Fig. 12–7), although the individual components differ with the function and size of the vessel. Accordingly, the authors distinguish between the large central or elastic

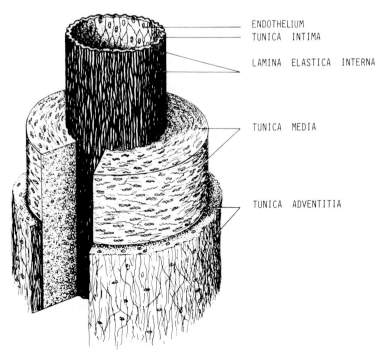

ENDOTHELIUM
TUNICA INTIMA

LAMINA ELASTICA INTERNA

TUNICA MEDIA

TUNICA ADVENTITIA

Fig. 12–7 Schematic drawing of medium-sized muscular artery showing its three distinct layers.

arteries, the distributing or muscular arteries, and the arterioles.

Tunica intima. The inner surface of the artery, toward the blood stream, is sealed by a flat endothelium that covers a layer of amorphous ground substance and longitudinal elastic fibers (Fig. 12–8). Occasionally, smooth muscle cells are present. The intima is separated from the media by a strong, fenestrated tube of elastic fibers, the internal elastic lamina (IEL), which limits the compliance of arteries and helps to reconstitute the original lumen after limited stretching of the wall.

Tunica media. The media is the thickest of the three layers of the arterial wall. It consists of principally concentric, fenestrated elastic laminae and circumferentially oriented smooth muscle fibers (Fig. 12–8). Between layers of elastic and muscle fibers, collagen fibers and an amorphous intercellular substance are found. According to the numbers of smooth muscle cells and elastic fibers, arteries of the elastic or muscular type are distinguished. Smooth muscle cells are pluripotent and probably produce not only elastin and collagen but also the intercel-

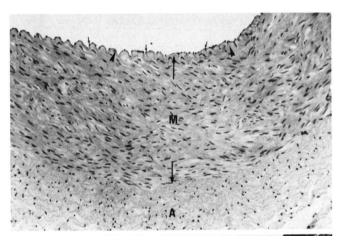

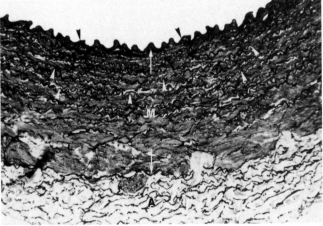

Fig. 12–8   Cross-section of a normal canine carotid artery (× 100). Hematoxylin and eosin (top) and Verhoeff–van Gieson (VVG) (bottom). Endothelium (small arrows) seals intima toward vessel lumen. Wavy IEL (black arrowheads) divides intima from media (M), which consists of predominantly circumferentially oriented smooth muscle fibers alternating with layers of elastic laminae. Elastic laminae are nearly continuous in spite of small fenestrations and ramifications (white arrowheads). Adventitia (A) forms outer layer of arterial wall toward loose surrounding connective tissue.

lular substance. The outer border of the media is formed by the external elastic lamina, which is usually developed to a lesser degree than is the IEL.

Tunica adventitia. The adventitia consists of fibrous connective tissue with collagen and elastic fibers oriented in a longitudinal or spiral fashion. In this layer, also, the vasa vasorum are found (more pronounced in the elastic and large muscular arteries), as are lymph vessels and nerves. Peripherally, the adventitia merges with the loose surrounding connective tissue.

Oxygenation of the Arterial Wall (Vasa Vasorum)

Oxygenation of the arterial wall is accomplished in two ways: first, by direct diffusion through the endothelium from the blood stream, and second, through the vasa vasorum, which are found in the elastic and the larger muscular arteries. The vasa vasorum are tiny vessels— about the size of arterioles or capillaries—that originate from the mother artery or its branches or from neighboring arteries.[41] In the aorta, the vasa vasorum originate mainly from intercostal and lumbar arteries. Newer studies using various methods to demonstrate the vasa vasorum[42–45] or to measure the blood flow in the arterial wall of humans and several animal species[46] have shown the intima and inner media to be without any vasa vasorum. That is, only the outer media and adventitia contain vasa vasorum in the normal animal, whereas the inner layers of the artery are oxygenated by diffusion from the blood stream.

MORPHOLOGIC CHANGES AFTER ANGIOPLASTY

In order to prove the hypothesis that transluminal angioplasty is effective primarily because of stretching of and controlled damage to the arterial layers, with subsequent healing, a series of experiments was performed on human cadaver arteries and on normal and atherosclerotic dog and rabbit arteries *in vivo*. On the basis of the radiologic, macroscopic, histologic, and ultrastructural changes seen in the dilated arteries, a new theory of the mechanism of PTA was proposed.

Experiments on Human Cadaver Arteries[47–50]

Material and methods. Fifty-six coronary, renal, mesenteric, and iliac arteries and abdominal aortas were removed at autopsy and dilated within 24 hr of death. Spot films in two projections of the arteries filled with a suspension of barium served to demonstrate the location and degree of stenoses. Because postmortem arteries have a tendency to shrink considerably due to the absence of blood pressure,[51–54] the arteries were dilated using a system that provided physiologic pressure (100 mm Hg)(Fig. 12–9). Under the same pressure, the dilated vessels were afterward fixed in Formalin. One group of arteries was dilated three times for 1 min each time using Grüntzig balloons 4–12 mm in diameter at 4–5 atm of pressure. A second group of 19 arteries was dilated using PVC balloons 12–21 mm in diameter (Fig. 12–10) at pressures of 2.5–11 atm. A third group was dilated using Foley

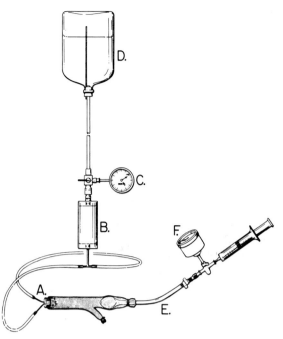

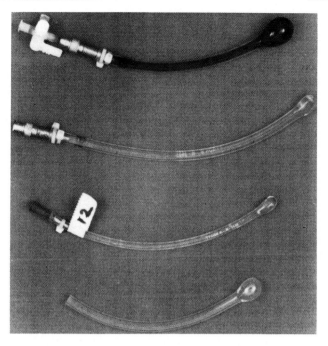

Fig. 12–9 Diagram of system for angioplasty under physiologic pressure. A. Stopper to seal vessel, with two small tubes that connect vessel to infusion system consisting of a small reservoir (B), manometer (C), and main reservoir (D). E,F. Balloon catheter with manometer for dilatation. (Reproduced from Laerum F, Vlodaver Z, Castañeda–Zuñiga WR, Edwards JE, Amplatz K: The mechanism of angioplasty: dilatation of iliac cadaver arteries with intravascular pressure control. *RöFo* 1982;136:573–576.)

Fig. 12–10   PVC balloons with diameters of 12–21 mm. (Reproduced from Laerum F, Vlodaver Z, Castañeda–Zuñiga WR, Edwards JE, Amplatz K: The mechanism of angioplasty: dilatation of iliac cadaver arteries with intravascular pressure control. *RöFo* 1982;136:573–576.)

catheters at 3 atm of pressure. The morphologic effects were assessed by the radiographic appearance, macroscopic alterations, including changes in outer diameter of the artery, and histologic changes.

Results.

Histologic changes. In the first group of arteries, dilatation caused intimal rupture, fragmentation, and partial dehiscence from the media. These changes generally were found at zones of transition from marked intimal thickening to areas with less plaque. In high-grade stenoses, additional rupture of the media was found (Fig. 12–11).

In the other two groups of arteries, analogous changes were seen in those vessels that had not completely ruptured. In addition, some areas of the media showed signs of compression, and other areas demonstrated partial or complete rupture of the media. Tears in the media were frequently combined with stretching of the adventitia (Fig. 12–12).

Changes of vessel diameter. The changes in external arterial diameter in response to polyethylene and PVC catheters are shown in Tables 12–1 and 12–2.

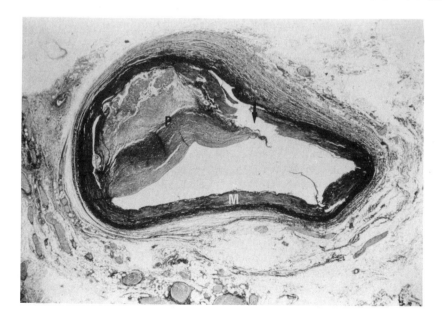

Fig. 12–11 Superior mesenteric artery after dilatation with 9-mm balloon for 3 min; there is a tear (arrow) at edge of plaque (P). Media (M) shows marked degenerative changes, mainly where it is covered by plaque. Tear also involves degenerative parts of media. Verhoeff–van Gieson; original magnification × 8. (Reproduced from Castañeda–Zuñiga WR, Formanek A, Tadavarthy M, et al: The mechanism of balloon angioplasty. *Radiology* 1980;135:565–571.)

Fig. 12–12 Iliac artery after dilatation with PVC balloon; rupture of intima and media where intima is only slightly thickened. Adventitia (A) has been stretched in this area. Media is partially detached from adventitia. P = plaque. Elastic stain; original amplification × 6.

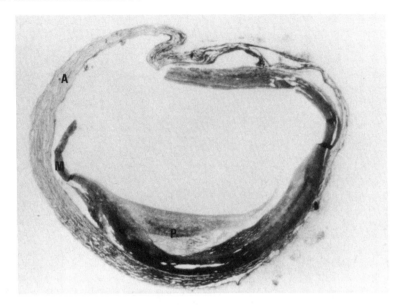

Table 12–1
Angioplasty of 10 Distal Abdominal Aortas and Iliac Arteries with PE Balloons of 8–12 mm Diameter (Inflation Pressure: 5 atm)

	No. of Dilatations		
	1	2	3
Increase of outer diameter in mm	0.5 (0–1.0)	0.6 (0–1.3)	0.8 (0–2.0)

Table 12–2
Angioplasty of 19 Iliac Arteries with PVC Balloons of 12–21 mm Diameter (Inflation Pressure: 5.5 atm (1.5–11))

	No. of Dilatations			
	1	2	3	4
Increase of outer diameter in mm	0.7 (0–2.5)	1.0 (0–2.5)	1.0 (0–2.5)	1.2 (0.5–3)
Number of arterial ruptures	5	1	3	1
Inflation pressure (atm) at arterial rupture	5.8 (2.5–11)	3.5	5.2 (2.5–8)	7.5

Table 12–3
Angioplasty of 6 Iliac Arteries with Foley Catheters (Inflation Pressure: 3 atm)

	No. of Dilatations			
	1	2	3	4
Increase in outer diameter in mm	0.7 (0.5–1.0)	0.8 (0.5–1.2)	1.2 (0.7–2.0)	1.4 (1.0–2.0)
Number of arterial ruptures	0	0	0	2

The increase in diameter in the first group was only 0.8 mm, and three arteries could not be dilated at all because of circumferential calcification. In the second group, which was dilated with large PVC balloons, several arteries could be dilated only by using increased pressures. The vessels that did not rupture completely showed an average increase in outer diameter of only 1.25 mm (12%). In the third group, the maximum average increase in diameter was 1.4 mm (Table 12–3). In all groups, the largest increase in diameter was achieved with the last or fourth dilatation. All arteries showed an inverse correlation between the amount of calcification and the increase in diameter—i.e., vessels with marked circumferential calcification could not be dilated measurably.

Radiographic changes. The increase in inner luminal diameter, as measured on x-ray films of the barium-filled arteries, was similar to the changes in the outer diameter. Again, heavily calcified arteries did not show a measurable increase in lumen (Fig. 12–13). All increases in lumen in the dilatable vessels resulted from rupture or tears in the plaques, with intimal dehiscence from the media, changes visible radiographically as radiolucent linear defects (Fig. 12–14A,B) that closely resembled those seen after clinical PTA (Fig. 12–14C). Histologically, these lucent lines matched the areas of intimal dehiscence or flaps. They were always oriented longitudinally. No signs of plaque redistribution could be found.

Discussion. The results of these first experiments confirmed the hypothesis that balloon dilatation does not compress atheromatous plaque but rather works by intimal rupture and partial dehiscence of this layer from the media, thus producing large clefts. These longitudinal clefts corresponded well with the radiolucent linear defects seen on postangioplasty arteriograms in clinical PTA. Noteworthy was the small increase in outside, and often also in luminal, diameter of the dilated arteries, a fact that was confirmed by LeVeen et al.[55] Circumferential plaque thickening resulted in especially limited luminal widening. On the other hand, asymmetric intimal thickening led to marked stretching and localized rupture of the media. Also, aneurysmal dilatation of the adventitia on the side opposite the plaque was found in these cases. Heavily calcified arteries could not be dilated at all unless the intimal plaque ruptured. This fact was again proved when dilating an atherosclerotic vessel within a test tube (Fig. 12–15), which prevents extension of the

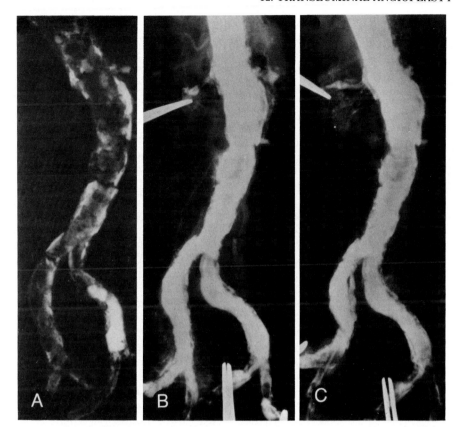

Fig. 12–13 Specimen of heavily calcified abdominal aorta including proximal pelvic arteries. A. Severe calcification. B. Specimen filled with suspension of barium; before dilatation. C. After dilatation of aortic bifurcation and common iliac arteries; no measurable dilatation because of the circumferential calcification.

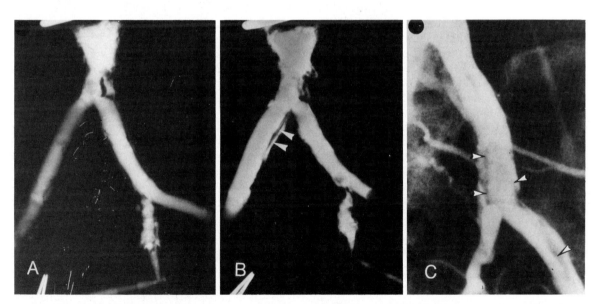

Fig. 12–14 Specimen (filled with barium suspension) of distal abdominal aorta with proximal pelvic arteries (A, B). Iliac angiogram of a patient after PTA of left pelvic axis (C). A. Before dilatation. B. After dilatation of bifurcation and right iliac artery; definite luminal widening, with a longitudinal lucent defect due to plaque dehiscence (arrowheads). C. Analogous findings *in vivo*, with linear contrast defects after dilatation (arrowheads).

outer diameter and thereby plaque rupture. Arteries with comparatively mild atheromatous disease often ruptured completely even when dilated with Foley catheters and pressures of only 3 atm (group 3; Table 12–3). Chin et al demonstrated that plaque dehiscence is already apparent at dilating pressures of 1–1.5 atm.[56]

Cadaver arteries obviously have a markedly reduced range of mechanical stretch as compared to living vessels, probably because of the lack of muscle tone and to autolytic changes that hasten rupture of the arterial wall. Nonetheless, even if experiments on cadaver arteries have limited value in defining optimal pressures and

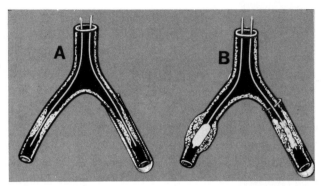

Fig. 12–15 Drawing of cadaver aortic–iliac specimen with severe bilateral iliac atherosclerosis. Left iliac artery has been placed in a glass test tube (A). With dilatation (B), right iliac artery expands at dilatation site, while the segment of left common iliac artery being dilated is restrained by test tube. (Reproduced from Wolinsky H, Glagov S: Nature of species differences in the medial distribution of aortic vasa vasorum in mammals. *Circ Res* 1967;20:409–421.)

duration of balloon inflation for dilating atherosclerotic vessels, the authors were able to draw some important conclusions from studying these specimens to confirm their hypothesis:

1. No significant compression or redistribution of the plaque takes place.
2. The mechanism for widening of the arterial lumen consists of a combination of rupture and tears in the intima, with consequent dehiscence of this layer from the media. Another important factor is stretching of the media and adventitia, which had already been mentioned by Hempel in 1969[34] and by Jester et al in 1976.[32] Thus, successful dilatation that leaves the endothelium and intima intact, as proposed by Baughman et al[37] and Simpson et al,[40] seems unlikely.
3. The longitudinal radiolucent defects in angiograms made after PTA and the transient intramural accumulations of contrast medium originally thought to represent complicating dissections[37,38] are a conse-

quence of this rupture and the dehiscence of the intima. This phenomenon is common, especially with fibrous, calcified lesions, and should be interpreted as a normal finding as long as there is no obstruction of flow or embolization.[57]

Animal Experiments

The authors further hypothesized that the extent of damage to the arterial wall depends on balloon size, the pressure applied, and the duration of balloon inflation. The time factor, especially, can be investigated appropriately only in living arteries. Therefore, a series of experiments was designed using normal canine and atherosclerotic rabbit arteries.

Angioplasty in normal canine arteries using inflation pressures of 4–5 atm.[47,48,58,59]

Materials and methods. As a pilot study, the infrarenal aorta and iliac arteries of three anesthetized mongrel dogs were dilated with 9-mm balloons (approximately 25% greater than the normal size for the abdominal aorta and more than 100% for the iliac arteries). In another dog, the aorta was dilated using a 15-mm balloon, and in a fifth dog, two 9-mm balloons were used simultaneously to dilate the aorta more than 100% oversize. Follow-up angiograms were taken immediately after and at intervals of 1 week to 4 months following PTA. The animals were killed 4 weeks to 4 months postangioplasty, and the dilated vessels, including normal control segments, were processed for histologic study.

Forty carotid and femoral arterial segments were dilated using 25% and 60%–80% oversized balloons, which were inflated for 1 min to 4.5 atm three times. Animals were killed for examination at 30 min; at 6, 18, 24, 48, and 72 hrs; at 1 and 2 weeks; and at 1 to 6 months after angioplasty. Follow-up angiograms were taken immediately after dilatation and before sacrificing the animals. Dilated and normal control segments were excised and prepared for histologic and electron microscopic examination. The arterial lumen was measured on the angiograms before and after dilatation.

Fig. 12–16 Abdominal aorta 4 months after > 100% overdilatation. Elastic stain; original magnification × 7. Media (M) is missing over a considerable area; thick neointima (I) composed of laminated fibrous tissue covers entire internal surface of vessel. Adventitia (A) appears intact. (Reproduced from Castañeda–Zuñiga WR, Formanek A, Tadavarthy M, et al: The mechanism of balloon angioplasty. *Radiology* 1980;135:565–571.)

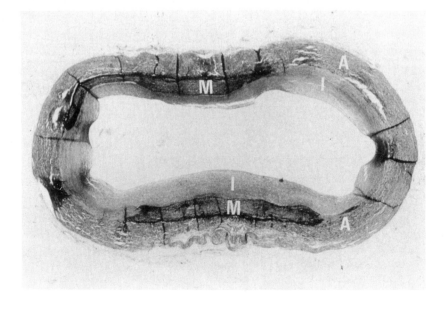

Results. Already in the pilot study, a correlation between the histologic changes in the abdominal aorta and iliac arteries and the balloon size or duration of inflation was suggested. With 25% overdilation at 5 atm for 3 min, histologic changes remained limited to the intima and endothelium, whereas with 100% or more overdilatation, the abdominal aortas showed extensive changes, with locally complete disruption of the media. At 3–4 months after angioplasty, the medial tears had been bridged by scar (neomedia) and there was extensive inti-

mal hyperplasia (Fig. 12–16). The adventitia was hyperplastic and intact, and there were no signs of local aneurysmal dilatation. In spite of this, after 4 months the aortas showed, both *in situ* and after excision, definite widening of the outer circumference (Fig. 12–17). The iliac arteries overdilated by more than 100% showed analogous changes, although the intimal hyperplasia tended to be localized rather than circumferential (Fig. 12–18).

Angiographically, 25% overdilatation of the aorta or

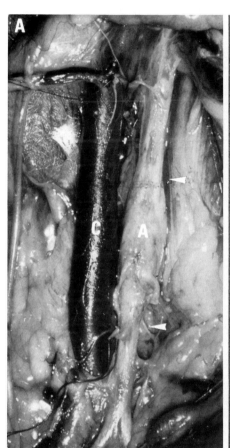
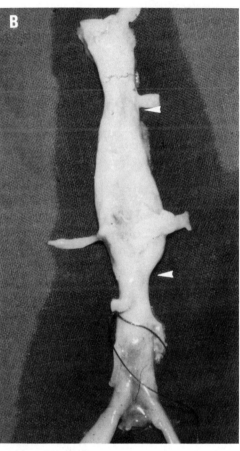

Fig. 12–17 Abdominal aorta 4 months after > 100% overdilatation. A. *In situ*. B. After excision. Marked widening of outer aortic contour (A) at area of previous dilatation (between arrowheads). C = vena cava.

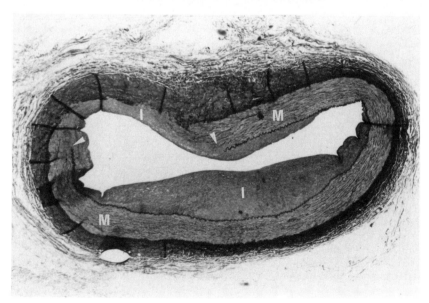

Fig. 12–18 Iliac artery from same animal 4 months after 100% overdilatation; media (M) and IEL show focal rupture (arrowheads). Defect is covered by neointima (I). Note irregular distribution of intimal hyperplasia. Adventitia shows proliferation particularly at area of medial rupture. Elastic stain; original magnification × 16.

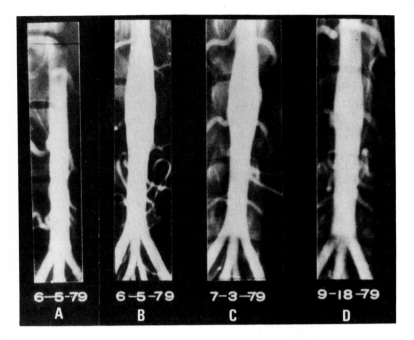

Fig. 12–19 Abdominal aortic angiograms of same animal after overdilatation with two 9-mm balloons. A. Before dilatation. B. After dilatation. C. Four weeks after dilatation; persistent luminal widening is apparent. D. At 3 1/2 months after dilatation, luminal widening has regressed.

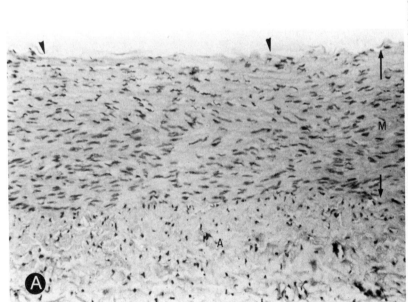

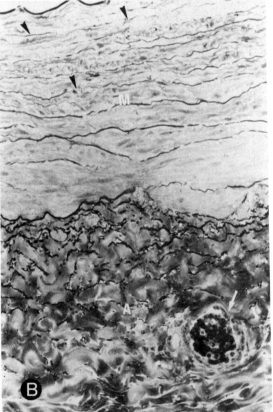

Fig. 12–20 A. Carotid artery 20 min after 80% overdilatation. Hematoxylin and eosin; original magification × 120. Endothelium is completely erased, and IEL (arrowheads) is partially detached. Inner media shows corkscrew-like deformation and pyknoses of smooth muscle nuclei. Inner media is edematous with multiple acellular areas. M = media, A = adventitia. B. Same vessel; note stretched elastic laminae (arrowheads) with increased fragmentation and thinning. There is a dilated vasa vasorum in adventitia containing several polymorphonuclear leukocytes (arrows). Toluidine blue; original magnification × 200.

iliac arteries did not cause any measurable widening of the lumen. Dilation of 100% or more resulted in marked widening of the arterial lumen lasting about 1 month and then slowly decreasing over the following 2–3 months (Fig. 12–19).

Histologic and electron microscopic examination of the carotid and femoral arteries revealed two important new observations: that significant stretching of normal arteries leads to intimal hyperplasia, which persists for at least 6 months, and that stretching causes irreversible changes in the medial architecture. These findings are in contrast to the results of studies on the significance of endothelial damage in the pathogenesis of atherosclerosis, the hallmark of which is intimal hyperplasia or "fibrous plaque formation" and the re-endothelialization of the luminal surface secondary to trauma to the endothelium but not to the underlying media.[60] These changes are limited to the intima and result from migration and proliferation of smooth muscle cells along with production of collagen and elastin.[61-64] In these studies, intimal hyperplasia was transient, with complete regression over 3–6 months.

The authors' light and electron microscopic studies showed endothelial abrasion with various degrees of medial damage in the acute stage, followed by intimal hyperplasia and medial fibrosis. Slight differences were noted according to balloon size. That is, balloons of 25% oversize caused focal fractures and stretching of the IEL, and damage to the media was limited to the inner third of this layer; whereas dilation with 60%–80% oversized balloons caused extensive destruction of the IEL and penetrating damage through more than half of the medial thickness (Figs. 12–20 and 12–21). After use of large balloons, separation of collagen and elastic fibers from the myocytes was common (Fig. 12–21). Within 18–48 hours, the damaged media had "empty" spaces filled with edema and debris but lacking any intact cellular elements (Fig. 12–22). It remains unclear how the cellular debris was removed, inasmuch as leukocytes and macrophages were present in large numbers only in those areas where blood had access to the interior of the arterial wall, i.e., in medial dissections.

Very soon after the dilatation injury, platelets could be observed attached to the denuded surface. These findings correspond closely to those reported after endothelial abrasion using the Baumgartner method[60,62-64] as well as to the studies of PTA in normal canine coronary arteries reported by Pasternak et al[65] and O'Gara et al.[66] These aggregated platelets could be followed for up to 3 days, at

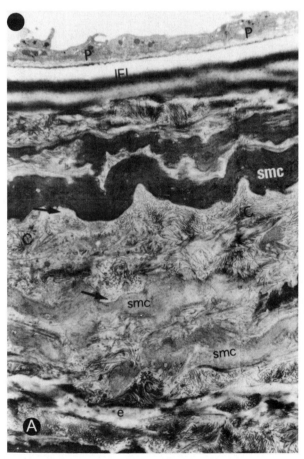

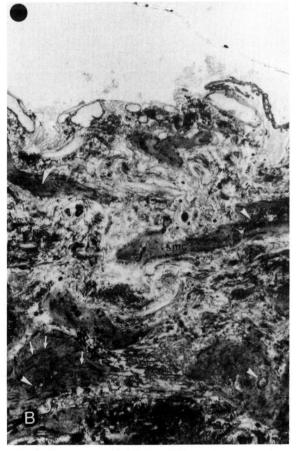

Fig. 12–21   Electron micrographs of carotid artery 30 min after dilatation. Original magnification × 5300. A. 25% dilatation; platelets (P) adhere to denuded and stretched IEL; note degenerating myocytes (smc) with corkscrew formation, loss of dense bodies, and loss of stainability. Collagen (C) and elastic fibers (e) have lost their close relation to smc (arrow). Edematous intercellular spaces are seen. B. 60% dilatation; complete destruction of IEL. Note chaotic structure and interstitial edema. Changes are much more severe than in A. Myocytes show myofilaments (arrows) and swollen mitochondria (arrowheads).

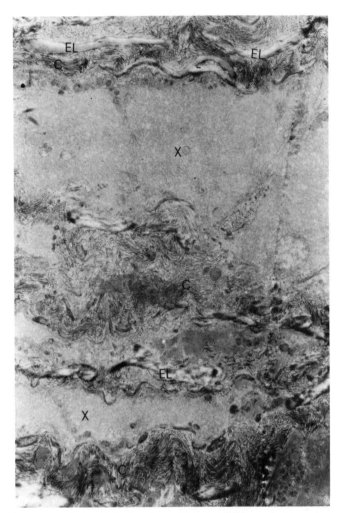

Fig. 12–22   Carotid artery 18 hr after 80% dilatation. Approximate original magnification × 5300. Transition of outer to middle third of media shows "empty" spaces (X) filled with edema and debris between original layers of collagen and elastic laminae (EL). Many EL are fragmented. Collagen fibers (C) remain in contact with EL. There are no cellular blood elements within the damaged wall. (Reproduced from Zollikofer CL, Salomonowitz E, Sibley R, et al: Transluminal angioplasty evaluated by electron microscopy. *Radiology* 1984;153:369–374.)

which time modified smooth muscle cells were seen invading the neointima, and re-endothelialization could be observed, which was complete at 1–3 weeks (Fig. 12–23). Intense proliferation and migration of smooth muscle cells and increased production of elastin and, especially, collagen caused marked intimal thickening at 1 month (Fig. 12–24). A similar repair process, with proliferation of smooth muscle cells and fibrosis secondary to irregular deposition of collagen and elastic fibers, was seen in the media. Reconstitution of the fractured or destroyed IEL was not seen (Fig. 12–24).

After 3–6 months, no significant regression of the irregular cushion-like intimal hyperplasia was noted. The fibrotic changes of the media with proliferation of collagen also persisted, and thus the irregular medial architecture correlated well with the degree of initial overdistension (Fig. 12–25).

The increase in the arterial lumen as measured on angiograms immediately after angioplasty was 0%–7% (average 2.6 ± 3.3) with overdilation of 25% and 8%–30% (average 17.4 ± 7.1) with overdilation of 60%–80% (Fig. 12–26). Two-thirds of the dilated arteries exhibited short, spasm-like luminal narrowings adjacent to the site of dilatation (Figs. 12–26 and 12–27). Occasionally, these spasms extended over several centimeters, (Fig. 12–27), and they appeared to have no correlation with the extent of arterial dilatation. They persisted for as long as 48 hr.

By 18–48 hr after 80% overdilation, the luminal widening had diminished to 10%–12% (Fig. 12–28), and 1–2 weeks later no increase in luminal diameter could be measured. Angiograms 4 weeks or more after angioplasty revealed no significant changes from the control films made before angioplasty. In cases of 25% overdilation, luminal widening persisted no longer than 18 hr.

Discussion.   These results prove that even dilatation of the normal vessel cannot be achieved without damage to the arterial wall structures. This damage is clearly dependent on the amount of wall stretching. The chron-

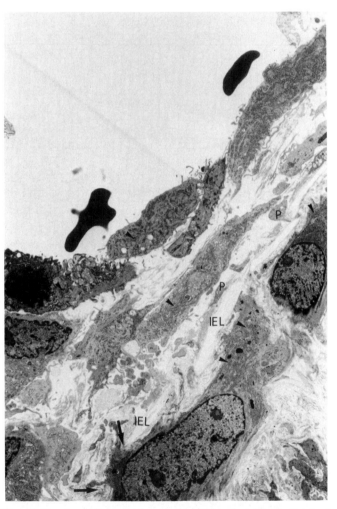

Fig. 12–23   Carotid artery 1 week after dilatation (75%). Original magnification × 4500. Electron micrograph shows intima and inner media. Two or three layers of modified smooth muscle cells (fibromyoblasts) with prominent endoplasmic reticulum (arrowheads) are seen on luminal side of IEL. Some platelets (P) are still visible close to IEL. A fibromyoblast seems to be migrating into intima through gap in IEL (between arrows).

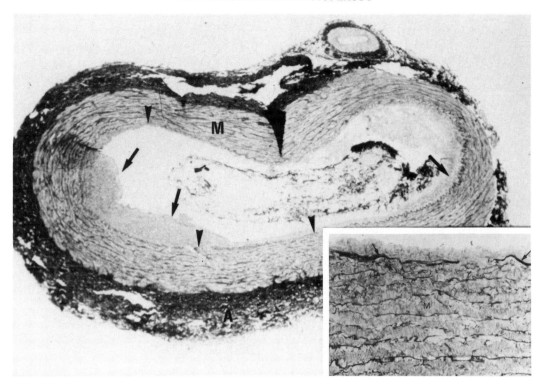

Fig. 12–24   Carotid artery 1 month after 60% dilatation. Verhoeff–van Gieson; original magnification × 20. Irregular intimal hyperplasia (arrows). Internal elastic lamina is interrupted in several areas (arrowheads). M = media, A = adventitia. Inset: Carotid artery 1 month after 60% dilatation. Toluidine blue; original magnification × 200. Intimal hyperplasia (I); IEL (arrows) is not reconstituted.

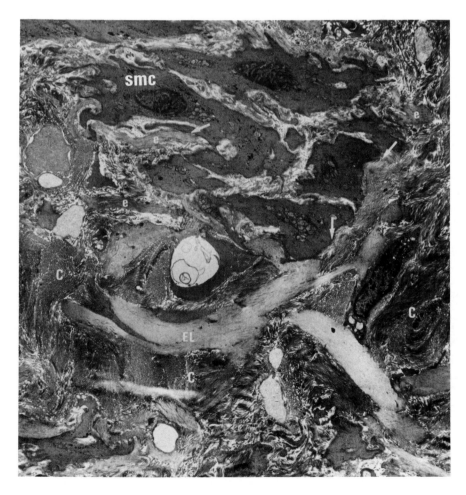

Fig. 12–25 Electron micrograph of carotid artery 3 months after 80% dilatation. Original magnification × 3700. Media exhibits irregular pattern with increased collagen (C). Elastic laminae (EL) are irregular and fragmented. Smooth muscle cells (smc) show prominence of mitochondria but no increase in rough endoplasmic reticulum. Note that close relation of collagen and elastin with smc has been reestablished (arrows). Overall, there is fibrosis from increase in collagen and irregular elastin. (Reproduced from Zollikofer CL, Salomonowitz E, Sibley R, et al: Transluminal angioplasty evaluated by electron microscopy. *Radiology* 1984;153:369–374.)

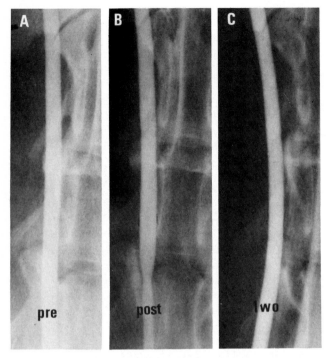

Fig. 12–26 Carotid artery angiogram before (A), immediately after (B), and 1 week after (C) 25% dilatation. Lumen increase in B amounts to 6%. Note local spasm at the proximal end of the dilated segment. One week after dilatation, there is no appreciable luminal widening.

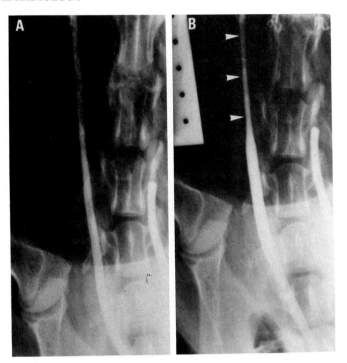

Fig. 12–27 Carotid artery angiogram before (A) and after (B) 80% dilatation. Note extensive spasm distal to the dilatation (arrowheads). Luminal widening of dilated segment is 23%.

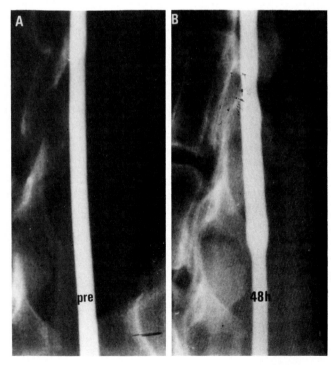

Fig. 12–28 Carotid artery angiogram before (A) and 48 hr after (B) 70% dilatation. Luminal widening in B is 10%; immediately after dilatation, the lumen increase had been 14%. Again, note spasm proximal and distal to dilatation.

ologic steps of platelet aggregation on the denuded inner vascular surface, followed by proliferation and invasion of smooth muscle cells that results in a hypertrophied neointima covered by a neoendothelium, support the theory that platelets play a major role in stimulating migration and proliferation of smooth muscle cells by releasing mitogenic factors leading to intimal hyperplasia.[62–64,67] In contrast to the results of Ross and Glomset,[62,68] Stemerman and colleagues,[64,69] and others,[61,63,70] the present authors did not find regression of this intimal hyperplasia. Also, Leu and Grüntzig, in their study of canine arteries, found persistent intimal thickening after a 7-month period.[36]

An 80% overdilation of nonaortic canine vessels caused widespread changes in the intima and media without definitely traumatizing the adventitia. Only dilated vasa vasorum were noted in the adventitia immediately after angioplasty. Complete medial destruction in excessively dilated (>100%) aortic and proximal iliac vessels resulted in healing with marked intimal hyperplasia. However, again, no signs of adventitial tears or localized, saccular aneurysm formation could be detected in areas of formerly complete medial rupture. The latter healed by scar formation resulting in a neomedia and proliferation of the adventitia which obviously compensate for the missing media after excessive dilation. A compensatory mechanism may also explain the persistence of intimal thickening as opposed to the findings of experiments where the arterial lesion was limited to the endothelium. Unlike the fibrosis in the media, the amount of intimal hyperplasia was not definitely dependent on the degree of overdilation and medial damage. This phenomenon may have some importance in the etiology of recurrent stenosis following balloon dilatation; *i.e.*, angioplasty with insufficient luminal widening may cause rapid recurrence of stenoses due to intimal hyperplasia, especially in nonatherosclerotic disease. Therefore, it seems noteworthy that experimentally, intimal hyperplasia may be reduced by antiplatelet therapy.[71]

Whether intimal hyperplasia occurs to the same degree in atherosclerotic vessels is not certain. Faxon et al have shown in atherosclerotic rabbits that restenosis occurs 4 weeks after angioplasty as a result of extensive intimal thickening.[72,73] Thrombotic occlusions also were found, suggesting that the intimal thickening may have been due to organization of thrombotic material rather than to genuine intimal hyperplasia.

Obviously, these findings in animals cannot simply be transferred to human atherosclerotic disease. The more complex condition of human atherosclerosis, with frequent necrosis and calcification, may respond differently to, and progress more slowly after, angioplasty. On the other hand, Waller et al found severe restenosis at areas of previous PTA at autopsy 2–5 months after successful clinical coronary angioplasty.[74,75] Possibly, the intimal proliferation stimulated after PTA in arteries of relatively small diameter is of greater importance and may explain the higher recurrence rate (approximately 30%) in coronary as compared to peripheral PTA. Furthermore, in the presence of hyperlipidemia, atherosclerosis may be accelerated by simple mechanical damage to the endothelium,[62,76–79] a fact also noted after the use of arterial clamps. Therefore, it is theoretically advisable to put patients on a low-cholesterol diet after PTA until re-endothelialization has occurred and to prescribe antiplatelet drugs. Indeed, Faxon et al showed in the atherosclerotic animal model that aspirin and dipyridamole or sulfinpyrazone significantly reduce intimal thickening and restenosis, as well as the rate of thrombotic occlusions, after PTA.[72]

In excessively dilated abdominal aortas, a long-lasting increase in arterial diameter could be demonstrated angiographically after angioplasty. The luminal widening tended to decrease simultaneously with the increasing intimal hyperplasia and scar formation. Nonetheless, the outer circumference was still definitely enlarged even after 4 months. To explain such an aneurysmal widening of the outer contour, adventitial stretching must take place in addition to medial damage.

The cause and significance of local spasm adjacent to the dilated arterial segments are discussed below under "Pharmacologic Phenomena and Metabolic Changes of the Arterial Wall after PTA."

In summary, these studies led to the following conclusions:

A long-lasting dilatation of the normal vessel can be achieved only by means of marked damage to the intima and media and stretching of the media and, to some degree, of the adventitia. As long as the adventitia is not severely damaged, healing without aneurysm formation can be expected. Intimal hyperplasia may compensate for medial destruction and therefore probably is irreversible.

Intimal thickening may also be important in the atherosclerotic vessel after PTA.

How antiplatelet drugs affect healing of the vessel wall, intimal thickening, and early reocclusion needs further investigation, if possible in primates.

Angioplasty in normal canine arteries using higher inflation pressures (8–12.5 atm).[50,80] In the previous studies of normal canine arteries, the authors noticed that balloons 50%–100% oversized, as compared to the arterial lumen, did not reach their full diameter at the usual inflation pressures of 4–5 atm (Fig. 12–29). They therefore studied the behavior of the balloons *in situ* and the histologic changes caused by higher inflation pressures. Of special interest were potential differences between balloons of differing compliances.[80]

Materials and methods. Twenty-five carotid and femoral arteries were dilated with balloon catheters with a diameter equal to that of the vessel, 30% larger, and 80%–100% larger than the original vessel diameter as measured on the angiogram (groups A, B, and C, respectively). The two brands of balloon catheters used were made from PVC or polyethylene. Spot films and cine films were taken of the balloon catheters filled with diluted contrast medium within the vessel at 4.5 atm as well as at inflation pressures of 6, 8, 10, and 12.5 atm. In this way, the diameters of the arterial lumen on the angiogram as well as the diameters of the balloons *in situ* could be compared with the aid of a micrometer caliper. After the animals were killed, the dilated arterial and normal vessel segments were excised and stained for histologic examination.

Results. Table 12–4 shows the diameters the balloons reached intravascularly, given as a percentage of their requested (inflated) diameter as stated by the manufacturer, at 4.5 atm and 8–12.5 atm (before possible rupture of the artery). At pressures of 4.5 atm, the diameters of the PVC balloons were less than those of the polyethylene balloons in the nine specimens overdilated by 80%–100%. Accordingly, the histologic changes were less penetrating with PVC balloons. At pressures of 8–10 atm, the differences in the diameters of the two types of balloons were again noted, although the differences in the histologic changes were less obvious (Fig. 12–30). With both balloons, extensive damage to the intima and media was noted, with focal stretching of the latter (Fig. 12–30). In addition, local thrombosis occurred, particularly in areas of complete medial rupture. Only one artery showed less penetrating lesions, and here the balloon catheter reached barely 70% of its requested diameter because of its relatively high compliance and elongation. In three cases (two polyethylene and one PVC balloon), complete rupture of the artery resulted at pressures of 10 atm. All three balloons reached 100% of their requested diameter after rupture of the vessel.

At 4.5 atm, neither the balloon diameters nor the histologic changes differed significantly for the two balloon materials in the eight cases of 30% overdilation (Table 12–4). At high pressures (10–12.5 atm), all of the polyethylene balloons reached their requested diameter (Fig. 12–31), whereas the PVC balloons showed a wide range in attained diameters, with two balloons not reaching their requested diameters while exhibiting severe deformation

Fig. 12–29 Effect of 80% dilatation of left carotid artery. A. Angiogram before dilatation; arterial diameter measures 4.5 mm. B. An 8-mm balloon catheter *in situ*; diameter is 5.7 mm at 4.5 atm. C. Angiogram postdilatation; dilated segment measures 5 mm (+12%). Note spasms proximal and distal to dilated segment (arrows).

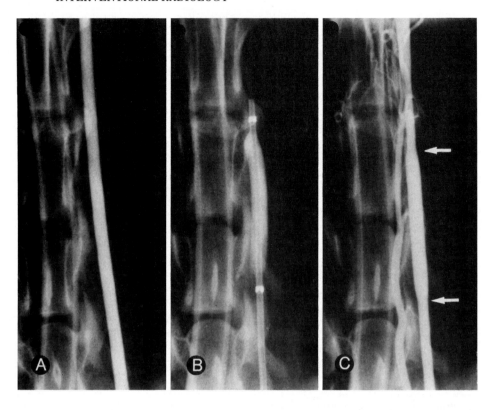

Table 12–4
Diameters of Balloons Attained Intravascularly (in % of Their Requested Diameter) at 4.5 and 8–12.5 atm—Comparison of PVC and PE Balloons

	4.5 atm		8–10 atm	
	PVC	PE	PCV	PE
A. Dilation 80%–100% (balloon diameter 8–9 mm)				
% of requested	68	82	80	95
diameter	(67–70)	(81–84)	(70–96)	(83–100)
B. Dilation 30% (balloon diameter 6 mm)				
% of requested	85	87	95	101
diameter	(78–96)	(77–92)	(85–114)	(100–101)
C. Dilation 0% (balloon diameter 4 mm):				
% of requested	131	110	150	121
diameter	(120–145)	(107–112)	(145–158)	(110–142)

and elongation (Fig. 12–32). Compared to group A, the arterial wall damage was less distinct in the areas of dilatation: only focal medial disruptions in two cases and no complete ruptures of the vessel (Fig. 12–31C). However, elongation and deformation of the PVC balloons, as shown in Figure 12–32, damaged the vessel wall far beyond the original balloon length.

As shown in Table 12–4, the range of attained diameters was much wider for PVC balloons at 4.5 atm as well as at 10–12.5 atm in the cases that were not overdilated. In addition, due to their greater compliance, the PVC balloons enlarged above the requested diameter more readily than did the polyethylene balloons (Figs. 12–33 and 12–34). Accordingly, the histologic changes were more penetrating with the PVC balloons (Fig. 12–35). Five of the eight balloons ruptured *in situ* at 10–12.5 atm.

However, there were no local histologic changes attributable to a jet of saline from the rupturing balloon.

Discussion. This study definitely demonstrated progressive histologic changes in the arterial wall with increasing balloon diameter as well as with increasing inflation pressure. Balloons oversized 30% and more do not reach their requested diameters at normal working pressures as suggested by the manufacturer; to achieve the requested diameter, the inflation pressure must be substantially increased. The study also showed that the result of angioplasty depends on the compliance of the balloon material. An oversized balloon of low compliance has more dilating strength and may even cause vessel rupture, whereas a balloon of the same size but with a comparatively large compliance may cause less local damage. However, because of the deformation and elongation of the balloon, the arterial wall may undergo changes far beyond the actual dilated segment, and this can lead to extensive vascular spasm and difficulties in retracting the balloon catheter. Balloons the diameter of the lumen or slightly larger that have large compliance, on the other hand, can cause more histologic damage than noncompliant balloons because of their considerable tendency to overinflate and "grow" at high pressures.

In addition, this study demonstrated that with high balloon pressures, rupture of the media may lead to focal stretching of the adventitia. Such aneurysmal outpouchings were also seen in the present authors' study on cadaver arteries (Fig. 12–12) and were described after PTA in atherosclerotic rabbits by Sanborn et al.[81]

A further important observation concerns the tendency to extensive local thrombus formation in areas of severe medial damage with complete rupture. Organization of such thrombi may play an important role in healing and

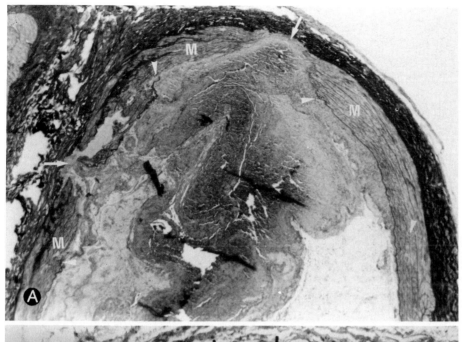

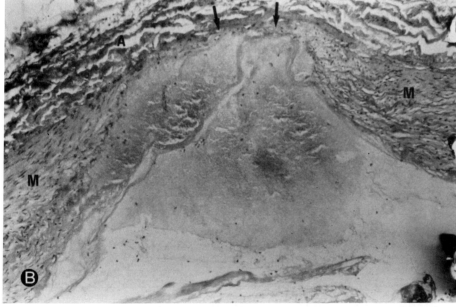

Fig. 12–30 Iliac artery 30 min after 80% dilatation at 10 atm. A. PE balloon. At two places, media has completely ruptured (arrows); adventitita bulges slightly in these areas. There is marked stretching of elastic lamina, and there are ruptures of the IEL (arrowheads). Adventitia prevents complete rupture of the artery. Thrombus is seen in lumen. Verhoeff–van Gieson; original magnification × 25. B. PVC balloon. Close-up view of area with medial rupture that reaches down to adventitia (arrows). There is severe damage to myocytes and elastic lamina of the media bordering the rupture, which is covered by thrombus. Hematoxylin and eosin; original magnification × 50. (Reproduced from Zollikofer CL, Salomonowitz E, Brühlmann WF, Castañeda–Zuñiga WR, Amplatz K: Dehnungs-, Verformungs und Berstungs-Charakteristika haufig verwendeter Balloon-Dilatationskatheter: in vivo Untersuchungen an Hundegefassen (Teil 2). *RöFo* 1986;144:189–195.)

in preventing aneurysm formation as a delayed complication. If the media was not completely destroyed and torn through to the adventitial layer (as shown in the previous study with inflation pressures limited to 4.5 atm), thrombus formation was much less prominent.

Angioplasty in atherosclerotic rabbits.[82] For clinical PTA, the often strictly followed rule of three dilations for 30–60 sec each with a balloon approximately equal in diameter to the original (nondiseased) lumen has been advocated without a solid scientific basis.[48,83,84] According to the authors' studies on canine arteries, a close correlation exists between the histologic alterations of the vessel wall and the diameter and inflation pressures of the balloon catheter. Healthy arteries were able to withstand >100% overdilation as long as inflation pressures were not above 4–5 atm. On the other hand, studies of atherosclerotic cadaver arteries have revealed

differences in behavior during angioplasty depending on the configuration and the amount of calcification of the atherosclerotic plaque.[47–50,85] However, the effects of various balloon sizes and inflation times had not been investigated in experimental animals by Block, Faxon, Sanborn, and their colleagues.[81,85–87] To gain better insight into the influence of balloon size and time of inflation on atherosclerotic arteries, the present authors studied normal and atherosclerotic rabbits.

Materials and methods. Two groups of eight 3.6-kg New Zealand rabbits were studied. The rabbits in group I served as controls and were fed standard rabbit chow, whereas those in group II were fed a 2% cholesterol-enriched diet. The thoracic and abdominal aortas were dilated with Grüntzig-type balloon catheters of 25% and 50% oversize, respectively, as compared to the original lumen of the aorta measured on the angiogram. The

Fig. 12–31 Carotid artery, 30% dilatation to maximum of 12.5 atm with 6-mm PE balloon. A. Balloon *in situ* at 4.5 atm attains 77% of full diameter. B. Balloon *in situ* at 12.5 atm is 100% inflated, to 6 mm. C. Histologic section (Verhoeff–van Gieson stain) of artery shows local rupture of media (arrow) with slight bulging of adventitia. Nonruptured parts of media (elastic laminae) seem less stretched and less compressed than in A.

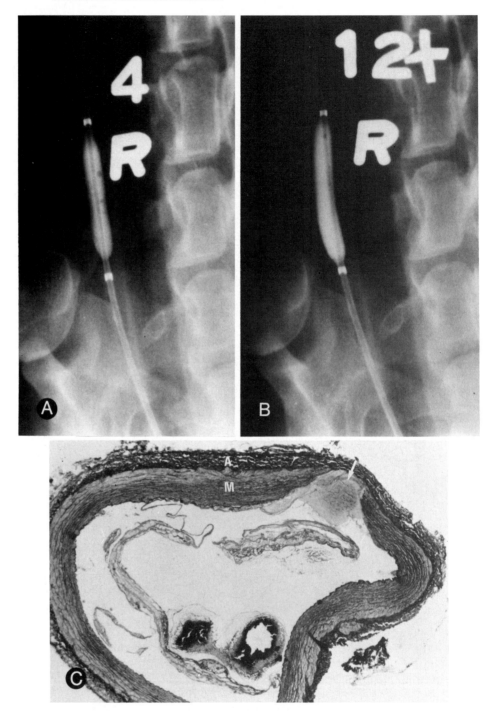

inflation time ranged from 15–60 sec. The animals were then killed, and dilated and nondilated aortic segments were prepared for histologic and electron microscopic examination.

Results. In nonatherosclerotic rabbits, there was a progressive increase in wall changes with time and balloon diameter (Table 12–5 and Fig. 12–36).

In the atherosclerotic rabbits, the atheromatous plaques were primarily fibrous and associated with both circumferential and focal plaques (Fig. 12–37). The histologic and electron microscopic studies revealed no linear correlation either with balloon size or with time of inflation (Table 12–6). Instead, the histologic changes

were governed by the thickness and location of the plaques. Fracture of plaque or dissection into the media, mainly at the edges of plaques or at sites of fracture, were seen with as little as 50% dilation for 15 sec and were accompanied by extensive damage to the smooth muscle cells (Fig. 12–38). These findings were even more pronounced and accompanied by local hematoma formation when multiple plaques were present (Fig. 12–37). The extent of dissection did not correlate linearly with either balloon size or inflation time. Segments with minor plaque formation exhibited more stretching and compression but less medial dissection. These changes were seen best with light microscopy, since the large field facil-

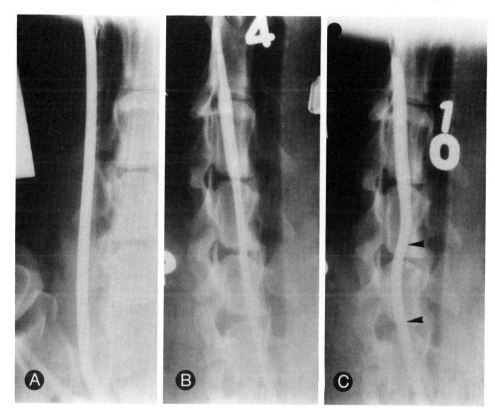

Fig. 12–32 Carotid artery, 30% dilatation to maximum of 10 atm with 6-mm PVC balloon. A. Angiogram before dilatation (arterial lumen = 5.1 mm). B. Balloon *in situ* at 4.5 atm attains 78% of its full diameter. C. Balloon *in situ* at 10 atm attains 85% of its full diameter. Severe elongation and deformation of balloon with marked dilatation of catheter shaft (arrowheads) are caused by spreading of injected fluid between inner and outer catheter sleeve (dissection between the two coaxial catheters). A further increase in the balloon pressure could not be achieved.

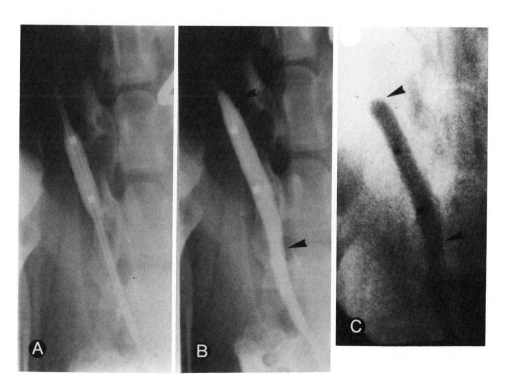

Fig. 12–33 Carotid artery (4.8-mm diameter) with 4-mm PVC balloon *in situ*. A. 4.5 atm; balloon diameter 5.8 mm. B. 8 atm; balloon diameter 6.3 mm (= 157%). There is severe deformation and elongation of balloon (arrowheads) and dissection of injected fluid between the inner and outer catheter sleeve at region of catheter shaft. C. 10 atm; no further increase in diameter. Balloon has extended toward tip of catheter and catheter shaft (arrowheads), causing enormous increase in diameter of shaft.

Fig. 12–34 Carotid artery (diameter = 4.6 mm) with 4-mm PE balloon *in situ*. A. 4.5 atm; balloon diameter = 4.3 mm. B. 8 atm; balloon diameter = 4.4 mm. C. 10 atm; balloon diameter = 4.6 mm (= 115%). No significant deformation or elongation of balloon is noted.

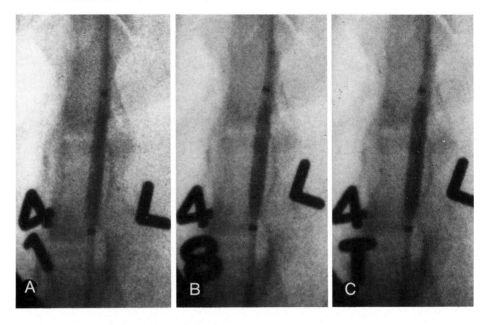

Fig. 12–35 Carotid artery after dilatation with 4-mm balloons (0% group). Hematoxylin and eosin; original magnification × 32. A. Dilatation with PVC balloon; dissection into media (M), with rupture and partial destruction of IEL (arrowheads). There is significant stretching of elastic laminae and pyknotic nuclei are seen within media. A = Adventitia. B. Dilatation with PE balloon; changes in media are significantly less penetrating than in A. There are no dissections, only interruptions, of IEL (arrowheads). (Reproduced from Zollikofer CL, Salomonowitz E, Brühlmann WF, Castañeda–Zuñiga WR, Amplatz K: Dehnungs-, Verformungs und Berstungs-Charakteristika haufig verwendeter Balloon-Dilatationskatheter: in vivo Untersuchungen an Hundegefassen (Teil 2). *RöFo* 1986;144:189–195.)

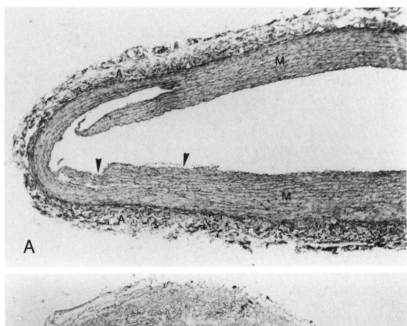

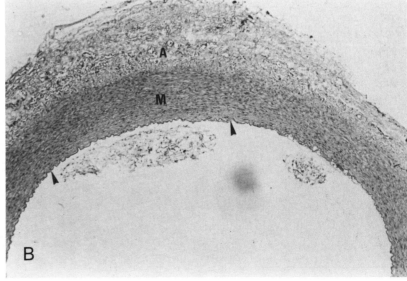

Table 12–5
Changes in Normal Rabbits after Vessel Dilatation[a]

	15 sec		30 sec		45 sec		60 sec	
	+25%	+50%	+25%	+50%	+25%	+50%	+25%	+50%
Intima								
Focal denudation	+	+	+	+	+	+	+	+
Complete denudation	−	−	−	−	−	+	−	+
IEL								
Stretching	+	+	+	+	++	++	++	++
Fractures	−	+	−	+	+	++	+	++
Dehiscence	−	−	−	+	−	+	++	++
Abrasion	−	−	−	−	−	+	+	++
Media								
Damage to smooth muscle cells	+1	+1	+1	+3	+3	++3	+3	++3
Intercellular edema	+1	+1	+1	+1	+3	++3	+3	++3
Destruction of the elastic lamina	−	−	−	+1	−	+1	−	+2
Separation of myocytes	−	−	−	−	−	+1	−	++2
Dissection	−	−	−	−	−	−	−	−

[a]Key: + = Present but limited; ++ = present and extensive; − = absent. 1 = inner one-third of media; 2 = inner two-thirds of media; 3 = entire media.

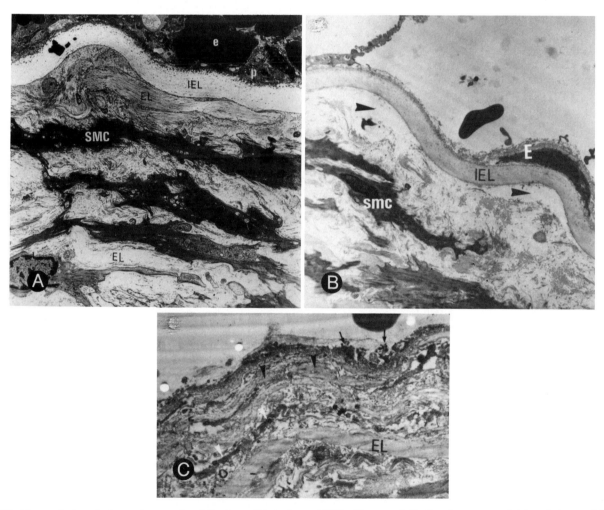

Fig. 12–36 Transmission electron micrographs of the inner third of nonatherosclerotic, dilated aorta. Original magnification × 3000. A. +50%, 15 sec; denuded endothelium is covered with thrombus. Smooth muscle cells (SMC) show hydropic changes, including swollen mitochondria. Otherwise, there are no definite changes in IEL and media. EL = elastic lamina; P = platelets; e = erythocyte. B. +50%, 30 sec; endothelium (E) is partially missing, and IEL has separated from media (arrowheads). Note marked interstitial edema. C. +50%, 45 sec; endothelium is now completely missing, and luminal surface is covered by platelets (arrows). Media shows marked compression as well as fragmentation of elastic fibers (black arrows). Note various grades of disintegration and other severe changes of smooth muscle cells (white arrowheads). (Reproduced from Zollikofer CL, Chain J, Salomonowitz E, et al: Percutaneous transluminal angioplasty of the aorta. *Radiology* 1984;151:355–363.)

Fig. 12–37 Dilated atherosclerotic aorta. Hematoxylin and eosin; original magnification × 20. A. +50%, 45 sec; several focal plaques (P) show dehiscence at edges (arrowheads). LA = lumbar artery. B. +50%, 30 sec; semicircular plaque with dissections at edges. Plaque-free wall shows marked stretching and thinning. Compression and stretching of plaque-free media (M) seems greater than in A. In both sections, there are no signs of plaque compression. (Reproduced from Zollikofer CL, Chain J, Salomonowitz E, et al: Percutaneous transluminal angioplasty of the aorta. *Radiology* 1984;151:355–363.)

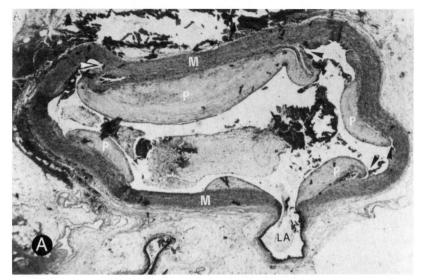

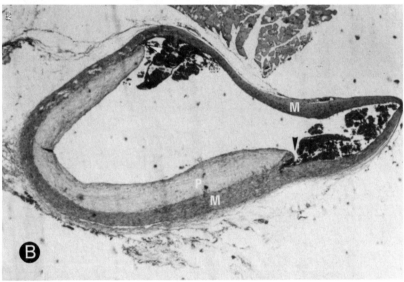

Table 12–6
Changes in Atherosclerotic Rabbits after Vessel Dilatation[a]

	15 sec		30 sec		45 sec		60 sec	
	+25%	+50%	+25%	+50%	+25%	+50%	+25%	+50%
Intima								
Focal denudation	+	−	−	−	−	−	−	−
Complete denudation	−	+	+	+	+	+	+	+
Plaque configuration	Circumferential	Circumferential	Circumferential	Semicircular ("horseshoe")	Semicircular ("horseshoe")	Multiple focal plaques	Multiple focal plaques	Multiple focal plaques
Plaque compression	−	−	−	−	−	−	−	−
Plaque fracture or splitting	−	+	−	−	−	−	−	−
Plaque dehiscence	−	+	++	+	−	+[c]	+[c]	+[c]
IEL								
Stretching	−	+	++	++	++	+[c]	+[c]	+[c]
Fractures	−	+	++	++	+	+[c]	+[c]	+[c]
Dehiscence	−	++	++	+	+[c]	+[c]	+[c]
Media[b]								
Damage to smooth muscle cells	−	++	++	++	+	+[c]	++[c]	++[c]
Compression	−	+	++	++	++	+[c]	+[c]	+[c]
Dissection	−	++	++	+	+	++[c]	++[c]	++[c]

[a]Key: + = Present but limited; ++ = present and extensive; − = absent.
[b]Multiple plaques.
[c]Changes seen only in areas of plaque and dehiscence or dissection or plaque-free areas.

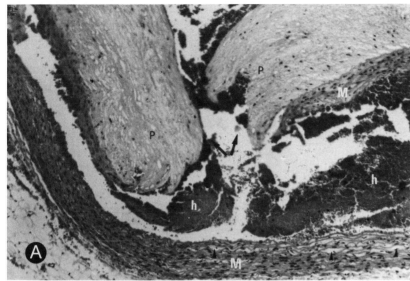

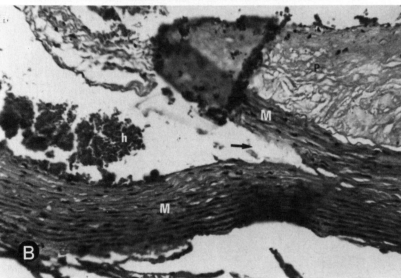

Fig. 12–38 Dilated atherosclerotic aorta. A. +50%, 15 sec; rupture of plaque (P; arrows), with dissection and compression of media (M). Note pyknosis of nuclei of smooth muscle cells and increased space between elastic laminae that is filled with edema fluid (arrowheads). There is a hematoma (h) within dissection. Hematoxylin and eosin; original magnification × 80. B. +25%, 30 sec; dissection into media (M) at edge of plaque (P, arrow). There are corkscrew nuclei in damaged smooth muscle cells and edema in medial layers. H = hematoma. Hematoxylin and eosin; original magnification × 150. (Reproduced from Zolliko-fer CL, Chain J, Salomonowitz E, et al: Percutaneous transluminal angioplasty of the aorta. *Radiology* 1984;151:355–363.)

itated comparison of various areas. Even with prolonged inflation, no plaque compression was seen; however, electron microscopy revealed superficial abrasion with production of plaque debris (Fig. 12–39).

Discussion. The current study again revealed that histologic changes in the nonatherosclerotic arterial wall after balloon dilatation are related to the size of the balloon and the duration of inflation, progressing in an approximately linear fashion as these factors increase. In contrast, histologic changes in atherosclerotic vessels are governed by the thickness and location of the plaques. That is, with a thick plaque, the underlying media remains unchanged. However, the wall is stretched in plaque-free areas and sites of dehiscence or rupture, and there is a tendency toward medial dissection, the extent of which correlates to only a limited degree with balloon size or length of inflation. This dissection is usually seen at the edges of the plaque or sites of rupture. Most likely, the force the dilating balloon exerts on the edge of the plaque causes dehiscence followed by rupture of the underlying tissues into the media. The wall of the atherosclerotic artery becomes stretched between the individual plaques, unlike normal arteries, in which the entire wall is stretched uniformly. This means that, in a way, the plaque protects the underlying media. Similar findings were described by Faxon et al in a study of three rabbit models of atherosclerosis.[87] The results of the current study also confirm the observations made in cadaver arteries, that in atherosclerotic disease with circumferential plaque, luminal widening can be accomplished only by cracking or rupture of the plaque. This study also clearly demonstrated that the wall of an atherosclerotic artery is more vulnerable than that of a normal vessel, as shown by the fact that changes penetrating into the media occur even with small balloons and short inflation times.

Although with extensive atherosclerosis, increased stretching results in greater plaque dehiscence and rupture accompanied by more pronounced medial dissection, which is in accord with observations in clinical PTA,[88-90] the current study showed that neither the amount nor the duration of the balloon dilatation necessarily correlated with the nature and extent of histologically visible damage to the wall of atherosclerotic arteries. In spite of the

Fig. 12–39 Transmission electron micrograph of dilated atherosclerotic aorta (+50%; 30 sec). Original magnification × 8000. Luminal surface of plaques show abrasion of superficial elements (arrowheads) and denudation of endothelium. No definite signs of compression. e = erythocytes. (Reproduced from Zollikofer CL, Chain J, Salomonowitz E, et al: Percutaneous transluminal angioplasty of the aorta. *Radiology* 1984;151:355–363.)

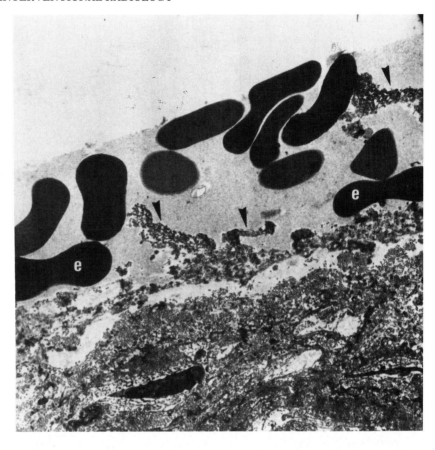

increased overall vulnerability of the atherosclerotic vessel, intimal and medial dissections remained limited to the dilated region; they measured 2–8 mm and were always oriented parallel to the long axis of the vessel. Occluding intimal flaps were not observed, and intramural hematomas remained localized, without formation of dissecting aneurysms. In accord with the authors' findings in atherosclerotic cadaver arteries, and also with the findings of other investigators,[85–87,91] no signs of plaque compression could be detected. However, the observation of endothelial abrasion and desquamation of superficial plaque elements is important because of the possibility of distal embolization, which is probably common, although silent. The incidence of embolization in peripheral angioplasty is only 3%–5%.[92,93] When clinically evident, it is probably the result of complete plaque dehiscence rather than of atherosclerotic debris.[94] Although marked intimal and medial splitting and partial plaque dehiscence were observed, neither peripheral embolization of the plaques nor true dissection producing an intimal hematoma large enough to obstruct the lumen were seen.

Because of the more complex conditions in human atherosclerosis, extrapolation of the findings in this animal model may legitimately be criticized. Human atherosclerotic lesions have significantly greater amounts of necrosis and calcifications. Also, the media often is involved to an extensive degree, with substantial alteration and thinning of this layer. No calcified lesions could be provoked in this model; the atheromas were mainly fibrous, similar to the models described by Faxon et al[72,73] and LeVeen et al.[95] In addition, the present authors were able to initiate focal, cushion-like atheromas by mechanically damaging

the endothelium prior to feeding the cholesterol diet. With this technique, the results of their animal experiments have closely paralleled the histologic findings after clinical angioplasty.

In summary, the following conclusions can be drawn from this study:

The mechanism of PTA is multifactorial, the result of a combination of rupture and dissection of the atheromatous plaque together with stretching of the plaque-free arterial wall segments. There is some desquamation of superficial plaque elements.

The wall of the atherosclerotic vessel is much more vulnerable than that of the normal artery.

Because of the limited correlation of balloon size and duration of inflation with the arterial wall damage in atherosclerosis and the difference in the tissue quality of the arterial wall in the animal model and human atherosclerosis, this study does not allow a definite recommendation on optimal balloon size and duration of inflation in clinical PTA.

Morphology of the Vasa Vasorum after PTA[50,96–98]

As stated earlier, the vasa vasorum are responsible for oxygenation of the outer layers of the media and adventitia in the central, elastic, and larger muscular arteries, whereas the intima and inner media are oxygenated by direct diffusion from the blood stream. This fact renders the middle media a critical area with regard to oxygenation, because thickening of the intima, as in atherosclerosis, must reduce this diffusion capacity. Geiringer found the maxium thickness of the intima at which the inner media is still adequately oxygenated by diffusion to be 0.5 mm.[99] Thereafter, further thickening leads to proliferation of the vasa vasorum into the intima, thus increasing the blood flow in the vessel wall.[99,100] This phenomenon of vascularization of the intima and media was confirmed in animal studies by Heistad et al.[101] The importance of the vasa vasorum was further substantiated by Wilens et al, who were able to induce medial necrosis of the aorta by blocking the blood supply to the vasa vasorum.[43] Possibly, atherosclerotic changes in the vasa vasorum are a causative factor in the pathogenesis of atherosclerotic aneurysm formation.[102] Because angioplasty induces severe changes in the intima and media, it is conceivable that the blood supply to the arterial wall could be jeopardized by this procedure. Therefore, theoretically, PTA-induced injury of the vasa vasorum could provoke late complications such as aneurysms or medial necrosis. To investigate the impact of PTA on the microcirculation of the blood vessel wall, the authors studied the morphology of the vasa vasorum using a latex infusion technique before and after angioplasty in normal canine arteries as well as in human cadaver arteries.

Materials and methods. Thoracic and abdominal aortic segments in three anesthetized dogs were dilated with 50%–100% oversized Grüntzig balloons at 4 atm of inflation pressure. An additional three dogs underwent dilatation of aortic segments to >100% oversize.

Three specimens of human cadaver abdominal aorta including the iliofemoral arteries were excised at autopsy. After roentgenologic location of the stenotic areas in the barium-filled specimens, the vessels were flushed clear with saline. The stenotic segments were then dilated using two 9-mm balloons for the aorta and a 12- or 8-mm balloon for the iliac vessels (>100%).

After death, the dilated vessels of the dogs were clamped proximally and distally, and large visceral branches of the aorta were ligated *in situ*. In the cadaver specimens, all visceral branches and lumbar arteries were ligated after angioplasty. A latex solution (Campton Biomedical Products, Inc.; Boulder, CO) was infused into the canine vessels *in situ* and into the cadaver specimens at 120 mm Hg during 10 min. After preparation, the latex-filled canine vessels were excised. Together with the cadaver arteries, the specimens were processed by the clearing technique of Spalteholz (alcohol dehydration and methylsalicylate) for macroscopic and microscopic examination.

Results.

Canine arteries. The morphology of the vasa vasorum of a nondilated aorta is shown in Figure 12–40. Most of the vasa vasorum originate from the lumbar arteries, close to the aorta. In cross-section, the vasa vasorum can be seen to run from the surface of the adventitia toward the outer third of the media, at which site they end in several ramifications (Fig. 12–40B).

In the specimens dilated to no more than 80% oversize, no definite alteration in the morphology or penetration of the vasa vasorum was noted. No tears were detectable in the small peripheral branches of the vasa vasorum (Fig. 12–41A). In contrast, overdilatation by 100% or more produced definite changes, with marked stretching or

rupture of the vasa vasorum in areas of significant thinning of the aortic wall (Fig. 12–41B).

Human cadaver arteries. Nondilated segments with pronounced intimal plaques showed abundant proliferation of the vasa vasorum, some of which penetrated through the intima into the lumen (Fig. 12–42A). The bush-like ramifications of the vasa vasorum were of irregular caliber with multiple ectasias (Fig. 12–42B). In the dilated segments, the findings were practically identical; but in addition, the vasa vasorum had been severed at sites where the intimal plaques had been ruptured by angioplasty (Fig. 12–43).

Discussion. Significant overdilatation of a nonatherosclerotic aortic wall may severely damage the integrity of the vasa vasorum. Nevertheless, follow-up angiograms as much as 6 weeks later did not show any evidence of aneurysm formation.

In spite of the lack of morphologic changes in the vasa vasorum in canine arteries dilated <100%, Cragg and coworkers found a significant change in vessel wall perfusion after PTA, with a striking increase in blood flow over more than 4 hr.[96–98] Similarly Train et al described

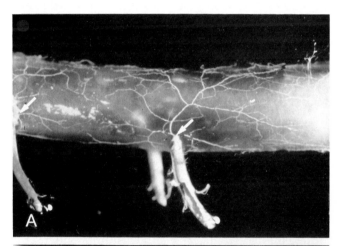

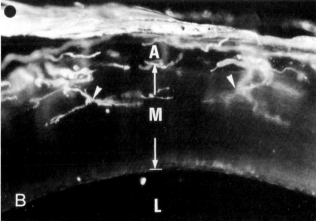

Fig. 12–40 Nondilated canine thoracic aorta after latex infusion. A. Extensive network of vasa vasorum arising from intercostal arteries (arrows). B. Cross-section shows adventitial vasa vasorum reaching and branching into outer media (arrowheads). A = adventitia; M = media; L = lumen. (Reproduced from Cragg AH, Einzig S, Rysavy JA, Castañeda–Zuñiga WR, Borgwardt B, Amplatz K: The vasa vasorum and angioplasty. *Radiology* 1983;148:75–80.)

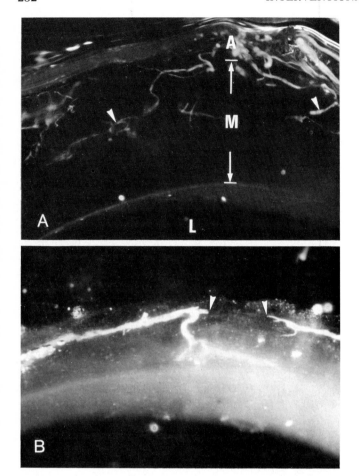

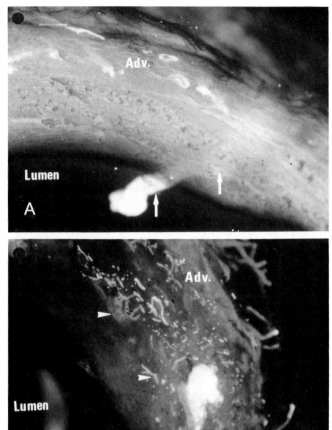

Fig. 12–41   Canine aorta after latex infusion. A. Cross-section after 80% dilatation shows adventitial vasa vasorum running into outer media. Branching and structure of vasa vasorum in outer media appear intact (arrowheads). A = adventitia; M = media; L = lumen. B. Thinning of wall and severe stretching of vasa vasorum with rupture (arrowheads) after >100% dilatation.

Fig. 12–42   Nondilated human abdominal aorta after latex infusion. A. Cross-section shows vasa vasorum penetrating from adventitia through to lumen (arrows). B. Cross-section shows bush-like ramifications and proliferation of vasa vasorum (arrowheads), which show marked caliber changes. Pl = calcified plaque; Adv = adventitia.

three cases of fine perivascular networks visible on angiography after clinical PTA, which they interpret as the vasa vasorum.[103] However, these minute vessels run at some distance along the mother artery and therefore may also represent adventitial collaterals. The present authors were never able, either in living canine or in human cadaver arteries, to demonstrate the intramural vasa vasorum angiographically after PTA. Indeed, the vasa vasorum of the inner adventitia and the media are below the limit of angiographic resolution. Nevertheless, it can be argued that through the same mediators that cause hyperemia of the vasa vasorum, dilatation of the adventitial collaterals also may be provoked.

The effects on the atherosclerotic cadaver vessels were difficult to distinguish. The nondilated atherosclerotic artery showed a very irregular pattern of the vasa vasorum, with vessel cut-offs, so only severance of the vasa vasorum at sites of plaque rupture could be definitely attributed to the dilating trauma. However, it is conceivable that advanced atherosclerosis with extensive proliferation of vasa vasorum throughout the arterial wall layers has a propensity for intramural hematoma formation after PTA. This, again, may be a cause of early reocclusion in clinical angioplasty.

Summary and conclusions.   The permanent widening of the arterial lumen by PTA could be the result of one or more of the following[104]:

1. Compression of the atherosclerotic plaque;
2. Redistribution of the plaque;
3. Embolization of the plaque;
4. Regression of plaque secondary to phagocytosis or metabolic changes; and
5. Stretching of the arterial wall.

In the authors' studies on cadaver arteries and atherosclerotic animals, no significant compression or redistribution was found. This has been confirmed by other investigators.[56,81,85–87] Compression of an atherosclerotic plaque is not possible without simultaneous extrusion of liquid constituents. This may be possible with "soft" edematous atheromas or relatively fresh thrombi[36,105,106]; however, according to the experimental results of Chin et al in atherosclerotic cadaver arteries, the expressible liquid contents of the plaque amount to no more than 12% of the total lumen increase, and the portion of the lumen increase attributable to plaque compression is <2%.[56] Hence, 87%–93% of the total lumen increase results from rupture of the plaque and stretching and tearing of

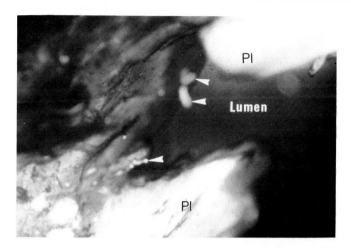

Fig. 12–43 Dilated human iliac artery after latex infusion. Cross-section shows area with rupture of plaque (Pl). Multiple vasa vasorum (arrowheads) end in lumen where plaque has been ruptured.

the media and adventitia. This rule does not apply to fibrinous thrombotic deposits with little cellular attachment to the intima; such deposits are pulverized by balloon compression and carried downstream by the blood without sequelae.[106] According the current experiments, redistribution of plaque occurs only with the use of dilating Teflon catheters according to the original Dotter method, but not when using balloon catheters. With the former, the axial (forward) force of the dilating catheter may displace atheromatous material by a snowplow effect.[8,13]

Peripheral embolization is encountered in 3%–5% of clinical PTA procedures and is often asymptomatic.[92,93,107] According to the authors' experimental studies, only superficial plaque elements are loosened, so their loss does not significantly increase the arterial lumen.[82,108] Clinically significant embolization, therefore, is the result of a completely detached atheromatous plaque or of dislocation of relatively fresh thrombi.

After dilatation of normal arteries, only occasional macrophages were encountered, and no significant phagocytosis of necrotic wall material could be detected.[59] Also, in long-term studies in atherosclerotic animals, there were no signs of significant phagocytosis of atherosclerotic wall constituents after PTA.[72,73,86]

Hence, stretching of the arterial wall is the principal mechanism for permanent widening of the arterial lumen after PTA. Since atheromatous plaques are essentially noncompressible and nonelastic, this stretching is possible only after rupture and partial detachment of the plaque. The increasing balloon diameter leads to tears and crevices in the plaque at its weakest point. Once the cuirass-like plaque has been torn, the freed parts of the media and adventitia are stretched by the further increase in the balloon diameter. This mechanism has been proved by the present authors' studies on cadavers and atherosclerotic animal arteries[47,49,82] and has been confirmed several times by other authors.[72,73,81,87,88] In addition, histologic findings in human arteries after successful clinical angioplasty parallel the findings in experimental angioplasty (Figs. 12–44 through 12–46). However, in severe atherosclerosis involving the entire wall

with thinning of the media, it is not always possible to recognize wall changes after clinical PTA.[75,109]

The dilating effect (wall stretching) in normal canine or rabbit artery is directly proportional to the size of the balloon as well as to the duration and pressure of balloon inflation. Unfortunately, this is not true in the atherosclerotic vessel. Although the authors found a general tendency toward progressive wall damage with increasing balloon diameter and inflation time, there was no predictable correlation due to the greater vulnerability and the heterogeneous behavior of the atherosclerotic vessel. They therefore can give no definite recommendation on the ideal balloon size and duration of inflation for clinical PTA, although there is a difference between treating circumferential and asymmetric, cushion-like atheromas (Fig. 12–47). That is, with an asymmetric, localized plaque, a comparatively low balloon pressure may significantly stretch those parts of the arterial wall with little atheromatous involvement, whereas in a severe circumferential stenosis, the plaque must be torn by the dilating balloon before the arterial wall can stretch (Fig. 12–47B,C). The smaller the plaque-free area of the arterial wall, the greater the local wall stretching at this site

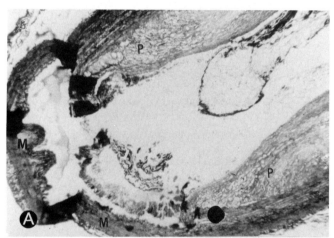

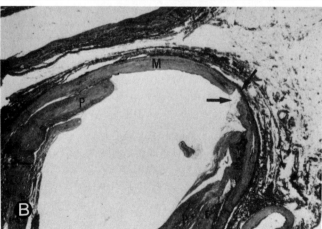

Fig. 12–44 Atherosclerotic rabbit aorta after 50% overdilatation for 60 sec (A) and human femoral artery 5 days after transluminal angioplasty (B). In both instances, there is stretching, with rupture of media at places where it is free of plaque (arrows). M = media, P = plaque. (Courtesy of PD. Dr. J. Schneider, Department of Pathology, University Hospital, Zurich.)

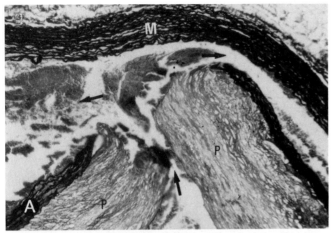

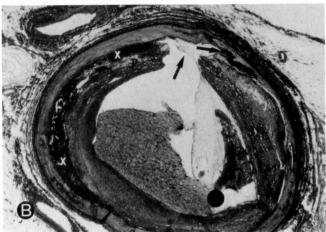

Fig. 12–45 Atherosclerotic rabbit aorta after 50% overdilatation for 15 sec (A) and human femoral artery 5 days after transluminal angioplasty (B). In both cases, there is rupture of plaque and dissection into media (arrows). In addition, the case of clinical PTA shows marked dehiscence of plaque from media. Spaces of dehiscence are filled with thrombi (x). (Courtesy of PD. Dr. J. Schneider, Department of Pathology, University Hospital, Zurich.)

needed to enlarge the arterial lumen to a given degree (Fig. 12–47B,C). Simultaneously, the danger of wall rupture increases. Therefore, careful analysis of the angiogram is important to avoid overstretching the artery.

As demonstrated in the authors' experiments in normal canine arteries,[47,59] postangioplasty healing of the arterial wall occurs with fibrotic scar formation in the media and hyperplasia in the intima secondary to widespread stimulation and migration of smooth muscle cells. Even severe stretching of the arterial wall with complete disruption of the medial layers does not result in significant localized aneurysm formation in the patent lumen, and healing without aneurysm formation can be expected as long as the adventitia is not too severely damaged.

The process of healing in the atherosclerotic vessel cannot be followed as easily, although it is apparent that scar formation and intimal hyperplasia are not of the same nature as in normal vessels. Faxon et al found the atherosclerotic process to be accelerated following angioplasty of rabbit arteries[72,73]; restenoses and thrombotic occlusion in various stages of organization were apparent 4

weeks after angioplasty. The thickened neointima was of a more complex nature than the intimal hyperplasia found in nonatherosclerotic vessels. The study also suggested that intraluminal thrombosis plays a significant role in reocclusion after angioplasty, because administration of antiplatelet drugs significantly reduced restenoses and reocclusions.[72] In clinical PTA, also, antiplatelet drugs and anticoagulants significantly improved the patency rate.[110–116]

In clinical practice, the higher stenosis recurrence rate after dilatation of smaller (e.g., coronary) arteries may be due to thrombosis or to an accelerated atherosclerotic process secondary to release of platelet factors. According to the authors' experimental findings, recurrence of stenosis may also be due to intimal hyperplasia; and this seems especially likely if a nonatherosclerotic stenosis has not been dilated sufficiently. Intimal hyperplasia causing restenosis after PTA of an atherosclerotic stenosis has not been definitely shown. However, occasionally, uncommonly long and rapidly occurring restenoses are found at

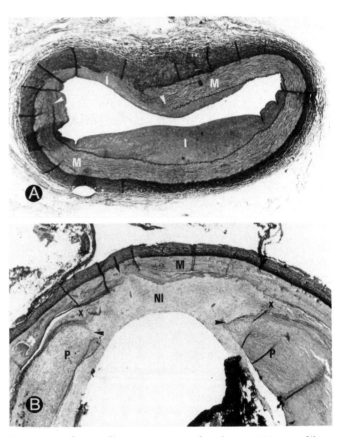

Fig. 12–46 Canine iliac artery 4 months after >100% overdilatation (A) and human superficial femoral artery 44 days after transluminal angioplasty (B). In the canine artery, there is focal rupture of media (M) and IEL (arrowheads). Defect is covered by neointima and medial scar (1), which merges with nonruptured medial areas. In the human artery, plaque rupture is clearly noticeable (arrowheads). Focally ossified media is partially torn (arrow). Rupture has been covered by thick neointima (NI), which has also filled spaces and crevices of original plaque (P) dehiscence (x), thereby smoothing luminal surface. Much as in the animal experiment, the new intima may serve as a compensatory layer where arterial wall had been partially ruptured. (Courtesy of PD. Dr. J. Schneider, Department of Pathology, University Hospital, Zurich.)

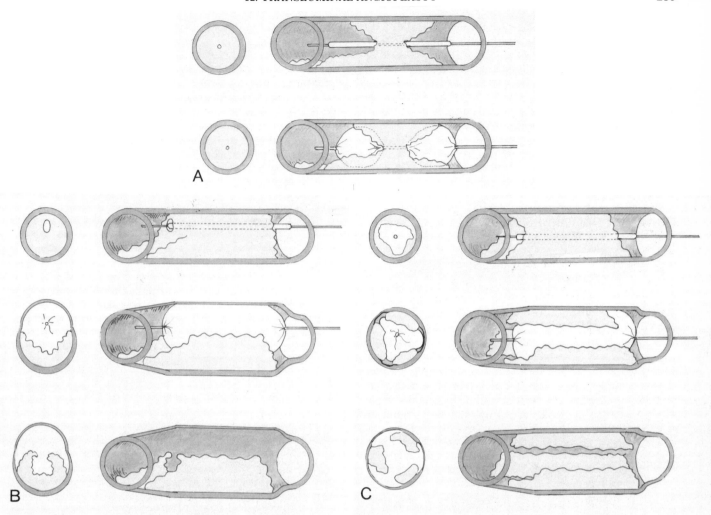

Fig. 12–47   Mechanisms of PTA. A. Schematic drawing of mechanism with high-grade circular stenosis. Above: High-grade circumferential stenosis has been crossed with dilating balloon. Below: Inflation of balloon. As long as atheromatous plaque cannot be torn, lumen cannot widen; balloon merely expands proximal and distal to stenosis, forming a waistline. B. Schematic drawing of mechanism with high-grade eccentric stenosis. Above: Stenosis has been crossed by dilatation catheter. Center: Inflated balloon has ruptured plaque at its weakest area; freed media and adventitia can now be stretched. Below: After dilatation, widened lumen stays open. Plaque shows longitudinal dehiscence at edges where plaque has been ruptured. C. Schematic drawing of mechanism with irregular stenosis. Above: Stenosis has been crossed by balloon catheter. Center: With inflation of balloon, there is rupture of plaque in several places, with local wall stretching. Below: Lumen increase after rupture and local dehiscence of plaque with stretching of wall in plaque-free areas.

the site of previous angioplasty. Such recurrences are attributed to a reaction of the intima and media.[117]

Extrapolation of the results of experimental atherosclerosis in rabbits to human atherosclerosis may be criticized because of the differences in the nature and complexity of the human disease. Therefore, in spite of the many animal experiments, the exact mechanism of healing and smoothing of the arterial wall after clinical PTA has not been clarified. The few examinations of human arteries following clinical PTA have revealed bridging of the plaque ruptures and medial tears by a neointima that probably represents organized thrombus (Fig. 12–46B).

The radiolucent linear filling defects seen in postdilatation angiograms could also be demonstrated *in vitro* after angioplasty of cadaver arteries. These radiolucent lines correspond to the crevices in the atherosclerotic plaque and sites of dehiscence of the thickened intima from the media. In advanced atherosclerosis, intima and media both may be partly dehisced from the adventitia. Similar filling defects were found in the animal experiments. In the atherosclerotic rabbits, a widening of the lumen was regularly accompanied by dehiscence or rupture of the plaque, proving that such dehiscence and rupture are integral parts of successful dilatation. Angiographically and histologically, these phenomena differ from true intraluminal dissections, because they are confined to the dilatation site and do not have a tendency to propagate. Therefore, rupture and dehiscence of plaques should not be interpreted as complications of PTA as long as there is no obstruction to flow or detachment of the plaque.[57] According to the histologic findings in the animal experiments, the degree of dehiscence of atherosclerotic plaques that is seen angiographically probably depends on both the amount of dilatation (balloon size, pressure, duration of inflation) and the nature and configuration of the atherosclerotic plaques. However, the present authors do not agree with Roth et al[117] that a rupture or dehiscence limited to the intimal plaque can be differentiated angiographically from a penetrating dehiscence that includes the media. In advanced atherosclerosis, the media is usually markedly thinned and involved in the pathologic process, so it is likely that this layer frequently is included to some extent in the rupture and dehiscence (Figs. 12–44 through 12–46).

Simultaneously with the healing process, at which time the crevices and clefts in the plaque are covered by a neointima (organized thrombi), smoothing of the contours is visible angiographically. Additional widening of the artery visible on follow-up angiograms over several months is probably caused by adaptation to blood flow. That is, once the media and adventitia are freed from the encasing atherosclerotic plaque (as after endarterectomy), the stretched arterial wall may dilate further as a response to the demand for increased blood flow. Enlargement of the lumen because of shrinkage (fibrosis) and metabolic degradation of atheromatous material are additional possible mechanisms for long-term patency.[36,106,118]

PHARMACOLOGIC PHENOMENA AND METABOLIC CHANGES OF THE ARTERIAL WALL AFTER PTA

It was the authors' hypothesis that the response of dilated arteries to vasoactive substances is altered by the destruction of contractile elements and by the scar formation and medial fibrosis seen in their animal experiments. To verify this hypothesis, vasoconstriction of dilated and nondilated canine arteries in response to vasopressin was tested. According to the studies of Cragg and coworkers, which showed significant hyperemia of the arterial wall after PTA,[96] they further postulated that metabolic changes as well as the direct mechanical trauma were responsible for paralysis of the arterial wall after angioplasty. Therefore, they investigated potential alterations in arachidonic acid metabolism in normal canine arteries.

Paralysis of the Arterial Wall after PTA[119]

MATERIALS AND METHODS

In this pilot study, carotid and iliac arteries in anesthetized dogs were dilated with Grüntzig balloons 80%–100% larger than the original lumen as measured on the angiogram. Dilatations were performed twice for 1 min at an inflation pressure of 4 atm. The arterial lumen was again measured, and 0.2–0.4 unit of vasopressin (Pitressin; Parke–Davis) was infused per minute until the mean arterial pressure had risen by 10 mm Hg. At this time, the angiogram was repeated, and the dilated lumen was compared with that on the postdilatation angiogram. In two dogs, angiography was repeated before and after administration of vasopressin 2 months after PTA.

RESULTS

As in the previously described studies, luminal widening was frequently accompanied by spasms adjacent to the dilated segments (Fig. 12–48A,B). After vasopressin administration, the dilated segments remained unchanged. However, the tendency toward proximal and distal constriction increased, and these areas now covered several centimeters (Fig. 12–48C). At follow-up, the wall paralysis persisted after administration of vasopressin (Fig. 12–49). Again, definite constriction of the nondilated areas was apparent.

DISCUSSION

As discussed earlier, the mechanism of luminal widening in PTA consists of a controlled injury to the arterial wall. The immediate trauma to the media obviously prevents vasoconstriction of the dilated segments. This condition may persist for months if there has been sufficient damage to the media, with fibrous scarring and permanent loss of elastic elements. The authors' results were recently confirmed by Wolf and coworkers,[120] who found

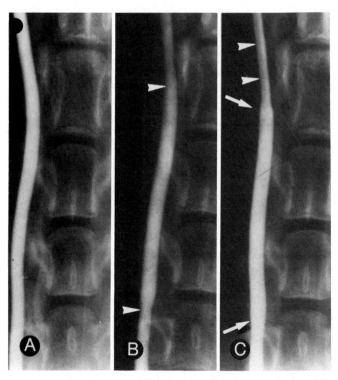

Fig. 12–48   Paralysis after PTA. A. Carotid arteriogram before dilatation. B. Angiogram immediately after dilatation; luminal widening is 22%. Note local vasoconstriction proximal and distal to dilated segment (arrowheads). C. Angiogram after dilatation and administration of vasopressin. No change in widening of dilated segment (between arrows); contraction in the adjacent segments, especially distally, has progressed (arrowheads). (Reproduced from Castañeda-Zuñiga WR, Laerum F, Rysavy J, Rusnak B, Amplatz K: Paralysis of arteries by intraluminal balloon dilatation. *Radiology* 1982;144:75–76.)

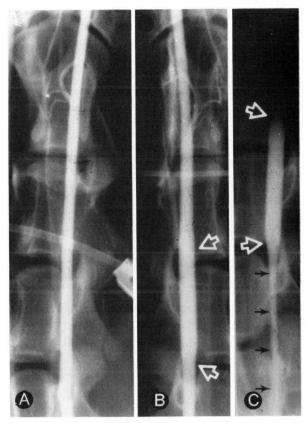

Fig. 12–49 Persisting paralysis after PTA. A. Carotid artery angiogram before dilatation. B. Angiogram immediately after dilatation shows widening of dilated segment (between arrows). C. Follow-up angiogram after 2 months shows persisting paralysis of dilated segment (between open arrows) during infusion of vasopressin. Note severe contraction of adjacent proximal nondilated segment (small arrows). (Reproduced from Castañeda–Zuñiga WR, Laerum F, Rysavy J, Rusnak B, Amplatz K: Paralysis of arteries by intraluminal balloon dilatation. *Radiology* 1982;144:75–76.)

that in rabbit aortas, wall paralysis depends on the extent of dilatation, with 50% overdilation abolishing vasoconstriction. However, these findings in normal animal vessels are difficult to confirm in human arteries.

The spontaneous spasm-like contractions proximal and distal to the dilated segments seen in this and earlier studies were unexpected. Histologically, these areas were damaged to a significantly lesser degree than the dilated segment itself and responded to vasoactive drugs. The phenomenon may be explained by the work of Price et al[121] and Tallaride et al,[122] who showed a direct correlation between the state of stretch of the arterial wall and the vasoconstrictor response. The studies of Wolf et al further showed that slight stretching *in vitro* enhances the vasoconstrictor response, whereas great stretching attenuates the vasoconstriction response to both depolarizing agents (potassium) and receptor-mediated agonists (norepinephrine).[123] It is therefore conceivable that with only limited stretching of the media in the areas adjacent to the dilated arterial segments, such a mechanism causes spontaneous vasoconstriction. These observations are also important with regard to clinical PTA, where spasms are not uncommon in spite of advanced atherosclerosis

with calcification and may lead to early thrombotic reocclusion.[24,83,107,112,124–126] For this reason, especially in renal and coronary angioplasty, prophylactic administration of vasodilating drugs (*i.e.,* nifedipin, nitroglycerin) is recommended.[83,125,127] Furthermore, on the basis of the authors' experimental findings and the study by Wolf and Lentini,[123] vasodilating drugs seem especially indicated in PTA of nonatherosclerotic disease.

Because the reduction of the vasoconstrictor response is roughly proportional to the effectiveness of the stretch, Wolf et al discuss the possibility that this response might be used to determine the endpoint of clinical PTA.[120] However, on the basis of the present authors' observations of frequent spontaneous spasms adjacent to sites of dilation, they consider this maneuver dangerous and contraindicated, especially for nonatherosclerotic vessels, where contractability is not compromised by atherosclerotic plaque.

Role of Prostaglandins after PTA[128]

In the animal studies by Cragg et al, an increase in vessel wall blood flow after PTA was demonstrated (Fig. 12–50).[97,98] The segments directly adjacent to the dilated areas also showed increasing flow although to a lesser degree and for a shorter time (Fig. 12–50). When acetylsalicylic acid (ASA) was given intravenously before angioplasty, vessel wall hyperemia was significantly attenuated when compared to the controls (283% *vs.* 2356%)(Fig. 12–51). On the basis of these studies, it was concluded that vessel wall hyperemia was caused by release of vasoactive compounds as well as by the effects of mechanical damage. Because post-PTA hyperemia could be influenced by ASA, which is a cyclooxygenase blocker, it was further hypothesized that prostaglandins play a key role in changing the vasoactive response. Such an effect is of particular clinical interest, because cyclooxygenase inhibitors such as ASA are recommended to prevent platelet aggregation after PTA.[23,28,116,127,129] Cyclooxygenase inhibitors prevent synthesis of the proaggregating thromboxane A_2 (TXA_2) in platelets by blocking the conversion of arachidonic acid into the unstable intermediate endoperoxide (PG) H_2. Likewise, PGI_2, which is formed in the blood vessels, is also synthesized from PGH_2.[130,131] Therefore, ASA blocks not only the formation of TXA_2, but also the antiaggregating and vasodilating effects of PGI_2 (Fig. 12–52). It may be postulated then, that the attenuation of post-PTA vessel wall hyperemia by ASA reflects a direct influence of this drug on PGI_2 production in the arterial wall. If indeed PGI_2 is produced and released by the damaged vessel wall after PTA, this would be beneficial and so should not be blocked. The following experiments were performed to investigate this hypothesis.

MATERIALS AND METHODS

Carotid arteries in anesthetized dogs were dilated with Grüntzig-type polyethylene balloon catheters three times for 1 min each time at 4.5 atm of inflation pressure. The balloon diameters were 25%–100% larger than the arte-

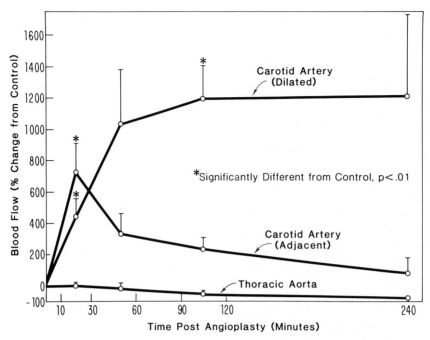

Fig. 12–50 Sequential vessel wall blood flow (VWBF) measurements up to 4 hr using radioactive microspheres (group 1). Dramatic increase (+1200%) in blood flow in dilated carotid artery persisted throughout experiment. Briefer rise in VWBF is also found in segrial lumen, as measured on a baseline angiogram. The dilated segments were divided into three groups:

ments directly adjacent to dilatation site. No elevation of blood flow in the thoracic aorta. (Reproduced from Cragg AH, Einzig S, Rysavy JA, Castañeda–Zuñiga WR, Borwardt B, Amplatz K: The vasa vasorum and angioplasty. *Radiology* 1983;148:75–80.)

rial lumen, as measured on a baseline angiogram. The dilated segments were divided into three groups:

Group A: Six arteries dilated to 50%–100% above normal size and studied within 6 hr;

Group B: Three arteries dilated to 25%–30% above

normal size, of which two were studied 24 hr after dilation and one after 1 week;

Group C: Four arteries dilated to 70%–100% above normal size, of which two were studied at 24 hr, one after 1 week, and one after 3 months.

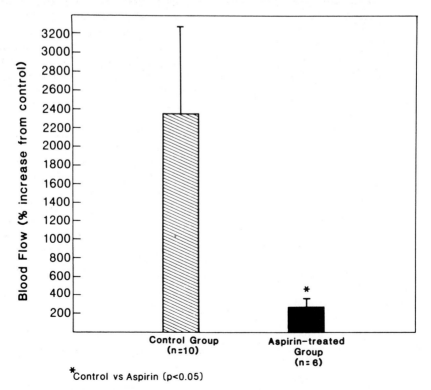

Fig. 12–51 Vessel wall blood flow measurement using radioactive microspheres 60 min after angioplasty. ASA significantly attenuates increase produced by angioplasty (2356% *vs.* 283%). (Reproduced from Cragg A, Einzig S, Rysavy J, Castañeda–Zuñiga WR, Borwardt B, Amplatz K: Effect of aspirin on angioplasty-induced vessel wall hypermia. *AJR* 1983;140:1233–1238.)

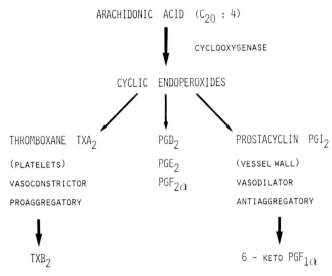

Fig. 12–52 Metabolism of arachidonic acid, showing synthesis of prostacyclin (PGI_2) and thomboxane (TXA_2) and their stable derivatives. (Reproduced from Zollikofer C, Cragg A, Einzig S, et al: Prostaglandins and angioplasty. *Radiology* 1983;149:681–685.)

Eight nondilated arteries served as controls (group D). Dilated and control segments were carefully excised and cut into rings 3 mm wide. These were attached to a transducer, which measures isometric contractile force (ICF)

in grams, and then suspended in an organ bath containing buffered Krebs' solution (Fig. 12–53). After sequential administration of 30 ng, 100 ng, and 1 μg of norepinephrine per milliliter to the bath, the ICF was measured. The bath was then changed, 3 μg of indomethacin were added per milliliter, and contraction was again measured after administration of the same norepinephrine doses. Any increased contraction following indomethacin administration was compared with short- and long-term studies and analyzed using Student's paired and unpaired t-tests.

RESULTS

As expected, the normal arterial rings exhibited progressive increases in ICF with increasing doses of norepinephrine. Contraction increased significantly when indomethacin was added (Fig. 12–54A), with the maximum ICF rising from a mean ($\pm$ SEM) of 3.71 $\pm$ 0.29 g to 4.63 $\pm$ 0.37 (p <0.02)(Table 12–7). Of the dilated arteries, those in group A showed significantly decreased contraction compared to the controls (0.95 $\pm$ 0.11 g *vs.* 3.71 $\pm$ 0.29 g; p <0.01). In the presence of indomethacin, contraction rose to 2.84 $\pm$ 0.25 g (p <0.001)(Fig. 12–54B and Table 12–7). Although the absolute contraction with indomethacin was lower than in the controls, the average

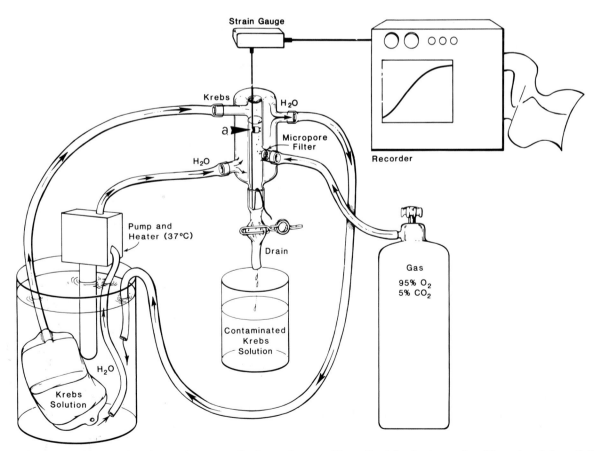

Fig. 12–53 System used to measure isometric contractile force of carotid arterial rings. Ring (a) is suspended in organ bath. Oxygenated Krebs' solution is kept at constant temperature of 37° C by perfusion pump. Contractions measured by strain gauge are displayed on fiberoptic strip-chart recorder. (Reproduced from Zollikofer C, Cragg A, Einzig S, et al: Prostaglandins and angioplasty. *Radiology* 1983;149:681–685.)

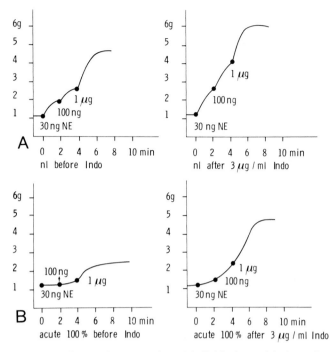

Fig. 12–54 Isometric contraction of individual arterial rings after sequential administration of 30 ng, 100 ng, and 1 μg of norepinephrine (indomethacin (Indo)) per milliliter. A. Normal nondilated artery; indomethacin moderately enhances contraction (right). B. Carotid artery overdilated by 100% in short-term study; contraction is decreased compared to control (A) and increases markedly after addition of indomethacin (right). (Reproduced from Zollikofer C, Cragg A, Einzig S, et al: Prostaglandins and angioplasty. *Radiology* 1983;149:681–685.)

percentage increase was 10 times greater in the dilated arteries (468% *vs.* 42%; p <0.01).

The percentage increase in contraction due to indomethacin in all groups is shown in Table 12–8 and Figure 12–55. In group B, there was no significant difference from the controls before or after indomethicin administration (Tables 12–7 and 12–8). Although not quite statistically significant, there was a distinct trend toward reduced contraction for arteries dilated 70%–100% and studied after 1 week to 3 months (Table 12–7 and Fig. 12–56). Similarly, ICF in group C tended to be lower than in group B. Arteries dilated to no more than 30% and studied 24 hr or more after angioplasty did not show a significant difference from the controls before and after indomethacin administration (Tables 12–7 and 12–8).

Table 12–7
Total Mean Contraction (±SEM) before and after Indomethacin

	Contraction (g)	
	Without Indomethacin	With Indomethacin
Normal (n = 8)	3.71 ± 0.29	4.63 ± 0.37[a]
Short-term (>50%) (n = 6)	0.95 ± 0.22[b]	2.84 ± 0.25[c]
Long-term		
≤30% (n = 3)	3.83 ± 0.60	4.51 ± 0.40
≥70% (n = 4)	2.88 ± 0.49	3.89 ± 0.27

[a]p < 0.02 for normal (with *vs.* without).
[b]p < 0.01 for with (normal *vs.* short-term).
[c]p < 0.001 for short-term (with *vs.* without).

The overall percentage increase in ICF after indomethacin was greater at lower doses of norepinephrine in all groups studied (Fig. 12–56).

DISCUSSION

These findings indicate that mechanical damage to carotid arteries dilated for a short time *in situ* reduces the responsiveness to exogenous norepinephrine *in vitro*. Treatment of damaged arterial rings with the cyclooxygenase inhibitor indomethacin significantly increased responsiveness to norepinephrine, although contraction was never completely restored. These results suggest that synthesis of PGI_2 by the damaged arterial wall is responsible for the decreased response to norepinephrine before cyclooxygenase blockade, because the local vasodilating effect of PGI_2 may have been sufficient to override the constrictor effect of norepinephrine. These effects lasted for at least 6 hr but less than 24 hr after dilatation, in accord with earlier flow studies of the vasa vasorum.[97] Although PGI_2 synthesis may certainly be a favorable side effect of PTA, preventing early reocclusion, these data indicate that this is an acute event. They are in general agreement with the fact that tissue damage may increase prostaglandin synthesis over the short term, whereas in the long term, synthesis at the site may actually be reduced. This is especially true of blood vessels, because cyclooxygenase is produced principally in the endothelium, with production gradually declining toward the peripheral media.[132,133] Damage to these layers by PTA may cause immediate local release of PGI_2, as suggested by these findings. Inasmuch as PGI_2 is a potent antiaggregatory and vasodilating drug and its

Table 12–8
Per Cent Increase in Contraction with Indomethacin (Mean ± SE)

	Short-term		Long-term	
	Normal (n = 8)	>50% (n = 6)	≤30% (n = 3)	≥70% (n = 4)
Norepinephrine				
30 ng	54.0 ± 27.0	699.0 ± 254.3	32.5 ± 42.5	81.4 ± 47.6
100 ng	43.6 ± 16.4	489.4 ± 108.9	44.2 ± 35.5	86.3 ± 33.1
1 μg	26.9 ± 10.1	216.6 ± 38.7	21.6 ± 13.8	41.1 ± 13.2
Average	42.0 ± 10.8	468.3 ± 99.7[a]	32.8 ± 16.8	69.6 ± 18.9

[a]p < 0.01 (normal *vs.* short-term).

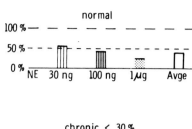

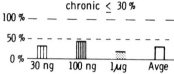

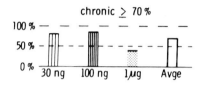

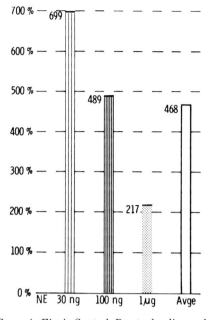

Fig. 12–55 Relative mean percentage increase in contractile force after indomethacin (norepinephrine (NE)) in the normal controls and the three groups of dilated arteries. (Reproduced from Zollikofer C, Cragg A, Einzig S, et al: Prostaglandins and angioplasty. *Radiology* 1983;149:681–685.)

release seems limited to a short time (at least 6, but less than 24 hr) ASA treatment may be delayed for 12–24 hr, in order not to affect PGI_2 synthesis. Nevertheless, it should be noted that platelets form aggregates *in vitro* in two distinct phases. The primary phase is initiated by adenosine diphosphate (ADP) or epinephrine; the second phase is due to TXA_2 synthesis, which initiates further release of ADP. Only the second phase is prevented by drugs such as ASA or indomethacin, that inhibit formation of TXA_2.[134] In contrast, substances such as adenosine and PGI_2, which elevate platelet levels of cylic adenosine monophosphate (cAMP), block primary as well as secondary aggregation.[135] Therefore, treatment with ASA alone will not eliminate all the factors responsible for platelet aggregation.

This experiment was performed in nonatherosclerotic canine carotid arteries, which may behave much differently from atherosclerotic human vessels. Whereas in normal vessels, synthesis of PGI_2 is greatest in the endothelium and gradually decreases toward the adventitia,[132] in atherosclerosis there is evidence that *in vitro*, PGI synthesis is generally reduced.[136,137] Therefore, the release of prostacyclin might also be reduced after PTA of atherosclerotic vessels. However, these results have been challenged. Probst et al demonstrated release of prostacyclin soon after coronary angioplasty,[138] and *in vivo* studies measuring excretion of urinary prostacyclin metabolites in patients with severe atherosclerosis showed a significant increase in endogenous biosynthesis of prostacyclin as compared with healthy subjects.[139] Furthermore, the vessel wall may synthesize prostacyclin not only from its endogenous endoperoxides, but also from exogenous endoperoxides released from platelets.[132] Consequently, platelet aggregation on the denuded surface of the dilated

segment may lead to increased prostacyclin synthesis in the arterial wall. Therefore, one must not rely on the ability of the blood vessels to produce prostacyclin, but rather on the ability of the platelets to adhere to the damaged surface.

This raises the question of whether a selective inhibitor of TXA_2 synthesis should be used instead of a cyclooxygenase inhibitor for PTA. Aiken et al[140] and Yarger et al[141] have shown that selective thromboxane synthetase inhibitors have a greater antiaggregating efficacy than do cyclooxygenase inhibitors due to the enhanced responsiveness of the platelets to endogenous PGI_2. Probably even more important is the fact that the antithrombotic action of these compounds can be blocked by previous treatment with ASA. Therefore, a selective thromboxane inhibitor may be preferable to ASA for preventing early reocclusion after PTA, because local PGI_2 synthesis would be unaffected and platelet aggregation at the damaged site would be impaired. On the other hand, it has recently been reported that the TXA_2 produced by platelets is more sensitive to ASA than to PGI_2 produced by the vessel wall, so that low-dose ASA has been advocated as having a lesser effect on PGI_2 synthesis.[142–146] Some authors have recommended giving one ASA tablet per day on the grounds that prostacyclin synthesis returns to normal within 24–36 hr after a single dose, whereas blockade of TXA_2 in the platelets is irreversible.[142,144] Weksler et al recently demonstrated differential inhibition of vascular and platelet prostaglandin synthesis by ASA in atherosclerotic patients undergoing aortocoronary bypass.[147] With low-dose (80 mg/day) ASA, a reliable blockade of TXA_2 was achieved, with only minor effects on prostacyclin synthesis. However, other investigators could not entirely confirm such beneficial differential effects of low-

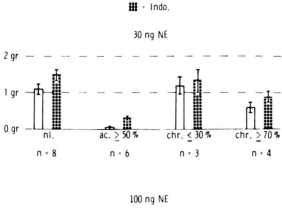

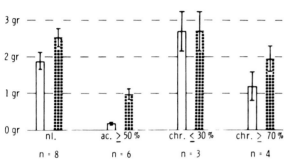

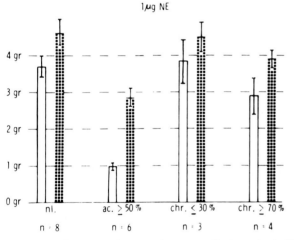

Fig. 12–56   Absolute mean increase in contractile force (g ± SE) after indomethacin (norephinephrine (NE)) administration in the controls and the three groups of dilated arteries. (Reproduced from Zollikofer C, Cragg A, Einzig S, et al: Prostaglandins and angioplasty. *Radiology* 1983;149:681–685.)

dose ASA on prostaglandin synthesis. Consequently, the response of PGI_2 synthesis to ASA and the appropriate dosage remain controversial, since there are wide *in vivo* differences in ASA sensitivity.[147–153]

Although the percentage of contraction increased 10-fold after indomethacin administration in the short-term study (Fig. 12–54), the arterial rings showed a decreased absolute response (Fig. 12–55). Therefore, in addition to the prostaglandin effect hypothesized above, there must be direct mechanical damage to the media that reduces responsiveness even after several weeks if the arterial wall has been stretched far enough. Such damage is obviously related to the amount of stretching by the balloon, as

shown by the authors' long-term studies (groups B and C) as well as by the histomorphologic investigations.[47,59,82]

SUMMARY AND CONCLUSIONS

Local paralysis and hyperemia of the arterial wall after PTA can now be explained by some combination of mechanical damage and release of vasoactive substances. These studies strongly suggest that prostaglandins are responsible for the pharmacologically induced vasodilation. Acetylcholine, ATP and ADP, histamines, and bradykinins are not active without an intact endothelium,[154] so one can logically conclude that cyclooxygenase inhibitors reduce vessel wall hyperemia by direct action on prostacyclin synthesis. Partial restitution of arterial contractility following administration of cyclooxygenase inhibitors can be similarly explained. Furthermore, it is tempting to speculate that cyclooxygenase inhibition with ASA or indomethacin might predispose a recently dilated vessel to spasm or amplify its response to circulating norepinephrine. It is known that inhibition of the cyclooxygenase pathway can shunt arachidonic acid metabolism into the lipoxygenase pathway (Fig. 12–57),[155] increasing the production of hydroxyeicosatetranoic acid (HPETE), a potent vasoconstrictor.

The local spasms proximal and distal to the dilated segments as seen on angiograms after experimental PTA can be explained by two mechanisms: increased release of HPETE in the dilated arterial segments and an enhanced vasoconstrictor response of those segments immediately adjacent to the dilation site that have been stretched only slightly.[123] Increased synthesis of HPETE after PTA of canine carotid arteries has recently been reported by Cragg et al.[156] Hence, the administration of ASA could, theoretically, cause vasospasm leading to early thrombotic occlusion by shunting arachidonic acid pathway metabolites into the lipoxygenase pathway. In addition, animal experiments have shown an ASA dosage of >10 mg/kg to enhance platelet deposition on the de-endothelialized vascular surface.[157,158]

In short, the problem of prophylactic ASA remains unsolved and controversial (at least for the common dose of 0.5–1.0 g/day).[142,147,151–153,159,160] Other means of preventing thrombosis after PTA must therefore be considered. Selective thromboxane inhibitors, stimulation of prostacyclin production by the vessel wall, development of inhibitors of phosphodiesterase (which might be potentiating endogenous prostacyclin production), and administration of synthetic prostacyclin offer new possibilities.[132] Because prostacyclin is the most powerful substance currently known for preventing platelet aggregation and simultaneously increasing cAMP production, it or a stable synthetic analog, alone or in combination with a phosphodiesterase inhibitor, should provide better prophylaxis against platelet aggregation.

However, one must be cautious in extrapolating these conclusions, derived from studies on normal canine arteries *in vitro* and *in vivo*, to the clinical situation in human atherosclerosis. Only detailed experiments on diseased vessels of primates and clinical trials with prostacyclin and TXA_2 inhibitors can validate these first experimental data.

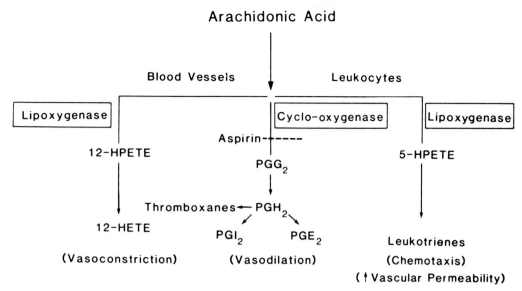

Fig. 12–57 Arachidonic acid metabolism and cyclooxygenase metabolites. Cyclooxygenase is blocked by ASA. Several other vasoactive substances are produced by the separate lipoxygenase pathway, including the potent vasoconstricting hydroxymetabolite hydroxyeicosatetranoic acid (HPETE). (Reproduced from Cragg A, Einzig S, Rysavy J, Castañeda–Zuñiga WR, Borgwardt B, Amplatz K: Effect of aspirin on angioplasty-induced vessel wall hypermia. *AJR* 1983;140:1233–1238.)

PHYSICAL BASIS OF PTA AND CHARACTERISTICS OF BALLOON CATHETERS

Successful dilatation and recanalization of vascular stenoses or occlusions requires not only correct interpretation of the angiogram and skilled hands for manipulating catheters and guidewires, but also a thorough knowledge of the available balloon materials and catheter designs. Although balloons are being advertised as nonelastic and nonexpandable at specified pressures, they exhibit differences in compliance and bursting characteristics that may considerably influence the results of dilatation, especially if hard, fibrous lesions are being treated with inflation pressures greater than those at which the balloon is guaranteed by the manufacturer. In addition, balloon dilatation is governed by a few basic principles of physics, which are discussed briefly below and which should always be borne in mind when performing transluminal balloon dilatation.[53,161–163]

Essential Physical Principles

DILATING FORCE *VS.* BALLOON DIAMETER AND INFLATION PRESSURE

The dilating force is the result of two factors: (1) the hydrostatic force produced by the inflating fluid and (2) the radial force vector. According to Laplace's law, the wall tension or hoop stress, T, is a function of pressure × radius. Because the inner surface of a balloon increases with the diameter, the dilating force at a given pressure is proportional to the radius. Therefore, a balloon double the radius of a smaller one produces twice the dilating force at a constant pressure. On the other hand, if the balloon diameter is kept constant, the dilating force increases linearly with the inflation pressure.

DILATING FORCE *VS.* LENGTH AND DEGREE OF STENOSIS

At a given pressure, the dilating force of the balloon is greater in a long (large area) stenosis than in a short one. Furthermore, at the same pressure, the dilating force will be greater in a short, high-grade stenosis than in a shallow, open one because of the "clothesline effect" (Fig. 12–58). Accordingly, in a short, high-grade stenosis, the dilating force is governed by the clothesline effect, whereas in a long, shallow stenosis, the hydrostatic pressure of the balloon is more important.

DILATING FORCE *VS.* BALLOON MATERIAL

Any balloon material tends to stretch when exposed to some particular pressure. The pressure *vs.* diameter curves not only depend on the balloon material, but also change with the temperature and the number and duration of balloon inflations. If the yield strength (the force that causes permanent deformation of the material) is close to the ultimate tensile strength (the force required to break the material), the diameter will change very little with increasing pressure. Therefore, balloons with the lowest compliance (least stretch) exert considerably higher dilating force. If, on the other hand, the balloon material begins to stretch and deform at low pressures, it cannot concentrate its dilating force on the stenosis and will stretch around the stenosis, producing a "waist" (Fig. 12–59). Therefore, for maximum dilating force, one should choose the balloon with the smallest compliance.

DILATING FORCE *VS.* BALLOON LENGTH

The dilating force of a material with a specific compliance will be considerably larger in a short balloon than a

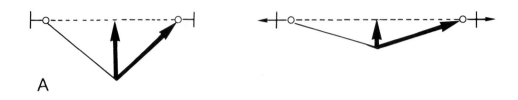

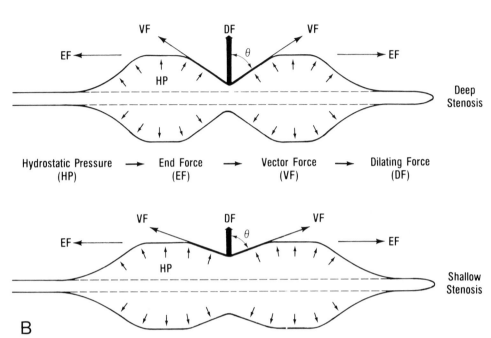

A

B

Hydrostatic Pressure → End Force → Vector Force → Dilating Force
(HP)   (EF)   (VF)   (DF)

Fig. 12–58 Clothesline effect. A. When weight hanging in center of clothesline is lifted by pulling on each end of the line, force vector pushing upward decreases as line straightens. B. Same principle applied to balloon dilatation. If balloon surface is indented by localized stenosis, component force pushing outward corresponds to dilating force. With progressive expansion of balloon or dilatation of stenosis, DF decreases.

Fig. 12–59 Demonstration of "waistline" with dilatation of a short, localized stenosis (coarctation of aorta). A. Dilatation with 6-mm PVC balloon exhibiting marked compliance at 4 and 6 atm. Balloon shows marked increase in diameter proximal and distal to stenosis without significant dilatation of stenosis itself (waistline). This may damage arterial wall distant from the stenosis. B. Dilatation with a 6-mm PE balloon exhibiting limited compliance at 6 and 8 atm. Result of dilatation is significantly better than in A. Despite increasing inflation pressure, there is no significant increase in balloon diameter proximal and distal to stenosis.

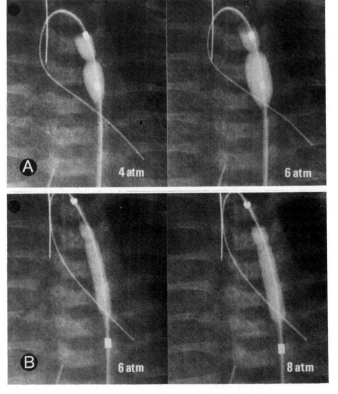

long one. With a noncompliant material, however, the length of the balloon is of minor importance. In an eccentric lesion, a larger balloon may even be more effective.[162] Other factors to be considered in angioplasty are the site, configuration, and nature of the stenotic lesion. Closely related are the following questions:

How much (balloon diameter);
How long (time of inflation); and
How often (should a lesion be dilated)?

Ideally, the nature or compliance of a stenotic lesion will be determined before or during dilatation. To investigate these problems and to test the characteristics of compliance and yield strength of different balloon materials, the authors performed several experimental studies *in vitro* and *in vivo* with the aim of optimizing the results of angioplasty.

Balloon Dilatation Catheters: Characteristics of Expansion, Deformation, and Rupture

In the European and Anglo-American literature, only a few reports on the mechanical properties of angioplasty balloon catheters had been published before 1983.[84,161,162,164–166] Therefore, the authors investigated the commonly used types of balloon-dilating catheters from the 1984 production line of four manufacturers. The balloons were tested *in vitro* and *in vivo* for compliance, deformation, and rupture, and the advantages and disadvantages of each type were noted. The possible differences in vessel wall alteration and the final outcome of angioplasty were also analyzed.

IN VITRO EXPERIMENTS[167]

Materials and Methods

Five types of angioplasty balloon catheters from four manufacturers were tested. (Cook, Inc.; Bloomington, IN: balloons designated PVC/C and PE/C; Schneider/Medintag; Zurich, Switzerland: PVC/S; Medi–Tech; Watertown, MA: PE/MT; Surgimed–Meadox; Glostrup, Denmark: PU/O). The balloons were made from three different materials, PVC, polyethylene (PE), and polyurethane (PU), and measured 4, 6, and 8 mm in diameter and 2–4 cm in length. The structural differences in the various brands are depicted schematically in Figures 12–60 and 12–61. The catheters were inflated in a 37° C water bath using a hand-driven balloon inflation device in combination with a pressure gauge.[168] Balloon diame-

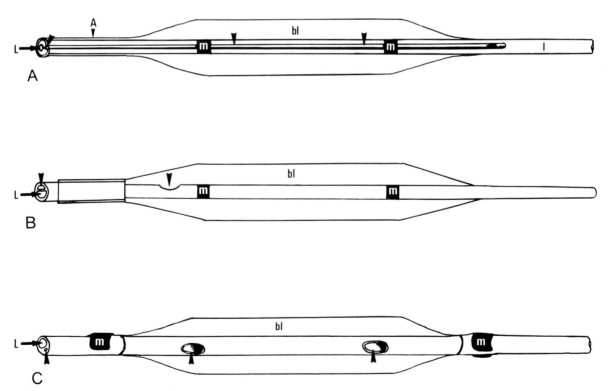

Fig. 12–60   Diagram of longitudinal section through balloon dilatation catheters. A. Coaxial system used by Cook consisting of central PE catheter and outer catheter sleeve, made of PVC or PE (A), which also includes the balloon segment (bl). Inner catheter (I) has central lumen (L) and one to three longitudinal side channels (arrowheads) through which balloon can be inflated. m = tantalum markers to indicate balloon segment. B. True double-lumen catheter system by Schneider/Medintag. Smaller lumen (arrowhead) is connected to balloon lumen (bl) via sidehole (arrowhead). Larger catheter lumen (L) takes guidewire or serves for injection of contrast medium into the vessel. The PVC balloon is glued to the catheter. m = tantalum markers. C. Double-lumen system used by Medi–Tech. Same principle as shown in B, with PE balloon being glued to double-lumen catheter. Small lumen (arrowheads) is connected to balloon lumen by two sideholes (arrowheads). The tantalum markers (m) are attached proximal and distal to balloon segment. (Reproduced from Zollikofer CL, Salomonowitz E, Brühlmann WF, Castañeda–Zuñiga WR, Amplatz K: Dehnungs-, Verformungs und Berstungs-Charakteristika haufig verwendeter Balloon-Dilatationskatheter: in vitro Untersuchungen. (Teil 1). *RöFo* 1986;140:40–46.)

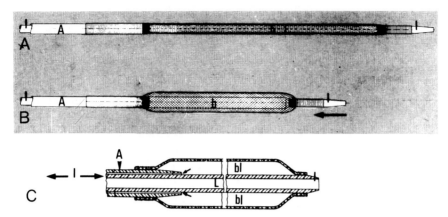

Fig. 12–61 Schematic diagram of balloon dilatation catheter according to Olbert/Surgimed system. A, B. Catheter empty and inflated. C. Coaxial system with two movable catheters (inner PE and outer Teflon); balloon (b) consists of PU reinforced with nylon mesh and is glued distally to inner catheter (I) and proximally to outer catheter (A), so that balloon lumen (bl) communicates with space between the two catheters (small arrows). When empty, inner catheter is fully extruded, and balloon wraps tightly around inner catheter without any folds. When balloon is inflated, inner catheter moves backward. (Reproduced from Zollikofer CL, Salomonowitz E, Brühlmann WF, Castañeda–Zuñiga WR, Amplatz K: Dehnungs-, Verformungs- und Berstungs-Charakteristika haufig verwendeter Balloon-Dilatationskatheter: in vitro Untersuchungen. (Teil 1). *RöFo* 1986;140:40–46.)

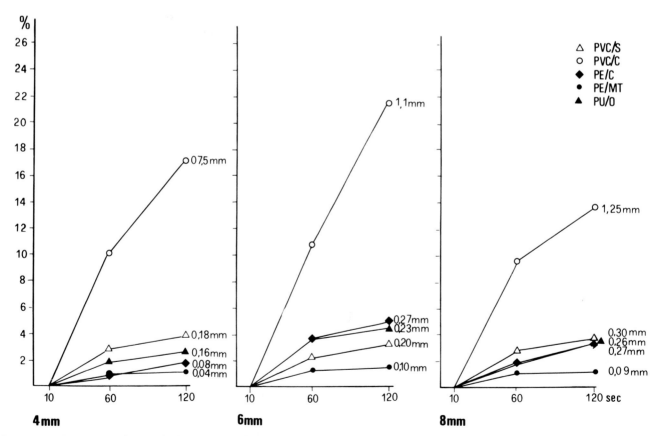

Fig. 12–62   Tests in 37° C water bath of 4-, 6-, and 8-mm balloons; increase in diameter is expressed as percentage of initial diameter after inflation for 10 sec with continued inflation at constant pressure of 4.5 atm. With the last reading, at 120 sec, absolute values in millimeters also are given. (Reproduced from Zollikofer CL, Salomonowitz E, Brühlmann WF, Castañeda–Zuñiga WR, Amplatz K: Dehnungs-, Verformungs- und Berstungs-Charakteristika haufig verwendeter Balloon-Dilatationskatheter: in vitro Untersuchungen. (Teil 1). *RöFo* 1986;140:40–46.)

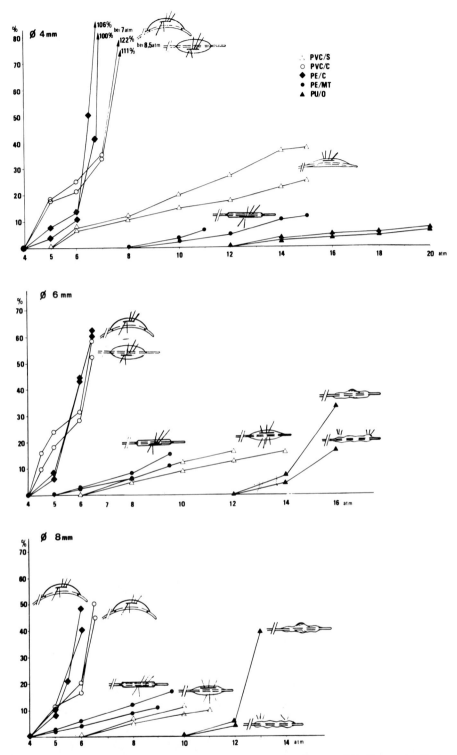

Fig. 12–63 Tests in 37° C water bath of 4-, 6-, and 8-mm balloons; increase in diameter is expressed as percentage of initial balloon diameter at 10 sec inflation time with increasing pressure until balloons burst. Balloon deformation immediately before bursting is drawn schematically. (Reproduced from Zollikofer CL, Salomono-witz E, Brühlmann WF, Castañeda–Zuñiga WR, Amplatz K: Dehn-ungs-, Verformungs- und Berstungs-Charakteristika haufig verwen-deter Balloon-Dilatationskatheter: in vitro Untersuchungen. (Teil 1). *RöFo* 1986;140:40–46.)

ters were measured using micrometer calipers. The following tests and measurements were performed:

1. Registration of balloon diameters at constant pressures of 4.5 atm;
2. Registration of balloon diameters and deformations at increasing pressures in increments of 1–2 atm every 20 sec;
3. Bursting pressures and the mode of balloon bursting, which was analyzed macroscopically and photographed.

In addition, balloon catheters of each brand and size were tested in Teflon tubing with inner diameters appropriate to the respective balloon diameters, *i.e.*, 4, 6, and 8 mm. Using contrast medium diluted 1:1, each balloon was inflated to the manufacturer's recommended pressure and then inflated further in increments of 2 atm at intervals of 20 sec to either a maximum pressure of 22 atm or bursting. The behavior of the balloons was documented by 100-mm spot films at each step.

Results

Tests in a 37° C water bath. Depending on the material and architecture, the balloon catheters showed different characteristics of compliance and deformity at constant pressure and with increasing inflation pressures (Figs. 12–62 and 12–63). It is noteworthy that the PVC/C balloons exhibited a significant compliance even at recommended working pressures. Larger balloons were more compliant than small ones (Table 12–9 and Fig. 12–62). Furthermore, balloon diameters increased from the first to the second inflation by 5%–15%. All other types of balloons showed only minor increases in diameter at constant suggested working pressures: 1.0%–2.8% for PV/S

Table 12–9

Maximum Inflation Pressure (atm) as Suggested by Manufacturers for Balloon Dilation Catheters (1984)

Balloon Type	4 mm	6 mm	8 mm
PVC/S	6	6	6
PVC/C	4.45	4.45	4.45
PE/C	4	4	4
PE/MT	6	4	4
PU/O	12	12	12

balloons, 0.4%–2% for PE/C balloons, 0.2%–0.8% for PE/MT balloons, and 1.2%–2.5% for PU/O balloons. While pressures were increasing, both types of Cook balloon showed greater deformity than the other brands, resulting in bulging and a banana shape (Fig. 12–63). The PU/O balloons showed comparatively little deformation, considering that their recommended working pressure is 4–8 atm higher than that of the other balloon types. Increasing the pressures above the suggested working pressure of 12 atm, however, resulted in rupture of the outer nylon mesh in a 6- and an 8-mm balloon, causing enormous ballooning of the inner PU part (Fig. 12–64F).

The modes of balloon bursting at elevated pressures are shown in Figure 12–64. The range of bursting pressures was limited to 1–3 atm. No significant differences were noted within the various groups (Table 12–10A). The PVC and PE products showed longitudinal tears when bursting. The PE/C balloons were characterized by stretched and wavy borders, whereas the enormous ballooning in the PVC/C design was largely reversible after rupture (Fig. 12–64B,C). The PVC/S and PE/MT balloons showed smooth, nondilated contours of the longitudinal tears, whereas PU/O balloons ruptured with a

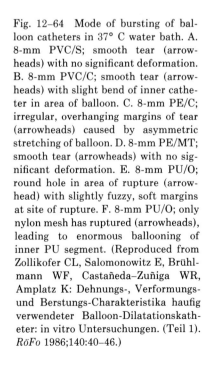
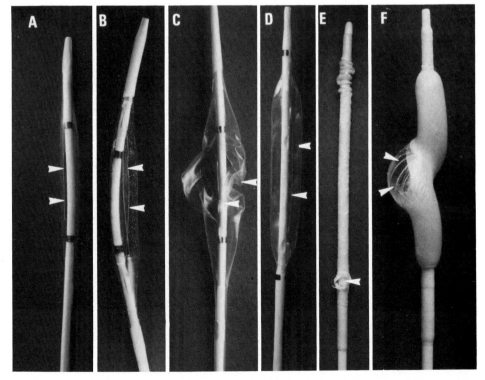

Fig. 12–64 Mode of bursting of balloon catheters in 37° C water bath. A. 8-mm PVC/S; smooth tear (arrowheads) with no significant deformation. B. 8-mm PVC/C; smooth tear (arrowheads) with slight bend of inner catheter in area of balloon. C. 8-mm PE/C; irregular, overhanging margins of tear (arrowheads) caused by asymmetric stretching of balloon. D. 8-mm PE/MT; smooth tear (arrowheads) with no significant deformation. E. 8-mm PU/O; round hole in area of rupture (arrowhead) with slightly fuzzy, soft margins at site of rupture. F. 8-mm PU/O; only nylon mesh has ruptured (arrowheads), leading to enormous ballooning of inner PU segment. (Reproduced from Zollikofer CL, Salomonowitz E, Brühlmann WF, Castañeda–Zuñiga WR, Amplatz K: Dehnungs-, Verformungs- und Berstungs-Charakteristika haufig verwendeter Balloon-Dilatationskatheter: in vitro Untersuchungen. (Teil 1). *RöFo* 1986;140:40–46.)

Table 12–10.
Comparison of Bursting Pressures (atm) of Different Balloon Types

Diameter	Balloon Type				
	PVC/S	PVC/C	PE/C	PE/MT	PU/O
A. Balloons in water bath					
4 mm	15	8.5	7	11–15	20–22
6 mm	12–14	6.5	6.5	9.5	16
8 mm	10–11	6.5	6	9	12–14
B. Balloons in Teflon tubing					
4 mm	>22	16[a]	22[b]	>22	>22
6 mm	19	16[a]	15	22	19[c]
8 mm	14	12.5	10	13	16–18[d]

[a]Massive dissection between central and outer catheter; dilatation of outer catheter up to catheter hub with compression of inner catheter.
[b]Elongation of balloon and compression of central catheter.
[c]Balloon leaks at catheter tip.
[d]Balloon leaks at catheter tip; in addition, rupture of outer nylon mesh at proximal balloon edge.

somewhat irregular, asterisk-like pattern unless the outer nylon mesh ruptured before the inner PU portion (Fig. 12–64E,F).

Tests within Teflon tubing. Testing the balloon catheters within tubing to simulate arteries markedly raised bursting pressures and diminished balloon deformation (Table 12–10B). In Figure 12–65A–E, typical sequences of balloon behavior for each type during increasing inflation pressures are shown. The nonelastic Teflon tubes limited radial expansion of the balloons, and the compliance of the balloon material resulted in a lengthening, which was greatest with PVC/C balloons. In these balloons of coaxial construction, the injected fluid dissected into the virtual lumen between the outer and inner catheter during pressure increases, causing overstretching of the outer catheter sleeve and simultaneous irreversible compression of the inner catheter. In some catheters, the dilatation of the shaft extended as far as the hub at the proximal end (Fig. 12–66A,B). One of the PE/C balloons displayed a similar phenomenon (Fig. 12–

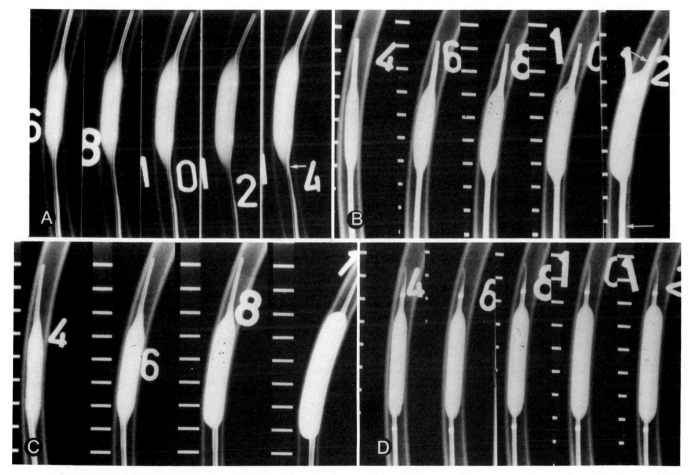

Fig. 12–65 Tests in 8-mm Teflon tubing. A. 8-mm PVC/S balloon; sequence with increasing pressure from 6 to 14 atm. There is moderate elongation (about 5 mm) of balloon, primarily when pressure increases from 12 to 14 atm. Local compression of catheter lumen (arrow 14 atm) was reversible with emptying of balloon. B. 8-mm PVC/C balloon; sequence of increasing pressure from 4 to 12 atm. Marked (>1 cm) elongation of balloon and beginning dissection between inner and outer catheter at 12 atm. C. 8-mm PE/C balloon; sequence at increasing pressure from 4 to 10 atm. Marked (>1 cm) elongation of balloon at 10 atm. D. 8-mm PE/MT balloon; sequence at increasing pressure from 4 to 12 atm. Moderate (<1 cm) elongation of balloon. E. 6-mm PU/O balloon in 6-mm Teflon tubing; sequence with increasing pressure from 12 to 18 atm. Practically no deformation or elongation of balloon. (Reproduced from Zollikofer CL, Salomonowitz E, Brühlmann WF, Castañeda–Zuñiga WR, Amplatz K: Dehnungs-, Verformungs- und Berstungs-Charakteristika haüfig verwendeter Ballon-Dilatationskatheter: in vitro Untersuchungen. (Teil 1). *RöFo* 1986;140:40–46.)

Fig. 12–66   The 4- (A) and 6-mm (B) PVC/C balloons in 4- and 6-mm Teflon tubing with balloon pressures of 4 and 16 atm, respectively. Striking elongation of balloons, with dissection of injected fluid between inner and outer catheter, increasing the diameter of the catheter shaft (arrows). Marked compression of inner catheter at 16 atm (small arrows). (Arrowheads mark balloon length at 4 atm.) C. 4-mm PE/C balloon in 4-mm Teflon tubing with inflation to 4 and 20 atm. Striking elongation of balloon (arrowheads) and compression of inner catheter (arrow) at 20 atm. (Reproduced from Zollikofer CL, Salomonowitz E, Brühlmann WF, Castañeda–Zuñiga WR, Amplatz K: Dehnungs-, Verformungs- und Berstungs-Charakteristika haufig verwendeter Balloon-Dilatationskatheter: in vitro Untersuchungen. (Teil 1). RöFo 1986;140:40–46.)

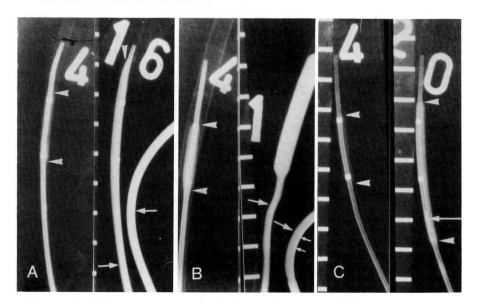

66C). In the other catheter types, the longitudinal extension of the balloons usually was much less, i.e., <1 cm (Fig. 12–65A,D,E). For example, only one of the PE/MT balloons increased in length more than 1 cm, its extension being limited by the proximal tantalum marker (Fig. 12–67A), whereas if the nylon mesh stayed intact, overall lengthening was smallest in the PU/O balloons. In one 8-mm PU/O balloon local rupture of the outer nylon mesh

led to expansion of the inner polyurethane balloon portion (Fig. 12–67B). Local compression of the central catheter lumen, seen in the PVC/S balloons, was always reversible and never impeded deflation (Fig. 12–65A).

Discussion

This study demonstrates significant differences in the behavior of the various balloon dilatation catheters in response to pressure and duration of inflation. All balloon types generally tolerated significantly higher pressures than the suggested working pressures guaranteed by the manufacturers, especially if they were tested within a retaining tube (Table 12–10).

Balloon catheter characteristics depend not only on the balloon and catheter material, but also on the structure. For example, the combination of a coaxial catheter system with high-compliance materials, as in the Cook catheters, results in suboptimal balloon stability relative to other brands, as evidenced by the potential overexpansion of the outer catheter sleeve proximal to the balloon at high inflation pressures. This overexpansion results in elongation of the balloon and compression of the inner catheter, which may jam the guidewire. Furthermore, deflation of the catheter may be impossible because of plastic overstretching of the outer catheter. The Olbert/Surgimed system[169,170] overcomes this disadvantage by using a coaxial system with an outer catheter made of nonexpandable Teflon tubing. Furthermore, the authors were able to show that the newest generation of PVC materials (PVC/S balloons) have a compliance as low as polyethylene, which had not been the case earlier.[161,164]

As expected, the bursting pressures of all balloons were significantly higher inside Teflon tubing than in the water bath. These tests clearly demonstrate the potential danger of balloon deformation in response to high inflation pressures in clinical PTA.[171] A significant compliance of the balloon and catheter material leads to a potentially dangerous deformation and elongation of the balloon and an irreversible increase in the diameter of the catheter shaft, as demonstrated by the PVC/C and PE/C balloons.

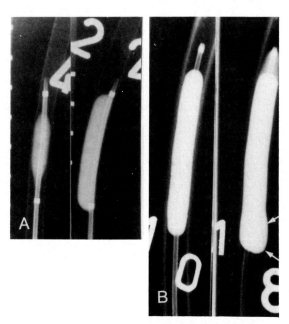

Fig. 12–67   Tests in Teflon tubing. A. 6-mm PE/MT balloon in 6-mm tubing with inflation to 4 and 22 atm. Striking (>1 cm) elongation of balloon is limited by tantalum markers. No compression of second catheter lumen. B. 8-mm PU/O balloon in 8-mm tubing with inflation to 10 and 18 atm. Elongation and local dilatation at proximal end (arrows) due to rupture of nylon mesh. In addition, there is a leakage at balloon tip. (Reproduced from Zollikofer CL, Salomonowitz E, Brühlmann WF, Castañeda–Zuñiga WR, Amplatz K: Dehnungs-, Verformungs- und Berstungs-Charakteristika haufig verwendeter Balloon-Dilatationskatheter: in vitro Untersuchungen. (Teil 1). RöFo 1986;140:40–46.)

In contrast, materials of low compliance generally allow a 3- to 5-fold elevation of pressures without significant deformity of the balloon shape before bursting. Only PU/O balloons generally tolerated pressure increases above the manufacturer's recommendation less well. On the other hand, these balloons offer the advantage of allowing dilatation at double or triple the working pressures of the other types.[172]

These tests also demonstrated that bursting pressures are related to balloon diameter. Bursting pressures of small balloons were significantly higher than those of larger balloons, a finding to be expected according to Laplace's law. The range between the suggested working pressure and the actual bursting pressure in balloon dilatation catheters of modern double-lumen or coaxial design (*e.g.*, Schneider, Medi–Tech, Olbert/Surgimed) is 2–3 times greater for 4-mm PVC or PE balloons and 1.5 times greater for those of PU than for the corresponding balloons 8 mm in diameter.

This study further proved that pressure–diameter curves obtained *in vitro* in a water bath, which often are printed in the literature enclosed in packaged catheter sets, are of limited value for clinical practice, because the characteristics of stretch and the pattern of balloon deformation and rupture are changed considerably if the balloon is sheathed by a tube simulating an artery.

IN VIVO EXPERIMENTS[80,173]

Materials and Methods

In this study, the same balloon catheters of three different sizes (with the exception of the PVC/S balloons) were used to dilate the common carotid, iliac, and femoral arteries of anesthesized dogs. The balloon diameters were equal to (0 group) or 30% or 80%–100% larger than the original arterial lumen as measured on a baseline angiogram. Balloon inflation with diluted contrast medium was controlled by a special apparatus that allows pressures of up to 12.5 atm (Medi–Tech) and simultaneous measurement and recording of inflation pressures and injected volumes (Fig. 12–68). Changes in the configuration and the bursting patterns of the balloons were documented on spot or cine films or both. Balloon and vessel diameters were measured using micrometer calipers. In some cases, the pressure curves and roentgen films were compared with the histologic findings in the dilated arteries.

Results

Balloon diameters obtained intravascularly (calculated as a percentage of their fully inflated diameter at 4.5 atm and at pressures of 8–12.5 atm before balloon rupture)

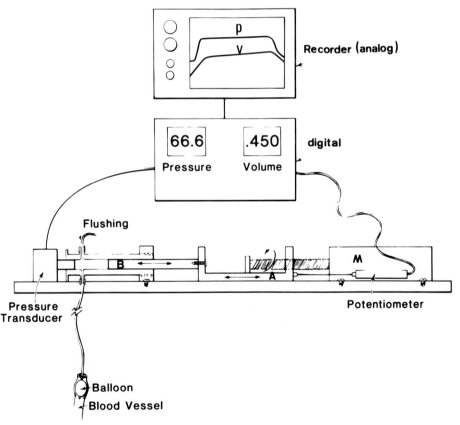

Fig. 12–68 Medi–Tech apparatus for recording balloon pressure to 12.5 atm and measuring volume and flow of saline into and out of balloon (potentiometer). Motor (M) turns lead screw (A) coupled to metal piston (B) of a noncompliant syringe. The syringe has two outlets, one for balloon catheter and one to allow flushing and refilling of syringe. For a given pressure setting, saline volume in balloon is adjusted automatically by the motor, which is controlled by an electronic feedback mechanism. Pressure (P) and volume (V) changes are recorded digitally on fiberoptic strip-chart recorder. (Reproduced from Zollikofer CL, Salomonowitz E, Castañeda–Zuñiga WR, Brühemann WF, Amplatz K: The relationship between arterial rupture and balloon bursting in experimental angioplasty. *AJR* 1985;144:777–779.)

Table 12–11
Balloon Bursting Pressures (atm) *in Vivo* Intra-arterially

Diameter	Balloon Type			
	PVC/C	PE/C	PE/MT	PU/O
4 mm	8	12	12	[a]
6 mm	10	10	[a]	[a]
8 mm	10[b]	10–12[b]	8–11[b]	12.5[b]

[a]Intra-arterially in balloon rupture up to 12.5 atm.
[b]Artery ruptured.

are listed in Table 12–11. In all three groups, the PVC/C balloons showed a growing deformation and elongation with increasing pressures (Fig. 12–69). In addition, there was a marked tendency for the injected fluid to penetrate into the virtual lumen between the inner and outer catheter, analogous to a dissection of the two coaxial catheters (Fig. 12–69C), which resulted in a growing outer diameter of the catheter shaft proximal to the balloon. This led to compression of the central catheter lumen, whereupon, in several cases, the guidewire could not be withdrawn. Furthermore, plastic deformation of the outer sleeve prevented deflation of the balloon, which then caused severe vasospasm that made retraction of the dilation catheter impossible. The large compliance of these balloons also reduced the dilating force of oversized balloons on one hand and caused undesired vascular dilatation by balloons in the 0 group on the other.

The PE/C balloons exhibited a relatively stable configuration (Fig. 12–70), and there was less tendency to dissection between the inner and outer catheter than in the PVC/C balloons. In the 80%–100% overdilations, these elevated pressures resulted several times in rupture of the artery, followed by bursting of the balloon. In the 0 group, high pressure caused an increase in diameter, with banana-shaped deformation (Fig. 12–71C).

The PE/MT balloons were stable in configuration (Figs. 12–71, and 12–72); only at very high pressures was a slight banana-shaped deformation noted, with no significant increase in diameter. In the 80%–100% group, high inflation pressures ruptured several arteries (Fig. 12–72). The PU/O balloons also showed little deformation (Fig. 12–73). The 8-mm balloon (normal working pressure 10–12 atm) caused rupture of a 4.6-mm artery at 12.5 atm (Fig. 12–73).

Table 12–12 clearly demonstrates the decreased unfolding of oversized balloons within the artery at normal working pressures of 4–5 atm. Even when applying elevated pressures (8–12 atm), some of the oversized balloons did not reach their full diameter unless the artery had ruptured (sequences in Figs. 12–72 and 12–73). The simultaneously recorded pressure and volume curves clearly displayed the reduced expansion of the dilatation balloons, resulting in a smaller than requested diameter as compared with the *in vitro* tests (Fig. 12–74). The pressure capacity of the balloons within the artery ranged from 8–12.5 atm (Table 12–11), *i.e.*, 1–6 atm higher than in the water bath (see Table 12–10A).

The most vigorous overdilation with elevated pressures caused the most pronounced histologic changes or rupture of the vessel wall. (Several arteries ruptured at pressures of 10–12.5 atm.) Histologic examination of nonrup-

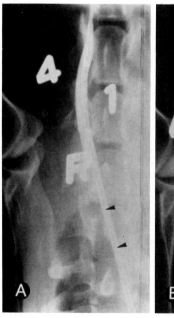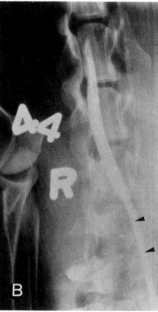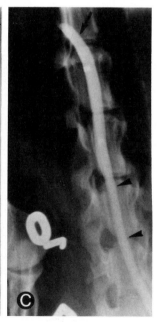

Fig. 12–69   An 8-mm PVC/C balloon in carotid artery 4.5 mm in diameter. A. First dilatation at 4.5 atm; balloon diameter = 5.4 mm. Note slight deformation of balloon tip. Central lumen of inner catheter is well seen (arrowheads). B. Fourth dilatation at 4.5 atm; balloon diameter = 5.4 mm. Discrete elongation of balloon at tip (arrowheads = central lumen of inner catheter). C. Dilatation at 10 atm; balloon diameter = 5.6 mm. Despite marked increase in inflation pressure, there is no significant increase in balloon diameter. However, there is marked elongation of balloon and sharp increase in catheter diameter proximal to balloon (arrowheads) secondary to penetration of injected fluid between inner and outer catheter. Central lumen of inner catheter is compressed and cannot be recognized. (Reproduced from Zollikofer CL, Salomonowitz E, Brühlmann WF, Castañeda–Zuñiga WR, Amplatz K: Dehnungs-, Verformungs- und Berstungs-Charakteristika haufig verwendeter Balloon-Dilatationskatheter: in vivo Untersuchungen an Hundegefassen (Teil 2). *RöFo* 1986;144:189–195.)

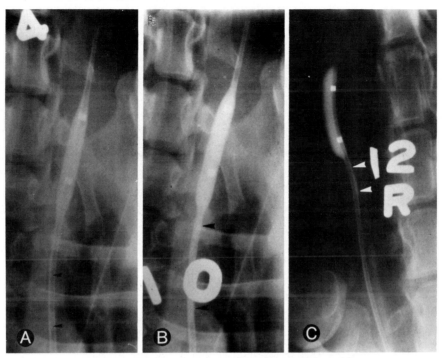

Fig. 12–70 A 6-mm PE/C balloon in carotid artery 4.7 mm in diameter, with dilatation at 4.5 atm (A) and 10 atm (B). Balloon diameter increases from 5.5 to 6 mm. There is little deformation of balloon; however, injected fluid penetrates between inner and outer catheter at 10 atm (arrowheads in B). Central lumen (arrowheads in A) is compressed in this segment. C. 4-mm PE/C balloon in carotid artery 4.5 mm in diameter. At 12 atm, balloon diameter is 5.7 mm. There is a slight banana-shaped deformation, with little dissection between inner and outer catheter (arrowheads). (Reproduced from Zollikofer CL, Salomonowitz E, Brühlmann WF, Castañeda–Zuñiga WR, Amplatz K: Dehnungs-, Verformungs- und Berstungs-Charakteristika haufig verwendeter Balloon-Dilatationskatheter: in vivo Untersuchungen an Hundegefassen (Teil 2). RöFo 1986;144:189–195.)

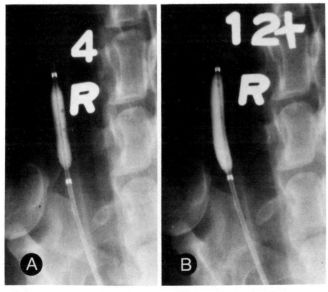

Fig. 12–71 A 6-mm PE/MT balloon in carotid artery 4.6 mm in diameter. A. At 4.5 atm, balloon diameter is 5.4 mm. B. At 12.5 atm, balloon diameter is 6 mm, and there is a slight banana-shaped deformation. Slight elongation of balloon is limited by tantalum markers. (Reproduced from Zollikofer CL, Salomonowitz E, Brühlmann WF, Castañeda–Zuñiga WR, Amplatz K: Dehnungs-, Verformungs- und Berstungs-Charakteristika haufig verwendeter Balloon-Dilatationskatheter: in vivo Untersuchungen an Hundegefassen (Teil 2). RöFo 1986;144:189–195.)

tured arteries showed marked destruction of the intima, IEL, and media. There were complete disruptions of the media, with focal stretching of the adventitia, frequently accompanied by thrombus formation (Fig. 12–75A). The PVC/C and PE/C balloons with 80%–100% overdilation caused arterial rupture only if no significant "dissection" of the coaxial catheter system occurred.

There were no arterial ruptures by any of the balloons of the 0 or 30% oversized groups. "Large" compliant balloons caused less penetrating damage to the arterial wall than did noncompliant balloons, exerting high radial forces on the wall (Fig. 12–75A,B). "Small" balloons, on the other hand, had the opposite effect, in that balloons of low compliance caused less damage than compliant ones due to their limited diameter increase (see Fig. 12–35).

Discussion

As shown in previous studies, increasing histologic damage is visible in the arterial wall with increasing balloon size and inflation pressure. Elevation of pressures to 12.5 atm and vigorous overdilation (80%–100%) led to severe traumatic changes, including complete rupture of the vessel wall. In some of these severely stretched arteries, rupture was limited to the media, but the beginning of aneurysmal dilatation of the adventitia was seen. These findings are similar to those seen in human cadaver arteries and in atherosclerotic rabbits.[48,49,82]

Fig. 12–72 An 8-mm PE/MT balloon in iliac artery 4.6 mm in diameter. A–D. Cine films of balloon at dilating pressures of 4.5, 6, 8, and 10 atm; balloon diameters are 6.6 mm at 4.5 atm and 6.9 at 10 atm. E, F. Cine films of balloon at 4.5 and 8 atm after rupture of artery. Balloon diameters now reach 7.5 mm (4.5 atm) and 8.5 mm (8 atm). (Reproduced from Zollikofer CL, Salomonowitz E, Brühlmann WF, Castañeda–Zuñiga WR, Amplatz K: Dehnungs-, Verformungs- und Berstungs-Charakteristika haufig verwendeter Balloon-Dilatationskatheter: in vivo Untersuchungen an Hundegefassen (Teil 2). RöFo 1986;144:189–195.)

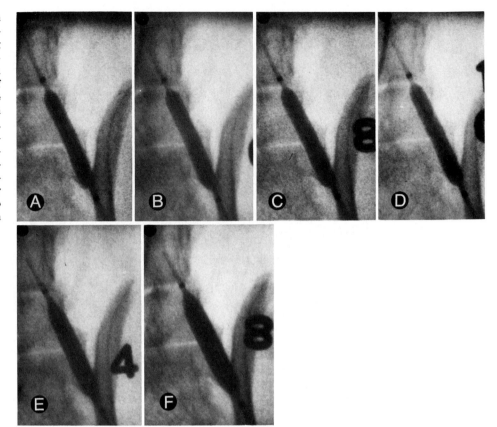

Deformation and elongation of the balloon catheters in the 0 and 30% groups caused extensive traumatic changes but no complete rupture. However, this does not necessarily mean that a 4-mm vessel can be dilated safely with a 6-mm balloon. Although this may be safe for healthy vessels, as discussed earlier, atherosclerotic arteries are more fragile, and their reaction to angioplasty is difficult to predict.[82]

As in the studies in Teflon tubes, balloon bursting pressures are significantly higher intra-arterially than in a water bath as long as the intact arterial wall limits overexpansion (Tables 12–11 and 12–12). Again, true double-lumen catheters (PE/MT) or coaxial catheters of the Olbert/Surgimed design exhibited the lowest compliance and hence the greatest radial dilating force. Coaxial catheters with PVC as the outer sleeve showed a tendency to dissection between the two parts by injected fluids, creating a risk of both failure of the balloon to deflate and trauma to the arterial wall beyond the balloon by the expanding catheter shaft. Clearly, for clinical PTA it is

Fig. 12–73 An 8-mm PU/O balloon in carotid artery 4.6 mm in diameter. A. Dilatation at 10 atm; no significant balloon deformation. Balloon diameter is 6.8 mm. B–D. Cine angiography at 12.5 atm reveals growing bulge in the balloon during rupture of artery (arrows) over 400 msec. After complete rupture of the vessel (D), balloon attains a diameter of 8.1 mm. Even after arterial rupture, there is only slight banana-shaped deformation of the balloon. (Reproduced from Zollikofer CL, Salomonowitz E, Brühlmann WF, Castañeda–Zuñiga WR, Amplatz K: Dehnungs-, Verformungs- und Berstungs-Charakteristika haufig verwendeter Balloon-Dilatationskatheter: in vivo Untersuchungen an Hundegefassen (Teil 2). RöFo 1986;144:189–195.)

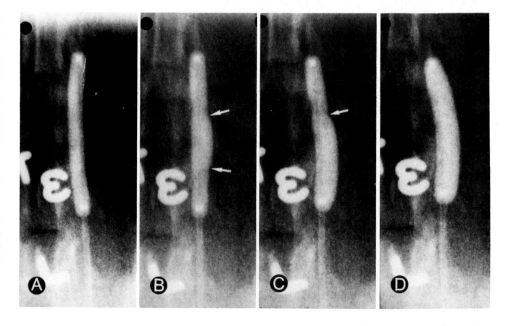

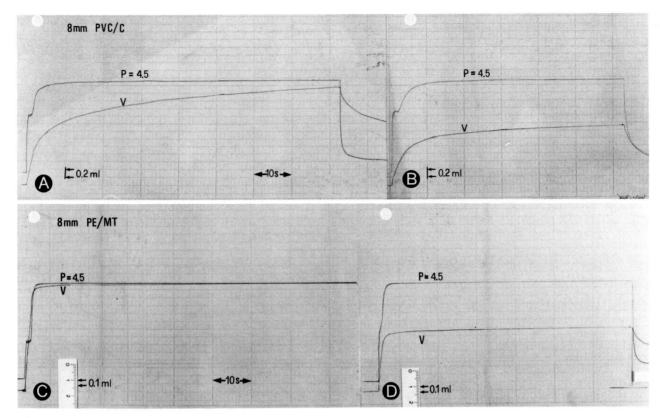

Fig. 12–74   Comparison of balloon compliance *in vitro* and *in vivo*. A, B. 8-mm PVC/C balloon; pressure–volume curves in 37° C water bath (A) and within carotid artery (B) at 4.5 atm of pressure. Note difference in volume curves, with shallower course in right curve (0.9 ml less after 60 sec). P = pressure curve; V = volume curve. C, D. 8-mm PE/MT balloon; pressure–volume curves in 37° C water bath (C) and in carotid artery (D) at 4.5 atm. With PE balloon, less volume (-0.8 ml) can be injected with balloon in artery at 4.5 atm. Because of the smaller compliance of this balloon compared with PVC balloon, however, there is no significant difference in slope of the two curves.

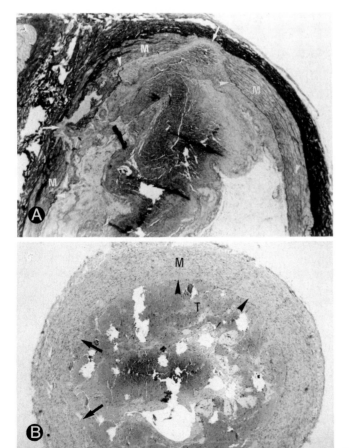

Fig. 12–75   A. Iliac artery 30 min after 80% overdilatation at 10 atm with PE/MT balloon. Verhoeff–van Geison; original magnification × 25. In two places, media (M) has completely ruptured (arrows); adventitia has bulged slightly in these areas. Marked stretching of elastic lamina and ruptures of IEL (arrowheads); adventitia prevents complete rupture of artery. A thrombus is seen within lumen. B. Carotid artery 30 min after 80% overdilatation at 10 atm with PVC/C balloon. Hematoxylin and eosin; original magnification × 25. Marked changes of inner media near lumen, with areas of reduced cellularity due to the destruction (arrowheads). In other areas, innermost layer of media is completely detached and destroyed (arrows). However, no completely penetrating medial ruptures are detectable, and outer layers of vessel are less damaged than in A. Lumen is filled with thrombus. M = media; T = thrombus. (Reproduced from Zollikofer CL, Salomonowitz E, Brühlmann WF, Castañeda–Zuñiga WR, Amplatz K: Dehnungs-, Verformungs- und Berstungs-Charakteristika haufig verwendeter Balloon-Dilatationskatheter: in vivo Untersuchungen an Hundegefassen (Teil 2). *RöFo* 1986;144:189–195.)

Table 12–12
Balloon Diameters Attained Intravascularly (in % of Their
Requested Diameter) at 4.5 and 12.5 atm Inflation Pressure

	4.5 atm (%)	8–12.5 atm (%)
Dilation 0% (4-mm balloons)		
PVC/C	131	150
PE/C	112	142
PE/MT	107	110
PU/O		108
Dilation 30% (6-mm balloons)		
PVC/C	78	85
PE/C	92	100
PE/MT	90	101
PU/O		102
Dilation 80–100% (8–9-mm balloons)		
PVC/C	65	68
PE/C	81	90
PE/MT	84	86
PU/O		85

vital to choose not only the correct balloon diameter and shape, but also the appropriate material and design of the balloon and catheter shaft.

This study also demonstrated that in the healthy artery, 30%–100% oversize balloons do not expand fully to their requested diameter at 4–5 atm. Only at elevated pressures (10–12 atm) do 30% oversize balloons attain their full diameter, and 80%–100% oversize balloons frequently expand that far only after rupture of the artery. The reduced, limited expansion of oversized balloons within a healthy artery could be demonstrated well on spot and cine films as well as on pressure–volume curves. The significance of recording such curves is discussed below. In clinical practice, inflation pressures of 4–5 atm are often sufficient because of the increased vulnerability of the atherosclerotic vessel,[82] yet hard (fibrotic and calcified) lesions require much higher pressures for significant dilation. Therefore, balloon catheters with the lowest compliance should be chosen to guarantee maximum concentration of the dilating force on the stenosis and an exactly defined balloon diameter without overexpansion. According to these studies, elevation of inflation pressures obviously carries the risk of vessel rupture, and this fact makes the choice of the balloon diameter even more crucial.

Significance of Balloon Pressure Recording and Relation between Arterial and Balloon Rupture in Experimental Angioplasty[171,174]

In clinical PTA, the number of repetitions of balloon inflations and their duration for a given lesion are still arbitrary.[84,161] Commonly, the balloon is inflated to an arbitrarily selected diameter for 15 sec to 1 min when treating renal or peripheral arteries; indeed, this "recipe" is often followed religiously despite the absence of scientific validation. Normal and atherosclerotic arteries differ considerably in their compliance and response to PTA, and this fact is of great importance in clinical practice, where careful fluoroscopic monitoring provides the only means of assessing the yielding of a lesion and where the

impending rupture of the artery cannot be detected directly. In order to define the moment of optimal dilation, and because the causal and temporal relations between vascular and balloon rupture were open to controversy,[84,164,175,176] an experiment was designed to characterize the compliance of a vascular lesion during dilatation.

MATERIALS AND METHODS

Three experiments were performed in atherosclerotic cadaver arteries and normal canine arteries. Volumes and pressures of the dilation balloons were monitored in digital and analog form using the special apparatus shown in Figure 12–68. In the experiments on cadaver vessels, atherosclerotic, stenotic lesions in iliac arteries were dilated. In addition to monitoring pressure–volume curves, volume was plotted against pressure during balloon inflation and deflation and the hysteresis cycle (difference in the pathways of the pressure–volume curves during inflation and deflation[53,177]) was recorded on an oscilloscope.

In the second series of experiments, normal carotid arteries of anesthetized dogs were dilated to 80% oversize, and the pressure and volume in the balloon were recorded. For assessment of possible stress effects on the arterial wall (changes in the viscoelastic property), dilations and recordings, including hysteresis cycles, were performed three or four times for each vessel at intervals of 5 min to permit stress relaxation in the artery.[177]

In the third series of experiments, carotid, iliac, and femoral arteries were dilated using PE balloon catheters with inflation pressures of 4.5 atm. Inflation pressures were then increased in 2-atm increments to a maximum pressure of 12.5 atm or until the balloon burst. Pressure and volume tracings of the balloons were recorded throughout. Deformation and bursting of the balloon during pressure increases were simultaneously recorded by cinefluorography at 30 frames/sec. The balloon sizes were selected according to the vessel diameters: equal to the arterial size (0 group), 50% larger, and 100% larger than the artery. Burst balloons remained in situ until after sacrifice of the dog and dissection of the artery. After the animals had been killed, the dilated vascular segments were examined macroscopically and by light microscopy.

RESULTS

Partial or total disruption of human atherosclerotic plaques could be clearly appreciated on the pressure recordings (Fig. 12–76). Partial intimal and medial tears, as well as rupture of intimal plaques, were seen better on the pressure curves than on the volume curves. Hysteresis cycles did not add any information but rather obscured significant pressure changes (Fig. 12–77).

Figure 12–78A shows a typical volume and pressure recording during dilatation of a normal canine carotid artery at a pressure of 4.5 atm. Repeated dilation of the same arterial segment did not alter the pattern of the curves (Fig. 12–78B), and the configuration of the hysteresis cycle did not change. The findings of increasing volume of the balloons with repeated dilations were incon-

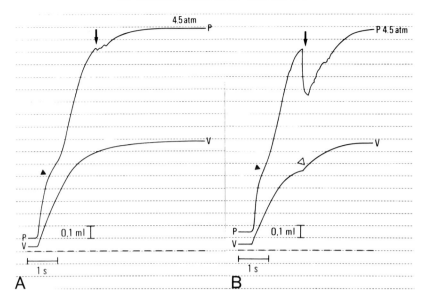

Fig. 12–76   Pressure (P) and volume (V) curves of angioplasty in cadaver iliac artery with 8-mm PE balloon at 4.5 atm. A. Discrete tear in atherosclerotic intimal plaque is shown as slight pressure drop (arrow) but cannot be appreciated on volume curve. Arrowhead indicates delay in pressure buildup due to unfolding of balloon. B. With rupture of plaque, there is a marked pressure drop (arrow). Note gradual change in slope of volume curve (open arrowhead) secondary to balloon expansion with injection of more fluid. (Reproduced from Zollikofer CL, Salomonowitz E, Brühlmann WF, Frick MP, Casta-ñeda–Zuñiga WR, Amplatz K: Significance of balloon pressure recording during angioplasty. *RöFo* 1985;142:526–530.)

sistent and could not be differentiated from the balloon's own compliance.

In a variation of the experimental set-up, using a non-compliant inflation system without the pressure–volume apparatus, a sudden yielding of human cadaver or normal canine arteries could be recorded faithfully simply by monitoring the pressure of the balloon with a high-pressure Statham transducer (Fig. 12–79).

In the dogs, with increasing pressures, arterial rupture with complete transmural tears could be demonstrated with 100% overdilation (Table 12–13). Rupture of the vessel preceded bursting of the balloon in every case, as shown on the pressure–volume tracings (Fig. 12–80). Arterial rupture allowed the balloon to expand suddenly, which caused a sharp pressure drop that activated the electronic servoloop feedback system to compensate for the pressure loss in the balloon; fluid was automatically injected until the original pressure was restored. Bursting

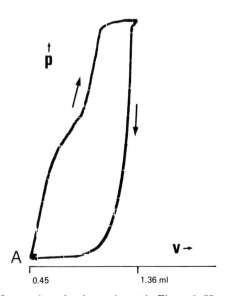

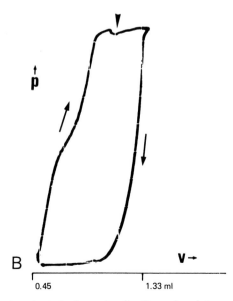

Fig. 12–77   Hysteresis cycle of experiment in Figure 5–77; pressure (P) *vs.* volume (V) during inflation (arrow up) and deflation (arrow down) of balloon. A. Discrete pressure drop in Figure 5–77A cannot be seen on hysteresis cycle during inflation. B. Marked pressure drop in Figure 5–77B is apparent only as a slight change in inflation curve of hysteresis cycle (arrowhead). (Reproduced from Zollikofer CL, Salomonowitz E, Brühlmann WF, Frick MP, Castañeda–Zuñiga WR, Amplatz K: Significance of balloon pressure recording during angioplasty. *RöFo* 1985;142:526–530.)

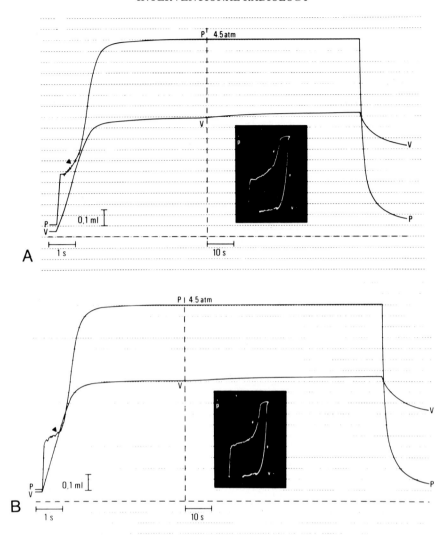

Fig. 12–78   Pressure (P)–volume (V) curves and corresponding hysteresis cycles at first (A) and third (B) dilatation of canine carotid artery at 4.5 atm; pressure–volume curves during inflation and deflation are practically identical. Arterial wall creep during progressive dilation from the first to the third inflation cannot be detected. Arrowhead indicates pressure curve "shoulder" due to unfolding of balloon. Broken vertical line indicates point at which paper speed changed from 25 to 2.5 mm/sec. (Reproduced from Zollikofer CL, Salomonowitz E, Brühlmann WF, Frick MP, Castañeda–Zuñiga WR, Amplatz K: Significance of balloon pressure recording during angioplasty. *RöFo* 1985;142:526–530.)

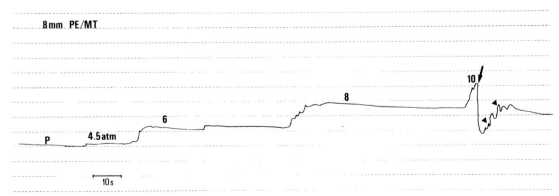

Fig. 12–79   Pressure curve during dilation of cadaver iliac artery with 8-mm PE balloon using a noncompliant injection system (noncompliant syringe, tubing, and high-pressure Statham transducer). Balloon inflation to 4.5 atm with sequential pressure increases up to 10 atm. The slight slope after each fractional pressure increase at 6 and 8 atm corresponds to compliance of balloon and artery. Sudden pressure drop at 10 atm (arrow) signals rupture of plaque. Under continuous balloon inflation, pressure buildup is irregular (arrowheads) due to stretching of arterial wall, which has been freed from the plaque.

Table 12–13
Number and Sequence of Arterial and Balloon Ruptures

	Rupture of:				
Overdilation	Artery Followed by Balloon	Balloon Followed by Artery	Balloon Only	Artery Only	No Rupture
0% (n = 8)	0	0	5	0	3
50% (n = 8)	0	0	3	0	5
100% (n = 10)	6	0	2	0	2

of the balloon was then signified by a complete pressure loss that could not be reversed by injection of saline (Fig. 12–80).

In both the 50% and the 0 groups, rupture of the balloon did not cause transmural rupture of the artery (Table 12–13). In the 50% group, intimal abrasion, medial stretching, and medial tears were seen, but the adventitia remained intact. In the 0 group, arterial wall damage was limited to intimal abrasion and stretch effects, which were restricted to the inner one-third to one-half of the media.

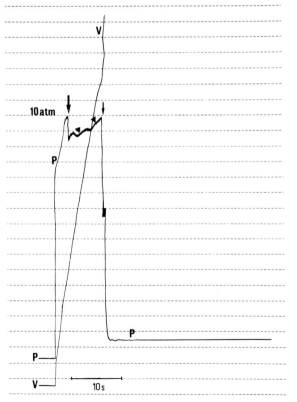

Fig. 12–80 Pressure (P)–volume (V) curve at inflation of 9-mm (100% oversized) PE balloon in canine iliac artery from 0 to 10 atm. Sudden pressure drop (large arrow) marks rupture of artery. With subsequent automatic injection of fluid, pressure in balloon is restored (arrowheads). Irregular wavy pressure buildup represents gradually increasing tear in the artery (see Fig. 12–81). With rupture of balloon (small arrow), there is complete pressure loss, and volume increases to infinity.

Balloon bursting pressures ranged from 8–12.5 atm (Table 12–14). Examination of burst balloons revealed longitudinal tears with smooth margins. The time between arterial rupture and balloon bursting ranged from 3–4 sec to 45 sec.

DISCUSSION

The author's experiments in atherosclerotic cadaver and normal canine arteries indicate that progress of angioplasty can be monitored by following pressure and volume changes in the balloon. With a sophisticated noncompliant system, a sudden yielding of the arterial wall can be recorded exactly. Sudden tears of the media and splitting or rupture of intimal plaques also are demonstrated on the pressure–volume curves of the dilating balloons.

In contrast, the assessment of viscoelastic properties of the dilated artery or the changing compliance of the slowly stretching arterial wall during repeated dilations could not be picked up by the pressure–volume curves; and the configurations of the curves could not be correlated with the nature of a lesion, as suggested by Abele.[161] Furthermore, the present authors were not able to demonstrate alterations in the hysteresis loops after repeated angioplasty, although they had expected that the changing compliance of the vessel wall would change the loop configuration.[177,178] Finally, the complicated recording of hysteresis loops proved unrewarding in detecting the sudden yielding of a lesion.

In this study, volume recordings were relatively insensitive when compared with the pressure curves. Hence, recording of the balloon pressure alone seems adequate. For clinical use, a noncompliant inflation system (syringe, connecting tubes, and balloon catheter) is necessary. Under laboratory conditions, such a system proved practical in picking up a sudden yielding of the vessel wall, such as a disruption of an atherosclerotic plaque. This system is more sensitive than looking for the famous "pop" of the lesion, as demonstrated by a sudden change of the balloon's shape on fluoroscopy. Therefore, a pressure-recording system should be valuable in determining when a procedure must be terminated to avoid overdistention of the vessel wall. This seems particularly important during use of high-pressure balloons.

With the advent of recording of balloon pressure and volume during PTA, the authors were able to demonstrate that arterial rupture occurs secondary to overdistention of the vessel and not *vice versa*.[163,172] With vascular rupture, the external restraint on the balloon is lost, allowing a sudden increase in the balloon diameter. Because of the lack of a retaining arterial sheath, the ten-

Table 12–14
Balloon Bursting Pressures

	Balloon Pressure		
Overdilation	≤8 atm	≤10 atm	≤12.5 atm
0% (n = 5)	0	1	4
50% (n = 3)	0	2	1
100% (n = 8)	1	5	2

sile strength of the balloon material is exceeded within seconds, and the balloon bursts even without a further pressure increase.

The authors did not observe a single case of arterial rupture caused by a bursting balloon. Further, the histologic changes could not be definitely attributed to a jet phenomenon caused by a rupturing balloon[164]; rather, diffuse changes of general overdistention were found. Localized ruptures in the medial layer were found irrespective of whether the balloon had ruptured *in situ*. If vascular ruptures were indeed caused by the jet from a rupturing balloon, the pressure curves should have dropped to zero and remained at this level. However, with activation of the pump and saline injection by the electronic feedback mechanism, balloon pressure was reconstituted, indicating an intact balloon.

During fluoroscopic observation, rupture of the nonopaque arterial wall cannot be seen, although cine recording may reveal an eccentric deformation of the balloon preceding extravasation of contrast medium at rupture (Fig. 12–81). However, the entire series of events, with the sequence and causal relations of arterial rupture and balloon bursting, was best displayed on the pressure–volume curves, with which the sequence was convincingly clarified.

An exception to these findings may occur with equatorial balloon ruptures, as described by Yune and Klatte[179] and Waltman et al.[84] Such ruptures produce irregular, sometimes sharp, edges that could harm the stretched arterial wall, especially when the balloon catheter is withdrawn. With today's improved balloon materials, however, such unusual and irregular ruptures should not occur.

SUMMARY AND CONCLUSIONS

The results of these tests of the various balloon dilation catheters support the use of the true double-lumen catheter or the Olbert system. The latter offers the potential advantage of high working pressures (10–12 atm). However, with these balloons, the operator should be reluctant to exceed the manufacturer's suggested pressures, especially with the larger (≥6-mm) balloons, because the outer nylon mesh may rupture, leading to significant expansion of the inner PU component. By contrast, in all the other balloons tested, the suggested working pressures are much lower, 4–6 atm. The PVC/S and PE/MT balloons, owing to their low compliance (an increase in diameter of no more than 1 mm) can exceed the manufacturer's suggested pressures by several atmospheres without the risk of untoward effects. Furthermore, these tests demonstrated that PE has no definite advantages over modern PVC materials with respect to compliance and tensile strength, as was formerly the case. Conventional PVC/C and PE/C balloons of the coaxial type should not be inflated above their suggested pressures, however, because of their considerable compliance. It should be stressed that there is a new balloon catheter, manufactured by Cook, Inc., that has a true double-lumen system that considerably improves the balloon's compliance.

In general, the results of angioplasty depend much less on the number of balloon inflations than on the inflation pressure and duration. Therefore, as a general rule (always bearing in mind that balloon characteristics and configuration must also be appropriate for the anatomic site and the nature of the vascular lesion), balloons with the lowest possible compliance should be used. In this way, maximum dilation force with exact definition of the balloon diameter should be achieved even with high inflation pressures.

As demonstrated, oversized balloons attained their full diameter in healthy arteries only at considerably increased inflation pressures. Accordingly, histologic changes increase and eventually culminate in rupture of the artery in parallel with increasing balloon diameter and inflation pressure. Applying high pressures in clinical PTA thus increases the risk of vascular rupture; sufficient attention must therefore be given to the selection of balloon diameter. Normally, balloon size is chosen according

Fig. 12–81 Cine film recording of rupture of canine iliac artery followed by balloon rupture at 10 atm (30 frames/sec; same experiment as in Fig. 12–80). A. Asymmetric bulging of balloon (arrowheads) caused by rupture of artery at dilation site. Distal half of balloon is still contained by intact part of arterial wall. B. 500 msec later, bulge is more prominent and has increased in length because of progressing arterial rupture. Note transition between balloon segments contained by the artery and unsupported expanded portion (arrow). C. Another 5 sec later, balloon has ruptured, with extravasation of contrast medium. (Reproduced from Zollikofer CL, Salomonowitz E, Castañeda-Zuñiga WR, Brühlmann WF, Amplatz K: The relationship between arterial rupture and balloon bursting in experimental angioplasty. *AJR* 1985;144:777–779.)

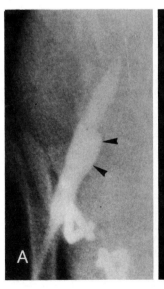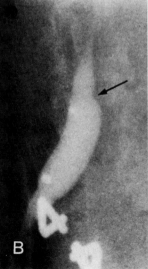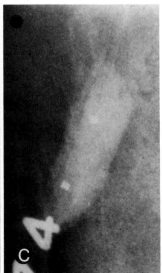

to the estimated diameter of the nondiseased vessel. As noted earlier, however, some experienced investigators always use slightly oversized (1- or 2-mm) balloons, whereas others oppose this tactic. In the present authors' opinion, use of a slightly oversized balloon seems justified as long as inflation pressures do not exceed 4–6 atm; but when high pressures (10–12 atm or more) are used, it is prudent not to use oversized balloons.

Despite the authors' extensive attempts to characterize the nature of stenotic lesions, they cannot give definite recommendations on optimal dilation because of the wide variation in compliance of atherosclerotic lesions. Generally, it seems that nonatherosclerotic disease, especially of the inflammatory and fibrous type, requires longer inflation times and higher pressures. Continuous monitoring of balloon pressure may demonstrate a gradual or abrupt yielding of a lesion to a much better degree than does fluoroscopic observation of the balloon shape, so pressure monitoring can help improve PTA results, particularly when using high inflation pressures. Furthermore, if one uses only state-of-the-art balloon dilatation catheters, arterial rupture secondary to a bursting balloon should not occur. Finally, the initial result of transluminal angioplasty still must be evaluated by follow-up angiograms, recording of pressure gradients, or both.

References

1. Dotter CT, Judkins MP: Transluminal treatment of arteriosclerotic obstruction. *Circulation* 1964;30:654

2. Dotter CT, Judkins MP: Percutaneous transluminal treatment of arteriosclerotic obstruction. *Radiology* 1965;84:631

3. Dotter CT, Judkins MP, Frische LH, Mueller R: The "nonsurgical" treatment of ilio-femoral arteriosclerotic obstruction. *Radiology* 1966;86:871

4. Dotter CT, Judkins MP, Frische LH, Rosch J: Nonoperative treatment of arterial occlusive disease: a radiologically facilitated technique. *Radiol Clin North Am* 1967;5:531

5. Dotter CT, Judkins MP, Rosch J: Nichtoperative transluminale Behandlung der arteriosklerotischen Verschlussaffektionen. *RöFo* 1968;109:125

6. Dotter CT, Rosch J, Judkins MP: Transluminal dilatation of atherosclerotic stenosis. *Surg Gynecol Obstet* 1968;127:794

7. Staple TW: Modified catheter for percutaneous transluminal treatment of atherosclerotic obstructions. *Radiology* 1968;91:1041

8. Van Andel GJ: *Percutaneous Transluminal Angioplasty: The Dotter Procedure.* Amsterdam, Excerpta Medica, 1976

9. Brahme F, Swedenborg J, Tibel B: Evaluation of transluminal recanalization of the femoral artery. *Acta Chir Scand* 1969;135:697

10. Berglund G, Bodvall B, Eldh J, Yden S: Nytt Behandlingsalternative vid Artiell insufficiens i benen. *Lakartidningen* 1969;66:129

11. Dow J, Hardwick C: Transluminal arterial recanalization. *Lancet* 1966;1:73

12. Grüntzig A, Bollinger A, Brunner U, Schlumpf M, Wellauer J: Perkutane rekanalisation chronischer arterieller Verschlusse nach Dotter: eine nicht-operative Kathetertechnik. *Schweiz Med Wochenschr* 1973;103:825

13. Zeitler E, Schoop W, Zahnow W: The treatment of occlusive arterial disease by transluminal catheter angioplasty. *Radiology* 1971;99:19

14. Brunner U, Grüntzig A: Das Dilatationsverfahren nach Dotter in gefässchirurgischer Sicht. *Vasa* 1975;4:334

15. Brunner U, Schneider E, Gygax P: Kombination der PTA mit chirurgischen Eingriffen im femoropoplitealen Bereich. *Vasa* 1982;11:278

16. Abbot WM: Percutaneous transluminal angioplasty: surgeon's view. *AJR* 1980;135:917

17. Alpert J: Grüntzig's plaque pressing: "verbum sapienti." *J Med Soc N Jersey* 1981;78:87

18. Vetto RM: Further comment (editorial). *JAMA* 1974;230:92

19. Vollmar J, Trede M, Laubach K, Forrest M: Principles of reconstructive procedures for chronic femoro-popliteal occlusion: report on 546 operations. *Ann Surg* 1968;168:215

20. Dotter CT, Rosch J, Anderson JM, Antonovic R, Robinson M: Transluminal iliac artery dilatation: nonsurgical catheter treatment of atheromatous narrowing. *JAMA* 1974;230:117

21. Grüntzig A, Hopff H: Perkutane rekanalisation chronischer arterieller Verschlusse mit einem neuen Dilatationskatheter. *Dtsch Med Wochenschr* 1974;99:2502

22. Porstmann W: Ein neuer Korsett-Ballonkatheter zur transluminalen Rekanalization nach Dotter unter besonderer Berücksichtigung von Obliterationen an den Beckenarterien. *Radiol Diagn* (Berl) 1973;2:239

23. Grüntzig A: Die perkutane Rekanalisation chronischer arterieller Verschlusse (Dotter–Prinzip) mit einem neuen doppellumigen Dilatationskatheter. *RöFo* 1976;124:80

24. Grüntzig A: *Die Perkutane Transluminale Rekanalisation Chronischer Arterienverschlusse mit einer Neuen Dilatationstechnik.* Baden–Baden, Witzstrock, 1977

25. Grüntzig A, Kuhlmann U, Vetter W, Lutolf U, Meier B, Siegenthaler W: Treatment of renovascular hypertension with percutaneous transluminal dilatation of a renal-artery stenosis. *Lancet* 1978;1:801

26. Dotter CT: Transluminal angioplasty: results and future outlook, in Dotter CT, Grüntzig A, Schoop W, Zeitler E (eds): *Percutaneous Transluminal Angioplasty.* Berlin, Springer–Verlag, 1983, pp 337

27. Doubilet P, Abrams HL: The cost of underutilization: percutaneous transluminal angioplasty for peripheral vascular disease. *N Engl J Med* 1984;310:95

28. Hall D, Grüntzig A: Percutaneous transluminal coronary angioplasty: current procedure and future direction. *AJR* 1984;142:13

29. Jang GC, Block PC, Cowley MJ, et al: Comparative cost analysis of coronary angioplasty and coronary bypass surgery: results from a national cooperative study. *Circulation* 1982;66(Suppl 2):123

30. Dotter CT: Clinical indications for transluminal dilatation in the management of atheromatous leg ischemia. *Cardiovasc Clin* 1971;3:104

31. Dotter CT: Transluminal angioplasty: pathologic basis, in Zeitler E, Grüntzig A, Schoop W (eds): *Percutaneous Vascular Recanalization.* Berlin, Springer–Verlag, 1978, pp 3

32. Jester HG, Sinapius D, Alexander K, Leitz KH: Morphologische Veranderungen nach transluminaler Rekanalisation chronischer arterieller Verschlusse, in Zeitler E (ed): *Hypertonie-Risikofaktor in der Angiologie.* Baden–Baden, Witzstrock, 1976

33. Jester HG, Sinapius D: Morphologic alterations after percutaneous transluminal recanalization of chronic femoral atherosclerosis, in Zeitler E, Grüntzig A, Schoop W (eds): *Percutaneous Vascular Recanalization.* Berlin, Springer–Verlag, 1978, p 51

34. Hempel KJ: Morphologische Befunde zur Kompressibilität atheromatoser und thrombotischer Intimaveranderungen, in *2. Angiologisches Symposiom.* Frankfurt, Aggertalklinik Engelskirchen, 1969

35. Hohn P, Wagner R, Zeitler E: Histologische Befunde nach der Katheterbehandlung arterieller Obliterationen nach Dotter und ihre Bedeutung. *Herz/Kreislaufforsch* 1975;7:13

36. Leu HJ, Grüntzig A: Histopathologic aspects of transluminal recanalization, in Zeitler E, Grüntzig A, Schoop W (eds): *Per-*

cutaneous Vascular Recanalization. Berlin, Springer–Verlag, 1978, pp 39

37. Baughman KL, Pasternak RC, Fallon JT, Block PC: Coronary transluminal angioplasty in autopsied human hearts (abstract). *Circulation* 1978;57/58(Suppl 2):II-80

38. Freudenberg H, Wefing H, Lichtlen PR: Risks of transluminal coronary angioplasty: a postmortal study (abstract). *Circulation* 1978;57/58(Suppl 2):II-80

39. Lee G, Ikeda R, Mason DT, et al. Effective dilatation of human coronary artery obstruction due to atherosclerosis utilizing a balloon-tip catheter. *Circulation* 1978;57/58 (Suppl 2):II-80

40. Simpson JB, Robert EW, Billingham ME, Myler RK, Harrison DC: Coronary transluminal angioplasty in human cadaver hearts (abstract). *Circulation* 1978;57/58(Suppl 2):II-80

41. Ramsey MR: Nutrition of the blood vessel wall: review of the literature. *Yale J Biol Med* 1936/37;9:14

42. Clarke JA: The vasa vasorum of normal human lower limb arteries. *Acta Anat* 1965;61:481

43. Wilens SL, Malcolm JA, Vazquez JM: Experimental infarction (medial necrosis) of the dog's aorta. *Am J Pathol* 1965;47:695

44. Woerner CA: Vasa vasorum of arteries: their demonstration and distribution, in Lansing AJ (ed): *The Arterial Wall.* Baltimore, Williams & Wilkins, 1959

45. Wolinsky H, Glagov S: Nature of species differences in the medial distribution of aortic vasa vasorum in mammals. *Circ Res* 1967;20:409

46. Heistad DD, Marcus ML, Law EG, Armstrong ML, Ehrhardt JC, Abboud FM: Regulation of blood flow to the aortic media in dogs. *J Clin Invest* 1978;62:133

47. Castañeda–Zuñiga WR, Formanek A, Tadavarthy M, et al: The mechanism of balloon angioplasty. *Radiology* 1980;135:565

48. Castañeda–Zuñiga WR, Amplatz K, Laerum F, et al: Mechanics of angioplasty: an experimental approach. *RadioGraphics* 1981;1:1

49. Laerum F, Vlodaver Z, Castañeda–Zuñiga WR, Edwards JE, Amplatz K: The mechanism of angioplasty: dilatation of iliac cadaver arteries with intravascular pressure control. *RöFo* 1982;136:573

50. Zollikofer CL: Experimentelle Grundlagen der perkutanen transluminalen Angioplastie. *Habilitationsschrift,* 1985

51. Bunce DF: Structural differences between distended and collapsed arteries, in *Atlas of Arterial Histology.* St. Louis, Green, 1974

52. Cook TA, Yates PO: A critical survey of techniques for arterial mensuration. *J Pathol* 1972;108:119

53. Dobrin PB: Mechanical properties of arteries. *Physiol Rev* 1978;58:397

54. Pesonen E, Martimo P, Rapola J: Histometry of the arterial wall. *Lab Invest* 1974;31:550

55. LeVeen RF, Wolf GL, Turco MA: Morphometric changes in normal arteries and those undergoing transluminal angioplasty. *Invest Radiol* 1983;18:63

56. Chin AK, Kinney TB, Rurik GW, Shoor PM, Fogarty TJ: A physical measurement of the mechanisms of transluminal angioplasty. *Surgery* 1984;95:196

57. Castañeda–Zuñiga WR, Tadavarthy SM, Laerum F, Amplatz K: "Pseudo" intramural injection following percutaneous transluminal angioplasty. *CardioVasc Intervent Radiol* 1984;7:104

58. Zollikofer CL, Castañeda–Zuñiga WR, Amplatz K: Results of animal experiments with balloon dilatation, in Dotter CT, Grüntzig A, Schoop W, Zeitler E (eds): *Percutaneous Transluminal Angioplasty.* Berlin, Springer–Verlag, 1983, p 60

59. Zollikofer CL, Salomonowitz E, Sibley R, et al: Transluminal angioplasty evaluated by electron microscopy. *Radiology* 1984;153:369

60. Baumgarter HR: Eine neue Methode zur Erzeugung von Thromben durch gezielte Überdehnung der Gefasswand. *Arch Ges Exp Med* 1963;137:227

61. Chidi CC, DePalma RG: Collagen formation by transformed smooth muscle cells after arterial injury. *Surg Gynecol Obstet* 1981;152:8

62. Ross R, Glomset JA: Atherosclerosis and the arterial smooth muscle cell. *Science* 1973;180:1332

63. Spaet TH, Stemerman MB, Veith FJ, Lejnieks I: Intimal injury and regrowth in the aorta: medial smooth muscle cells as a source of neointima. *Circ Res* 1975;36:58

64. Stemerman MB, Ross R: Experimental arteriosclerosis: fibrous plaque formation in primates: an electron microscopic study. *J Exp Med* 1972;136:769

65. Pasternak RC, Baughman KL, Fallon JT, Block PC: Scanning electron microscopy after coronary transluminal angioplasty of normal canine coronary arteries. *Am J Cardiol* 1980;45:592

66. O'Gara PT, Guerrero JL, Feldman B, Fallon JT, Block PC: Effect of dextran and aspirin on platelet adherence after transluminal angioplasty of normal canine coronary arteries. *Am J Cardiol* 1984;53:1695

67. Fishman JA, Ryan GB, Karnovsky MJ: Endothelial regeneration in the rat carotid artery and the significance of endothelial denudation in the pathogenesis of neointimal thickening. *Lab Invest* 1975;32:339

68. Ross R, Glomset JA: The pathogenesis of atherosclerosis. *N Engl J Med* 1976;295:369

69. Stermerman MB, Spaet TH, Pitlick F, Clintron J, Lejnieks I, Tiell ML: Intimal healing: the pattern of reendothelialization and intimal thickening. *Am J Pathol* 1977;87:125

70. Nam SC, Lee WM, Jarmolych J, Lee KT, Thomas WA: Rapid production of advanced atherosclerosis in swine by a combination of endothelial injury and cholesterol feeding. *Exp Mol Pathol* 1973;18:369

71. Hagen P, Wang Z, Mikat EM, Hackel DB: Antiplatelet therapy reduces aortic intimal hyperplasia distal to small diameter vascular prostheses (PTFE) in non-human primates. *Ann Surg* 1981;195:328

72. Faxon DP, Sanborn TA, Haudenschild CC, Ryan TJ: Effect of antiplatelet therapy on restenosis after experimental angioplasty. *Am J Cardiol* 1984;53:72C

73. Faxon DP, Sanborn TA, Weber JV, et al: Restenosis following transluminal angioplasty in experimental atherosclerosis. *Arteriosclerosis* 1984;4:189

74. Waller BF: Early and later morphologic changes in human coronary arteries after percutaneous transluminal coronary angioplasty. *Clin Cardiol* 1983;6:363

75. Waller BF, Gorfinkel HJ, Rogers FJ, Kent KM, Roberts WC: Early and late morphologic changes in major epicardial coronary arteries after percutaneous transluminal coronary angioplasty. *Am J Cardiol* 1984;53:42C

76. DePalma RG: Atherosclerosis in vascular grafts. *Atheroscleros Rev* 1979;5:147

77. Lee WM, Lee KT: Advanced coronary atherosclerosis in swine produced by combination of balloon catheter injury and cholesterol feeding. *Exp Mol Pathol* 1975;23:492

78. Ross R, Harker L: Hyperlipidemia and atherosclerosis: chronic hyperlipidemia initiates and maintains lesions by endothelial cell desquamation and lipid accumulation. *Science* 1976;193:1094

79. Scott RF, Imai H, Makita T, Thomas WA, Reiner JM: Lining cell and intimal smooth muscle cell response and Evans blue staining in abdominal aorta of young swine after denudation by balloon catheter. *Exp Mol Pathol* 1980;33:185

80. Zollikofer CL, Salomonowitz E, Brühlmann WF, Castañeda–Zuñiga WR, Amplatz K: Dehnungs-, Verformungs, und Berstungs-Charakteristika haufig verwendeter Balloon-Dilatationskatheter: in vivo Untersuchungen an Hundegefassen (Teil 2). *RöFo* 1986;144:189

81. Sanborn TA, Faxon DP, Haudenschild C, Gottsman SB, Ryan TJ: The mechanism of intraluminal angioplasty: evidence for formation of aneurysms in experimental atherosclerosis. *Circulation* 1983;68:1136

82. Zollikofer CL, Chain J, Salomonowitz E, et al: Percutaneous transluminal angioplasty of the aorta. *Radiology* 1984;151:355

83. Levin DC, Harrington DP, Bettmann MA, et al: Equipment choices, technical aspects and pitfalls of percutaneous transluminal angioplasty. *CardioVasc Intervent Radiol* 1984;7:1

84. Waltman AC, Greenfield AJ, Athanasoulis CA: Transluminal angioplasty: general rules and basic considerations, in Athanasoulis CA, Pfister RC, Greene RE, Roberson GH (eds): *Interventional Radiology.* Philadelphia, WB Saunders, 1982, p 253

85. Block PC, Fallon JT, Elmer D: Experimental angioplasty: lessons from the laboratory. *AJR* 1980;135:907

86. Block PC, Baughman KL, Pasternak RC, Fallon JT: Transluminal angioplasty: correlation of morphologic and angiographic findings in an experimental model. *Circulation* 1980;61:778

87. Faxon DP, Weber VJ, Haudenschild C, Gottsman SB, McGovern WZ, Ryan TJ: Acute effects of transluminal angioplasty in three experimental models of atherosclerosis. *Arteriosclerosis* 1982;2:125

88. Block PC, Myler RK, Stertzer S, Fallon JT: Morphology after transluminal angioplasty in human beings. *N Engl J Med* 1981;305:382

89. Clouse ME, Tomashefski JF Jr, Reinhold RE, Costello P: Mechanical effect of balloon angioplasty: case report with histology. *AJR* 1981;137:869

90. Hoffman MA, Fallon JT, Greenfield AJ, Waltman AC, Athanasoulis CA, Block PC: Arterial pathology after percutaneous transluminal angioplasty. *AJR* 1981;137:147

91. Saffitz JE, Totty WG, McClennan BL, Gilula LA: Percutaneous transluminal angioplasty: radiological–pathologic correlation. *Radiology* 1981;141:651

92. Grüntzig A, Kumpe DA: Technique of percutaneous transluminal angioplasty with the Grüntzig balloon catheter. *AJR* 1979;132:547

93. Zeitler E, Ernsting M, Richter EI, Seyferth W: Komplikationen nach PTA femoraler und iliakaler Obstruktionen. *Vasa* 1982;11:270

94. Katzen BT, Chang J, Knox WG: Percutaneous transluminal angioplasty with the Grüntzig balloon catheter: a review of 70 cases. *Arch Surg* 1979;114:1389

95. LeVeen RF, Wolf GL, Villanueva TG: New rabbit atherosclerosis model for the investigation of transluminal angioplasty. *Invest Radiol* 1982;17:470

96. Cragg A, Einzig S, Rysavy J, Borgwardt B, Castañeda W, Amplatz K: Arterial wall hyperemia following transluminal angioplasty (abstract). *Am J Cardiol* 1982;49

97. Cragg AH, Einzig S, Rysavy JA, Castañeda–Zuñiga WR, Borgwardt B, Amplatz K: The vasa vasorum and angioplasty. *Radiology* 1983;148:75

98. Cragg A, Einzig S, Rysavy J, Castañeda–Zuñiga W, Borgwardt B, Amplatz K: Effect of Aspirin on angioplasty-induced vessel wall hyperemia. *AJR* 1983;140:1233

99. Geiringer E: Intimal vascularization and atherosclerosis. *J Pathol Bacteriol* 1951;63:201

100. Schutte HE: Plaque localization and distribution of vasa vasorum. *Angiologica* 1966;3:21

101. Heistad DD, Armstrong ML, Marcus ML: Hyperemia of the aortic wall in atherosclerotic monkeys. *Circ Res* 1981;48:669

102. Schutte HE: Changes in the vasa vasorum of the atherosclerotic aortic wall. *Angiologica* 1968;5:210

103. Train JS, Mitty HA, Efremidis SC, Rabinowitz JG: Visualization of a fine periluminal vascular network following transluminal angioplasty: possible demonstration of the vasa vasorum. *Radiology* 1982;143:399

104. Wolf GL, LeVeen RF, Ring EJ: Potential mechanism of angioplasty. *CardioVasc Intervent Radiol* 1984;7:11

105. Leu HJ: Morphologie der Arterienwand nach perkutaner transluminaler Dilatation. *Vasa* 1982;11:265

106. Leu HJ: The morphological concept of percutaneous transluminal angioplasty, in Dotter CT, Grüntzig A, Schoop W, Zeitler E (eds): *Percutaneous Transluminal Angioplasty.* Berlin, Springer–Verlag, 1983, p 46

107. Seyfert W, Ernsting M, Grosse–Vorholt R, Zeitler E: Complications during and after percutaneous transluminal angioplasty, in Dotter CT, Grüntzig A, Schoop W, Zeitler E (eds): *Percutaneous Transluminal Angioplasty.* Berlin, Springer–Verlag, 1983, p 161

108. Block PC, Elmer D, Fallon JT: Release of atherosclerotic debris after transluminal angioplasty. *Circulation* 1982;65:950

109. Sinapius D: Pathological basis for percutaneous catheter balloon revascularization, in Dotter CT, Grüntzig A, Schoop W, Zeitler E (eds): *Percutaneous Transluminal Angioplasty.* Berlin, Springer–Verlag, 1983, p 56

110. Hess H, Muller–Fassbender H, Ingrisch H, Mietaschk A: Verhutung von Wiederverschlussen nach Rekanalisation obliterierter Arterien mit der Kathetermethode. *Dtsch Med Wochenschr* 1978;103:1994

111. Hess H, Mietaschk A: Rezidivprophylaxe nach PTA: Antikoagulatien oder Aggregationshemmer. *Vasa* 1982;11:344

112. Horvath L, Illes I, Fendler K: Prevention of complications in percutaneous transluminal angioplasty, in Dotter CT, Grüntzig A, Schoop W, Zeitler E (eds): *Percutaneous Transluminal Angioplasty.* Berlin, Springer–Verlag, 1983, p 170

113. Schneider E, Grüntzig A, Bollinger A: Langzeitergebnisse nach perkutaner transluminaler Angioplastie (PTA) bei 882 konsekutiven Patienten mit iliakalen und femoropopliteualen Obstrucktionen. *Vasa* 1982;11:322

114. Schneider E, Grüntzig A, Bollinger A: Long-term patency rates after percutaneous transluminal angioplasty for iliac and femoropopliteal obstructions,in Dotter CT, Grüntzig A, Schoop W, Zeitler E (eds): *Percutaneous Transluminal Angioplasty.* Berlin, Springer–Verlag, 1983, p 175

115. Zeitler E, Reichold J, Schoop W, Loew D: Einfluss von Acetylesalicylsaure auf das Fruhergebnis nach perkutaner Rekanalization arterieller Obliterationen nach Dotter. *Dtsch Med Wochenschr* 1973;98:1285

116. Zeitler E: Percutaneous dilatation and recanalization of iliac and femoral arteries, in Athanasoulis CA, Abrams HL, Zeitler E (eds): *Therapeutic Angiography.* New York, Springer–Verlag, 1981, p 11

117. Roth FJ, Cappius G, Fingerhut E: Radiological pattern at and after angioplasty, in Dotter CT, Grüntzig A, Schoop W, Zeitler E (eds): *Percutaneous Transluminal Angioplasty.* Berlin, Springer–Verlag, 1983, p 73

118. Block PC: Mechanism of transluminal angioplasty. *Am J Cardiol* 1984;53:69C

119. Castañeda–Zuñiga WR, Laerum F, Rysavy J, Rusnak B, Amplatz K: Paralysis of arteries by intraluminal balloon dilatation. *Radiology* 1982;144:75

120. Wolf GL, Lentini EA, LeVeen RF: Reduced vasoconstrictor response after angioplasty in normal rabbit aortas. *AJR* 1984;141:1023

121. Price JM, Davis DL, Knauss EB: Length-dependent sensitivity in vascular smooth muscle. *Am J Physiol* 1981;241:H557

122. Tallaride RJ, Sevy RW, Harakal C, Bendrick J, Faust R: The effect of preload on the dissociation constant of norepinephrine in isolated strips of rabbit thoracic aorta. *Arch Int Pharmacodyn Ther* 1974;210:67

123. Wolf GL, Lentini EA: The influence of short duration stretch on vasoconstrictor response in rabbit aortas. *Invest Radiol* 1984;19:269

124. Cowley M, Bentivoglio L, Block P, et al: Emergency coronary artery bypass surgery for complications of coronary angioplasty: NHLBI PTCA Registry experience (abstract). *Circulation* 1981;64(Suppl 4):IV-193

125. Holmes DR, Vliestra RE, Mock MB, et al: Angiographic changes produced by percutaneous transluminal coronary angioplasty. *Am J Cardiol* 1983;51:676

126. Sos TA, Sniderman KW: Percutaneous transluminal angioplasty. *Semin Roentgenol* 1981;16:26

127. Sos TA, Pickering TG, Sniderman KW, et al: Percutaneous transluminal renal angioplasty in renovascular hypertension due to atheroma or fibromuscular dysplasia. *Semin Intervent Radiol* 1984;1:237

128. Zollikofer C, Cragg A, Einzig S, et al: Prostaglandins and angioplasty. *Radiology* 1983;149:681

129. Richter EI, Zeitler E: Percutaneous transluminal angioplasty: adjunct drug therapy, in Dotter CT, Grüntzig A, Schoop W, Zeitler E (eds): *Percutaneous Transluminal Angioplasty.* Berlin, Springer–Verlag, 1983, p 84

130. Moncada S, Higgs EA, Vane JR: Human arterial and venous tissues generate prostacyclin (prostaglandin x), a potent inhibitor of platelet aggregation. *Lancet* 1977;1:18

131. Weksler BB, Marcus AJ, Jaffe EA: Synthesis of prostaglandin I_2 (prostacyclin) by cultured human and bovine endothelial cells. *Proc Natl Acad Sci USA* 1977;74:3922

132. Moncada S: Prostacyclin and arterial wall biology. *Arteriosclerosis* 1982;2:193

133. Smith WL, Bell TG: Immunohistochemical localization of the prostaglandin forming cyclooxygenase in renal cortex. *Am J Physiol* 1978;235:F451

134. Gorman RR, Bundy GL, Peterson DC, Sun FF, Miller OV, Fitzpatrick FA: Inhibition of human platelet thromboxane synthetase by 9,11-azoprosta-5,13-dienoic acid. *Proc Natl Acad Sci USA* 1977;74:4007

135. Gorman RR: Modulation of human platelet function by prostacyclin and thromboxane A_2. *Fed Proc* 1979;38:83

136. Dembinskia–Kiec A, Gryglewska T, Zmuda A, Gryglewski RJ: The generation of prostacyclin by arteries and the coronary vascular beds is reduced in experimental atherosclerosis in rabbits. *Prostaglandins* 1977;14:1025

137. Sinzinger H, Feigl W, Silberbauer K: Prostacyclin generation in atherosclerotic arteries. *Lancet* 1979;2:469

138. Probst P, Pachinger O, Sinzinger H, Kaliman J: Release of prostaglandins after percutaneous transluminal coronary angioplasty. *Circulation* 1983;68(Suppl 3):144

139. Fitzgerald GA, Smith B, Pedersen AK, Brash AR: Increased prostacyclin biosynthesis in patients with severe atherosclerosis and platelet activation. *N Engl J Med* 1984;310:1065

140. Aiken JW, Shebuski RJ, Miller OV, Gorman RR: Endogenous prostacyclin contributes to the efficacy of a thromboxane synthetase inhibitor for preventing coronary artery thombosis. *J Pharmacol Exp Ther* 1981;219:299

141. Yarger WE, Schocken DD, Harris RH, et al: Obstructive nephropathy in the rat: possible roles for the renin-angiotensin system, prostaglandins, and thromboxanes in post-obstructive renal function. *J Clin Invest* 1980;65:400

142. Harter HR, Burch JW, Majerus PW, et al: Prevention of thrombosis in patients on hemodialysis by low-dose aspirin. *N Engl J Med* 1979;301:577

143. Lorenz R, Siess W, Weber PC: Effects of very low versus standard dose acetyl salicylic acid, dipyridamole and sulfinpyrazone on platelet function and thromboxane formation in man. *Eur J Pharmacol* 1981;70:511

144. Masotti G, Galanti G, Poggesi L, Abbate R, Neri Serneri GG: Differential inhibition of prostacyclin production and platelet aggregation by aspirin. *Lancet* 1979;2:1213

145. Shaikh BS, Bott SJ, Demers LM: The differential inhibition of prostaglandin synthesis in platelets and vascular tissue in response to aspirin. *Prostagland Med* 1980;4:439

146. Jaffe EA, Weksler BB: Recovery of endothelial cell prostacyclin production after inhibition by low doses of aspirin. *J Clin Invest* 1979;63:532

147. Weksler BB, Pett SB, Alonso D, et al: Differential inhibition by aspirin of vascular and platelet prostaglandin synthesis in atherosclerotic patients. *N Engl J Med* 1983;308:800

148. Burch JW, Stanford N, Majerus PW: Inhibition of platelet prostaglandin synthetase by oral aspirin. *J Clin Invest* 1978;61:314

149. Kelton JG: Antiplatelet agents: rationale and results. *Clin Hematol* 1983;12:311

150. Killackey JJ, Killackey BA, Philp RB: Structure–activity studies of aspirin and related compounds on platelet aggregation, arachidonic acid metabolism in platelets and artery, and arterial prostacyclin activity. *Prostagland Leukotrienes Med* 1982;9:9

151. Marcus AJ: Aspirin as an antithrombotic medication. *N Engl J Med* 1983;24:1515

152. O'Brien JR: Platelets and the vessel wall: how much aspirin? (letter). *Lancet* 1980;1:372

153. Preston FE, Whipps S, Jackson CA, French AJ, Wyld PJ, Stoddard CJ: Inhibition of prostacyclin and platelet thromboxane A_2 after low dose aspirin. *N Engl J Med* 1981;304:76

154. Furchgott RF: Role of endothelium in responses of vascular smooth muscle. *Circ Res* 1983;53:558

155. Hamberg M, Svensson J, Samuelsson B: Prostaglandin endoperoxides: a new concept concerning the mode of action and release of prostaglandins. *Proc Natl Acad Sci USA* 1974;71:3824

156. Cragg A, Einzig S, Castañeda–Zuñiga WR, Amplatz K, White JG, Rao GHR: Vessel wall arachidonate metabolism after angioplasty: possible mediators of postangioplasty vasospasm. *Am J Cardiol* 1983;51:1441

157. Buchanan MR, Dejana E, Gent M, Mustard JF, Hirsh J: Enhanced platelet accumulation onto injured carotid arteries in rabbits after aspirin treatment. *J Clin Invest* 1981;67:503

158. Buchanan MR, Hirsch J: Effect of aspirin and salicylate on platelet–vessel wall interactions in rabbits. *Arteriosclerosis* 1984;4:403

159. Lewis HD, Davis JW, Archibald DG, et al: Protective effect of aspirin against acute myocardial infarction and death in men with unstable angina. *N Engl J Med* 1983;309:396

160. Lorenz RL, Weber M, Kotzur J, et al: Improved aortocoronary bypass patency by low-dose aspirin (100 mg daily). *Lancet* 1984;1:1261

161. Abele JE: Balloon catheters and transluminal dilatation. *AJR* 1980;135:901

162. Abele JE: Basic technology of balloon catheters, in Dotter CT, Grüntzig A, Schoop W, Zeitler E (eds): *Percutaneous Transluminal Angioplasty.* Berlin, Springer–Verlag, 1983, p 31

163. Burton AC: *Physiology and Biophysics of the Circulation.* Chicago, Year Book Medical Publishers, 1972, p 67

164. Athanasoulis CA, Abbott WM, Fidrych AM, et al: Balloon catheters for transluminal angioplasty: balloon bursting characteristics and clinical significance (abstract). Presented at 66th Scientific Meeting of the Radiological Society of North America, Dallas, TX, 1980

165. Athanasoulis CA: Percutaneous transluminal angioplasty: general principles. *AJR* 1980;135:893

166. Gerlock AJ, Regen DM, Shaff MI: An examination of the physical characteristics leading to angioplasty balloon rupture. *Radiology* 1982;144:421

167. Zollikofer CL, Salomonowitz E, Brühlmann WF, Castañeda–Zuñiga WR, Amplatz K: Dehnungs-, Verformungs- und Berstungs-Charakteristika haufig verwendeter Balloon-dilatationkatheter: in vitro Untersuchungen (Teil 1). *RöFo* 1986;144:40

168. Cragg AH, Kotula F, Castañeda–Zuñiga WR, Amplatz K: A simple mechanical device for inflation of dilating balloons. *Radiology* 1983;147

169. Olbert F, Hanecka L: Transluminale Gefassdilatation mit einem modifizierten Dilatationskatheter. *Wien Klin Wochenschr* 1977;89:281

170. Olbert F, Hanecka L: Transluminal vascular dilatation with a modified dilatation catheter, in Zeitler E, Grüntzig A, Schoop W (eds): *Percutaneous Vascular Recanalization.* Berlin, Springer–Verlag, 1978, p 32

171. Zollikofer CL, Salomonowitz E, Castañeda–Zuñiga WR, Brühl-

mann WF, Amplatz K: The relationship between arterial rupture and balloon bursting in experimental angioplasty. *AJR* 1985;144:777

172. Olbert F, Kasparzak Muzika N, Schlegl A: Percutaneous transluminal dilatation and recanalization: long-term results and report on experience with a new catheter system. *Ann Radiol* 1984;27:349

173. Zollikofer CL, Brühlmann W, Castañeda–Zuñiga WR, Sibly R, Amplatz K: Vergleich von polyaethylen (PEB) und Polyvinylchlorid (PVCB) Balloonkatheter in der perkutanen transluminalen Angioplastie (PTA) (abstract). Dtsch Röntgenkongress Hannover, June 1983

174. Zollikofer CL, Salomonowitz E, Brühlmann WF, Frick MP, Castañeda–Zuñiga WR, Amplatz K: Sigificance of balloon pressure recording during angioplasty. *RöFo* 1985;142:526

175. Waltman AC: Percutaneous transluminal angioplasty: iliac and deep femoral arteries. *AJR* 1980;135:921

176. Simonetti G, Rossi P, Passariello R, et al: Iliac artery rupture: a complication of transluminal angioplasty. *AJR* 1983;140:989

177. McDonald DA: *Blood Flow in Arteries*. Baltimore, Williams & Wilkins, 1960, p 153

178. Altose MD: Pulmonary mechanics, in Fishman AP (ed): *Pulmonary Diseases and Disorders*. New York, McGraw–Hill, 1980, p 359

179. Yune HY, Klatte EC:. Circumferential tear of percutaneous transluminal angioplasty catheter balloon. *AJR* 1980;135:395

13

Noninvasive Evaluation of Peripheral Vascular Disease

DAVID W. HUNTER, M.D.

Noninvasive methods for evaluating peripheral vascular disease are an important adjunct to physical examination, because they provide a variety of anatomic and physiologic information. The quantitative and reproducible nature of the data offers interventional radiologists an excellent means of planning an angioplasty and of assessing its immediate and long-term effectiveness. Continuing advances in digital angiography, videodensi-tometry, and magnetic resonance imaging (MRI) promise even further expansion of our ability to assess vascular anatomy and physiology with little or no vascular invasion.

Most of the noninvasive methods available today fall into three categories: intravenous digital subtraction angiography (IVDSA), plethysmography, and ultrasound.

INTRAVENOUS DIGITAL SUBTRACTION ANGIOPLASTY

This type of angiography has several advantages. First, it is a radiologic procedure, which means that evaluations before and after angioplasty will be made in the radiology department. This ensures that the follow-up information will reach the radiologist who performed the procedure. Also, IVDSA can provide reasonably accurate anatomic information and, with newer software, generate quantified numeric and graphic flow curves.

However, IVDSA has some important disadvantages. It is more expensive and time consuming than the other methods. It requires a physician's supervision, if not participation, whereas other methods can be done entirely by a technologist. Moreover, it is not truly noninvasive, because it requires a venipuncture and injection of contrast medium.

PLETHYSMOGRAPHY

Plethysmography, in its several forms, depends on the sensing of the slight volume or pressure changes created in an extremity by arterial pulsation. The sensing device can be an air-filled cuff (pulse-volume recorder), a fluid-filled cuff, or a thin mercury-filled Silastic tube strain gauge. The cuffs respond to pressure–volume changes and the strain gauge to changes in diameter. With any of the methods, the normal pulse contour tracing has a sharp upstroke, a narrow peak, a dicrotic notch, and a lower tricrotic wave (Fig. 13–1). When a vascular lesion reduces arterial inflow and pressure, the wave becomes broader and lower, and the notch and wave disappear (Fig. 13–1). Plethysmography can be combined with venous occlusion to give a relative measure of arterial inflow.

The advantages of plethysmography are primarily ones of ease of performance and low cost. The record is easily readable, understandable, and, because the technique is standardized, reproducible.

The disadvantages are primarily two. The first, which is critical in the follow-up of patients with peripheral vascular disease, is that the results give only a qualitative view of the extent of disease. This feature makes accurate assessment of hemodynamic changes difficult. The second, which is important in planning the approach to angioplasty, is that the lesion cannot be accurately located with plethysmography.

ULTRASOUND

Ultrasound can be used in both of its capacities: as a two-dimensional imager and as a one-dimensional Doppler flow analyzer. A duplex imager has both func-tions in one machine. This technology has been applied primarily to the carotid arteries, because problems with resolution, depth of penetration, and ability to assess cal-

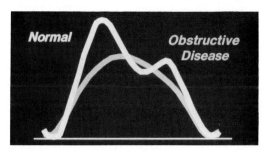

Fig. 13–1 Plethysmography pulse waveform on normal and obstructive disease status.

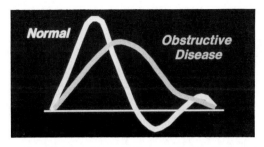

Fig. 13–2 Doppler waveform maximum velocity display in normal and diseased status.

cified arteries accurately have limited its use in the periphery. Mathematical analysis of the complicated Doppler waveforms is also possible, permitting quantitative assessment of flow and, therefore, of the degree of stenosis. The technique requires accurate sampling in the vicinity of the stenosis, however, which severely limits its usefulness.

The most widely used noninvasive method is a simple continuous-wave Doppler detection of flow. A sphygmomanometer cuff is placed around the extremity immediately proximal to the area being evaluated, inflated to a suprasystemic pressure, and slowly deflated. The pressure at which flow is first detected by the Doppler probe is the local systolic pressure. The measurement can be used as a single value but is more often expressed as an index or fraction that compares the systolic pressure in the affected extremity with that in the contralateral (one hopes normal) extremity (Fig. 13–2). The measurement provides a highly accurate evaluation of both the severity of disease and any changes that result from angioplasty.

The small, hand-held instrument is inexpensive, and the test may be done with the patient in the resting state with accuracy equal to that of exercise testing and with superior reproducibility. Indeed, some radiology departments have begun including Doppler indices obtained before and after peripheral angioplasty as part of the procedure covered by the single procedural fee.

The method does have its drawbacks. Even with careful segmental pressure measurements and qualitative Doppler waveform analysis, it may be difficult to pinpoint a stenosis. The pressure reading may be falsely elevated (*i.e.,* normal) in extremities with calcified, noncompressible arteries. There may be a second, adjacent artery beneath the probe, which is nonselective and will therefore "hear" the higher (more normal) pressure. The supposedly normal reference extremity may also be diseased, which would give a spurious index, although the absolute value of the extremity being studied would, of course, not be affected.

OTHER METHODS

MRI has a promising future in vascular imaging but will probably never be cost effective for serial peripheral artery examinations. Other methods, such as thermography, optical skin blood flow detection, nuclear angiography, and audible (bruit) spectral analysis, have not achieved the accuracy or simplicity of the other methods and are currently only investigative tools.

14

Aortic, Iliac, and Peripheral Arterial Angioplasty

DONALD E. SCHWARTEN, M.D.

Nonsurgical restoration of normal, or near normal, hemodynamics in the presence of arteriosclerotic stenotic or occlusive disease was first described by Dotter and Judkins in 1964,[1] the first description of the procedure now known as percutaneous transluminal angioplasty (PTA). Modification of the original Dotter–Judkins coaxial Teflon catheter system was described by Staple in 1968,[2] and further modifications were described by Van Andel, who chose to use a gradually tapered catheter rather than a more cumbersome coaxial system.[3] Several theoretical benefits accrued from Van Andel's design, including a diminution in the (undesirable) longitudinal shear force on the intima, which predisposes to acute thrombosis of the angioplasty site, and elimination of the possibility of entrapment of the intima between the two coaxial catheters, causing the "snowplow effect," which also predisposes to acute postangioplasty thrombosis. One further addition to the nonballoon-type catheters was made by Zeitler, who added a sidehole for contrast injection.[4] Both the Dotter and the Van Andel types of systems were utilized extensively in Europe for PTA of midsize and relatively small arteries but were used only sparingly in the United States for a number of reasons, not the least of which was consciousness of the potential for complications in the groin because of the large puncture wounds needed in the femoral artery.

The Dotter- and Van Andel-type catheters were too small to alter the hemodynamics in the common iliac arteries. Therefore, Porstmann designed a "caged" or "corset" catheter comprising a latex balloon enclosed in Teflon strips that helped minimize the propensity of the elastic latex to deform around the lesion rather than to dilate it.[5] However, Porstmann's balloon catheter caused little change in the prevailing attitude of angiographers and surgeons toward management of arteriosclerotic occlusive disease by PTA.

In 1974, Grüntzig and Hopff introduced an angioplasty catheter with a balloon made of a relatively nonelastic material, polyvinyl chloride.[6] This balloon could be inflated to a consistent predetermined diameter over a modest range of pressures without fear of balloon overdistention and vessel rupture. The advantages of such a device are obvious: (1) the balloon exerts almost exclusively radial forces against the plaque and the arterial wall, thereby minimizing the unwanted shear forces; (2) the balloon can be placed on a smaller catheter shaft (2.5F–9F); and (3) balloons can be made in various diameters (3.0–25.0 mm at present), thus permitting dilatation of the aorta, iliac arteries, superficial and deep femoral arteries, popliteal arteries, and tibial vessels. Also, since Grüntzig's initial reports of coronary and renal angioplasty,[7,8] other reports have confirmed the value of PTA in a wide variety of applications.[9–12]

It is now clear that polyvinyl chloride is not the ideal material for angioplasty balloons, and numerous studies are in progress to determine the ideal material as well as which balloon configuration optimizes the immediate and long-term results of PTA. (See Chapter 12 for an extensive discussion of catheter materials, properties, and actions.) Today, it appears that the most widely used material is irradiated polyethylene. Polyethylene terephthalate (*e.g.*, Mylar) materials tolerate enormous pressures (15–20 atm) with little, if any, tendency toward deformity or bursting; but whether such high pressures are necessary or beneficial in a significant percentage of patients with atherosclerotic disease remains unresolved. These high-pressure balloons may be of more value in treating nonatherosclerotic disease.

The long-term results of PTA in a variety of vessels in properly selected patients are as good as the results achieved with traditional surgical methods,[13] and the advantages of the percutaneous method are obvious. First, the procedure is safe, simple, and relatively painless. Second, in nearly all cases, the procedure can be performed with the patient in the hospital for little more than 24 hr. Third, unsuccessful angioplasty does not preclude surgical revascularization. Fourth, recurrent or worsening disease after an initially successful PTA can be managed with another angioplasty without the necessity of dealing with postoperative scarring. Finally, there is no risk of loss of sexual function as a consequence of aortoiliac angioplasty, as there is when the surgical procedures are used.

Perhaps, then, the time has come for an aggressive approach to patients with even mild lower extremity claudication, who, because their symptoms are not severe or for other reasons might not be surgical candidates. Rather than give these patients medical therapy until claudication limits their life style and their disease becomes too extensive for angioplasty, so that operation is the only way to restore relatively normal hemodynamics, one should consider early accurate anatomic evaluation and, perhaps, PTA.

PATIENT SELECTION

Indications and Contraindications

Selecting patients for aortoiliac and peripheral angioplasty requires assessment of both clinical and anatomic features. Angioplasty is more dependent than is surgery on certain anatomic criteria as predictors of both primary and long-term success. Therefore, both the clinical and the anatomic indications and contraindications are discussed here.

PTA is a cooperative effort, and although the burden of performing the diagnostic and dilatation procedures falls upon the angiographer, the decision to do PTA should be made jointly by a qualified vascular surgeon, the angiographer, and, usually, an internist. It is imperative to refrain from attempting PTA where surgical cooperation is not available; although the procedure is relatively safe, complications are inevitable in any series, and immediate availability of a capable vascular surgeon will be essential to avert catastrophes.

CLINICAL INDICATIONS

At this time, the clinical indications for PTA are essentially those guidelines observed by many moderately aggressive vascular surgeons. As a rule, patients with intermittent claudication who desire symptom relief will be considered candidates for arteriography and possible angioplasty provided that data from noninvasive studies suggest that the principal hemodynamic abnormalities are proximal to the popliteal artery.[14] However, when limb salvage is the goal, patients are considered for arteriography and angioplasty regardless of the site of disease predicted by noninvasive studies.[15]

CLINICAL CONTRAINDICATIONS

The presence of symptoms for <6–8 weeks, or sudden worsening of lower extremity symptoms within this time, is a relative contraindication to angioplasty.[16] Because fresh thrombus is likely to be present in these cases, PTA should not be performed unless the radiologist is thoroughly familiar with thrombolytic agents and uses them before PTA to lyse any relatively fresh thrombus and so minimize the risk of downstream embolization. The patient presenting with the "trash-foot" syndrome, indicative of peripheral embolization, likewise must be considered to have at least a relative contraindication to angioplasty,[17] although some unpublished work suggests that angioplasty is an appropriate alternative to operation in some of these patients as well (BT Katzen, A Van Breda; personal communication).

ANATOMIC INDICATIONS AND PROCEDURE PLANNING

Doppler data are invaluable in planning the approach for diagnostic arteriography in anticipation of angioplasty performed either in conjunction with the arteriogram or later. Furthermore, a baseline Doppler study obtained at approximately the same time as the arteriogram, when considered in conjunction with a study obtained 24–48 hr after successful angioplasty, permits objective assessment of the immediate and long-term results of the procedure.[18]

For the author's first 1000 lower extremity angioplasty procedures, postprocedural Doppler examinations were routinely obtained at quarterly intervals during the first year and semiannually for the next year. The efficacy of the procedure in the author's hands is now well established, and he no longer performs such frequent noninvasive studies. Instead, patients are carefully instructed about the implications of even minor recurrent symptoms, particularly within the first year, and are asked to see their referring physician immediately for a Doppler examination should symptoms return. Certainly as a quality control measure during the development of a PTA program at an institution, it is helpful to obtain regular noninvasive examinations of the first several hundred patients for comparison with the results of reported large series.

Perhaps the single most important factor in deciding whether a patient is a candidate for PTA is the diagnostic arteriogram. No other information is as valuable as the appearance of the pathologic anatomy in predicting the likelihood of success. It stands to reason, then, that the arteriogram, whether obtained by conventional screen film techniques or by digital techniques, must be of the highest quality to permit identification of ulcerations, mural thrombus, or thread-like patent channels within high-grade stenoses if the appropriate therapeutic decision is to be made. Oblique views are needed for examination of such areas as the orifices of the common iliac arteries, the origins of the hypogastric arteries, and the bifurcation of the common femoral artery.

ANATOMIC CONTRAINDICATIONS

Certain angiographic features are said to diminish the likelihood of success or to increase the likelihood of recurrent disease at the angioplasty site. Thus, these findings may be considered relative anatomic contraindications[19,20]:

Aorta: eccentric lesions in the proximal infrarenal region, particularly those of nonatherosclerotic etiology;

Iliac arteries: stenoses longer than 2.0–3.0 cm, eccentric stenoses, heavy calcification (particularly if eccentric), total occlusion of the common iliac artery, or stenosis at the origin of the common iliac artery;

Superficial and deep femoral artery: stenoses longer than 2.0–3.0 cm, occlusions longer than 10–15 cm, or heavy calcification of the stenotic or occlusive lesion;

Popliteal, tibial, and peroneal arteries: long segments of disease where there is a large patent vessel at the ankle, because the latter vessel is suitable for bypass grafting, and good results are likely to be obtained, particularly in institutions where in situ grafting is utilized;

In general, at this time the author considers ulcerative

disease in the presence of evidence of distal embolization a contraindication;

Complete occlusion of the superficial femoral artery in the presence of morbid obesity (relative contraindication);

Extensive disease in any segment of the aortoiliac or femoral vasculature, because long segments of intimal–medial disruption predispose to recurrent disease and distal complications.

The demonstration of fresh mural thrombus is an absolute contraindication unless thrombolysis is successful. This anatomic contraindication points out the necessity for performing a diagnostic arteriogram immediately before attempting any angioplasty procedure: even an overnight interval may permit thrombus to develop in an area of high-grade stenosis in a low-flow system. If such a thrombus is overlooked, the risk of embolization is increased.

Poor runoff diminishes the likelihood of long-term benefit from PTA. Zeitler et al found, in patients who had had a successful common iliac angioplasty, that if runoff was good to excellent, the patency rate at 5 years was approximately 85%, whereas in patients with poor runoff it was 50%.[21] The same limitation confronts the surgeon, however, so even if poor runoff is apparent in a patient who probably will have severe symptoms and, possibly, tissue loss, PTA may be the treatment of choice because of its simplicity and safety.

The foregoing list of anatomic contraindications must be considered in light of the patient's clinical condition; in general, they are relative contraindications. It is clear that long occluded segments of the superficial femoral artery can be recanalized using balloon catheter techniques (Fig. 14–1). Likewise, calcification is not always a predictor of failure, nor is eccentricity of a lesion. The radiologist must recognize that these anatomic situations are merely less than optimal for PTA; they do not preclude it. Because angioplasty failures rarely cause significant deterioration in the patient's clinical status, the author attempts PTA in the presence of unfavorable anatomy in these circumstances:

When the patient is at high operative risk;

When preservation of a saphenous vein is desirable;

When operation would be technically compromised because of an inadequate saphenous vein;

When the patient is not expected to live much longer;

Whenever limb salvage is the primary goal; that is, when an amputation is expected, angioplasty is attempted regardless of the anatomy if for no other reason than that it may alter the level of amputation even if it is only partially successful;

As an adjunct to surgery, such as in patients who may be at high risk in a major intra-abdominal operation.

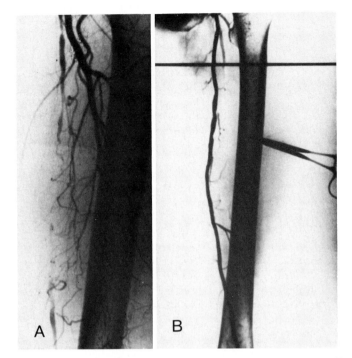

Fig. 14–1   A. Complete occlusion of superficial femoral artery. B. Successful recanalization of long-segment occlusion of superficial femoral artery.

Here, angioplasty of a flow-limiting aortoiliac segment lesion to provide inflow to the groin in preparation for a femoral–popliteal bypass graft, profundoplasty, or femoral–femoral bypass graft may obviate the intra-abdominal procedure.

Lesions for which the author never performs PTA are stenoses below the knee (except for limb salvage) and occlusions of the origin of the superficial femoral artery flush with the common femoral artery bifurcation. In the latter instance, there is no reasonable way to catheterize the superficial femoral artery.

LESIONS IDEAL FOR ANGIOPLASTY

The lesions that are ideal for PTA are:

Focal distal aortic stenoses of atherosclerotic origin;

1.0–2.0-cm concentric, high-grade stenoses of the iliac arteries located some distance from a major bifurcation;

2.0–4.0-cm stenoses or occlusions of the superficial and deep femoral arteries;

Relatively short isolated stenoses or occlusions in the popliteal and tibial arteries.

PERIPROCEDURAL PATIENT CARE

Preangioplasty Care

Well before the procedure, at a minimum, the following laboratory data should be available: blood urea nitrogen, serum creatinine, platelet count, prothrombin time, and partial thromboplastin time. If the patient has compromised renal function and a diagnostic arteriogram is obtained near the time of the planned angioplasty, the serum creatinine level should be ascertained immediately prior to PTA to ensure that the procedure is not begun on a patient with failing kidneys.

All patients receiving intravascular contrast medium should be well hydrated, so intravenous fluids should be begun the evening before angioplasty and continued at a rate of 50–100 ml/hr at least until the evening after the procedure.

Patients who are to undergo PTA should be seen well in advance of the procedure and be apprised of the primary success rate for the vessel to be treated as well as of the expected long-term success rate, the complication rate at that institution, and in general of what factors influence the results. More specifically, the patient should be informed about the use of antiplatelet agents, the probable value of an exercise program (the guidelines for which are best determined by the patient's internist or cardiologist), and the necessity of abstinence from tobacco use.

It is best not to premedicate heavily if narcotic analgesics are to be used, not only because of the risk of complications but because of the value of having the patient able to communicate the degree of discomfort as the balloon is inflated within the vessel. It has been the author's experience, as well as that of Katzen (personal communication) and others, that a patient who feels no discomfort during inflation of the balloon in the distal aorta, common or external iliac arteries, or hypogastric arteries may have an anatomically unsatisfactory result unless a larger balloon is used. Conversely, the patient who experiences excruciating pain with minimal inflation of a balloon may be at risk of excessive arterial trauma and perhaps should be treated with a smaller balloon. Therefore, the author believes it is ideal for a patient to feel moderate discomfort and to communicate this during the procedure. Obviously, a patient under the influence of substantial doses of narcotics is not likely to be communicative.

Intraprocedural Care

BALLOON SELECTION AND USE

The many and varied effects of balloon inflation within a vessel range from initiation of an aggressive atherosclerotic process to the creation of an atonic, somewhat ectatic, vessel.[22–24] Probst and coworkers have shown that the likelihood of the vessel remaining patent after successful angioplasty is greater if the treated site is slightly greater in diameter than the adjacent normal caliber vessel.[25] This finding suggests that use of a balloon slightly larger than the actual diameter of the vessel would produce the ideal result; in practice, it is the author's belief that the size of the balloon used should depend on the size of the nearest segment of normal caliber artery. In general, the author uses a balloon equal to the measured diameter of the nearest normal caliber segment of vessel without correction for magnification. The balloon should be slightly longer than the lesion. It is important to optimize the anatomic result because, as Tegtmeyer and colleagues have shown, recurrent stenoses are most likely after incomplete dilatation.[26] If the author has performed

angioplasty on a common iliac artery, for example, and finds an unsatisfactory arteriographic appearance, indicating incomplete dilatation of the vessel, in a patient who experienced mild to modest discomfort during balloon inflation, the procedure is repeated with a balloon one size larger, stopping only if the patient experiences severe pain (Fig. 14–2).

The duration of balloon inflation may have some bearing on the outcome of the angioplasty. For example, Kaltenbach and colleagues showed that, by prolonging the inflation, "nondilatable" lesions frequently can be dilated adequately.[27] The author routinely inflates the balloon to its maximum diameter and pressure and leaves it in this state for 60–120 sec. With this technique, a single inflation usually produces the desired result. Balloons should be inflated with a 3–12-ml syringe with contrast medium diluted 1:3, because smaller syringes generate unacceptably high pressures, predisposing to balloon rupture. Intraballoon pressures should be monitored. Deflation of balloons is best performed with large-bore syringes, which can generate maximum negative pressure (see Chapter 12).

PRESSURE MEASUREMENTS

The author does not routinely measure pressures before angioplasty in patients with lesions that obviously are hemodynamically significant; it is only in questionable lesions that pressure measurements are of value in determining whether to perform angioplasty. Under these circumstances, pressures are measured with the patient at rest and after maximizing lower extremity flow with tolazoline (15 mg intra-arterially), nitroglycerin (100 μg intra-arterially), or contrast medium. The author believes that any pressure gradient at rest is significant and that a gradient of ≥15 mm Hg after flow augmentation warrants angioplasty of the offending lesion.

PHARMACOLOGIC CONSIDERATIONS

During angioplasty, all of the author's patients are systemically heparinized. Some angiographers believe that heparin is not essential during angioplasty in high-flow vessels—e.g., the aorta and the iliac and, in many cases, the superficial femoral arteries—but the author believes heparin is of value, not only for its properties as an anticoagulant, but because of its antithromboxane A effect and thus its antispasm properties. He therefore uses this versatile drug routinely. Wolf has shown that the duration of the angioplasty procedure is adequately covered by systemic heparinzation with 2500 units, which the author uses routinely except when dealing with the distal vasculature, when he occasionally uses 5000 units.[28] With high-flow vessels, if postprocedure bleeding at the groin is a problem, systemic heparinization can be reversed with intravenous protamine on a milligram-for-milligram basis with allowance for the amount of heparin already metabolized. Protamine must be given slowly intravenously. The author frequently reverses the effects of systemic heparin in patients undergoing angioplasty of large and medium-sized vessels, whereas patients undergoing angioplasty of vessels below the knee, particularly when

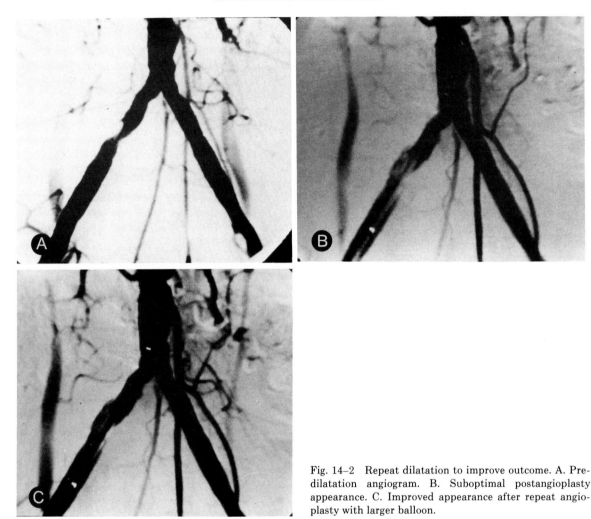

Fig. 14–2 Repeat dilatation to improve outcome. A. Pre-dilatation angiogram. B. Suboptimal postangioplasty appearance. C. Improved appearance after repeat angioplasty with larger balloon.

the disease is extensive, continue to receive systemic heparin for 48–72 hr afterward. The goal is to maintain the partial thromboplastin time in the therapeutic range of 60–90 sec. Similarly, whenever flow is compromised after angioplasty, heparin therapy is extended.

Pharmacologic manipulation plays a more important role in angioplasty than is generally appreciated, certainly a more important role than in general diagnostic arteriography. In certain circumstances, drugs other than heparin are invaluable. Useful agents include the following:

1. Lidocaine (Xylocaine);
2. Nitroglycerin (sublingual, transdermal, or as a 100-μg intra-arterial bolus);
3. Sublingual or oral nifedipine (10–20 mg);
4. Tolazoline (15-mg bolus);
5. Papaverine;
6. Prostaglandins;
7. Intravascular verapamil (2.5 mg).

Peripheral vessels are surprisingly agile structures, even those one would expect to be relatively rigid and thick-walled secondary to the arteriosclerotic process. Therefore, it is not uncommon to see severe vasospasm obliterating the vascular lumen around the catheter in

the external iliac artery, particularly in women. This phenomenon is also seen in the common femoral artery, and, to some degree, in the superficial femoral artery. Zeitler et al have noted that significant vasospasm occurred in more than half of their patients in whom a guidewire was placed in the popliteal artery or tibial vessels.[4] To combat such catheter-induced vasospasm, the drug of first choice is nitroglycerin given as a 100-μg intra-arterial bolus. This dose may be repeated several times unless systemic hypotension appears. The stimulus to vasospasm is the presence of the catheter and guidewire; once the spasm is broken with nitroglycerin or other drug and the stimulus is removed, it is unlikely that vasospasm will recur. If the operator is concerned about incomplete resolution of vasospasm, transdermal nitroglycerin may be given. Sublingual nitroglycerin also is useful, but its short duration of action makes it less effective than the transdermal form when the patient is away from the cardiovascular laboratory. In the cardiovascular laboratory, the availability and the almost immediate onset of action of intra-arterial nitroglycerin make this agent more attractive than the sublingual form.

Because of the propensity of the popliteal and tibial vessels to respond with spasm to the presence of the guidewire and catheter, the author routinely premedicates patients scheduled for angioplasty of these vessels with 10–20 mg of nifedipine unless there is a contraindication to its use. If the dose is to be given on an on-call basis, it may be given orally; if the drug is to be given when the patient arrives in the cardiovascular laboratory, it is given sublingually. Adequate blood levels are then reached in approximately 10 min. The duration of action of nifedipine is 4–6 hr, which is enough for even the most tedious below-the-knee procedures. Patients undergoing below-the-knee procedures also are given at least one 100-μg bolus of nitroglycerin as soon as the catheter is placed in the proximal popliteal artery. Nitroglycerin is utilized liberally whenever a spasm is noted.

In the unlikely event that severe vasospasm cannot be controlled with nitroglycerin, intravascular verapamil may be given if one exercises the utmost care. Verapamil is contraindicated in the presence of congestive heart failure or bradyarrhythmias.

The author has had little success in blocking or reversing vasospasm with papaverine or tolazoline. He has had no experience with prostaglandins as antispasm agents. Intravascular lidocaine has been utilized as an antispasm drug, but the present author, like Wolf, believes that this drug is of little value in the vascular system, although it is of substantial value as a local anesthetic in the groin.[28] The purpose of lidocaine is to prevent pain, and it belongs where the pain is generated.

Postangioplasty Care

Postangioplasty care in patients treated for lower extremity arterial insufficiency is similar to that given after routine diagnostic arteriography. The patient who has had a groin puncture is returned to a general medical or surgical bed and maintained at bed rest with the leg extended for 6 hr. The groin is monitored for bleeding, vital signs are monitored, and pulses are checked at frequent, regular intervals. If it was necessary to utilize an axillary approach, the patient is likewise maintained at bed rest, with the arm kept in a sling for 24–48 hr. The axilla is monitored, and the neurologic function of the arm is checked regularly for evidence of brachial plexus dysfunction secondary to an axillary hematoma which, if not promptly cared for, could cause devastating permanent brachial plexus palsy.

ANTIPLATELET THERAPY

All patients receive salicylates for at least 6 months postangioplasty; the author believes that salicylates should be maintained indefinitely. He administers 80 mg of acetylsalicylic acid (ASA) once daily in combination with 50–75 mg of dipyridamole. The optimum dose of ASA is uncertain, particularly when used in combination with dipyridamole, and the results of some current clinical studies are being awaited.

EQUIPMENT FOR ANGIOPLASTY

Dilatation Catheters

Although almost all angioplasty today is performed with balloon catheters, other angioplasty catheters are still manufactured and, in certain circumstances, are useful adjuncts. In particular, the Van Andel-type catheter should be available in the cardiovascular laboratory for special situations.

In general, three types of balloon catheters are available from various manufacturers. Balloons are constructed of polyvinyl chloride, polyethylene, or Mylar, and the shafts of the catheters are available in woven Dacron, polyethylene, and polyvinyl chloride.

At present, the author approaches distal popliteal and tibial angioplasty with the catheters designated as coronary angioplasty catheters. These catheters are currently available only in 125-cm lengths, and for this reason are somewhat cumbersome to use via an antegrade puncture down the relatively short superficial femoral artery. The author has, as prototypes, 60–85-cm variations of these small angioplasty catheters that have recently become available. Although in the past the author used a Van Andel-type angioplasty system for these distal vessels almost exclusively, he is now dedicated to the small ($\leq$5F) balloon catheters.

Guidewires and Sheaths

Guidewires used for angioplasty are the same as those used for diagnostic angiography, with some additions. Which guidewire to use in a specific situation depends in part on the angiographer's preference. Versatility and the use of meticulous, gentle technique in the manipulation of these guidewires are vital in negotiating lesions, preventing subintimal guidewire passage, and achieving a successful angioplasty.

Sheaths occasionally are valuable. The author does not routinely use them for what appear to be straightforward aortic, iliac, and femoral angioplasties. However, if the groin is scarred, if entrance through graft material is necessary, or if several catheter exchanges are expected, a sheath is used. Sheaths are routinely used for angioplasty of the vessels below the knee.

TECHNIQUES FOR ANGIOPLASTY IN SPECIFIC LOCATIONS

Abdominal Aorta

Aortic angioplasty has been attempted in atherosclerosis, retroperitoneal fibrosis, Takayasu's arteritis, neurofibromatosis, and anastomotic stenoses. Success has

been obtained consistently with atherosclerosis and anastomotic stenoses.[29]

Angioplasty of distal aortic lesions may be accomplished via retrograde catheterization of a single common femoral artery utilizing a large balloon designed specifically for aortic angioplasty (Fig. 14–3). Aortic angioplasty may also be accomplished with a pair of smaller balloon catheters introduced from the right and left common femoral arteries and advanced over soft guidewires into the lesion, with the balloons being inflated simultaneously with diluted contrast medium (Fig. 14.4). If the lesion is at the aortic bifurcation, the recommended approach is the retrograde use of bilateral catheters with balloons whose total diameter equals that of the adjacent normal caliber aorta. This method avoids possible occlusion of the orifice of one iliac artery.

There may be some theoretical advantage to inflation of several balloons simultaneously within an aortic stenosis. For example, in an 18-mm aorta with a relatively focal stenosis proximal to the bifurcation, three 6.0-mm balloon catheters may be placed, one from the right femoral artery, one from the left femoral artery, and one from the left axillary artery. The configuration of the inflated balloons conforms better to the configuration of the adjacent normal aorta than would be achieved with two balloons placed side by side and inflated simultaneously. The author has undertaken angioplasty in several patients using three or more catheters but believes it is unnecessary to achieve a closer approximation of the aortic configuration. Therefore, he no longer risks axillary catheterization for aortic angioplasty.

Common and External Iliac Artery Stenoses

The common and external iliac arteries are ideal for angioplasty. The best approach is the most direct approach, which, in most cases, is ipsilateral retrograde

catheterization. As noted previously, the author utilizes Doppler data to select the approach for diagnostic arteriography. When the Doppler data indicate a common or external iliac artery stenosis, the diagnostic arteriogram is performed from the ipsilateral approach in expectation of an angioplasty procedure immediately after the diagnostic procedure provided renal function is not severely compromised. If the diagnostic arteriogram reveals a long segment of external iliac artery that appears severely narrowed, to the degree that the lumen of the vessel is filled by the diagnostic catheter and no contrast medium is visible until the level of the common femoral artery, the diagnostic catheter is retracted over a 0.025-inch guidewire with a Y adapter, and 100 μg of intra-arterial nitroglycerin is administered via the catheter at the origin of the external iliac artery. A small volume of diluted contrast medium is then injected with the catheter parked in the common iliac artery, and digital images are acquired; these usually reveal a relatively focal stenosis uncovered by the ablation of vasospasm by the nitroglycerin (Fig. 14–5). Once an iliac artery stenosis has been demonstrated, provided the lesion does not involve the origin of the common iliac artery or the common iliac bifurcation and clearly is hemodynamically significant, a single appropriate-size balloon catheter is placed within the distal aorta after exchange over a soft guidewire for the diagnostic catheter.

With the balloon catheter in the distal aorta, 2500 units of heparin is administered intra-arterially. The soft-tip guidewire is then placed in the distal aorta below the renal arteries but well above the aortic bifurcation. The radiopaque markers designating the balloon position are placed within the stenosis, which, in the iliac system, usually is easy to locate without contrast medium because of the available bony landmarks. The balloon is inflated slowly to its maximum diameter and then to its maximum permissible pressure with diluted contrast medium and maintained in this state for 1–2 min even if there is

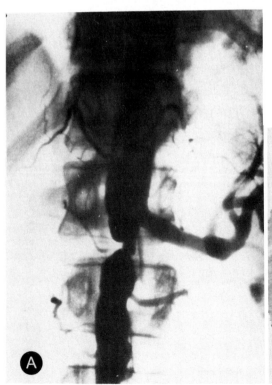
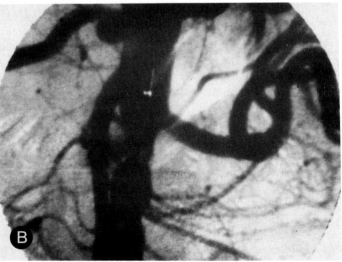

Fig. 14–3 Appearance of aortic stenosis before (A) and after (B) dilatation with single (15-mm) aortic angioplasty catheter.

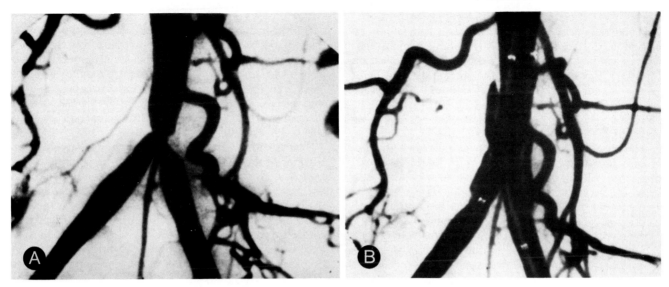

Fig. 14–4 Appearance of distal aortic disease before (A) and after (B) dilatation with two balloon catheters.

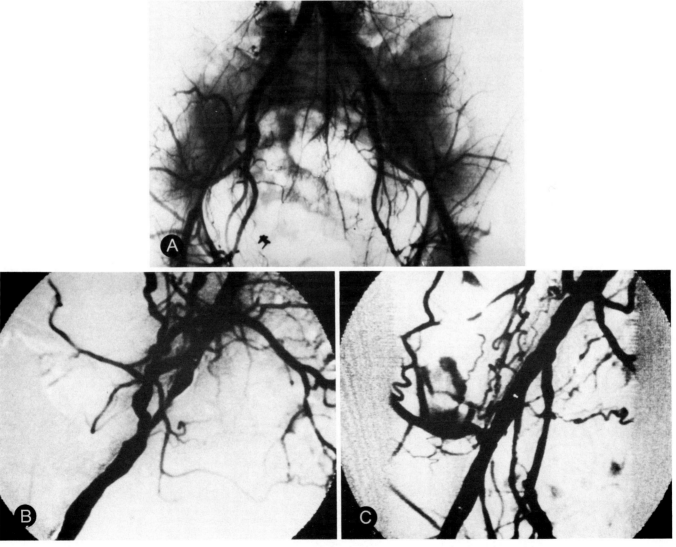

Fig. 14–5 Spasm giving false impression of extent of disease. A. Apparent long-segment obstruction of external iliac artery. B. After relief of spasm with 100µg of nitroglycerin, focal stenosis is revealed. C. Postangioplasty appearance.

an initial "waist" in the balloon that "pops." After deflation of the balloon, a documentary arteriogram should be obtained. If digital capabilities are available, a high-quality study can be obtained with a simple manual injection of contrast medium through the angioplasty catheter (Figs. 14–6 and 14–7). If digital techniques are not available, it is advisable to place a multihole catheter in the distal aorta and obtain a spot-film or cut-film arteriogram.

Never inject through an end-hole catheter in the vicinity of an angioplasty site. The risk of lifting the fractured intima–media is significant and may convert a successful angioplasty procedure into a catastrophe (Fig. 14–8). The documentary arteriogram should always be obtained with the catheter tip remote from the angioplasty site.

If the stenosis revealed by arteriography is of uncertain hemodynamic significance by anatomic criteria, then it is appropriate to obtain pressure measurements to confirm

the significance of the lesion before angioplasty. This is accomplished by placing a 0.025-inch guidewire in the distal aorta and retracting the catheter across the stenosis into the iliac artery. Pressure measurements are particularly useful after flow augmentation to maximize any gradient that may be present. If a gradient cannot be documented, angioplasty should not be performed. There is no justification for prophylactic angioplasty of lesions without hemodynamic significance.

The author is less likely to use pressure measurements to determine if an angioplasty procedure is complete. The goal is to create a normal, or near normal, lumen caliber, and he therefore relies on angiographic data to determine if there is need for additional dilatation. A residual stenosis of >30% in any projection in a patient who experienced only mild discomfort during balloon inflation is enough to warrant exchanging the original angioplasty catheter for one with a balloon 1.0 mm larger and repeat-

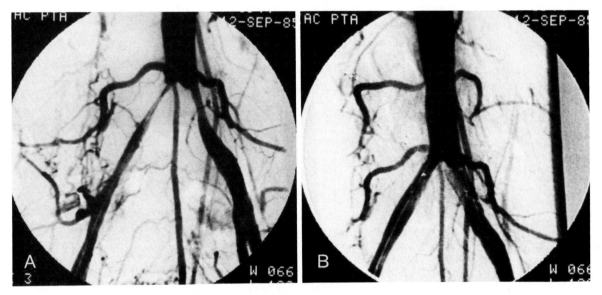

Fig. 14–6   A. Long stenosis of right common iliac. B. Successful common iliac angioplasty; injections made by hand through angioplasty catheter.

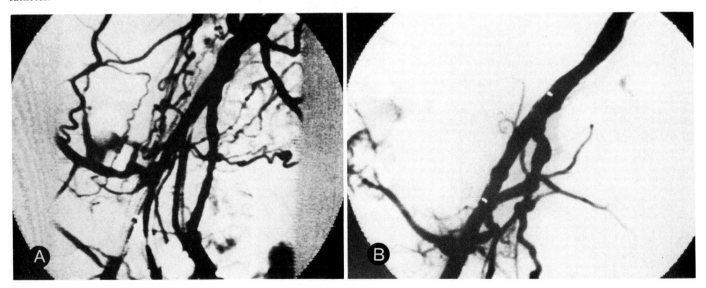

Fig. 14–7   Digital subtraction examinations made during manual injection of contrast medium documenting appearance of external iliac lesion before (A) and after (B) angioplasty.

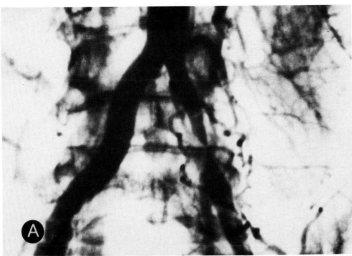

Fig. 14–8 Possible complication of postangioplasty radiographic study. A. Preangioplasty appearance of high-grade iliac stenosis. B. Postangioplasty injection of contrast medium creates extensive dis- section secondary to elevation of intima–media at angioplasty site by jet of fluid.

ing the procedure. In this case, it is important to inflate the balloon slowly; if the patient experiences severe discomfort, further inflation should be approached with exceptional care. Excruciating pain is highly suggestive of excessive vessel trauma, and the goal of an optimum anatomic result probably should be abandoned.

Iliac angioplasty can be a quick (<10 min) procedure, or it can be an extremely time-consuming, tedious procedure. Difficulties in performing iliac angioplasty are largely the result of the need to traverse complex, tortuous, ulcerated, highly diseased segments of the artery. Many solutions to this common problem have been offered. The author prefers one of the following. The initial attempt to negotiate the artery is made with a standard 0.035- or 0.038-inch 15-mm J-guidewire. These wires are, to some degree, "steerable" and may traverse the vessel with relative ease. If this fails, the author generally places a simple curved catheter with a "hockey-stick" configuration in combination with a 15-mm J-wire and attempts to steer through the diseased segment(s) of vessel (Fig. 14–9). If the vessel is severely ulcerated with multiple eccentric lesions, a Bentson wire is used in combination with the catheter because of its soft distal seg-

ment (Fig. 14–10). The author has recently begun to use the Wholey steerable guidewire (Advanced Cardiovascular Systems; Mountain View, CA) to negotiate highly diseased iliac arteries and has found it extremely useful. It is available in several configurations. He would use it more often were it not for its high cost. When dealing with near occlusions and with vessels that are severely ulcerated and tortuous, the author has used a combination of the hockey-stick catheter and a guidewire tapered from 0.035 inch at its base to 0.018 inch at its distal 4.0-cm segment (Advanced Cardiovascular Systems). This tip is not of the traditional "safety wire" configuration but has a densely opaque platinum tip. It is ultrasoft and appears to be the least traumatic guidewire available today (Fig. 14–11), but, again, its expense precludes its routine use. When all else fails, this guidewire may salvage the procedure. An alternative to the tapered wire is a combination of a 0.018-inch floppy platinum-tip guidewire as the core of a "injectable" guidewire (USCI; Billerica, MA). This guidewire is used in a 0.038-inch configuration, providing the needed rigidity for the passage of iliac angioplasty catheters.

Negotiation of complex pathologic anatomy in the iliac

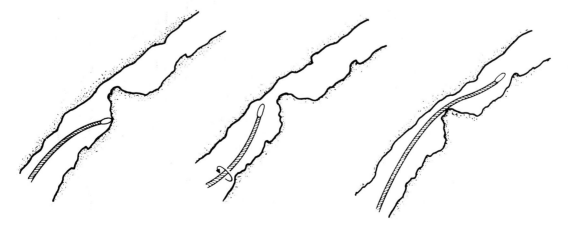

Fig. 14–9 Use of 15-mm J-guidewire to negotiate simple iliac stenosis.

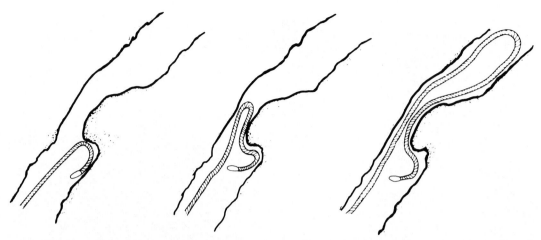

Fig. 14-10   Bentson wire is so soft that it will deflect off eccentric, undermined lesions with little risk of intimal elevation or subintimal passage.

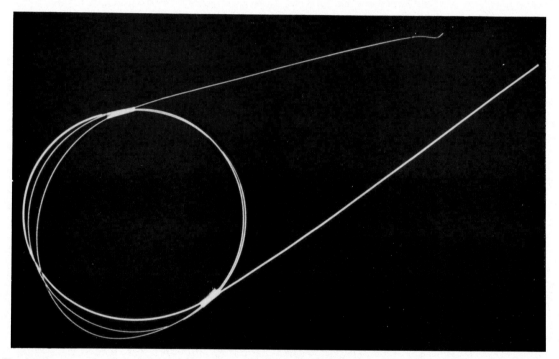

Fig. 14-11   Torsional attenuating diameter guidewire; at base, wire is 0.035 inch; tip tapers to 0.018-inch floppy segment (Advanced Cardiovascular Systems; Mountain View, CA).

system or femoral–popliteal–tibial system is greatly facilitated by digital roadmapping.

Lesions at the orifice of the common iliac artery may be dealt with using a single balloon catheter and the ipsilateral retrograde approach (Fig. 14–12). However, many of these lesions resist angioplasty, and it appears that placement of a second, contralateral balloon catheter and simultaneous inflation of the two balloons in the orifices of the common iliac arteries buttresses the balloon on the diseased side, helping to create the desired intimal–medial cleft and produce a successful angioplasty (Fig. 14–13). The author has not encountered occlusion of the nonstenotic common iliac artery when using the ipsilateral approach with a single catheter for a common iliac artery orifice lesion, although published experiences would indicate that this occurs.[30] If the radiologist is con-

cerned about the risk of occluding the contralateral iliac artery, it may be reasonable to pass a small diagnostic catheter into the distal abdominal aorta from the contralateral vessel to provide access in the event that angioplasty of one iliac artery orifice results in occlusion of the opposite side. With this access, any occlusion can be reversed quickly merely by exchange for an angioplasty catheter and simultaneous balloon inflation within the iliac artery orifices.

Upon completion of an iliac angioplasty, it is the author's habit to reverse part of the effect of the systemic heparinization. This is accomplished, as previously noted, with intravenous protamine, allowing for a 30% drop in heparin activity within the first hour after its administration.

Insertion and removal of the large-caliber balloon cath-

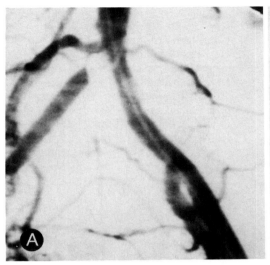

Fig. 14–12   Single-catheter approach to lesion at orifice of common iliac artery. A. Preangioplasty appearance of high-grade focal stenosis at orifice of common iliac artery. B. Appearance after angioplasty with single catheter from ipsilateral approach.

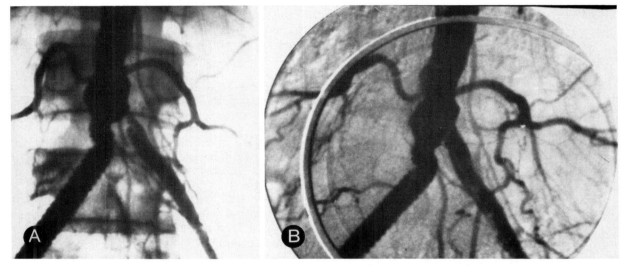

Fig. 14–13   Two-catheter approach to lesion at orifice of iliac artery. A. Preangioplasty appearance of iliac orifice lesion. B. Appearance after angioplasty utilizing bilateral catheters.

eters should be done with considerable care. The catheter should be inserted and extracted while suction is applied with a large-bore syringe to ensure that the balloon hugs the catheter shaft as tightly as possible. Some manufacturers wrap the "wings" of the balloon around the catheter shaft and designate that catheter as wrapped for clockwise or counterclockwise insertion. Be aware of the design of the catheter of your choice, and if it is appropriate to rotate it as it is passed through the groin tissue and vessel wall, be sure it is being rotated in the proper direction (Fig. 14–14).

Hypogastric Artery and Common Iliac Bifurcation

Angioplasty at any bifurcation may create a noncolinear intimal–medial cleft that spirals an intimal flap into the orifice of the untreated vessel, causing a tempo-

rary, or even a permanent, occlusion (Fig. 14–15). In the case of the common iliac artery bifurcation, the author feels that it is optimal to protect the hypogastric artery even if it does not have a significant stenosis at its origin. To do this, angioplasty is accomplished by bilateral retrograde catheterization of the common femoral arteries. On the ipsilateral side, the appropriate size balloon catheter is placed within the stenosis using bony landmarks as guide. The contralateral femoral artery is catheterized with a catheter suitable for passage of a guidewire and catheter system around the aortic bifurcation. This crossover technique can be accomplished in at least three ways:

1. A pigtail catheter is used to engage the orifice of the contralateral common iliac artery. The guidewire is then passed down the contralateral iliac system.[31] Occasionally, it may be passed directly into the hypo-

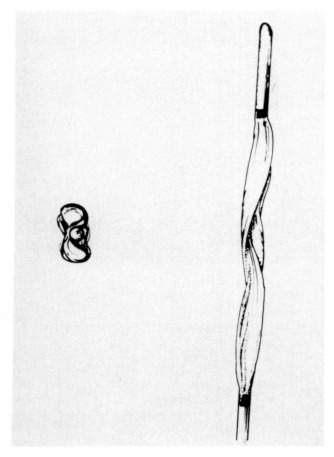

Fig. 14–14 Large balloons, when not tightly wrapped around shaft of catheter, will have "wings," which are designed to be tightly wrapped in clockwise or counterclockwise fashion around shaft. This will minimize trauma at puncture site.

gastric artery, greatly facilitating quick placement of a balloon catheter there (Fig. 14–16).

2. A Simmons-type curved catheter is used to engage the contralateral common iliac artery origin after the catheter has been reformed in a more proximal branch of the abdominal aorta or in the descending thoracic aorta.[32] However, the primary segment of the Simmons catheter may not be long enough to facilitate passage into the hypogastric artery (Fig. 14–17). Therefore, we prefer to:

3. Form a loop with a cobra catheter[33] and use this in conjunction with a Bentson wire to negotiate the orifice of the contralateral common iliac artery and ultimately the hypogastric artery (Fig 14–18).

Once the hypogastric artery has been entered, if the aortic bifurcation is not extremely acute, a heavy-duty, 15-mm, 0.038-inch J-guidewire is placed in the hypogastric artery. Angioplasty of the diseased common iliac bifurcation is performed, and a control arteriogram is obtained using digital techniques and injecting through the angioplasty catheter while a guidewire is left in the hypogastric artery (Fig. 14–19). If there is no evidence of compromise of the orifice of the hypogastric artery, the procedure is considered complete, heparinization is reversed, and the catheters are removed. If there is a stenosis of the hypogastric artery, or if there is evidence of compromise of the hypogastric artery after angioplasty of the iliac bifurcation, an appropriate size balloon catheter is placed around the aortic bifurcation over the heavy-duty guidewire and inflated simultaneously with the catheter in the common iliac artery bifurcation. Digitally acquired images are again reviewed, and if the angioplasty result is satisfactory, heparinization is reversed and the catheters are removed as previously described (Fig. 14–20).

If the aortic bifurcation is acute and the contralateral approach is being used for whatever reason—be it for hypogastric angioplasty or because the angiographer

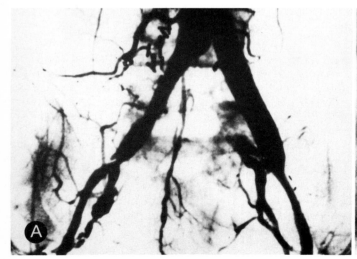

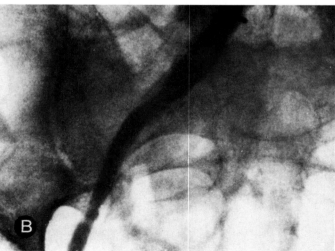

Fig. 14–15 Insufficient extent of dilatation leading to arterial occlusion. A. Preangioplasty arteriogram demonstrating stenosis at bifurcation of common iliac artery in patient after aortoiliac bypass surgery. B. Failure to perform angioplasty on both the hypogastric and iliac arteries results in occlusion of hypogastric artery.

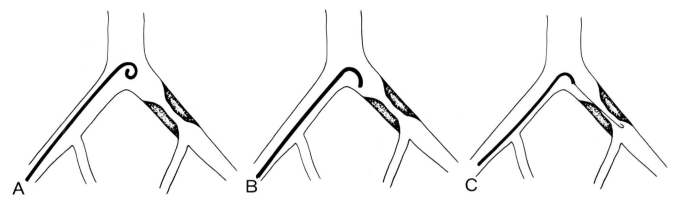

Fig. 14–16   Use of pigtail catheter to engage contralateral iliac orifice.

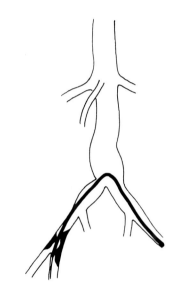

Fig. 14–17   Use of Simmons-type catheter to engage a contralateral iliac orifice.

desires, for anatomic reasons, to approach a common external iliac artery this way—the author finds either the Amplatz wire (Cook, Inc.; Bloomington, IN) or the Wholey wire to be very helpful. The stiffness of the shaft of these wires greatly facilitates passage of catheters around an acute aortic bifurcation. The Wholey wire offers the additional advantage of being steerable and permitting relatively easy negotiation of stenotic lesions.

When the contralateral approach is used for iliac disease in general, and the catheter tends to buckle into the abdominal aorta rather than to follow the guidewire around the aortic bifurcation, if the guidewire can be advanced to the groin, manual compression of the common femoral artery will entrap the guidewire and reduce the likelihood of such buckling (Fig. 14–21).

When the contralateral approach is used for angioplasty of the common iliac bifurcation and there is a rigid stenosis at the hypogastric origin, the balloon placed ipsilaterally may be inflated gently at the orifice of the common iliac artery and pulled down slightly to force the hypogastric catheter through the stenotic origin (Fig 14–22).

The interventional radiologist is uniquely equipped to revascularize the hypogastric system for patients who suf-

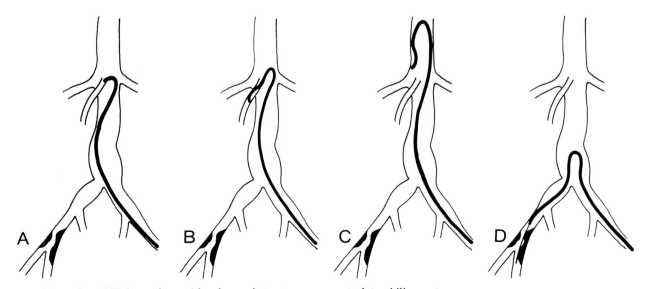

Fig. 14–18   Formation of Waltman loop with cobra catheter to engage contralateral iliac system.

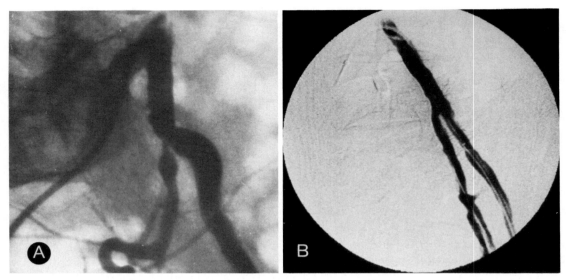

Fig. 14–19   A. Preangioplasty appearance of hypogastric orifice lesion viewed in oblique position. B. Intra-angioplasty examination with guidewire in hypogastric artery and angioplasty catheter retracted.

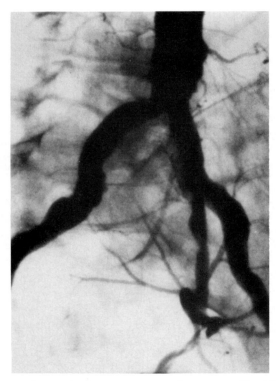

Fig. 14–20   Postangioplasty appearance of a common iliac bifurcation–hypogastric orifice lesion.

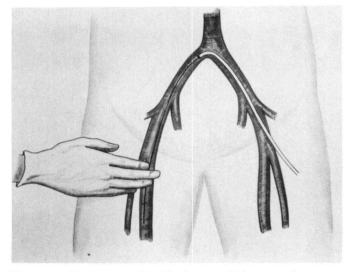

Fig. 14–21   Entrapment of guidewire at groin by manual compression provides more rigid track for catheter to follow and decreases likelihood of buckling in aorta.

Occluded Common Iliac Arteries

Ring et al have reported contralateral embolization during attempts at direct recanalization of occluded common iliac arteries.[34] Although the author has not had this experience in >100 patients in whom he has performed direct recanalization, patients considered for this procedure are highly selected. That is, this procedure is attempted only in patients with what appear to be relatively straight iliac arteries with short-segment occlusions and relatively nondiseased distal abdominal aortas (Fig. 14–23). The author has been successful in approximately 60% of attempted direct recanalizations using the Rosen

fer hip and buttock claudication. In addition, angioplasty of the proximal hypogastric artery or its pudendal branch has, in a few patients, helped in the management of vasculogenic impotence. It is unreasonable to perform angioplasty at the common iliac bifurcation and to ignore a diseased hypogastric artery.

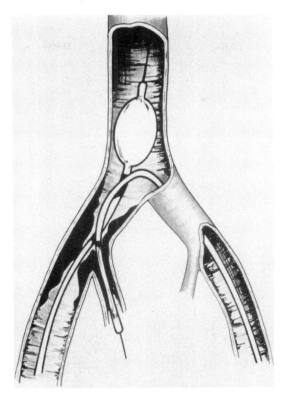

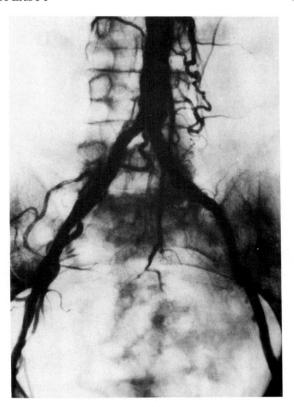

Fig. 14–22 Gentle traction on ipsilateral catheter with balloon inflated forces contralateral catheter to pass into hypogastric artery.

Fig. 14–24 Postangioplasty appearance following direct recanalization using a 6F straight Teflon catheter advanced in combination with a Rosen guidewire through the occluded segment.

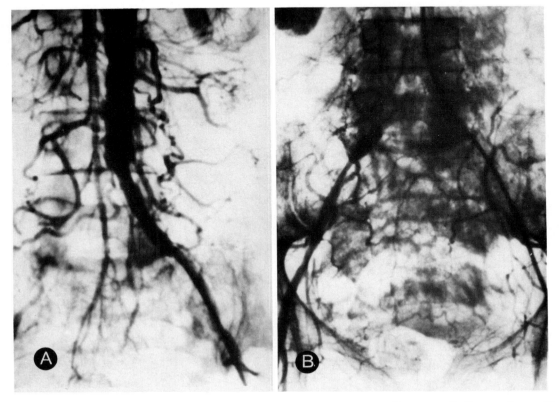

Fig. 14–23 Recanalization of iliac artery. A. Preangioplasty appearance of occluded common iliac artery. B. Retrograde opacification of common iliac artery through collaterals.

guidewire introduced by the ipsilateral approach in combination with a straight Teflon catheter. The catheter and guidewire are advanced as a unit through the occluded segment (Fig. 14–24). Failure to achieve recanalization is almost invariably secondary to subintimal passage of the guidewire, which has not, in the author's hands to date, caused significant complications.

Puncture of the "pulseless" common femoral artery in the presence of occlusive or stenotic iliac disease can be accomplished with relative ease by:

Palpation of the nonpulsatile thick-walled artery (in slender patients);

Fluoroscopic observation of the femoral head and puncture of the artery, which is almost always located over the medial third of the femoral head. Any calcification in the vessel wall may facilitate the puncture;

Doppler localization of the vessel[35]; or

Injection of contrast medium, if a catheter is present in the distal aorta from a diagnostic procedure per-

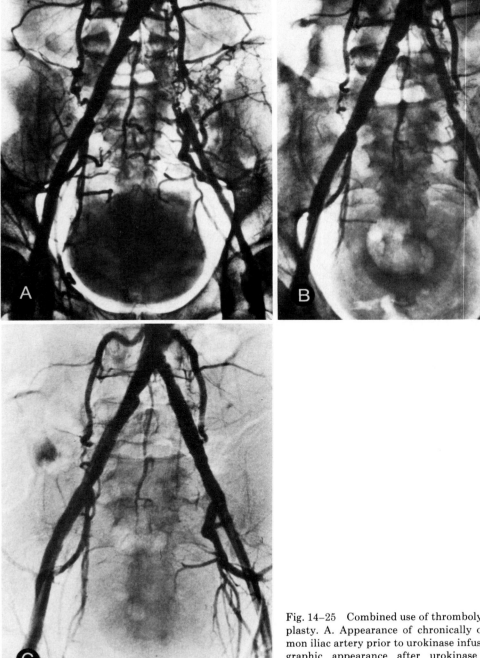

Fig. 14–25 Combined use of thrombolysis and angioplasty. A. Appearance of chronically occluded common iliac artery prior to urokinase infusion. B. Angiographic appearance after urokinase infusion. C. Postangioplasty arteriogram. (Courtesy of Barry T. Katzen, M.D.)

formed via the contralateral approach, to cause collateral opacification of the common femoral artery, which can then be punctured.

Although the author has had modest success with direct recanalization of the occluded common iliac artery, the incidence of contralateral embolization cannot be ignored. Thus, it would appear that the best approach to angioplasty of the common iliac artery is to catheterize the contralateral common femoral artery, place a small (4F–5F) Simmons configuration catheter in the abdominal aorta, reform the catheter, wedge its tip in the orifice of the occluded vessel, and infuse a thrombolytic agent in an attempt to uncover the stenosis, which may be suitable for angioplasty (Fig. 14–25).[36] It goes without saying that this should not be attempted unless the angiographer is thoroughly familiar with the use of thrombolytic agents.

There are angiographers who believe that the occluded common iliac artery should not be treated by transluminal angioplasty but rather surgically.

Common Femoral Artery

Lesions of the common femoral artery are frequently related to previous surgery. When atherosclerosis is present, the lesions are frequently thick, heavily calcified, and eccentric and may not yield optimally to balloon angioplasty. In contrast, lesions at graft anastomoses are usually caused by intimal hyperplasia and respond readily to angioplasty.

Transluminal angioplasty of the common femoral artery usually requires a contralateral approach with passage of a catheter around the aortic bifurcation using one of the methods previously described. This approach is not unreasonable for stenotic disease of the proximal and mid common femoral artery, particularly in patients who are high surgical risks. The author is reluctant to undertake angioplasty of the bifurcation of the common femoral artery with a single catheter because of the potential for occlusion of either the superficial or the deep femoral

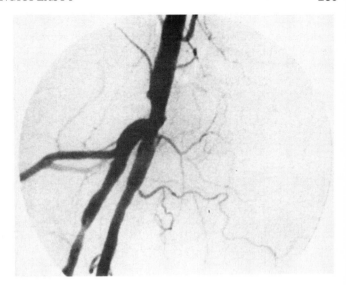

Fig. 14–27 Postangioplasty appearance; two balloon catheters were used.

artery if the procedure creates a noncolinear intimal–medial cleft (Fig. 14–26). The occluded common femoral artery is not suitable for angioplasty because it is unlikely that the forces necessary to traverse the occlusion can be generated via the contralateral approach, inasmuch as the catheter tends to buckle into the abdominal aorta when forward force is applied in the groin (Fig. 14–27).

Surgical management of common femoral artery disease is a well-established procedure that usually can be done at low risk.[37] Thus, it seems unwise to attempt angioplasty of this vessel in most circumstances.

Superficial and Deep Femoral Artery Stenoses

The optimal approach to stenoses of the superficial and deep femoral arteries is an ipsilateral antegrade common femoral puncture, which may be the most difficult

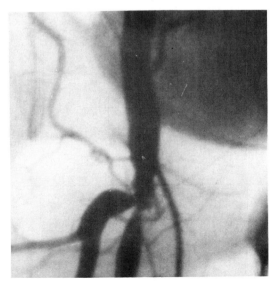

Fig. 14–26 Dilatation at common femoral bifurcation. Preangioplasty appearance of common femoral bifurcation lesion.

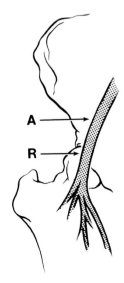

Fig. 14–28 Bony landmarks and their relations to skin entrance sites for antegrade (A) and retrograde (R) punctures.

maneuver for the interventional radiologist with little experience. Antegrade puncture requires that the skin of the abdominal wall be entered above the inguinal ligament, whereas the needle enters the common femoral artery below the ligament (Fig. 14–28). In obese patients, this can be extremely difficult; it is frequently helpful to retract the panniculus cephalad and medially. For angiographers beginning their experience, it may be beneficial to observe the groin area fluoroscopically with the needle poised for puncture to ascertain the level at which the needle tip will enter the artery in order to avoid puncturing the vessel proximal to the inguinal ligament. Puncture below the common femoral bifurcation increases the risk of a groin hematoma. Of necessity, the angle of puncture of the common femoral artery is steeper when using the antegrade than the retrograde approach (Fig. 14–29). Once the common femoral artery has been entered, it is helpful to depress the hub of the needle against the abdominal wall to elevate the tip when it is the angiographer's desire to enter the superficial femoral artery. If the needle hub is not depressed, the natural tendency of the guidewire will be to enter the deep femoral artery (Fig. 14–30). Other maneuvers for entering the desired vessel have been described, including placing the patient in the frog-leg lateral position to observe the direction of passage of the guidewire,[38] modification of the Cope method,[38] and use of catheters with short curves to direct the guidewire.[39] The author has found that simply depressing the abdominal wall and manipulating the needle hub and tip consistently allow passage of a guidewire into the desired vessel.

Angioplasty of the deep femoral artery should be performed with renal tip catheters, which have the balloon located as close as possible to the tip, thus minimizing the chance of trauma to distal branches of the deep femoral artery beyond the treated area. One should give careful consideration to deep femoral angioplasty when that artery is the sole collateral source in a nonthreatened limb in a patient with an occluded superficial femoral artery. Angioplasty of the deep femoral artery also may

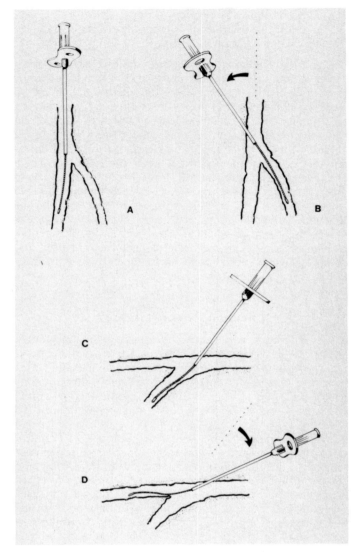

Fig. 14–30 Manipulations of needle hub permits angiographer to direct needle tip toward superficial or deep femoral artery.

Fig. 14–29 Comparative angles for needle approach for antegrade (A) and retrograde (R) punctures.

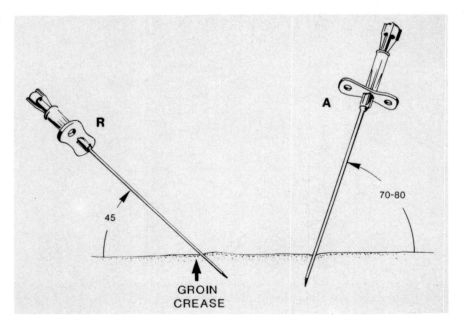

be a useful adjunct to iliac angioplasty, particularly in high-risk patients with peripheral ischemia.

Bony landmarks may be of some help in angioplasty of the superficial and deep femoral arteries, as may calcification observed at fluoroscopy. When these landmarks are not available for locating the stenotic lesion, it is necessary to place towel clips or other opaque markers at the site of the stenosis, as determined by injection of a small volume of contrast medium through the first dilator placed in the vessel to be treated. An opaque ruler also may be used to mark the lesion(s).

Once the stenosis has been located in either the superficial or the deep femoral artery, angioplasty is accomplished by negotiating the lesion with the guidewire of choice. As in the iliac system, our first choice is the 15-mm, 0.035-inch or 0.038-inch J-guidewire (Fig. 14–31).[20] This somewhat steerable wire frequently negotiates uncomplicated stenoses with surprising ease. Alternatives

include the Bentson wire, the Wholey wire, and the Amplatz wire. The author has found the previously described 0.035-inch wire tapered to a 0.018-inch soft platinum tip useful in negotiating extremely high-grade ulcerated lesions, where the risk of subintimal wire passage is high (Fig. 14–32).

After the stenosis has been negotiated, a catheter with a balloon of appropriate diameter and length is advanced over the guidewire and positioned within the lesion. The guidewire is removed, and a small volume of contrast medium is injected to ensure intraluminal position. Hep-

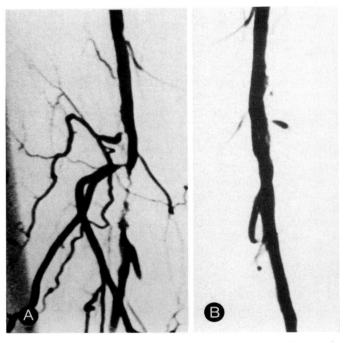

Fig. 14–32 Dilatation of irregular segment lesion. A. High-grade irregular segment superficial femoral artery stenosis negotiated with torsional attenuating diameter guidewire. B. Postangioplasty appearance.

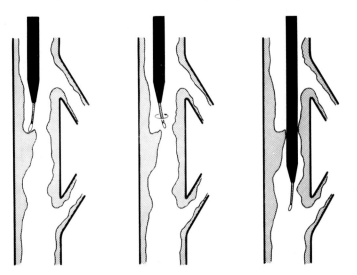

Fig. 14–31 Use of 15-mm J-curve guidewire to negotiate superficial femoral stenosis.

Fig. 14–33 Appearance of focal superficial femoral artery stenosis before (A) and after (B) angioplasty.

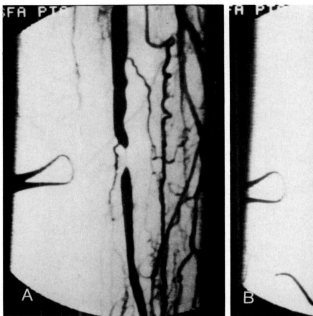
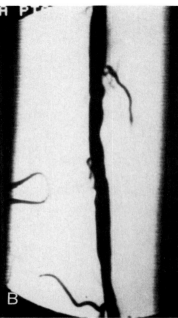

arin is administered, and the guidewire is reinserted and parked in the distal superficial femoral artery or the distal deep femoral artery. The balloon is inflated slowly to its maximum diameter with diluted contrast medium and then to its maximum pressure, and inflation is maintained for 60–120 sec. If a standard end-hole angioplasty catheter is used and the angiographer desires to document the appearance of the angioplasty site before removing the dilating system, a 0.025-inch guidewire may be parked in the distal vessel during the angioplasty. Alternatively, after angioplasty, the dilating catheter may be retracted and, with the use of a Y adapter, contrast medium can be injected manually and images acquired to assess the immediate appearance of the vessel (Fig. 14–33). If the result is satisfactory, the system can be removed, the heparin reversed, and hemostasis obtained at the groin. If the result is not satisfactory, the catheter can be advanced over the 0.025-inch wire to a point distal to the angioplasty site. The wire is then replaced with a larger diameter wire to facilitate exchange for an angioplasty catheter with a larger balloon or for a catheter permitting higher pressures for repetition of the procedure. It is essential that a guidewire be left well distal to the angioplasty site until the angiographer is certain that the procedure is complete (Fig. 14–34), because any attempt to recross a freshly dilated site risks intimal dissection and vessel occlusion.

When dealing with multiple stenoses in the same vessel, all of the Lesions should be negotiated with the guidewire; angioplasty should begin with the most distal lesion, working toward the most proximal lesion. More than one catheter may be necessary because of the increasing diameter of the vessel.

Two angioplasty catheters are available that permit injection of contrast medium without the necessity of inserting a 0.025-inch guidewire. Barth's design[40] has two sideholes distal to the balloon and a relatively long catheter tip (Fig. 14–35).[31] He believes that this catheter is useful, not only for postangioplasty angiographic checks, but also for negotiating lesions while injecting contrast medium. The other catheter, devised by Ricketts, has a sidehole proximal to the balloon (Fig. 14–36). Simple use of a sidearm adapter over a conventional 0.035- or 0.038-

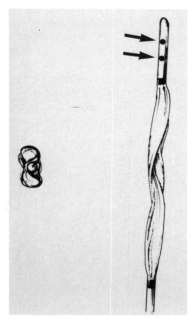

Fig. 14–35 Angioplasty catheter with sideholes distal to balloon (arrows).

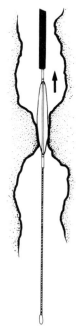

Fig. 14–34 If balloon is not centered precisely, it may retract or advance spontaneously during inflation. For this reason, among others, it is always wise to leave guidewire well distal to angioplasty site until procedure is complete.

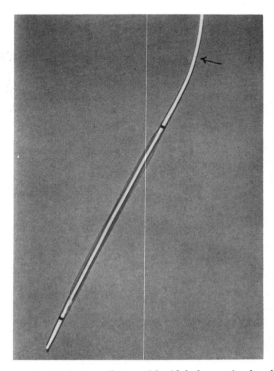

Fig. 14–36 Angioplasty catheter with sidehole proximal to balloon (arrow).

inch guidewire also permits injection of contrast medium, which will exit through the sidehole and provide adequate images of the angioplasty site, particularly if digital techniques are used.[41] In this way, the anatomic result can be ascertained before catheter removal.

Occasionally, it is nearly impossible to advance the angioplasty catheter over a conventional guidewire through an extremely tight, rigid femoral artery stenosis; the catheter and guidewire buckle in the groin, and no forward progress can be made. This is a particular problem in the obese patient. In this circumstance, it may be helpful to:

Insert a sheath into the femoral artery to provide additional support for the catheter to prevent buckling in the groin;

Use a heavy-duty Amplatz- or Wholey-type guidewire for additional support;

Manually support and compress the groin tissues;

Advance a heavy-duty guidewire into the popliteal artery and then manually compress the artery, entrapping the guidewire and providing a more rigid system for the catheter to follow.

The same maneuvers may be helpful if the initial insertion of the angioplasty catheter is difficult, *e.g.*, because of groin obesity or scar tissue. If these measures fail, it may be useful to attempt PTA with a Van Andel-type catheter, which has a more rigid shaft.

Rarely, it is necessary to approach femoral artery stenoses contralaterally around the aortic bifurcation. Any of the techniques for passing a catheter around the bifurcation can be employed. A catheter with a longer shaft may be necessary to reach a distal lesion. In general, the author avoids this approach, utilizing it only in extremely obese patients.

Occluded Superficial Femoral Arteries

Successful angioplasty of occluded superficial femoral arteries requires ipsilateral antegrade femoral artery puncture, inasmuch as it generally is impossible to achieve the desired forward forces from the contralateral approach because of catheter buckling in the abdominal aorta. Antegrade catheterization is performed, and a 6F straight Teflon catheter is advanced into the proximal superficial femoral artery over a flexible-tip guidewire. The proximal and distal limits of the occluded segment are identified with opaque markers or other landmarks.

Several methods for recanalizing occluded segments of the superficial femoral artery have been described, including attempts to pass a Bentson- or a Newton-type straight guidewire through the occluded segment and the use of a movable core straight guidewire, alternately advancing and retracting the core to stiffen the tip of the wire as it passes through the occluded segment. The author prefers to use a Rosen-type guidewire advanced as a unit with a catheter through the occluded segment (Fig. 14–37), because he has tried all the above-mentioned methods and believes that the incidence of subintimal passage is lowest with the Rosen wire–catheter combination. Once the occluded segment has been bridged, the guidewire is removed, and, after confirmation of the posi-

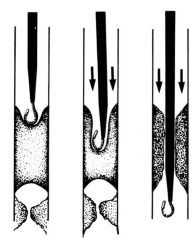

Fig. 14–37 Method of advancing guidewire–catheter combination through superficial femoral artery occlusions.

tion of the catheter tip with a small volume of contrast medium, heparin is administered. The guidewire is inserted and parked in the distal superficial femoral artery, and the procedure is completed as when dealing with a simple stenosis (Fig. 14–38). As with previously described procedures, after completion of the angioplasty, the heparin is usually partly reversed unless runoff is poor or a low-flow state exists, and hemostasis is obtained at the groin.

Distal Popliteal and Tibial Artery Stenoses

Angioplasty below the knee is reserved for patients with threatened limbs. The procedure mandates an ipsilateral antegrade puncture of the common femoral artery. The author believes that balloon angioplasty is a better choice than the use of a Van Andel-type catheter or a series of long tapered catheters of increasing diameter, because these cause more shear trauma to the intima. To accomplish the angioplasty, after the common femoral artery has been punctured, a sheath is placed in the superficial femoral artery. A small-bore catheter with an appropriate diameter balloon is advanced over a 0.014–0.018-inch guidewire with a soft, floppy platinum tip. The catheter is advanced to the popliteal artery, where the guidewire is removed, and 5000 units of heparin and 100 μg of nitroglycerin are administered through the catheter. (The patient is premedicated with 10–20 mg of nifedipine.) Contrast medium is injected through either the catheter or the flushing port of the sheath to locate the stenosis. Bony landmarks may be helpful, but other opaque markers may be necessary to pinpoint the lesion for placement of the balloon. The guidewire is then reinserted and advanced into the vessel of interest, and the catheter is advanced over the guidewire. The progress of this system can be monitored via small injections of contrast medium through the flushing port of the sheath. Once the balloon markers are placed appropriately within an area of stenosis, the balloon is inflated to its maximum diameter and maintained at its maximum diameter/pressure for 90–120 sec (Fig. 14–39). As in the superficial femoral artery, if several stenoses are to be dealt with, the

Fig. 14–38 Appearance of occluded superficial femoral artery before (A) and after (B) recanalization and angioplasty.

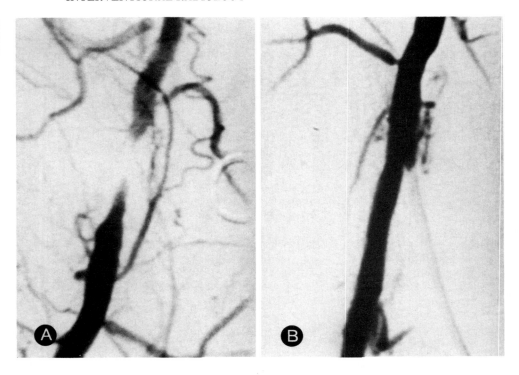

Fig. 14–39 Appearance of focal peroneal–tibial trunk stenosis before (A) and after (B) angioplasty with 3.5-mm balloon.

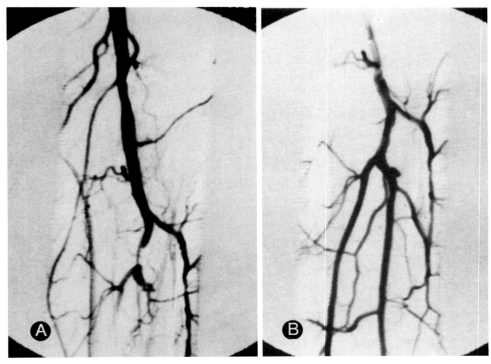

most distal lesion is dilated first and then the more proximal lesions (Fig. 14–40). The catheter tip can be retracted over the small guidewire and the guidewire left distally in the vessel while a documentary arteriogram is obtained by injecting contrast medium through the flushing port of the sheath.

If vasospasm is a problem despite nifedipine and nitroglycerin, multiple boluses of intra-arterial nitroglycerin can be administered, bearing in mind that the patient should be monitored constantly for systemic hypotension (Fig. 14–41). For the rare spasm that is not relieved by

nitroglycerin, intravascular verapamil may be administered if there is no contraindication to its use.

Upon completion of the procedure, the balloon catheter and guidewire are removed. Systemic heparinization is maintained for 48–72 hr.

Occlusions of the Distal Popliteal and Tibial Arteries

Angioplasty of distal vascular occlusions is considered only for limb salvage. The patient is premedicated with

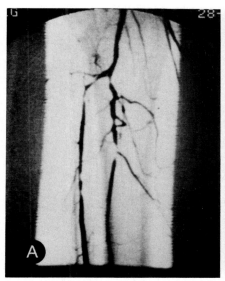
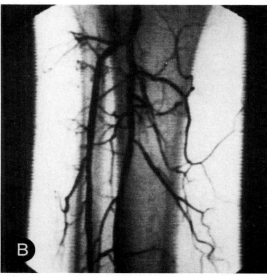

Fig. 14–40 Appearance before (A) and after (B) balloon angioplasty of multiple tibial lesions.

nifedipine, and the procedure is begun in the same fashion as for stenotic disease. Once the sheath is in the superficial femoral artery, a straight 5F Teflon catheter is advanced into the popliteal artery. With the catheter tip in this artery, a 100-μg bolus of nitroglycerin is administered. A tight-J small-diameter guidewire is advanced together with the catheter through the occluded segment of the vessel. The guidewire is removed, and intraluminal position is confirmed with a small volume of contrast medium. Heparin is administered via the arterial cathe-

ter, and an exchange is made for the angioplasty catheter over a 0.018-inch exchange guidewire. Angioplasty is completed as in the case of stenotic disease (Fig. 14–42). Once again, the patient is maintained on systemic heparin for 48–72 hr.

Anastomotic and Graft Stenoses

Szilagyi et al described the changes in reversed saphenous vein grafts used for peripheral bypass grafting.[42]

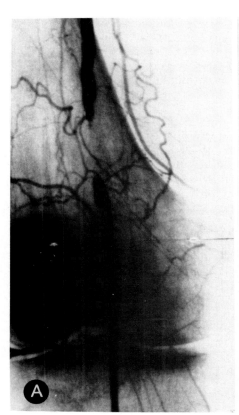
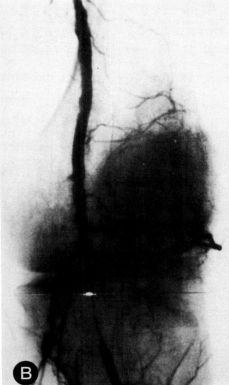
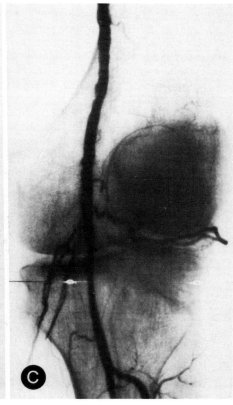

Fig. 14–41 Spasm compromising angioplasty result. A. Preangioplasty appearance of short-segment occlusion of proximal popliteal artery. B. Severe spasm after successful angioplasty compromises angioplasty site. C. Marked improvement in appearance of popliteal artery after bolus of 100 μg of intra-arterial nitroglycerin.

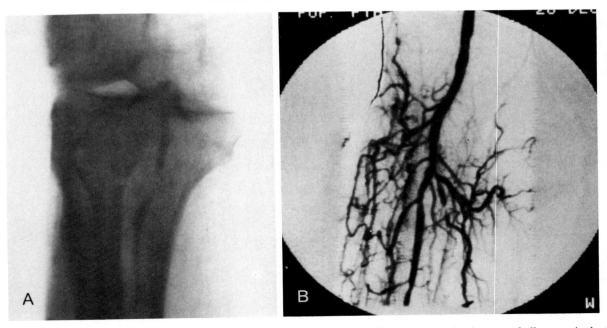

Fig. 14–42   Appearance before (A) and after (B) recanalization of occluded distal popliteal artery and subsequent balloon angioplasty.

Serial angiography revealed wavy narrowings of the vessel lumen that were attributed to intimal thickening, atherosclerosis, fibrotic valves, traumatic stenoses, suture stenoses, and aneurysmal dilatation. Intimal thickening and atherosclerosis were the most common findings, with atherosclerosis appearing similar to that in native arteries. All of the lesions observed by these investigators were progressive. Angioplasty is ideal for the management of stenoses at anastomoses of aortoiliac or aortofemoral bypass grafts, at anastomoses of reverse saphenous vein bypass grafts, or stenoses within saphenous vein bypass grafts, whereas reoperation through scar tissue is technically more difficult than the original procedure and carries greater risk.

Proximal and distal anastomotic stenoses associated with aortoiliac bypass grafts are approached in the same fashion as lesions in the native iliac arteries or abdominal aorta. The distal lesions are frequently secondary to clamp injury to the native vessel and the development of intimal thickening and will yield to PTA, although dilatation may require use of a high-pressure balloon. Restenoses are common, so repeated dilatations may be necessary.

Stenoses at the distal anastomosis of an aortofemoral bypass graft can be approached from the contralateral groin around the graft bifurcation. This requires the use of a sheath for introduction of the balloon catheter. Graft bifurcations are frequently acute, and it is usually technically difficult to reach the stenoses for angioplasty. Once again, the lesions may prove difficult but probably will yield, particularly when balloons of Mylar-type material are used.

Stenoses related to autogenous vein bypass grafts are suitable for angioplasty. The proper approach to a lesion at an anastomosis or within a graft depends on the location of the lesion. Proximal anastomotic lesions may be approached ipsilaterally or contralaterally, whereas lesions within the graft or at the distal anastomosis may be approached by antegrade puncture of the ipsilateral common femoral artery using a technique similar to that for stenotic disease of the native superficial femoral artery. Alternatively, the graft may be punctured directly (Fig. 14–43). Whenever scar tissue is traversed, a sheath is used to permit easy introduction and withdrawal of the balloon catheter.

COMPLICATIONS OF ANGIOPLASTY

Nearly every conceivable complication has been reported, but a list of likely problems includes the following:

1. Significant groin hematomas (2%–4% of angioplasty procedures);
2. Distal embolic complications (2%–5%); distal embolization *should not* occur except in occlusive vascular disease;
3. Elevation of intimal flaps (≤4%);
4. False aneurysms (≤2%);
5. Arterial rupture secondary to catheter or balloon trauma (rare in the iliac artery; approximately 3% in the superficial femoral artery);
6. Burst balloon with a circumferential tear (rare).

Hematomas at the puncture site can be minimized by consistently puncturing the common femoral artery, using the smallest suitable catheter, and using a sheath when several catheter exchanges are expected.

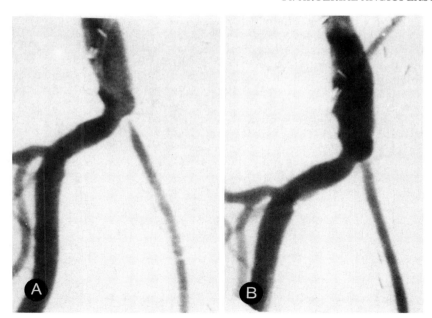

Fig. 14–43 Appearance of femoral–popliteal saphenous vein bypass graft stenoses before (A) and after (B) angioplasty.

Distal embolization is unavoidable in attempts to recanalize occluded native vessels. The incidence can be minimized by passing through occlusions with small-bore catheters and by not undertaking direct angioplasty of possibly recent occlusions, such that fresh thrombus will be present. The appropriate management of the embolism depends on the clinical status of the leg. If the limb remains viable, with intact sensation and motor function, attempts to deal with the embolism in the cardiovascular laboratory may be reasonable. Thrombolysis is unlikely to be of value, because the offending material is probably old, organized clot. However, it may be possible to aspirate the embolus into a nontapered large-bore catheter. Percutaneous Fogarty embolectomy also has been successful.[43] If these methods fail and the distal extremity remains viable, semielective surgical removal may be

planned. If distal embolization causes acute ischemia of the leg, spending time with percutaneous techniques is inappropriate, and the patient is best managed by urgent surgical removal of the embolism to decrease the risk of a compartment syndrome or loss of the limb.

Acute postangioplasty occlusion can be prevented by creating the optimum anatomic result whenever possible to maximize flow. When flow cannot be optimized, either because of a large intimal–medial disruption at the angioplasty site or because of poor runoff, systemic heparinization may avert acute thrombosis. Prevention of acute postangioplasty thrombosis is of particular value in patients with below-the-knee disease who are candidates for angioplasty for limb salvage, because these patients do not need long-term patency rates equivalent to those achieved in the more proximal vessels. That is, the goal

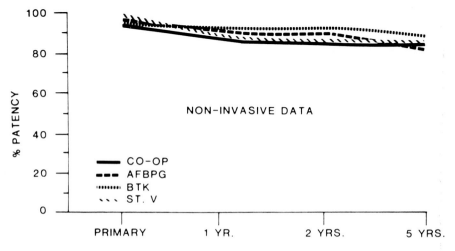

—Results in iliac PTA (short stenoses). CO-OP = cooperative study group; AFBPG = aortofemoral bypass graft; BTK = Barry T. Katzen, M.D.; ST.V. = St. Vincent's Hospital, Indianapolis.

Fig. 14–44 Results of angioplasty for short iliac stenoses.

is tissue healing, and this may occur in a relatively short time. Thereafter, even if the vessel reoccludes or restenoses, tissue breakdown will not necessarily recur.

When a balloon ruptures, the tear is usually longitudinal, and the balloon can be removed without difficulty. However, when the tear is circumferential, it is difficult to remove the balloon without excessive trauma at the site of insertion and extraction: therefore, the hub of the balloon catheter should be cut off and a sheath 1F–2F larger than the shaft of the catheter should be inserted to permit atraumatic extraction.[44]

Occasionally, immediately after an apparently successful angioplasty, the patient's foot will appear cold, mottled, and pale, suggesting distal embolization. Before catheter removal, an angiographic check of the distal vasculature should be made. If no evidence of distal embolization is observed, a 100-μg bolus of nitroglycerin should be administered through the catheter in an attempt to relieve what is probably distal vasospasm causing the "ugly foot" syndrome. Additional boluses of nitroglycerin may be necessary; occasionally, transdermal nitroglycerin is beneficial.

Restenoses may reasonably be considered a complication of angioplasty, and it appears that they are best avoided by using balloon catheters that produce the optimum anatomic result and by giving patients antiplatelet drugs postangioplasty. The patient who is motivated will refrain from cigarette smoking, will exercise appropriately, and, in general, will reduce his or her risk factors for atherosclerosis as much as possible.

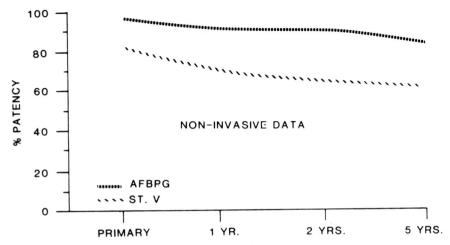

—Results in iliac PTA (long stenoses/occlusion). AFBPG = aortofemoral bypass graft; ST. V. = St. Vincent's Hospital, Indianapolis.

Fig. 14–45   Results of angioplasty for long iliac stenoses.

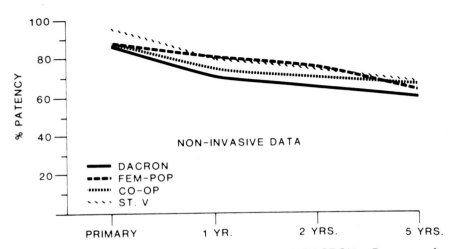

—Results in femoral PTA (short stenoses). DACRON = Dacron graft; FEM-POP = femoral-popliteal artery bypass graft; CO-OP = cooperative study group; ST.V = St. Vincent's Hospital, Indianapolis.

Fig. 14–46   Results of angioplasty for short superficial femoral stenoses.

RESULTS

The results of PTA are, as previously described, influenced by the preangioplasty anatomy. The 5-year patency rate in initially successful procedures involving the iliac arteries with short focal, concentric stenoses should approximate 90% given a 95% primary success rate. When longer segments of the iliac artery are subjected to angioplasty, the primary success rate drops to approximately 89% for stenotic lesions, and the 5-year patency rate drops to approximately 65% (Figs. 14–44 and 14–45).

Short stenoses of the superficial femoral and popliteal arteries can be dilated >90% of the time and will remain patent 5 years later in approximately 75% of patients

(Fig. 14–46). When longer or multiple stenoses are treated, a high primary success rate may be obtained, but the 5-year patency rate is only about 60% (Fig. 14–47).

Short occlusions of the superficial femoral and proximal popliteal arteries can be recanalized in 85%–90% of patients and will have a 70%–75% 5-year patency rate (Fig. 14–48). When longer occlusions are dilated, the primary success rate diminishes to approximately 80% and the 5-year patency rate to 60% (Fig. 14–49). In the author's experience, distal popliteal and tibial–peroneal angioplasty with the techniques described here has a primary success rate of 90% and an initial limb-healing rate of 92%.

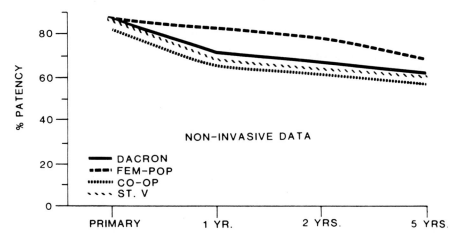

—Results in femoral PTA (long stenoses). DACRON = Dacron graft; FEM-POP = femoral-popliteal artery bypass graft; CO-OP = cooperative study group; ST. V. = St. Vincent's Hospital, Indianapolis.

Fig. 14–47 Results of angioplasty for long or multiple superficial femoral stenoses.

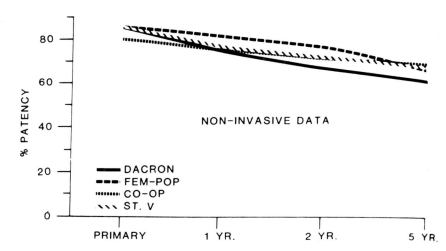

—Results in femoral PTA (short occlusion). DACRON = Dacron graft; FEM-POP = femoral-popliteal artery bypass graft; CO-OP = cooperative study group; ST. V. = St. Vincent's Hospital, Indianapolis.

Fig. 14–48 Results of angioplasty for short-segment occlusions in superficial femoral artery.

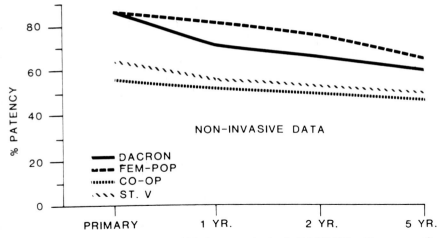

—Results in femoral PTA (long occlusion). DACRON = Dacron graft; FEM-POP = femoral -popliteal artery bypass graft; CO-OP = cooperative study group; ST. V. = St. Vincent's Hospital, Indianapolis.

Fig. 14–49 Results of angioplasty for long-segment occlusions in superficial femoral artery.

References

1. Dotter CT, Judkins MP: Transluminal treatment of arteriosclerotic obstruction: description of a new technique and a preliminary report of its application. *Circulation* 1964;36:654
2. Staple TW: Modified catheter for percutaneous transluminal treatment of arteriosclerotic obstructions. *Radiology* 1968; 91:1041
3. Van Andel GJ: *Percutaneous Transluminal Angioplasty: The Dotter Procedure.* Amsterdam, Excerpta Medica, 1976
4. Zeitler E, Grüntzig A, Schoop W (eds): *Percutaneous Vascular Recanalization: Technology, Application, Clinical Results.* Berlin, Springer–Verlag, 1978
5. Porstmann W: Ein neur Korsett-Balloon-Katheter zur transluminalen Rekanalisation nach Dotter unter besonderer Berucksichtigung von obliterationen an den Beckenarterien. *Radiol Diag (Berl)* 1973;14:239
6. Grüntzig A, Hopff M: Perkutane Rekanalisation chronischer arterieller Verschlusse mit einem neuer Dilatations Katheter: Modifikation der Dotter-Technik. *Dtsch Med Wochenschr* 1974;99:2502
7. Grüntzig A, Vetter W, Meier B, Kuhlman U, Lotoff U, Sigenthaler W: Treatment of renovascular hypertension with percutaneous transluminal dilatation of renal-artery stenosis. *Lancet* 1978;1:801
8. Grüntzig A: Transluminal dilatation of coronary-artery stenosis (letter). *Lancet* 1978;1:263
9. Tegtmeyer CJ, Kellum CD, Ayers C: Percutaneous transluminal angioplasty of the renal artery: results and long term follow-up. *Radiology* 1984;153:77
10. Spence RK, Freiman DB, Gatenby R, et al: Long term results of transluminal angioplasty of the iliac and femoral arteries. *Arch Surg* 1981;116:1377
11. Grüntzig A: Percutaneous transluminal angioplasty: six years experience. *Am Heart J* 1984;107:818
12. Motarjeme A, Kiefer JW, Zuska AJ: Percutaneous transluminal angioplasty of the brachiocephalic arteries. *AJR* 1982;138:457
13. Schwarten DE: Transluminal angioplasty: overview of complications and long term results. *ARRS Categorical Course on Interventional Radiology,* April 21, 1985
14. Waltman AC, Greenfield AJ, Novelline RA, et al: Transluminal angioplasty of iliac and femoropopliteal arteries. *Arch Surg* 1982;117:1218
15. Tamura S, Sniderman KW, Beinart C, Sos TA: Percutaneous transluminal angioplasty of the popliteal artery and its branches. *Radiology* 1982;143:645
16. Greenfield AJ: Femoral, popliteal and tibial arteries: percutaneous transluminal angioplasty. *AJR* 1980;135:927
17. Katzen BT: Transluminal angioplasty of the iliac arteries, in Castañeda–Zuñiga WR (ed): *Transluminal Angioplasty.* New York, Thieme–Stratton, 1983, p 93
18. Friedman MH, Katzen BT: Noninvasive evaluation procedures, in Castañeda–Zuñiga WR (ed): *Transluminal Angioplasty.* New York, Thieme–Stratton, 1983, p 48
19. Motarjeme A, Keiger JW, Zuska AK: Percutaneous transluminal angioplasty and case selection. *Radiology* 1980;135:573
20. Schoop W: Indications for PTA from the angiologic point of view, in Zeitler E, Grüntzig A, Schoop W (eds): *Percutaneous Vascular Recanalization.* Berlin, Springer–Verlag, 1978
21. Zeitler E, Richter EL, Roth FJ, Schoop W: *Results of Percutaneous Transluminal Angioplasty.* Berlin, Springer–Verlag, 1985
22. Block PC, Fallon JT, Elmer D: Experimental angioplasty: lessons from the laboratory. *AJR* 1980;135:907
23. Castañeda–Zuñiga WR, Formanek AG, Tadavarthy SM, et al: Mechanism of balloon angioplasty. *Radiology* 1980;135:565
24. Castañeda–Zuñiga WR, Laerum F, Rysavy JA, Rusnak BW, Amplatz K: Paralysis of arteries by intraluminal balloon dilatation: an experimental study. *Radiology* 1982;144:74
25. Probst P, Cerny P, Owen A, Mahler F: Patency after femoral angioplasty: correlation of angiographic appearance with clinical findings. *AJR* 1983;140:1227
26. Tegtmeyer CT, Kellum CD, Ayers C: Percutaneous transluminal angioplasty of the renal artery. *Radiology* 1984;153:77
27. Kaltenbach M, Beyer J, Walter S, et al: Prolonged application of pressure in transluminal coronary angioplasty. *Catheter Cardiovasc Diagn* 1984;10:213
28. Wolf GL: Pharmacology of angioplasty. Presented at the 10th Annual Course on Diagnostic Angiography and Interventional Radiology, Society of Cardiovascular and Interventional Radiology, Orlando, FL, March 1985
29. Grollman JR Jr, Delvicario M, Mittal AK: Percutaneous transluminal abdominal aortic angioplasty. *AJR* 1980;134:1053

30. Velasquez G, Castañeda–Zuñiga W, Formanek A, et al: Nonsurgical angioplasty in Leriche syndrome. *Radiology* 1980;134:359

31. Bachman DM, Casarella WJ, Sos TA: Percutaneous iliofemoral angioplasty via the contralateral femoral artery. *Radiology* 1979;130:61

32. Katzen BT, Chang J, Knox WG: Percutaneous transluminal angioplasty with the Grüntzig balloon catheter: a review of 70 cases. *Arch Surg* 1979;114:1389

33. Waltman AC, Courey WR, Athanasoulis C, et al: Technique for left gastric artery catheterization. *Radiology* 1973;109:732

34. Ring EJ, Freiman DB, McLean GK, et al: Percutaneous recanalization of common iliac artery occlusion: an unacceptable complication rate? *AJR* 1982;139:587

35. Kaufman SL: Femoral puncture using Doppler ultrasound guidance: aid to transluminal angioplasty and other applications. *AJR* 1980;134:402

36. Auster M, Kadir S, Mitchell SE, et al: Iliac artery occlusion: management with intrathrombus streptokinase infusion and angioplasty. *Radiology* 1984;153:385

37. Greenfield AJ: Percutaneous transluminal angioplasty of the femoral, popliteal and tibial vessels, in Athanasoulis CA, Pfister RC, Greene RE, Roberson GH (eds): *Interventional Radiology.* Philadelphia, WB Saunders, 1982

38. Sos TA: The influence of recent advances in equipment and techniques on indications and results of angioplasty of the popliteal artery and its branches. *Intervention USCI,* Spring 1985

39. Freiman DB, McLean GK, Oleaga JA, Ring EJ: Percutaneous transluminal angioplasty, in Ring EJ, McLean GK (eds): *Interventional Radiology: Principles and Techniques.* Boston, Little, Brown & Co, 1981

40. Barth KH: Modified catheter for transluminal angioplasty of the femoral popliteal artery. *Radiology* 1983;149:598

41. Ricketts HJ: Presented at the Members Meeting, Society of Cardiovascular and Interventional Radiology, Napa, CA, February 1984

42. Szilagyi DE, Elliott JP, Hageman SH, et al: Biologic fate of autogenous vein grafts implanted as arterial substitutes. *Ann Surg* 1973;78:232

43. Hayden W: Presented at a Round Table discussion on distal percutaneous transluminal angioplasty. Washington, DC, November 1984

44. Tegtmeyer CJ, Bezirdjian DR: Removing the stuck, ruptured angioplasty balloon catheter. *Radiology* 1981;139:231

15

Percutaneous Transluminal Angioplasty of the Renal Arteries

CHARLES J. TEGTMEYER, M.D., AND CHARLES D. KELLUM, M.D.

Data from the United States National Health Examination Survey indicate that hypertension (blood pressure ≥160/95 mm Hg) occurs in 10%–15% of the adult population.[1] Of this group of approximately 23 million persons, 1 million (≃4%) have potentially correctable renovascular hypertension.[2] Coronary artery disease, stroke, and renal failure have all been unequivocally related to uncontrolled hypertension,[3,4] and hypertension of the renovascular type poses the additional threat of progressive renal insufficiency.

Pharmacotherapy and surgical revascularization, the traditional modes of treatment for renovascular hypertension, have significant shortcomings. For example, in many cases, drugs only partially control blood pressure; and when several drugs are combined, side effects and poor patient compliance can become a problem.[5–7] Also, if the renal artery is severely stenotic, lowering the blood pressure with drugs further reduces renal blood flow, sometimes leading to ischemic atrophy or even renal infarction. Hunt et al proved that surgical correction of renovascular hypertension was superior to medical therapy. With 7–14 years of follow-up, 84% of their surgically treated patients were alive, in contrast to only 60% of those treated medically.[8] Therefore, whenever possible, the treatment of choice for renovascular hypertension is correction of the renal artery stenosis. However, operation requires general anesthesia, and many patients are poor risks because of severe diffuse atherosclerotic disease, renal insufficiency, or both. Moreover, surgical results vary, there is considerable morbidity, and the mortality rate can be as high as 5.9%.[9] Therefore, although surgery and medical therapy have significant benefits in spite of these shortcomings,[10,11] there is no question that alternative treatments are desirable.

Grüntzig reported the first successful balloon dilatation of renal artery stenosis in 1978.[12] In the relatively short period since then, several articles detailing the results of percutaneous transluminal angioplasty (PTA) in large series have been published.[13–21] The preliminary data suggest that PTA is highly successful in correcting renal artery stenosis. Only a few series have described the long-term results of renal angioplasty,[22–25] but more definitive analyses of the long-term results are now emerging.[26,27]

RENAL ARTERY STENOSES

Etiology

There are many causes of stenoses in the renal arteries, but the majority of the lesions are atherosclerotic in origin and most of the remainder are due to fibromuscular dysplasia. For example, in the 884 hypertensive patients with renal artery lesions among the 2442 patients in the Cooperative Study on Hypertension, atherosclerosis was the cause in 557 (63.0%), fibromuscular hyperplasia in 286 (32.4%), and miscellaneous diseases in 41 (4.6%).[10] In the University of Virginia series, atherosclerosis was the cause of the stenosis or occlusion in 75 patients, who had 93 lesions dilated, and fibromuscular dysplasia was the cause of 30 stenoses in 27 patients. Seven patients had stenoses in the arteries to renal allografts, and three patients had lesions in saphenous vein bypass grafts. One patient had his native artery dilated after his saphenous bypass graft occluded, and one patient had three stenoses due to previous irradiation.[26]

Significance

Renovascular hypertension can be defined as hypertension caused by obstruction of the main renal artery or one of its branches. The difficulty in making the diagnosis of true renovascular hypertension only begins with identification of an anatomic obstruction, however. The temptation to dilate a renal artery stenosis once discovered is great, especially because the absence of lateralization of renin production does not preclude a response to correction of the stenosis in 21% of patients.[28] However, in 1956, Homer Smith pointed out that only 26% of patients undergoing a nephrectomy for apparently unilateral renovascular hypertension were normotensive at the end of 1 year.[29] Eyler et al studied the arteriograms of normotensive and hypertensive adults and found significant renal artery stenoses in both groups,[30] and Holley and associates found renal artery stenosis at autopsy in 49% of patients who had been normotensive during life.[31]

Therefore, once renal artery stenosis is identified in a hypertensive patient, the physiologic importance of the lesion should be assessed. If the physiologic significance of the lesion is not ascertained, optimal angioplasty results will not be achieved.

INDICATIONS FOR RENOVASCULAR EVALUATION

It is not feasible or cost effective to evaluate completely all patients who have hypertension for renovascular disease. The criteria for workup vary from one medical center to another; however, certain patients have an increased risk of renovascular hypertension and should be evaluated:

1. Those with a documented sudden onset of hypertension;
2. Those without a family history of hypertension or other identifiable secondary causes;
3. Young women who develop hypertension and are not taking oral contraceptives;
4. Patients, especially whites, who develop malignant hypertension;
5. Those with long-standing hypertension who suddenly develop accelerated hypertension;
6. Those who are refractory, or who become refractory, to antihypertensive drugs other than blockers of the renin–angiotensin system;
7. Those with a flank bruit;
8. Those who suffer renal insufficiency while taking captopril.

The evaluation protocol also varies with the institution. Initially, peripheral blood may be assayed for renin; if the concentration is elevated, selective samples are obtained from both renal veins and from the inferior vena cava. This test can be performed on an outpatient basis, and an intravenous digital subtraction angiography (DSA) study can be obtained at the same time. However, intravenous radiologic studies may miss subtle lesions caused by fibromuscular dysplasia or branch stenoses. Therefore, if the renin concentrations are elevated and the DSA study is negative, an arteriogram should be obtained. Alternatively, in patients strongly suspected of having angiotensiogenic hypertension, renal vein renin sampling and an arteriogram can be performed on the same day. If the patient has impaired renal function, an intra-arterial digital study can be performed. Intra-arterial digital studies are far superior to intravenous ones, as they have better resolution and require less contrast medium.

INDICATIONS FOR RENAL ANGIOPLASTY

The indications for renal angioplasty include relief of proved renovascular hypertension or of the angiotensiogenic component in patients with both essential and renovascular hypertension. Many of the patients in the University of Virginia series have a long history of hypertension with recent acceleration due to superimposed renal disease. In patients with deteriorating renal function, renal angioplasty may be indicated, because if there are underlying renal artery stenoses, correction of these lesions may preserve or improve renal function.

TECHNIQUES

Since the introduction of renal angioplasty by Grüntzig et al in 1978, the technique has been refined and simplified.[19] Nonetheless, renal angioplasty remains more complex than peripheral angioplasty. It is far from innocuous and should be performed only by angiographers who have considerable experience dilating peripheral vessels. Inflating the balloon is simple, but crossing a tight renal stenosis with a balloon catheter requires great skill; and selection of the proper size balloon requires experience.

A high-quality preliminary midstream arteriogram is necessary to determine the approach. Unless an abdominal arteriogram has been obtained within the previous month, this study should always be obtained before catheterizing the renal arteries, because profound changes may occur in a short time in the presence of a tight renal artery stenosis.

There are four percutaneous angiographic approaches to the treatment of stenoses in the renal arteries with Grüntzig-type balloons:

1. Guided coaxial balloon catheter system;
2. Femoral balloon catheter system via a femoral approach;
3. Femoral balloon catheter system via an axillary approach;
4. Femoral balloon catheter system with the sidewinder approach.

Each will be discussed.

Guided Coaxial Balloon Catheter System

The Grüntzig-type guided coaxial balloon catheter system utilizes an 8F or 9F renal guiding catheter and a 4.3F or 4.5F coaxial balloon catheter (Fig. 15–1). The renal guiding catheter is available in three configurations (Fig.15–2). It is inserted by a femoral approach, and the orifice of the renal artery is carefully selected. The small coaxial catheter is then passed through the guiding catheter across the stenosis. The balloon catheter will accept a 0.014- or 0.016-inch guidewire, which can be passed across the stenosis before advancing the coaxial catheter to facilitate traversing a tight stenosis. With the advent of the new platinum wires, which are easily visible radiologically, this is a very effective technique. In the presence of a tortuous renal vessel, a tight stenosis, or a ste-

Fig. 15-1 Technique of renal dilatation with the coaxial balloon catheter
system. A. Stenosis in left renal artery.
B. Orifice of renal artery is selected
with guiding catheter. C. The 4.5F dilatation catheter is directed through stenosis by guiding catheter and inflated,
dilating the stenosis. D. Intima is split,
and portion of media is stretched or
spilt, relieving the obstruction in the
renal artery. (Reproduced from Tegtmeyer CJ, Dyer R, Teates CD, et al:
Percutaneous transluminal dilatation
of the renal arteries: techniques and
results. *Radiology* 1980;135:589–599.)

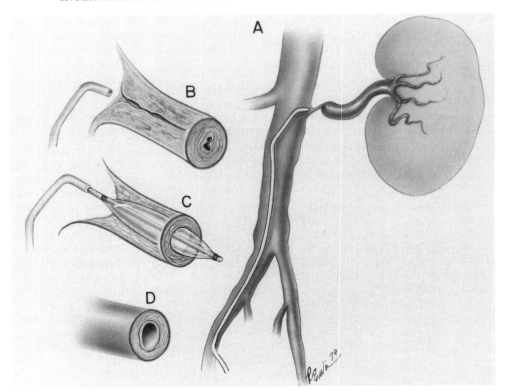

Fig. 15-2 The renal guiding catheter is
available in three basic configurations; the
choice for a particular procedure depends on
size of aorta and angle that renal artery
takes as it branches from aorta.

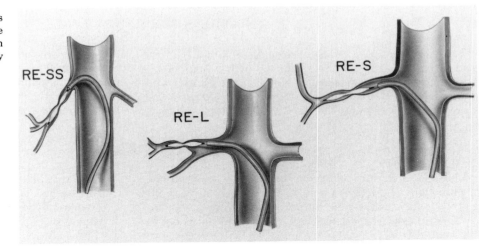

nosis in a branch, the fine guidewire greatly facilitates passage of the balloon catheter. If the stenosis is not too tight, the coaxial catheter can be advanced across it without the guidewire while injecting a small amount of contrast medium.

The advantage of this coaxial technique is that the small catheter passes through the tight stenosis more readily than does the 7F balloon catheter. It is also easy to steer this catheter out into the branches of the renal artery. Therefore, this catheter system is usually used for a tight stenosis that cannot be passed by other techniques or for the treatment of distal or branch stenoses. There are several disadvantages to the technique, however. For example, the catheters are expensive, and it is necessary to make an 8F or 9F puncture wound in the femoral

artery. Also, the guiding catheter is stiff and may damage the aortic wall, and it is inserted over a 0.063-inch guidewire that also is quite stiff and thus potentially traumatic. Balloons are available from 2–5 mm, but if an 8F guiding system is used, the balloon catheter can be no larger than 3 mm.

This technique is more complex than the standard femoral balloon catheter technique. The common femoral artery is punctured, and a two-part sheath is introduced over a 0.038-inch guidewire. The sheath is advanced into the distal abdominal aorta, its inner cannula is removed, and the 0.063-inch guidewire is advanced into the aorta as far as the diaphragm. The guiding catheter is then advanced over the guidewire through the sheath and into the abdominal aorta. The guidewire is removed, and the guiding catheter is used to select the renal artery orifice. The balloon catheter is then advanced through the guiding catheter and across the stenosis. The small diameter of the balloon makes it possible to measure the pressure gradient across the stenosis. The balloon is inflated with a 1:1 mixture of contrast medium and in (0.9%) saline. Balloon inflation and the progress of the angioplasty can be monitored by injecting contrast medium through either the balloon catheter or the guiding catheter, which is a definite advantage. However, because of the dilatation injury to the intima, caution should be exercised when injecting contrast medium near the dilatation site.

Femoral Balloon Catheter System via a Femoral Approach

This technique involves a modification of the double-lumen balloon catheter designed by Grüntzig for angioplasty of superficial arteries (Fig. 15–3). Only catheters with a low-profile balloon located close to the catheter tip should be utilized in the renal arteries. In tight stenoses, it is important not to prepare the balloon before inserting it, because this may interfere with passage through the stenosis. The 7F Grüntzig-type balloon catheters are most often used, although in children or in other patients with small arteries, a 5F catheter system may be preferable.

The femoral artery is punctured, and the appropriate

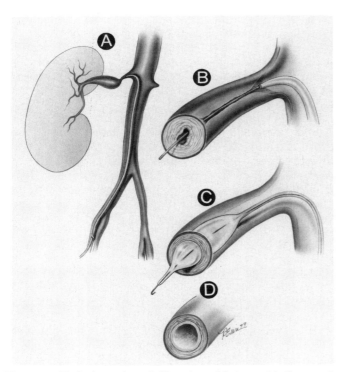

Fig. 15–3 Technique of renal dilatation with femoral balloon catheter system via femoral approach. A. Stenotic right renal artery is catheterized selectively with cobra catheter. B. Guidewire is passed through stenosis. C. Selective catheter is exchanged for dilation catheter, and balloon is inflated, compressing stenosis. D. Obstruction is now relieved. (Reproduced from Tegtmeyer CJ, Dyer R, Teates CD, et al: Percutaneous transluminal dilatation of the renal arteries: techniques and results. *Radiology* 1980;135:589–599.)

5F diagnostic catheter is advanced into the abdominal aorta using the Seldinger technique. The orifice of the renal artery is carefully selected, and contrast medium is injected to locate the lesion. Under fluoroscopic guidance, a 0.035-inch tight-J or a 0.035-inch Bentson guidewire is advanced beyond the stenosis. If these guidewires will not pass, the lesion can often be traversed with a 15-mm J-guidewire. It is imperative to avoid subintimal passage of the guidewire. Once the stenosis has been crossed, the 5F selective catheter should be passed across it, because this facilitates subsequent passage of the balloon catheter. A small amount of contrast medium is injected to confirm the intraluminal position of the catheter, and 2000–3000 units of heparin are injected through the catheter. A movable-core type-J or a Rosen wire is then inserted through the catheter beyond the stenosis, and the diagnostic catheter is replaced with the appropriate size renal balloon catheter, chosen by measuring the renal artery proximal and distal to the stenosis (Fig. 15–4) and estimating the original size of the renal artery. If the artery is estimated to have been 5 mm in diameter, this is the balloon size that should be used. Because this method does not take radiographic magnification into account, the renal arteries are being slightly (approximately 1 mm) overdilated. The guidewire must not be moved back and forth in the branches of the renal artery when exchanging the catheters, because this may induce spasm or cause occlusion of the segmental branches.

If the balloon catheter will not cross the stenosis, a 5F catheter with a 3-mm balloon is passed across the lesion and inflated, partially dilating the stenosis. The proper size balloon catheter can then be advanced easily across the stenosis.

The balloon catheter is positioned in the lesion under fluoroscopic control, and the balloon is inflated, either with a USCI inflation device or with a syringe. If a syringe is used, a 10-ml type is probably ideal, because it is capable of generating approximately 9.4 atm of pressure during inflation and sufficient negative pressure to deflate the balloon rapidly. A pressure gauge should always be used. The balloon is first inflated to 2 atm of pressure to determine its position in relation to the stenosis. When it is properly positioned, it is inflated to 4–6 atm and left inflated for 30–40 sec. It may be necessary to repeat this several times. The progress can be monitored by watching the configuration of the balloon as it is inflated. The 0.035-inch wire is then replaced with a 0.025-inch wire, and a Tuohy–Borst connector is attached. The balloon is carefully pulled back, and contrast medium is injected to assess the results. With a 0.025-inch wire in place, the balloon catheter can be readvanced if the lesion requires further dilatation. Immediately after angioplasty, an arteriogram is performed to assess the results. Before removing the balloon catheter, it is important to deflate the balloon completely and to apply suction as it is being removed from the femoral artery.

The primary advantage of this technique is that only a 5F or 7F puncture wound is needed in the femoral artery. If the stenosis permits easy passage of the balloon, this is the simplest approach. However, if the stenosis is tight or the renal artery branches from the aorta at an acute angle, the balloon catheter may be reluctant to follow the

Fig. 15–4 Balloon catheter is selected to correspond to original diameter of stenotic renal artery; post-stenotic dilatation must be taken into account. Because renal arteries are magnified by 15%–20% on standard angiograms, arteries will be overdilated by approximately 1 mm. (Reproduced from Tegtmeyer CJ, Kellum CD, Ayers C: Percutaneous transluminal angioplasty of the renal arteries. *Radiology* 1984;153:77–84.)

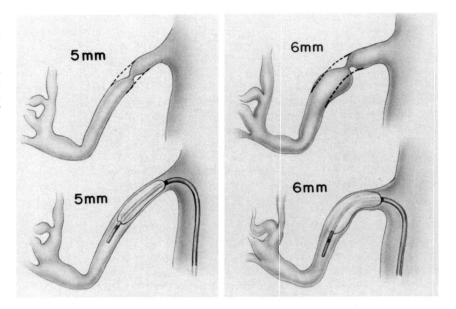

guidewire across the lesion, because it has a tendency to buckle in the aorta when pressure is applied. This difficulty may often be overcome by advancing the 5F diagnostic catheter first and then either a 7F tapered Van Andel or the 3-mm balloon catheter as described, and then reinserting the balloon catheter.

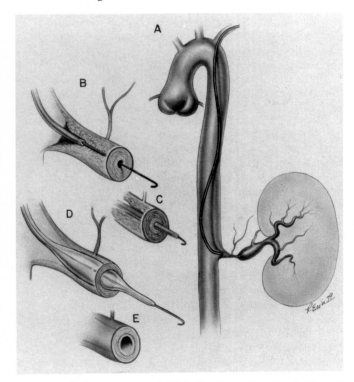

Fig. 15–5 Technique of renal dilatation through axilla. A. Stenotic left renal artery is selected with diagnostic cobra catheter. B. Guidewire is passed through stenosis. C. Cobra catheter is advanced through stenosis. D. Selective catheter is replaced with dilatation catheter, which is inflated. E. Stenosis is now relieved. (Reproduced from Tegtmeyer CJ, Dyer R, Teates CD, et al: Percutaneous transluminal dilatation of the renal arteries: techniques and results. *Radiology* 1980;135:589–599.)

Femoral Balloon Catheter System via an Axillary Approach

The axillary approach may also be used to dilate the renal arteries (Fig. 15–5).[32] This approach greatly simplifies the procedure when the renal arteries originate from the aorta at a sharp angle, because the stenotic artery is easily selected. Once the guidewire is in place across the lesion, the dilatation catheter has a natural tendency to follow its gentle downward curve. Passage of the guidewire and then the catheter through the stenosis is often facilitated by having the patient take a deep breath. The axillary approach is also useful when severe atherosclerotic disease or a bypass graft is present in the pelvic or abdominal vessels.

This technique also uses the double-lumen balloon catheter designed by Grüntzig for superficial femoral artery angioplasty. The balloon is available for renal angioplasty in 4-mm through 8-mm sizes and in several lengths. The 2-cm-long balloon is the most popular. A left axillary approach is usually taken because it offers the straightest approach to the descending aorta and because the catheter has a tendency to buckle in the ascending aorta when the right axillary approach is attempted. The technique is otherwise similar to that of the femoral approach.

Theoretically, there is an increased risk of damage to the smaller axillary artery; however, this can be minimized by deflating the balloon carefully and rotating it as it is being inserted and removed. There is also the possibility of brachial plexus injury, the chances of which can be minimized by using the high brachial approach, in which the artery is entered just distal to the axillary crease. The artery is easier to control in this area because it can be compressed against the humerus.

Femoral Balloon Catheter System via a Sidewinder Approach

The sidewinder approach combines the advantages of the femoral and axillary approaches (Fig. 15–6). The

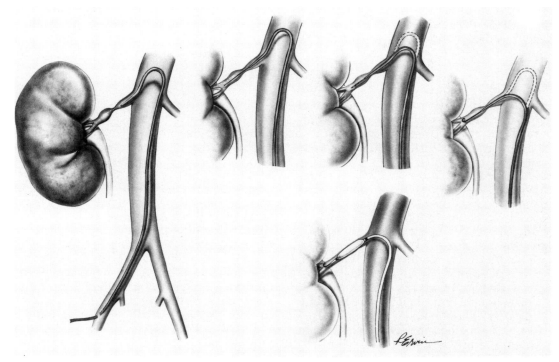

Fig. 15–6 Technique of renal angioplasty using shepherd's crook catheter. After selection of appropriate renal artery, flexible-tip guidewire is advanced through lesion under fluoroscopic control. Catheter is advanced across stenosis by withdrawing the catheter at the puncture site. The guidewire is then exchanged for heavy-duty tight-J wire, and appropriate balloon catheter is inserted to dilate lesion.

same 7F Grüntzig-type double-lumen balloon catheter used in the femoral approach is again used. The femoral artery is punctured, but the renal artery is approached from above in order to take advantage of its natural curve. It is selected with a 5F "shepherd's crook" or "sidewinder" catheter, which is advanced across the lesion under fluoroscopic control as contrast medium is injected, with care to keep the tip within the lumen of the artery. Alternatively, a flexible-tip guidewire is advanced across the stenosis and followed by the catheter. Once the catheter is across the lesion, 2000–3000 units of heparin are injected through it. The guidewire is replaced with a movable-core J-guidewire or a Rosen wire. The diagnostic catheter is then exchanged for the appropriate size renal balloon catheter. After the sidewinder catheter has crossed the lesion, the balloon catheter will usually cross with ease. After dilatation, a midstream arteriogram is obtained to document the results.

The principal advantage of this technique is that withdrawing the sidewinder catheter advances the diagnostic catheter even across a tight stenosis because the configuration of the catheter exerts considerable downward force as it is withdrawn over the guidewire. This technique is very helpful in traversing tight stenoses.

PERIPROCEDURAL MANAGEMENT

Proper management of candidates for renal angioplasty requires a team approach. The proper selection of patients and the management of the blood pressure require the close cooperation of a hypertension specialist. Also, inadvertent occlusion of the renal artery may create a surgical emergency, so the procedure should be performed only when a skilled vascular surgeon is available.

The blood pressure must be monitored especially carefully during the first 24–48 hr after angioplasty because profound changes may occur. It is important to discontinue the antihypertensive drugs before angioplasty, thereby helping to prevent a precipitous drop in the blood pressure. If the diastolic pressure rises above 110 mm Hg, the blood pressure should be controlled by cap-topril or short-acting antihypertensive drugs. A drop in blood pressure can usually be controlled by rapid intravenous infusion of saline. Therefore, all patients undergoing renal angioplasty should have an intravenous line in place.

If not contraindicated, the patient receives 2000 units of heparin subcutaneously every 6 hr beginning 8 hr after the procedure and continuing for 2 days. The patient also receives 75 mg of dipyridamole (Persantine) orally twice a day and 325 mg of acetylsalicylic acid once a day beginning the day before angioplasty and continuing for at least 6 months. The patients are strongly encouraged to stop smoking. After angioplasty, the patients should be monitored by a cardiologist or nephrologist who specializes in the control of high blood pressure. The patient's need for antihypertensive drugs changes after a successful procedure, so blood pressure must be monitored closely. If the blood pressure rises in the ensuing months, arteriography or DSA should be repeated.

COMPLICATIONS

Because renal angioplasty is more complex than peripheral angioplasty, and because the potential complications are serious, the procedure should be performed only in hospitals where a skilled vascular surgeon is immediately available.

The complication rate of renal angioplasty ranges from 5%–10%, with most complications being minor. The most frequent major complication is transient renal insufficiency, which clearly is related to the contrast medium. The frequency can be reduced by performing the diagnostic arteriogram several days before the therapeutic procedure in patients with renal insufficiency. Subintimal dissection with the guidewire or the diagnostic catheter may result when attempting to cross the stenosis. A small intimal flap will usually heal, but angioplasty should be postponed for 4–6 weeks. Thrombosis of the renal artery infrequently follows balloon dilatation. This complication is sometimes treated by infusing streptokinase into the renal artery, but it is vital that sufficient collateral vessels be present if this approach is selected so that renal ischemia does not develop while one is waiting for the enzyme to work. Another, rare, major complication is rupture of the renal artery, which may result from weakening of the wall or from subintimal placement of the balloon catheter. If rupture is noted immediately after deflation of the balloon, the balloon should be reinflated to occlude the proximal renal artery, and the patient should be operated on immediately. Distal embolization is an infrequent complication, but a recently occluded renal artery should be approached with caution, because thrombi may be dislodged by the catheter to occlude segmental branches.

The most frequent minor complication is spasm or occlusion of a renal arterial branch (Fig 15–7), usually caused by movement of the tip of the guidewire back and forth within the vessel. If possible, the guidewire should not be placed within the segmental branches. Focal spasm may also be produced in the area immediately adjacent to the angioplasty site. Calcium channel blockers prevent and reverse spasm in the renal arteries. Nifedipine is the most potent vasodilator among the calcium antagonist drugs and can be given in a dose of 20 mg sublingually at the outset of the procedure. If spasm occurs, verapamil may be given through the arterial catheter in a dose of 2.5–5 mg. Also, because the mechanism of action of nitroglycerin differs from that of the calcium antagonists, and since it has an additive effect with the calcium channel blockers, it may be useful against spasm in the renal arteries. It is either injected directly into the affected renal artery (50–200 μg) or given sublingually (0.4–0.6 mg). Calcium channel blockers may induce hypotension and should be used with caution in patients with known cardiac conduction defects.

In addition to these complications unique to renal angioplasty, there may be complications at the puncture site. The principal complication is formation of a large hematoma. Because the patient is receiving anticoagulants and there are frequent catheter exchanges when using the axillary approach, the operator should be careful to puncture high in the brachial artery and not in the axilla itself to avoid the devastating effects, including brachial plexus injury, of a large hematoma in the axilla.

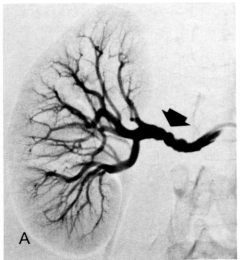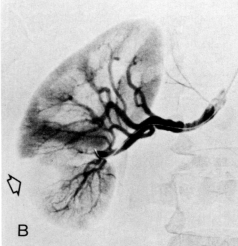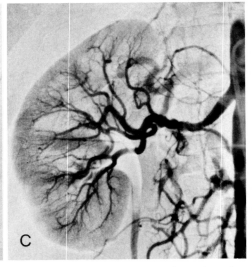

Fig. 15–7 Renal parenchymal defect caused by guidewire during angioplasty procedure. A. Selective renal arteriogram reveals changes consistent with fibromuscular dysplasia (arrow). B. Immediately after dilatation, angiogram demonstrates defect in lower pole of kidney (arrow), apparently caused by guidewire, which is still in place. C. Arteriogram obtained 3 months later shows resolution of defect. Renal arteries are widely patent. (Reproduced from Tegtmeyer CJ, Teates CD, Crigler N: Percutaneous transluminal angioplasty in patients with renal artery stenosis: follow-up studies. *Radiology* 1981;140:323–330.)

RESULTS

In experienced hands, renal angioplasty is highly effective in correcting renal artery lesions. An initial success rate of >90% should be achieved when dilating stenoses (Table 15–1). Technical failures usually result from an inability to cross the lesion or insufficient dilatation.

The long-term results of renal angioplasty can be assessed in three ways: the effect on vessel patency, on blood pressure, and on renal function. The effect of the procedure on vessel patency is related to the cause and characteristics of the lesion. The patients can be divided into five distinct groups:

1. Those with atherosclerotic renal artery stenoses or occlusions;
2. Those with fibromuscular dysplasia;
3. Those with renal allografts;
4. Those with saphenous bypass grafts;
5. Those treated primarily for renal insufficiency.

Atherosclerotic Lesions

Atherosclerotic disease is the most frequent cause of stenoses subjected to renal dilatation. In the University of Virginia series, 94% of the 65 hypertensive patients with atherosclerotic lesions were helped by the procedure: 15 were cured, and 46 improved.

Analysis of the results in these patients revealed some factors that are important to the success of renal angioplasty. First, better results are achieved with unilateral renal artery stenoses than with bilateral stenoses, because the restenosis rate is higher in patients with severe bilateral disease than in those with unilateral stenosis.[26] Sos et al[25] and Martin and associates[27] also showed that suc-cess was more frequent in patients with unilateral lesions. Second, it is becoming increasingly clear that certain lesions are more amenable to balloon dilatation than are others. For example, good results can be expected in short isolated lesions (Fig. 15–8), whereas when the stenosis is caused by a large plaque in the abdominal aorta that engulfs the origin of the renal artery (Fig. 15–9), the chances of success are diminished. Figure 15–10 illustrates the type of lesion in which this diminished response is often obtained. Cicuto et al,[33] Sos et al,[25] and Schwarten[34] all reported similar results. In the University of Virginia series, one-third of the lesions requiring redilation were caused by aortic plaques that engulfed the origin of the renal artery. Finally, complete blocks are more difficult to dilate than are stenoses, and one should not try to dilate complete blocks that are not perfectly straight.

Table 15–1
Results of Percutaneous Transluminal Renal Angioplasty

No. of Patients	Initial Success (% of Patients)	Patency Rate after Initial Success (% Patients)	Follow-up (Years)
68	85	81	3
17	94[a]	74[a]	1
54	96	70	1
70	93[a]	71	0.5
101	79	–	1
109	95	93[b]	5
100	88	70	3
519	79–95	70–90	

[a]Percentage of lesions.
[b]Includes successful redilations.

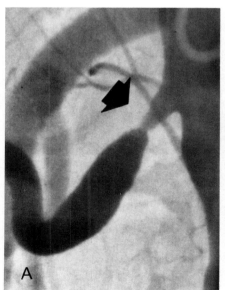
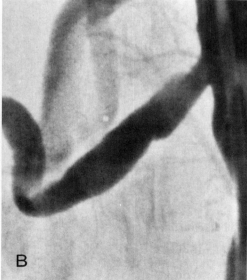
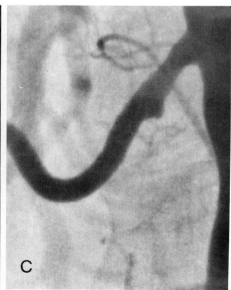

Fig. 15–8 Successful dilatation of short atherosclerotic lesion in 51-year-old woman with 12-year history of hypertension. A. Midstream arteriogram reveals tight stenosis in right renal artery (arrow). B. Immediately after PTA, stenosis is ablated but post-stenotic dilatation remains. C. Arteriogram obtained 14 1/2 months later reveals that vessel is widely patent. The patient still requires antihypertensive drugs, however, illustrating the difficulty in curing long-standing hypertension despite correction of the renal artery stenosis. (Reproduced from Tegtmeyer CJ, Kellum CD, Ayers C: Percutaneous transluminal angioplasty of the renal arteries. *Radiology* 1984;153:77–84.)

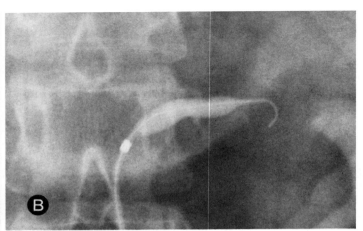

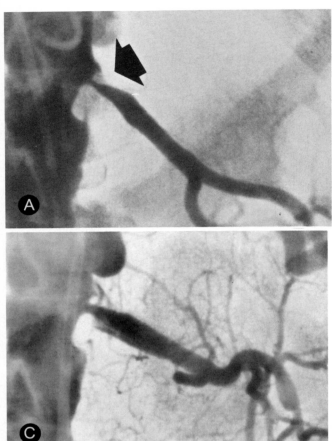

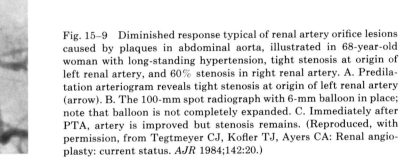

Fig. 15–9   Diminished response typical of renal artery orifice lesions caused by plaques in abdominal aorta, illustrated in 68-year-old woman with long-standing hypertension, tight stenosis at origin of left renal artery, and 60% stenosis in right renal artery. A. Predilatation arteriogram reveals tight stenosis at origin of left renal artery (arrow). B. The 100-mm spot radiograph with 6-mm balloon in place; note that balloon is not completely expanded. C. Immediately after PTA, artery is improved but stenosis remains. (Reproduced, with permission, from Tegtmeyer CJ, Kofler TJ, Ayers CA: Renal angioplasty: current status. *AJR* 1984;142:20.)

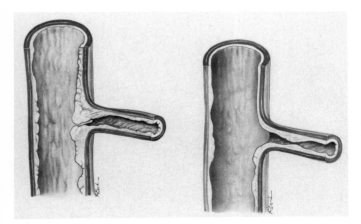

Fig. 15–10   This is the type of atherosclerotic lesion in which diminshed response to balloon dilatation can be expected. Lesion on left is caused by atherosclerotic plaque in abdominal aorta that engulfs orifice of renal artery. Occasionally, a good result is obtained, but usually results are poor when compared with other types of lesions. A good response can be expected in short stenoses within renal artery (right). (Reproduced, with permission, from Tegtmeyer CJ, Kofler TJ, Ayers CA: Renal angioplasty: current status. *AJR* 1984;142:20.)

Fibromuscular Dysplasia

The best results in renal angioplasty are achieved in patients with fibromuscular lesions (Fig. 15–11), which respond well to balloon dilatation, usually at pressures of ≤4 atm. Thus, if the lesion can be crossed, a good result can be expected. There were 27 hypertensive patients with 30 lesions caused by fibromuscular dysplasia in the authors' series, and all of the patients benefited from renal angioplasty, with only one patient requiring a second dilatation.[26] Similar results have been achieved by several other authors. Geyskes et al performed PTA in 21 patients with fibromuscular dysplasia, and all but one were either cured or improved.[24] Sos et al achieved technical success in 27 of their 31 patients.[25]

Stenoses in Renal Allografts

Seven patients with stenoses in the arteries of renal allografts underwent dilation (Fig. 15–12). Five patients improved, and there were two failures, one of which was caused by inability to dilate the lesion, probably because of the use of a polyvinyl chloride balloon. With the polyethylene balloons now available, a better result probably would have been achieved in this patient. In another patient, a tight stenosis at the anastomosis of the allograft vessel with the hypogastric artery recurred after 7 months despite three dilatations with pressures as high

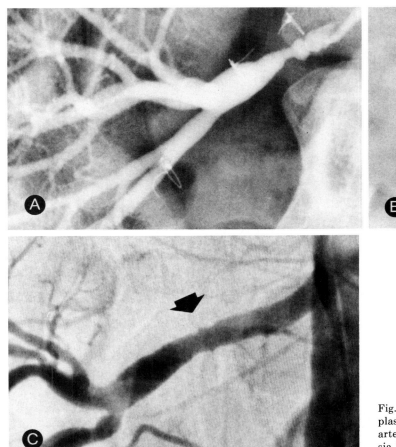

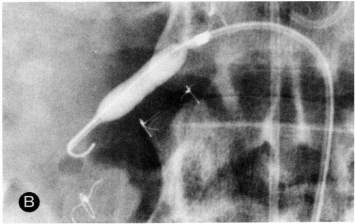

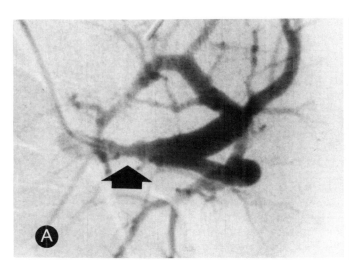

Fig. 15-11 Balloon dilatation of lesion caused by fibromuscular dysplasia in 24-year-old hypertensive woman. A. Selective right renal arteriogram reveals stenosis in the artery. B. Fibromuscular dysplasia is usually easy to dilate; 5-mm balloon expands easily, dilating lesion. C. Immediately after dilation, lesion has disappeared (arrow).

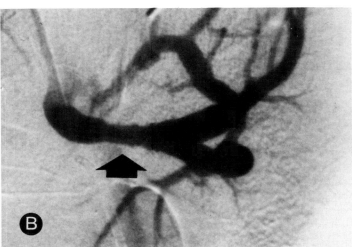

Fig. 15-12 Percutaneous transluminal angioplasty in a 23-year-old woman with a renal allograft. A. Selective renal arteriogram demonstrates tight stenosis (arrow) at anastomosis between renal and hypogastric arteries. B. Lumen of vessel is much improved after balloon angioplasty via axillary approach. (Reproduced from Tegtmeyer CJ, Brown J, Ayers CA, Wellons HA, Stanton LW: Percutaneous transluminal angioplasty for the treatment of renovascular hypertension. *JAMA* 1981;246:2068–2070.)

as 14 atm. Sniderman et al attempted to dilate stenoses in the arteries of renal allografts in 15 patients, 3 of whom underwent repeat dilatations. The procedure was technically successful in 15 of the 18 attempts in 13 of the 15 patients.[35] Gerlock et al were successful in all seven patients in their series with allograft stenoses.[36]

Caution should be exercised when dilating lesions of renal allografts, because there are no collateral vessels to the kidney. Therefore, if the vessel is occluded, operation must be undertaken immediately. It follows that wherever allograft dilatation is done, a surgeon should be readily available.

Stenoses in Saphenous Bypass Grafts

In the University of Virginia series, three patients had PTA of stenoses in their saphenous bypass grafts. The procedure was successful in all cases.[26]

Renal Insufficiency

Under certain circumstances, alleviation of renal artery stenosis is important to preserve renal function. Correction of stenosis is probably worthwhile in unilateral disease if kidney size indicates potentially significant preservation of functional tissue or if bilateral renal artery stenoses are present. In the latter case, an attempt to alleviate obstruction of the larger kidney should be given priority even if the smaller kidney is secreting all the renin.

The results of angioplasty are not as dramatic in patients treated primarily for renal insufficiency as in patients treated primarily for hypertension, but they are nonetheless encouraging. In the present authors' series, 10 patients were treated primarily for renal insufficiency, all with atherosclerotic lesions, the mean serum creatinine being 5.2 mg/dl before dilation. After angioplasty, this average decreased to 2.3 mg/dl,[26] with five of the patients having a positive response to PTA. Five of the patients have not been helped. Twenty-nine of the patients treated primarily for hypertension also had renal insufficiency, and nine of these patients now have better

renal function, with four having normal blood urea nitrogen (BUN) and creatinine values. In some patients, the improvement was gradual, so that the full benefit of the procedure was not apparent for several months.

Summary of Results

Renal angioplasty is an effective means of treating renovascular hypertension. In the present authors' series, the blood pressure response was analyzed in the 92 hypertensive patients whose initial dilatation was successful, who have been followed from 1–60 months (mean 23.7 months). The mean systolic pressure was 199.74 mm Hg before angioplasty and 140.34 mm Hg afterward; the mean diastolic pressure was 117.05 mm Hg before angioplasty and 83.74 mm Hg afterward. Analysis of the long-term clinical results in the 98 hypertensive patients who underwent renal angioplasty to control their blood pressure reveals that 26% were cured (defined by the Cooperative Study of Renovascular Hypertension[37] as having an average diastolic pressure of ≤90 mm Hg with at least a 10 mm Hg decrease from the predilatation level). Sixty-seven per cent were improved, in that their blood pressure was easier to control with drugs as a result of angioplasty, and 7% were nonresponders, although one of these was helped for several months. A review of the large series in the world literature (Table 15–1) shows that if the initial dilatation is successful, the vessels can be expected to remain patent in 70%–90% of the patients and that if the vessel remains patent for at least 8 months, it is likely to remain patent for at least 5 years.

The recurrence rate has been variously reported as 12.9%[26] to 22.5%.[34] The rate is clearly higher for atherosclerotic stenoses than for other types. A significant factor is the success of the initial dilatation: lesions with a ≥30% residual stenosis on the immediate postdilatation films are more likely to recur than are lesions in which a better result has been obtained.[20,26] Therefore, it is essential that a good result be obtained initially. However, restenoses can usually be redilated, and the procedure is often easier than the initial one.

CONCLUSION

The results of the University of Virginia series and published series show that TA of the renal arteries is a versatile and reliable procedure. Excellent results can be obtained in the control of hypertension if the patients are carefully selected. It is encouraging to note that the procedure also has the potential for stabilizing or reversing renal insufficiency. In the University of Virginia series, of the 39 patients who had high BUN and creatinine levels before TA, 18 currently have better renal function, and four of these have normal BUN and creatinine values.

In experienced hands, the results of renal angioplasty compare favorably with surgical results in the treatment of renovascular hypertension. The success so far has changed the original skepticism to tempered enthusiasm. If the renal artery remains patent for at least 8 months after PTA, a good long-term result can be expected.

Renal angioplasty should be considered the treatment of choice in patients with hypertension and renal artery stenoses caused by fibromuscular dysplasia or short isolated atherosclerotic lesions. Good results can also be obtained in patients with stenoses in the arteries of renal allografts and in patients with stenoses in bypass grafts.

The procedure is enticing because it offers many advantages. It is relatively simple compared with surgery, and it preserves renal tissue. It avoids general anesthesia and intra-abdominal surgery, and the patient experiences less pain. The procedure is relatively inexpensive and reduces the hospital stay.[38] For the more than 1 million Americans who suffer from renovascular hypertension, renal angioplasty indeed provides an excellent alternative to operation.

References

1. Stokes JB III, Payne GH, Cooper T: Hypertension control: the challenge of patient education (editorial). *N Engl J Med* 1973;289:1369

2. Gifford RW Jr: Evaluation of the hypertensive patient with emphasis on detecting curable causes. *Milbank Mem Fund Q* 1969;47:170

3. Kaplan NM: *Clinical Hypertension.* New York, Medcom, 1973, pp 1, 173

4. Janeway TC: A clinical study of hypertensive cardiovascular disease. *Arch Intern Med* 1913;12:755

5. Genest J, Boucher R, Rojo–Ortega JM, et al: Renovascular hypertension, in Genest J, Koiw E, Kuchel O (eds): *Hypertension: Physiopathology and Treatment.* New York, McGraw–Hill, 1977, p 815

6. Youngberg SP, Sheps SG, Strong CG: Fibromuscular disease of the renal arteries. *Med Clin North Am* 1977;61:623

7. Dollery CT, Bulpitt CJ: Management of hypertension, in Genest J, Koiw E, Kuchel O (eds): *Hypertension: Physiopathology and Treatment.* New York, McGraw–Hill, 1977, p 1038

8. Hunt JC, Sheps SG, Harrison EG Jr, Strong CG, Bernatz PE: Renal and renovascular hypertension: a reasoned approach to diagnosis and management. *Arch Intern Med* 1974;133:988

9. Foster JH, Maxwell MH, Franklin SS, et al: Renovascular occlusive disease: results of operative treatment. *JAMA* 1975;231:1043

10. Veterans Administration Cooperative Study Group on Antihypertensive Agents: Effects of treatment of morbidity in hypertension: results in patients with diastolic blood pressures averaging 115 through 129 mm Hg. *JAMA* 1967;202:1028

11. Veterans Administration Cooperative Study Group on Antihypertensive Agents: Effects of treatment on morbidity in hypertension: results in patients with diastolic blood pressure averaging 90 through 114 mm Hg. *JAMA* 1970;213:1143

12. Grüntzig A, Kuhlmann U, Vetter W, Lutolf U, Meier B, Siegenthaler W: Treatment of renovascular hypertension with percutaneous transluminal dilatation of a renal artery stenosis. *Lancet* 1978;1:801

13. Boomsma JHB: *Percutaneous Transluminal Dilatation of Stenotic Renal Arteries in Hypertension.* Groningen, The Netherlands, Drukkerij van Denderen B.V., 1982, p 103

14. Katzen BT, Chang J, Knox WG: Percutaneous transluminal angioplasty with the Grüntzig balloon catheter: a review of 70 cases. *Arch Surg* 1979;114:1389

15. Martin EC, Mattern RF, Baer L, Fankuchen EI, Casarella WJ: Renal angioplasty for hypertension: predictive factors for long term success. *AJR* 1981;137:921

16. Puijlaert CBAJ, Boomsma JHB, Ruijs JHJ, et al: Transluminal renal artery dilatation in hypertension: technique, results and complications in 60 cases. *Urol Radiol* 1981;2:201

17. Schwarten DE: Percutaneous transluminal renal angioplasty. *Urol Radiol* 1981;2:193

18. Sos TA, Saddekni S, Sniderman KW, et al: Renal artery angioplasty: techniques and early results. *Urol Radiol* 1982;3:223

19. Tegtmeyer CJ, Dyer R, Teates CD, et al: Percutaneous transluminal dilatation of the renal arteries: techniques and results. *Radiology* 1980;135:589

20. Tegtmeyer CJ, Teates CD, Crigler N: Percutaneous transluminal angioplasty in patients with renal artery stenosis: follow-up studies. *Radiology* 1981;140:323

21. Tegtmeyer CJ, Brown J, Ayers CA, Wellons HA, Stanton LW: Percutaneous transluminal angioplasty for the treatment of renovascular hypertension. *JAMA* 1981;246:2068

22. Tegtmeyer CJ, Elson J, Glass TA, et al: Percutaneous transluminal angioplasty: the treatment of choice for renovascular hypertension due to fibromuscular dysplasia. *Radiology* 1982;143:631

23. Colapinto RF, Stronell RD, Harries–Jones EP, et al: Percutaneous transluminal dilatation of the renal artery: follow-up studies on renovascular hypertension. *AJR* 1982;139:727

24. Geyskes GG, Puylaert CBAJ, Oei HY, Mees EJD: Follow up study of 70 patients with renal artery stenosis treated by percutaneous transluminal dilatation. *Br Med J (Clin Res)* 1983;287:333

25. Sos TA, Pickering TG, Sniderman K, et al: Percutaneous transluminal renal angioplasty in renovascular hypertension due to atheroma or fibromuscular dysplasia. *N Engl J Med* 1983;309:274

26. Tegtmeyer CJ, Kellum CD, Ayers C: Percutaneous transluminal angioplasty of the renal arteries. *Radiology* 1984;153:77

27. Martin LG, Price RB, Casarella WJ, et al: Percutaneous angioplasty in clinical management of renovascular hypertension: initial and long-term results. *Radiology* 1985;155:629

28. Bourgoignie J, Jurz S, Catanzaro FJ, Serirat P, Perry HM: Renal venous renin in hypertension. *Am J Med* 1970;48:332

29. Smith HW: Unilateral nephrectomy in hypertensive disease. *J Urol* 1956;76:685

30. Eyler WR, Clark MD, Garman JE, et al: Angiography of the renal areas including comparative study of renal artery stenoses in patients with and without hypertension. *Radiology* 1962;78:879

31. Holley KE, Hunt JC, Brown AL Jr, et al: Renal artery stenosis: a clinical pathologic study in normotensive and hypertensive patients. *Am J Med* 1964;37:14

32. Tegtmeyer CJ, Ayers CA, Wellons HA: The axillary approach to percutaneous renal artery dilatation. *Radiology* 1980;135:77

33. Cicuto KP, McLean GK, Oleaga JA, et al: Renal artery stenosis: anatomic classification for percutaneous transluminal angioplasty. *AJR* 1981;137:599

34. Schwarten DE: Percutaneous transluminal angioplasty of the renal arteries: intravenous digital subtraction angiography for follow-up. *Radiology* 1984;150:369

35. Sniderman KW, Sos TA, Sprayregen S: Postrenal transplantation, in Castañeda–Zuñiga WR (ed): *Transluminal Angioplasty.* New York, Thieme–Stratton, 1983, p 80

36. Gerlock AJ Jr, MacDonnell RC Jr, Smith CW, et al: Renal transplant arterial stenosis: percutaneous transluminal angioplasty. *AJR* 1983;140:325

37. Simon N, Franklin SS, Bleifer KH, Maxwell MH: Clinical characteristics of renovascular hypertension. *JAMA* 1972;220:1209

38. Doubilet P, Abrams H: The cost of underutilization: percutaneous transluminal angioplasty for peripheral vascular disease. *N Engl J Med* 1984;310:95

16

Vascular Access for Long-Term Hemodialysis: an Integrated Approach to the Management of Failing and Thrombosed Accesses

SAMUEL K. S. SO, M.B., B.S., AND DAVID W. HUNTER, M.D.

This chapter is written in two parts. The first part provides a synopsis of the basic principles and choice of access for long-term hemodialysis. The second part deals with the role of radiographic evaluation in assisting the surgeon in the preoperative and postoperative assessment of the patient and with the management of the complications associated with each access device.

BASIC CONSIDERATIONS

Vascular access is appropriately described as the Achilles' heel of dialysis patients, because problems associated with these accesses are a significant cause of morbidity and even death.[1-3] Nonetheless, if the initial access is carefully tailored to the needs of the individual patient, high long-term patency rates usually can be achieved with few complications.

Surgeons strive to provide reliable vascular accesses without compromising the perfusion of the extremity. The access should provide adequate flow for efficient dialysis with the greatest likelihood of long-term function and the fewest complications. The initial access should be constructed with the most distal suitable vessels in order to preserve valuable proximal lengths of vessels for future access needs. Together with the nephrologist, the surgeon must make sure that the type of access is matched to the needs of the patient and the capabilities of the particular dialysis unit. Therefore, the surgeon must be familiar with the needs of the patient and with the advantages, limitations, and possible complications of each type of access procedure and of dialysis. Access procedures for immediate (short-term) and long-term hemodialysis are often different and require different strategies.[4,5]

Long-term hemodialysis accesses, such as the Brescia–Cimino fistula and bridge grafts, usually must mature for 3 weeks before being used. Therefore, an access route must be chosen for all patients with end-stage renal disease in whom a need for maintenance dialysis is expected within a few months. Such planning will minimize the need for a temporary access procedure to be added to that required for maintenance hemodialysis and will help ensure that the vessels to be used are protected from venipuncture.

CHOICE OF ACCESS FOR LONG-TERM HEMODIALYSIS

A low incidence of complications, high long-term patency rates, and patient acceptance are the key features of an ideal angioaccess for long-term hemodialysis (Fig. 16–1). The Brescia–Cimino fistula, introduced in 1966, is constructed between the distal radial artery and the cephalic vein and is still the best access for long-term hemodialysis.[2,4-6] Its complications are minor and few. For example, in 1049 patients followed for >1 year, the chances of hospitalization for an access-related problem was 5 times greater in patients with shunts or bovine grafts than in patients with Brescia–Cimino fistulae.[2] The 1-year and 3-year cumulative patency rates are estimated at 85%–90% and 60%–85%, respectively.[7-9] If the distal vessels are unsuitable for an access, the next best choice is an internal fistula higher in the forearm, such as between the more proximal radial artery and the cephalic vein or an adjacent suitable superficial vein. The Scribner shunt, introduced by Quinton et al in 1960, is now seldom used for long-term hemodialysis because of its low long-term patency rate.[8,10]

In patients who have no suitable forearm vessels, the best access is usually a proximal antecubital arteriovenous (AV) fistula or a bridge graft. However, a proximal internal fistula[11] is suitable only for patients with a patent and easily accessible upper arm cephalic vein. The short superficial course of the basilic vein above the elbow

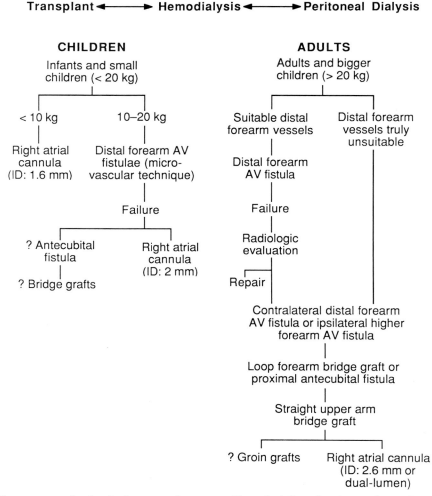

Fig. 16–1 A practical guide to access selection for long-term hemodialysis. (Modified from So SKS: General principles of access surgery, in Simmons RL, Finch ME, Ascher, NL, Najarian JS (eds): *Manual of Vascular Access, Organ Donation, and Transplantation.* New York, Springer–Verlag, 1984, pp 3–87.)

generally makes this vessel unsuitable, because extensive dissection is needed to elevate it to a superficial subcutaneous position for easy puncture by dialysis needles.

For patients with no suitable forearm vessels who are not candidates for an antecubital AV fistula, either a straight (radial artery–antecubital vein) or looped (brachial artery–antecubital vein) bridge graft can be used. Because the distal radial artery is often not available or is unsuitable for graft placement, the authors prefer to use the loop forearm graft from the brachial artery to an antecubital vein. If no suitable antecubital vessel is available, an excellent alternative is a straight brachial artery to axillary or basilic vein bridge graft. There is no ideal graft material, but in most dialysis centers, expanded polytetrafluoroethylene (E-PTFE) has performed better than any other material, including autogenous veins, as determined by the patency and complication rates.[4,12–14]

Bridge grafts in the groin are associated with a high incidence of infectious complications and should be considered only for the rare patient who has no suitable vessels in the arms and in whom peritoneal dialysis is not feasible.[3] Even then, these grafts may be unnecessary if the adult Silastic right atrial catheter with an internal

diameter of 2.6 mm, or the more recently introduced dual-lumen Silastic central venous catheter, can be used.[4,15]

In children weighing between 10 and 20 kg, the authors advocate a similar approach but with some modifications. Microvascular techniques are mandatory in the construction of AV fistulae in children of this weight. Distal forearm fistulae in such small children usually require 4–8 weeks to mature. Because little vein is available for needle puncture, the repeated punctures often cause venous stenoses; use of single-needle dialysis may help to prolong the problem-free lifespan of these small fistulae. Small children will often tolerate a distal ulnar artery–basilic vein fistula when no suitable radiocephalic vessels are found. The short, narrow extremities of small thin children render them poor candidates for bridge graft placement, and groin grafts should be avoided because of the high incidence of infection and leg swelling.

For infants weighing <10 kg, long-term access is a difficult problem.[16] Distal forearm fistulae have a high early failure rate and may take 4 months to mature,[17] so internal access is limited to antecubital fistulae and bridge grafts placed in the groin. Many dialysis centers prefer peritoneal dialysis for these tiny infants. Since June 1980, the authors have taken a new appraoch to this problem: hemodialysis with a Hickman catheter (internal diameter: 1.6 mm) or the larger bore (2.0-mm) Silastic catheter placed in the right atrium.[4,18-20] This method creates a painless and reliable access for dialysis and spares the peripheral vessels for future access sites. The catheter is usually left in place until the child is sent home after renal transplantation. Children who might not receive an allograft for some time—*e.g.*, because of a high antibody titer—can be maintained on hemodialysis with the Silastic catheter until they are big enough for a more suitable angioaccess.

CHOICE OF ACCESS SITE

When selecting a vascular access site, the following factors should be taken into consideration.[4,21] First, the nondominant arm should be chosen if the vessels are suitable bilaterally. Second, the most distal site is chosen so a longer segment of the proximal vessel can be used for needle puncture and the proximal vessels can be preserved for any necessary revision. Third, use of the groin vessels should be avoided because the incidence of infection is extremely high, and septic complications in the groin can cause serious morbidity and even death. Fourth, use of the more proximal major arteries for access generally increases the risk of ischemic complications and high-output cardiac failure. Fifth, use of extremites with poor collateral circulation should be avoided. Also, the popliteal artery and the brachial artery at the bifurcation are particularly vulnerable to ischemic complications and should be avoided as vascular access sites. Sixth, when hemodialysis is required in a patient whose long-term access site is not ready for use, a temporary access, such as a subclavian venous cannula, should be placed in the opposite extremity to avoid jeopardizing the long-term access. Seventh, the thin-walled veins on the volar surface of the forearm are generally unsuitable for construction of an AV fistula. Finally, patients with two functioning AV fistulae are at a higher risk of congestive heart failure.

Venipunctures *must* be prohibited above the wrist of the arm chosen for access. While the patient is in the hospital, the chosen extremity should be kept in Ace wraps and labeled so that other medical staff members do not accidently use it for injections or venipunctures.

PREOPERATIVE EVALUATION

It cannot be overemphasized that the key to creating a long-lasting reliable access for hemodialysis is careful planning. This includes obtaining a thorough medical and surgical history, with particular attention to past access procedures; a thorough physical examination of the arterial and venous system bilaterally; and, if necessary, a preoperative venogram. This information provides a map of the patient's available vasculature and helps the surgeon select the best site as well as the best form of access. A high incidence of primary nonfunction is frequently a hallmark of poor planning rather than of poor surgical technique.

The arterial system is assessed simply by palpation of the pulses in both upper and lower extremities. The possibilty of limb ischemia after arterial interruption is evaluated by selective occlusion of the major vessels and by performing the Allen test to check the adequacy of collateral perfusion to the hand. To perform the Allen test, the hand is drained of blood by repeated digital flexion. Both the ulnar and the radial arteries are then occluded at the wrist by the thumbs of the examiner. Color should return to all fingers within 6 sec after each artery is individually released.[22] If digital circulation returns promptly after release, either artery can be ligated safely. In the authors' experience, any artery with a palpable pulse, even if the vessel is calcified, generally provides adequate blood flow and is suitable for construction of an internal fistula. A preoperative brachial or axillary arteriogram is unnecessary.

The venous system is often the limiting factor in the flow through any AV fistula. The veins must be assessed by applying a tourniquet over each extremity. Even though a distal vein is distended, a more proximal stenotic segment may be present. Therefore, it is important to palpate and percuss the vein along its entire length to check for proximal stenosis that can result from previous venipuncture or cannulation. In difficult circumstances, a preoperative venogram will identify distal veins and help rule out proximal stenosis and obstruction. A preoperative venogram is particularly useful in the evaluation of children and in adult patients who have bilateral venipuncture bruises along their forearms and antecubital fossae. A venogram is also useful in assessing patients who have had indwelling subclavian vein or jugular vein catheters, who may have developed thrombosis of the subclavian or innominate veins. An AV fistula inadvertently placed on the side with a tight stenosis or thrombosis of the central veins will cause severe venous hypertension and will quickly fail.

To minimize the risk of nephrotoxicity in the uremic patient, it is important to use the minimum amount of intravenous contrast medium in performing the venogram. In the authors' experience, the veins of the arm are best evaluated as shown in Figure 16–2. Access to the venous system is obtained by cannulation of a superficial vein over the dorsum of the hand. A rubber tourniquet or blood pressure cuff is then placed around the upper arm to occlude venous outflow, so that the vessels can be filled with just 10–20 ml of 30% diatrizoate. Anteroposterior and lateral views of the forearm and upper arm vessels are then obtained. As the tourniquet is released, rapid sequential films or cine radiographs should be taken of the upper arm or shoulder to rule out a more proximal lesion. Proximal obstruction may either be evident radiologically or be suggested by a delay in the clearance of the contrast medium.

EVALUATION AND MANAGEMENT OF ACCESS PROBLEMS

Complications related to the vascular access are the most frequent cause of hospitalization of patients on long-term hemodialysis. In a 1-year, five-center study of 1049 patients on dialysis for at least 3 months, 26% of the initial hospitalizations were necessitated by access problems. In addition, patients with xenogeneic bridge grafts or external prosthetic shunts had a 5-fold greater frequency of hospitalization than did patients with internal AV fistulae.[2]

Most complications are preventable if the patient is thoroughly evaluated preoperatively and if the procedures are well planned and carefully performed. However, all dialysis staff members and physicians must be aware of the possible complications so they can be recognized early and treated promptly to prevent both access loss and morbidity.

There are, essentially, five complications: infection, bleeding, aneurysm, partial or complete obstruction, and hemodynamic problems.[1,4] Infection is the second most common cause of access failure. The primary principle for the management of access-related infection is prophylaxis; it is important to give prophylactic antibiotics and to use strict aseptic techniques whenever invasive radiologic procedures are used. Bleeding is primarily a problem of external AV shunts; fatal hemorrhage may result from disconnection of the external cannulas. Brescia–Cimino fistulae may appear aneurysmal, with dilated, tortuous veins, but these rarely reach a size that requires excision. True aneurysms are uncommon in E-PTFE grafts, although repeated traumatic punctures may create

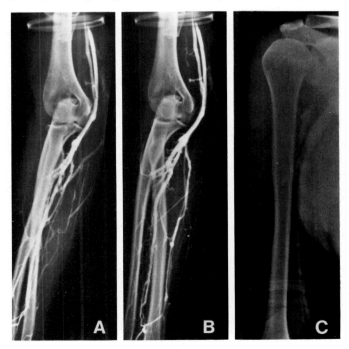

Fig. 16–2 A venogram of upper extremity can be obtained with minimum contrast medium by using tourniquet to occlude venous outflow. After anteroposterior (A) and lateral (B) views of the forearm and arm have been obtained, proximal venous runoff is assessed by rapid sequential films or cine radiograph of the upper arm and shoulder (C) as the tourniquet is released.

a small hole in the graft, leading to formation of a pseudoaneurysm. Arterial insufficiency following creation of an AV access is uncommon if the adequacy of collateral perfusion has been carefully assessed preoperatively and if the diameter of the bridge graft does not exceed 6 mm. Ischemic complications are best assessed by physical examination and Doppler studies[4]; contrast studies are seldom indicated.

The most common cause of access failure is thrombosis, which is often preceded by increasing problems during dialysis, such as difficult cannulation, frequent withdrawal of clots, and high venous resistance or poor arterial flow. In addition, patients with AV communications may have a diminished bruit or thrill. It is often difficult or impossible to salvage a thrombosed access, so evaluation of all access problems should be prompt.

Radiographic evaluation is invaluable in the management of a failing access, because it helps confirm the presence and locate the site of the lesion. Simple roentgenograms of the chest confirm the positioning of right atrial Silastic catheters. Angiography is the best way to assess the lumen of the access device and the caliber of the venous outflow. Assuming that the study is carefully planned, reliable information can be obtained with a low risk and a small volume of contrast medium. Needle puncture of the graft or fistula for radiologic study is no more invasive than needle puncture for dialysis and almost always yields more useful information than does ultrasonography or thermography. Operative angiography is absolutely necessary during repair of the occlusive defects.

Radiocephalic and Other Internal AV Fistulae

The Brescia–Cimino internal fistula is the best access for maintenance hemodialysis because of its low incidence of complications and the high long-term patency rate.[2,7–9] Ideally, the distal radial artery is anastomosed to the distal cephalic vein just above the wrist so a long segment of arterialized cephalic vein can be used for insertion of dialysis needles. Because thrombosis is still the most common cause of early failure, the authors prefer to use the side-to-side anastomosis described by Brescia et al, because it produces the highest blood flow[23] (Fig. 16–3). However, some surgeons prefer to construct an end-to-side or end-to-end fistula with ligation of the distal cephalic vein and radial artery to minimize the risk of distal venous hypertension or arterial steal (Fig. 16–3).[24–26]

Failure of an internal AV fistula is often signaled by difficulties in dialysis, with low flow rates or high venous resistance; an apparent diminution of the thrill or bruit; or failure of a recently created fistula to mature despite the presence of a thrill or bruit. Some patients with a stenosis in the proximal outflow vein may suffer venous hypertension, characterized by swelling of the arm and hand distal to the fistula that may be associated with stasis ulceration and throbbing pain over the thumb.[24,25] The common causes of failing Brescia–Cimino fistulae are stenoses of either the proximal artery or the vein at

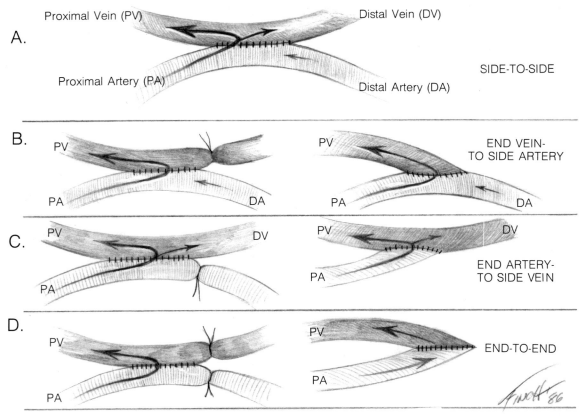

Fig. 16–3   Types of anastomoses used in construction of radiocephalic fistula; side-to-side anastomosis is used in the original Brescia–Cimino fistula.

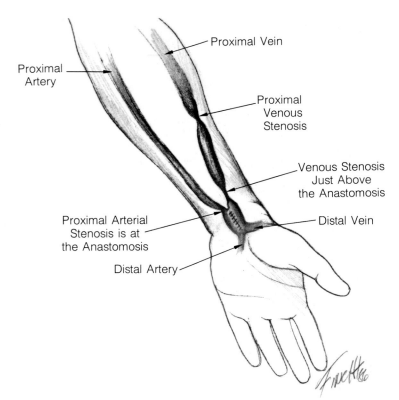

Fig. 16–4   Common lesions found in association with failing or thrombosed Brescia–Cimino fistula.

or just above the anastomosis or stenoses of the proximal vein at the puncture sites (Fig. 16–4).[4,27–30] The most common problem, stenosis of the vein just above the anastomosis, can be the result of a technical error, a fibrous band, or intimal hyperplasia from turbulent flow. Stenosis of the artery at the anastomosis is often the result of technical error.

EVALUATION OF FAILING FISTULAE

It is most important and informative to analyze the clinical information and perform a thorough physical examination. Insight into the problem is often obtained by talking to the dialysis staff. It is helpful to remember that high venous resistance during dialysis is suggestive of proximal venous stenosis or occlusion of the major venous outflow channel, whereas poor arterial flow is indicative of proximal arterial stenosis or stenosis of the fistula distal to the arterial needle. Venous hypertension with swelling of the hand is usually associated with proximal venous stenosis or occlusion. Loss of the thrill and bruit on compression of the distal vein is a sign of proximal obstruction. If the thrill is replaced by a prominent pulsation, venous runoff is probably compromised.

With these data alone one can often locate the lesion, and they are of utmost value to the access surgeon or the radiologist. For example, the patient in Figure 16–5 had a normal venous fistulogram up to the elbow; but since he had high venous pressure during dialysis, contrast flow was followed above the elbow, revealing complete occlusion of his major venous outflow tract.

A failing fistula is best evaluated by a venous fistulogram.[4,5,27–29] A clear picture of the vessels is usually obtained with a small amount of contrast medium if both arterial and venous flow are temporarily occluded in the upper arm with a tourniquet. Although Glanz and associates used the brachial artery and reported few complications,[30] the present authors prefer to cannulate the distal vein of the fistula, which allows easy access to both the proximal artery and the vein for balloon angioplasty[27,31–33](Fig. 16–6). Furthermore, even if stenosis develops at the puncture site, flow through the fistula will not be compromised. In an end-to-side fistula when the distal vein has been ligated, the distal artery or the proximal vein can be cannulated.

The authors do fistulograms of failing Brescia–Cimino fistulae on an outpatient basis after obtaining permission to perform percutaneous balloon dilation also should it prove appropriate. A blood pressure cuff is placed close to the axilla, and the extremity is prepared with antiseptic solution and draped from the hand to 6 cm above the elbow. After venous distention has been obtained by inflating the cuff to 60 mm Hg, the distal vein of the fistula is punctured with a 19-gauge butterfly infusion needle 3–5 cm below the fistula (Fig. 16–6). The cuff is then deflated, and the needle is replaced with a 5F angiocatheter threaded over a 0.022-inch guidewire to avoid inadvertent displacement of the needle during subsequent manipulation. The catheter is advanced 2–3 cm beyond the puncture site so that the tip lies below the level of the proximal vessels of the fistula. Small doses of contrast medium are infused to verify the catheter position and to make a preliminary assessment of the proximal venous anatomy. A cine fistulogram is made with 15–30 ml of 30% contrast medium (60% diatrizoate in a 1:1 dilution) infused at the rate of 2–5 ml/sec with the blood pressure

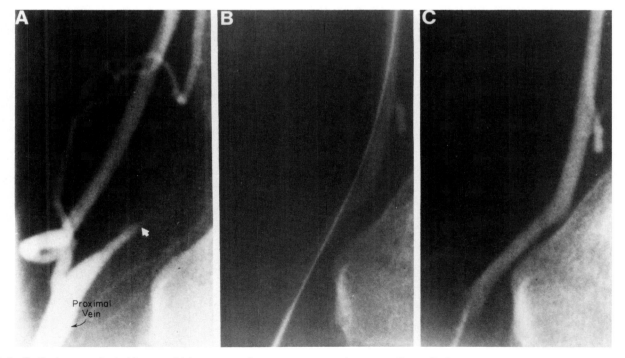

Fig. 16–5 Patient was evaluated because high venous resistance was persistently encountered at dialysis. A. Cine fistulogram shows high proximal venous stenosis with occlusion above elbow at site w̵ patient normally applied tourniquet to train fistula. B. Occlusion has been traversed by guidewire. C. Normal caliber vessel after balloon angioplasty.

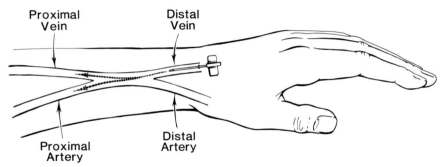

Fig. 16–6   Cine fistulography and manipulation through distal vein of fistula provides easy access to fistula, proximal artery, and vein.

cuff inflated 20 mm Hg above systolic pressure to obtain arterial as well as venous filling. Rapid clearing of the contrast when the cuff is deflated and the anatomic distribution distinguish the arteries from the veins. Oblique and lateral views are obtained by rotation of the arm slowly through 90° to evaluate lesions that may otherwise by obscured by contrast-filled vessels. One or two injections may be necessary. The vessels should be traced to the axilla to avoid overlooking a proximal stenosis (Fig. 16–5).

This technique is simple and no more invasive than is venipuncture of the fistula for dialysis. A cine fistulogram

Furthermore, if stenosis occurs at distal artery or vein, it has almost no functional significance.

with video recording permits a more dynamic study with instant replay and reduces the expense.

Pressure gradients are measured across the fistula to assess the functional significance of any stenoses and to reveal any lesions not appreciated on angiography (Fig. 16–7). The lesions most difficult to assess by contrast study are those at the junction of the proximal vessels and the anastomosis. For this reason, the authors now routinely measure the pressure within the fistula by positioning the catheter just below the proximal vessels. This value is compared with the systemic cuff pressure; a pressure gradient of ≥20 mm Hg suggests significant proxi-

Fig. 16–7   Value of pressure gradient measurement. A. Pressure measurements across seemingly insignificant arterial stenosis show impressive gradient of 110 mm Hg. B. After balloon dilation of proximal artery, there is marked morphologic improvement as well a drop in pressure gradient to only 20 mm Hg. The systolic pressure at the fistula or the proximal vein rose from 40 mm Hg to 130 mm Hg after dilation. PV = proximal vein; PA = proximal artery.

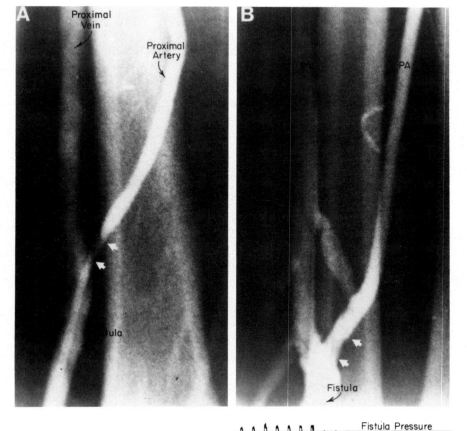

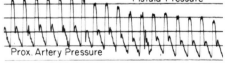

mal arterial stenosis. The catheter is then positioned in the proximal artery, and pull-back pressures across the fistula are measured to confirm the presence of a significant gradient and the site of narrowing. Pull-back pressures are also measured across the fistula from the proximal vein and across gross stenotic lesions. Although a gradual change in pressure may occur without indicating a lesion, an abrupt change of >20 mm Hg is considered significant. Pressure gradient measurement is an essential part of the evaluation and may predict the outcome of the dilation.

On completion of the contrast study and pressure measurements, the vascular access surgeon should review the findings with the radiologist and plan therapy.

PERCUTANEOUS TRANSLUMINAL ANGIOPLASTY

If dilation of the stenotic lesion is chosen, 5000 units of heparin are given intravenously through the catheter placed proximal to the stenotic segment. The stenosis is then repeatedly stretched with Teflon dilators as large as 8F that are passed over a 0.038-inch guidewire. A Grüntzig catheter with a 4–10-mm balloon is then centered across the stenosis, and several (usually 4–6) inflations to 4–6 atm are performed at 1.5-min intervals until the narrowing around the balloon is relieved (Figs. 16–5, 16–7, and 16–8). The result is assessed by contrast injection and pull-back pressure measurements. Successful dilation is invariably accompanied by the return of a prominent thrill or bruit.

In the authors' experience, transluminal angioplasty will salvage a failing fistula caused by proximal venous or arterial stenosis and is well tolerated by the patient, with no need for hospitalization.[27,33] Complications are few and often minor, and dialysis can be resumed immediately after the procedure,[27] although as a precaution against traumatic restenosis, the authors generally request that the dialysis staff not insert the needles directly over the dilated segment for at least 2 weeks. In contrast, critical stenosis near the anastomosis of an end-to-end fistula is difficult or impossible to dilate and should be managed by surgical revision and an operative fistulogram. Also, if more than two dilations are required within 12 months, surgical revision is recommended: venous patch angioplasty, interposition graft, or reconstruction of the fistula just proximal to the stenosis.[4,34]

FISTULA THROMBOSIS

When a bruit or thrill can no longer be detected over the fistula, thrombosis has occurred. The standard treatment for a previously well-functioning fistula is surgical exploration, thrombectomy with Fogerty balloon catheters, and, if necessary, revision of the fistula.[4,32,34] After clot removal, an intraoperative fistulogram is essential to locate any unsuspected stenotic lesions, which predispose the fistula to thrombosis. These lesions can be treated by balloon angioplasty or surgical repair.[27] However, if the fistula thrombosed immediately after or within a few days of construction because an unsuitable site was chosen, re-exploration and attempts to evaluate the fistula radiologically are usually futile. Another access site should be planned in these cases.

Arteriovenous Bridge Grafts

If a Brescia–Cimino fistula cannot be constructed, a looped forearm graft is a well-accepted alternative. The U-shaped graft is positioned in a subcutaneous tunnel to allow easy access for dialysis, and the ends of the graft are anastomosed end to side to the brachial artery and an antecubital vein. In patients who have no suitable antecubital veins, a straight bridge graft between the brachial artery and the axillary or basilic vein is an excellent alternative (Fig. 16–9). All newly constructed bridge grafts

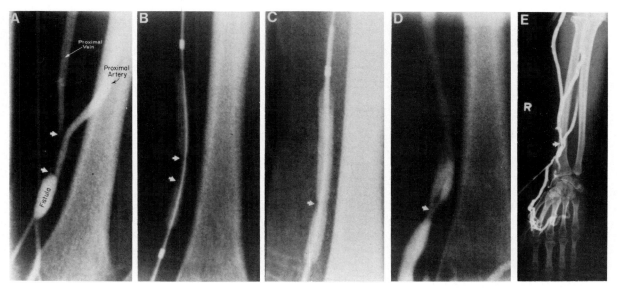

Fig. 16–8 Balloon angioplasty of AV fistula. A. Cine fistulogram shows tight proximal venous stenosis. B. Deformity of balloon at site of stenosis. C. Correction of balloon deformity with progressive and repeated dilation. D. Significant morphologic improvement after dilation. E. Follow-up angiography with portable equipment at dialysis 6 weeks later shows that dilated proximal vein has remained wide open.

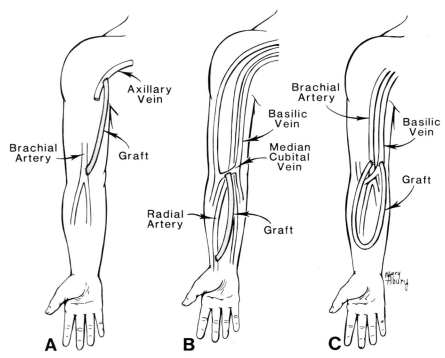

Fig. 16–9   Common types of bridge grafts used for long-term hemodialysis.

should be allowed to heal for 3 weeks to minimize the risk of early failure due to bleeding and infection.[1,4]

There are two types of graft materials. Biologic grafts include autogenous or homologous saphenous vein, bovine carotid artery, and human umbilical cord veins.[14] These grafts are more susceptible to the formation of aneurysms, and, over time, the incorporation of the graft into the adjacent soft tissues makes revision difficult or impossible. Infected biologic grafts, with the exception of those of autogenous saphenous vein, generally require removal, so these grafts have a relatively poor salvage rate. The autogenous saphenous vein graft is the least susceptible to infection, but it has a high incidence of diffuse stenosis and aneurysm formation.

Among the synthetic graft materials is E-PTFE, which is the most popular graft material in North America.[4,12,13,35] Despite the propensity of prosthetic material to infection, suture line disruption is rare compared with bovine grafts. The graft withstands repeated needle punctures, has a low incidence of aneurysm formation, and is relatively easy to revise because it can be removed easily from its fibrous tract. Arterial–arterial bridge grafts enjoyed a brief popularity but were abandoned because of aneurysm formation and the risks of ischemic and embolic complications.

Stenosis at or just above the venous anastomosis is a common finding in failing bridge grafts no matter what material was used (Fig. 16–10). Stenosis probably results from the intimal damage with reactive hyperplasia caused by the turbulence associated with the progressive increase in flow over time. Critical stenosis can be managed with a trial of transluminal angioplasty, although the venous anastomotic narrowing associated with bridge grafts often resists dilation and often recurs if it does

respond.[36] It is important to stress that all invasive procedures in patients with bridge grafts, as with other types of dialysis access, must be performed with appropriate antibiotic coverage and strict aseptic techniques.

Operative repair is the best treatment for a thrombosed bridge graft. Because the most common lesion is a stenosis near the venous anastomosis,[32,36,37] the authors advocate making an incision at the venous end of the graft to perform thrombectomy and an intraoperative contrast study. After the stenosis has been located, it can be repaired by patch angioplasty or bypassed by a short-segment interposition graft. Intraoperative balloon angioplasty may be useful in some cases, particularly when a high proximal venous stenosis is found. The authors do not recommend use of fibrinolytic agents such as streptokinase and urokinase because of the resulting need for many days of hospitalization for infusion and monitoring and because of the risk of infection and bleeding through old needle holes in the graft[37] (Fig. 16–11).

Arteriovenous External Shunts

Although the artificial kidney was invented in 1944,[38] its clinical application was restricted for the next 16 years by the lack of a reliable vascular access. The breakthrough came in 1960, when Quinton, Dillard, and Scribner introduced the Teflon–Silastic AV shunt.[10] The Scribner shunt and other external AV shunts are seldom used for long-term hemodialysis now, however, because they are plagued by relatively low long-term patency rates as a result of infection and clotting, the average shunt lifespan in an adult being 7–10 months.[39] Nonetheless, the Scribner shunt is still effective for temporary hemodialysis and may be indicated when placement of a

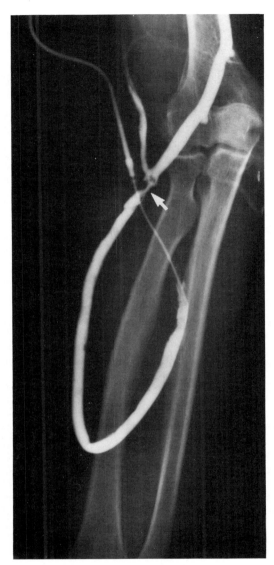

Fig. 16–10 High venous resistance during dialysis caused by tight stenosis at venous anastomosis of an E-PTFE bridge graft.

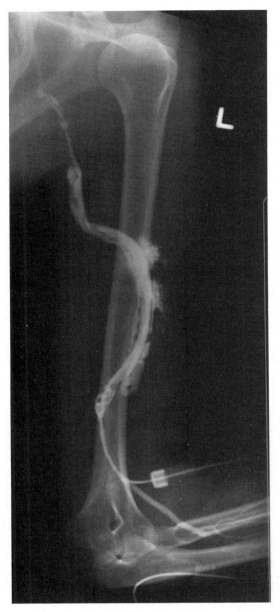

Fig. 16–11 Bleeding through old puncture sites on an E-PTFE graft after infusion of streptokinase; note tight stenosis at venous anastomosis.

subclavian cannula for short-term hemodialysis is considered hazardous or difficult.[4] Use of the Scribner shunt requires ligation of the distal artery and vein, and preoperative assessment therefore must include the Allen test of the adequacy of collateral perfusion. The common sites for shunt placement are similar to those used for internal AV fistulae.

The Scribner shunt has two components, a radiolucent Teflon vessel tip and a silicone rubber shunt cannula. An appropriate size vessel tip is tied to the shunt cannula before being secured within the lumen of the vessel (Fig. 16–12). The two ends of the shunt cannulas are then brought out through separate incisions and connected externally with a straight or a T-shaped connecting piece. Patency is assured if a bruit or a thrill is detected over the proximal vein. A clotted shunt is easily recognized, because blood separates into distinct serum and red cell layers in the external tubing.

Stenosis at the vessel–Teflon tip junction due to excessive motion or angulation of the tip is the most frequent finding in a thrombosed shunt or a shunt inadequate for dialysis. Any clots are removed by aspiration with a syringe and, if necessary, a small polyethylene catheter is passed beyond the obstruction to flush out the clots with heparinized (10 units/ml) saline as the catheter is withdrawn.[4] A shuntogram can be obtained using 10–20 ml of 30% diatrizoate infused through the arterial or venous cannula after temporarily occluding the proximal flow with a tourniquet applied to the upper arm (Fig. 16–13). Infusion through the artery must not be forceful, or retrograde cerebral embolization can result. If the shuntogram shows a critical mechanical obstruction, surgical revision

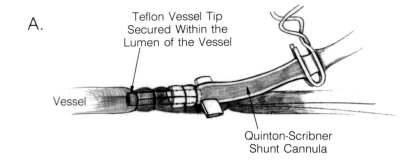

A.

Teflon Vessel Tip
Secured Within the
Lumen of the Vessel

Vessel

Quinton-Scribner
Shunt Cannula

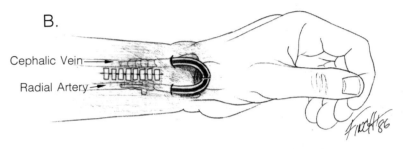

B.

Cephalic Vein

Radial Artery

Fig. 16–12 In the construction of a Scribner shunt, both the distal artery and vein are ligated.

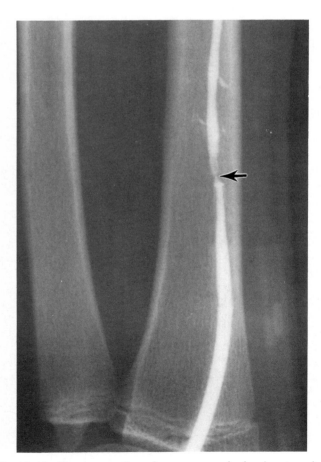

Fig. 16–13 Shuntogram through venous cannula showing stenosis at Teflon tip–vessel junction and partial occlusion with thrombus (arrow).

is the best treatment. If only residual thrombus is seen, however, the clot can be removed by further aspiration and flushing with a polyethylene catheter or by gentle Fogarty thrombectomy. After declotting the shunt, the authors prefer to use an intermittent or continuous heparin infusion until the next dialysis session, the heparin being infused directly into the shunt through a T-shaped connector.

Right Atrial Cannulas

Single- or dual-lumen cannulas positioned in the right atrium are becoming more common as access for both immediate and long-term hemodialysis. The more rigid polyethylene or polyurethane catheters are inserted percutaneously through the subclavian vein and have largely replaced the Scribner shunt for immediate or short-term dialysis.[40] The less thrombogenic and more flexible silicone rubber catheters with internal diameters of 1.6 mm (regular Hickman catheter) and 2.0–2.6 mm, as well as the large dual-lumen catheter, can be used for long-term dialysis. The larger single-lumen or dual-lumen silicone rubber catheters are particularly useful in managing adult patients in whom almost all the available vessels in the arms have been exhausted in previous access procedures and in those who are likely to suffer ischemic complications if the proximal arteries are used.[15] The smaller single-lumen silicone rubber catheter is invaluable as a reliable and painless access for dialysis in small children.[18–20] Except for the small Hickman catheter, which can be placed percutaneously through the subclavian vein, most silicone rubber dialysis catheters are positioned through a direct cut-down into the external or internal jugular vein[4] (Fig. 16–14).

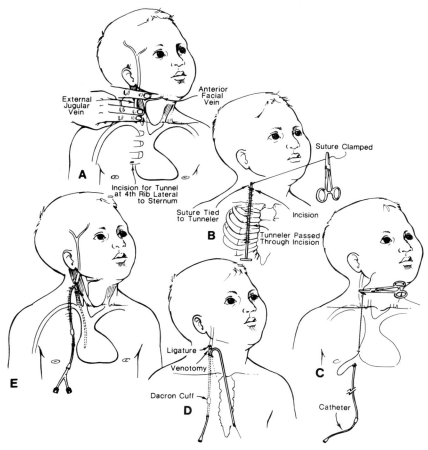

Fig. 16–14 The right atrial silicone rubber dialysis catheter is usually inserted through cut-down into external or internal jugular vein or anterior facial vein.

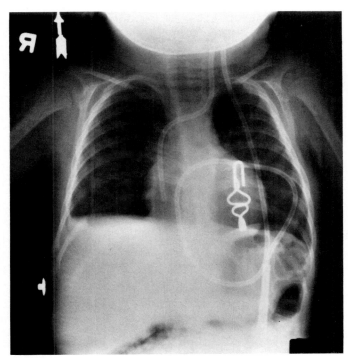

Fig. 16–15 Chest film obtained after catheter placement to check position of radiopaque catheter in right atrium and to rule out pneumothorax and hemothorax.

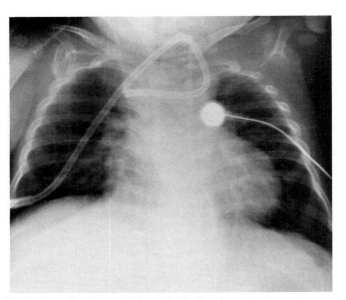

Fig. 16–16 Acute angulation of catheter tip against superior vena cava may occur when catheter is introduced through left-sided vessels; this catheter must be repositioned immediately to prevent erosion of vessel.

Flow inadequate for efficient dialysis may occur when: (1) the catheter is too small for the patient; (2) the catheter tip is not positioned correctly in the right atrium; (3) the lumen of the catheter is compromised by a tight suture; or (4) the catheter is kinked along its subcutaneous course. A roentgenogram of the chest is essential after catheter placement to assess the position and course and to rule out technical complications such as pneumothorax or hemothorax (Fig. 16–15). Radiologic evidence of acute angulation of the catheter against the superior vena cava is sometimes seen when the catheter is introduced from the left side (Fig. 16–16). These catheters must be repositioned to prevent erosion of the catheter tip through the vena cava. Thrombosis of the silicone rubber catheters does not appear to be a significant problem as long as the catheter is aspirated and then filled with heparinized saline every 6–12 hr. When the catheter does become obstructed by thrombosis, and the clot cannot be dislodged by aspiration, infusion of several milliliters of urokinase solution (5000 units/ml), or a volume just great enough to fill the catheter every 8 hr, often lyses the clot.[4]

References

1. Wilson SE: Complications of vascular access procedures, in Wilson SE, Owens ML (eds): *Vascular Access Surgery*. Chicago, Year Book Medical Publishers, 1980, p 185
2. Hirschman GH, Wolfson M, Mosimann JE, Clark CB, Dante ML, Wineman RJ: Complications of dialysis. *Clin Nephrol* 1981;15:66
3. Morgan AP, Knight DC, Tilney NL, Lazarus JM: Femoral triangle sepsis in dialysis patients: frequency, management, and outcome. *Ann Surg* 1980;191:460
4. So SKS: Access for dialysis, in Simmons RL, Finch ME, Ascher NL, Najarian JS (eds): *Manual of Vascular Access, Organ Donation and Transplantation*. New York, Springer–Verlag, 1984, pp 3–87
5. So SKS, Sutherland DER: Vascular access procedures, in Najarian JS, Delaney JP (eds): *Advances in Vascular Surgery*. Chicago, Year Book Medical Publishers, 1980, p 185
6. Brescia MJ, Cimino JE, Appel K, Hurwich BJ: Chronic hemodialysis using venipuncture and a surgically created arteriovenous fistula. *N Engl J Med* 1966;275:1089
7. Kinneart P, Vereerstraeten P, Toussaint C, Van Geertruyden J: Nine years' experience with internal arteriovenous fistulas for haemodialysis: a study of some factors influencing the results. *Br J Surg* 1977;64:242
8. Ishihara AM: The current state-of-the-art for vascular access in hemodialysis. *Controv Dialysis* 1980;1:9–29
9. Reilly DT, Wood RFM, Bell PRF: Prospective study of dialysis fistulas: problem patients and their treatment. *Br J Surg* 1982;69(9);549
10. Quinton WE, Dillard D, Scribner BH: Cannulation of blood vessels for prolonged hemodialysis. *Trans Am Soc Artif Intern Organs* 1960;6:104
11. Gracz KC, Ing TS, Soung LS, Armbruster KFW, Seim SK, Merkel FK: Proximal forearm fistula for maintenance hemodialysis. *Kidney Int* 1977;11:71
12. Haimov M, Slifkin R: Experience with the PTFE graft in the construction of vascular access for hemodialysis, in Kootstra G, Jorning PJG (eds): *Access Surgery*. Lancaster, MTP Press, 1983, p 113
13. Sabanayagam P, Schwartz AB, Soricelli RR, Lyons P, Chinitz J: A comparative study of 402 bovine heterografts and 225 reinforced expanded PTFE grafts as AVF in the ESRD patient. *Trans Am Soc Artif Intern Organs* 1980; 26:88
14. Akhondzadeh L, Wilson SE, Williams R, Owen ML: Infection of materials used in vascular access surgery: an evaluation of Dacron, bovine heterograft, Teflon, and human umbilical vein grafts. *Dialysis Transplant* 1980;9:697
15. McGonigle DJ, Schrock LG, Hickman RO: Experience using central venous access for long-term hemodialysis: a new concept. *Am J Surg* 1983;45:571
16. Buselmeier TJ, Santiago EA, Simmons RL, Najarian JS, Kjellstrand CM: Arteriovenous shunts for pediatric hemodialysis. *Surgery* 1971;70:638
17. Bourquelot P, Wolfeler L, Lamy L: Microsurgery for hemodialysis distal arteriovenous fistulas in children weighing less than 10 kg. *Proc Eur Dialysis Transplant Assoc* 1981;18:537
18. Mahan JD Fr, Mauer SM, Nevins TE: The Hickman catheter: a new hemodialysis access device for infants and small children. *Kidney Int* 1983;24:694
19. So SKS, Mahan JD Jr, Mauer SM, Sutherland DER, Nevins TE: Hickman catheter for pediatric hemodialysis: a 3-year experience. *Trans Am Soc Artif Intern Organs* 1984;30:619
20. Nevins TE: A new Hickman catheter for hemodialysis access in children (abstract). *Trans Am Soc Artif Intern Organs*, 1984
21. Humphries AL, Nesbit RR, Caruana RJ, Hutchins RS, Heimburger RA, Wray CH: Thirty-six recommendations for vascular access operations: lessons learned from our first thousand operations. *Am Surg* 1981;47:145
22. Kamienski RW, Barnes RW: Critique of the Allen test for continuity of the palmar arch assessed by Doppler ultrasound. *Surg Gynecol Obstet* 1976;142:861
23. Forsberg G, Forsberg L, Lindstedt E, Westling H, White T: Side-to-side, side-to-end, end-to-end anastomosis for Cimino–Brescia fistula: preliminary report of a randomized study, in Kootstra G, Jorning PJP (eds): *Access Surgery*. Lancaster, MTP Press, 1983, p 21
24. Butt KMH, Friedman EA, Kountz SL: Angioaccess. *Curr Probl Surg* 1976;13:3
25. Wood RFM, Reilly DT: Hyperemia of the hand in side-to-side arteriovenous fistulas, in Kootstra G, Jorning PJG (eds): *Access Surgery*. Lancaster, MTP Press, 1983, p 147
26. Bussell JA, Abbott JA, Lim RC: A radial steal syndrome with arteriovenous fistula or hemodialysis. *Ann Intern Med* 1971;75:387
27. Hunter D, So SKS, Castañeda–Zuñiga W, Coleman C, Sutherland DER, Amplatz K: Angiographic evaluation and percutaneous transluminal angioplasty in failing or thrombosed Brescia–Cimino arteriovenous dialysis fistulas. *Radiology* 1983;149:105
28. Gilula LA, Staple TW, Anderson CB, Anderson LS: Venous angiography of hemodialysis fistulas. *Radiology* 1975;115:555
29. Lawrence PF, Miller FJ, Minean DE: Balloon catheter dilatation in patients with failing arteriovenous fistulas. *Surgery* 1985;89:439
30. Glanz S, Bashist B, Gordon DH, Butt K, Adamsons R: Angiography of upper extremity access fistulas for dialysis. *Radiology* 1982;143:45
31. Heidler R, Zeitler E, Gessler U: Percutaneous transluminal dilatation of stenosis behind A-V fistulas in hemodialysis patients, in Zeitler E, Grüntzig A, Schoop H (eds): *Percutaneous Vascular Recanalization*. New York, Springer–Verlag, 1978, pp 142–144
32. Bone GE, Pomijzl MJ: Management of dialysis fistula thrombosis. *Am J Surg* 1979;138:901
33. So SKS, Castañeda–Zuñiga, WR, Hunter D, Sutherland DER, Amplatz K: Percutaneous transluminal angioplasty in failing arteriovenous fistula, in Kootstra G, Jorning PJP (eds): *Access Surgery*. Lancaster, MTP Press, 1983 p 225
34. Silcott GR, Vannix RS, DePalma JR: Repair versus new arteriovenous fistulae. *Trans Am Soc Artif Intern Organs* 1980;26:99
35. Palder SB, Kirkman RL, Whittemore AD, Hakim RM, Lazarus JM, Tilney NL: Vascular access for hemodialysis: patency rates and results of revisions. *Ann Surg* 1985;202:235

36. Tortolani EC, Tan AHS, Butchart S: Percutaneous transluminal angioplasty: an ineffective approach to the failing vascular access. *Arch Surg* 1984;119:221

37. Young AT, Hunter DW, Castañeda–Zuñiga WR, So SKS, Mercado S, Cardella JF, Amplatz K: Thrombosed synthetic hemodialysis fistulas: failure of fibrinolytic therapy. *Radiology* 1985;154:639

38. Kolff WJ, Berk HTJ: The artificial kidney: a dialyser with a great area. *Acta Med Scand* 1944;117:121

39. Cross AS, Steigbigel RT: Infective endocarditis and access site infections in patients on hemodialysis. *Medicine* 1976; 55:453

40. Dorner DB, Stubbs DH, Shadur CA, Flynn CT: Percutaneous subclavian vein catheter hemodialysis impact on vascular access surgery. *Surgery* 1982;91:712

17

Problems in the Management of Hemodialysis Accesses

ROBERT M. ZEIT, M.D., AND CONSTANTIN COPE, M.D.

The continued well-being of uremic patients undergoing hemodialysis is dependent on the functional integrity of their arteriovenous accesses. An adequately functioning hemodialysis access should have a flow rate of at least 250–300 ml/min (ideally, 400–500 ml/min)[1] and be able to withstand two 14-gauge needle punctures at least 150 times each year.[2] These are stringent requirements, and the usual patient experiences the creation and subsequent loss of a series of cannulation sites. It has been estimated that 18% of these individuals die because of a lack of adequate vascular access,[3] usually following exhaustion of all feasible locations.

The availability of thrombolytic enzymes and transluminal angioplasty has enabled the interventional radiologist to participate in the preservation of these accesses and in their salvage when compromised. This chapter describes the historical development of the various hemodialysis approaches and the complications of each. Techniques of shunt evaluation are described, the therapeutic use of thrombolytic enzymes and transluminal angioplasty detailed, and the results discussed.

DEVELOPMENT OF HEMODIALYSIS ACCESSES AND REVIEW OF THEIR COMPLICATIONS

Practical hemodialysis was initiated by Kolff and colleagues in 1965.[4] However, their vascular access was obtained by surgically cannulating an artery and a vein for each dialysis and ligating both vessels at the end of the session; obviously this attrition of vessels could not be long maintained. Dialysis was therefore limited to short-term use.

Scribner Shunt

Long-term patency of a glass arteriovenous shunt with continuous heparinization was reported in 1949. Obviously, however, this device was impractical. In 1960, Quinton and coworkers developed a shunt using polytetrafluoroethylene (PTFE; Teflon) for the intravascular portion of the cannulas, permitting long-term placement without a need for systemic anticoagulation.[6] Various modifications of the original rigid Teflon design were produced, eventually resulting in a shunt in which the two intravascular PTFE components were connected by a Silastic bridge. This Scribner shunt made short-term dialysis much more practical.

When used for long-term hemodialysis, however, Scribner shunts engendered numerous complications, most commonly thrombosis and infection,[7] but also pseudoaneurysm formation, hemorrhage, and erosion of the overlying skin.[8] Alignment of the cannula tips relative to the wall was critical, because an angulated cannula could traumatize the vessel wall, resulting in occlusive endarteritis and subsequent thrombosis (Fig. 17–1). Another

consequence of improper tip placement was the creation of a "dead space," also implicated in arterial limb thrombosis.[9] Trauma caused by motion of the rigid catheter tip was thought to cause aneurysms at the site of cannulation (Fig. 17–2). Other factors contributing to shunt thrombosis included a circumferential arterial stenosis at the tip of the cannula, variously ascribed to the interaction of Teflon with the surrounding endothelium, to the Bernoulli effect, or to rubbing of the cannula against the vessel wall.[10] Also, venous outflow stenosis (Fig. 17–3), often distant from the venous cannula, was noted in most patients within 14 days of shunt placement. Histologically, this lesion contained both intimal and adventitial fibrosis and was progressive, eventually causing venous occlusion.[9] (This problem has been characteristic of all chronic dialysis accesses, from the earliest cannulas to the present time.) Another cause of thrombosis affecting all vascular accesses is arterial hypotension, usually occurring during a dialysis session. Infection occurred in 17%–50% of Quinton–Scribner shunts[11] and was associated occasionally with phlebitis, embolism, septicemia, endocarditis, and pulmonary abscesses. Pseudoaneurysms, especially of the arterial limb, are an additional complication.

Because of all these complications, the average patency of a Scribner shunt is measured in months,[8,9] with the longest reported patency being 2 years.[12] Further, because of the shunt's external location, there is a constant danger of dislodgment, which limits the patient's activities and therefore acceptance of the device.

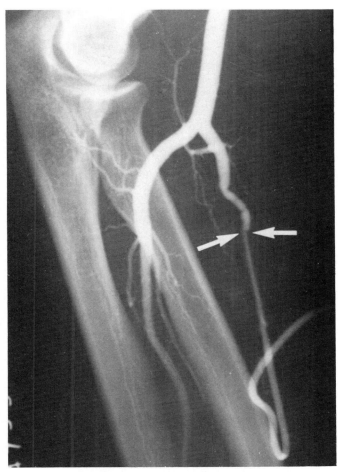

Fig. 17–1 Scribner shunt with angulation of arterial cannula tip against vessel wall (arrows). This was associated with poor shunt longevity.

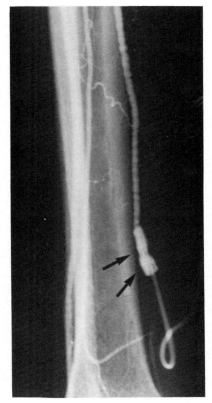

Fig. 17–2 Scribner shunt with aneurysm at tip of Teflon cannula (arrows).

Other External Shunts

Another early external shunt was the Sheldon femoral artery–femoral vein shunt, developed in 1961.

Newer external devices, such as the Shiley and Sorenson catheters, which are inserted into the subclavian or femoral vein, have replaced the Scribner shunt for short-term hemodialysis. Also, 11F–12F double-lumen subclavian catheters have recently become popular for short- and intermediate-term hemodialysis, although occasionally they are difficult to insert because of fibrosis from previous subclavian catheterizations. Further, the small inner diameter of these catheters, which must be divided into two discrete lumens, creates suboptimal flow rates, whereas the large outer diameter of the catheter and the bleeding tendency found in uremic patients may create hemorrhagic complications during insertion. These problems may be minimized by using the fine 22-gauge needle and 0.018-inch guidewire popularized by Cope[13] and by slightly (1F–2F) overdilating the soft tissues. Other complications associated with these double-lumen subclavian catheters include thrombosis of one or both lumens, thrombus formation at the tip, infection, and perforation of the superior vena cava by the stiff tubing. In addition, some patients have become anemic as a result of red cell fragmentation during passage of blood through the catheter lumens during dialysis. External arteriovenous accesses still have an average useful life of only 3–8 months[14] and usually are used only to gain time for a more permanent access to mature.

SURGICALLY CREATED ARTERIOVENOUS FISTULAE

Currently, the preferred long-term hemodialysis access is the primary arteriovenous fistula, an internal shunt, usually between the radial artery and the cephalic vein, introduced by Brescia and associates in 1966.[15] In patients in whom the venous outflow tract is sufficient to dilate eventually with the increased flow and be used as the dialysis puncture site, the Brescia–Cimino fistula has been the most trouble-free and longest lived access, with numerous fistulae remaining in use for 5 years or more.[16] This longevity may be attributed both to the absence of foreign prosthetic materials and to the progressive hypertrophy of the venous drainage channel, which eventually permits puncture of collateral veins as well as the primary draining vein, thus creating additional sites for dialysis needle insertion and providing alternative drainage in case of thrombosis of the original vein. However, the

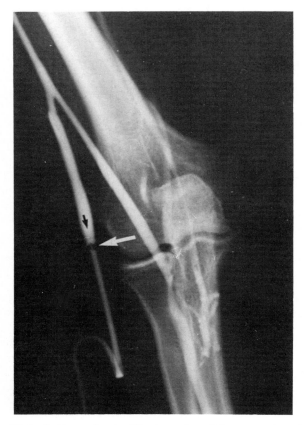

Fig. 17–3 Scribner shunt with circumferential venous stenosis at cannula tip (arrows).

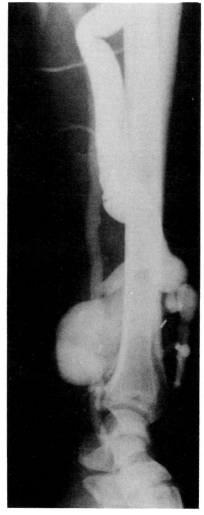

Fig. 17–4 Venous aneurysms in Brescia–Cimino fistula.

necessity for adequate venous drainage requires a period of "maturation" of the fistula, usually 4 weeks, before it can be used and precludes placement of these fistulae in the leg because of the fear of venous hypertension.[8,13]

Despite the advantages of the Brescia–Cimino fistula, it is subject to the usual access complications: infection, development of true aneurysms (Fig. 17–4) and pseudo-aneurysms (Fig. 17–5),[1] thrombosis secondary to hypotensive episodes, and arterial (Fig. 17–6) and venous intimal hyperplasia. In addition, there are complications specific to the arteriovenous fistula. Both excessive shunting of blood through the fistula at the expense of the arterial supply of the hand ("steal syndrome") and venous hypertension of the hand or digits have been reported. In a series of 346 fistulae treated by Giacchino and associates, arterial insufficiency of the hand, manifested by symptoms of ischemia that worsened during dialysis, appeared in three patients, and venous hypertension appeared in eight.[2] Digital gangrene secondary to fistula steal has been reported,[17] and the severity of the resultant ischemia, like most other vascular complications of dialysis, is more severe in diabetic patients.[18]

Venous hypertension, indicated by swelling, cyanosis, and ulceration of the hand, usually is secondary to venous outlet obstruction and may involve the entire hand or be limited to one[1] or more[19] digits (Fig. 17–7). Fistulae created by side-to-side anastomosis seem more likely to result in both steal syndrome and venous hypertension.

Congestive heart failure secondary to a high-output fis-

tula has occasionally been reported.[20] It is more common in patients who have two simultaneously functioning fistulae.

Outflow stenosis, occurring anywhere between the venous anastomosis and the subclavian vein, has been noted in all dialysis accesses from the Scribner shunt to the Brescia–Cimino fistula and current prosthetic shunts. Subclavian venous stenosis may occur spontaneously but is particularly likely if a catheter is allowed to remain in the vein longer than 15 days.[21] Severe swelling of the ipsilateral arm appears weeks to months later and may render the entire extremity unsuitable for dialysis access.[21,22] In the authors' experience, it has occasionally been possible to dilate subclavian venous stenoses by balloon angioplasty, with symptomatic relief.

Aneurysmal dilatation of outflow veins occasionally occurs in fistulae and has produced atrophic changes in the overlying skin.[8]

A variant shunt, usually created surgically when a Brescia–Cimino access has failed, is the "reverse fistula," in which the brachial artery is anastomosed to the basilic vein, with plication of the basilic vein cephalad, thus forcing blood to flow retrograde down the antecubital veins.[23]

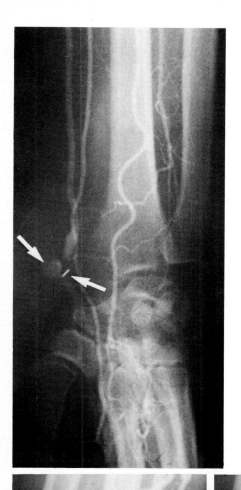

Fig. 17–5 Pseudoaneurysm (arrows) of Brescia–Cimino anteriovenous fistula.

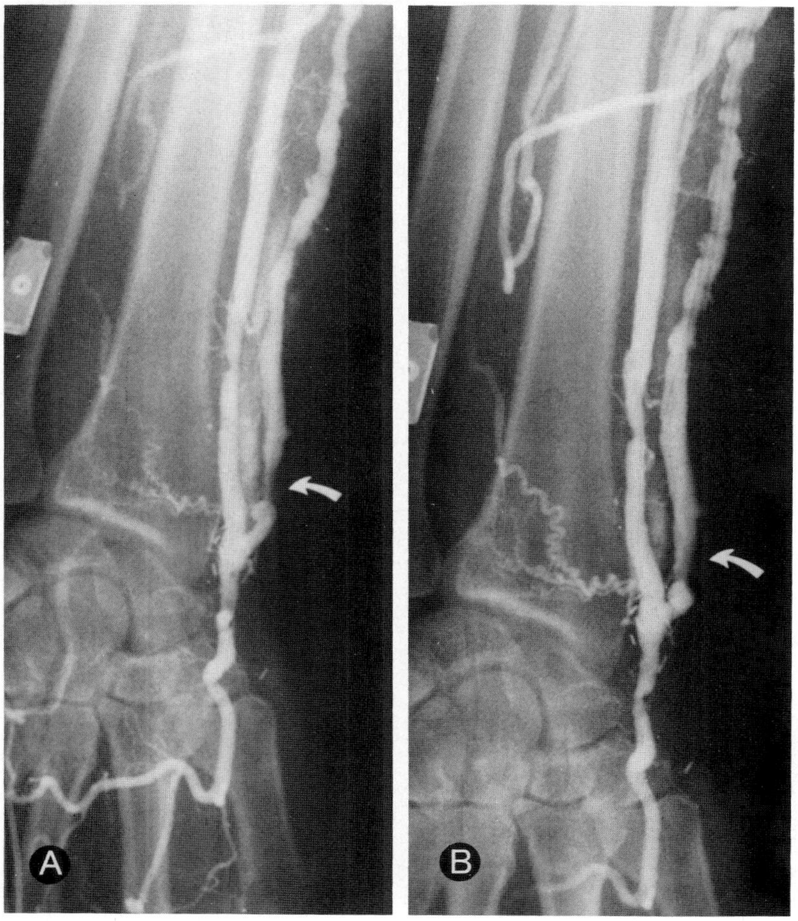

Fig. 17–6 Brescia–Cimino shunt with intimal hyperplasia (arrows) 1 cm from arterial anastomosis. A. Before dilatation. B. After Dotter dilatation with 7F sheath; good result was obtained.

ARTERIOVENOUS GRAFTS

Because many patients do not have good enough venous drainage to allow creation of a radiocephalic fistula, various materials have been interposed between the radial or brachial artery and a large draining vein. These grafts are punctured during dialysis in the same manner as the arterialized vein of the Brescia–Cimino shunt. Both biologic materials (autogenous saphenous vein, bovine carotid artery, human umbilical vein) and nonbiologic materials (Dacron velour, expanded polytetrafluoroethylene (E-PTFE)) have been used. All have lower patency rates and a higher incidence of complications than the Brescia–Cimino fistula. Because of their widespread use and their amenability to clearance with thrombolytic enzymes and to dilatation with percutaneous transluminal angioplasty, they are of great interest to the interventional radiologist.

Because of its success in vascular surgery, autogenous saphenous vein was regarded as a likely material for dialysis grafts. However, results were extremely poor, with only a 51% 1-year graft survival rate.[24] In addition, it was difficult to free these grafts of thrombi because of the presence of valve remnants, and the grafts had a tendency to develop endothelial thickening along their entire length. The additional operative effort required for harvesting and the desire to preserve the saphenous vein for possible use later in coronary or femoral–popliteal bypass have also discouraged use of the saphenous vein.[25]

Another biologic graft material that excited considerable interest but proved unsuitable was the Sparks mandril graft, in which living tissue was grown over Dacron mesh. In use, the Dacron fibers tended to separate, resulting in a 20% incidence of aneurysm formation. There also was a high rate of intimal hyperplasia.[26]

Bovine carotid artery modified by treatment with glutaraldehyde[27] has a better patency rate, as high as 70%–80% 1 year after implantation.[24] However, bovine heterografts undergo degenerative changes,[28] resulting in aneurysm formation in 21% of implants[29] (Fig. 17–8) and loss of integrity of the entire graft wall in 9%.[24] Later bovine prostheses were covered with Dacron mesh to guard against this. Bovine implants are also extremely susceptible to the consequences of infection, which was responsible for the loss of 38% of these grafts in one series.[30] Even a localized infection at a puncture site necessitates removal of the entire prosthesis. Moreover, thrombectomy of clotted bovine shunts is usually unsuc-

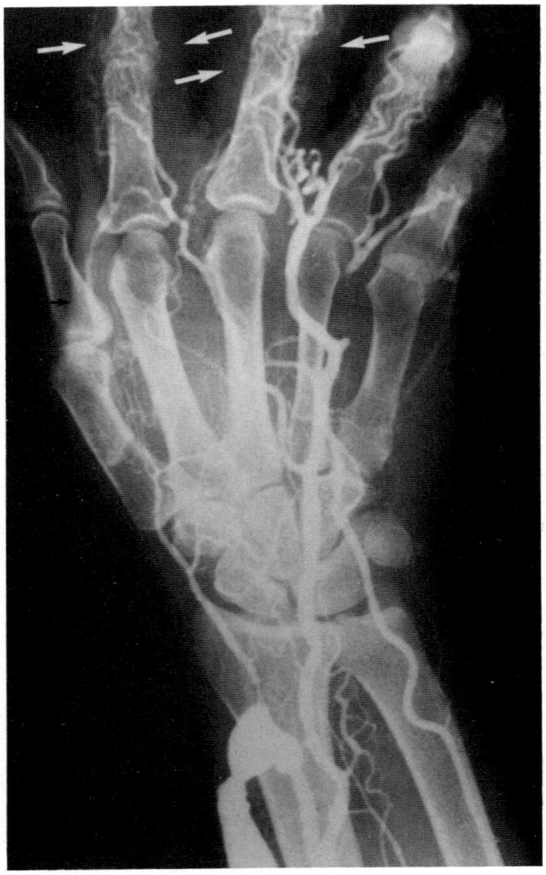

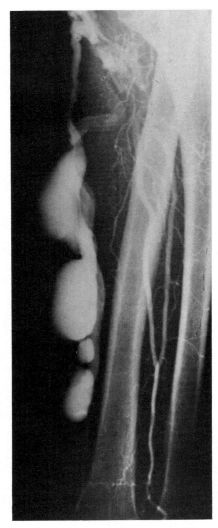

Fig. 17–7 Digital venous hypertension in patient with Brescia–Cimino fistula; note retrograde venous flow and swelling of fingers (arrows).

Fig. 17–8 Bovine carotid heterograft with multiple aneurysms.

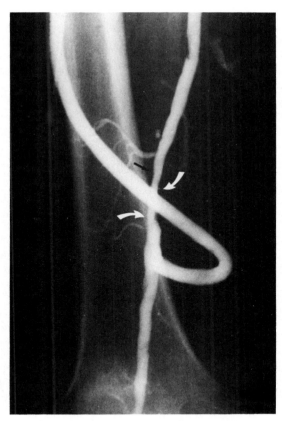

Fig. 17–9 Atherosclerotic narrowing (arrows) of superficial femoral artery proximal to arterial anastomosis of lower-extremity shunt. Significant narrowing of proximal artery will decrease flow through shunt.

cessful, patency being restored in less than one-third of cases.[27]

The newest and most promising biologic shunt material is human umbilical vein, usually covered with Dacron mesh. Rubio and DelGuercio have reported an 88% patency rate 4 years after implantation.[31] Complications of this access are similar to those of the Brescia–Cimino shunt, the most common being hyperplastic stenosis of the venous outflow tract.

Dacron velour gave disappointing results because of a high incidence of thrombosis and infection.[31]

Expanded polytetrafluoroethylene currently is the prosthetic material most widely used for dialysis access. Numerous studies have documented longer graft survival and diminished complications compared to saphenous vein or bovine carotid artery.[24,28–31] In part, this superiority is attributed to the unique structural and physical characteristics of E-PTFE, in which nodes of PTFE are interconnected with fibrils, resulting in 10–30-μm pores that allow tissue ingrowth and eventual production of a true neointima.[32,33] These grafts also have a 17 mV electronegative potential, which reduces their thrombogenicity.[32,33] The presence of a true neointima results in a higher success rate in thrombectomy of E-PTFE than in bovine grafts, 50%[34] and 32%, respectively. The E-PTFE shunts also require only half as many revisions per dialysis month as do bovine prostheses.[30]

Nevertheless, E-PTFE accesses are subject to the same types of complications as those grafts previously described. Early (1975–1976) E-PTFE grafts were prone to aneurysm formation,[35] although subsequent reinforcement of these grafts with Dacron mesh has reduced the rate of aneurysm formation far below that of bovine implants. Bacterial and even fungal[36] infection of E-PTFE prostheses occurs, occasionally leading to fatal sepsis.[37] As with all vascular accesses, the skin overlying the shunt may erode, and surgical transposition of skin or muscle[38] may be required to re-cover the prosthesis. Occasionally, the anastomosis between the artery and the E-PTFE shunt is too wide, causing excessive flow; the use of a tapered prosthesis reduces the likelihood of this problem.[39]

DIABETES, LOWER EXTREMITY ACCESSES, AND INFECTION

Three interrelated factors deserve special mention in any review of the complications of hemodialysis accesses: diabetes, access placement in the leg, and infection.

Diabetic uremic patients develop atherosclerosis at an accelerated rate[2] and experience more vascular complications than do nondiabetics.[18,34] Placement of hemodialysis access in the leg is undesirable because the arterial supply is more subject to atherosclerotic narrowing (Fig. 17–9) and because the venous outflow is less developed than in the arm. In addition, there is a greatly increased incidence of infection in leg accesses of all types.[31] Infection is second only to heart disease as a cause of morbidity and death in these patients,[3] and 75% of septic episodes are attributable to infected vascular accesses.[40]

ANGIOGRAPHIC EVALUATION OF DIALYSIS ACCESSES

The use of angiography in the anatomic and functional evaluation of dialysis accesses closely parallelled their development. Thus, arterial and venous opacification was used to define the anatomy for shunt and fistula placement.[41,42] Management of the complications of Scribner shunts was aided by contrast studies,[43,44] and a prospective angiographic study of Scribner shunts from the day of insertion over a period of several months documented the gradual onset of outflow stenosis.[9] With the advent of the radiocephalic arteriovenous fistula, angiography was used in the evaluation of this access as well.[45]

Accesses may be studied either by direct injection of contrast medium into the feeding artery[45,46] or by injection into the venous limb of the shunt during interruption of outflow by a tourniquet or inflated cuff. (See also Chapter 16.[1,47]) Because it avoids the trauma of arterial puncture, the present authors use the latter technique (Fig. 17–4). An interesting variation of the venous approach is described by Hunter et al.[48] They approach Brescia–Cimino fistulae from the distal venous limb, which allows them to measure pressure gradients across the fistula or to probe the stump of an occluded fistula with a guidewire, possibly allowing percutaneous recanalization.

Both conventional[49] and real-time[50] sonography have been used to evaluate the complications of arteriovenous fistulae and prosthetic shunts.

Regardless of the technique used, a complete examination should image the flow from the arterial anastomosis to the mediastinum. In addition, the possibility of atherosclerotic disease proximally in the feeding artery should be considered. Doppler wave studies of the artery proximal to the anastomosis might be useful in documenting normal triphasic flow, with arteriography if the results are abnormal.

INTERVENTIONAL RADIOLOGIC SALVAGE OF DIALYSIS ACCESSES

The recent widespread availability of thrombolytic enzymes and percutaneous transluminal angioplasty with balloon catheters has allowed the interventional radiologist to play a significant role in the salvage of hemodialysis accesses. In 1970, Hartley and colleagues used urokinase to declot thrombosed Quinton–Scribner shunts that had not responded to the usual heparin irrigation.[51] Although the initial results were encouraging, the study was discontinued because of the cost of the enzyme. Gordon and colleagues performed transluminal angioplasty on 16 stenotic accesses, with restoration of function in 10.[52] Hunter et al approached nine nonfunctional Brescia–Cimino fistulae from the distal venous limb, as previously described.[48] Despite the complete occlusion present in five fistulae, good results were obtained. In a series of 56 angioplasties of dialysis access fistulae, Glanz et al treated 44 venous anastomotic stenoses, 9 venous outflow stenoses, and 3 arterial stenoses, with initial success in 70%. Of those patients with a successful result, 80% had patent accesses after 3 months, 70% after 6 months, and 55%, 50%, and 33% after 1, 2, and 3 years, respectively.[53] The preponderance of stenoses at the venous anastomosis and along the outflow tract also has been true in the present authors' experience[54] and in that of others.

Thrombolysis of clotted dialysis accesses has been accomplished both by the continuous infusion of dilute streptokinase solution into the shunt[55,56] and by injection of streptokinase directly into the clot.[54,57] Rodkin and colleagues administered a loading dose of 40,000 units of streptokinase, followed by the hourly infusion of 5000–7500 units through a multihole catheter. Clinical benefit was obtained in seven of nine patients. One graft bled

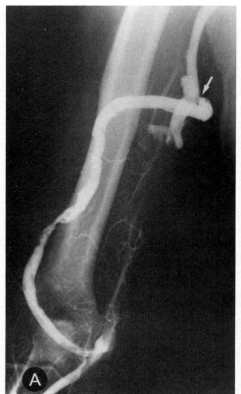
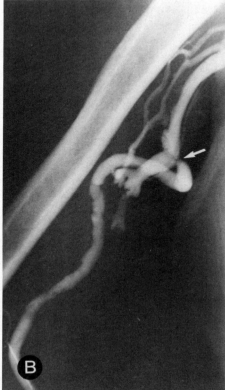
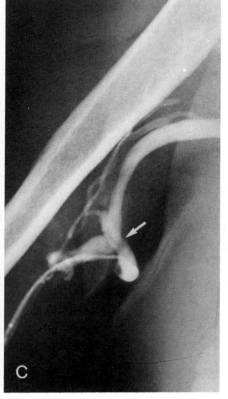

Fig. 17–10   Thrombosed E-PTFE shunt declotted with 50,000 units of streptokinase injected over a period of 45 min. Balloon angioplasty was performed the following day with good result. A. Angiogram obtained during thrombolysis. B. Predilation angiogram. C. Postdilation angiogram. Note venous anastomosis narrowing (arrows) in all images.

from previous puncture sites.[55] Graor et al treated 50 thrombosed dialysis accesses, with a 68% success rate, by a similar infusion technique.[56]

By alternately injecting dilute streptokinase solution percutaneously into the clot and massaging the shunt, Zeit and Cope were able to declot 77% of 33 dialysis accesses.[54] Most shunts were reopened in an hour with streptokinase doses of 15,000–100,000 units, and long-term infusions of streptokinase were avoided. With trans-luminal angioplasty after thrombolysis, 52% of the shunts treated were restored to function without surgery (Fig. 17–10), and an additional 21% were declotted and restored to function after minor operations. Two accesses bled severely enough from sites of previous dialysis punctures to force termination of thrombolysis. A similar technique of injection of small amounts of streptokinase has been useful in declotting double-lumen subclavian dialysis catheters.

COMPLICATIONS OF THROMBOLYSIS AND ANGIOPLASTY

Bleeding from previous puncture sites is the most frequent complication of, and the greatest obstacle to success in, access thrombolysis. Young et al showed that punctures in E-PTFE grafts are sealed with a collagenous plug, presumably the result of organization within a thrombus, and postulated that recently thrombosed puncture sites are themselves susceptible to fibrinolytic effects.[58] Certainly hemorrhage from previous puncture sites can be most impressive (Fig. 17–11), but it can be controlled as described below, usually allowing thrombolysis to proceed.

Other complications of thrombolysis by either infusion or direct injection include embolization of the partially lysed clot (Fig. 17–12)[56]; extravasation through graft interstices (usually with knitted Dacron grafts but also seen in an E-PTFE graft treated with urokinase)[59]; induction of sepsis if the clotted shunt is infected; and immunologic responses to streptokinase, usually only low fever,[56] although "serum sickness" also has been reported. Complications of access angioplasty include intimal shearing,[52] thrombosis of the shunt,[53] and late development of a pseudoaneurysm at the catheterization site.[53]

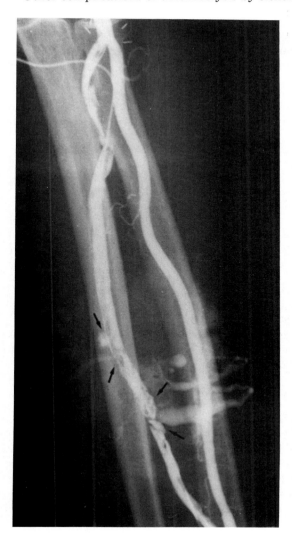

Fig. 17–11 Extravasation from sites of multiple previous dialysis punctures (arrows) during streptokinase thrombolysis by direct injection.

PRACTICAL SUGGESTIONS FOR THE MANAGEMENT OF FAILED ACCESSES

The timely treatment of stenotic lesions by angioplasty can be performed on an outpatient basis and is greatly preferable to treating a thrombosed shunt. Elevated venous resistance during dialysis should initiate a search for outflow stenosis (Fig. 17–13). Complete evaluations must include study of the subclavian vein.

Bleeding from previous puncture sites during thrombolysis can usually be controlled by placing purse-string sutures through the skin overlying the bleeding site. Thrombolysis has been obtained in shunts that required suturing of multiple bleeding sites. One advantage of the direct injection over infusion of thrombolytic enzymes is that the material is administered over a short time under direct physician observation, allowing immediate recognition and treatment of puncture site bleeding.

Thrombolysis must be complete before angioplasty can be attempted, because the introduction of a dilating catheter into a shunt containing even a small residual thrombus usually precipitates immediate total rethrombosis. Although this problem can be treated by a second course of thrombolytic enzymes, an overnight delay after initial declotting usually results in lysis of small residual clot fragments and allows uneventful angioplasty the following day. If necessary, low-dose heparin may be infused into the access to prevent rethrombosis until angioplasty can be performed.

Adequate balloon dilatation of access stenoses may require inflation pressures much higher than usually needed for the treatment of atherosclerotic disease. Balloons have been developed that may safely be inflated to pressures well above 10 atm, and these have given good dilatation results.

Infected accesses are not candidates for thrombolysis or angioplasty because of the risk of inducing sepsis and the probable necessity for eventual surgical removal.

DISCUSSION AND CONCLUSIONS

The interventional radiologist is currently able to treat the stenosed access shunt cheaply, easily, and, usually,

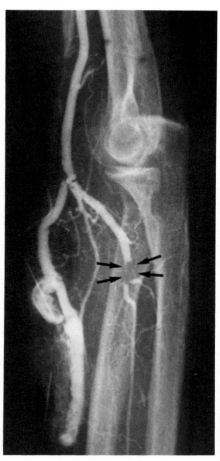

Fig. 17–12   Embolization of fragment of partially lysed clot (arrows) during thrombolysis by direct injection of streptokinase. Patient remained asymptomatic.

successfully. Even a modest radiographic improvement may translate into several months or even years of additional use of a shunt (Fig. 17–14). Once a shunt has thrombosed, however, the prognosis for return of function depends on the underlying cause. For example, accesses that have clotted because of hypotension or excessive postdialysis compression respond well to thrombolysis.[54] Shunts that thrombose because of an underlying stenosis may be declotted and used for some time, but their ultimate longevity will depend on the ability to treat the underlying stenosis by angioplasty or surgery. Accesses that fail within the first few weeks probably suffer from technical problems (Fig. 17–15),[60] and although they, too, may be usable after thrombolysis, eventual surgical revision is inevitable.

Ultimately, the safety, efficacy, and cost of thrombolysis and angioplasty must be compared with that of thrombectomy and surgical revision. No such comparison has yet been published, to the authors' knowledge. It should be noted that thrombectomy and surgical revision are not invariably successful in salvaging an access.[33] For example, Wilson cites an operative failure rate of 17%, with an additional 23% of thrombectomized and revised shunts failing within the first postoperative month.[3]

No systematic study of shunt survival after thrombolysis and angioplasty or angioplasty alone has yet been published. However, numerous such shunts have remained useful longer than a year,[52,55] and the patient in Figure 17–14 has had 31 months of trouble-free use of his shunt. It is therefore apparent that significant benefit may be obtained by nonoperative treatment.

The range of transcatheter treatment will be greatly expanded if the intravascular metal sleeves currently under development[61,62] become available for clinical use. An obvious role for these would be in the prevention of recurrence of outflow tract stenosis after angioplasty. Their use in the treatment of shunt aneurysms and pseudoaneurysms also might prove practical.

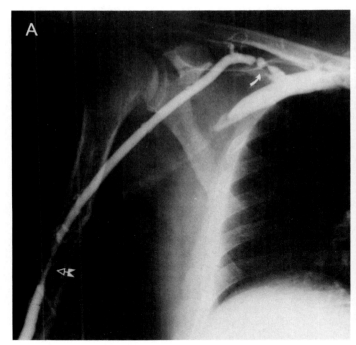

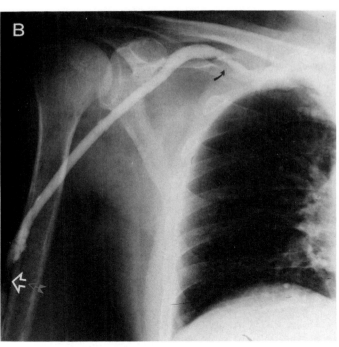

Fig. 17–13 Prophylactic dilatation of venous outflow stenosis affecting both anastomosis and cephalic vein. A. Before dilatation, venous resistance during dialysis ranged from 250–300 mm Hg. B. After dilatation with 10-mm high-pressure balloon, venous resistance dropped to 125–150 mm Hg (normal range).

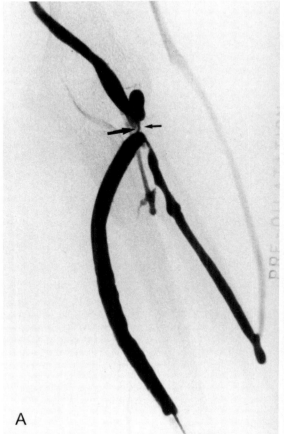

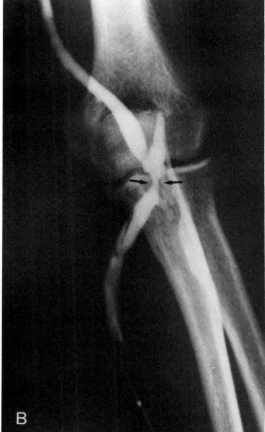

Fig. 17–14 Dilatation of venous outflow stenosis after streptokinase thrombolysis. Only modest radiographic improvement was obtained, but shunt has functioned without further difficulty for 31 months. A. Before dilatation; marked outflow stenosis (arrows). B. After dilatation; considerable residual narrowing is still present (arrows).

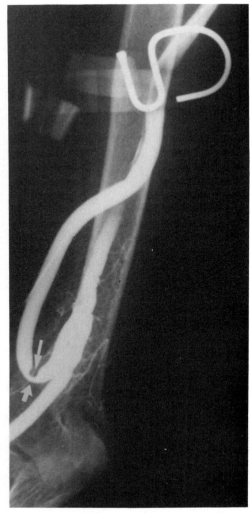

Fig. 17–15 Kinking of E-PTFE shunt (arrows) produced occlusion 9 days after implantation. Shunt was declotted with 25,000 units of streptokinase. Surprisingly, shunt remained open for 1 month and was used for dialysis during that period. Surgical revision was performed after reclotting.

In this review, the historical development of dialysis accesses and their problems have been outlined. Although some of the complications described are beyond the ministrations of the interventional radiologist, many, including the common venous outflow stenosis, are treatable by transcatheter techniques. With methods now readily available, and with the close cooperation of clinical colleagues, radiologists can effect significant improvements in access longevity.

References

1. Gilula LA, Staple TW, Anderson CB, Anderson LS: Venous angiography of hemodialysis fistulae. *Radiology* 1975;115:555
2. Giacchino JL, Geis WP, Buckingham JM, et al: Vascular access: long term results, new techniques. *Arch Surg* 1979;114:403
3. Wilson SE: Complications of vascular assess, in Wilson SE, Owens ML (eds): *Vascular Access Surgery*. Chicago, Year Book Medical Publishers, 1980, p 185
4. Kolff WF: The first clinical experience with the artificial kidney. *Ann Intern Med* 1965;62:608
5. Alwall N, Norviit L, Steins AM: On the artificial kidney: clinical experience of dialytic treatment of uremia. *Acta Med Scand* 1949;132:587
6. Quinton W, Dillard D, Scribner BH: Cannulation of blood vessels for prolonged hemodialysis. *Trans Am Soc Artif Intern Organs* 1960;6:104
7. Pendras JP, Smith MP: The Silastic–Teflon arterio-venous cannula. *Trans Am Soc Artif Intern Organs* 1966;12:222
8. Haimov M: Vascular access for hemodialysis. *Surg Gynecol Obstet* 1975;141:619
9. Moskowitz H, Gerber NA, McDonald HP Jr, et al: Angiographic study of arteriovenous shunt in hemodialysis patients. *Radiology* 1969;93:72
10. Glashan RW, Walker FA: A histological examination of veins used in artificial arteriovenous (Quinton–Scribner) shunts. *Br J Surg* 1968;55:189
11. Foran RF, Golding AL, Treiman RL, DePalma JR: Quinton–Scribner cannulas for hemodialysis: review of four years' experience. *Calif Med* 1970;112:8
12. Mandel SR: Vascular access in a university transplant and dialysis program. *Arch Surg* 1977;112:1375
13. Cope C: An improved fine needle catheter introducing set for safer central vein cannulation. *Parent Enteral Nutr* 1983;7:296
14. Butt KMH, Riedman EA, Kountz SL: Angioaccess. *Curr Probl Surg* 1976;13:1
15. Brescia MJ, Cimino JE, Appel K, et al: Chronic hemodialysis using venopuncture and surgically created arteriovenous fistula. *N Engl J Med* 1966;275:1089
16. Haimov M, Burrows L, Casey JD, Schupak E: Vascular access for hemodialysis: experience with 214 patients: special problems and causes for early and late failures. *Proc Eur Dial Transplant Assoc* 1973;9:173
17. Matolo W, Kastigir B, Stevens L, et al: Neurovascular complications of brachial arteriovenous fistula. *Am J Surg* 1971;121:716
18. Buselmeier TJ, Najarian JS, Simmons R, et al: A-V fistulae and the diabetic: ischemia and gangrene may result in amputation. *Trans Am Soc Artif Intern Organs* 1973;19:49
19. Swayne LC, Manstein C, Somers R, Cope C: Selective digital venous hypertension: a rare complication of hemodialysis arteriovenous fistula. *CardioVasc Intervent Radiol* 1983;10:61
20. Ahern D, Maher J: Heart failure as a complication of hemodialysis arteriovenous fistula. *Ann Intern Med* 1972;77:201
21. Davis D, Petersen J, Feldman R, et al: Subclavian vein stenosis: a complication of subclavian dialysis. *JAMA* 1984;252:3404
22. Watlington, J, Contes G, Yium J, et al: Arm edema due to subclavian vein occlusion and vascular access placement in maintenance hemodialysis patients with previous subclavian vein temporary catheters (abstract). *33rd Annual Scientific Meeting of the National Kidney Foundation*. New York, Grune and Stratton, 1983, p 33
23. Geis WP, Giacchino JL, Iwatsuki S, et al: The reverse fistula for vascular access. *Surg Gynecol Obstet* 1977;144:901
24. Haimov M, Burrows L, Schanzer H, et al: Experience with arterial substitutes in the construction of vascular access for hemodialysis. *Cardiovasc Surg* 1980;21:149
25. Giardet RE, Hacket RE, Goodwin NJ, et al: Thirteen months' experience with the saphenous vein graft arteriovenous fistula for maintenance hemodialysis. *Trans Am Soc Artif Intern Organs* 1970;16:285
26. Beemer RK, Hayes JF: Hemodialysis using a mandril grown graft. *Trans Am Soc Artif Intern Organs* 1973;19:43
27. Chintz JL, Yoloyama T, Bower R: Self-sealing prosthesis for arteriovenous fistula in man. *Trans Am Soc Artif Intern Organs* 1972;18:452
28. Tellis VA, Kohlberg WI, Bhat DJ, et al: Expanded polytetrafluoroethylene fistula for chronic hemodialysis. *Ann Surg* 1970;189:101

29. Mohaideen AH, Tanchajja S, Avram MM, Mainzer RA: Arteriovenous access for hemodialysis utilizing polytetrafluoroethylene grafts. *N Y State J Med* 1980;80:190

30. Anderson CB, Sicard GA, Etheredge EE: Bovine carotid artery and expanded polytetrafluoroethylene grafts for hemodialysis vascular access. *Surg Res* 1980;29:184

31. Rubio PA, DelGuercio LRM: Vascular access: methods, maintenance and management of complications. *Infect Surg* 1985;26:355

32. Sabanayagam P, Schwartz AB, Soricelli RR, et al: A comparative study of 402 bovine heterografts and 225 reinforced expanded PTFE grafts as AVF in the ESRD patient. *Trans Am Soc Artif Intern Organs* 1980;26:88

33. Shack RB, Neblett W, Richie RE, Dean RH: Expanded polytetrafluoroethylene as dialysis access grafts: serial study of histology and fibrinolytic activity. *Am Surg* 1977;44:817

34. Anderson CB, Etheredge EE, Sicard GA: One hundred polytetrafluoroethylene vascular access grafts. *Dial Transplant* 1980;9:237

35. Mohr LL, Smith LL: Polytetrafluoroethylene graft aneurysms: a report of five aneurysms. *Arch Surg* 1980;115:1467

36. Pasternak BM, Samson R, Karp MP: Fungal infection of a vascular prosthesis. *Surgery* 1979;85:586

37. Rendl KH, Prenner KV: The redo-surgery of expanded polytetrafluoroethylene (PTFE) arteriovenous fistulae for hemodialysis. *Vasc Surg* 1984;18:261

38. Hodgkinson DJ, Shepard GH: Coverage of exposed Gore-tex dialysis access graft with local sublimis myocutaneous flap. *Plast Reconstr Surg* 1982;69:1010

39. Rosental JJ, Bell DD, Gaspar MR, et al: Prevention of high flow problems of arteriovenous grafts. *Am J Surg* 1980;140:231

40. Dobkin JF, Miller RH, Steigbigel NH: Septicemia in patients on chronic hemodialysis. *Ann Intern Med* 1978;88:28

41. Chintz J, Onesti G, Brest AH, Swartz C: Radiography of A-V shunt in hemodialysis. *JAMA* 1969;207:2286

42. Wing AJ, Jones NF, Lea–Thomas M, Thompson AE: Peripheral angiography of arms and legs as aid to planning shunt and fistula operations. *Proc Eur Dial Transplant Assoc* 1971;7:510

43. Dathan JR, Thompson JMA, Worthington BS: Angiographic studies of Quinton–Scribner arterio-venous cannulae. *Br Med J* 1969;4:20

44. Smalley RH, Klinger EL Jr, Blakeley WR: Angiographic evaluation in external arteriovenous shunt management. *AJR* 1969;107:434

45. Hurwich BJ: Brachial arteriography of the surgically created radial arteriovenous fistula in patients undergoing chronic intermittent hemodialysis by venipuncture technique. *AJR* 1968;104:394

46. Glanz S, Bashist B, Gordon DH, et al: Angiography of upper extremity access fistulae for dialysis. *Radiology* 1982;143:45

47. Anderson CB, Gilula LA, Sicard GA, Etheredge EE: Venous angiography of subcutaneous hemodialysis fistulae. *Arch Surg* 1979;114:1320

48. Hunter DW, So SKS, Castañeda–Zuñiga WR, et al: Failing or thrombosed Brescia–Cimino arterio-venous dialysis fistulae: angiographic evaluation and percutaneous transluminal angioplasty. *Radiology* 1983;149:105

49. Kottle SP, Gonzalez AC, Macon EJ, Fellner SK: Ultrasonographic evaluation of vascular access complications. *Radiology* 1978;129:751

50. Scheible W, Skram C, Leopold GR: High resolution real-time sonography of hemodialysis vascular access complications. *AJR* 1980;134:1173

51. Hartley LCJ, Ellis FG, Rendall M, et al: The use of urokinase in Scribner shunts. *Br J Urol* 1980;42:246

52. Gordon DH, Glanz S, Butt KM, et al: Treatment of stenotic lesions in dialysis access fistulae and shunts by transluminal angioplasty. *Radiology* 1982;143:53

53. Glanz S, Gordon D, Butt KMH, et al: Treatment of stenoses by transluminal angioplasty. *Radiology* 1984;152:637

54. Zeit RM, Cope C: Failed hemodialysis shunts: one year of experience with aggressive treatment. *Radiology* 1985;154:353

55. Rodkin RS, Bookstein JJ, Heeney DJ, Davis GR: Streptokinase and transluminal angioplasty in the treatment of acutely thrombosed hemodialysis access fistulae. *Radiology* 1983;149:425

56. Graor RA, Risius B, Young JR, et al: Low dose streptokinase for selective thrombolysis: systemic effects and complications. *Radiology* 1984;152:35

57. Zeit RM: Clearing of clotted dialysis shunts by streptokinase injection at multiple sites. *AJR* 1983;141:1053

58. Young AT, Hunter DW, Castañeda–Zuñiga WR, et al: Thrombosed synthetic hemodialysis access fistulae: failure of fibrinolytic therapy. *Radiology* 1985;154:639

59. Becker GJ, Holden RW, Rabe FE: Contrast extravasation from a Gore-tex graft: a complication of thrombolytic therapy. *AJR* 1984;142:573

60. Rohr MS, Browder W, Frentz GD, McDonald JC: Arteriovenous fistulae for long term dialysis. *Arch Surg* 1978;113:153

61. Cragg AH, Lund G, Rysavy JA, et al: Percutaneous arterial grafting. *Radiology* 1984;150:45

62. Maass D, Zollikofer CL, Largiader F, Senning A: Radiological follow-up of transluminally inserted vascular endoprostheses: an experimental study using expanding spirals. *Radiology* 1984;152:659

18

Catheter-Directed Interventional Procedures in Children

JOHN L. BASS, M.D.

Cardiac catheterization originally developed as a diagnostic procedure. However, catheters have since been modified for therapeutic use, either by attaching inflatable balloons to their tips or by using them to deliver or remove objects or substances. Catheters are now used to enlarge openings, obstruct abnormal communications, or remove unwanted fluid accumulations. This discussion addresses several such uses, namely balloon and blade atrial septostomy, balloon valvuloplasty and angioplasty, embolization of abnormal vascular communications, and percutaneous drainage of the pericardium. A number of other catheter-directed interventional procedures, such as nonoperative closure of atrial septal defects,[1] catheter ablation to control arrhythmias,[2] and destruction of tissue using laser energy,[3] will not be covered. The last-mentioned procedure is discussed in Chapter 19.

BALLOON ATRIAL SEPTOSTOMY

Balloon atrial septostomy (BAS) was one of the first catheter-directed interventional procedures.[4] Tearing a hole in the atrial septum with a balloon-tipped catheter provides palliation for infants with complete transposition of the great arteries by decompressing the left atrium and allowing mixing of pulmonary and systemic venous blood. Although operative correction of complete transposition has been used in some newborn infants,[5] BAS remains the mainstay of early palliation.

Technique

As with most effective procedures, BAS remains relatively unchanged from the original description.[4] Venous access is now usually obtained percutaneously rather than by cutdown of the femoral vein. Newer balloons with larger capacities are available, with a dog-leg tip to facilitate entrance into the left atrium. These require large-bore (e.g., 7F) sheaths for insertion, and care must be taken that the sheaths are not inserted too far, because they may obstruct renal venous return or protrude into the right atrium and strip the balloon from the catheter during the procedure.

The catheter is inserted and directed into the left atrium. Positioning within the left atrium is traditionally confirmed with fluoroscopy or sometimes by advancing the catheter tip into a pulmonary vein. More recently, confirmation of catheter positions, and sometimes positioning of the catheter, has been accomplished with the aid of 2-dimensional echocardiography.[6,7] The advantage of ultrasound is that the precise positions of the catheter and the inflated balloon are easily determined, and withdrawing the balloon across an atrioventricular valve can be avoided. In addition, radiation exposure is reduced. In some infants, the procedure has been performed using cross-sectional echocardiography without leaving the neonatal intensive care unit.[8] The balloon is inflated either with dilute contrast medium (to allow observation by fluoroscopy and rapid deflation) or simply with normal intravenous fluid (when using ultrasound imaging). There is some evidence that using a volume of ≥ 2 ml on the initial pullback is more likely to produce a tear rather than simple stretching of the foramen ovale.[9] Obviously, however, the size of the infant must be taken into account when selecting the volume for inflation. Once inflated, the balloon is sharply withdrawn into the right atrium (Fig. 18–1), stopping short of withdrawing it into the inferior vena cava. Vigorous withdrawal of the balloon is thought to increase the chances of producing a tear, leading Dr. William Rashkind to remark that success is related to the size of the "jerk at the end of the catheter."[10] Subsequent withdrawal of the balloon inflated to diameters of >3 ml may also be related to successful palliation.[7] Success can be judged by measuring the size of the interatrial communication with 2-dimensional ultrasound,[11] by measuring the right and left atrial pressures or the arterial oxygen saturation before and after the procedure, and by observing the clinical course of the infant.

Complications

Avulsion of the atrioventricular valves or inferior vena cava and atrial rupture have been reported.[9,12] However, these complications are unlikely with careful technique and monitoring with echocardiography. Thrombosis of the femoral or iliac vein through which the catheter is inserted, or even of the inferior vena cava, may occur.[13] Inadequacy of the interatrial communication can usually be avoided by vigorous withdrawal of a large balloon.

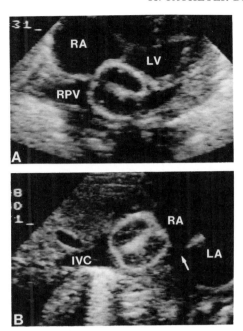

Fig. 18–1 Two-dimensional echocardiogram of balloon atrial septostomy recorded from subcostal window. A. Septostomy catheter is positioned in left atrium and balloon is inflated. B. Inflated balloon is withdrawn sharply into right atrium. Resulting hole in interatrial septum is indicated by arrow. IVC = inferior vena cava; LA = left atrium; LV = left ventricle; RA = right atrium; RPV = right pulmonary vein.

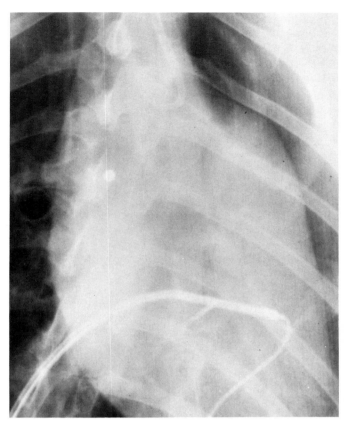

Fig. 18–2 Anteroposterior roentgenogram of blade atrial septostomy catheter. Tip of catheter is positioned in left atrium with blade opened inferiorly.

BALLOON ATRIAL SEPTOSTOMY WITH A BLADE CATHETER

Balloon septostomy remains the most common palliative procedure for infants with complete transposition of the great arteries and usually improves arterial oxygen saturation and the patient's clinical condition. However, after the first few weeks of life, the procedure is less successful, leading Park and associates to develop a blade catheter that can be withdrawn across the atrial septum to create an incision.[14] Left atrial size and anatomy should be evaluated using 2-dimensional echocardiography before attempting blade atrial septostomy, particularly when left atrioventricular valve stenosis or atresia is an indication for the procedure. A small left atrium or an inferior location of the foramen ovale may predispose to complications.

The blade catheter is introduced into the left atrium from a femoral venous approach. Use of a Mullins long sheath (USCI) may facilitate placement. The sheath is withdrawn and the blade extended in an inferior–anterior position (Fig. 18–2). Resistance to opening may indicate that the blade tip is buried in the atrial wall, and it should not then be opened. Once open, the blade is withdrawn firmly but gently into the right atrium but not into the inferior vena cava. Attempts to make additional cuts may be made by varying the angle of the blade. A BAS is performed after blade septostomy to enlarge the tear. Immediate enlargement of interatrial communications in the presence of a thick atrial septum has been reported, but long-term results are unknown. Potential complications include laceration of the posterior left atrial wall, the atrioventricular valves, or the pulmonary or systemic veins.

BALLOON DILATION VALVULOPLASTY (BDV) AND BALLOON DILATION ANGIOPLASTY (BDA)

Both these techniques involve inflation of a balloon positioned across a stenotic lesion; the force applied to the relatively rigid, distended balloon is transmitted to the surrounding tissue.[15] The degree of relief of the obstruction and the mechanism by which it occurs depend on the characteristics of the tissue forming the stenosis. The appeal of this technique is that it avoids the large incision, long hospitalization, exposure to blood products, and expense of surgery. Its success, however, must be interpreted, not only in terms of the degree and permanency of the enlargement of the stenosis, but also in relation to the results of current operations. BDV was initially applied to stenoses of the coronary,[16,17] renal,[18] and peripheral systemic arteries,[19,20] so it was natural that BDV and BDA be applied to stenotic intracardiac valves and to central systemic and pulmonary venous stenoses.

Pulmonic Stenosis

Perhaps the largest number of patients to whom BDV has been applied are those with valvar pulmonic stenosis. Inspired by the success of operative relief of pulmonary stenosis by passage of progressively larger bougies during inflow stasis,[21] Kan and associates reported an initial case of BDV in 1982.[22] Since then, there have been experimental studies of safety[23,24] as well as numerous reported series with good short- and long-term results.[23,25–29]

MECHANISM

The enlargement of the narrowed pulmonary valve orifice is produced by tearing of valve tissue. Ideally, all tearing would occur along the commissures, but postmortem[30] and surgical[27] observations suggest that the tearing may also occur by disruption or avulsion of valve cusps. There is considerable variability in the anatomy of the stenotic pulmonary valve, from fusion of the commissures to dysplasia,[30] and it is probable that the morphology of the valve tissue determines the effects of dilation. Some reports suggest that the truly dysplastic pulmonary valve is refractory to BDV.[25] Because the increase in valve area after dilation results from tearing of valve tissue, the effect should be permanent. One would expect that pulmonary insufficiency would be a frequent complication of BDV, although it should be well tolerated if pulmonary artery pressure is low.

TECHNIQUE

Selection of patients for BDV of the pulmonary valve is based on clinical criteria as well as on estimates of severity made by cardiac ultrasound. In addition to Doppler estimates of the pressure gradient across the valve and the presence of pulmonary regurgitation, it is possible to estimate the anulus diameter before cardiac catheterization.[31] Application of BDV to the infant with valvar pulmonic stenosis is limited by the large size of the available catheters (8F–9F for 10–25-mm balloons), which may be difficult to insert without avulsion of the femoral vein. In the small patient with severe stenosis, the catheter itself may obstruct right ventricular outflow. In some patients with a single ventricle or a ventricular septal defect and limitation of pulmonary blood flow by valvar pulmonic stenosis, BDV could be considered an alternative to shunting procedures for palliation. The following discussion, however, considers only those patients with congenital valvar pulmonic stenosis and an intact ventricular septum.

Cardiac catheterization is performed to exclude associated defects, measure the pressure difference across the valve, and provide angiographic assessment of the pul-

monary anulus. Usually, a pulmonary arteriogram is performed in addition to a right ventriculogram to assess pulmonary regurgitation. Angiograms are performed with 45° of cranial angulation to place the pulmonary anulus parallel to both the vertical and horizontal tubes. The angiograms are examined for associated lesions such as muscular right ventricular outflow obstruction or supravalvar pulmonic stenosis. The diameter of the pulmonary anulus is measured on each of the projections, correcting for magnification using the known diameter of the catheter.

The optimal size of the dilating balloon in most of the reported cases has been 1 mm less than[27] or 1–2 mm larger than[23,29] the anulus diameter. However, animal studies by Ring and associates demonstrated that, in lambs without right ventricular hypertrophy, a balloon with a diameter 20%–30% larger than the anulus produces no more damage to the right ventricle than do smaller balloons, whereas a balloon ≥40% larger than the anulus causes significant hemorrhage into the right ventricular outflow tract.[24] In order to achieve the maximum enlargement of the valve orifice during dilation, the present author uses balloons 20%–30% larger than the valve anulus.

At this time, the largest balloon available is 25 mm (Mansfield Scientific). Thus, if the diameter of the pulmonary anulus exceeds 21 mm, no adequate balloon is available. To overcome this limitation, some interven-

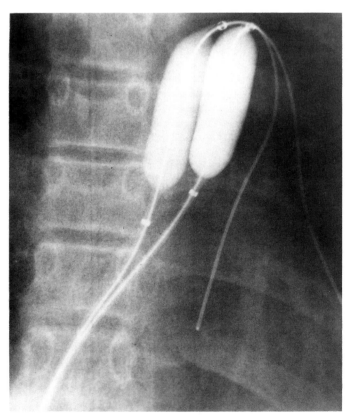

Fig. 18–3 Anteroposterior cine angiogram performed during BDV of stenotic pulmonary valve. Two balloons are positioned across pulmonary anulus and inflated to a pressure of 5 atm. Indentation produced by stenotic valve has disappeared.

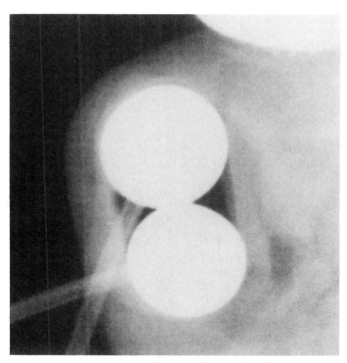

Fig. 18–4 Roentgenogram of two balloons inflated across pulmonary anulus of canine heart. The balloons, viewed in cross-section, are of equal diameter and inflated to equal pressures. There is no effacement of two balloons against each other. Small radiolucent spaces are evident where balloons are not in contact with pulmonary anulus; these spaces may allow partial decompression of right ventricle while balloons are inflated.

tional radiologists have used two balloons simultaneously[29] (Fig. 18–3). Whether the combined diameter of the two balloons should not exceed the anulus diameter by more than 30%, or whether the cross-sectional area of the anulus during dilation should equal that of a single balloon 30% larger than the anulus has not been determined. It has been shown that if the two balloons are nearly equal in size, there is no distortion of their circular shapes[32] (Fig. 18–4). If two balloons with diameters equal to 86% of the pulmonary anulus are used, the resulting cross-sectional area of the anulus will be equal to that of a single balloon 30% larger than the anulus. The benefits of dilating with two balloons include the smaller venotomies needed and the possibility of partial ventricular decompression through the gaps between the balloons.

Arterial access is established to allow monitoring of pressure during the dilation procedure. Once the appropriate sized balloon has been chosen, a 0.038-inch Teflon-coated exchange guidewire is positioned in the distal left pulmonary artery. The introducing catheter and sheath are removed, and the deflated dilating balloon catheter is advanced over the guidewire. Dilute (half-strength or less) contrast medium is used to inflate the balloon, allowing fluoroscopic observation of the balloon as well as rapid inflation and deflation. All air bubbles are removed. Under fluoroscopic control, the balloon is positioned with its midpoint across the stenotic valve and inflated to 2 atm of pressure so that the position of the valve is seen, then immediately inflated to a maximum pressure of 3.5–8 atm (depending on the balloon diameter) so that the indentation ("waist") produced by the stenotic orifice disappears (Fig. 18–5). The balloon is then rapidly deflated. The author avoids rupturing the balloon during the inflation because of the large balloon size and the possibility that a jet through the rupture could injure the right ventricle or pulmonary artery.[33] Total inflation time should be no longer than 10–12 sec and with experience may be reduced to 5–6 sec. While the right ventricular outflow is obstructed, the systemic arterial pressure falls precipitously unless there is an interatrial communication to allow right-to-left shunting during the procedure.[34,35] Ventricular ectopy may also occur, as may sinus or junctional bradycardia, but these arrythmias usually stop promptly when the balloon is deflated. Patients who are awake during the procedure experience a sensation of fullness or pressure when the balloon is inflated. If inflation is prolonged, low cardiac output during obstruction of venous return may result in loss of consciousness.

RESULTS

Immediately after the procedure, the hemodynamic state is not stable. Nevertheless, there is usually an

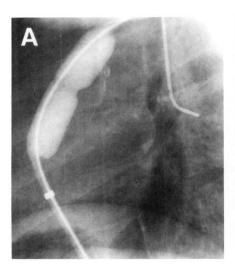
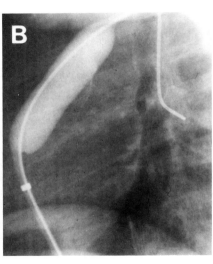

Fig. 18–5 Cine angiograms performed during BDV of stenotic pulmonary valve. A. Balloon is inflated to low pressure; indentation by stenotic valve is evident. B. After inflation to 6 atm, indentation has disappeared.

Fig. 18–6 Right ventriculograms performed immediately after (A) and 3 months after (B) BDV of stenotic pulmonary valve. Both demonstrate minimum infundibular diameter during systole. In A, there is severe infundibular narrowing associated with unchanged right ventricular peak systolic pressure. In B, residual gradient has fallen to 35 mm Hg, and infundibular narrowing has regressed significantly.

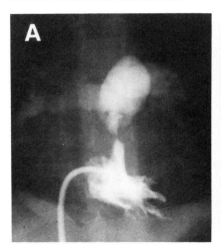 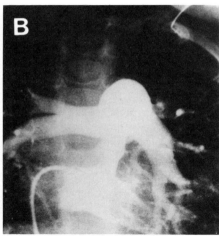

immediate fall in right ventricular systolic pressure and the right ventricular outflow pressure gradient (51%–65%)[27,29] that approach the immediate results of operation.[36,37] If there is significant infundibular hypertrophy, however, right ventricular pressure may not fall immediately. For example, in a 6-month-old child with a predilation gradient of 115 mm Hg and severe infundibular obstruction, the author observed no change in the gradient immediately after dilation. However, cardiac catheterization at 9 months of age revealed that the gradient had fallen to 35 mm Hg, with a reduction in systolic infundibular narrowing (Fig. 18–6). This change parallels surgical experience.[36,38]

Reported long-term (1 year) follow-up by cardiac catheterization has shown persistence of improvement or a further decrease in the right ventricular pressure and pressure gradient.[25,29] An additional decrease in pressure may be a result of regression of infundibular hypertrophy. An immediate "failure" of the dilation attempt is not necessarily an indication for surgical intervention,[39] and enough time should be allowed for regression of subvalvar obstruction. Noninvasive evaluation of residual obstruction can be performed using Doppler ultrasound. Recurrent stenosis has not been reported.

COMPLICATIONS

Pulmonary regurgitation has been infrequent after BDV of the pulmonary valve.[25,29] All 16 of the author's patients have had trace to 2+ pulmonary regurgitation detectable angiographically (with a catheter across the pulmonary valve) before BDV, and this remained unchanged in all but one patient, in whom it increased from 1+ to 2+. As pulmonary artery pressure is low in these patients, the regurgitation should be well tolerated. The incidence is no different from that reported with surgical valvotomy.[38] Prolonged arrhythmias have been uncommon.[29] The author has cared for one patient in whom the femoral vein through which the dilating catheter had been inserted was occluded at the time of recatheterization, an experience also reported by Kveselis and associates.[29]

SUMMARY

Balloon valvuloplasty of the pulmonary valve is a significant improvement over surgical valvotomy in terms of cost and patient convenience and also avoids the surgical scar and exposure to blood products. The true test of success, however, is the adequacy of gradient relief and the incidence of complications in comparison with those of surgical valvotomy. No deaths have been reported, and gradients have been reduced an average of 60%.[27,29] Pulmonary regurgitation has been mild and hemodynamically insignificant. Late follow-up has shown persistent or further improvement.[29] These results are nearly as good as those of surgical valvotomy.[37,38] If efforts with balloons significantly larger than the valve anulus further decrease the gradients, and if long-term follow-up reveals no unexpected complications, BDV may replace operation for many patients with valvar pulmonic stenosis.

Aortic Stenosis

Postmortem and experimental studies of the safety or efficacy of BDA of the stenotic aortic valve have only recently been reported.[33,40] Nevertheless, inspired by success with other lesions, Lababidi and associates reported an initial series of 23 patients[41] and later an additional four patients[27] with excellent results.

MECHANISM

Enlargement of the stenotic aortic valve orifice must be produced by a mechanism similar to that of the pulmonary valve, i.e, by tearing of the commissures or disruption or avulsion of valve leaflets. Destruction of valve tissue may result in significant aortic regurgitation. In two infants, observations at the time of surgical valvotomy of stenotic aortic valves that had previously been dilated revealed 1–4-mm tears at the free margins of the commissures.[27,41] No other reports describing the postdilation appearance of stenotic aortic valves are available.

TECHNIQUE

Indications for BDV of a stenotic aortic valve are not clear cut. Despite the initially excellent results reported by Lababidi and associates,[41] many institutions have adopted a conservative approach, including only those patients who have undergone an unsuccessful surgical aortic valvotomy that did not produce significant aortic regurgitation or infants who would not otherwise be considered good surgical candidates. Certainly, those patients with significant aortic regurgitation should be excluded. Application of the technique to infants may be limited by the availability of suitable catheters. Five- and 6-mm balloons are available on a 4.5F catheter; the next largest balloon size is on an 8F shaft (Mansfield Scientific, Inc.). Improvements in catheter design, such as larger balloons on small shafts or low profiles of the deflated balloon to reduce the risk to a small femoral artery, are needed.

Cardiac catheterization is performed to determine the severity of obstruction and the presence of any other defects. An aortogram is performed to allow measurement of the aortic anulus and ascending aorta as well as to assess the degree of any aortic insufficiency.

The diameter of the dilation balloon in the reported large clinical series was arbitrarily chosen as 1–2 mm less than that of the anulus.[27,41] Dilation of the normal aortic anulus in lambs showed that balloons with diameters 90%–110% of the aortic root diameter produced no cardiac damage other than superficial abrasions, whereas balloons 120%–150% larger than the aortic root produced root or leaflet tears and hemorrhage into the mitral valve.[40] This finding suggests that the aortic root is more susceptible to damage by very large balloons than is the pulmonary anulus. Nevertheless, to reduce the pressure gradient as much as possible, the largest available balloon whose diameter does not exceed 100% of that of the aortic anulus should be used.

Both venous and arterial access should be obtained to allow monitoring of the patient and to provide a route for administration of drugs. To position the balloon, a guidewire is advanced across the aortic anulus with its tip in the left ventricle. A J-tip guidewire may minimize irritation of the myocardium during manipulation of the balloon. The introducing catheter and sheath are removed, and the deflated dilating balloon is advanced over the guidewire. All air bubbles are aspirated from the balloon, which is then advanced until its midpoint is across the aortic anulus. The balloon is inflated to 2 atm with dilute contrast medium to confirm its location in the valve and then rapidly inflated to maximum dilation pressure for 5–15 sec (Fig. 18–7). The balloon is then deflated and withdrawn over the guidewire into the ascending aorta. The primary difficulty during dilation is maintaining position across the valve, because the inflated balloon tends to be ejected from the left ventricle. Ventricular ectopy and the transient fall in cardiac output, which occur during the obstruction of left ventricular outflow, are usually limited to the period of inflation. Lababidi and associates remove the guidewire so that the central lumen of the dilating catheter can be connected to a venous catheter during

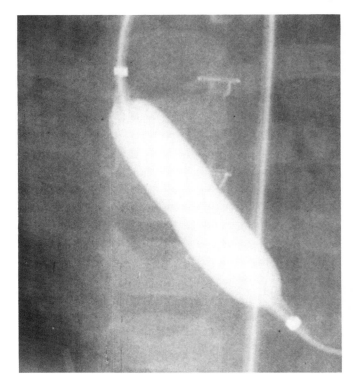

Fig. 18–7 Cine angiogram performed during BDV of congenitally stenotic aortic valve. Indentation produced by stenotic valve has almost disappeared with inflation to high pressure.

inflation of the balloon in an attempt to decompress the left ventricle.[41] The resulting reduction in peak left ventricular pressure and the amount of blood that actually flows through this communication have not been documented. Care should be taken that the balloon is not inflated to the point of rupturing, because dissection or aortic rupture may result if the balloon is the same size as or larger than the aorta.[33]

RESULTS

The immediate fall in the peak systolic pressure gradient across the aortic valve after dilation has been reported to be 60%[40] to 70%,[27] with average postdilation gradients of 25–32 mm Hg. Follow-up cardiac catheterization in 14 patients 7 months after dilation revealed lasting gradient relief.[27] These results should be considered palliative, because the number of patients in whom subsequent operation will be necessary is not known. Nevertheless, the results are similar to reported surgical results,[42,43] suggesting that there is a significant place for BDV of the stenotic aortic valve. However, if the valve is significantly thickened and obstruction results from the bulk of leaflet tissue rather than from commissural fusion, BDV may have limited efficacy.

COMPLICATIONS

Significant aortic regurgitation after BDV of the aortic valve has been a concern. In the 27 patients reported by Walls and associates, only one developed more than mild aortic regurgitation, whereas 10 apparently had no insufficiency either before or after BDV.[27] However, Helgason et al found that BDV resulted in aortic regurgitation in all patients in their smaller group.[40] The other reported complication has been thrombosis of the femoral artery through which the valvuloplasty balloon was introduced. The use of intravenous streptokinase has restored the pulse in the affected extremity.[40] There are no published reports of death associated with BDV of the aortic valve.

SUMMARY

The place of BDV in the management of patients with congenital valvar aortic stenosis has not been completely defined. Because of the risk of significant aortic insufficiency, many institutions have limited their candidates to patients who have failed surgical aortic valvotomy without developing significant aortic regurgitation or to patients who would otherwise be at great risk during cardiopulmonary bypass. Comparison with surgical experience in a large series needs to be done (and could probably best be accomplished in a cooperative study), but it already is clear that there is a real potential for BDV of the aortic valve.

Mitral Stenosis

Only preliminary results are available on the efficacy of BDV of the stenotic mitral valve. Since the initial case report of dilation of rheumatic mitral stenosis using a specially modified balloon dilation catheter,[44] two reports of use of the technique in rheumatic and congenital mitral stenosis have been published.[45,46]

MECHANISM

Enlargement of the stenotic orifice in rheumatic mitral disease might be expected to occur in a fashion similar to that described in pulmonic and aortic stenosis: by commissural tears or by disruption of leaflet tissue. The mechanism of gradient reduction in congenital mitral stenosis is more obscure. For instance, in parachute mitral valve, blood passes through interchordal spaces to enter the left ventricle, and operation to relieve obstruction is usually accomplished by removing some of the chordae. Therefore, BDV of this lesion may not be successful.

TECHNIQUE

Patients with symptomatic mitral stenosis are potential candidates for BDV. Contraindications would include active rheumatic disease, associated mitral regurgitation, or thrombus within the left atrium.

Cardiac catheterization is performed from a percutaneous femoral arterial and venous approach. Lock and associates enter the femoral vein as proximally as possible to allow passage of a large valvuloplasty catheter.[46] Cardiac output is measured while pulmonary venous and left ventricular end-diastolic pressures are recorded simultaneously. Left ventriculography is performed to assess mitral regurgitation. A balloon-tipped catheter is introduced into the left atrium through a Mullins sheath posi-

tioned across the atrial septum using a Brockenbrough technique. The transmitral pressure gradient is confirmed, and the flow-directed catheter is advanced into the left ventricle, across the aortic valve, and into the descending aorta. A Teflon-coated exchange guidewire is inserted through the catheter, and the sheath and catheter are removed. Dilation of the atrial septum and, if necessary, the venotomy with an 8-mm dilation balloon advanced over the guidewire may be performed to allow passage of the valvuloplasty balloon. Specially designed short, distally located valvuloplasty balloons have been developed by Mansfield Scientific, Inc., with diameters of 18, 20, and 25 mm. The valvuloplasty balloon is advanced over the guidewire and across the atrial septum and mitral valve, and the guidewire is withdrawn into the left ventricle. The balloon is inflated to a pressure of 3 atm with its midpoint across the anulus until the indentation produced by the stenotic valve disappears (8–15 sec). Hemodynamic measurements and left ventriculography are repeated, and a right-sided oximetry series is performed to look for a left-to-right atrial level shunt.

RESULTS

Clinical experience with BDV of the mitral valve is not extensive. Lock and associates reported treating eight patients who had rheumatic mitral stenosis. After BDV, there was an 84% increase in the mitral valve area and a 52% fall in the gradient, in spite of an increase in the cardiac output. The improvement persisted in all but one patient after 2–8 weeks.[46] Kveselis, Rocchini and associates reported two patients, one with congenital mitral stenosis, who had a significant fall in pressure gradient and an increase in valve area after BDV.[45] No long-term follow-up data are available.

POSSIBLE COMPLICATIONS

Significant mitral regurgitation was not found in the reported cases. Left-to-right shunting detectable by oximetry did not occur after dilation of the atrial septum with an 8-mm balloon. There was no acute hemoptysis or evidence of pulmonary edema or thromboembolic events.

SUMMARY

BDV of the stenotic mitral valve, at least in rheumatic mitral stenosis, may be important in the management of some patients. The exact part that it will play must await use in a larger population, as well as the long-term results.

Coarctation of the Aorta

Coarctation of the aorta was one of the first lesions successfully treated by surgery. However, there is a high incidence of persistent or recurrent gradients, especially after repair in infancy.[47,48] This led to consideration of BDA as the initial procedure in infants, who have a high mortality rate with surgical treatment,[49] or as a means of relieving residual gradients postoperatively.

The feasibility of using BDA was first evaluated by dilation of early postmortem[50] and excised human coarctations.[51] Tears in the intima extending into the media, with an increase in the circumference resulting from stretching of the remaining media and adventitia, were found. This work was followed by evaluation of experimental models of coarctation,[52,53] from which it was determined that large balloons (2.5 times the size of the coarctation) and high dilating pressures (6–7 atm) produced the best results, with persistent increases in diameter and decreased gradients. The mechanism of improvement was similar to that in excised human specimens, with intimal and medial tears. Healing left areas of medial thinning with regrowth of the intima. Attempts to dilate end-to-end anastomoses in dogs and excised human specimens were unsuccessful. Since these initial attempts, a number of reports of the application of BDA in humans with coarctation of the aorta have appeared.

TECHNIQUE

Catheterization with measurement of proximal and distal pressures is performed. An aortogram is performed to measure the diameter of the coarctation and of the aorta proximal and distal to the narrowing. The dilating balloon is chosen with a diameter 2.5–3.0 times that of the narrowed area but <1.5 times the diameter of the aorta proximal to the coarctation. A Teflon-coated exchange guidewire is positioned across the coarctation with its tip in the ascending aorta, and the positioning catheter and sheath are removed. The dilating catheter is advanced through the femoral artery over the guidewire and positioned with its midpoint across the narrowed segment. The position of the balloon is confirmed by inflation to 1–2 atm. Care is taken that the catheter is not within the left subclavian artery and not too distal in the transverse arch. The balloon is then inflated to 3.5–8 atm, depending on its diameter (Fig. 18–8). Inflation is maintained for 10–20 sec until the indentation from the stenosis disappears. Protracted occlusion of a carotid artery should be avoided. The dilating catheter is removed, leaving the guidewire in place across the dilated area. If the guidewire is inadvertently withdrawn below the coarctation, it should not be readvanced, because it or a catheter may produce a dissection of the freshly dilated area with its tip.[53,54] A catheter is advanced over the guidewire,

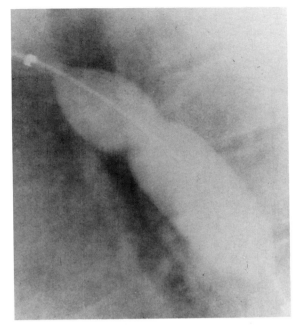

Fig. 18–8 Cine angiogram performed during BDA of stenosis of surgically repaired coarctation of aorta; balloon is inflated to maximum pressure. Indentation remains at site of stenosis.

which can then be withdrawn. An angiogram in the ascending aorta is performed (Fig. 18–9), with measurement of any residual gradient. The patient is monitored overnight in the intensive care unit. Long-term follow-up may be accomplished by exercise testing of gradients, ultrasound, or magnetic resonance imaging (Fig. 18–10).

RESULTS

There are many published reports of clinical experience with balloon dilation of coarctations. The patients can be divided into three principal categories, which will be discussed in turn: (1) infants younger than 8 weeks with no previous coarctation repair; (2) older children and adults who have not undergone surgery for coarctation; and (3) patients with residual or recurrent gradients after repair of coarctation.

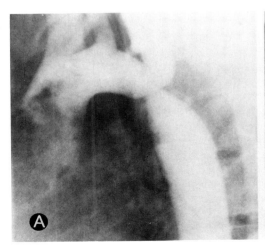

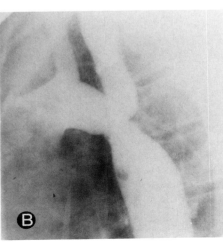

Fig. 18–9 Lateral aortogram before and after BDA in Figure 18–8. A. Narrowing distal to left subclavian artery is at site of previous end-to-end repair. B. After BDA, narrowed area is enlarged; small amount of contrast medium is seen outside lumen, presumably due to intimal and medial rupture.

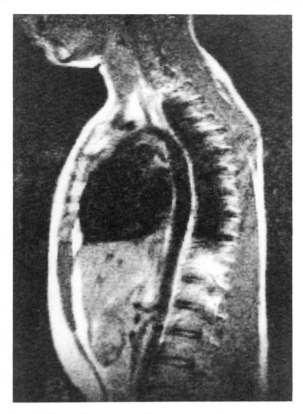

Fig. 18–10   Magnetic resonance image 1 year after BDA of stenosis of surgically repaired coarctation of aorta (same patient as in Figures 18–8 and 18–9). There is no significant residual narrowing or evidence of aneurysm formation at site of BDA.

The results of BDA in infants with coarctation who have not previously had operative repair are disappointing. Of 19 infants from the author's own and published experience, 11 had either no improvement or recurrence of gradients or symptoms, often within 48 hr of dilation.[54–59] Three infants died, one with perforation of the aorta, possibly resulting from passage of an angiographic catheter across the coarctation immediately after BDA; one at operation for associated valvar aortic stenosis, who was found to have a large dissection of the transverse aortic arch, presumably from the tip of the straightened dilating catheter during balloon inflation; and one with ventricular fibrillation 4 hr after dilation and no other apparent cause of death. The remaining five infants had lasting improvement over a 3–5-month follow-up. It is important to recognize that transient improvement may be enough in some infants to allow management of associated cardiac lesions.

At least 26 cases of BDA of coarctation of the aorta in older patients (8 months to 27 years) who had not been operated on have been reported.[58,60] A significant immediate decrease (55%–80%) in their gradients has been found. Follow-up 4–17 months later demonstrated persistent improvement or a further decrease in gradient in 14 of the 18; the other 4 had a slight increase in the gradient. However, Marvin and associates, in their 11 patients, discovered enlarging areas of dilation in the wall of the aorta at the site of BDA 1 year later.[60]

Application of BDA to recurrent or residual stenosis after surgical repair of coarctation has met with good success. There are at least 22 reported patients who had earlier undergone end-to-end anastomosis, patch angioplasty, or subclavian flap repair. These patients had an immediate 68%–80% reduction in their gradients that persisted over a 1–24-month follow-up period.[56,58,61,62] Thus far, there have been no reports of dilated areas in the aorta. One patient collapsed 6 hr after BDA while trying to void, was found to have ventricular fibrillation, and could not be resuscitated. Autopsy revealed no anatomic cause.

COMPLICATIONS

Paradoxical hypertension associated with elevated plasma renin activity sometimes follows surgical relief of coarctation of the aorta. Although transient early hypertension has occurred after BDA of coarctation,[60] prolonged hypertension associated with elevated plasma renin activity has not been found.[63] The reason for this difference is not clear. Although prolonged cross-clamping of the aorta is avoided by BDA, abnormal renal perfusion is known to persist acutely after BDA in lambs.[64] Occlusion of the femoral artery through which a dilation catheter is inserted may occur but can often be relieved by intravenous streptokinase.[40,65] Perforation or dissection of the aorta has been reported in infants after passage of a catheter across a freshly dilated site, use of overlarge balloons, or incorrect positioning of the balloon within the aorta. Sudden death associated with ventricular fibrillation has been reported in infants and older children within hours of the procedure. The cause of these deaths is uncertain, but careful post-BDA monitoring is clearly indicated. Finally, the report of dilated areas within the aorta associated with BDA of coarctation raises questions about the long-term prognosis of this group. No central nervous system complication of BDA of coarctation has been reported.

SUMMARY

The role of BDA of coarctation of the aorta is evolving. Clearly, at least in patients with incomplete operative relief of the obstruction, the procedure can be performed safely, with enlargement of the aortic lumen and a fall in gradient approaching that after operation. In most infants, however, the results will be transient, although in some of these patients, even transient relief of obstruction may be useful in that it allows improvement of the clinical condition and initiation of other therapy. It must be remembered, however, that surgery attempts to model the normal internal shape of the aorta, whereas BDA produces intimal and medial tears to enlarge the internal diameter. These tears may weaken areas of the aorta, which could lead to later aneurysms, particularly if a previous operation has not reinforced the adventitia with scar tissue, or to accelerated atherosclerosis.[66] The lifetime prognosis of coarctation after BDA remains unknown, and only controlled application of the technique with careful long-term follow-up will provide the answers.

Peripheral Pulmonary Artery Stenosis

Stenosis or hypoplasia of a branch pulmonary artery may occur as an isolated lesion, in assocation with tetralogy of Fallot, or as a result of shunts surgically placed to increase pulmonary blood flow.[67] Application of BDA to this lesion was first reported in 1980 by Martin and associates.[68] Lock et al devised an experimental model of surgically induced branch pulmonary artery stenosis in lambs in order to evaluate the safety and optimal method of applying this technique.[69] Since then, several clinical series have demonstrated the safety and efficacy of BDA in relieving branch pulmonary artery stenosis.[62,67,70]

One goal of relieving obstruction is to reduce right ventricular pressure, because severe elevation produces right ventricular fibrosis in patients with valvar pulmonary stenosis.[71] In addition, maldistribution of pulmonary blood flow sometimes produces symptoms.[72] Decreased flow during the first 2 years of life may influence the growth of intra-acinar pulmonary arteries,[73] known to be fewer in patients with peripheral pulmonary artery stenosis.[74] Thus, BDA might be expected to be most beneficial before the age of 2 years.

MECHANISM

Although surgically induced ovine branch pulmonary artery stenosis differs somewhat pathologically from the congenital lesion in humans, the enlargement resulting from BDA occurs by the same mechanism observed in human postmortem specimens.[30] The intima and media are split, with vascular integrity maintained by the adventitia, which stretches to allow enlargement of the lumen. These gaps heal in the open position by filling with collagen and elastic fibers, and the adventitia is thickened by collagen. This mechanism is similar to that observed with BDA of coarctation of the aorta.

TECHNIQUE

Selection criteria include: (1) stenosis or segmental hypoplasia of a branch pulmonary artery that is ≤8 mm in diameter; (2) elevation of right ventricular or main pulmonary artery systolic pressure to ≥50% of that of systemic arteries or at least 60 mm Hg; and (3) no significant left-to-right interventricular shunt.

Venous access is usually obtained from the femoral vein and an arterial catheter maintained for monitoring. Hemodynamic measurements are performed, followed by angiography to delineate the location, extent, and diameter of the stenotic area(s). A Teflon-coated exchange guidewire is introduced across the narrowed area and advanced into the distal pulmonary artery. Specially formed catheters may be necessary to enter the stenotic vessel.

The diameter of the dilating balloon is 3–4 times the diameter of the narrowed segment. A second catheter is available that could be inserted over the guidewire to tamponade a ruptured vessel. Dilute contrast medium is used to inflate the balloon to facilitate rapid deflation. The dilating catheter is advanced over the guidewire until the balloon is positioned across the narrowed area, and the guidewire is left in position. The balloon is initially inflated to 1–2 atm to be certain the indentation produced by the stenotic area is in the center of the balloon. If no indentation is seen, the balloon is repositioned or replaced with the next larger balloon. When the balloon is in a good position, it is inflated to 3.5–8 atm until the indentation produced by the stenosis disappears (Fig. 18–11) (a maximum of 20–30 sec) and then rapidly deflated. Successful dilation is usually accompanied by disappearance of the indentation in the balloon. The dilating catheter is withdrawn, leaving the guidewire in place. As in treating coarctation, no guidewire or catheter should be advanced past a freshly dilated area because of the possibility of dissecting through intimal and medial tears. A postdilation pulmonary arteriogram is performed to evaluate the changes in diameter (Fig. 18–12). The patient is monitored overnight in an intensive care unit, with follow-up hemoglobin and hematocrit measurements and a chest roentgenogram. Discharge is frequently possible the day after the procedure.

RESULTS

Several methods of evaluating the success of BDA are available. The most obvious is to measure the increase in the diameter of the dilated area. A small increase can produced significant improvement in flow and pressure gradient, because the cross-sectional area is proportional to the square of the radius. A decrease in the pressure gradient also indicates improvement. However, the hemodynamic state in the immediate postdilation period is not always stable, so the pressures during this time may not reflect the actual results. If dilation is attempted on only one side, an increase in the ipsilateral pulmonary blood flow would indicate success. Relative right and left lung blood flows may be quantitated by injecting [99m]technetium-labeled macroaggregated albumin into a

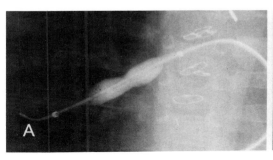
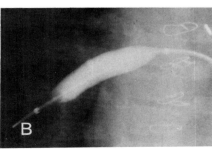

Fig. 18–11 Cine angiogram of dilating balloon during BDA of peripheral pulmonary artery stenosis. A. Balloon is positioned in right pulmonary artery and inflated to 2 atm. Indentation from stenotic area is located in midportion of balloon. B. Balloon has been inflated to maximum pressure; indentation from stenotic area has disappeared.

Fig. 18–12 Right pulmonary arteriogram before (A) and after (B) the BDA seen in Figure 18–11. Diameter of stenotic area (arrows) has increased substantially.

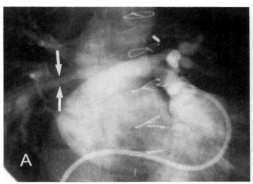
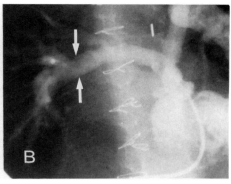

peripheral vein and comparing the counts obtained from the lungs with a gamma camera.

Of the 52 dilations reported by Ring and associates, 26 were successful, with an average increase in the diameter of the narrowed segment of 76%, an average of a 40% fall in the pressure gradient, a 20% decrease in the pressure proximal to the obstruction, and an average increase in flow to the lung supplied by the dilated vessel of 28%.[70] Kveselis and Rocchini had improvement in 6 of 12 patients.[62]

Failure resulting from technical limitations, such as the inability to advance a guidewire or the dilating catheter across the narrowed area, may occur in 18%[70] to 25%[62] of patients. Migration of the balloon away from the obstruction may also occur. Direct placement of the balloon at operation may be possible in some patients with technical failure.[75] An undilatable lesion is defined as one in which balloon indentation persists and there is no change in the diameter of the narrowed area. Although the number of reported cases is small, it appears that such lesions are more common after the age of 2 years, in isolated congenital stenosis of the pulmonary artery, and when the stenosis is associated with a surgically created shunt (although most of this latter group were older than 8 years of age). Extended follow-up data are available for only 10 patients, in 9 of whom there was persistent or further enlargement. The obstruction had returned to predilation diameter in the other patient. Additional dilation 2 or 3 months later was attempted in four patients and was successful in two.[62,70]

COMPLICATIONS

Rupture of the pulmonary artery associated with rupture of the dilating balloon followed by death from exsanguination has occurred in one patient,[70] as has rupture of the pulmonary artery by a guidewire causing hemorrhage necessitating surgical repair.[62] Care must be taken in positioning the balloon, because the right ventricular outflow tract may become obstructed during inflation. Thrombosis of the iliac vein through which the dilating catheter is inserted has also been reported.[70] Late aneurysm formation and atherosclerosis remain potential problems.

SUMMARY

BDA of branch pulmonary artery stenosis appears to be a safe and effective means of treating many patients in whom traditional surgical management has often proved unsatisfactory.[76] Dilation should be attempted before the age of 2 years, but the procedure should not be withheld from older patients or those with surgically induced narrowing. Long-term results are still unknown.

Pulmonary and Systemic Venous Obstructions

PULMONARY VEINS

Stenosis of the pulmonary veins may occur congenitally as an isolated lesion or in combination with anomalous pulmonary venous connection. It may also occur as the result of previous operation or develop after birth. Operative relief of these narrowings has been disappointing, and death has usually occurred in infancy or childhood.[77] As a result of this poor prognosis with surgery, attempts have been made to palliate or relieve this condition with BDA.

Technique

A quantitative lung perfusion scan frequently is obtained before dilation to aid in evaluating improvement. Assessment of the severity of obstruction is made by entering the pulmonary veins directly and measuring any gradient, as well as by angiography to measure the diameter and length of stenoses. Selective pulmonary arteriography may be helpful in delineating the pulmonary veins. A guidewire is introduced across the stenotic area. A dilating balloon at least 2 times the diameter of the stenotic area is positioned with its midpoint across the area and inflated to 1–2 atm to locate the indentation formed by the stenosis. If no indentation is seen, the lesion is assumed to be compliant, and the next largest balloon is chosen. The balloon is inflated to a pressure of 3.5–8 atm, depending on the balloon diameter. Balloon indentation by the stenotic area should disappear with successful dilation. The guidewire is left in place during and after dilation to allow catheter passage without risk of dissection. When the dilating catheter is removed, an end-hole angiocatheter is advanced over the guidewire; and angiography and pressure measurements are performed to assess the immediate results. Follow-up quantitative lung perfusion scans should show improved flow to the area drained by a successfully dilated pulmonary vein.

Results

At least 11 attempts to dilate stenotic pulmonary veins have been reported.[62,78–80] Eight of these lesions were congenital, four of which were associated with total anomalous pulmonary venous connection.[77,79,80] In the four cases of isolated congenital stenosis, the indentation disappeared, with enlargement of the stenotic area on angiography and a fall in the pressure gradient.[62,77] However, the improvement was followed by restenosis or lack of clinical improvement. No medial tears were demonstrated, suggesting that the lesions were extremely compliant. In the four patients with anomalous pulmonary venous connection, the lesion was so rigid that the indentation in the balloon remained in three, with no angiographic improvement being apparent.[79] In the remaining patient, there was enlargement of the narrowing, but surgical reanastomosis of the pulmonary veins to the left atrium was performed 10 days later, so the permanence of improvement could not be assessed.[80] Thus, in this group of patients, results of dilation of congenital narrowings of the pulmonary veins were not impressive, with the cause of failure depending on the etiology of the obstruction.

SYSTEMIC VEINS

Only two cases of BDA for true vena caval obstruction are reported in the literature.[79,81] In one, there was organized thrombosis in the superior vena cava[81] and in the other, narrowing of the inferior vena cava after orthotopic liver transplantation.[79] In both, the stenosis was enlarged using balloons 3–5 times the diameter of the narrowing. However, death occurred 4 hr and 7 days later.

After a Mustard operation to correct complete transposition of the great arteries, obstruction of systemic venous return through the superior or inferior limbs of the baffle may occur. An initial report by Waldman and associates described two attempts to relieve such obstruction by BDA of the systemic venous baffle.[82] Although there was initial improvement, with enlargement of the narrowing and a decrease in the pressure gradient, obstruction had recurred by 3 and 6 months after the procedures, and there was persistent indentation of the balloon at the second dilation attempt. Subsequently, Lock and associates reported BDA of obstruction of the superior (two cases) or inferior (two cases) limbs of a Mustard baffle. Using huge balloons (2.5–15 times the diameter of the narrowing), those operators produced significant enlargement of the stenosis in three patients, with resolution of symptoms and an average of a 75% reduction in the gradient.[79] The fourth patient had dynamic obstruction that did not improve with dilation. Follow-up information was available in two patients 6–7 months postdilation, with persistent improvement in both.

Mechanism

The mechanism by which obstruction of venous narrowing is relieved is not clear. Medial disruption, which occurs in successful BDA of pulmonary artery or aortic stenosis, is unlikely in venous or baffle obstructions, because there is little media in veins. It is possible that there is intimal disruption with stretching of the adventitia, but pathologic evidence is not available.

Summary

BDA of congenital or acquired pulmonary venous obstructions has generally been unsuccessful. However, postoperative caval or baffle narrowings can be enlarged with large dilating balloons. Long-term follow-up information is not yet available.

Patent Ductus Arteriosus

Closure of the patent ductus arteriosus (PDA) in the newborn infant is usually performed because of congestive heart failure or complications of respiratory problems. In the older child, closure is usually indicated because of a large shunt or the risks of bacterial endocarditis. Although this operation is safe, it requires hospitalization and a thoracotomy. This has stimulated efforts to devise a method of transcatheter closure.

TECHNIQUE

One of the first efforts at transcatheter closure was described by Porstmann and associates.[83] Their method involved placement of a guidewire from the femoral artery to the femoral vein, over which a plug was advanced into the PDA. The technique is complicated and involves creation of a considerable arteriotomy. Rashkind and Cuaso developed a device that could be inserted percutaneously through the femoral vein.[84] The most recent modification of their device is a double umbrella, the arms of which locate it within the PDA.

Cardiac catheterization is performed to measure pulmonary artery pressure and the amount of shunting, and aortography is performed to locate and measure the PDA. An end-hole venous catheter is used to position an exchange guidewire across the PDA into the descending thoracic aorta. The catheter and sheath are exchanged for an 8F Mullins transseptal introducer (USCI), the sheath of the introducer being positioned across the PDA in the descending aorta. The guidewire is withdrawn and the Rashkind ductus occluder device is advanced through the sheath to the tricuspid orifice. Because of the sharp anatomic bend at that point, it is easiest to advance the occluder out of its delivery pod and use the sheath as the delivery system. The device is advanced until the distal arms open in the aortic end of the PDA. The sheath is then withdrawn with the device in place until the proximal arms open within the PDA, and the device is released. Once the proximal arms are released, the device can no longer be collapsed within the sheath. It is not safe to withdraw the opened device across the tricuspid and pulmonary valves. If the device dislodges within the pulmonary vascular tree, it should be positioned within the left pulmonary artery so that it can be easily reached during routine PDA ligation. Repeat aortography is performed to confirm the position of the device.

RESULTS

Utilizing the femoral arterial to venous loop technique of placing a plug into the PDA, a 90%[83] to 95%[85] occlusion rate has been reported in 122 patients.

In 10 piglets in which a PDA had been created by balloon dilation of the probe-patent ductus, placement of the Rashkind double-umbrella device occluded the PDA in nine.[86] Bash and Mullins reported their experience using the same device in 34 patients over the age of 1 year. The device could be inserted into the PDA in 30, with total occlusion of the PDA in 14.[87] The device was modified during this study, and the authors speculated that the success rate would be much higher with additional clinical experience.

COMPLICATIONS

There was a 3% incidence of systemic arterial embolization with the femoral loop technique.[83,85] One of these patients suffered acute renal failure. There was an 11% incidence of stenosis or occlusion of the iliac artery through which the plug had been inserted,[83] leading to a recommendation that the technique be limited to children older than 3 years. Two of the 62 patients reported by Porstmann et al were treated for suspected endocarditis immediately after occlusion of the PDA.[83]

In the experimental study of the Rashkind device in 10 pigs, embolization into the left pulmonary artery or aorta occurred in two animals.[86] Retrieval of the device led to destruction of a pulmonary valve cusp in two instances,

so a device that embolizes should not be withdrawn across a valve. The devices were not inserted aseptically, and endocarditis developed in two pigs. The device protruded into the aorta in two additional pigs, which may not be a problem, because complete endothelialization of the device has been reported in calves.[10] In the 34 patients reported by Bash and Mullins, there was a 23% incidence of embolization into the pulmonary artery or aorta, although the release mechanism has since been redesigned.[87] All of these migratory devices were removed at PDA ligation without complications.

SUMMARY

The femoral loop method of inserting a ductus occlusion plug has not enjoyed widespread use in this country because of the complexity of the technique, as well as the need for a large femoral artery. However, because one of the principal indications for occluding a PDA in older patients is to eliminate the risk of endocarditis, the high incidence of residual shunts, protrusion of the device into the aorta, and endocarditis observed when the Rashkind device was inserted nonaseptically raise questions that must be answered before widespread use can be advocated. The incidence of incomplete occlusion and of embolization of the device may fall with additional experience and advances in design. Closure of a PDA with the Rashkind device has been reported in a 3.5-kg infant,[84] and this holds the greatest hope for nonsurgical closure in smaller patients.

THORACIC VASCULAR EMBOLIZATION

Children with systemic or pulmonary arteriovenous malformations or systemic to pulmonary artery communications may be candidates for occlusion. Methods of transcatheter delivery of occluding substances or devices have been developed to avoid hospitalization, thoracotomy, and anesthesia. In some instances, operation may be impractical because of the location or extent of the anomaly, and transcatheter occlusion may be the only alternative.

Various devices and substances have been injected to cause thrombosis of vascular communications, including absorbable gelatin sponge[88] and isobutyl-2-cyanoacrylate (Bucrylate) adhesive.[89] Particulate matter carries a risk of nonselective or distal embolization, particularly with large vascular communications. Detachable silicone balloons also have been developed that can be delivered to a specific area and are flow directed. When inflated with a hyperosmotic contrast agent, many will not remain inflated for the minimum 21-day period necessary to induce permanent thrombosis of the vessel they occlude,[90,91] whereas if the radiopaque material used to inflate them is isosmotic with blood, they may remain inflated for as long as 5 months, leading to permanent vascular occlusion.[92] Balloons with a 4-mm inflated diameter (1 mm deflated) can be delivered through a 4F or 5F catheter; however, those with the larger (8–9-mm) inflated diameter (2 mm deflated) require a 9F catheter.

The disadvantages of this system include the risk of premature balloon detachment in high flow velocity areas, the large catheters necessary to deliver balloons >4 mm, and the possibility of premature deflation. Nevertheless, there is a large successful experience with embolization of pulmonary arteriovenous malformations in older children and adults using detachable silicone balloons[93,94] (see Chapter 3). A miniature stainless-steel coil has been developed that can be delivered through a 5F catheter.[95] These Gianturco coils are coated with thrombogenic Dacron and are available in loose diameters of 3, 5, and 8 mm. The diameter of the coil when packed for delivery is 0.083 inch. A method of delivery has been developed that prevents the device from coiling prematurely.[96,97]

Technique

The precise arterial (or venous) supply of the area to be embolized is defined angiographically, as is the diameter of the vessel. A device is chosen with a loose diameter 30%–50% greater than the estimated lumen diameter. The delivery catheter is positioned distally in the vessel so that the extruded coil will not protrude into a vascular lumen that supplies normal tissue. The catheter may be shaped over steam to facilitate stable distal positioning. The packed coils are fed into the catheter lumen and advanced using a floppy-tip guidewire. The flexibility of this guidewire tip helps prevent displacement of the catheter during coil delivery. After placement of the coil, occlusion by thrombosis usually occurs within 10 min (Fig. 18–13). If angiographically demonstrable occlusion has not occurred within this period, smaller coils may be delivered to the residual lumen to further obstruct the vessel.

Results

Using this method, Bass et al have attempted to occlude 27 vessels in six children,[98] including two infants weighing <6.5 kg in whom the coils were delivered intra-arterially. Twenty-five vessels were totally occluded via 5F or 6F catheters. In two patients, 20 of 21 pulmonary

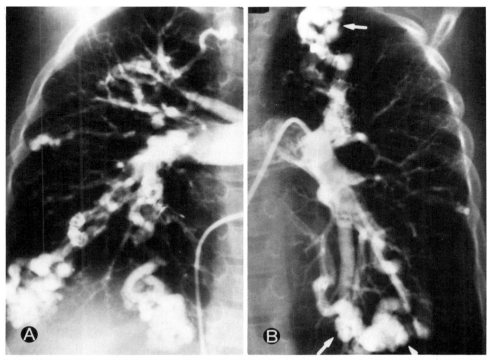

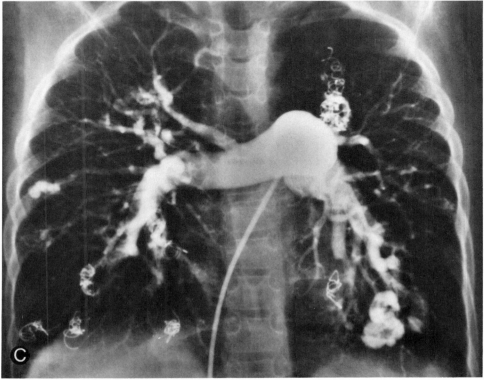

Fig. 18–13 A, B. Pulmonary arteriogram revealing multiple large pulmonary arteriovenous malformations (arrows) bilaterally. C. Postembolization biplane left pulmonary arteriogram demonstrates occlusion of multiple fistulae (arrows) performed in several procedures. There was marked clinical and symptomatic improvement.

arteriovenous malformations were embolized. To reduce pulmonary venous return during cardiopulmonary bypass, all of three bronchial arteries and a PDA were occluded in two patients with tetralogy of Fallot before surgical correction. An attempt in an infant with an aberrant systemic to pulmonary artery communication and associated disseminated intravascular coagulation was unsuccessful. Finally, occlusion of a persistent left superior vena cava prior to a right-sided Glenn anastomosis was successful.

Complications

None of the possible complications occurred in Bass et al's series. Unintentional embolization of normal vascular structures with or without infarction did not occur, nor did any coil embolize through the vessel into which it was inserted. There was neither late migration nor recanalization of occluded vessels, and there was no thrombosis of the vessel through which the delivering catheter was inserted.

Summary

Transcatheter occlusion of thoracic vascular abnormalities with miniature Gianturco steel coils is safe and effective in infants and children. The small catheter diameters that can be used for delivery make the method especially attractive in the small patient. Transcatheter occlusion may be useful as primary therapy, as in pulmonary arteriovenous malformations, or as an adjunct to operative correction of congenital heart disease.

PERCUTANEOUS DRAINAGE OF PERICARDIAL EFFUSIONS

Needle aspiration of pericardial effusions provides both fluid for diagnostic evaluation and acute relief of tamponade. Until recently, operation or repeated aspirations were necessary to provide the long-term drainage needed to treat purulent pericarditis and, possibly, to prevent a constrictive process,[99] as well as to provide access for instillation of drugs. Percutaneous placement of the catheters normally used in cardiac catheterization has been performed, but early clotting prevented long-term drainage.[100,101]

Larger (0.05-inch) sideholes in the catheters allow such drainage.[102] A pigtail catheter was chosen because the tapered tip facilitates percutaneous insertion. Location of the holes along the inner and outer curve of the pigtail prevents obstruction, because the plane of the curve tends to lie parallel to the pericardial surfaces. These features have been incorporated into a commercially available set (Cook, Inc.) that includes a 40-cm-long, 8.3F pig-

tail catheter with six 0.05-inch holes. The relative sizes of the catheter and the holes maintain catheter integrity.

Technique

The greatest accumulation of pericardial fluid is located by ultrasound so that the best entry site in the pericardium can be selected. This site may be either subcostal or through the chest wall. The patient is sedated and sat up 30°, and the site is prepared aseptically. Local anesthesia is obtained with lidocaine. The needle is inserted to the left of the midline below the lower rib (subcostal approach) or over the top of the rib (transthoracic approach). The needle is connected to a V lead of an electrocardiograph that is monitored for an injury current as the needle is advanced into the pericardial space. Sterilizable guides are available which can be attached to the ultrasound transducer so that the needle can be

Fig. 18–14 Anteroposterior thoracic roentgenogram after placement of pericardial drainage catheter. Catheter lies along posterior cardiac border with its tip positioned superiorly.

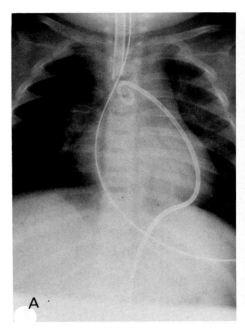
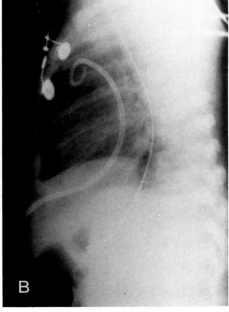

observed entering the pericardial space. Enough fluid is aspirated to demonstrate free communication, the syringe is removed, and a 0.038-inch J-tip guidewire is advanced through the needle, which is then removed. The wire provides stable access to the pericardial space and guides the catheter. Contact of the guidewire with the epicardial surface produces an injury current that is picked up by the exploring electrode. If the fluid is hemorrhagic, the intrapericardial location of the needle tip can be confirmed by reinjecting the fluid and noting the resulting contrast effect within the effusion. A stab wound is made in the skin over the guidewire, and a dilator is inserted over the guidewire while keeping it taut. The dilator is removed, and the catheter is advanced over the guidewire into the pericardial space (Fig. 18–14) and connected to continuous suction at 20 cm H_2O until no fluid has been obtained for at least 6 hr and there is no further need for access to the pericardial space.

Results

This technique has provided adequate drainage of even purulent fluid for as long as 15 days. With recurrent effusions—for example, with malignancies—the tube can be reinserted. The youngest patient in whom an 8.3F catheter has been inserted was 6 months old and weighed 5 kg[98]; this catheter size may not be appropriate for use in a newborn infant. The author has also found this technique useful for the treatment of pleural effusion and pneumothorax.

SUMMARY

The success of catheter-directed interventional procedures will lead to their use in more and more conditions. Initially restricted to patients with lesions inaccessible surgically, where operation carried an extremely high risk or where palliation to defer an operation was beneficial, the indications for nonsurgical interventional techniques are shifting toward ease and cost effectiveness. In valvar pulmonary stenosis, for which perhaps the largest experience is available, most patients in many medical centers undergo BDV rather than surgical valvotomy. It is critical to continue to compare these new forms of therapy with the existing treatment and follow the long-term results, lest a population of partially treated patients be created. The procedures must be applied systematically, rather than haphazardly by many different groups.[103] Multicenter cooperative studies are necessary for all to benefit from the experiences of others, especially when there is only a small number of patients with a particular indication.

References

1. King TD, Mills NL: Nonoperative closure of atrial septal defects. *Surgery* 1974;75:383
2. Scheinman MM, Davis JC: Catheter ablation for treatment of tachyarrhythmias: present role and potential promise. *Circulation* 1986;73:10
3. Riemenschneider TA, Lee G, Ikeda RM, et al: Laser irradiation of congenital heart disease: potential for palliation and correction of intracardiac and intravascular defects. *Am Heart J* 1983;106:1389
4. Rashkind WJ, Miller WW: Creation of an atrial septal defect without thoracotomy: palliative approach to complete transposition of the great arteries. *JAMA* 1966;196:991
5. Coto ED, Norwood WI, Lang P, Castaneda AD: Modified Senning operation for treatment of transposition of the great arteries. *J Thorac Surg* 1979;78:721
6. Allan LD, Leanage R, Wainwright R, Joseph MD, Tynan M: Balloon septostomy under two-dimensional echocardiographic control. *Br Heart J* 1982;47:41
7. Perry LW, Ruchman RN, Galioto FM Jr, et al: Echocardiographically assisted balloon atrial septostomy. *Pediatrics* 1982;70:403
8. Powell TG, Dewey M, West CR, Arnold R: Fate of infants with

9. Rashkind WJ: Transcatheter treatment of congenital heart disease. *Circulation* 1983;67:711
10. Baker EJ, Allan LD, Tynan MJ, et al: Balloon atrial septostomy in the neonatal intensive care unit. *Br Heart J* 1984;51:377
11. Bierman FZ, Williams RG: Subxiphoid two-dimensional imaging of the interatrial septum in infants and neonates with congenital heart disease. *Circulation* 1979;60:80
12. Rashkind WJ, Miller WW: Transposition of the great arteries—results of palliation by balloon atrioseptostomy in thirty-one infants. *Circulation* 1968;38:453
13. Keane JF, Lang P, Newburger J, Fyler DC: Iliac vein–inferior caval thrombosis after cardiac catheterization in infancy. *Pediatr Cardiol* 1980;1:257
14. Park SC, Neches WH, Zuberbuhler JR, et al: Clinical use of blade atrial septostomy. *Circulation* 1978;58:600
15. Abele JE: Balloon catheters and transluminal dilation: technical considerations. *AJR* 1980;135:901
16. Dotter CT, Judkins MP: Transluminal treatment of arteriosclerotic obstruction: description of a new technique and a preliminary report of its application. *Circulation* 1964;30:654
17. Grüntzig AR, Senning A, Siegenthaler WE: Nonoperative dilatation of coronary artery stenosis: percutaneosu transluminal coronary angioplasty. *N Engl J Med* 1979;301:61
18. Tegtmeyer CJ, Dyer R, Teates CD, et al: Percutaneous transluminal dilation of the renal arteries: technique and results. *Radiology* 1980;135:589
19. Spence RK, Freiman DB, Gatenby R, et al: Long-term results of transluminal angioplasty of the iliac and femoral arteries. *Arch Surg* 1981;116:1377
20. Athanasoulis CA: Percutaneous transluminal angioplasty: general principles. *AJR* 1980;135:891
21. Brock RC, Campbell M: Valvulotomy for pulmonary valvular stenosis. *Br Heart J* 1950;12:377
22. Kan JS, White RI, Mitchell SE, Gardner TJ: Percutaneous balloon valvuloplasty: a new method for treating congenital pulmonary valve stenosis. *N Engl J Med* 1982;307:540
23. Kan JS, White RI Jr, Mitchell SE, Anderson, Gardner TJ: Percutaneous transluminal balloon valvuloplasty for pulmonary valve stenosis. *Circulation* 1984;69:554
24. Ring JC, Kulik TJ, Burke BA, Lock JE: Morphologic changes induced by dilation of the pulmonary valve anulus with overlarge balloons in normal newborn lambs. *Am J Cardiol* 1985;55:210
25. Kan JS, White RI Jr, Mitchell SE, Anderson JH: Transluminal balloon valvuloplasty for the treatment of pulmonary and aortic valvular stenosis. *Semin Intervent Radiol* 1984;1:217

26. Lababidi Z, Jiunn-Ren W: Percutaneous balloon pulmonary valvuloplasty. *Am J Cardiol* 1983;52:560

27. Walls JT, Lababidi Z, Curtis JJ, Silver D: Assessment of percutaneous balloon pulmonary and aortic valvuloplasty. *J Thorac Cardiovasc Surg* 1984;88:352

28. Rocchini AP, Kveselis DA, Crowley D, Dick M II, Rosenthal A: Percutaneous balloon valvuloplasty for treatment of congenital pulmonary valvular stenosis in children. *J Am Coll Cardiol* 1984;3:1005

29. Kveselis DA, Rocchini AP, Snider AR, et al: Results of balloon valvuloplasty in the treatment of congenital valvar pulmonary stenosis in children. *Am J Cardiol* 1985;56:528

30. Lucas RV Jr, Burke BA, Edwards JE: Anatomic sequelae of balloon angioplasty in congenital heart disease. *Semin Intervent Radiol* 1984;1:225

31. Latson L, Caha D, Cheatham J, et al: Echocardiographic vs. angiographic measurements of pulmonary annulus diameter in patients undergoing successful balloon pulmonary valvuloplasty (abstract). *J Am Coll Cardiol* 1985;5:405

32. Butto F, Amplatz K, Bass JL: Geometry of the pulmonary anulus in dilation with 2 balloons. *Am J Cardiol* 1986;58:380

33. Waller BF, Girod DA, Dillon JC: Transverse aortic wall tears in infants after balloon angioplasty for aortic valve stenosis: relation of aortic wall damage to diameter of inflated angioplasty balloon and aortic lumen in seven necropsy cases. *J Am Coll Cardiol* 1984;4:1235

34. Pepine CJ, Gessner IH, Feldman RL: Percutaneous balloon valvuloplasty for pulmonic valve stenosis in the adult. *Am J Cardiol* 1982;50:1442

35. Shuck JW, McCormick DJ, Cohen IS, Getgen WJ, Brinker JA: Percutaneous balloon valvuloplasty of the pulmonary valve: role of right to left shunting through a patent foramen ovale. *J Am Coll Cardiol* 1984;4:132

36. Engel MA, Holswade GR, Goldberg HP, Lukas DS, Glenn F: Regression after open valvulotomy of infundibular stenosis accompanying severe valvular pulmonary stenosis. *Circulation* 1958;17:862

37. Nugent EW, Freedom RM, Nora JJ, Ellison RC, Rowe RD, Nadas AS: Clinical source in pulmonary stenosis. *Circulation* 1977;56(Suppl I):38

38. Griffith BP, Hardesty RL, Siewers RD, Lerberg DB, Ferson PF, Bahnson HT: Pulmonary valvulotomy alone for pulmonary stenosis: results in children with and without muscular infundibular hypertrophy. *J Thorac Cardiovasc Surg* 1982;83:577

39. Ben Shachar G, Cohen MH, Sivakoff MC, Portman MA, Riemenschneider TA, Van Heeckeran DW: Development of infundibular obstruction after percutaneous pulmonary balloon valvuloplasty. *J Am Coll Cardiol* 1985;5:754

40. Helgason H, Keane JF, Kulik TJ, Lock JE: Balloon dilation of aortic root in lambs and of valvar aortic stenosis in children (abstract). *Circulation* 1985;72:II-260

41. Lababidi Z, Wu J, Walls JT: Percutaneous balloon aortic valvuloplasty: results in 23 patients. *Am J Cardiol* 1984;53:194

42. Lawson RM, Bonchek LI, Menashe V, Starr A: Late results of surgery for left ventricular outflow tract obstruction in children. *J Thorac Cardiovasc Surg* 1976;71:334

43. Presbitero P, Somerville J, Revel-Chion R, Ross D: Open aortic valvulotomy for congenital aortic stenosis: late results. *Br Heart J* 1982;47:26

44. Inoue K, Owaki T, Nakamura T, Kitamura F, Miyamoto N: Clinical application of transvenous mitral commissurotomy by a new balloon catheter. *J Thorac Cardiovasc Surg* 1984;87:394

45. Kveselis DA, Rocchini AP, Beekman R, et al: Balloon angioplasty for congenital and rheumatic mitral stenosis. *Am J Cardiol* 1986;57:348

46. Lock JE, Khalilullah M, Shrivistava S, Bahl V, Keane JF: Percutaneous catheter commissurotomy in rheumatic mitral stenosis. *N Engl J Med* 1985;313:1515

47. Williams WG, Shindo G, Trusler GA, Dische MR, Olley PM: Results of repair of coarctation of the aorta during infancy. *J Thorac Cardiovasc Surg* 1980;79:603

48. Beekman RH, Rocchini AP, Behrendt DM, Rosenthal A: Reoperation for coarctation of the aorta. *Am J Cardiol* 1981;48:1108

49. Shinebourne EA, Tam ASY, Elseed AM, et al: Coarctation of the aorta in infancy and childhood. *Br Heart J* 1976;38:375

50. Sos T, Sniderman KW, Rettek-Sos B, Strupp A, Alonso DR: Percutaneous transluminal dilatation of coarctation of thoracic aorta post mortem. *Lancet* 1979;2:970

51. Lock JE, Castañeda-Zuñiga WR, Bass JL, et al: Balloon dilatation of excised aortic coarctations. *Radiology* 1982;143:689

52. Castañeda-Zuñiga WR, Lock JE, Vlodaver Z, et al: Transluminal dilatation of coarctation of the abdominal aorta. *Radiology* 1982;143:693

53. Lock JE, Niemi T, Burke BA, Einzig S, Castañeda-Zuñiga WR: Transcutaneous angioplasty of experimental aortic coarctation. *Circulation* 1982;66:1280

54. Finley JP, Beaulieu RG, Nanton MA, Roy DL: Balloon catheter dilatation of coarctation of the aorta in young infants. *Br Heart J* 1983;50:411

55. Sperling SR, Dorsey TJ, Rowen M, Gazzaniga AB: Percutaneous transluminal angioplasty of congenital coarctation of the aorta. *Am J Cardiol* 1983;51:562

56. Lock JE, Bass JL, Amplatz K, Fuhrman BP, Castañeda-Zuñiga WR: Balloon dilation angioplasty of aortic coarctations in infants and children. *Circulation* 1983;68:109

57. deLezo JS, Fernandez R, Sancho M, et al: Percutaneous transluminal angioplasty for aortic isthmic coarctation in infancy. *Am J Cardiol* 1984;54:1147

58. Lababidi ZA, Daskalopoulos DA, Stoeckle H: Transluminal balloon coarctation angioplasty: experience with 27 patients. *Am J Cardiol* 1984;54:1288

59. Singer MI, Rowen M, Dorsey TJ: Transluminal aortic balloon angioplasty for coarctation of the aorta in the newborn. *Am Heart J* 1982;103:131

60. Marvin WJ, Mahoney LT, Rose EF: Pathologic sequelae of balloon dilation angioplasty for unoperated coarctation of the aorta in children (abstract). *J Am Coll Cardiol* 1986;7:117

61. Kan JS, White RI, Mitchell SE, Farmlett EJ, Donahoo JS, Gardner TJ: Treatment of restenosis of coarctation by percutaneous transluminal angioplasty. *Circulation* 1983;68:1087

62. Kveselis D, Rocchini AP: Percutaneous transluminal angioplasty of peripheral pulmonary arterial stenosis, coarctation of the aorta, superior vena caval and pulmonary venous stenosis, and other great-artery stenoses. *Semin Intervent Radiol* 1984;1:201

63. Choy M, Rocchini AP, Beekman RH, Kveselis DA, Rosenthal A: No paradoxical hypertension after balloon angioplasty of coarctation of the aorta (abstract). *Circulation* 1985;72:III-260

64. Lock JE, Kulik TJ, Green TP, Neimi T, Einzig S: Resting and exercise renal blood flows in immature ovine aortic coarctation—impact of gradient relief. *Circ Res* 1983;53:644

65. Gagnon R-M, Goudreau E, Joyal F, Morissette M, Roussin A: The role of intravenous streptokinase in acute arterial occlusions after cardiac catheterization. *Cathet Cardiovasc Diagn* 1985;11:409

66. Lock JE: Now that we can dilate, should we? (editorial). *Am J Cardiol* 1984;54:1360

67. Lock JE, Castañeda-Zuñiga WR, Fuhrman BP, Bass JL: Balloon dilation angioplasty of hypoplastic and stenotic pulmonary arteries. *Circulation* 1983;67:962

68. Martin EC, Diamond NG, Casarella WJ: Percutaneous transluminal angioplasty in non-atherosclerotic disease. *Radiology* 1980;135:27

69. Lock JE, Niemi T, Einzig S, Amplatz K, Burke B, Bass JL: Transvenous angioplasty of experimental branch pulmonary artery stenosis in newborn lambs. *Circulation* 1981;64:886

70. Ring JE, Bass JL, Marvin W, et al: Management of congenital stenosis of a branch pulmonary artery with balloon dilation angioplasty: report of 52 procedures. *J Thorac Cardiovasc Surg* 1984;90:35

71. Lucas RV Jr, Moller JH: Pulmonary valvular stenosis, in Downing DF (ed): *Cardiovascular Clinics: Congenital Heart Disease, Vol. 2.* Philadelphia, FA Davis, 1970, p 156

72. Furhman BP, Pokora TJ, Bessinger FB, Lucas RV Jr: Hypercarbia in the infant with congenital cardiac disease. *Pediatr Cardiol* 1982;2:245

73. Hislop A, Reid A: Pulmonary arterial development during childhood: branching pattern and structure. *Thorax* 1973;28:129

74. Haworth SG, Reid L: Quantitative structural study of pulmonary circulation in the newborn with pulmonary atresia. *Thorax* 1977;32:129

75. Foker JE, Turley K, Lock JE, Ring WS, Stanger P: Intraoperative balloon dilation of stenotic and hypoplastic pulmonary arteries. *Circulation* 1983;68(Suppl III):III-213

76. Fuster V, McGoon DC, Kennedy MA, Ritter DG, Kirklin JW: Long-term evaluation (12–22 years) of open heart surgery for tetralogy of Fallot. *Am J Cardiol* 1980;46:635

77. Driscoll DJ, Hesslein PS, Mullins CE: Congenital stenosis of individual pulmonary veins: clinical spectrum and unsuccessful treatment by transvenous balloon dilation. *Am J Cardiol* 1982;49:1767

78. Massumi A, Woods L, Mullins CE, Nasser WK, Hall RJ: Pulmonary venous dilation in pulmonary veno-occlusive disease. *Am J Cardiol* 1981;48:585

79. Lock JE, Bass JL, Castañeda–Zuñiga WR, et al: Dilation angioplasty of congenital or operative narrowings of venous channels. *Circulation* 1984;70:457

80. Rey C, Marache P, Francart C, Dupuis C: Percutaneous balloon angioplasty in an infant with obstructed total anomalous pulmonary vein return. *J Am Coll Cardiol* 1985;6:894

81. Rocchini AP, Cho KJ, Byrum C, Heidelberger K: Transluminal angioplasty of superior vena cava obstruction in a 15-month-old child. *Chest* 1982;82:506

82. Waldman JD, Waldman J, Jones MC: Failure of balloon dilatation in mid-cavity obstruction of the systemic venous atrium after the Mustard operation. *Pediatr Cardiol* 1983;4:151

83. Porstmann W, Wierny L, Warnke H, Gerstberger G, Romaniuk PA: Catheter closure of patent ductus arteriosus—62 cases treated without thoracotomy. *Radiol Clin North Am* 1971;9:203

84. Rashkind WJ, Cuaso CC: Transcatheter closure of patent ductus arteriosus—successful use in a 3.5-kilogram infant. *Pediatr Cardiol* 1979;1:1

85. Sato K, Fujino M, Kozuka T, et al: Transfemoral plug closure of patent ductus arteriosus—experiences in 61 consecutive cases treated without thoracotomy. *Circulation* 1975;51:337

86. Lock JE, Bass JL, Lund G, Rysavy JA, Lucas RV Jr: Trans-

catheter closure of patent ductus arteriosus in piglets. *Am J Cardiol* 1985;55:826

87. Bash SE, Mullins CE: Insertion of patent ductus arteriosus occluder by transvenous approach: a new technique (abstract). *Circulation* 1984;70(Suppl II):II-285

88. Fellows KE, Shaw KT, Schuster S, Shwachman H: Bronchial artery embolization in cystic fibrosis: technique and long-term results. *J Pediatr* 1979;95:959

89. Zuberbuhler JR, Dankner E, Zoltun R, Burkholder J, Bahnson HT: Tissue adhesive closure of aortic–pulmonary artery communications. *Am Heart J* 1974;88:41

90. White RI, Ursic TA, Kaufman SL, et al: Therapeutic embolization with detachable balloons: physical factors influencing permanent occlusion. *Radiology* 1978;126:521

91. Kaufman SL, Strandberg JD, Barth KH, Gross GS, White RI: Therapeutic embolization with detachable silicone balloons: long-term effects in swine. *Invest Radiol* 1979;14:156

92. Barth KH, White RI, Kaufman SL, Strandberg JD: Metrizamide, the ideal radiopaque filling material for detachable silicone balloon embolization. *Invest Radiol* 1979;14:35

93. White RI, Mitchell SE, Barth KH, et al: Angioarchitecture of pulmonary arteriovenous malformations: an important consideration before embolotherapy. *AJR* 1983;140:681

94. Terry PB, White RI, Barth KH, Kaufman SL, Mitchell SE: Pulmonary arteriovenous malformations: physiologic observations and results of therapeutic balloon embolization. *N Engl J Med* 1983;308:1197

95. Anderson JH, Wallace S, Gianturco C, Gerson LP: "Mini" Gianturco stainless steel coils for transcatheter vascular occlusion. *Radiology* 1979;132:301

96. Castañeda–Zuñiga WR, Zollikofer C, Barreto A, Formanek A, Amplatz K: A new device for the safe delivery of stainless steel coils. *Radiology* 1980;136:230

97. Furman BP, Bass JL, Castañeda–Zuñiga WR, Amplatz K, Lock JE: Coil embolization of congenital thoracic vascular anomalies in infants and children. *Circulation* 1984;70:285

98. Bass JL, Fuhrman BP, Kulik TJ, Lock JE: Interventional thoracic procedures in children. *Semin Intervent Radiol* 1984;1:195

99. Rubenstein JJ, Goldblatt A, Daggett WM: Acute constriction complicating purulent pericarditis in infancy. *Am J Cardiol* 1961;124:591

100. Owens WC, Schaeler RA, Rahimtoola SH: Pericardiocentesis: insertion of a pericardial catheter. *Cathet Cardiovasc Diagn* 1975;1:317

101. Glancy DL, Richter MA: Catheter drainage of the pericardial space. *Cathet Cardiovasc Diagn* 1975;1:311

102. Lock JE, Bass JL, Kulik TJ, Fuhrman BP: Chronic percutaneous pericardial drainage with modified pigtail catheters in children. *Am J Cardiol* 1984;53:1179

103. Shinebourne EA: Ethics of innovative cardiac surgery. *Br Heart J* 1984;52:597

19

Transluminal and Intraoperative Laser Angioplasty

WILSON GREATBATCH, Ph.D., F.I.E.E.E., AND T. J. BOWKER, M.A., M.R.C.P.

The laser (*l*ight *a*mplification by *s*timulated *e*mission of *r*adiation) is the fulfillment of one of humanity's oldest technologic dreams—a beam of light that removes even the hardest and most heat-resistant materials. The laser provides a beam of electromagnetic radiation that is parallel, coherent, monochromatic, and of high intensity, a beam that can be delivered to a precisely defined target. Lasers will perform microsurgery on subcellular structures, weld the retina to its supports, and drill holes in diamonds. In the last few years, lasers have become a useful tool in many medical specialties, and increasingly they are being investigated by interventional radiologists.

THE NATURE OF LASERS

A laser is a hollow tube with mirrors at each end that is filled with a lasable material—glass, crystal, gas, liquid, or a dye—which is capable of being excited (pumped) briefly to a higher energy state by some other energy source, such as an intense flash of light or an electrical discharge. This reaction creates a new light beam that is amplified as it is reflected back and forth between two mirrors. As the electrons of each atom fall back to their ground energy level, light is emitted that releases other nearby atoms, creating more light, which oscillates back and forth between the mirrors, building in intensity. If one of the mirrors reflects only 99% of the light, the remaining 1% passes through as a brilliant beam of monochromatic, coherent light, which can have a wavelength throughout the visible spectrum, or may be invisible, such as ultraviolet or infrared.

MECHANISMS OF LASER ACTION

The distinctive characteristics of a laser are directly determined by its wavelength, by the range of its power, and by whether its light is emitted in pulses or as a continuous wave (CW).

If laser energy is absorbed by tissue, that tissue may react in several ways. It may itself emit energy; this is the mechanism of laser-induced fluorescence. Alternatively, it may dissipate the energy through atomic vibration, rotation, or collision, thus generating heat. If sufficient laser energy is delivered, this heating will vaporize the water in the tissue. Such *photothermal* ablation appears to be responsible for the action of lasers in the infrared and visible parts of the spectrum, such as the Nd:YAG (neodymium:yttrium–aluminum–garnet) and carbon dioxide (CO_2) lasers. Excimer (*exci*ted *d*imer) lasers, which operate in the far ultraviolet, appear to break molecular bonds, producing dissociation products with a larger volume than the original tissue; this leads to vaporization of tissue with little production of heat.[1] Such *photochemical* ablation may have clinical applications in interventional radiology. Lasers of very short wavelength, such as those of gamma rays and x-rays, ionize their targets. These lasers have no clinical applications at present.

Another type of laser action is *photodynamic*, in which a tissue-toxic dye that has been taken up selectively by the undesired tissue is activated by laser. The classic example is tumor photodynamic therapy with hematoporphyrin derivative.[2] Some of the investigation of laser angioplasty has been devoted to finding substances that are taken up specifically by atherosclerotic plaque; presumably, such substances would enhance the effect of laser energy.[2-4]

Argon Lasers

The argon (Ar) laser produces blue-green light at 488 and 514.5 nm at powers as high as 20 watts (W). These wavelengths are intensely absorbed by heme-containing tissue, making the Ar laser ideal for photocoagulation and selective ablation of blood-containing tissues such as port-wine stains. The Ar laser beam is readily transmitted through fiberoptics and has been used extensively in ophthalmology. This laser requires a high power input and a very high discharge current, typically 30 A. Further, its efficiency is very low, so an 18-W output laser will require a 20,000-W power supply. Such machines are not very portable. Further, special wiring and water cooling are usually required, and the laser laboratory thus becomes a permanent installation to which patients must be brought.

Nd:YAG Lasers

The Nd:YAG laser produces a near infrared beam at 1060 nm at powers as great as 100 W. This laser has a longer extinction length than the Ar laser, and it is scattered diffusely in tissue. These properties cause deep heating and coagulation of tissue. It is poorly absorbed, and this property, in addition to its scattering and its facility for transmission through fiberoptics, make the Nd:YAG laser useful for both ablation and coagulation. It has shown great promise in reducing the frequency of recurrence of superficial bladder tumors.

Carbon Dioxide Lasers

The CO_2 laser is the most efficient of all the lasers, converting some 30% of its input energy into useful light. It is available in power outputs from 10 mW to 5 kW in the CW mode or from 0.1–1000 J in the pulsed mode. The CO_2 laser has the longest wavelength of the lasers in clinical use, 10,600 nm. It also has the shortest extinction length, which means that its effect is virtually confined to the tissue surface (0.1 mm). It does not transmit well through available fiberoptics, and thus its clinical use has been restricted to vaporization of surface lesions under direct vision. Because its beam is invisible, the CO_2 laser is commonly used in conjunction with a helium–neon laser operating at 632.8 nm in the visible red portion of the spectrum.

Limitations of Ar, Nd:YAG, and CO_2 Lasers

These lasers have two potential limitations in clinical use. First, they may cause substantial thermal injury to nearby normal tissues. However, this effect can be minimized by delivering a pulse of energy sufficiently short to vaporize a lesion before much lateral heat conduction has occurred. Second, none of these lasers can ablate densely calcified tissue.

Excimer Lasers

Excimer lasers are composed of halides of noble gases. Among the commercially available excimer lasers are ArF (193 nm), KrF (248 nm), XeCl (308 nm), and XeF (351 nm), all in the ultraviolet. The average power output ranges from 4–100 W. The excimer laser has a relatively high efficiency, at about 4%. Helium is added as a buffer gas and is essential for stabilization of the discharge. It acts as a collision partner in the three-body recombination. The laser is operated at a pressure of 2–4 atm. A typical gas mixture of KrF will contain 4 torr of F_2, 120 torr of Kr, and 2400 torr of He. The output is decreased if impurity levels in the gases are too high, so gas purity should exceed 99.99%. Gas lifetimes have been improved markedly during recent years, and XeCl lifetimes now exceed 10^7 shots. The pulse width of excimer lasers is narrow, on the order of 10–25 nsec, and a peak pulse power of 10^7 W is obtainable. These properties permit excimer lasers to ablate calcified and other tissue with little or no thermal injury.

Excimer lasers are still highly experimental for medical use, although Grundfest et al have reported impressive results.[5] The XeF laser may be usable with quartz fiberoptic wave guides. Grundfest et al suggested that excimer lasers operate by breaking chemical bonds in the long-chain proteins, resulting in accurately controllable disintegration of tissue without burning or charring.[5] It is questionable whether the shorter wavelength excimers can be used with flexible fibers, but much work is proceeding in this area.

Isner and Clarke stress the clean-cutting capability of the excimer laser, both in air and under fluids.[6] Trokel et al have used this laser in radial keratotomy, in which several clean, fine incisions are made in the cornea to reshape the lens, dramatically correcting certain vision defects in some cases. The precision and quality of laser incisions far exceed those obtainable with a standard diamond knife.

There has been concern about the toxic and mutagenic effect of the ultraviolet laser beam on treated tissue. The magnitude of this risk remains to be defined.

FIBEROPTIC CONDUCTORS

Glass fibers for fiberoptic systems are made of a core with a high index of refraction coated by a cladding with a lower index of refraction. Because of this design, light is continually bent from the periphery toward the core and cannot escape unless it encounters some discontinuity such as a scratch or a slag inclusion. Fibers may be made entirely of glass or of plastic-cladded silica or plastic. Fiberoptics for therapeutic lasers use all-glass construction, because plastics would be destroyed at the power levels necessary.[7] Connectors for optical fibers are a problem, inasmuch as any discontinuity will instantly develop destructive temperatures. Ideally, the ends to be joined should be polished, mated, and fused. A number of mechanical connection schemes are now commercially available, but one must exercise great care in using them,

because a loose connection or a spot of dirt could destroy the connector and the fiber.

The CO_2 infrared laser has been limited to open procedures because of the absence of satisfactory nontoxic fiberoptics to guide the laser beam to closed areas. However, infrared-transmitting glasses may become the next generation of optical communications, and if this happens, medical usage will soon follow.[8]

A number of new fibers have been suggested. Poulain described a heavy-metal fluoride glass (HMFG) that transmits well in a 2.5–5-μm window but not at 10.6 μm.[9] Polycrystalline fibers extruded from KRS-5 (thallium bromoiodide) transmit at 5–20 μm and have losses of 1 db/km at 10.6 μm. Chalcogenide glasses (As_2S_3) have historically been good for short runs.[10] Unfortunately, thallium and arsenic are probably too toxic for medical work.[7] White describes KRS-5 chalcogenide fibers by Galileo, based on Texas Instruments 1173 glass, which have been drawn in diameters as small as 25 μm.[10] Transmission is good in the 8–12-μm (CO_2 laser) range.

CARDIOVASCULAR APPLICATIONS OF ANGIOPLASTY

Lasers have been used to measure coronary blood flow, to map the propagation of myocardial depolarization, and to ablate atrioventricular conduction tissue.[11–23] However, most of the interest has been in their use to recanalize blood vessels, either alone or in conjunction with balloon angioplasty. The first experimental studies of such use were published in the early 1980s.[14,19,24–31]

Intraoperative Experience

Choy et al attempted Ar laser recanalization of a proximal coronary artery stenosis in five patients during distal saphenous vein–coronary artery bypass surgery. Under direct vision, three vessels were recanalized, but only one remained angiographically patent approximately 1 month later. One mechanical vessel perforation occurred from the protruding quartz fiber.[11] Livesay et al reported CO_2 laser angioplasty of coronary arteries at bypass surgery in six patients, in five of whom recanalization was achieved. There were no perforations, and all five arteries were patent 1 week later.[12] This procedure must be considered highly experimental and does not have the approval of the Food and Drug Administration.

Laser and Laser-Assisted Peripheral Angioplasty

The Ar laser passes through fiberoptic wave guides with little attenuation and thus is attractive for laser angioplasty of occluded blood vessels. Some investigators combine angioplasty with angioscopy to observe the intra-arterial operative field.[11,13] Other proposed systems use laser angioplasty to make conventional balloon angioplasty possible when the balloon will not pass initially, the Ar beam being used to create a hole large enough to permit insertion of the balloon.[13–15] The synergy of the two systems should permit extension of balloon angioplasty to cases where surgical bypass is now the only option. There is some evidence that restenosis of the treated vessels will be less frequent if balloon angioplasty is also used, although contradictory data also have been obtained.

Ginsburg et al utilized an Ar laser in 16 patients with occlusive peripheral vascular disease of the legs.[29] A fiberoptic wave guide, through which the laser energy was delivered, was passed under fluoroscopic control, and the laser energy usually was delivered as the laser catheter was being pulled back across a partially obstructing atherosclerotic lesion. Of the 16 vessels, eight were partially recanalized; however, the diameter of the recanalized segment was routinely <1.0 mm by angiographic measurement. Seven patients suffered significant discomfort and intense vascular spasm during laser delivery, and there were three perforations and one dissection during the procedure. Several of the recanalized vessels quickly occluded. Geschwind et al have obtained similar results, having partially recanalized an obstructive femoral–popliteal system in three patients using an Nd:YAG laser.[14,15]

Another approach to laser recanalization uses the laser indirectly to heat a metal probe that is applied to the lesion.[17] Sanborn et al performed percutaneous laser-assisted recanalization in the peripheral arteries of 40 patients, using the Ar laser-heated tip probe. Preliminary results appear promising, in that with the additional assistance of balloon angioplasty, these investigators achieved some improvement in patency in approximately 90% of patients.[13]

PROBLEMS AND QUESTIONS

Before laser or laser-assisted angioplasty can be considered for routine use, numerous questions need to be answered.

What Type of Energy Should Be Delivered?

The power, exposure time (pulse duration), and wavelength of the laser energy determine the immediate damage to the vessel wall, which presumably differs depending on the nature of that wall—e.g., normal or atherosclerotic tissue. Studies of these factors—the physical mechanisms of laser ablation and the optical and thermal properties of atherosclerotic and healthy vascular tissue—are only now beginning.

What Is the Best Way to Deliver Laser Energy?

Several variables are involved in answering this question. One group of variables concerns the orientation of the laser fiber in relation to the target tissue. For example, the core diameter of the optical fiber determines the diameter of the beam as it strikes the target (spot size), which, in turn, determines the power density at each set of energy parameters. There also are questions about the proximity of the optical fiber to the target: the closer the tip, the smaller the spot and thus the greater the power density. At the same time, it must be remembered that the optical fiber can easily perforate a vessel, either mechanically or by lasing. It was in an attempt to avoid this complication that balloon catheter systems have been designed to maintain the optical fiber in the center of the vessel lumen.[18] Finally, the effect of intra-arterial fluid cannot be ignored, especially for laser wavelengths readily absorbed by hemoglobin.

The second group of delivery variables involves the delivery system itself. Most percutaneous laser treatments have been delivered by classic angiographic techniques with fluoroscopic monitoring. An alternative system, still in the early stages of development, involves passage of a fine intravascular endoscope (angioscope) through which the optical fiber of the laser is passed. This technique necessitates removal of most of the blood from the operating field. Production of such an instrument has proved to be a significant challenge. A third option, already mentioned, is the use of a laser-heated metal cap to ablate the lesion.[13,17]

How Can the Uptake of Laser Energy by Atheroma Be Enhanced?

It would be ideal if atheroma and normal vascular tissue differed in their optical absorption characteristics or could be made to do so. Some preliminary results are encouraging.[2-4] For example, tetracyclines localize in atherosclerotic tissue, presumably because of their interaction with calcium. Hematoporphyrin derivative also is taken up selectively by atheroma and has been an effective enhancer of the action of a tunable-dye laser driven by an Ar laser in animal models. Unfortunately, animal models of atherosclerosis differ considerably from the human disease, so the clinical applicability of these findings is in doubt. *In vitro*, fluorescein and Sudan black enhance the action of Ar lasers on atherosclerotic arteries.

How Dangerous Is the Debris Created by Laser Angioplasty?

Two by-products of laser treatment must be considered: vaporization products and particulate debris. Available information suggests that neither will be a significant problem.[18] For example, Nordstrom et al isolated the products of *in vitro* laser application to human atheroma and found that ambient air and CO_2 were the most abundant vaporization products. Tetrafluoroethylene was present in concentrations of ≤100 ppm, and there were trace amounts of short carbon chain gases such as ethane.[18] Most of the particles were in the 10-20-μm range and had little or no cytotoxicity. No toxic reactions or embolizations have been apparent in the clinical trials of laser angioplasty.

Is There Significant Long-Term Damage to the Vessel Wall?

In atherosclerotic rabbits fed an atherogenic diet, lasers can damage the vascular wall. Application of 3-6 J to aortic plaques invariably caused damages to the medial layer of the vessel wall, and in follow-up studies areas of aneurysmal dilatation were apparent. Histologically, these outpouchings were thinned, necrotic, and disorganized.[19-21] Again, there is some question of the applicability of these findings to the human disease, because rabbit atheroma is considerably softer than the human type.

FUTURE DIRECTIONS

Clearly, much work remains to be done even though it is apparent that lasers can vaporize atherosclerotic plaque. First, the incidence of vascular perforation is unacceptably high. Second, to date, laser-treated vessels have shown a disconcerting tendency to reocclude, often within days; and investigation of the mechanism has been severely hampered by the lack of a good animal model. Third, spasm in the treated vessels has been a significant problem in some clinical trials, and this response may limit the use of lasers unless a way can be found to prevent it. Fourth, many problems remain in equipment, laser energy, and delivery. Finally, the long-term effects of laser energy on normal tissue remain unknown. Until these probems are solved, laser angioplasty can be only an experimental procedure.

References

1. Srinivasan R, Leigh WJ: Ablative photodecomposition: action of far-ultraviolet (193 nm) laser radiation on poly(ethylene terephthalate) films. *J Am Chem Soc* 1982;104:6784
2. Dougherty TJ, Kaufman JE, Goldfarb A, Weiskaupt KR, Boyle D, Mittleman A: Photoradiation therapy for treatment of malignant tumors. *Cancer Res* 1978;38:2628
3. Chan MC, Lee G, Seckinger DI, et al: Pretreatment with vital dyes to enhance or attenuate argon laser energy absorption in blood vessels (abstract). *Circulation* 1984;70(suppl II):298
4. Kelley JF, Snell ME: Hematoporphyrin derivative: a possible aid in the diagnosis and therapy of carcinoma of the bladder. *J Urol* 1976;115:150
5. Grundfest WS, Litwack F, Forrester JS, et al: Laser injury of human atherosclerotic plaque without adjacent tissue injury. *J Am Coll Cardiol* 1985;5:929
6. Isner JM, Clarke RL: *IEEE J Quantum Electron* 1984; QE20:1406
7. Haavind R: Lighting the way with lasers. *High Technology* 1985;5:39
8. Tick PA, Thompson DA: IR fibres: at the frontier. *Photon Spectra* 1985;19:65
9. Poulain M: The paths ahead for fluoride fibres. *Photon Spectra* 1985;19:68
10. White P: Chalcogenide fibres make their debut. *Photon Spectra* 1985;19:70
11. Choy DSJ, Stertzer SH, Myler RK, Marco J, Fournial G: Human coronary laser recanalization. *Clin Cardiol* 1984;7:377
12. Livesay JJ, Leachman DR, Hogan PJ, et al: Preliminary report on laser coronary endarterectomy in patients (abstract). *Circulation* 1985;72(suppl III):III-302
13. Litwack F, Grundfest W, Beeder C, Forrester JS: Laser angioplasty: status and prospects. *Semin Intervent Radiol* 1986;3:75
14. Geschwind H, Boussignac G, Teisseire B, et al: Percutaneous transluminal laser angioplasty in man. *Lancet* 1984;1:844

15. Geschwind H, Boussignac G, Teisseire B, Benhaiem N, Bittoun R, Laurent D: Conditions for effective Nd-YAG laser angioplasty. *Br Heart J* 1984;52:484

16. Murphy–Chutorian D, Selzer P, Wexler L, et al: Cardiovascular laser research at Stanford University. *Semin Intervent Radiol* 1986;3:51

17. Sanborn TA, Faxon DP, Haudenschild CC, Ryan TJ: Experimental angioplasty: circumferential distribution of laser thermal energy with a laser probe. *J Am Coll Cardiol* 1985;5:934

18. Nordstrom LA, Castañeda–Zuñiga WR, Grewe DD, Schoster JV: Laser enhanced transluminal angioplasty: the role of coaxial fiber placement. *Semin Intervent Radiol* 1986;3:47

19. Gerrity RG, Loop FD, Golding LAR, Erhart LA, Argenyl ZB: Arterial response to laser operation for removal of atherosclerotic plaques. *J Thorac Cardiovasc Surg* 1983;85:409

20. Abela G, Franzini D, Crea F, Pepine CJ, Conti CR: No evidence of accelerated atherosclerosis following laser radiation (abstract). *Circulation* 1984;70(suppl II):323

21. Abela GS, Conti CR: Laser revascularization: what are its prospects? *J Cardiovasc Med* 1983;8:977

22. LeeBI, Fletcher RD, Cohen AI, Cutler DJ, Del Negro AA, Singh SN: Transcatheter endocardial ablation: comparison of laser photo ablation and electode shock ablation (abstract). *J Am Coll Cardiol* 1984;3:536

23. Narula OS, Bharati S, Chan MC, Embi AA, Lev M: Laser microtransection of the His bundle: a pervenous catheter technique (abstract). *J Am Coll Cardiol* 1984;3:537

24. Choy DSJ: Fiberoptic laser tunneling device: the laser catheter, in *Beijin/Shanghai Proceedings of an International Conference on Lasers.* New York, Wiley Interscience, 1980, p 685

25. Macruz R, Martins JRM, Tupinamba AS, et al: Possibilidades terapeuticas do raio laser em ateromas. *Arq Bras Cardiol* 1980;34:9

26. Abela GS, Normann S, Cohen D, Feldman RL, Geiser EA, Conti CR: Effects of carbon dioxide, Nd:YAG, and argon laser radiation on coronary atheromatous plaques. *Am J Cardiol* 1982;50:1199

27. Choy DSJ, Stertzer SH, Rotterdam HZ, Sharrock N, Kaminow IP: Transluminal laser catheter angioplasty. *Am J Cardiol* 1982;50:1206

28. Lee G, Ikeda RM, Kozina J, Mason DT: Laser dissolution of coronary atherosclerotic obstruction. *Am Heart J* 1981; 102:1074

29. Ginsburg R, Wexler L, Mitchell RS, Profitt D: Percutaneous transluminal laser angioplasty for treatment of peripheral vascular disease: clinical experience with sixteen patients. *Radiology* 1985;156:619

30. Lee G, Ikeda RM, Stobbe D, et al: Intraoperative use of dual fiberoptic catheter for simultaneous in vivo visualization and laser vaporization of peripheral atherosclerotic obstructive disease. *Cath Cardiovasc Diag* 1984;10:11

31. Ginsburg R, Kim DS, Cuthener D, Toth J, Mitchell RS: Salvage of an ischemic limb by laser angioplasty: description of a new technique. *Clin Cardiol* 1984;7:54

20

Fibrinolytic Therapy

GARY J. BECKER, M.D., AND ROBERT W. HOLDEN, M.D.

The discovery of streptokinase (SK) by Tillett and Garner[1] and the elucidation of its interaction with the human fibrinolytic system by Sherry[2] have led to a wide variety of clinical applications. Fibrinolytic therapy has produced dramatic successes, dismal failures, and serious, even life-threatening, hemorrhage. A lack of predictive laboratory tests has made the hemorrhagic complications difficult to avoid. In this chapter, the authors provide the reader with insight into fibrinolysis: past, present, and future.

PATHOPHYSIOLOGY OF THROMBOSIS AND FIBRINOLYSIS

To understand fibrinolysis and thrombolysis, one must first grasp the core concepts in thrombosis. (The terms "fibrinolysis" and "thrombolysis" are almost interchangeable. When one uses thrombolytic therapy, one lyses the fibrin component of thrombi, not the cellular components. However, these terms are not completely interchangeable because of the difference between thrombus and blood clot. Blood clot may be formed *in vitro*, whereas thrombi are *in vivo* products of the coagulation cascade. Therefore, although one can produce fibrinolysis of an *in vitro* clot or an *in vivo* thrombus, one cannot produce thrombolysis of an *in vitro* clot.) Welch defined a thrombus as a solid plug formed in the living heart or blood vessels from constituents of blood.[3] Thrombosis is the process of thrombus generation. Venous and arterial thrombi have distinctive structures. Arterial (white) thrombi, which form in a higher flow circulation, are characterized by closely packed, aggregated platelets and a small amount of fibrin, whereas venous (red) thrombi consist primarily of a fibrin–red blood cell coagulum. Mixed thrombi—a white head with a red tail—are frequently found in stenotic arteries. The pathologic events leading to thrombosis are different in the arterial and venous circulations.

Arterial Thrombosis

Atheromatous roughening of the arterial endothelium can produce thrombosis, particularly where accompanying stenosis and altered blood flow are involved. Under such circumstances, platelets adhere, aggregate, and initiate thrombosis. Moncada and Vane,[4] Bunting et al,[5] and others have shown the importance of prostaglandin endoperoxide metabolism to both the homeostatic condition of normal blood flow and under conditions of disease.

Prostaglandin endoperoxide metabolism occurs in both platelets and endothelial cells. In the latter, the endoperoxides (substrate) are converted by prostacyclin synthetase to prostacyclin (PGI_2), which is the most potent known inhibitor of platelet aggregation. It is also a disaggregator of extant platelet clumps and a potent vasodilator. Platelets utilize the same endoperoxides to synthesize thromboxane A_2 (TXA_2), which induces platelet aggregation[6–9] and constricts arterial smooth muscle.[10] This constriction may result from the opening of cellular calcium entry channels when TXA_2 binds to its receptor sites.[11] Obviously, vascular patency cannot be maintained when the TXA_2 mechanisms predominate. How can an injured vessel produce a hemostatic plug in its outer wall if PGI_2 synthesis predominates in this location? Interestingly, PGI_2 probably does not predominate under such circumstances. Not only does the vascular injury promote platelet aggregation and TXA_2-mediated events, but the ratios of proaggregatory and antiaggregatory elements are different in the various layers of the vessel wall.[12] That is, proaggregatory elements increase in concentration from the endothelium to the adventitia, whereas prostacyclin synthetase progressively decreases from the intima to the adventitia.

Although this balance is important in normal vessels, conditions are altered in the presence of atheroma. Atherosclerotic plaques contain lipid peroxides,[13] which are potent selective inhibitors of prostacyclin synthesis.[12,14] This factor alone could tip the balance in favor of TXA_2 and result in thrombosis. It has been shown in a few patients that plaques may be incapable of producing sufficient quantities of prostacyclin.[15] Differences between early and advanced plaque have not been demonstrated. Therefore, it would seem that even in early lesions, the normal protective mechanism of prostacyclin production is absent.

Venous Thrombosis

In the venous system, Virchow's triad of factors predisposing to thrombosis—changes in the vein wall, venous stasis (abnormally increased contact time of venous blood with the endothelium), and a hypercoagulable state[16]—

has endured. Morphologic changes in the vessel wall are less important in venous thrombosis than they are in arterial thrombosis. We know this is true because most deep venous thromboses begin in the absence of a primary acute intimal lesion or inflammatory process.[17,18] Therefore, the term "deep venous thrombosis" (DVT) is preferable to "thrombophlebitis." Thrombus formation usually starts in the apex and vein wall of a valve pocket, but the thrombus is not attached to the valve cusp.[18,19] Growing out of the pocket and into the main channel, the thrombus produces turbulence, which increases fibrin formation and the entrapment of red blood cells. With increasing obstruction, stasis becomes nearly complete, and rapid and extensive proximal and retrograde thrombosis ensues. Edema, venous distention, pain, and tenderness result. The soleal veins of the calf are the most frequent sites of early venous thrombosis,[20,21] and stasis is the most important predisposing factor.[22]

What about the role of hypercoagulable states? In 1947, Astrup and Permin described the existence of a chemical agent in tissue that is capable of activating plasminogen.[23] Subsequently, it has been shown that human veins have a highly fibrinolytic endothelium, whereas arteries are low in fibrinolytic activity. Astrup later postulated that an imbalance between the fibrinolytic mechanism and the coagulation pathways may be causative in venous thrombosis.[24] It is now known that blood vessels are the main source of tissue plasminogen activator (tPA), and tissue culture studies have shown that plasminogen activator is synthesized and stored in endothelial cells.[25] It also appears that plasminogen activator is continuously released from normal endothelial cells into the blood stream,[26] and that immunologically, vascular plasminogen activator is the same as tPA.[27,28] The absence of tPA in valve pockets[29] and its presence in the remainder of the venous endothelium may explain why thrombi originate in valve sinuses yet remain unattached to the vein wall as they propagate. There is evidence for fibrinolytic "shutdown" postoperatively,[30] in that a decrease in circulating tPA has been reported in patients with postoperative DVT. It is possible that this is related to a lack of activity, because exercise increases fibrinolytic activity by causing a release of tPA.[26] Other studies have revealed decreased plasminogen activator in the blood and venous walls of patients with recurrent DVT.

INTERRELATED HOMEOSTATIC MECHANISMS

Coagulation and Fibrin

Notwithstanding the obvious importance of the balances described above, they are not the sole mechanisms maintaining normal blood flow and the vascular response to injury or disease. The coagulation mechanism (clotting cascade), which involves the sequential activation of at least 13 different factors, is extremely important. Figure 20–1 is a simple representation of both the intrinsic and the extrinsic coagulation pathways. The extrinsic pathway is activated when tissue substances from outside the blood stream, known as thromboplastin, are exposed to the blood stream after vascular injury. The intrinsic pathway is activated when factor XII is converted to active form (XII$_a$). The latter process, which can be demonstrated in blood isolated from tissues (for example, in a test tube), also occurs in vivo. Excellent discussions of the complex interrelations between the coagulation pathways and the kallikrein and complement systems may be found in most standard textbooks of internal medicine.

Whatever the initial stimulus (intrinsic or extrinsic), the final common pathway of the two cascades is the conversion of soluble fibrinogen to fibrin by the action of the enzyme thrombin. Insoluble fibrin forms the matrix for hemostatic plugs in instances of vascular injury and the matrix which solidifies thrombi in the process of thrombosis. Fibrin also provides the framework for the reparative connective tissue. Upon this framework, healing proceeds, with fibroblastic proliferation and ingrowth of capillaries.

If the activated coagulation mechanisms were allowed to operate unchecked, the entire human circulation might coagulate after a single vascular injury. This is avoided, at least in part, through the action of various plasma coagulation factor inhibitors. These include alpha$_2$-mac-roglobulin, alpha$_2$-antiplasmin, antithrombin III, alpha$_1$-antitrypsin, and C1 inactivator.[31] The coagulation mechanism may also be inhibited by various other means[32]: (1) dicoumarols, which are vitamin K antagonists which interfere with the hepatic synthesis of the vitamin K-dependent clotting factors (II, VII, IX, and X); (2) heparin, which blocks the action of thrombin on fibrinogen; (3) antiplatelet agents such as acetylsalicylic acid and dipyridamole, which decrease platelet function; (4) fibrinolytic agents such as urokinase and streptokinase (mechanism to be discussed below); and (5) certain snake venoms, which cause fibrinogen depletion.

Fibrin and Fibrinolysis

Another system providing a balance against the formation of fibrin, the fibrinolytic system, is the major topic of this chapter. The principal function of this system is to maintain the fluidity of blood by dissolving the fibrin in arterial and venous thrombi. In normal persons, there is a constant dynamic balance between fibrin formation and dissolution. Fibrin dissolution, a proteolytic process, results in the formation of soluble fibrin degradation products or FDPs (fragments X, Y, D, and E). The process is mediated by plasmin, a relatively nonspecific plasma protease formed from the zymogen (inactive precursor) plasminogen (Fig. 20–2). Normally, plasminogen is found in the circulation in concentrations of 12–25 mg/dl, whereas plasmin is not detectable.[31] The latter may, however, be detected in certain disease states.

Several substances promote the initial conversion of plasminogen to plasmin. These include urokinase (UK), which is produced by the human kidney and circulates as

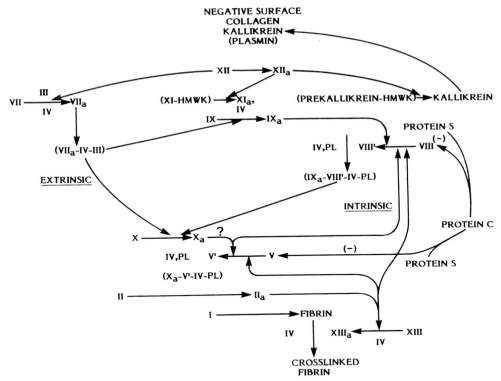

Fig. 20–1 Extrinsic and intrinsic coagulation cascades. Inactive clotting factors are denoted by Roman numerals; activated clotting factors are indicated by Roman numeral plus subscript "a." Active complexes are enclosed in parentheses. A prime sign (') after clotting factor V or VIII signifies special form with enhanced activity. The identities of the clotting factors are listed below. All factors promote coagulation with the exceptions of proteins C and S. Protein C inhibits factors V and VIII, and protein S serves as a cofactor in this inhibition. These inhibitory functions are indicated by a minus sign (−).

I: Fibrinogen; II: Prothrombin; III: Tissue factor; IV: Calcium (Ca^{++}); V: Proaccelerin (labile factor); VI: Not assigned; VII: Proconvertin (stable factor); VIII: Antihemophilic factor; IX: Christmas factor; X: Stuart factor; XI: Plasma thromboplastin antecedent; XII: Hageman factor; XIII: Fibrin-stabilizing factor; Prekallikrein; HMWK: High molecular weight kininogen; von Willebrand factor; Protein C; Protein S; PL: phospholipid.

a trace protein; plasma activators; tissue activator (tPA); and bacterial enzymes, such as streptokinase (SK). Plasma activator is present in the circulation in increased concentrations in response to exercise, physical trauma, shock, ischemia, and chemicals such as nicotinic acid and epinephrine. Part of the balance provided against these activators derives from a number of inhibitors present in endothelial cells[33,34] and in plasma.[35-37] Furthermore, the

plasma protein alpha$_2$-antiplasmin is a potent inhibitor of plasmin, and there are other, less rapidly acting, ones such as alpha$_2$-macroglobulin and alpha$_1$-antitrypsin.[31]

Importantly, there are significant influences of the activated fibrinolytic system on the coagulation cascade. The nonspecific protease plasmin cleaves not only fibrin, but also factors V and VIII and fibrinogen. Thus, plasmin exerts a direct anticoagulant effect. In addition, FDPs have their own inhibitory effect on the clotting cascade, which amplifies the anticoagulant effect.

Plasminogen, which has a high affinity for fibrin, probably becomes intimately bound within thrombi during the polymerization of fibrin. Because plasma activator and tPA also have high fibrin affinity, the binding processes bring plasminogen substrate close to activator molecules, which tends to localize the process of plasmin generation to sites where fibrinolysis is needed. The activators UK and SK are not nearly so specific, and as a result, administration of these agents frequently results in activation of large amounts of circulating (unbound) plasminogen, with production of high levels of circulating plasmin. The rare patients with congenital abnormalities of the fibrinolytic system have enhanced our understanding of these processes.[38-45] A few patients with recurrent DVT have proved to have functionally defective plas-

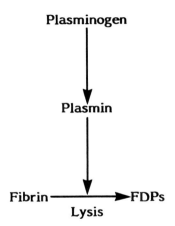

Fig. 20–2 Final common pathway in fibrinolysis.

minogen,[38,39] and others have a familial defect in the synthesis or release of plasminogen activator from vascular endothelial cells.[40,41] Congenital deficiency of alpha$_2$-antiplasmin leads to excessive fibrinolysis,[42–44] and a hemorrhagic disorder caused by excessive plasminogen has been described.[45]

It is apparent that the fibrinolytic mechanism is pro-

tective. However, in many instances of intravascular coagulation (DVT, arterial thrombosis), this endogenous mechanism is inadequate to restore patency of the involved blood vessel. Efforts to hasten or amplify the fibrinolytic process have led to the administration of exogenous fibrinolytic agents.

STREPTOKINASE AND UROKINASE

Streptokinase

Streptokinase is a single-chain, antigenic protein product of beta-hemolytic streptococci. Teleologically, streptococci are able to survive and proliferate in the face of the human healing process in part because of their capacity to synthesize this substance. Streptokinase, when coupled with human plasminogen, results in the formation of plasmin, which dissolves fibrin in the reparative framework, preventing the infection from being walled off.

Alkjaersig et al elucidated the mechanism of clot lysis by plasmin in 1959,[46] and in the same year, Johnson and McCarty reported the lysis of human clots by intravenous infusion of SK.[47] The latter report marked the beginning of first-generation fibrinolytic therapy, a generation of high-dose intravenous systemic administration for lysing thrombi and thromboemboli remote from the site of infusion.[48]

The mechanism of action of SK is shown diagrammatically in Figure 20–3. Basically, SK forms a one-to-one stoichiometric complex with plasminogen. This enzymatically active complex controls the conversion of additional plasminogen molecules to plasmin. Plasmin is then available to lyse the fibrin component of thrombi. In addition, SK may form active complexes with plasmin molecules. With increasing dose or duration of therapy, the active SK–plasminogen complexes are gradually replaced by SK–plasmin active complexes, which are also capable of activating plasminogen. Importantly, SK does not have the high affinity for fibrin characteristic of plasma activator and tPA; therefore, it activates not only the plasminogen molecules within thrombus, but also those circulating in the plasma. This activity creates high levels of circulating plasmin, with all of the aforementioned effects on the coagulation cascade.

Urokinase

In 1946, Macfarlane and Pilling first isolated UK from human urine.[49] The work of Sherry et al helped bring the substance into clinical use.[50] It is a protein product of the normal human kidney which is found in trace quantities in the circulation and is available commercially for exogenous administration as a fibrinolytic agent. Commercial laboratories derive the substance from cultures of human fetal kidney cells.

The mechanism of action of UK is diagrammed in Figure 20–4. Unlike SK, UK does not form active complexes with plasminogen in order to produce its fibrinolytic effect. Rather, it acts directly on plasminogen to produce plasmin. Importantly, like SK, it does not have the high affinity for fibrin that is characteristic of plasma activator and tPA. Therefore, it also activates circulating plasminogen molecules to produce plasmin. The action of circulating plasmin, in turn, results in the anticoagulant effects described above. When the circulating plasmin level is high, its effects on the coagulation cascade are evident, and the fibrinogen level is decreased (normal approximately 350–400 mg/dl), a "systemic fibrinolytic state" is said to exist.

Streptokinase and Urokinase: A Comparison

The most obvious, and one of the most significant, differences between SK and UK is that the former is a foreign and therefore antigenic protein, whereas the latter is human derived. The antigenicity of SK has had important clinical manifestations (to be described below), whereas UK has had no such ill effects. The prevalence of SK antibody in the general population led Verstraete et al to investigate and eventually to describe a standard

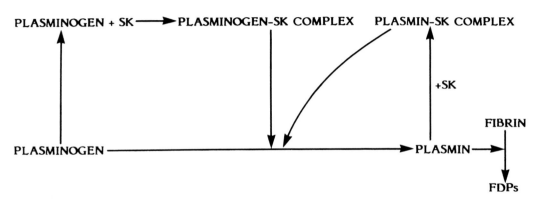

Fig. 20–3   Mechanism of action of SK. As plasmin becomes more plentiful and plasminogen is depleted, the SK–plasminogen active complexes are replaced by SK–plasmin active complexes.

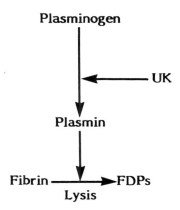

Fig. 20-4 Mechanism of action of UK. UK is a nonantigenic, enzymatic protein that does not require formation of active complexes in order to activate plasminogen.

dosage regimen that includes a 250,000-unit bolus administered over 1/2 hour (an amount sufficient to neutralize existing SK antibody in approximately 90% of the population) prior to initiating the continuous intravenous systemic infusion.[51] In addition, because of its antigeni-city, SK retreatment within 6 months is not advisable because of the potential for an anamnestic immune response. UK, on the other hand, may be readministered at any time. SK is slightly pyrogenic, whereas UK is nonpyrogenic. SK has a half-life of 10–12 min (not the same as the fibrinolytic half-life that results from its adminis-

tration), and UK has a half-life of 11–16 min. There is evidence that SK produces a slightly higher fibrinogen-olytic:fibrinolytic ratio than does UK.[52] Both produce markedly higher ratios than does tPA, as one would expect from the more specific mechanism of action of the latter. The ratios are important in that the higher one resulting from SK would seem to indicate that SK is more likely than UK to produce a systemic fibrinolytic state and therefore is conceivably more likely to cause hemorrhage when administered in therapeutically similar amounts. Clinical experience with local infusion methods since 1981 has indeed shown more hemorrhagic complications with SK than with UK.[53-55] The likelihood of hemorrhagic complication is also related to infusion duration. In an effort to hasten lysis with increasing enzyme concentrations while minimizing hemorrhagic complications, high dose-rate, short infusion duration UK protocols have become a favorite method. SK is stable when stored at room temperature, but UK must be stored at 4° C until use. Finally, and importantly, UK costs approximately six times as much as SK on a per-unit basis. Worse still, most UK regimens require far more units than do comparable SK regimens (four times as many units in most low-dose local regimens and three to four times as many in the systemic or intravenous regimens). These factors combine to make UK therapy as much as 24 times as expensive as therapeutically similar SK therapy. Manufacturers have recently increased the availability of UK by increasing their production capacity.

CLINICAL EXPERIENCE

First-Generation Therapy

In two previous works, the cumulative clinical experience with SK and UK was described as having evolved in generations.[48,53] The first generation of therapy was characterized by high-dose intravenous infusion of fibrinolytic agents aimed at lysing thrombi or thromboemboli that usually were remote from the site of infusion. SK was used for a variety of vascular occlusive problems in this early period,[56-58] but the true momentum in first-generation therapy developed only when the National Institutes of Health (NIH) formed its Committee on Thrombolytic Agents. This committee identified UK, derived from human urine and recently purified sufficiently,[59] as the most suitable thrombolytic agent for clinical trials.

Large-scale investigation into the clinical use of UK and SK came when the National Heart, Lung, and Blood Institute (NHLBI) began the first national cooperative trial comparing UK with heparin in the treatment of pulmonary thromboembolic disease (Urokinase Pulmonary Embolism Trial; UPET).[60] This multicenter study used pulmonary angiography, perfusion lung scanning, and hemodynamic measurements in the right side of the heart and the pulmonary circulation to assess the rate and degree of dissolution of emboli. UK-treated patients received an intravenous loading dose of 4400 units/kg and a maintenance infusion of 4400 units/kg/hr for 12 hr.

Heparin-treated patients received a loading dose of 165 IU/kg and a maintenance infusion of 22 IU/kg/hr. There were 160 patients. At the end of the 12 hr, all patients received heparin in therapeutic doses for at least 5 days, then oral anticoagulants. In the follow-up period, patients had interval histories, physical examinations, and lung scans at 3, 6, and 12 months. Trial results revealed: (1) greater resolution of emboli with UK; (2) greater return of blood pressures toward normal with UK; (3) greater return of perfusion (by lung scanning) with UK; and (4) greatest improvement in patients with large pulmonary emboli.

Subsequently, the Urokinase–Streptokinase Pulmonary Embolism Trial (USPET) was undertaken.[61] In this multicenter study, UK, administered with two infusion durations (12 hr and 24 hr), was compared with SK. The results revealed no significant differences between UK-treated and SK-treated patients with respect to the measures used in the UPET trial.

Although UPET and USPET did not examine the long-term differences between fibrinolytic-treated and heparin-treated patients with pulmonary embolic disease, other studies did. In 40 patients without heart or lung disease who had pulmonary emboli, Sharma et al proved that heparin-treated patients have abnormally low pulmonary capillary blood volumes both in the immediate convalescent period and at 1-year follow-up,[62] whereas patients in the fibrinolytic group have normal pulmonary capillary blood volumes at both of these times. The significance of these measurements is not yet fully appreciated. It may well be that recurrent pulmonary emboli in patients with compromised pulmonary capillary volumes cause higher morbidity and mortality rates than similar recurrences in patients with normal pulmonary capillary blood volumes. It may also be that patients with abnormally low pulmonary capillary blood volumes have limited capacity for capillary recruitment and therefore have an inherent inability to respond to stresses such as exercise and illness (e.g., myocardial infarction with pulmonary edema). These hypotheses have not been adequately tested.

If thrombolytic agents are responsible for all of the beneficial effects described above, why did their use ever fall into disfavor? The answer is simply that physicians typically weigh the risk:benefit ratios of all forms of therapy, and many believe that the risks of hemorrhage attending systemic fibrinolytic therapy outweigh the potential benefits. This feeling stems principally from the UPET results, so it is essential to examine these findings in more detail; they provided the impetus for second-generation fibrinolytic therapy.

In the UPET study, a "moderate" hemorrhage was said to be loss of 500–1500 ml with an associated decrease in hematocrit of 5–10 points. A "severe" hemorrhage was a loss of >1500 ml with a hematocrit decrease of >10 points or a transfusion requirement of more than 2 units of blood. The frequency of moderate or severe hemorrhage was 27% for the heparin-treated group and 45% for the UK-treated group. Since the numbers of moderate hemorrhages were similar, the difference was accounted for almost entirely by a higher incidence of severe hemorrhage in the UK-treated patients. However, the UPET protocol was invasive by design (pulmonary angiography, arterial blood gas studies, etc.), and hemorrhage from the resulting puncture sites was definitely responsible for the difference in the overall incidences of hemorrhagic complications in the two groups. Stated simply, the incidence of spontaneous hemorrhage was the same (19%) in both groups. It seems that in the absence of invasive procedures, there is no difference in hemorrhagic complications between heparin-treated and UK-treated patients. However, when one examines the spontaneous hemorrhages that occurred in UPET, it is clear that the proportion of severe ones is higher in the UK-treated group than in the heparin-treated group (88% and 53%, respectively). One may conclude that *systemic doses* of fibrinolytic agents are more dangerous than systemic doses of heparin.[63] Bleeding complications occurred with equal frequency in all three study groups of USPET (UK for 12 hr, UK for 24 hr, SK for 24 hr).

Second-Generation Therapy

In an effort to avoid hemorrhagic complications while effectively dissolving thrombi and thromboemboli, Dotter et al began to use a transcatheter method of directing SK into peripheral vascular occlusions at a dose rate of approximately 1/20th the systemic dose rate (5,000 units/hr without a loading dose instead of 100,000 units/hr following a 250,000-unit loading dose).[64] As little as 1% of

the usual systemic dose was given to some of their 17 patients, 15 of whom had lower extremity arterial occlusions and two of whom had upper extremity occlusions. Treatment lasted from less than 1 day to 2 weeks. The best results were achieved in patients with recent occlusions.

Even in this earliest series, the authors recognized several of the important features of the local infusion method. First, they realized that lysis is not curative. In most instances, it merely restores patency and uncovers an underlying structural problem that requires treatment. Indeed, Dotter et al treated several of their patients with transluminal dilatation after identifying an underlying stenosis. Second, those authors cautioned readers about the potential for remote hemorrhages, particularly intracerebral ones, even with the local method. Third, they suggested that indwelling arterial lines may encourage thrombus formation along the catheter shaft, a problem that has since proved significant.[65]

Although the report of Dotter et al initiated second-generation therapy—a generation of percutaneous transcatheter low-dose fibrinolytic therapy given by the interventional angiographer and the intensive care unit (ICU) nurses—enthusiasm was lacking until Katzen and van Breda reported its use in the peripheral vasculature[66] and Rentrop et al reported a relatively high-dose, short-duration form of therapy for coronary artery occlusion.[67]

In the past few years, a number of authors have described the efficacy and complications of the local infusion method. The following sections review these reports, noting the indications, methods, and results according to anatomic region or specific type of vessel treated. Contraindications, complications, and laboratory monitoring are dealt with in separate sections that follow.

ABDOMINAL AORTA AND LOWER EXTREMITIES

It would be counterproductive to list all of the different methods utilized and presumptuous to detail a "preferred" method for local transcatheter fibrinolytic therapy for thrombotic and thromboembolic occlusive disease of the legs. Instead, the basic methods used in the earliest series will be explained, and important variations on those themes will be covered by brief descriptions.

The series of Katzen and van Breda included 12 patients, eight of whom were treated for common iliac or more distal lower extremity arterial occlusions through a 5F catheter with 5000 units/hr of SK in 50 ml of normal saline.[66] Five of these eight patients subsequently underwent percutaneous transluminal angioplasty (PTA), and most of the eight had a good long-term result. The authors used simultaneous heparin in two of their patients, but bleeding complications supervened, and the heparin infusions were terminated. Most importantly, Katzen and van Breda emphasized the need for proper patient selection. For example, they stated that fibrinolytic therapy should be reserved for patients tolerating their ischemia, whereas those who are not tolerating their ischemia are better candidates for operation. The present authors have found this concept invaluable when discussing therapeutic options with the vascular surgeons. Obviously, in other anatomic areas, such as the coronary circulation (and potentially in the cerebral vasculature), this concept does not apply as intuitively as it does in the extremities.

Totty et al described 26 infusions in 22 patients. Nineteen patients (22 infusions) were treated for lower extremity arterial occlusions, 13 of which followed PTA.[68] The authors used SK (19 infusions) in doses ranging from 2,500 units/hr (one patient) to 10,000 units/hr, with 5,000 units/hr being used most frequently; UK was used in doses ranging from 40,000–80,000 units/hr in the remaining patients. Of the 13 PTA-associated infusions, eight produced complete or nearly complete lysis, whereas five resulted in partial lysis, with only one of the latter patients requiring no further treatment. Of the 10 lower extremity infusions for spontaneous thrombi or thromboemboli, nine resulted in partial lysis, but none produced complete lysis. The authors concluded that low-dose fibrinolytic therapy has a definite role in PTA-associated vascular occlusions but a less well-defined, perhaps adjunctive, role (together with operation) in spontaneous occlusions.

Becker et al reported 57 local infusions in 50 patients in their original series.[69] They used 5,000 units/hr of SK in most patients and 20,000 units/hr of UK in two. In order to avoid catheter-related thrombosis (to be discussed), they simultaneously administered enough heparin by intravenous infusion to maintain the partial thromboplastin time (PTT) at 1.5 times normal. Catheters as small as 3F were occasionally introduced coaxially through larger angiographic catheters for the infusion, and catheters as large as 6.5F were frequently used alone. The coaxial system was generally used when the popliteal or trifurcation branches were occluded; in these instances, the larger angiographic catheter was withdrawn to the most proximal position possible. Patients were managed in the surgical ICU and monitored by physical examination, bedside Doppler examinations, and serial angiograms made via the infusion catheter in the angiography suite. When partial lysis was observed, a catheter exchange was made over a guidewire (following rescrubbing and administration of local anesthetic), and the new catheter was advanced to the level of occlusion. Only 16 of these infusions were performed for occlusion of native arteries in the legs. In each case, the catheter was positioned within or as near to the thrombus as possible. Partial lysis occurred in 50% of the infusions, complete lysis in 25%, and no lysis in 25%. The relatively small success in these vessels led the authors to postulate that native arterial occlusions have many collateral or alternate egress pathways for the fibrinolytic solution. This hypothesis also seemed to explain the small success in hemodialysis fistulae and veins in contrast to the great success in dialysis shunts and in lower extremity grafts, which have no branches. These results alerted the authors to the importance of placing the infusion catheter within the occlusion. It now seems that such intrathrombus positioning is important not only in avoiding loss of fibrinolytic agent through collateral channels but also in increasing the surface area of thrombus exposed to the fibrinolytic solution and thus hastening thrombolysis.

Hess et al reported their use of a modified technique for low-dose intra-arterial infusion in 136 patients with lower extremity arterial occlusions.[70] Their technique involved positioning a double-lumen polyvinyl balloon catheter in the occluded vessel with the tip embedded 1 cm into the thrombus or thromboembolus (eight of their patients were thought to have embolic occlusions). One to 3 ml of SK (1,000 units/ml in normal saline) were then injected. After 5–15 min, the catheter was advanced under fluoroscopy, and the procedure was repeated. This continued until the catheter reached the patent lumen distal to the occlusion. Residual stenoses were detected by angiography through the infusion catheter and treated with PTA. The total dose of SK required per patient ranged from 4,000–180,000 units. Patients were given acetylsalicylic acid, 500 mg two or three times daily, after the initial treatment. Ninety-four recanalizations were achieved in 136 attempts (69%), but only 70 (51%) lasted 2 weeks according to follow-up angiography. The cumulative patency rate at 16 months was still close to 50%, however. Importantly, the method of Hess et al requires less SK than those techniques previously reported, which may help lower the frequency of hemorrhagic complications secondary to the systemic fibrinolytic state. In addition, the procedure times were considerably shorter than those reported by others (1–5 hr). Another important observation was that patients with chronic occlusions (6 months or longer) still had a 50% recanalization frequency with the new method, whereas acute occlusions responded with an 80% frequency. The success indicated for chronic occlusions is higher than expected on the basis of the previous literature but agrees with Rabe et al's observation that SK can lyse chronic fibrin deposits.[71]

In the series of 159 infusions reported by Graor et al, patients were divided into groups with atherosclerotic occlusions, postprocedural occlusions, and peripheral arterial emboli.[72] The number of infusions performed for lower extremity native arterial occlusions is unclear. Atherosclerotic occlusions were opened in 56% of cases and postprocedural occlusions in 79%, and arterial emboli were lysed in 70%. Infusions were made through 5F end-hole catheters embedded in the occlusions; heparinization was not used. Empiric cefamandole antibiotic prophylaxis was used (1 g intravenously every 6 hr throughout treatment and for 24 hr afterward). Clinical estimates of the durations of the occlusions were from 1 hr to 1 year. Infusion durations ranged from 12–120 hr.

Dardik et al reported their experience with SK in 38 patients, nine of whom were managed with local infusions for lower extremity native arterial occlusions.[73] Although all infusions were begun at 5,000 units/hr, the dose rates were sequentially increased to 15,000 units/hr and continued for 48–72 hr in slow responders. Recanalization was achieved in all of these patients, and a distal bypass operation was subsequently required in only one.

In his article on the complications of intra-arterial use of SK, Lang reported 35 patients treated for lower extremity vascular occlusions, 23 of whom had occlusions in native arteries rather than grafts.[74] The SK dose of 5000 units/hr was infused through a 5F catheter embedded in the occlusions, with heparin (200–1000 units/hr) being given to maintain the PTT at 1.5–2.0 times normal. The catheters were advanced as lysis proceeded until patency was completely restored. Sixteen of the 23 infusions resulted in complete lysis.

In the series of Mori et al, 50 infusions of SK were made for a variety of thrombotic and thromboembolic conditions.[75] Of these, 24 involved treatment for native arterial occlusions in the legs. The most common regimen was a local infusion of SK at 5000 units/hr plus simultaneous heparin infusion at 250–500 units/hr. Infusions were terminated when: (1) significant lysis had occurred; (2) no lysis was observed after 24–48 hr; (3) the symptoms worsened; or (4) hemorrhagic complications supervened. Infusion durations were 1–20 hr. Although clinical benefit from SK infusion alone was observed in only approximately half the cases, combinations of SK plus operation or SK plus PTA produced clinical benefit in another 30%. Therefore, some benefit was obtained by approximately 80% of the patients, with slightly better results being noted for embolic occlusions than for thrombotic ones.

On the basis of evidence that high-dose local UK infusion for a short time is efficacious for coronary thrombolysis,[76] McNamara and Fischer used a similar high-dose regimen in 93 peripheral arterial and graft occlusions in 85 patients.[77] The method involves infusing 4000 units/min of UK until antegrade blood flow is re-established, then 2000 units/min until lysis is complete. Although the authors did not separate their results according to graft *versus* native artery infusions, they did report clinical improvement in 75 (81%) of the patients. After an initial experience with catheter-related thrombosis (two of seven patients early in the series not treated with concomitant heparin), McNamara and Fischer began to use simultaneous heparin infusion in dose rates sufficient to maintain the PTT at approximately 3 times normal, after which the frequency of catheter-related thrombosis decreased to 3%. Those authors also found a low frequency of hemorrhagic complications and, of course, no allergic complications. The lower frequency of hemorrhage probably reflects the importance of the lower fibrinogenolytic:fibrinolytic ratio that UK has relative to SK. The authors concluded that the high-dose local UK regimen is superior to all local SK regimens previously used. This infusion regimen has now become the most popular one used by interventional angiographers in the United States.

Finally, Bean et al recently reported successful treatment of a patient with a 4-week history of Leriche syndrome by means of local SK infusion and PTA.[78] They used the blind femoral angiogram technique[79,80] to catheterize the aorta retrograde. After an arteriogram revealed thrombotic occlusion of the distal abdominal aorta, they infused SK at 5000 units/hr for 26 hr until lysis was complete and stenosis of the aorta due to atherosclerotic plaque was identified. A PTA was performed using two balloon catheters ("kissing balloon" technique).

Representative cases of local thrombolytic therapy for occlusion of native arteries in the legs are illustrated in Figures 20–5 and 20–6.

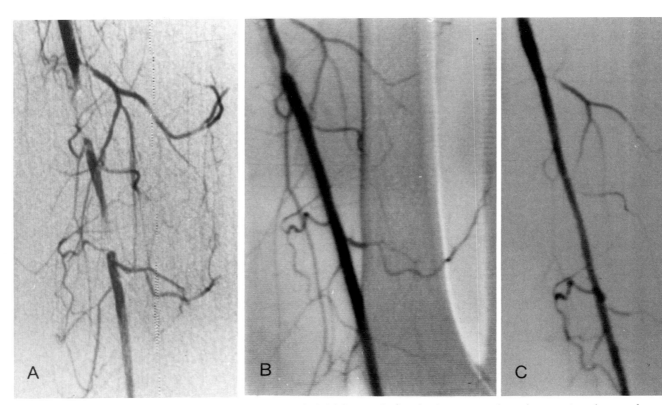

Fig. 20–5 Patient with acute lower extremity ischemia. A. Initial digital subtraction angiogram shows two segments of superficial femoral artery (SFA) occlusion. B. After 24 hr of local UK at 20,000 units/hr plus intravenous heparin, repeat angiogram shows patency of SFA and atheromatous plaque in region of previous occlusion. C. SFA after PTA of stenotic segment.

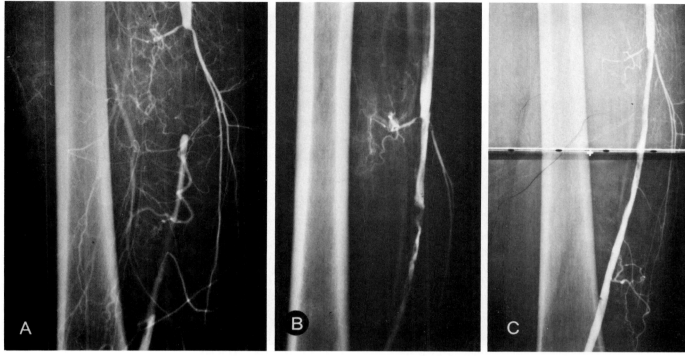

Fig. 20–6 A 49-year-old diabetic man with acute right lower extremity ischemia complicating long-standing claudication. A. Initial right lower extremity arteriogram shows superficial femoral artery occlusion. B. After 1 day of transcatheter SK at 5000 units/hr plus intravenous heparin, most of thrombus has been lysed, and an underlying stenosis is identified. C. Angiogram after PTA.

GRAFTS

Twenty-one infusions reported in Becker et al's initial series were for graft occlusions.[69] They were most successful in this group, with complete lysis occurring in 15 patients and partial lysis in an additional 4. In some patients, stenoses were identified at graft anastomotic sites and a few of these were treated with PTA. Figures 20–7 and 20–8 are illustrations of two patients with graft occlusions treated with local fibrinolysis. As stated above, the high degree of success noted in this group was attributed to the lack of collateral pathways or alternate egress channels available to divert the fibrinolytic solution.

The present authors' experience is not unique. In the series of Wolfson et al, 27 infusions of SK were given for a variety of thrombotic and thromboembolic conditions.[81] Graft occlusions lysed faster than native arterial ones (35 hr and 62 hr, respectively) and more frequently (seven of nine cases *versus* 11 of 18). Most patients were treated with local infusions of 5000 units/hr. Those authors also believed that concomitant heparin administration was important in preventing catheter-related thrombosis.

None of the patients in the original series of Dotter et al[64] was treated for graft occlusion, nor were the patients reported by Katzen and van Breda[66] with the exception of one with an occluded dialysis graft. The latter case is discussed under "Hemodialysis Accesses." In their series, Hess et al did not state that any patients were treated for graft occlusions.[70]

Four of the infusions reported by Totty et al were for graft occlusion, and although all patients had some clinical improvement, only three had angiographically demonstrable improvement.[68] In the series of Dardik et al, 26 of the 38 patients had graft thromboses. Sixteen were treated with intra-arterial SK and the remainder with intravenous SK; lysis occurred in five of the former and three of the latter.[73] In Lang's series, thrombolytic therapy was most efficacious in cases of thrombosed synthetic grafts (11 of 12).[74] Of the 50 local infusions in the series of Mori et al, 10 were performed for thrombosed arterial bypass grafts to the lower extremities. Although SK infusion alone was beneficial in only 30%, SK plus operation or SK plus PTA proved beneficial in another 20%.[75] Of the 93 infusions in the series of McNamara and Fischer, 22 were performed for occlusions of grafts to the legs, but it is impossible to ascertain from the data the percentage resulting in complete lysis.[77]

In the series of Graor et al, 35 patients were treated for graft thrombosis. Of these, 11 were Dacron aortic bifurcation grafts, 12 were polytetrafluoroethylene (PTFE) grafts, and 12 were saphenous vein grafts in the legs. Although these patients were grouped with three post-PTA occlusions, for a total of 38 postprocedural occlusions, the results in this category were remarkable, with 79% of patients achieving thrombolysis—complete dissolution of thrombus and clinical improvement.[72]

UPPER EXTREMITIES

In the original series reported by Dotter et al, two patients were treated for vascular occlusions in the hands and arms.[64] The first was a patient with a 2-week history of occlusion in the left digital arteries of uncertain etiology, who was treated with SK 5000 units/hr administered via a transfemoral catheter positioned in the brachial

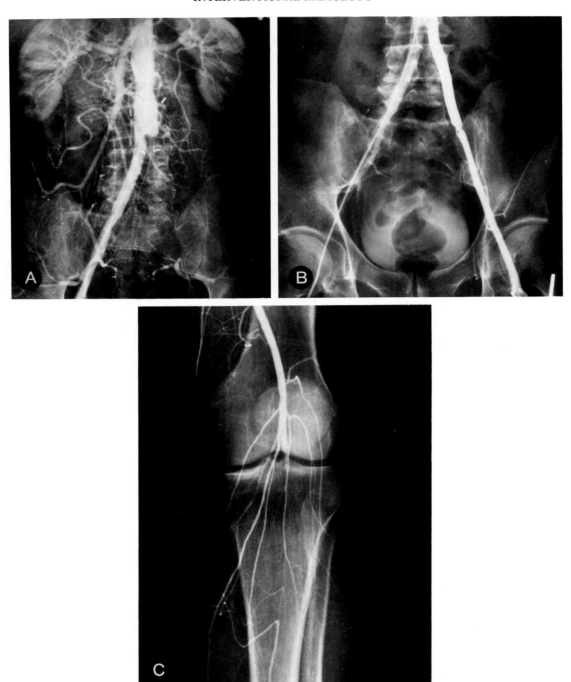

Fig. 20–7 This 56-year-old man with a 5-year-old knitted-Dacron aortobi-iliac graft presented with new left lower extremity ischemia. A. Initial angiogram discloses complete occlusion of left limb of graft. A catheter was placed over the bifurcation into the occlusion, and SK infusion of 5000 units/hr was started. The patient also received heparin. B. Angiogram through infusion catheter after 19 hr of SK shows patency of left limb of graft and stenosis at distal anastomotic site.

C. This angiogram, also made after 19 hr of SK, shows complete midpopliteal occlusion (embolic). D. Angioplasty was performed, and this angiogram was made. E. After PTA, 3F coaxial catheter was placed into popliteal occlusion, and SK infusion was restarted. F. Angiogram after another 24 hr shows patency of popliteal and trifurcation arteries.

artery. There was no change in the clinical findings or the angiographic appearance after 19 hr of infusion. The second was a patient with an ulnar artery occlusion treated with SK 2500 units/hr administered via a transaxillary catheter positioned in the brachial artery. There was no change after 23 hr of infusion, and no surgical or other

confirmation of the presence of thrombus or thromboembolus was ever obtained.

Only one patient in the original series of Katzen and van Breda was treated for vascular occlusion of an arm vessel. The patient had mitral valve disease and an embolic occlusion of the left distal brachial artery. The

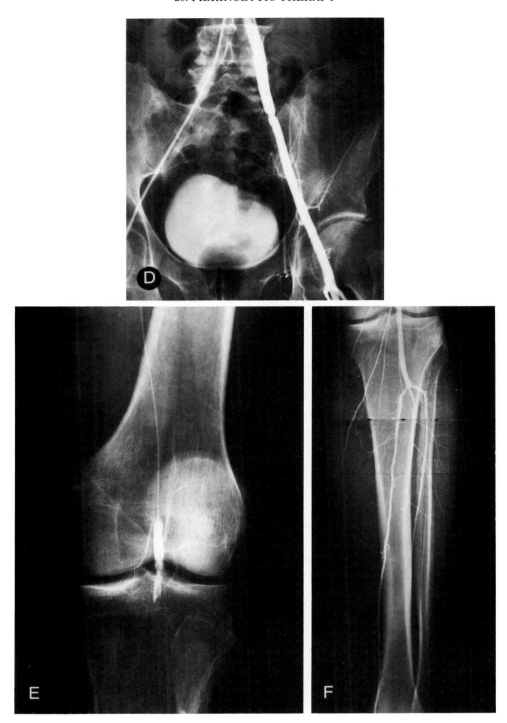

Fig. 20-7D-F

offending thromboembolus was lysed with 7 hr of trans-catheter local SK at 5000 units/hr.[66]

None of the patients in Becker et al's original series of 57 infusions was treated for upper extremity arterial occlusion,[69] but Totty et al had two upper extremity cases in their series.[68] The first was an 80-year-old woman with an axillary artery thrombus and symptoms of 1 day's duration, who was treated with transcatheter SK at 5,000 units/hr for 90 hr. Although this treatment lysed the thrombus, small brachial thrombi or thromboemboli required surgical removal. The second patient was a 45-year-old woman who presented with right axillary, brachial, radial, and ulnar occlusions and symptoms of 1 week's duration. Despite treatment with SK 10,000 units/hr for 45 hr that lysed the axillary thrombus, the patient ultimately required amputation below the elbow.

None of the patients in the large series of Hess et al[70] was treated for upper extremity arterial occlusions, and it is impossible to ascertain from the data of Dardik et al[73] whether any of their patients was treated for this

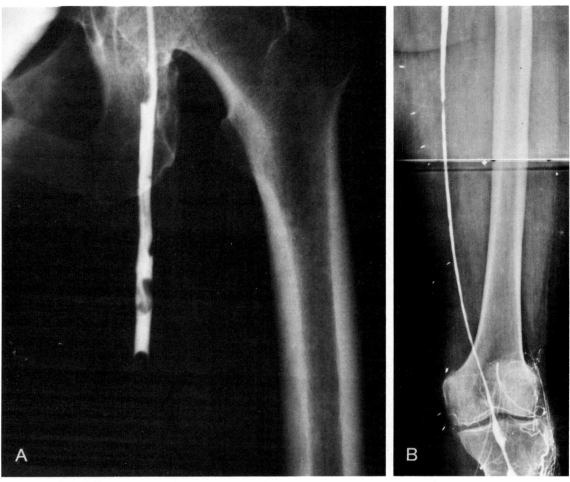

Fig. 20–8 A 72-year-old woman with occluded saphenous femoro-popliteal graft. A. Initial angiogram showing occlusion. B. Angiogram after local SK and intravenous heparin shows graft patency and severe midgraft stenosis that was probably responsible for thrombotic occlusion.

problem. It appears from Lang's report that none of his patients was treated for upper extremity arterial occlusions.

Mori et al treated one patient for axillary artery thrombosis, two for brachial artery emboli, and three for emboli to the hand, but it is impossible to ascertain their success in these cases because of the manner in which the data are grouped.[75] It can be stated that considering arterial thrombi as a group (upper and lower extremity data together) in this series, only 24% of the patients had no clinical benefit; considering arterial emboli as a group, only 10% had no clinical benefit. Likewise, although McNamara and Fischer had several patients who were treated for upper extremity arterial occlusions, because of the method of grouping the data, the exact number and treatment results are not evident.[77] Eighteen of the 27 patients of Wolfson et al were treated for native arterial rather than graft occlusions, but in this study, too, the number of upper extremity cases is not specified.[81] The number of patients with upper-extremity arterial occlusions likewise cannot be ascertained in the series of Graor et al.[72]

Tisnado et al reported the use of local SK infusion in the treatment of hand ischemia.[82] This series has now been expanded to include nine cases of acute and one case of chronic hand ischemia treated with local SK infusion.[83] The authors make the following important points. First, most cases of hand ischemia are caused by atherosclerotic occlusion, emboli, or trauma, whereas only a small number are due to Raynaud's disease, connective tissue disorders, or thoracic outlet syndrome.[84–89] Second, although two-thirds of cases are due to occlusions proximal to the wrist, which are potentially amenable to operation, the remaining one-third are due to occlusion of the small arteries of the hand and fingers, a type in which surgical reconstruction is often difficult or impossible.[89–91] Spasm is rarely an important factor, and cervicodorsal sympathectomy is of little value. Third, occlusive disease limited to the midpalm and fingers is not amenable to vascular surgery, and the results of conservative therapy with vasodilators, anticoagulants, and dextran have been disappointing; many of these patients eventually require amputation.[89] In one previous report, nine patients with arterial occlusions in the arm were treated with local SK using a technique much like that of Hess et al, described earlier in this chapter. The SK (1000 units) was infused by hand injection every 1–3 min, and the catheter was advanced stepwise through the occlusion until the patent distal segment of the artery was reached.[92]

The method of Tisnado et al involves complete upper

extremity angiography, including arch aortography, as an initial step. A 5F transfemoral selective catheter is used for the SK infusion, and the catheter is advanced to the distal brachial artery for infusion of all forearm arteries or to the level of the distal brachial artery occlusion if one is present. This avoids placement of the catheter directly in the forearm vessels, which are small and prone to spasm. In addition, it permits simultaneous infusion of all three forearm arteries. Pharmacoangiography using 25–50 mg of tolazoline, 50 mg of papaverine, 0.1 mg of nitroglycerin, or 50–100 mg of lidocaine is used to identify fixed vascular occlusions. Vasodilators are not needed when initial forearm angiography demonstrates intraluminal filling defects. Tisnado et al typically use a loading dose of SK of 50,000 units administered through the catheter over 30 min, but other investigators have not used loading doses in local low-dose therapy. In fact, some believe strongly that the concept of loading doses is diametrically opposed to the principal aim of fibrinolytic therapy—successful lysis without induction of a systemic fibrinolytic state. The SK infusion is then continued at 5,000 units/hr in the ICU. Heparin is administered concomitantly in doses sufficient to maintain the PTT at 1.5 times normal. Followup arteriograms are obtained every 6–12 hr through the infusion catheter. In the present authors' experience, angiograms with portable equipment in the ICU are often inadequate for assessing fibrinolytic therapy and less likely to detect complications such as catheter-related thrombosis than is a conventional study in the angiography suite.

During the infusion, patients may experience transient pain and changes in pulse, color, and temperature in the extremity. All of these findings are probably due to distal emboli, which tend to lyse with continued infusion, and are identical to findings in the present authors' original series. Importantly, Tisnado et al relate that clinical improvement in the hand may precede angiographic evidence of lysis by a day or more. After fibrinolytic therapy and catheter removal, patients are maintained on heparin for 1–3 days and then on oral anticoagulants for 3–6 months. To date, Tisnado et al have treated nine patients with acute and one patient with chronic hand ischemia successfully. None of the patients required further vascular procedures to restore flow to the hand. In the few instances of tissue loss in the hand or digital amputations, it was believed that SK decreased the extent of amputation necessary. The authors concluded that local low-dose SK infusion should be considered the treatment of choice for patients with hand ischemia who are not candidates for vascular reconstruction because of the anatomic distribution of disease.

Recently, Rapaport et al reported the successful use of an aggressive approach combining vasodilators, intraarterial SK, and simultaneous heparin to salvage a vein graft and an acutely ischemic reattached index finger.[93]

HEMODIALYSIS ACCESSES

In Becker et al's series, 14 patients underwent local fibrinolytic therapy for occluded dialysis accesses.[69] The six patients with fistulae were treated with the local transcatheter method described earlier in this chapter, whereas the eight patients with shunts received SK infusions of 5000 units/hr directly into the shunt and therefore did not require a catheter or simultaneous heparinization. Although complete lysis occurred in only six patients overall, there was a great discrepancy between the results for shunts (six patients had complete lysis) and those for fistulae (five patients had no change). The authors interpret this outcome as further support for the hypothesis that local therapy is less effective when there are numerous alternative egress channels. Figure 20–9 illustrates a representative case from this series.

In the series of Katzen and van Breda, one patient was treated for an occluded dialysis access.[66] After successful fibrinolysis, an underlying stenosis was identified. The series of Totty et al included a single case of a thrombosed forearm dialysis access shunt. Nearly complete lysis was achieved with 19 hr of SK local therapy, and no further treatment was necessary.[68] Mori et al treated nine patients for dialysis access thrombosis.[75] Therapeutic benefit was derived from SK alone or in combination with PTA or operation in seven cases. Ten of the patients of McNamara and Fischer were treated for occluded forearm dialysis accesses,[77] but from the presentation of the data, the degree of success cannot be ascertained.

In the series of Graor et al, 50 patients were treated for thrombosed hemodialysis fistulae.[72] Lysis was successful in 68% overall and in 84% of occlusions no more than 4 days old. The issue of the response to fibrinolytic therapy as a function of the duration of vascular obstruction is considered below.

Zeit reported an unusual approach to fibrinolysis for clotted dialysis accesses.[94] In two patients with thrombosed PTFE hemodialysis fistulae, following failure of more conventional infusion methods, SK was infused locally through needles placed in the occluded portion of the shunts. In one patient, a stenosis of the venous anastomosis identified after successful thrombolysis was managed with PTA.

Rodkin et al reported their experience with local SK infusion for thrombosed PTFE dialysis accesses in nine occlusions in eight patients.[95] After diagnostic angiography, the vessels were treated through a catheter positioned in the proximal portion of the occlusion. In most cases, 40,000 units of SK were infused over 20 min and patients were then maintained on 5,000–7,500 units/hr in the ICU. Lysis was achieved in all but one case, and definite clinical benefit was obtained in seven of the eight patients. Three patients also underwent PTA.

Young et al reported dismal results in treating seven episodes of acute thrombosis of PTFE dialysis fistulae in five patients.[96] After diagnostic angiography, patients underwent local transcatheter infusions of SK at dose rates ranging from 2,500–10,000 units/hr. Patients were monitored in an ICU and examined by angiography at 8-hr intervals. Infusions were terminated following either successful thrombolysis or the appearance of pain and swelling. The only two patients whose infusions resulted in lysis also underwent PTA, and only one PTA was successful. Therefore, all patients ultimately required additional surgical intervention except for one who began peritoneal dialysis when failed PTA of the venous anastomosis resulted in immediate rethrombosis.

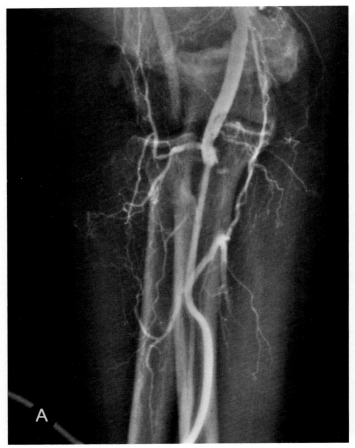

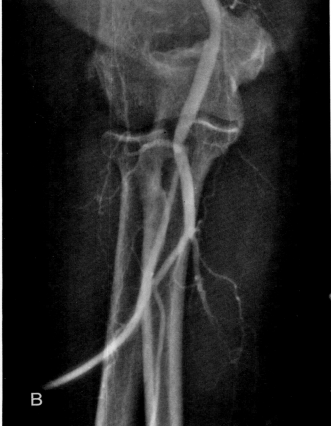

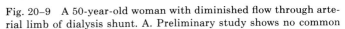

Fig. 20–9 A 50-year-old woman with diminished flow through arterial limb of dialysis shunt. A. Preliminary study shows no common interosseous artery. B. Study after local SK through shunt without concomitant heparin shows normal common interosseous artery.

MESENTERIC ARTERIES

Flickinger et al reported a patient with a superior mesenteric artery embolic occlusion due to atrial fibrillation who was treated with local low-dose transcatheter SK infusion.[97] The patient was thought to be a poor operative candidate because of poor cardiopulmonary status, including three previous myocardial infarctions. At the time of diagnostic angiography, ischemic bowel symptoms had been present for only 3 hr. Although the infusion was started at 5,000 units/hr, a repeat arteriogram after 3 hr of therapy showed minimal improvement, and the catheter was advanced and the infusion rate increased to 10,000 units/hr. After much clinical improvement and evidence of significant thrombolysis on the 60-hr angiogram, the dose rate was decreased to 5,000 units/hr. After a total of 80 hr of infusion and resolution of the symptoms, angiography showed nearly normal vessels, and the infusion was terminated. The authors emphasized that patients with findings of bowel infarction require rapid diagnosis and surgical intervention but that certain patients with ischemic bowel may respond nicely to local SK infusion.

Pillari et al reported a patient with congestive heart failure and transvenous pacing who had embolic occlusions of both the celiac and the superior mesenteric arteries.[98] Bilateral transfemoral catheters were placed selectively, one in the celiac and the other in the superior mesenteric artery. Each catheter provided an infusion dose rate of 5000 units/hr of SK, and the patient's ischemic bowel recovered without surgical intervention.

With so few cases reported, the role of fibrinolytic therapy in the management of ischemic bowel has not yet been adequately defined.

Local SK has been successful in treating hepatic artery thrombosis resulting from intra-arterial chemotherapy.[99]

RENAL ARTERIES

One patient in the series of Katzen and van Breda underwent local transcatheter SK infusion for renal artery occlusion. Successful lysis in this case allowed subsequent PTA.[66] Three patients in the series of Dardik et al were treated with local transcatheter SK for acute renal artery thrombosis. All achieved successful thrombolysis, and all required PTA for correction of an underlying stenosis.[73] One of the patients in the series of Mori et al was treated for embolic occlusion of a renal artery, but the results are not evident from the grouping of the data.[75] Lang's series includes four patients with occluded synthetic aortorenal grafts and one patient with an occluded renal artery in a cadaveric allograft kidney who were treated with local transcatheter SK. Although the author does not specify the percentage of responders in this group, he does state that his greatest degree of success was in patients with thrombosed synthetic grafts (lysis in 11 of 12 cases).[74]

As with mesenteric thrombolysis, the experience with local trancatheter renal artery thrombolysis is not sufficient to define its role.

VEINS

There is much information attesting to the value of systemic SK therapy for acute DVT of the legs.[58,100-110] These studies indicate that SK improves the potential for early restoration of normal blood flow in addition to preventing thrombus extension and embolization and make systemic SK therapy appear more attractive than anticoagulation with heparin. However, little has been done to evaluate local (second-generation) therapy with SK and UK in venous occlusive disease, and most of the available information is anecdotal. The following sections review much of the accumulated clinical experience.

Lower Extremities

The present authors' experience with second-generation therapy in lower extremity DVT is entirely anecdotal. They have treated two patients, both of whom had extensive iliofemoral and calf DVT. The first was treated with a dorsal pedal vein infusion of SK at 5000 units/hr and semiupright positioning. The patient suffered mild superficial phlebitis on the dorsum of the foot but had no improvement on his venogram the following day, so the infusion was terminated. The second patient was treated as follows. A transfemoral arterial catheter was passed over the aortic bifurcation and into the contralateral common femoral artery (ipsilateral to the venous thrombi). An infusion of 5000 units/hr of SK was started, and the patient was observed in the ICU. Tourniquets were applied at the ankle and knee in an effort to promote deep venous drainage and routing of the fibrinolytic solution. There was no clinically or radiographically demonstrable benefit.

Inferior Vena Cava (IVC)

Greenwood et al reported a patient with Budd–Chiari syndrome following viral perimyocarditis.[111] Peritoneoscopy with liver biopsy revealed dilatation of central lobular sinusoids and fibrosis surrounding the central lobular veins, but no evidence of cirrhosis. Computed tomography (CT) and inferior venacavography disclosed intraluminal filling defects in the IVC between the level of the renal veins and the right atrium. Urokinase was given through the IVC catheter as a local infusion in large doses, the patient being given 308,000 units (4,400 units/kg) as a loading dose and then 4,400 units/hr as a continuous infusion (systemic doses). After 55 hr of infusion, there was marked improvement in flow in the IVC. The patient's pain, ascites, and edema rapidly resolved.

Prior to this report, SK had been used to treat hepatic vein thrombosis in a patient on oral contraceptives.[112] Pulmonary emboli occurred. Because of this potential for life-threatening pulmonary emboli during thromobolytic therapy,[113] the danger of such emboli must always be considered. However, Greenwood et al cite evidence that the risk of this complication does not appear higher for thrombolytic therapy than for treatment with heparin alone, at least in peripheral DVT.[111]

Superior Vena Cava (SVC)

In 1981, SK treatment of a patient with idiopathic SVC thrombosis was reported.[114] The largest experience with local low-dose thrombolytic therapy using SK in cases of SVC occlusion has been reported by Graor et al, who successfully treated six patients with this problem.[72] All of the occlusions were <72 hr old. Catheters were introduced through an arm vein and positioned within the most distally occluded segment.

The danger of pulmonary embolization during thrombolytic therapy for SVC obstruction should parallel that of IVC obstruction.

Axillary and Subclavian Veins

This is one area in the venous system in which local transcatheter low-dose fibrinolytic therapy is rapidly becoming the treatment of choice. Idiopathic axillary and subclavian vein thrombosis is known by a variety of names, including "gouty phlebitis," "spontaneous subclavian vein thrombosis," "effort thrombosis of the subclavian vein," and "primary axillary–subclavian vein thrombosis." Since Paget originally described the disease,[115] none of the available therapeutic options, including bed rest, bed rest with anticoagulation, thrombectomy, thrombectomy with rib resection, and stellate ganglion blockade, has proved entirely satisfactory.[116,117] Chronic disability may result from pain with use of the arm (venous claudication), recurrent swelling, or nonfatal pulmonary emboli (5%–10%).

Becker et al's original small series of patients treated with transcatheter local thrombolytic therapy for this disorder[118] has expanded to 11 patients,[119] and review of the clinical entity and this experience is in order. Primary axillary–subclavian vein thrombosis is an entity distinct from subclavian vein thrombosis secondary to central venous catheterization, malignancy, and other causes. Two-thirds of the patients are male and 40 years of age or less. Two-thirds give a history of unusual or vigorous exercise prior to the onset of symptoms. In Becker et al's series, all patients had better than average upper extremity strength, and most were able to relate a particularly strenuous or unusual exercise that led to thrombosis. Weight lifting was common. Cyanosis of the extremity (which may be present only upon exertion), swelling, and prominent venous collaterals about the shoulder and anterior chest are important physical findings, which were present, to various degrees, in these patients. There are two venographic patterns. One is a long-segment obstruction of the axillary and subclavian veins, and the other is a short-segment obstruction of the axillary–subclavian venous segment at the level of the first rib–clavicle junction anteriorly.

Catheterization of an antecubital vein in a patient with significant upper extremity edema can be time-consum-

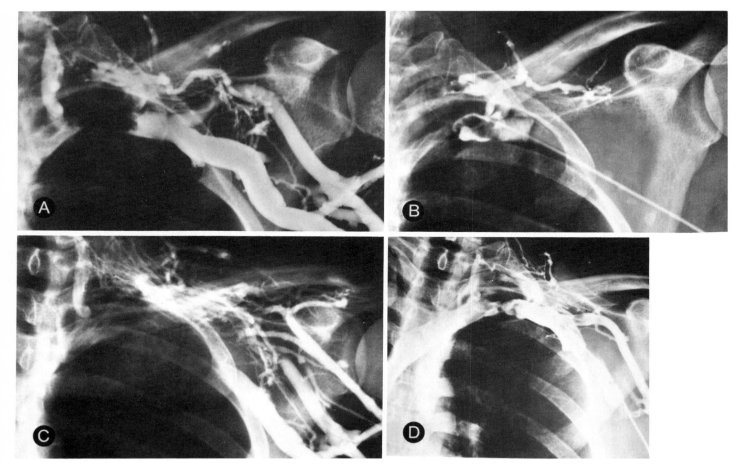

Fig. 20–10 This 35-year-old amateur weight lifter presented with left upper extremity swelling and pain after attempting to lift his car from underneath. A. Venogram shows short-segment subclavian vein occlusion in the region of first rib–clavicle junction anteriorly. B. Catheter tip positioned in occlusion for local SK. C. Venogram after SK shows worsened occlusion. Patient's SK resistance (blood drawn before infusion started) was later found to be markedly elevated, so infusion was changed to UK. D. After local UK, thrombus has been almost entirely cleared, and residual stenosis is identified in the typical location (first rib–clavicle junction anteriorly). Patient subsequently underwent venous bypass.

ing and frustrating. The difficulty can be overcome by injecting the contrast medium into a hand vein, then puncturing the antecubital vein under fluoroscopic guidance. Once the vein has been cannulated, a guidewire is positioned in the subclavian vein at the level of occlusion and followed with a 5F catheter for venography and infusion. Patients with recent streptococcal infection or a high SK antibody titer are poor candidates for SK therapy. One of the authors' patients initially treated with SK suffered propagation of the thrombus but then responded promptly when the infusion solution was changed to UK. These problems, and the fact that 3 of their 11 patients had drug-related fevers while on SK, make them feel that UK is the drug of choice for this condition.

Once the catheter has been embedded within the thrombus, UK at 20,000 units/hr is started via infusion pump. A second infusion pump is required for concomitant intravenous heparin administration at a dose rate sufficient to maintain the PTT at 1.5 times normal. Progress is monitored with serial transcatheter venograms in the radiology department. In all of the present authors' cases, complete or nearly complete lysis was achieved

using these methods. Figure 20–10 illustrates one of the cases.

Importantly, in each case, after successful thrombolysis, they were able to demonstrate irregularity, stenosis, or both phlebographically in the subclavian vein at the first rib–clavicle junction anteriorly. The authors have hypothesized that this abnormality is the important structural causative factor in this disorder and therefore have chosen to call it by another name: the "thoracic inlet syndrome." The anatomic (Fig. 20–11) and functional etiologic factors in the development of this syndrome are not completely understood. Subclavian and axillary vein compression by the costocoracoid ligament, subclavius muscle, and clavicle against the first rib may all be important. Stasis, recurrent trauma, and venospasm have been implicated. Regardless of the precise mechanisms involved, the venographic abnormality is consistently present.

Two patients in this series with only small stenoses improved symptomatically after fibrinolytic therapy and were maintained for a time on oral anticoagulants as outpatients. One had PTA of the subclavian vein, which

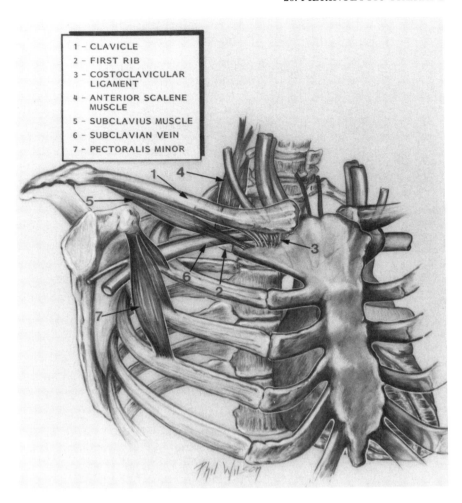

1 – CLAVICLE
2 – FIRST RIB
3 – COSTOCLAVICULAR
     LIGAMENT
4 – ANTERIOR SCALENE
     MUSCLE
5 – SUBCLAVIUS MUSCLE
6 – SUBCLAVIAN VEIN
7 – PECTORALIS MINOR

Fig. 20–11   Important anatomic features of thoracic inlet.

resulted in venographic evidence of partial resolution of the stenosis. Five underwent venous bypass procedures, the efficacy of which has not yet been determined. Three had significant residual stenosis but have had no further treatment except oral anticoagulants. Perivascular fibrosis and mural abnormalities in the subclavian vein were found consistently in the patients who went to surgery. None of the patients in this series had hemorrhagic complications or clinical evidence of pulmonary emboli.

Patients with venous infusion catheters frequently suffer local inflammatory reactions to the catheter, fibrinolytic agent, or contrast medium. Reactions may be manifest as pain and local tenderness with or without rubor. Some authors have suggested simultaneous administration of corticosteriods to alleviate or prevent this problem, but the present authors have no experience with this.

Central Venous Lines

Double-lumen Hickman central venous catheters have been used for long-term access for transfusions and chemotherapy in patients with malignancy (JJ Reilly Jr, DL Steed, PS Ritter, unpublished data). Although a twice-daily flush with heparin solution usually preserves patency, occlusions do occur, and fibrin sheaths around the catheter tip and shaft may prevent effective venous access.[120,121]

Zajko et al reported a series of 16 episodes of Hickman catheter occlusions in 14 patients.[122] In three instances, a mechanical problem was responsible; in the remaining 13, venography performed by direct injection of contrast medium into the catheter disclosed a fibrin sheath occluding its distal end. In each of these 13 instances, SK infusion was started using 3000 units/lumen/hr. This was continued for 12 hr, at which time venography was repeated. In 12 cases, venography revealed catheter patency. In the remaining case, infusion was continued for another 12 hr without therapeutic benefit. In this case, the catheter had been occluded for longer than 2 weeks.

Although others have used fibrinolytic therapy to restore patency to central venous catheters, the results are difficult to assess because venography was not used.[123,124]

PULMONARY ARTERIES

Human Studies

The large experience with systemic (first-generation) fibrinolytic therapy for pulmonary thromboembolic disease (PTE) that resulted from UPET and USPET was described above. Recently, several authors have described their experiences with transcatheter local fibrinolytic therapy for PTE.

Barbarena reported 11 patients who were treated with local transcatheter UK for acute PTE.[125] All patients had had symptoms for <12 hr. All had symptoms of acute PTE, but only one presented with shock. Six PTE were postoperative events (3–26 days). All patients underwent pulmonary angiography with an 8F, 100-cm NIH cardiovascular catheter positioned in the main trunk of the pulmonary artery regardless of the location or suspected location of the embolus. Follow-up angiograms to assess therapeutic benefit were obtained at 48 hr in nine patients, 24 hr in one, and 72 hr in one. Infusions of UK were made through the angiography catheter, which was not moved after the diagnostic study. A loading dose of 2700 units/kg was administered over 5–10 min, then a continuous infusion of 2700 units/kg/hr was maintained for 12 hr. Longer infusions were not attempted because data from UPET do not suggest that longer systemic UK infusions provide additional benefit. After fibrinolytic therapy, all patients were given intravenous heparin. All 11 patients improved clinically, and nine improved electrocardiographically. One patient who showed evidence of only partial improvement on ECG later underwent embolectomy. Angiographically demonstrable improvement, assessed by the objective scoring method of Miller et al,[126] was seen in all cases, with a somewhat greater improvement noted in perfusion than in the grade of obstruction. Complications, which were frequent in this series, are discussed below.

Vujic et al treated three patients who had severe pulmonary emboli using full heparinization in combination with transcatheter low-dose SK.[127] In each case, the diagnosis was confirmed by angiography and the decision to use SK instead of operation was made because of severe or terminal underlying disease. Two patients had only acute emboli and one had had recurrent emboli over a 3-week period. Pulmonary angiography and SK infusion were accomplished using a 6.7F Grollman pulmonary angiography catheter placed via a transfemoral approach. In one case, the catheter was positioned as near to the embolus as possible, in another within the embolus, and in the remaining patient, who had large bilateral emboli, at the bifurcation of the main pulmonary artery. The dose rate of SK was 10,000 units/hr, and simultaneous heparin was administered intravenously at 1000 units/hr. Pulmonary artery pressure and arterial PaO$_2$ were monitored, and shrinkage of the embolus was evaluated by follow-up pulmonary arteriography. All three patients responded favorably to this regimen. In the first case, the pulmonary artery pressure decreased from 40/19 mm Hg before treatment to 22/12 mm Hg after 16 hr of treatment, while the PaO$_2$ increased from 56 torr to 76 torr within 6 hr. In the second case, the pulmonary artery pressure decreased from 56/24 mm Hg to 35/22 mm Hg by 6 hr and 32/16 mm Hg by 30 hr, while the PaO$_2$ went from 40 torr on 100% FiO$_2$ to 69 torr on 40% FiO$_2$. In the patient with recurrent emboli the PaO$_2$ increased from 38 torr to 85 torr after 16 hr of infusion. Although the pulmonary artery pressure did not change significantly in

this patient, it had been only minimally elevated before treatment (28/10 mm Hg).

The authors of this report make several interesting points about the method and their findings, as well as about the findings of others. They state that direct delivery of SK to the embolus enhances SK–plasminogen interaction by minimizing exposure of the drug to antibodies and endogenous inhibitors. At the same time, bleeding due to systemic fibrinolytic states can be avoided, because the drug can be given at much lower dose rates. The authors also think that patients with severe obstruction due to PTE have faster and more extensive lytic responses to local therapy, because severe obstruction provides more time for SK–plasminogen interaction. (As we shall see, more rapid lysis is not necessarily better lysis.) Finally, Vujic et al think that mechanical fragmentation of the embolus by the catheter tip may enhance the lytic response by creating a larger surface for SK–plasminogen interaction.

Of the 159 patients in the series of Graor et al, 10 were treated for severe pulmonary emboli involving a main or two or more lobar pulmonary arteries.[72] This experience has now expanded to include 13 patients.[128] In 10, emboli were <72 hr old; in three, they were 1 week old. Mean pulmonary artery pressures were elevated (>30 mm Hg), and all patients were hemodynamically unstable and in need of 100% FiO$_2$ to maintain normal arterial oxygenation. The first 10 had pulmonary angiography and local SK infusion through a 6F Grollman pulmonary angiography catheter or a 7F cardiovascular catheter at 5,000–10,000 units/hr plus concomitant systemic heparinization until the next daily pulmonary angiogram. At angiography, if no lysis had occurred, SK was discontinued. If lysis was incomplete and there were no signs of bleeding, the heparin was discontinued and the SK dose rate was increased to 100,000 units/hr. Infusions were continued until there was complete lysis or lack of further progress. In the last three patients, SK was started at 100,000 units/hr without systemic heparinization. If follow-up angiography showed either complete or no lysis, the infusion was terminated, whereas if angiography disclosed partial lysis, the infusion was continued at the same dose rate until lysis was complete. All patients received conventional anticoagulant therapy after the SK regimen was completed. As in the other patients, these patients received intravenous cephalosporins every 6 hr during and for 24 hr after therapy. Patients were monitored with Swan–Ganz catheters in the ICU.

Lytic therapy was successful in 11 of these 13 patients. Blood pressures, pulse, and respiratory rates returned to normal, and patients became increasingly comfortable. These clinical signs of improvement occurred between 6 and 18 hr after the start of local SK. By 24 hr, pulmonary artery pressures and arterial PaO$_2$ were normal or near baseline. One of the failures was in a patient 8 days postresection of an abdominal aortic aneurysm; this patient's low-dose infusion was terminated when a retroperitoneal hemorrhage occurred. In the high-dose group, two of the three patients had complete lysis, one after 24 hr of therapy and the other after 48 hr. The remaining patient was a treatment failure who eventually required embolectomy. Seven of the 11 successfully treated patients had follow-up ventilation–perfusion lung scans showing complete resolution of the perfusion abnormalities.

Figure 20–12 illustrates the use of local fibrinolytic therapy in a patient with PTE.

Animal Studies

Over the past 2 years, Holden et al have developed an animal model for comparing systemic and local fibrinolytic therapy for PTE.[129] Although the details of this work are not relevent here, a few of the salient features must be described, if only to temper enthusiasm for local fibrinolytic therapy in the pulmonary circulation. The authors' model involves adult New Zealand white rabbits, transcatheter embolization of autologous clot prepared *in vitro*, and a multiparametric assessment of the effects of fibrinolytic infusions. Animals were treated with high-dose SK infused in a peripheral vein, in the pulmonary artery with the catheter tip above the clot, or in the pulmonary artery with the catheter tip embedded in the clot.

All pulmonary arterial infusions (intraclot and above the clot) resulted in more rapid and thorough lysis (more lysis of intraluminal clot within the time of the experiment) than did peripheral intravenous infusions. Although rapid lysis would appear to be desirable, this is not necessarily the case. These results indicate that rapid lysis with intraclot infusion produces extensive obstruction of small pulmonary vessels, with obliteration of capillary perfusion (Fig. 20–13), in contrast to the relatively preserved pulmonary capillary perfusion that may be seen with intravenous infusion. The return of pulmonary capillary perfusion in obstructed portions of the lung in some of the animals during continued infusion suggests that blockade of small pulmonary vessels is an intermediate phenomenon resulting from fragmentation of clot during infusion and that perfusion is restored as clot fragments are lysed. It is important to remember, however, that many patients probably cannot tolerate this extent of capillary blockade even for a short time. The critical point is that although fibrinolytic therapy for PTE can be lifesaving, there are instances in which it can be life threatening.

It appears from this model that one of the most important differences between central (pulmonary artery) infusions and peripheral (intravenous) infusions is the higher enzyme concentration bathing the clot with the former. Rapid fibrinolysis produced by infusion of higher enzyme concentrations increases the frequency of clot fragmentation, whereas the slower fibrinolysis produced by lower enzyme concentrations creates more soluble FDPs and relatively little pulmonary capillary blockade. There are many patients with lung disease, a diminished pulmonary capillary bed, or elevated right-sided intracardiac pressures who probably cannot tolerate clot fragmentation with pulmonary capillary blockade even as an intermediate phase. In these patients, the authors suggest monitoring right atrial and pulmonary artery pressures during therapy.

These findings and the limited clincial experience with

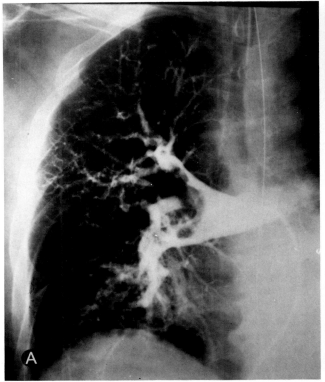 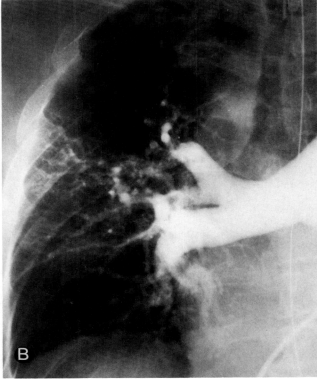

Fig. 20–12 Patient with severe pulmonary embolus. A. Initial pulmonary angiogram reveals large embolus at bifurcation of right pulmonary artery. Note that upper lobe perfusion is intact. B. Angiogram after 24 hr of local SK at 60,000 units/hr shows that extensive lysis has occurred. However, note lack of perfusion in right upper lobe. This change is probably due to fragmentation and peripheral embolization.

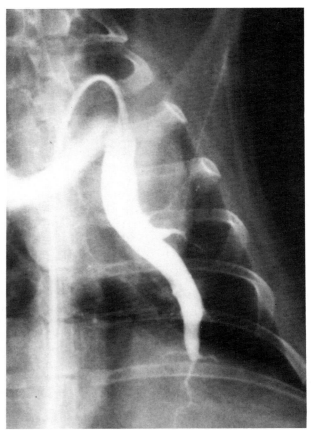

Fig. 20–13   Rabbit pulmonary angiogram after 4 ½ hr of transcatheter infusion of a total of 125,000 units of SK. Extensive rapid fibrinolysis has resulted in dissolution of all previously visible clot in left main pulmonary artery. Note absence of pulmonary capillary perfusion; this is caused by fragmentation of the clot as a result of rapid lysis.

second-generation fibrinolytic therapy in PTE serve to underscore the fact that the role of this method in the pulmonary arterial circulation is just beginning to be defined.

CORONARY ARTERIES

Since the original report of Rentrop et al on the use of local fibrinolytic therapy for coronary occlusion,[67] many additional series have appeared in the literature.

Coronary artery thrombosis is present in approximately 90% of patients with acute myocardial infarction (AMI).[130] Prior to the elucidation of this fact, there was no pathophysiologic basis for taking aggressive measures to alleviate coronary obstruction in cases of AMI. Rather, most treatments focused on administering coronary vasodilators, decreasing myocardial oxygen demand, and improving myocardial oxygenation. Although the first use of selective SK administration for coronary occlusion was reported in 1960,[131] the method did not gain wide acceptance because of several problems. First, the reported success of those first authors was not documented by angiography. Second, the hemorrhagic risks were thought to be unacceptably high. Third, even though it was known that coronary angiography could easily be used to

document coronary occlusion and resolution, most investigators were reluctant to subject their patients to coronary angiography in the acute phase of AMI.

In 1976, Chazov et al reported the first angiographically documented selective fibrinolysis-mediated coronary recanalization.[132] Widespread enthusiasm developed after the report of Rentrop et al.[67] Because most interventional radiologists do not do selective coronary thrombolysis, and since the literature is too extensive to review thoroughly in this chapter, only a few comments will be made on this topic.

Patients selected for intracoronary thrombolysis must present within the first few hours of the onset of symptoms of AMI for there to be any likelihood of myocardial salvage by coronary recanalization. The procedure requires a 24-hr on-call emergency angiography team, and a backup cardiovascular surgical team is advisable, if not essential. Once the diagnosis is established by ECG and clinical impression, the patient is moved to the catheterization laboratory as quickly as possible. During that time, oxygen, nitroglycerin, and other standard supportive measures are given.

According to the methods outlined by Paulin and Als,[133] patients are given 5,000 units of prophylactic heparin intravenously, and selective coronary catheterization, with or without preliminary ventriculography, is performed for diagnostic angiography in both coronary arteries in at least two projections via a transfemoral approach. Repeat angiography after 0.2 mg of intracoronary nitroglycerin has been given documents the fixed nature of the occlusion. Following a hand-injected bolus of 20,000 units of SK in 20 ml, Paulin and Als use a continuous intracoronary infusion of 4,000 units/min (4 ml/min) administered via infusion pump. Signs of improvement include abatement of symptoms, lowering of ST segments on continuous ECG monitoring, mild hypotension, and new onset of arrhythmias. These indicators of success generally occur within ½ hr of the start of the infusion.

Other specific actions can be taken during the ½-hr delay, including placement of a mobile gamma camera for ventricular function studies, repeat full 12-lead ECG, etc. Angiographic monitoring is achieved by selective injections of contrast medium at 15-min intervals. If patency is re-established but flow velocity is less than normal, the infusion is slowed to 2,000 units/min (2 ml/min). Generally, this can be continued for as long as an hour without exceeding a total dose of 250,000 units. After the fibrinolytic infusion is completed, a complete coronary arteriogram is performed. Repeat ECG and assessment of left ventricular function by radionuclide scanning can be done at this time as well. Heparinization is continued, and the patient is sent to the ICU with the sheath still in place at the puncture site; this provides hemostasis in the immediate post-treatment period and provides immediate easy access if repeat coronary arteriography becomes necessary.

In the experience of Paulin and Als, as well as that of others, successful reperfusion (not identical to myocardial salvage) occurs in approximately 70%–75% of cases. Often, the flow is slow initially, possibly indicating distal emboli in the coronary circulation that lyse with continued infusion. It has been known for some time that this occurs during fibrinolytic therapy for other types of thromboembolic disease, and there now is evidence that it also occurs with significant frequency in the coronary circulation.[134] In the report of Paulin and Als, reperfusion was said to be complete when the velocity and pattern of contrast flow in the involved vessel paralleled that in uninvolved coronary arteries. When flow appeared ineffective or incomplete, the authors were able to demonstrate persistent defects on thallium-201 myocardial scans.

Successful reperfusion often leads to the discovery of underlying stenosis, just as it does in the peripheral vasculature, and some of these lesions are amenable to percutaneous transluminal coronary angioplasty (PTCA). Definitive measures, such as coronary bypass grafting and PTCA, must be applied to individual patients on the basis of the clinical circumstances, expected outcomes, and analysis of treatment alternatives. Angioplasty may be considered in the immediate postfibrinolysis period if clinical and ECG evidence of persistent ischemia is present.

Predischarge follow-up angiography, practiced by many, often discloses further resolution of an area of "stenosis." This finding probably indicates continued lysis of thrombus that is adherent to the vessel wall immediately after treatment.

What is the correlation between reperfusion and myocardial salvage? Coronary occlusion leads to decreased myocardial contractility within minutes,[135] yet short-lived occlusions do not necessarily damage myocardial cells.[136,137] In dogs, hypokinesia can persist for 30 min after restoration of coronary flow in instances of transient occlusion ("stunned myocardium"),[138] and the longer the duration of occlusion, the smaller the degree of recovery after re-establishment of normal flow. In the same canine models, occlusions for ≥6 hr are followed by little if any myocardial recovery. Paulin and Als suggest, however, that these results cannot readily be extrapolated to coronary occlusion in man, because of the usual presence there of atheromatous disease and variably developed collaterals. That is, it is theoretically possible that patients with atherosclerotic coronary disease would be able to tolerate longer durations of coronary occlusion than the dogs because of the presence of these collaterals.

There is evidence that left ventricular function studies are not as sensitive for determinating the degree of myocardial salvage as is thallium-201 myocardial scanning.[139]

Currently, local thrombolytic therapy for AMI must be viewed as being in the stage of clinical investigation.

Nevertheless, strong support for its use may be found in the results of the Western Washington Randomized Trial in which 250 patients who were treated with selective intracoronary SK had a significant reduction in group 30-day mortality.[140] High-dose intravenous SK infusion for AMI has its proponents[141] and must be considered seriously as an alternative to second-generation therapy, especially in view of the fact that only the minority of hospitals have the cardiac catheterization laboratories needed to institute the selective method. Nonetheless, although the results of intravenous infusion are encouraging, they have not been as favorable as those achieved with the selective method.

Recently, results of clinical trials using tPA for AMI have been reported.[142,143] Although the percentage of patients responding has been extremely high, hemorrhagic complications have occurred.

CENTRAL NERVOUS SYSTEM

Investigators are working on methods of infusing UK directly into acutely occluded middle cerebral arteries in humans with the aid of flow-directed balloon catheters. Although these endeavors to recanalize acutely occluded carotid arteries appear exciting, one must remember that acute cerebral reperfusion may carry a high morbidity and mortality rate as a result of cerebral hemorrhage.[144]

To test the potential of local fibrinolytic therapy in acute carotid occlusion resulting from operation or angiography, Eskridge et al recently studied transcatheter local fibrinolysis in a canine model of acute carotid occlusion.[145] They found the risk of hemorrhage from reperfusion to be unacceptably high, and it is with these data in mind that they discourage the use of local fibrinolytic therapy for acute carotid occlusion. Perhaps further studies will not corroborate this impression, but for now, extreme caution is recommended.

In a recent study with New Zealand white rabbits, Narayan et al tested the safety and efficacy of UK in lysing intracranial hematomas.[146] Using stereotactically guided equipment, the authors injected clotted human blood into the frontal lobes and lateral ventricles of these animals. A direct injection of 50,000 units of UK was then given to the test animals and saline was administered to the controls. Hematomas were lysed in 90% of the experimental animals, whereas only 14% of the control hematomas were lysed. The possible future application of this method in neurosurgery or in CT-guided interventional neuroradiology is unclear.

LABORATORY MONITORING

In first-generation fibrinolytic therapy with SK or UK, a systemic fibrinolytic state, characterized by conversion of circulating plasminogen to plasmin, is required for success. This is not to say that activation of plasminogen that is bound within the thrombus or embolus is inadequate; rather, the method of administration and the doses required entail generalized plasminogen activation. Remember that circulating plasmin is a nonspecific protease, which cleaves and inactivates not only fibrin, but

also fibrinogen, factors V and VIII, and other proteins. This has an obvious anticoagulant effect. Remember, too, that FDPs resulting from cleavage of fibrin and fibrinogen have their own inhibitory effect on the coagulation cascade. This, in turn, results in further anticoagulation. In second-generation therapy, on the other hand, one attempts to activate the plasminogen that is bound within the thrombus or embolus, and a systemic fibrinolytic state is therefore considered a side effect. The available laboratory tests for monitoring the fibrinolytic state have been reviewed in detail by Ramchandani and Soulen.[147] A summary is provided here.

Free circulating plasmin may be measured directly by radioimmunoassay (RIA), by the fibrin plate method, or by euglobulin lysis time. The RIA is complex and not widely available. The fibrin plate method takes 16–20 hr, making it impractical for guiding clinical decisions. Therefore, euglobulin lysis time is the most widely utilized direct method. In this test, acidification of the patient's blood precipitates fibrinogen and the fibrinolytically active plasma components (euglobulin precipitate). Thrombin is added to the precipitate, and the clot lysis time is measured. A normal value is 3–4 hr; during fibrinolytic therapy, the time is usually much less than 1 hr. Although it is sensitive, the euglobulin lysis test is an exacting method and is not widely available on a 24-hr basis. Therefore, indirect tests are often indicated.

The blood fibrinogen level is the most useful and widely used indirect test. Since fibrinogen is a major substrate of plasmin that can be measured, it provides a useful index of fibrinolytic activity. Whereas normal levels are approximately 300–400 mg/dl, most experts believe that 100 mg/dl are required for adequate hemostasis. In this test, thrombin is added to a sample of the patient's blood, and thrombin clotting time is measured; the value obtained is inversely proportional to the fibrinogen concentration. A normal thrombin time must be within 5 sec of control, and typical control values are 18–22 sec. This test can be utilized in most cases of systemic fibrinolytic therapy, but if the patient is receiving local therapy with heparin, the test is invalid, because heparin increases the thrombin (clotting) time.

A second useful indirect test is the measurement of FDPs. These products accumulate in the blood during systemic fibrinolytic therapy and are specific for lysis of fibrinogen or fibrin by plasmin. A normal value is <10 µg/ml. One must appreciate an interrelation between the laboratory measures; increased FDPs prolong thrombin time through their anticoagulant effect.

The PTT is insensitive in detecting a systemic fibrinolytic state but is a good screen for the intrinsic coagulation pathway. The authors have recently used only the PTT, measured every 4 hr, to monitor patients on local low-dose fibrinolytic therapy given concomitant heparin to prevent pericatheter thrombosis. The authors attempt to keep the PTT at approximately 1.5 times normal,

whereas others attempt to keep it even higher (2.0–3.0 times normal). If the PTT is longer than desired, the heparin infusion rate is decreased or the heparin is replaced with saline until the next measurement but the SK or UK infusion rate is not altered. It should be remembered that during administration of this combination form of therapy, there generally is a decrease in the dose rate of heparin required to maintain the PTT at the desired value because of the anticoagulant effects of plasmin and FDPs.

Why are the fibrinolytic values not measured in such cases? There are two reasons. First, there are insufficient data showing that abnormal values correspond to a tendency for patients to hemorrhage. Second, as detailed above, in the presence of heparin, the common measures are rendered invalid. The reptilase clotting time can be used to monitor the systemic fibrinolytic state in the presence of heparin anticoagulation, but it is expensive and not readily available, particularly on a 24-hr basis.

To reiterate, no single laboratory test is a reliable predictor of the degree of lysis or of the likelihood of a hemorrhagic complication.[148–150] Therefore, the laboratory tests used to assess the systemic fibrinolytic state can only warn of severe hypofibrinogenemia and fibrinolysis.

It is probably useful to obtain certain laboratory data before beginning fibrinolytic therapy. A complete blood count, including platelets, plus PT and PTT constitutes a readily available standard screen. In addition, if SK is to be used, an anti-SK antibody titer (SK resistance test) can be obtained. In systemic fibrinolytic therapy, it is desirable to neutralize existing antibody before starting the maintenance infusion. This was the logic that led to the development of the loading dose concept. A 250,000-unit bolus of SK administered over 30 min is sufficient to neutralize existing antibody in approximately 90% of patients.[51] The intravenous systemic maintenance infusion can then begin. Such a large bolus seems counterproductive in cases of local therapy, and in fact, the importance of anti-SK antibody in such cases is poorly understood. However, the authors have seen patients fail on local SK infusion yet respond beautifully to UK infusion and therefore suspect that anti-SK antibodies can influence the outcome of this therapy. Obviously, patient selection is important: one need not measure SK resistance in a patient recently (within the preceding 6 months) treated with SK to know that UK is the preferred drug.

COMPLICATIONS

The hemorrhagic complications of systemic infusion of fibrinolytic agents have been amply covered already; this section deals with the complications of local infusion.

The reader need only review the variety of second-generation treatment regimens to appreciate the complexity in understanding the complications and the frequencies of their occurrence. Palaskas et al have reviewed this topic,[63] and the information in the following sections derives from their work, as well as from a review of several series.

Hemorrhage

It is safe to say that local transcatheter fibrinolytic therapy has not done away with hemorrhagic complications, even though it was hoped that it might. However, it probably has reduced their frequency. In the original series of Dotter et al, 17 patients received SK at the rate of 5000 units/hr, and four had significant bleeding complications.[64] Although this frequency seems to compare favorably with that in UPET (45%), Dotter et al did not report data on hemoglobin or hematocrit, so there may have been undetected bleeding. This deficiency is noted in almost all reports of second-generation therapy. Importantly, hemorrhage during fibrinolytic therapy is usually due to dissolution of hemostatic plugs at sites of recent vascular trauma, although gastrointestinal, intracranial, and retroperitoneal bleeding and other serious hemorrhagic complications can occur.

Feissinger et al identified six intracranial hemorrhages or emboli and 18 other bleeding complications in a series of 194 patients treated with systemic UK.[151] They also reported a series of 25 patients treated with local UK[152] in whom there were no serious hemorrhagic complications, although three patients bled slightly from the catheter insertion site. In the series of 12 local infusions reported by Katzen and van Breda, two patients who bled at the puncture site did so only after the addition of heparin, and the bleeding ceased when heparin was stopped.[66] In the series of 26 local infusions reported by Totty et al, SK was used in dose rates of 2,500–10,000 units/hr and UK in dose rates of 40,000–80,000 units/hr. All five patients with serious complications had bleeding at the catheter insertion site, although only two required transfusion with packed red cells or whole blood. In this series, cryoprecipitate was administered to patients whose fibrinogen levels dropped to <100 mg/dl.[68]

In Becker et al's original series of 57 local infusions plus concomitant intravenous heparin, significant hemorrhagic complications occurred in 12.2% of the patients, and only one of these patients required operation because of the bleeding. One of the other major hemorrhages was intracerebral, but it developed in a patient whose markedly prolonged PTT had gone unrecognized for an inordinately long time. Three of the serious hemorrhages were gastrointestinal. Another 14% of patients suffered minor hemorrhagic complications not necessitating intervention.[69]

In the series of Hess et al, whose method requires a total SK dose much lower than in most other methods, only 3 of 136 patients receiving local infusion had hematomas at the catheter insertion site. No serious hemorrhagic complications occurred.[70] In the series of 159 local infusions reported by Graor et al serious hemorrhagic complications, defined as those necessitating blood transfusion or operation or resulting in clinical deterioration, occurred in 17 patients (10.7%). Only 3.8% of these hemorrhages were at sites remote from the catheter insertion. Another 27 patients (17%) had slight bleeding at the catheter entry site.[72]

In the series of 50 local infusions of SK reported by Mori et al minor bleeding, usually from the arterial puncture site, occurred in 30% of patients, and serious hemorrhage necessitating transfusion or operation occurred in 8%.[75] Only three hematomas (one retroperitoneal) occurred in the 38 infusions (28 local) reported by Dardik et al.[73] In a series of complications reported by Lang, 7 of 35 patients had bleeding at the catheter entry site.[74] In the series of 27 infusions reported by Wolfson et al only one patient had a serious hemorrhagic complication. Slight bleeding not mandating discontinuation of SK occurred in another two patients.[81] In the series of 93 high-dose local UK infusions reported by McNamara and

Fischer, significant bleeding necessitating transfusion occurred in 4%.[77]

It is clear that there can be hemorrhagic complications of local transcatheter fibrinolytic therapy. When they occur, they are most frequently at the catheter insertion site. Other, more serious, local and remote hemorrhages occur during local therapy with a much lower frequency. Particular attention should be paid to the methods of Hess et al because it appears that their use of a smaller total dose of fibrinolytic agent results in a very small frequency of bleeding complications.[70]

Local fibrinolytic therapy must sometimes be given when hemorrhage ensues or when laboratory results dictate use of local therapy without concomitant heparin. When overt hemorrhage occurs during local transcatheter SK or UK infusion, the drug should be stopped and catheter patency maintained with saline infusion. Cryoprecipitate or fresh-frozen plasma (3–6 units) should be administered. For continued unresponsive bleeding, ε-aminocaproic acid (Amicar) can be given; it inhibits plasminogen activator and may stimulate antiplasmin. The initial dose is 5 g followed by hourly doses of 1.0–1.25 g to maintain the plasma level at 0.13 mg/ml. Obviously, packed red blood cells or whole blood should be administered in many of these cases.

Allergic Reactions

No serious allergic reactions to local low-dose SK and UK have been reported, but anaphylactic reactions have occurred with systemic SK. Local SK infusions may result in nausea, vomiting, and mild hypotension. A case of serum sickness syndrome caused by local low-dose SK infusion has been reported.[153] Allergic reactions are not expected with UK.

Fever

Fever may occur in 10%–40% of patients receiving local SK. Fever occurred with approximately this frequency in the present authors' series of patients treated for axillary and subclavian vein occlusion. However, in their experience and that of others,[63] fever is truly a minor complication associated with no other ill effects and is easily managed with antipyretics. With local transcatheter therapy, sepsis must be excluded as an etiology for any fever, and blood probably should be cultured.

Distal Emboli

Distal embolizations during transcatheter local infusion for thromboembolic disease have been reported in most of the large series reviewed in this chapter. Emboli also occur with systemic intravenous infusion therapy. They are probably secondary to uneven dissolution, which weakens the thrombus in certain areas, resulting in fragmentation. In peripheral embolization, the patient may suffer abrupt onset of pain or paresthesia. Cyanosis or pallor and coolness may be noted in the extremity, and pulses may be diminished or absent. Such emboli have been demonstrated angiographically in some of these patients. Fortunately, these emboli usually dissolve with continued fibrinolytic infusion, although in some cases, they must be surgically removed.

Emboli remote from the thrombus being treated have been reported with systemic infusion therapy, so the potential for such phenomena cannot be ignored. For instance, patients with embolic occlusion of a leg secondary to mural thrombi or other cardiac etiology may release additional emboli to other portions of the systemic circulation during fibrinolytic therapy. Sicard et al recently reported four patients who had pulmonary emboli during or shortly after local infusion therapy.[154] One explanation offered by those authors is that the emboli may have originated in DVT partially lysed during the infusion. The other possible explanation is that the pulmonary emboli may be due to a relatively hypercoagulable state.[155]

Catheter-Related Thrombosis

Although catheters indwelling for such maneuvers as vasopressin infusion do not often cause thromboembolic complications, those placed for fibrinolytic therapy often do. This may be simply because the diminished flow proximal to the occlusion enhances the potential for thrombus formation around the catheter shaft. Eskridge et al reported a 26% frequency of this phenomenon in 57 local infusions.[65] Although other authors report a lower incidence, many of the evaluations were performed by hand injection of contrast medium and a single film obtained in the ICU. The present authors' arteriograms are all performed in the angiography suite with multiple films, and they believe that pericatheter thrombosis is much more likely to be detected with this method.

Concomitant heparin administration for prevention of this complication has already been discussed. Pila et al described a modification of the local transcatheter infusion technique that also may help prevent pericatheter thrombosis.[156] Those authors use a 5F Teflon sheath and a coaxial 2.5F catheter for their infusions. The smaller catheter may prove less thrombogenic for two reasons. First, it provides less surface area for thrombus formation than does a standard 5.0F–7.0F angiographic catheter. Second, the smaller diameter may cause less diminution of flow in the vessel proximal to the occlusion. Small heparin-bonded catheters for infusion are available.

Extravasation through Graft Interstices

This phenomenon may be seen on serial angiograms (Fig. 20–14) during local fibrinolytic therapy with either SK or UK.[71] The authors' first report of this problem included four patients with occluded knitted-Dacron grafts, all of whom were treated with SK and none of whom became symptomatic during infusion. Since one of these grafts was 6 years old, it was apparent to us that SK can lyse long-term fibrin deposits in the "pseudointima" of grafts. There is much other supportive evidence that SK is efficacious in chronic occlusions.[157,158] Additional

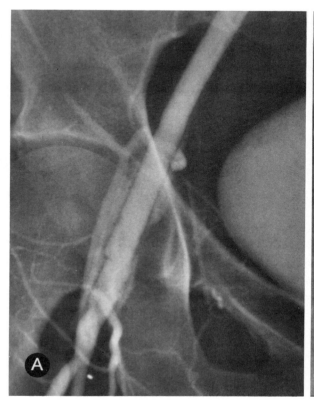
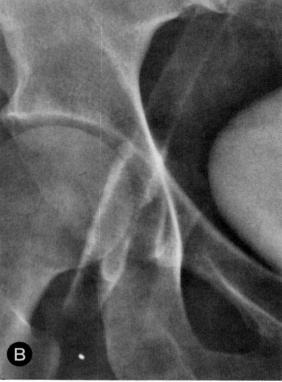

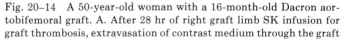

Fig. 20–14   A 50-year-old woman with a 16-month-old Dacron aortobifemoral graft. A. After 28 hr of right graft limb SK infusion for graft thrombosis, extravasation of contrast medium through the graft is seen. B. Later phase of same angiogram sequence; negative cast of graft is result of extravasated contrast medium.

reports have confirmed that both UK and SK can permeate graft interstices; that PTFE grafts, like Dacron ones, are susceptible; and that the angiographic findings of permeation may also be associated with symptomatic perigraft hematoma formation.[159,160] In one of Becker et al's patients with a PTFE graft, a hematoma formed in the popliteal fossa during low-dose transcatheter UK therapy.[159] Figure 20–14 illustrates contrast extravasation through graft interstices. The authors suggest that patients with angiographic evidence of extravasation, particularly those with aortofemoral or aortoiliac grafts, undergo CT examination to search for an "occult" hematoma. In some patients, it is likely that hematoma will be found, and fibrinolytic therapy may have to be stopped.

Myoglobinuria and Renal Failure

Lang's article on the complications of intra-arterial use of SK reminds us that reperfusion of ischemic-necrotic muscle achieved by operation or other means of revascularization, including fibrinolytic therapy, can lead to the "crush syndrome."[74] This syndrome is characterized by shock, myoglobinuria that may cause renal failure, hyperkalemia, and cardiac conduction abnormalities, including bundle branch block, complete heart block, and asystole. In 17 patients who presented with neither ischemic necrosis nor compartment syndrome in the involved extremity, Lang observed no instances of myoglobinuria. However, significant myoglobinuria did occur in 10 of 18 patients who presented with compartment syndrome. Fasciotomy appears efficacious but may not prevent myoglobinuria once perfusion has been re-established. Three patients in this series whose myoglobinuria intensified after thrombolytic therapy developed acute tubular necrosis. Lang concluded that attempts at limb salvage by means of revascularization when tissue is already compromised are unjustified and carry an unacceptable risk of renal complications as well as a threat to the patient's life.

CONTRAINDICATIONS

Most of the contraindications to fibrinolytic therapy relate to the risk of hemorrhage. Some relate to the allergenic potential of SK. See Table 20–1 for a complete list of contraindications.

THIRD-GENERATION THERAPY: PRESENT AND FUTURE

There are several formidable challenges in fibrinolytic therapy today. First, it needs to be less invasive. Second-generation therapy has brought both improvements in the results and a lower frequency of hemorrhagic complications, but the methods still lead to a significant frequency of hemorrhage and to new complications, such as pericatheter thrombosis, not seen with first-generation therapy. Second, one or more "magic bullets" are needed which, upon intravenous or oral administration, will lyse thrombi without creating high levels of circulating plasmin (third-generation therapy). With such agents, thromboembolic disorders could be treated effectively yet the systemic fibrinolytic state and its accompanying hemorrhagic complications could be avoided. In addition, the setting for patient management would once again be the medical ward instead of the angiography suite and the ICU. Third, the magic bullets need to be widely available and affordable so they can be used on an emergency basis. For instance, such agents might be administered intravenously by ambulance crews or other emergency specialists to abort myocardial infarctions or cerebrovascular accidents. Finally, radiologists need to keep up with all the changes in medicine that are relevant to their practice and use their growing knowledge to increase their participation in overall patient management. The latter challenge is fundamental to interventional radiologic practice.

The preceding challenges have been addressed to some extent and continue to be addressed in biochemical and microbiologic research laboratories around the world. Tissue plasminogen activator is a magic bullet capable of lysing remote thrombi upon intravenous administration without inducing a systemic fibrinolytic state. Its fibrinogenolytic:fibrinolytic ratio is markedly lower than that of UK *in vitro*.[161] This highly specific activity is related to its great affinity for fibrin-bound plasminogen and its relatively low affinity for circulating free plasminogen (Fig. 20–15). tPA has been isolated from normal human tissues,[162] as well as from the culture fluid of a cell line derived from human melanoma.[163] The derivation of tPA from melanoma is a tedious, time-consuming, and expensive process, with an extremely low yield. Therefore, researchers have sought other sources. Recently, the protein was purified and sequenced so that its messenger RNA (mRNA), together with reverse transcriptase, could

Table 20–1
Contraindications to Fibrinolytic Therapy

Hemorrhagic
  Recent major operation
  Recent gastrointestinal bleeding
  Severe hypertension
  Hemostatic defects
  Diabetic hemorrhagic retinopathy
  Cerebrovascular disease
Embolic
  Subacute bacterial endocarditis
  Left-sided cardiac thrombus
Allergic (SK)
  Known allergy to SK
  Recent SK infusion
  Recent streptococcal infection
  Rheumatic fever
  Post-streptococcal glomerulonephritis

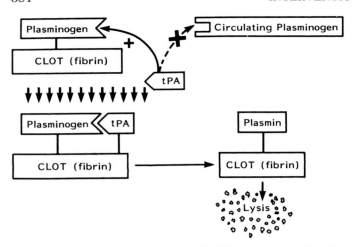

Fig. 20–15 Mechanism of action of tPA. This agent's specific affinity for fibrin-bound plasminogen is probably due to a conformational difference between fibrin-bound and circulating free plasminogen. This special affinity allows the formation of a trimolecular complex between tPA, plasminogen, and fibrin. The activity of this complex results in fibrinolysis. The observable consequences of lack of activation of circulating plasminogen include very little circulating plasmin and no systemic fibrinolytic state.

be used to generate the DNA sequence that codes for the enzyme. Armed with the sequence, investigators produced a plasmid, which, when inserted into *Escherichia coli,* directed synthesis of a polypeptide with the same fibrinolytic activity as authentic human tPA.[164] This recombinant DNA product has coronary fibrinolytic activity similar to that of tPA in a canine model of coronary occlusion.[142] The biosynthetic process or one like it should provide larger quantities of tPA for clinical use.

Weimar et al used melanoma-derived tPA to lyse iliofemoral and renal vein thrombi in a 30-year-old recipient of a cadaveric renal allograft.[165] More recently, Van de Werf et al reported successful lytic therapy of human coronary thrombi within 20–50 min in six of seven attempts with melanoma-derived tPA.[166] Since that time, several medical centers have instituted clinical trials of tPA in both the coronary circulation[142,143] and the peripheral circulation.[167,168]

There is another potential agent for clinical fibrinolytic therapy. One of the vitamin K-dependent, hepatic-synthesized factors mentioned in earlier discussion of the basic coagulation cascade was protein C. Unlike the other factors, activated protein C has an anticoagulant effect. It inactivates the activated forms of factors V and VIII by limited proteolysis.[31,169] In addition, a stimulating effect of protein C on the fibrinolytic mechanism has been described, and apparently it is capable of increasing the levels of circulating plasminogen activator.[31] Future studies of this substance will determine its precise roles in inhibiting thrombus formation and in thrombolysis.

Acylated SK-plasminogen complex does not activate circulating plasminogen. Upon binding to fibrin, deacylation occurs and activator complexes activate fibrin-bound plasminogen. The result is selective clot lysis without a systemic lytic state.

Prourokinase offers potential as an endogenously administered fibrinolytic agent, because it has little or no activity while circulating, but it activates plasminogen in the presence of a fibrin clot.

Finally, a report by Bode et al describes another important potential new avenue of therapeutic approach. The authors produced a highly specific fibrinolytic agent by covalently coupling urokinase to a fibrin-specific monoclonal antibody that did not cross-react with fibrinogen.[170] The newly created fibrinolytic agent showed a 100-fold increase in fibrinolysis over unmodified urokinase *in vitro.* This exciting new concept provides a means by which fibrin-specific action of the administered agent may be achieved while the systemic fibrinolytic state is avoided. Commercial laboratories are working on this murine antibody product.

SUMMARY

Fibrinolytic therapy is a tool increasingly utilized by the interventional angiographer. Its successful use depends on the cooperation of the angiographer, surgeon, nurses, and others involved in the total care of the patient. The techniques and agents are evolving rapidly, and it is incumbent on interventional radiologists to stay abreast of changes and to increase their participation in patient management.

References

1. Tillett WS, Garner RL: The fibrinolytic activity of hemolytic streptococci. *J Exp Med* 1933;58:485
2. Sherry S: The fibrinolytic activity of streptokinase activated human plasmin. *J Clin Invest* 1954;33:1054
3. Welch WH: Thrombosis and embolism, in Albutt TC (ed): *A System of Medicine.* London, Macmillan and Co. Ltd, 1899, p 155
4. Moncada S, Vane JR: The discovery of prostacyclin: a fresh insight into arachidonic acid metabolism, in Kharasch K, Fried J (eds): *Biochemical Aspects of Prostaglandins and Thromboxanes.* New York, Academic Press, 1977, p 155
5. Bunting S, Gryglewski RJ, Moncada S, et al: Arterial walls generate from prostaglandin endoperoxides a substance (prostaglandin X) which relaxes strips of mesenteric and coeliac arteries and inhibits platelet aggregation. *Prostaglandins* 1976;12:897
6. Willis AL, Kuhn DC: A new potential mediator of arterial thrombosis whose biosynthesis is inhibited by aspirin. *Prostaglandins* 1973;4:127
7. Hamberg M, Samuelsson B: Detection and isolation of an endoperoxide intermediate in prostaglandin biosynthesis. *Proc Natl Acad Sci USA* 1973;70:899
8. Smith JB, Ingerman C, Kocsis JJ, et al: Formation of an intermediate in prostaglandin biosynthesis and its association with platelet release reaction. *J Clin Invest* 1974;53:1468
9. Hamberg M, Svensson J, Samuelsson B: Thromboxanes: a new group of biologically active compounds derived from prostaglandin endoperoxides. *Proc Natl Acad Sci USA* 1975;72:2994
10. Bunting S, Moncada S, Vane JR: The effects of prostaglandin endoperoxides and thromboxane A$_2$ on strips of rabbit coeliac

artery and other smooth muscle preparations. *Br J Pharmacol* 1976;57:462P

11. Smith EF III, Lefer AM, Nicolaou KC: Mechanism of coronary vascoconstriction induced by carbocyclic thromboxane A_2. *Am J Physiol* 1981;240:H493

12. Moncada S, Herman AG, Higgs EA, et al: Differential formation of prostacyclin (PGX or PGI_2) by layers of the arterial wall: an explanation for the anti-thrombotic properties of vascular endothelium. *Thromb Res* 1977;11:323

13. Glavind J, Hartmann S, Clemmesen J, et al: Studies on the role of lipoperoxides in human pathology: the presence of peroxidized lipids in the atherosclerotic aorta. *Acta Pathol Microbiol Scand* 1952;30:1

14. Moncada S, Gryglewski RJ, Bunting S, et al: A lipid peroxide inhibits the enzyme in blood vessel microsomes that generates from prostaglandin endoperoxides the substance (prostaglandin X) which prevents platelet aggregation. *Prostaglandins* 1976;12:715

15. D'Angelo V, Villa S, Mysliewic M, et al: Defective fibrinolytic and prostacyclin like activity in human atheromatous plaques. *Thromb Haemost* 1978;39:535

16. Virchow R: *Cellular Pathology as Based upon Physiological and Pathological Histology.* London, Churchill, 1860, p 197

17. Beckering RE, Titus JL: Femoral-popliteal venous thrombosis and pulmonary embolism. *Am J Pathol* 1969;52:530

18. Paterson JC: The pathology of venous thrombi, in Sherry S, Brinkhous KM, Genton E, et al (eds): *Thrombosis.* Washington, DC, US National Academy of Sciences, 1969, p 321

19. Sevitt S: The structure and growth of valve-pocket thrombi in femoral veins. *J Clin Pathol* 1974;27:517

20. Nicolaides AN, Kakkar VV, Renney JTG: The soleal sinuses. *Br J Surg* 1970;57:860

21. Nicolaides AN, Kakkar VV, Renney JTG: Soleal sinuses and stasis. *Br J Surg* 1971;58:307

22. McLachlin AD, McLachlin JA, Jory TA, et al: Venous stasis in the lower extremities. *Ann Surg* 1960;152:678

23. Astrup T, Permin PM: Fibrinolysis in animal organism. *Nature* 1947;159:681

24. Astrup T: The biological significance of fibrinolysis. *Lancet* 1956;2:565

25. Todd AS: The histological localization of fibrinolysin activator. *J Pathol Bacteriol* 1959;78:281

26. Rjken DC, Wijngaards G, Welbergen J: Relationship between tissue plasminogen activator and the activators in blood and vascular wall. *Thromb Res* 1980;18:815

27. Ljungner J, Holmberg L, Kjeldgaard A, et al: Immunological characterization of plasminogen activators in the human vessel wall. *J Clin Pathol* 1983;36:1046

28. Levin EG: Latent tissue plasminogen activator produced by human endothelial cells in culture: evidence for an enzyme–inhibitor complex. *Proc Natl Acad Sci USA* 1983;80:6804

29. Ljunger J, Bergqvist D: Decreased fibrinolytic activity in the bottom of human vein valve pockets. *Vasa* 1983;12:333

30. Ljunger J, Bergqvist D, von Hebel I, et al: Influence of major surgery on plasminogen activator activity in superficial hand veins. *Eur Surg Res* 1983;15:161

31. McKee PA: Disorders of blood coagulation, in Wyngaarden JB, Smith LH Jr (eds): *Cecil Textbook of Medicine.* Philadelphia, WB Saunders, 1985, p 1040

32. Bookstein JJ, Moser KM, Hougie C: Coagulative interventions during angiography. *CardioVasc Intervent Radiol* 1982;5:46

33. Loskutoff DJ, Edgington TS: An inhibitor of plasminogen activator in rabbit endothelial cells. *J Biol Chem* 1981;256:4142

34. Emeiss JJ, van Hinsbergh VMW, Verheijen JH, et al: Inhibition of tissue-type plasminogen activator by conditioned medium from cultured human and porcine vascular endothelial cells. *Biochem Biophys Res Commun* 1983;110:392

35. Chmielewska J, Ranby M, Wiman B: Evidence for a rapid

inhibitor to tissue plasminogen activator in plasma. *Thromb Res* 1983;31:427

36. Kruithop EKO, Ransijn A, Bachmann F: Inhibition of tissue plasminogen activator by human plasma, in Davidson JF, Bachmann F, Bouvier CA, Kruithop EKO (eds): *Progress in Fibrinolysis.* Edinburgh, Churchill Livingstone, 1983, p 365

37. Verheijen JH, Chang GTG, Kluft C: Evidence for the occurrence of a fast-acting inhibitor for tissue-type plasminogen activator in human plasma. *Thromb Haemost* 1984;51:392

38. Aoki N, Moroi M, Sakata Y, et al: Abnormal plasminogen: a hereditary molecular abnormality found in a patient with recurrent thrombosis. *J Clin Invest* 1978;61:1186

39. Wohl RC, Summaria L, Robbins KC: Physiological activation of the human fibrinolytic system: isolation and characterization of human plasminogen variants, Chicago I and Chicago II. *J Biol Chem* 1979;254:9063

40. Johansson L, Hedner U, Nilsson IM: A family with thromboembolic disease associated with deficient fibrinolytic activity in vessel wall. *Acta Med Scand* 1978;203;477

41. Jorgensen M, Mortensen JZ, Madsen AG, et al: A family with reduced plasminogen activator activity in blood associated with recurrent venous thrombosis. *Scand J Haematol* 1982;29:217

42. Aoki N, Saito H, Kamiya T, et al: Congenital deficiency of alpha-2-plasmin inhibitor associated with severe hemorrhagic tendency. *J Clin Invest* 1979;63:877

43. Miles LA, Plow EF, Donnelly KJ, et al: A bleeding disorder due to deficiency of alpha-2-antiplasmin. *Blood* 1982;59:1246

44. Kluft C, Vallenga E, Brommer EJP, et al: A familial hemorrhagic diathesis in a Dutch family: an inherited deficiency of alpha-2-antiplasmin. *Blood* 1982;59:1169

45. Booth NA, Bennett B, Wijngaards G, et al: A new life-long hemorrhagic disorder due to excess plasminogen activator. *Blood* 1983;61:267

46. Alkjaersig N, Fletcher AP, Sherry S: The mechanism of clot dissolution by plasmin. *J Clin Invest* 1959;38:1086

47. Johnson AJ, McCarty WR: The lysis of artificially induced intravascular clots in man by intravenous infusions of streptokinase. *J Clin Invest* 1959;38:1627

48. Becker GJ: Local thrombolytic therapy: bridging the "generation gap." *AJR* 1983;140:403

49. Macfarlane RG, Pilling J: Observations on fibrinolysis: plasminogen, plasmin and antiplasmin content of human blood. *Lancet* 1946;2:562

50. Sherry S, Lindemeyer RI, Fletcher AP, Alkjaersig N: Studies on enhanced fibrinolytic activity in man. *J Clin Invest* 1959;38:810

51. Verstraete M, Vermylen J, Amery A, et al: Thrombolytic therapy with streptokinase using a standard dosage scheme. *Br Med J* 1966;1:454

52. Mattsson C, Nyberg–Arrhenius V, Wallen P: Dissolution of thrombi by tissue plasminogen activator, urokinase and streptokinase in an artifical circulating system. *Thromb Res* 1981;21:535

53. Becker GJ: Second-generation fibrinolytic therapy: state of the art. *Semin Intervent Radiol* 1985;2:409

54. Katzen BT: Mechanism and clinical application of fibrinolysis. *Proceedings of the Joint Meeting of the European and American Societies of Cardiovascular and Interventional Radiology,* 1987, p 10

55. Tennant SN, Dixon J, Venable TC, et al: Intracoronary thrombolysis in patients with acute myocardial infarction: comparison of the efficacy of urokinase with streptokinase. *Circulation* 1984;69:756

56. Browse NL, Thomas ML, Pim HP: Streptokinase and deep vein thrombosis. *Br Med J* 1968;4:421

57. Den Ottolander GJH, Craandjik A: Treatment of thrombosis of the central retinal vein with streptokinases. *Thromb Diath Haemorrh* 1968;20:41

58. Kakkar VV, Flanc C, Howe CT, et al: Treatment of deep vein

thrombosis: a trial of heparin, streptokinase, and Arvin. *Br Med J* 1969;1:806

59. Ploug J, Kjeldgaard NO: Urokinase: an activator of plasminogen from human urine: isolation and properties. *Biochim Biophys Acta* 1957;24:278

60. Sasahara AA, Hyers TM, Cole CM, et al (eds): The Urokinase Pulmonary Embolism Trial: a national cooperative study. *Circulation* 1973;47(suppl 2):1

61. Urokinase-Streptokinase Pulmonary Embolism Trial (Phase II): Results: a cooperative study. *JAMA* 1974;229:1606

62. Sharma GVRK, Burleson VA, Sasahara AA: Effect of thrombolytic therapy on pulmonary capillary blood volume in patients with pulmonary embolism. *N Engl J Med* 1980;303:842

63. Palaskas C, Totty WG, Gilula LA, Reinus WR: Complications of local intra-arterial fibrinolytic therapy. *Semin Intervent Radiol* 1985;2:396

64. Dotter CT, Rosch J, Seaman AJ: Selective clot lysis with low-dose streptokinase. *Radiology* 1974;111:31

65. Eskridge JM, Becker GJ, Rabe FE, et al: Catheter-related thrombosis and fibrinolytic therapy. *Radiology* 1983;149:429

66. Katzen BT, van Breda A: Low dose streptokinase in the treatment of arterial occlusions. *AJR* 1981;136:1171

67. Rentrop P, Blanke H, Karsch KR, et al: Acute myocardial infarction: intracoronary application of nitroglycerin and streptokinase. *Clin Cardiol* 1979;2:354

68. Totty WG, Gilula LA, McClennan BL, Ahmed P, Sherman L: Low-dose intravascular fibrinolytic therapy. *Radiology* 1982;143:59

69. Becker GJ, Rabe FE, Richmond BD, et al: Low-dose fibrinolytic therapy: results and new concepts. *Radiology* 1982;148:663

70. Hess J, Ingrisch H, Mietaschk A, Rath H: Local low-dose thrombolytic therapy of peripheral arterial occlusions. *N Engl J Med* 1982;307:1627

71. Rabe FE, Becker GJ, Richmond BD, et al: Contrast extravasation through Dacron grafts: a sequela of low dose streptokinase therapy. *AJR* 1982;138:917

72. Graor RA, Risius B, Young JR, et al: Low-dose streptokinase for selective thrombolysis: systemic effects and complications. *Radiology* 1984;152:35

73. Dardik H, Sussman BC, Kahn M, et al: Lysis of arterial clot by intravenous or intra-arterial administration of streptokinase. *Surg Gynecol Obstet* 1984;158:137

74. Lang EK: Streptokinase therapy: complications of intra-arterial use. *Radiology* 1985;154:75

75. Mori KW, Bookstein JJ, Heeney DJ, et al: Selective streptokinase infusion: clinical and laboratory correlates. *Radiology* 1983;148:677

76. Tennant SN, Dixon J, Venable TC, et al: Intracoronary thrombolysis in patients with acute myocardial infarction: comparison of the efficacy of urokinase with streptokinase. *Circulation* 1984;69:756

77. McNamara TO, Fischer JR: Thrombolysis of peripheral arterial and graft occlusions: improved results using high-dose urokinase. *AJR* 1985;144:769

78. Bean WJ, Rodan BA, Thebaut AL: Leriche syndrome: treatment with streptokinase and angioplasty. *AJR* 1985;144:1285

79. Lynch WA, Westcott JL: "Blind" femoral angiography. *Radiology* 1977;125:379

80. Dotter CT, Rosch J, Robinson M: Fluoroscopic guidance in femoral artery puncture. *Radiology* 1978;127:266

81. Wolfson RH, Kumpe DA, Rutherford RB: Role of intra-arterial streptokinase in treatment of arterial thromboembolism. *Arch Surg* 1984;119:697

82. Tisnado J, Bartol DT, Cho S-R, et al: Low-dose fibrinolytic therapy in hand ischemia. *Radiology* 1984;150:375

83. Tisnado J, Cho S-R, Beachley MC, Vines FS: Low-dose fibrinolytic therapy in hand ischemia. *Semin Intervent Radiol* 1985;2:367

84. Gross WS, Flanigan DP, Kraft RO, et al: Chronic upper extremity arterial insufficiency: etiology, manifestations and operative managament. *Arch Surg* 1978;113:419

85. Erlandson EE, Forrest ME, Shields JJ, et al: Discriminant arteriographic criteria in the management of forearm and hand ischemia. *Surgery* 1981;90:1025

86. Schmidt FE, Hewitt RL: Severe upper limb ischemia. *Arch Surg* 1980;115;1188

87. Baur GM, Porter JM, Bardana EJ Jr, et al: Rapid onset of hand ischemia of unknown etiology: clinical evaluation and follow-up in ten patients. *Ann Surg* 1977;186:184

88. Holleman JH, Hardy JD, Williamson JW, et al: Arterial surgery for arm ischemia: a survey of 136 patients. *Ann Surg* 1980;191:727

89. Taylor LM Jr, Baur GM, Porter JM: Finger gangrene caused by small artery occlusive disease. *Ann Surg* 1981;193:453

90. McNamara MF, Takaki HS, Yao JST, et al: A systemic approach to severe hand ischemia. *Surgery* 1978;83:1

91. Silcott GR, Polich VL: Palmar arch arterial reconstruction for the salvage of ischemic fingers. *Am J Surg* 1981;142:219

92. Slany J, Enzenhofer V, Karnik R: Local thrombolysis in arterial occlusive disease. *Angiology* 1984;35:231

93. Rapoport S, Glickman MG, Salomon JC, Cuono CB: Aggressive postoperative pharmacotherapy for vascular compromise of replanted digits. *AJR* 1985;144:1065

94. Zeit RM: Clearing of clotted dialysis shunts by streptokinase injection at multiple sites. *AJR* 1983;141:1053

95. Rodkin RS, Bookstein JJ, Heeney DJ, Davis GB: Streptokinase and transluminal angioplasty in the treatment of acutely thrombosed hemodialysis access fistulas. *Radiology* 1983;149:425

96. Young AT, Hunter DW, Castañeda–Zuñiga WR, et al: Thrombosed synthetic hemodialysis access fistulas: failure of fibrinolytic therapy. *Radiology* 1985;154:639

97. Flickinger EG, Johnsrude IS, Ogburn NL, Weaver MD, Pories WJ: Local streptokinase infusion for superior mesenteric artery thromboembolism. *AJR* 1983;140:771

98. Pillari G, Doscher W, Fierstein J, Ross W, Loh G, Berkowitz BJ: Low-dose streptokinase in the treatment of celiac and superior mesenteric artery occlusion. *Arch Surg* 1983;118:1340

99. Ziessman HA, Juni JE, Gyves JW, Brady TM, Ensminger WD: Thrombosis and streptokinase lysis during hepatic intraarterial chemotherapy: the value of perfusion scintigraphy. *AJR* 1985;144:1067

100. Gormsen J: Thrombolytic therapy of acute phlebothrombosis, in Hiemeyer V, Schattauer FE (eds): *Therapeutische und Experimentelle Fibrinolyse*. Stuttgart, Verlag, 1969, p 267

101. Browse NL, Thomas ML, Pim HP: Streptokinase and deep vein thrombosis. *Br Med J* 1968;3:707

102. Robertson BR, Nillson IM, Nylander G: Value of streptokinase and heparin in therapy of acute deep vein thrombosis. *Acta Chir Scand* 1968;134:203

103. Robertson BR, Nillson IM, Nylander G: Thrombolytic effect of streptokinase as evaluated by phlebography of deep vein thrombosis of the leg. *Acta Chir Scand* 1970;136:173

104. Tsapogas MJ, Peabody RA, Wu KT, et al: Controlled study of thrombolytic therapy in deep vein thrombosis. *Surgery* 1973;74:973

105. Duckert F, Muller G, Nyman D, et al: Treatment of deep vein thrombosis with streptokinase. *Br Med J* 1975;1:479

106. Rosch JJ, Dotter CT, Seaman AJ, et al: Healing of deep vein thrombosis: venographic findings in a randomized study comparing streptokinase and heparin. *AJR* 1976;127:533

107. Marder VJ, Soulen RL, Atichartakarn V: Quantitative venographic assessment of deep vein thrombosis in the evaluation of streptokinase and heparin therapy. *J Lab Clin Med* 1977;89:1018

108. Arnesen H, Heilo A, Jakobsen E, et al: A prospective study of

streptokinase and heparin in the treatment of venous thrombosis. *Acta Med Scand* 1978;203:457

109. Elliot MS, Immelman EJ, Jeffery P, et al: A comparative randomized trial of heparin versus streptokinaase in the treatment of acute proximal venous thrombosis: an interim report of a prospective trial. *Br J Surg* 1979;66:838

110. Watz R, Savidge GF: Rapid thrombolysis and preservation of venous valvular function in high deep vein thrombosis. *Acta Med Scand* 1979;205:293

111. Greenwood LH, Yrizarry JM, Hallett JW Jr, Scoville GS Jr: Urokinase treatment of Budd–Chiari syndrome. *AJR* 1983;141:1057

112. Warren RL, Schlant RC, Wenger NK, Galambos JT: Treatment of Budd–Chiari syndrome with streptokinase. *Gastroenterology* 1972;62:200

113. Goldsmith JC, Lollar P, Hoak JC: Massive fatal pulmonary emboli with fibrinolytic therapy. *Circulation* 1982;64:1068

114. Herrera JL, Willis SM, Williams TH: Successful streptokinase therapy of acute idiopathic superior vena cava thrombosis. *Am Heart J* 1981;102:1063

115. Paget J: *Clinical Lectures and Essays.* London, Longmans Green and Co, 1875

116. Swinton NW, Edgett JW, Hall RJ: Primary subclavian–axillary vein thrombosis. *Circulation* 1968;38:737

117. Adams JT, McEvoy RK, DeWeese JA: Primary deep venous thrombosis of upper extremity. *Arch Surg* 1965;91:29

118. Becker GJ, Holden RW, Rabe FE, et al: Local thrombolytic therapy for subclavian and axillary vein thrombosis: treatment of the thoracic inlet syndrome. *Radiology* 1983;149:419

119. Becker GK, Holden RW, Mail JT, Olson EW, Castañeda–Zuñiga WR: Local thrombolytic therapy for "thoracic inlet syndrome." *Semin Intervent Radiol* 1985;2:349

120. Hoshal VL Jr, Ause RG, Hoskins PA: Fibrin sleeve formation on indwelling subclavian central venous catheters. *Arch Surg* 1971;102:353

121. Peters WR, Bush WH Jr, McIntyre RD, Hill LD: The development of fibrin sheath on indwelling venous catheters. *Surg Gynecol Obstet* 1973;137:43

122. Zajko AB, Reilly JJ Jr, Bron KM, Desai R, Steed DL: Low-dose streptokinase for occluded Hickman catheters. *AJR* 1983;141:1311

123. Hurtubise MR, Bottino JC, Lawson M, McCredie KB: Restoring patency of occluded central venous catheters. *Arch Surg* 1980;115:212

124. Glynn MFX, Langer B, Jeejeebhoy KN: Therapy for thrombotic occlusion of long term intravenous alimentation catheters. *J Parent Enteral Nutr* 1980;4:387

125. Barbarena J: Intraarterial infusion of urokinase in the treatment of acute pulmonary thromboembolism: preliminary observations. *AJR* 1983;140:883

126. Miller GAH, Sutton GC, Karr IH, Gibson RV, Honey M: Comparison of streptokinase and heparin in treatment of isolated acute massive pulmonary embolism. *Br Med J* 1971;2:681

127. Vujic I, Young JWR, Gobien RP, Dawson WT, Liebscher L, Shelley BE Jr: Massive pulmonary embolism: treatment with full heparinization and topical low-dose streptokinase. *Radiology* 1983;148:671

128. Risius B, Graor RA: Fibrinolyic therapy in pulmonary thromboembolic disease. *Semin Intervent Radiol* 1985,2:338

129. Holden RW, Becker GJ, Schauwecker DS, et al: Capillary blockade due to rapid clot lysis in an experimental rabbit pulmonary thomboembolism mode (poster session). Tenth Congress of the International Society on Thrombosis and Hemostasis, San Diego, CA, July 1985

130. DeWood MA, Spores J, Notske R, et al: Prevalence of total coronary occlusion during the early hours of transmural myocardial infarction. *N Engl J Med* 1980;303:897

131. Boucek RJ, Murphy WP Jr: Segmental perfusion of the coronary arteries with fibrinolysis in man following a myocardial infarction. *Am J Cardiol* 1960;6:525

132. Chazov EI, Mateeva LS, Mazaev AV, et al: Intracoronary administration of fibrinolysis in acute myocardial infarction. *Ter Arkh* 1976;48:8

133. Paulin S, Als AV: Thrombolytic therapy in coronary artery occlusion. *Semin Intervent Radiol* 1985;2:381

134. Terrosu P, Ibba GV, Contini GM, Franceschino V: Angiographic features of the coronary arteries during intracoronary thrombolysis. *Br Heart J* 1984;52:154

135. Tennant R, Wiggers C: The effect of coronary occlusion on myocardial contraction. *Am J Physiol* 1935;112:351

136. Blumgart H, Gilligan R, Schlesinger M: Experimental studies on the effect of temporary occlusion of coronary arteries. *Am Heart J* 1941;22:374

137. Jennings R, Summers J, Smyth G, et al: Myocardial necrosis induced by temporary occlusion of a coronary artery in the dog. *Arch Pathol* 1960;70:82

138. Braunwald E, Kloner RA: The stunned myocardium: prolonged, post-ischemic ventricular dysfunction. *Circulation* 1982;66:1146

139. Silverman KJ, Becker LC, Bulkley BH, et al: Value of early thallium 201 scintigraphy for predicting mortality in patients with acute myocardial infarction. *Circulation* 1980;61:996

140. Kennedy JW, Ritchie JL, Davis KB, Fritz JK: Western Washington Randomized Trial of Intracoronary Streptokinase in Acute Myocardial Infarction. *N Engl J Med* 1983;309:1477

141. Schroder R, Biamino G, Von Leitner ER, Linderer TH: Intravenous streptokinase infusions in acute myocardial infarction. *Dtsch Med Wochenschr* 1981;106:294

142. Van de Werf F, Bergmann SR, Fox KAA, et al: Coronary thrombolysis with intravenously administered human tissue-type plasminogen activator produced by recombinant DNA technology. *Circulation* 1984;69:605

143. Gold HK, Fallon JT, Yasuda T, et al: Coronary thrombolysis with recombinant human tissue-type plasminogen activator. *Circulation* 1984;70:700

144. Blaisdell WF, Clauss RH, Galbraith JG, et al: Joint study of extracranial arterial occlusion: review of surgical complications. *JAMA* 1969;209:1889

145. Eskridge JM, Becker GJ, Rabe FE, Holden RW: Local fibrinolytic therapy for acute carotid occlusion in a canine model. *Semin Intervent Radiol* 1985;2:405

146. Narayan RK, Narayan TM, Katz DA, Kornblith PL, Murano G: Lysis of intracranial hematomas with urokinase in a rabbit model. *J Neurosurg* 1985;62:580

147. Ramchandani P, Soulen RL: Laboratory monitoring in fibrinolytic therapy. *Semin Intervent Radiol* 1985;2:391

148. Marder VJ: The use of thrombolytic agents: choice of patient, drug administration, laboratory monitoring. *Ann Intern Med* 1979;90:802

149. Rutkowsky DM, Burkle WS: Advances in thrombolytic therapy. *Drug Intell Clin Pharm* 1982;96:115

150. Brogden RN, Speight TM, Avery GS: Streptokinase: review of its clinical pharmacology, mechanism of action and therapeutic uses. *Drugs* 1973;5:357

151. Feissinger JN, Aiach M, Vaysariat M, et al: Traitment thrombolytique des arteriopathies. *Ann Anesthesiol Fr* 1978;19:739

152. Feissinger JN, Vayssariat M, Juillet Y, et al: Local urokinase in arterial thromboembolism. *Angiology* 1980;31:715

153. Totty WG, Romano T, Benian G, et al: Serum sickness following streptokinase therapy. *AJR* 1982;138:143

154. Sicard GA, Schier JJ, Totty WG, et al: Thrombolytic therapy for acute arterial occlusion. *J Vasc Surg*, in press

155. Sherry S: Thrombolytic therapy in surgical patients. *Curr Surg* 1981;38:75

156. Pila T, Fantana S, Peterson G, et al: A modified technique for the infusion of low-dose streptokinase. *AJR* 1984;142:1213

157. Berkman WA, White RI Jr, Parandian BB: Lysis of a chronic arterial occlusion with streptokinase. *AJR* 1983;141:40

158. Martin M: *Streptokinase in Chronic Arterial Disease.* Boca Raton, FL, CRC Press, 1982

159. Becker GJ, Holden RW, Rabe FE: Contrast extravasation from a Gore–Tex graft: a complication of thrombolytic therapy. *AJR* 1984;142:573

160. Rosner NH, Doris PE: Contrast extravasation through a Gore–Tex graft: a sequela of low dose streptokinase therapy. *AJR* 1984;143:633

161. Matsuo O, Collen DC: Comparison of the relative fibrinogenolytic, fibrinolytic and thrombolytic properties of tissue plasminogen activator and urokinase in vitro. *Thromb Haemost* 1981;45:225

162. Rijken DC, Wijngaards G, Zall–de Jong M, Welbergen J: Purification and partial characterization of plasminogen activator from human uterine tissue. *Biochim Biophys Acta* 1979;580:140

163. Rijken DC, Collen D: Purification and characterization of the plasminogen activator secreted by human melanoma cells in culture. *J Biol Chem* 1981;256:7035

164. Pennica D, Holmes WE, Kohr WJ, et al: Cloning and expression of human tissue-type plasminogen activator cDNA in E. coli. *Nature* 1983;301:214

165. Weimar W, Stibbe J, van Seyen AJ, Billiau A, Somer P, Collen D: Specific lysis of an iliofemoral thrombus by administration of extrinsic (tissue-type) plasminogen activator. *Lancet* 1981;2:1018

166. Van de Werf F, Ludbrook PA, Bergmann SR, et al: Coronary thrombolysis with tissue-type plasminogen activator in patients with evolving myocardial infarction. *N Engl J Med* 1984;310:609

167. Risius B, Graor RA, Geisinger MA, et al: Recombinant human tissue-type plasminogen activator for thrombolysis in peripheral arteries and bypass grafts. *Radiology* 1986;160;183

168. Graor RA, Risius B, Denny KM, et al: Local thrombolysis in the treatment of thrombosed arteries, bypass grafts and arteriovenous fistulas. *J Vasc Surg* 1985;2:406

169. Esmon CT: Protein-C biochemistry, physiology and clinical implications. *Blood* 1983;62:1155

170. Bode C, Matsueda GR, Hui KY, Haber E: Antibody-directed urokinase: a specific fibrinolytic agent. *Science* 1985;229:765

21

Intravascular Foreign Body Removal

S. MURTHY TADAVARTHY, M.D., CAROL C. COLEMAN, M.D., FLAVIO CASTAÑEDA, M.D., MICHAEL D. DARCY, M.D., ANDREW H. CRAGG, M.D., GUNNAR LUND, M.D., TONY P. SMITH, M.D., DAVID W. HUNTER, M.D., KURT AMPLATZ, M.D., AND WILFRIDO R. CASTAÑEDA-ZUÑIGA, M.D., M.Sc.

Since the first report by Turner and Sommers in 1954 of an embolized intravenous polyethylene catheter,[1] well over 200 similar cases have been reported in the English-language literature, most of them as single case reports commonly associated with a complication or a successful percutaneous removal. The true incidence of this problem is believed to be much higher than the number of reports would suggest, however, as it is reasonable to assume that most cases are not published. Recent surveys estimate the incidence of catheter embolism in the venous circulation during angiography, cardiac catheterization, intensive care monitoring, and cardiac pacing at 0.1%.[2–6] The incidence is directly related to the site of the puncture, catheter introduction technique, duration of placement *in situ*, size of catheter used, type of catheter material, and experience of the operator.[3]

The most common mechanism of catheter embolization is puncture of the polyethylene tubing by the sharp bevel of the needle housing the indwelling venous line. Additional causes are the breakage of the catheter without preceding needle injury, detachment from the connector, and accidental severance of the catheter during dressing changes.[7] Most reported cases concern embolization in the venous circulation, but there are a few cases of arterial embolization during angiographic procedures[3,8–12] or vascular interventional techniques.[13–21]

Intravascular foreign bodies should be removed as soon as possible to prevent such serious complications as thrombus formation with pulmonary or peripheral arterial embolization,[1,22,23] to remove a source of infections such as endocarditis and septicemia,[7,24,25] and to prevent myocardial damage leading to arrhythmias and myocardial perforation.[26–31] A 71% incidence of serious morbidity or death directly attributable to the retained foreign body has been reported by Fischer and Ferreyro.[32] This high incidence of complications is probably related to the high incidence (52%) of bacterial contamination (defined as positive cultures) in catheter tips left in place longer than 48 hr.[33]

FOREIGN BODY LOCATION

In an international cooperative study of 180 cases, Bloomfield found that in most cases, fragments that have embolized in the venous circulation lie with their proximal end in the superior inflow area of the right atrium and their distal end lodged in the inferior right atrial or ventricular wall. In the next largest group, the fragments lie totally within the pulmonary arterial system.[34] The site was predictable from the entry point and the length of the fragment. Eighty per cent of the fragments in this series were polyethylene central venous pressure catheters cut in two by the needle introducer.

REMOVAL TECHNIQUES

Forceps

Rigid forceps were used by Thomas and coworkers for the first successful intravascular foreign body removal.[25] This technique has the obvious risk that the rigid instrument will cause vascular and cardiac perforation. Endoscopic forceps of the alligator type were used by Smyth et al,[35] and myocardial biopsy forceps have been used by others.[36–38] Bronchoscopic three-pronged forceps introduced through 12F plastic tubing were used for removal of a catheter fragment from the right pulmonary artery, but they were unsuccessful in removing a second fragment due to their lack of maneuverability.[38] Modified bronchoscopic four-pronged forceps have been used in six cases for intravascular foreign body removal with the help of a steerable catheter and an external steering handle (Medi–Tech) to overcome maneuverability problems.[39] Bivalvar round-edged flexible forceps (Fig. 21–1) have recently been described for removal of obstructed urinary stents, and the authors have adapted this device for the retrieval of intravascular foreign bodies.

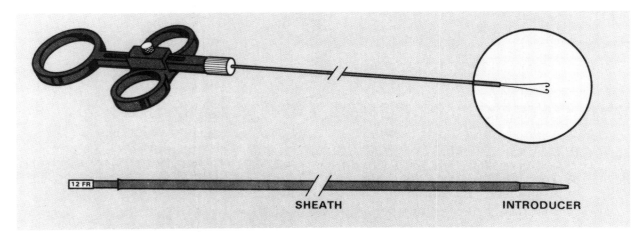

Fig. 21–1   Boren–McKinney retriever set consists of 5F radiopaque sheath; 3-ring handle with thumb screw; stainless-steel double-lobe retriever, which opens to 2.5 cm long and 3.3 mm diameter; and 12F radiopaque polyethylene introducer with radiopaque Teflon sheath. (Courtesy of Cook Urological, Inc.)

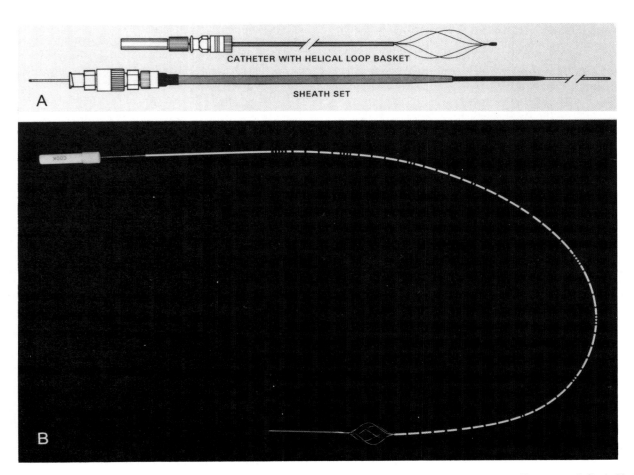

Fig. 21–2   A. Dotter intravascular retrieval set consists of catheter with helical loop basket and introducer sheath. (Courtesy of Cook, Inc.) B. Five-wire helical stone extractor with 5-cm filiform tip and 5F radiopaque introducer catheter. (Courtesy of Cook Urological, Inc.)

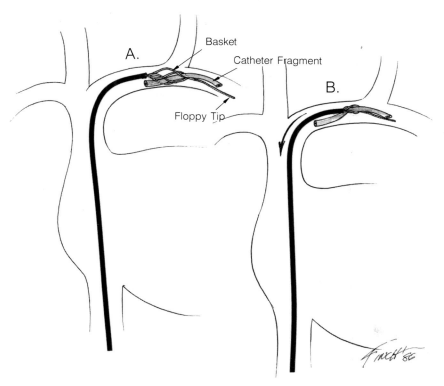

Fig. 21–3 Diagram showing removal of catheter fragment from innominate–subclavian veins using helical loop basket with floppy tip. A. Fragment has been embraced by open basket. B. Basket is closed around fragment, which is slowly withdrawn.

Baskets

Lassers and Pickering described the use of a helical ureteric stone basket for the removal of a catheter fragment from the descending aorta.[8] Several other cases have been reported since (Fig. 21–2A).[38,40–42] Better designed baskets specifically for intravascular use, which have a long floppy tip (Fig. 21–2B) to prevent vascular or cardiac perforation, are now available (Cook Urological). They have limited value in large-caliber vessels such as the vena cava or the aorta because of their small maximum diameter. However, they are ideal for manipulation in children or in small vessels. This instrument can be effective only when one end of the foreign body is free in the lumen of the vessel (Fig. 21–3).

Loop Snares

This technique was first used for the removal of a transvenous pacing catheter from the right side of the heart.[43] Hammermeister used a thinner guidewire (0.025-mm) snare, getting easier manipulation of the loop snare through a 12F Lehman catheter.[44] Ramos et al modified the snare by adding a metal stylus to its external end to facilitate advancement and withdrawal of the loop.[6]

Snares are usually made of guidewire-like material folded in its end section and accompanied by an introducer catheter, commonly made of Teflon (Fig. 21–4). The early snares had the loop oriented in the same axis as the introducer catheter (Fig. 21–5A), but in tubular structures like the great vessels, a loop of this design has dif-

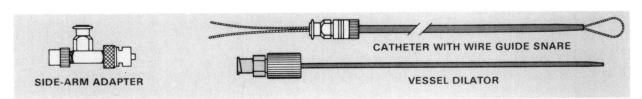

Fig. 21–4 Curry intravascular retriever set: snare loop with radiopaque sheath and sidearm adapter to allow flushing during manipulations and at same time control bleeding along wires. (Courtesy of Cook, Inc.)

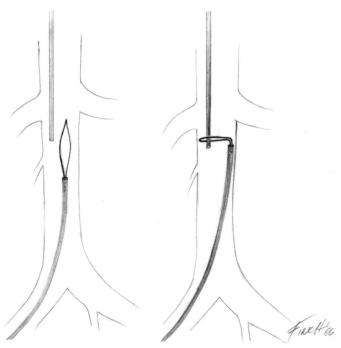

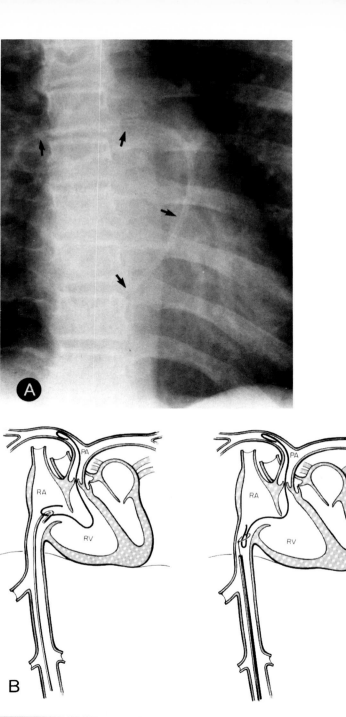

Fig. 21–5   Retrieval problem and its solution. Left. Diagram of difficulties in snaring intravascular foreign body using Curry loop retriever: snare loop lies in same plane as catheter fragment. Right. Modified snare loop with 90° angle to facilitate trapping of catheter fragments in tubular vascular structures.

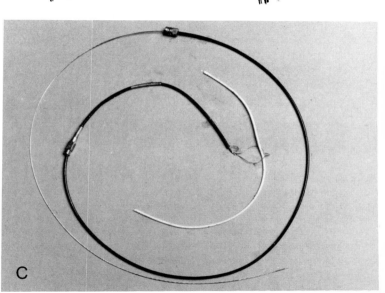

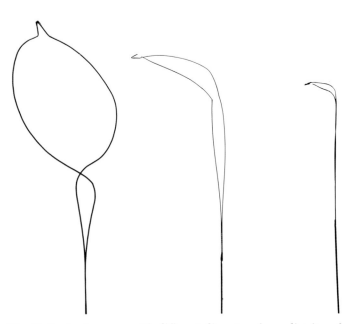

Fig. 21–6   Angle snares with different diameters for pediatric and adult uses. (From Zollikofer C, Nath PH, Castaneda WR, et al: Nonsurgical removal of intravascular foreign bodies. *Fortschr Röntgenstr* 1979;1301:590.)

Fig. 21-7 Retrieval of broken LeVeen shunt. A. Distal end of shunt, broken during manipulations, is seen with its distal end lodged in right pulmonary artery and proximal end in right atrium (arrows). B. Diagram of removal technique. Hooked catheter has been used to snare one loop of catheter fragment within right atrium (RA); loop is then pulled down into inferior vena cava, where it can be trapped with snare. PA = pulmonary artery; RV = right ventricle. C. Catheter fragment after percutaneous removal photographed with snare loop and introducer sheath.

ficulty engaging the foreign body (Fig. 21-5B). Moreover, snares made of guidewire-like material are either too rigid or too soft, and their bulkiness makes them bind to the catheter wall during introduction, necessitating use of larger French sizes for the introducer catheter.

Because of these problems, Randall and Amplatz proposed making the snare loop of soft, pliable, braided stainless steel 0.018 inch in diameter and mounting it at a right angle to the axis of the catheter, thus creating a larger loop that would make direct contact with the entire circumference of the vessel to facilitate snaring[45] and at the same time eliminating the sharply kinked guidewire loop described by Curry,[46] which may perforate the vessel as it exits through the distal end of the introducer catheter. Right-angle snare loops of different diameters (Fig. 21-6) have subsequently been described for use in children and adults (Figs. 21-7 and 21-8).[47] Loops fashioned

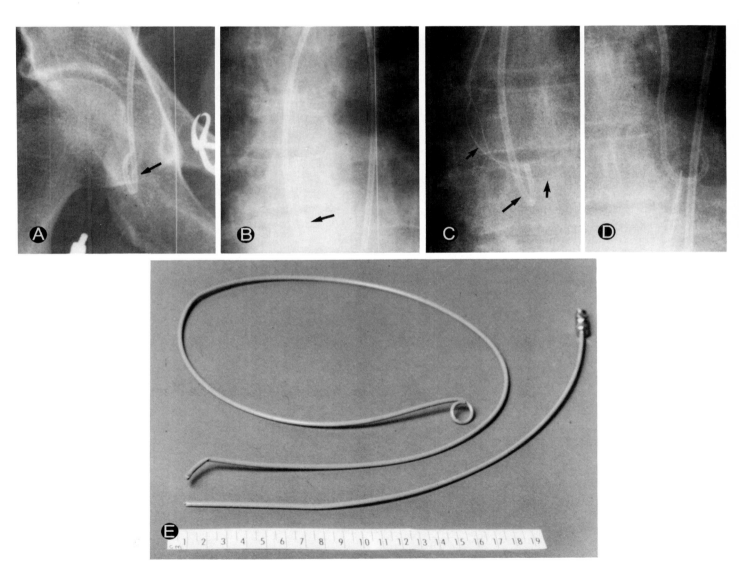

Fig. 21-8 Removal of broken pigtail catheter. A, B. During manipulations, 8F wire mesh pigtail catheter was broken, leaving distal end of pigtail near aortic valve (A, arrow) and proximal end in right common femoral artery (B, arrow). C. Through puncture of left femoral artery, snare loop (small black arrows) was introduced and passed around pigtail end of catheter (long black arrow). D. Loop has been closed around catheter, which is being withdrawn slowly through descending aorta. E. Removed fragment of pigtail catheter, together with proximal fragment.

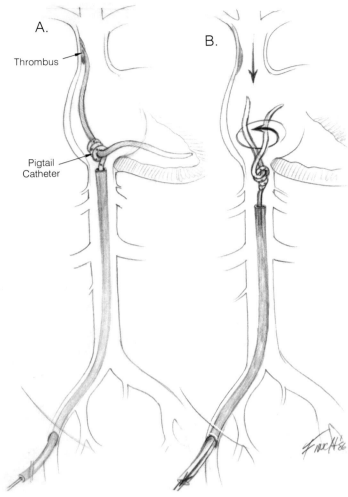

Fig. 21–9 Diagram of technique for removing intracardiac foreign bodies with help of pigtail catheter. Fragment of catheter lodged with distal tip at apex of right ventricle and proximal tip embedded in thrombus in superior vena cava. A. Pigtail catheter passed through long introducing sheath has been looped around fragment. B. By gentle rotation of pigtail, fragment has been detached from superior vena cava and is carefully and slowly withdrawn into the inferior vena cava.

by tying a suture to the flexible end of the guidewire and inserting guidewire and suture through the introducing catheter also have been described.[48–52]

The loop technique can be effective only when one of the ends of the catheter fragment or wire is free floating within a vessel or the heart, so several maneuvers to dislodge and mobilize foreign bodies into more suitable locations have been described.[34,47,53–55] Basically, these maneuvers involve using a hooked catheter to engage the fragment somewhere along its shaft, wrapping the fragment around the hook or pigtail catheter if possible (Fig. 21–9A,B), and then pulling the fragment either to a more favorable position for snaring or completely out of the patient.[53,55] A deflector wire can be used to mobilize a catheter fragment from the right atrium into the right common iliac vein, from which it can be extracted with a J-shaped probe.[54]

A modification of the intra-arterial snare loop retrieval of foreign bodies was proposed by Smith to reduce the blood loss through the introducing catheter during the manipulation.[56] A Check-Flo sheath set assembly (Cook, Inc.) with a sidearm is attached to the hub of the retrieval catheter, with the snare loop passed through the check valve. This inhibits bleeding during manipulations of the snare (Fig. 21–10), and the sidearm assembly allows flushing of the catheter or injection of contrast medium, which is sometimes needed to see the catheter fragments. (Poor radiopacity generally creates a problem during manipulations.)

Balloon Catheters

Balloon catheters, such as the Fogerty, have been used for retrieval of catheter fragments from smaller peripheral vessels[57] or as an adjunct to mobilize the fragment into a better location for snaring.

OTHER USES OF SNARE TECHNIQUES

Management of Complications of Embolization

Systemic embolization or misplacement of Gianturco spring coils can complicate arterial occlusion with this device.[13–19] Successful snaring (Fig. 21–11) or basketing of the coil allowed percutaneous extraction, either through a sheath introducer or directly through the puncture site, in most cases.[13,17–19] In some cases, the coil was removed through an arteriotomy after snaring.[14,16] A coilon (stainless-steel coil with an attached 8-mm Ivalon plug) was removed from the venous circulation through an 18F Teflon coaxial dilator introduced percutaneously over the 8F Teflon catheter of the snare loop.[20] Such a large lumen was needed for removal of the embolic device, because the re-expanded Ivalon plug precluded

retrieval through the puncture site (Fig. 21–12A,B) or through a standard sheath introducer. The Ivalon might have been stripped off and might have embolized to the lungs.[20]

Retrieval of Pacemaker Wires

Broken pacemaker electrodes commonly remain fixed to the vein wall or surrounding soft tissues. The retained fragment at the vein entry site is usually not considered a threat to the patient. However, the fragments can migrate (Fig. 21–13),[6,58–63] an event that entails the risk of caval thrombosis, iliofemoral phlebitis, venous perforation, or pulmonary embolism secondary to thrombosis. Percutaneous removal of these migrating wires should be

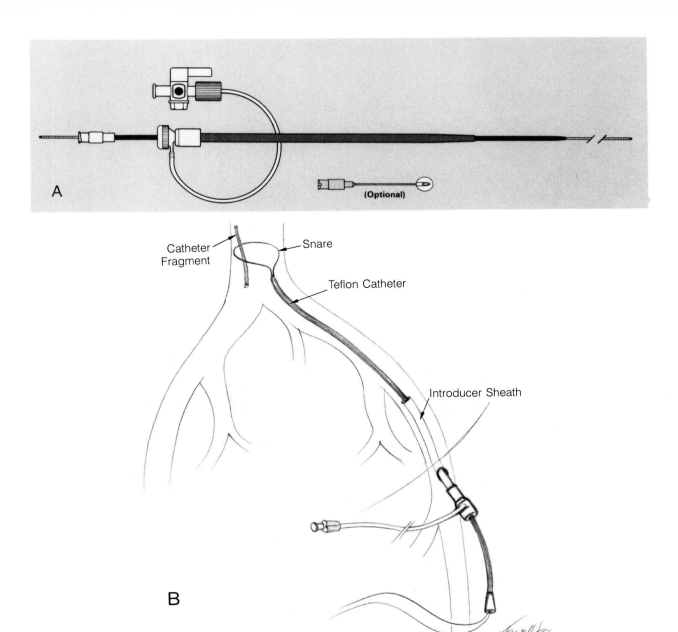

Fig. 21–10 A. Check-Flo sheath. A. Rubber seal within hub prevents blood leakage during manipulations; sidearm fitting allows flushing around catheter. (Courtesy of Cook, Inc.) B. Diagram of snare loop introduced through Check-Flo sheath to entrap fragment of catheter in aorta.

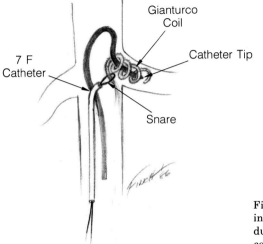

Fig. 21–11 Diagram of misplaced Gianturco spring coil protruding into lumen of aorta from left renal artery and held in place by introducing catheter. Snare loop is being used to grab one end of spring coil for percutaneous removal.

Fig. 21–12 Coilon retrieval. A. During embolization of right spermatic vein, coilon (arrow) stuck in distal end of introducer catheter. Catheter was therefore removed from right spermatic vein and advanced through inferior vena cava into right iliac vein for percutaneous removal. B. Spot film showing coilon trapped by snare (arrow) being pulled through 18F Teflon dilator. C. Coilon trapped by snare introduced through 8F/18F coaxial dilator system. Observe size of expanded Ivalon plug (arrows), which made it necessary to introduce 18F Teflon dilator for percutaneous removal.

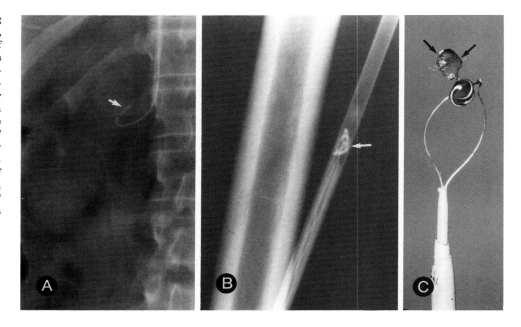

Fig. 21–13 A. Chest radiograph shows fragment of broken pacemaker leads in right subclavian vein area (arrow). B. Fragment of pacemaker leads in left popliteal vein (arrow).

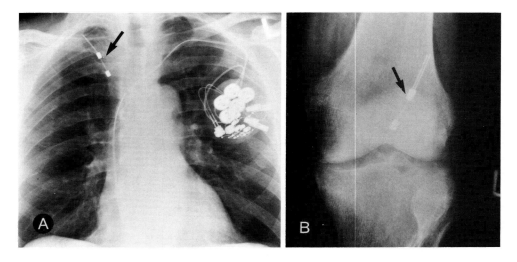

considered either as an alternative to surgical removal or as a complement to operation in cases where the wire cannot be detached from the myocardium by simple pulling.

In these instances, grasping the wire close to the myocardial implant site with a snare will provide the safest traction.

REASONS FOR FAILURE

The most common causes of retrieval failure are as follows:

No free ends are available for snaring. This problem can be overcome by manipulating the fragment into a more suitable location with a hooked catheter or wire.[34,47,53–55]

The catheter fragment is lodged in peripheral pulmonary artery branches, where manipulation of the snare onto the free end of the fragment can be extremely difficult, particularly if biplane fluoroscopy is not used.

The catheter fragment is nonopaque. This problem can

be solved by injecting contrast medium to locate the fragment and then performing blind manipulations. As an alternative, real-time ultrasound can be used for the entire procedure.[64]

Inability to remove the catheter fragment intact due to the extreme friability of its walls. This complication usually arises only if a catheter is being reused. If this problem is suspected after direct inspection of the proximal fragment, it probably is better either to remove the retained fragment surgically or to leave it alone, because further attempts at percutaneous removal might create additional fragments (Fig. 21–14).

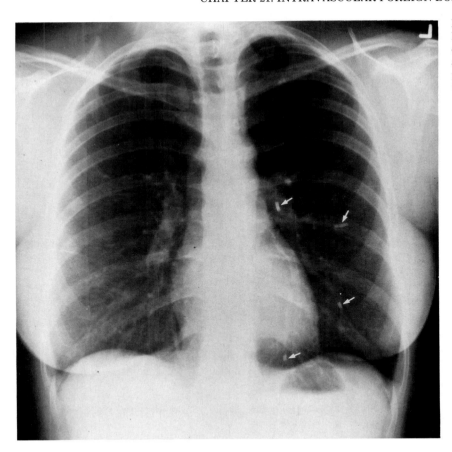

Fig. 21–14 Patient with fragment of catheter lodged in left pulmonary artery. Because of extreme fragility of repeatedly sterilized catheter, attempts to remove fragment produced multiple pieces of catheter, which embolized into lung (white arrows).

COMPLICATIONS

The most common complication of percutaneous intravascular retrieval of foreign bodies is cardiac arrhythmia.[34,41] Vascular or cardiac perforation is a potential complication, particularly with the use of flexible forceps. No deaths have been associated with the procedure.

References

1. Turner DC, Sommers SC: Accidental passage of a polyethylene catheter from a cubital vein to right atrium: fatal case. *N Engl J Med* 1954;251:744
2. Block PC: Transvenous retrieval of foreign bodies in the cardiac circulation. *JAMA* 1973;224:241
3. Burri C, Ahnefeld FW: *The Caval Catheter.* Berlin, Springer, 1978, p 39
4. Dhingra RC, Rosen KM, Rahimtoola SM: Transvenous removal of catheter fragments from the heart and pulmonary artery. *Arch Intern Med* 1973;105:894
5. Drabinsky M: Retrieval of embolized central venous catheter by a Dormia ureteral stone basket with straight filiform tip. *Chest* 1976;69:435
6. Ramos BW, Peter RH, Kong Y, Morris JJ Jr: Migration of a severed transvenous pacing catheter and its successful removal. *Am J Cardiol* 1968;22:880
7. Wellman KF, Reinhard A, Salazar EP: Polyethylene catheter embolism. *Circulation* 1968;37:380
8. Lassers BW, Pickering D: Removal of iatrogenic foreign body from aorta by means of ureteric stone catheter. *Am Heart J* 1967;73:375
9. Rao VR, Rout D, Sapru RP: Retrieval of a broken catheter from the aorta without operation. *Neuroradiology* 1982;22:263
10. Dotter CT, Rösch J, Bilbao MK: Transluminal extraction of catheter and guide fragments from the heart and great vessels: 29 collected cases. *AJR* 1971;111:467
11. Rubinstein ZJ, Morag B, Itzchak Y: Percutaneous removal of intravascular foreign bodies. *CardioVasc Intervent Radiol* 1982;5:64
12. Fjälling M, List AR: Transvascular retrieval of an accidentally ejected tip occluder and wire. *CardioVasc Intervent Radiol* 1982;5:34
13. Chuang VP: Nonoperative retrieval of Gianturco coils from abdominal aorta. *AJR* 1979;132:996
14. Tisnado J, Beachely MC, Cho SR, Amendola M: Peripheral embolization of a stainless steel coil. *AJR* 1979;133:324
15. Wallace S, Gianturco C, Anderson JH, Goldstein HM, Davis LJ, Bree RL: Therapeutic vascular occlusion utilizing steel coil technique: clinical applications. *AJR* 1976;127:381
16. Habighorst LV, Kreutz W, Klug B, Sparwasser HH, Göbel EA: Spiralembolization der Nierenarterie nach Gianturco. *RöFo* 1978;128:47

17. Radojkovic S, Kamenica S, Jasovic M, Draganic M: Catheter-aided extraction of a steel coil accidentally lodged in the right ventricle. *CardioVasc Intervent Radiol* 1980;3:153

18. Weber J: A complication with the Gianturco coil and its non-surgical management. *CardioVasc Intervent Radiol* 1980;3:156

19. Chuang VP, Wallace S, Gianturco C, Soo CS: Complication of coil embolization: prevention and management. *AJR* 1981; 137:809

20. Castañeda–Zuñiga WR, Herrera M, Rusnak B, Amplatz K: Coilon removal. *CardioVasc Intervent Radiol* 1982;5:69

21. Kim MS, Horton JA: Intra-arterial foreign body retrieved using endoscopic biopsy forceps. *Radiology* 1983;149:597

22. Knutson H, Steinberg K: Pulmonary embolus with foreign body. *Nord Med* 1959;62:1491

23. Scebat L, Renais J, Meeus–Bithe L, Lenegre J: Accidents, indications et contreindicaitons du catheterisme des cavites droits du coeur. *Arch Mal Coeur* 1957;50:943

24. Harken DE, Zoll PM: Foreign bodies in and in relation to thoracic blood vessels and heart. *Am Heart J* 1946;32:1

25. Thomas J, Sinclair–Smith B, Bloomfield D, Davachi A: Nonsurgical retrieval of broken segment of steel spring guide from right atrium to superior vena cava. *Circulation* 1964;30:106

26. Nathan DA, Center S, Mina RE, Medow A, Keller W Jr: Perforation during indwelling catheter pacing. *Circulation* 1966;33:128

27. Johnston CE: Perforation of the right atrium by a polyethylene catheter. *JAMA* 1966;195:584

28. Brown CA, Kent A: Perforation of right ventricle by polyethylene catheter. *South Med J* 1956;49:466

29. Decker HR: Foreign bodies in heart and pericardium—should they be removed? *J Thorac Surg* 1939;9:62

30. Swan H, Forsee JH, Goyette EM: Foreign bodies in heart. *Ann Surg* 1952;135:314

31. Doering RB, Stemmer EA, Connolly JE: Complications of indwelling venous catheters. *Am J Surg* 1967;114:259

32. Fischer RG, Ferreyro R: Evaluation of current techniques for nonsurgical removal of intravascular iatrogenic foreign bodies. *AJR* 1978;130:541

33. Druskin MS, Seigel PD: Bacterial contamination of indwelling intravenous polyethylene catheters. *JAMA* 1963;185:966

34. Bloomfield DA: The nonsurgical retrieval of intracardiac foreign bodies: an international survey. *Cathet Cardiovasc Diagn* 1978;4:1

35. Smyth NPD, Boivin MR, Bacos JM: Transjugular removal of foreign body from right atrium by endoscopic forceps. *J Thorac Cardiovasc Surg* 1968;55:594

36. Bashour TT, Banks T, Cheng TO: Retrieval of lost catheters by a myocardial biopsy catheter device. *Chest* 1974;66:395

37. Kurita A, Kanazawa M, et al: Successful removal of a foreign body from the caval vein by use of endomyocardial bioptome. *Jpn Heart J* 1972;13:464

38. Tanaka M, Iyomasa Y: Nonsurgical technique for removal of catheter fragments from the pulmonary artery. *Cathet Cardiovasc Diagn* 1983;9:109

39. Millan VG: Retrieval of intravascular foreign bodies using a modified bronchoscopic forceps. *Radiology* 1978;129:587

40. Harnick E, Rohmer J: Atraumatic retrieval of catheter fragments from the central circulation of children. *Eur J Cardiol* 1974;1:421

41. Pickering E, Gaasch WH: Nonsurgical removal of intracardiac polyethylene catheter emboli. *J Am Osteopath Assoc* 1975;74:489

42. Noe HN: Removal of intravascular foreign body with stone retriever. *Urology* 1981;17:184

43. Massumi RA, Ross AM: Atraumatic nonsurgical technic for removal of broken catheters from cardiac chamber. *N Engl J Med* 1967;227:195

44. Hammermeister KE: Removal of broken cardiac catheters. *N Engl J Med* 1968;278:911

45. Randall PA: Percutaneous removal of iatrogenic intracardiac foreign body. *Radiology* 1972;102:591

46. Curry JL: Recovery of detached intravascular catheter or guidewire fragments: a proposed method. *AJR* 1969;105:894

47. Zollikofer C, Nath PH, Castañeda–Zuñiga WR, et al: Nonsurgical removal of intravascular foreign bodies. *Fortschr Röntgenstr* 1979;130:590

48. Barman PC: A simple method for removal of polyethylene catheters from the pulmonary artery. *J Thorac Cardiovasc Surg* 1973;65:792

49. Geraci AT, Selman MW: Pulmonary artery catheter emboli: successful nonsurgical removal. *Ann Intern Med* 1973;78:353

50. Hyman AL: An improved snare catheter for retrieving embolized fragments of polyethylene tubing. *Chest* 1972;62:98

51. Marlon AM, Cohn LH, Fogarty TH, Harrison DC: Retrieval of catheter fragments. *Calif Med* 1971;115:61

52. Vaeusorn N, Burodom N, Harnchonboth A, Noiklang P, Viranuvatti J: Modified loopsnare for percutaneous removal of intravascular catheter fragments. *Radiology* 1982;145:839

53. Rossi P: "Hook catheter" technique for transfemoral removal of foreign body from the right side of the heart. *AJR* 1970; 109:101

54. McSweeney WJ, Schwarts DC: Retrieval of a catheter foreign body from the right side of the heart using a guidewire deflector system. *Radiology* 1971;100:61

55. Rossi P, Passariello R, Simonetti G: Intravascular iatrogenic foreign body retrieval: experience in 13 cases. *Ann Radiol* 1980;23:286

56. Smith PL: An improved method for intra-arterial foreign body retrieval. *Radiology* 1982;145:539

57. Mathur AP, Pochaczevsky R, Levowitz BS, Feraru F: Fogarty balloon catheter for removal of catheter fragment in subclavian vein. *JAMA* 1971;217:481

58. Tallury VK, DePasquale NP, Bruno MS, et al: Migration of retained transvenous electrode catheter. *Arch Intern Med* 1972;130:390

59. Tuna N, Nicoloff DM: Unusual migration of a piece of pacemaker electrode. *JAMA* 1978;239:2240

60. Toumbouras M, Spanos P, Konstantaras C, et al: Inferior vena cava thrombosis due to migration of retained functionless pacemaker electrode. *Chest* 1982;82:785

61. Drizin GS, Fein AM, Lippmann ML: Clinical pulmonary embolism from migration of a retained transvenous permanent pacemaker electrode. *Crit Care Med* 1982;10:788

62. Widmann WD, Edoga JK, Garfias D, McLean ER Jr: Peripheral migration of pacemaker electrodes. *PACE* 1984;7:227

63. Gould L, Maghazeh P, Giovanniello J: Successful removal of a severed transvenous pacemaker electrode. *PACE* 1981;4:713

64. Woo VL, Gerber AM, et al: Real-time ultrasound for percutaneous transluminal retrieval of nonopaque intravascular catheter fragement. *AJR* 1979;133:760

22

Inferior Vena Cava Filters

S. MURTHY TADAVARTHY, M.D., CAROL C. COLEMAN, M.D., FLAVIO CASTAÑEDA, M.D.,
MICHAEL D. DARCY, M.D. ANDREW H. CRAGG, M.D., GUNNAR LUND, M.D., TONY P. SMITH, M.D.,
DAVID W. HUNTER, M.D., KURT AMPLATZ, M.D., AND WILFRIDO R. CASTAÑEDA-ZUÑIGA, M.D.,
M.Sc.

Pulmonary embolism is one of the principal causes of hospital morbidity and mortality and accounts for approximately 200,000 deaths annually in the U.S.[1] In another series, it was reported that 140,000 patients per year suffer fatal pulmonary embolism, and nonlethal embolism was estimated to occur in 570,000 patients per year.[2]

In most cases, pulmonary embolism is effectively treated by heparin. However, certain situations do require mechanical interruption of the inferior vena cava. For example, in patients whose response to anticoagulants has been inadequate, or in patients in whom anticoagulation is contraindicated, the placement of an inferior vena cava filter is an effective alternative. The inferior vena cava is interrupted because in 75%–90% of the cases pulmonary emboli originate in the legs and pelvis. The other sources of pulmonary emboli are the arms and the right atrium, and these emboli probably account for some of the apparent failures of filter placement.

Surgical techniques to prevent pulmonary emboli include inferior vena cava ligation and clipping,[3–9] which are major procedures necessitating extensive extraperitoneal dissection. Less drastic surgical procedures, such as ligation of the superficial and common femoral veins, are ineffective, being associated with a 10%–26% incidence of recurrent pulmonary emboli and complications attributable to venous stasis.[10] Furthermore, open operations have a 10%–15% mortality rate,[11] and emboli recur in 5.9% of patients.[12]

To decrease the mortality rate and avoid general anesthesia in patients with severely compromised cardiac and pulmonary reserves, several transluminal approaches to interruption of the inferior vena cava have been used.[13–19] The Eichelter sieve[15] and the Moser balloon[16] offered temporary protection but had significant drawbacks, namely dislodgment and migration of trapped emboli at the time of catheter removal. Another group of devices are the detachable type, including the Pate clip,[17] the Hunter balloon,[18] the Mobin–Uddin (MU) umbrella filter,[19] and the Kimray–Greenfield (KG) filter.[13,14] In most institutions, the popular MU and KG filters are placed under local anesthesia through a venotomy in either the jugular or the femoral vein.

Transluminal placement through a venous cutdown under local anesthesia avoids major operations that require extensive retroperitoneal dissection. A mortality rate of 4% for the transluminal placement of filters has been reported, with deaths being related to the underlying disease rather than to the placement of filters.[11] This is a striking improvement over the 10%–15% operative mortality rate for vena caval ligation and the 8% rate for partial interruption.[11,20,21] Techniques for percutaneous introduction of the MU and KG filters, developed at the University of Minnesota,[22–24] further reduce morbidity and mortality rates.[24,25] However, the principal drawback of these methods was the need to use large dilators to enlarge the venipuncture in order to introduce the filters. Continued research for new alternatives has led to the development of several new devices,[26–32] which will be discussed.

INFERIOR VENACAVOGRAPHY

Before operative or percutaneous placement of inferior vena cava filters, inferior venacavography should be performed to demonstrate the size of the vessel, any anatomic variations, and the location of the renal veins.[33] The position of the latter is marked with metallic markers on the abdominal wall with reference to the lumbar vertebral bodies. Filters can then be placed below the level of the renal veins by placing them below the metallic marker, thus minimizing interference with renal venous return. The size of the inferior vena cava is determined directly from the angiogram, the transverse diameter of the vessel below the renal veins being measured with correction for magnification (Fig. 22–1). Accurate measurement is essential, because if the vena cava is larger than the transverse diameter of the filter, secure placement is unlikely. If the vena cava is larger than the available filters, one filter can be placed in each iliac vein, but surgical interruption should be considered.

The presence of iliac or low inferior vena caval thrombi is a contraindication to the placement of the filter by the femoral approach. An internal jugular entry is the only effective route in these cases.

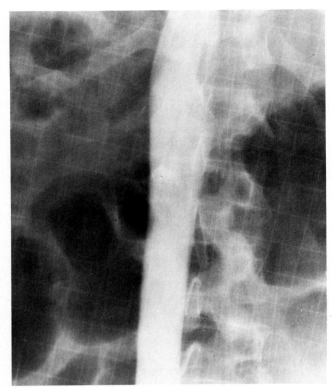

Fig. 22–1 Inferior venacavography performed with grid for determining magnification prior to filter placement.

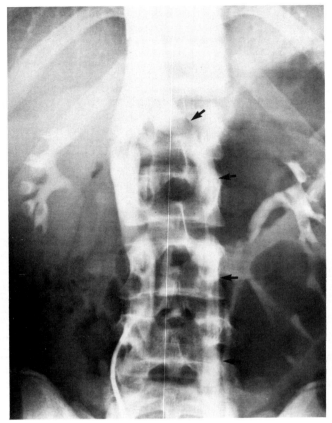

Fig. 22–2 Persistent left-sided inferior vena cava (arrows) is demonstrated following Valsalva maneuver during inferior venacavogram.

Anomalies of the Vena Cava

Several congenital anomalies of the inferior vena cava can interfere with the placement of filters:

1. Double inferior vena cava;
2. Circumaortic left renal vein;
3. Left-sided inferior vena cava.

DOUBLE INFERIOR VENA CAVA

Embryologic persistence of the right and left cardinal veins results in a double inferior vena cava.[34] The two vessels may be the same size, but more commonly the left is smaller than the right. After joining with the left renal vein, the left vena cava passes in front of the aorta to join the right inferior vena cava (Fig. 22–2).

CIRCUMAORTIC LEFT RENAL VEIN

A circumaortic left renal vein is seen in 8.7% of the population.[34] The anterior half ring of the left renal vein joins the inferior vena cava at the usual level, whereas the posterior half follows a right downward course posterior to the aorta to join the inferior vena cava at a lower level. Location of the posterior branch is important, because the filter should be placed below the ostia of both renal veins.

LEFT-SIDED INFERIOR VENA CAVA

A left-sided inferior vena cava occurs with an incidence of 0.2%–0.5%.[34] The vessel courses along the left side of the lumbar spine, and, after receiving the left renal vein, it crosses in front of the spine to the right and then continues upward in the normal location of the inferior vena cava. The placement of KG or MU filters in a left-sided infrarenal vena cava is practically impossible from a jugular approach because of the stiffness of the introducing systems. The bulky capsules that carry the filters may not be able to angle to the left despite preshaping of the introducer. Forceful advancement should be avoided, because the inferior vena cava may be perforated at the site where the intrahepatic straight segment of the vessel joins the transverse segment of the left vena cava. With the KG filter, advancement of a stiff leading guidewire may help to advance the system toward the left, but this obviously cannot be done with the MU filter, because it does not admit a wire. In this situation, placement of the KG filter[24] or the modified MU filter[22] via the left groin is the most logical approach.

Postprocedure Films

Venacavography after filter placement is helpful in the diagnosis of complications such as perforation or filter migration and, later, in the evaluation of the source of recurrent embolism. For example, a large left ovarian pre-

vertebral vein may serve as a conduit for emboli in spite of an adequately positioned filter.

INDICATIONS FOR INTRALUMINAL INTERRUPTION OF THE INFERIOR VENA CAVA

Contraindications to Anticoagulants

Patients with pulmonary emboli associated with bleeding peptic ulcer, intracranial hemorrhage, or recent major operation cannot be given anticoagulants. Also, there is a 50% risk of hemorrhagic complications if women older than 60 years receive anticoagulants.[35] Such contraindications to anticoagulants are one of the chief indications for transluminal interruption of the inferior vena cava by a mechanical device.[14,35]

Documented Recurrent Thromboembolism in Patients Adequately Treated with Anticoagulants

In patients who have received adequate anticoagulation, there is an 18% incidence of recurrent emboli, half of which are fatal.[2,36] This incidence is not surprising if one remembers that heparin is only thrombostatic and that final lysis of clots already formed depends on fibrinolytic activity. Inferior vena cava interruption is indicated in patients who have recurrent pulmonary embolism in spite of adequate anticoagulation.[14,35,37] This is a common problem in patients with congestive heart failure.[35]

Complications of Anticoagulation

Patients with such complications as intracerebral or retroperitoneal hemorrhage or severe oozing from a recent incision require discontinuation of anticoagulants. These patients are ideal candidates for intraluminal interruption with filters.

Chronic Pulmonary Hypertension

Pulmonary hypertension can have many causes, such as left-to-right intracardiac shunts, left-sided intracardiac obstruction such as that caused by mitral stenosis, recurrent pulmonary emboli, and hypoxic states of the lung. Primary pulmonary hypertension has no demonstrable cause. All of these patients have poor prognoses, often dying within 2–3 years of complications such as right-sided heart failure or recurrent embolism. These

patients can be managed prophylactically with anticoagulants and inferior vena cava interruption with devices such as filters.[38] There are no large-scale trials of filters with long-term follow-up and comparison with control groups, but the inability of many of these patients to tolerate even a single episode of pulmonary embolism suggests the advisability of filter placement.

Septic Thromboemboli

The conventional treatment for septic thromboemboli has been ligation of the inferior vena cava to prevent migration of emboli to the lungs. In dog experiments, KG filter placement plus antibiotic administration proved superior to vena caval ligation, because the former treatment prevented the infected emboli from reaching the lungs while the antibiotics sterilized the clots trapped within the KG device.[39]

Postembolectomy

After surgical or catheter pulmonary embolectomy, further episodes of pulmonary emboli can be prevented by placing filters in the infrarenal segment of the inferior vena cava.

Prophylactic Interruption

In patients with documented deep iliofemoral vein thrombi loosely adherent to the walls and free floating in the iliac veins or lower inferior vena cava, prophylactic filter placement may well be warranted.[2,14,37] Free-floating clots that are loosely attached to the inferior vena cava have a higher chance of detachment than do thrombotic clots and may result in fatal complications. Anticoagulation probably will not prevent detachment and migration of such clots.[35]

Elderly Persons with Recurrent Thromboemboli

Filters may be superior to anticoagulation in this group.[12] Indeed, this is the third most common indication for filter insertion, accounting for 18% of procedures in one series.[14]

TYPES OF DEVICES AND THEIR USE

Mobin–Uddin Umbrella Filter

One of the earliest devices to filter the inferior vena caval blood is the MU filter, which was released for clinical use in 1970.[35] It was designed for introduction through a venotomy under local anesthesia[2,5,35,36,40–42] and its use reduced the prohibitive operative mortality

rate of 5%–39%[36] to 0.[41] Up to 1982, it was estimated that approximately 10,000 MU filters had been implanted.[35] At present, only a 28-mm umbrella filter impregnated with heparin is available, the 23-mm filter having been discontinued because of its high migration rate.

Patency rates of the inferior vena cava ranging from

33%–40%[42] to 60%–68%[35,43] have been reported with the MU filter. The heparin reportedly inhibits thrombus formation on the undersurface of the device, and within 6–8 weeks, endothelialization can occur.[35] Migration has been reported in 0.4% of patients and recurrent pulmonary emboli in 0.5%.[35,36,42] Leg edema and stasis complications such as dermatitis and ulcerations have occurred in 16%–75% of patients.[42] The incidence of leg edema was reported to be as high as 50% even in patients with a patent inferior vena cava,[44] so this is a highly controversial "complication." That is, some authors maintain that the problem is not a complication of filter placement but rather a consequence of pre-existing thrombi in the leg veins and of poor development of collateral vessels after filter placement.[36]

DESIGN OF THE MU FILTER

The MU filter consists of a central hub, from which six cobalt–chromium spokes radiate (Fig. 22–3). This framework makes the device visible on plain radiographs (Fig. 22–2). A thin layer of silicone rubber covers each side of the metallic spokes and extends like a web, leaving only the distal 2 mm of the spokes bare. By its design, the uncovered 2 mm of the sharp spokes limit their penetration of the inferior vena cava to about 1–2 mm. There are eighteen 3-mm perforations in the silicone webbing to maintain the return through the inferior vena cava. The

Silastic covering is bonded to a heparin coating to minimize clotting and to augment endothelialization.

The center of the hub has a 1-mm hole to receive the threaded tip of the stylet. The filter is loaded on either a 90-cm-long regular applicator or the modified angiography applicator–catheter. The modified carrier capsule has a sideport for injection of contrast medium, and the capsule is designed with perforations so that contrast escapes at the base, allowing performance of an inferior venacavogram before and after the delivery of the filter without resort to a conventional angiographic catheter. The capsule is 32 mm long and 7 mm wide, with a bullet "nose" for easier insertion through small hypoplastic jugular veins. The stiff nylon catheter, along with the stylet, have good torque control and can be bent sideways to negotiate prominent eustachian valves. This maneuver avoids repeated entry of the applicator into the hepatic or renal veins.

If it proves difficult to advance the carrier capsule from the right atrium, the patient can be turned to the left lateral decubitus position to free the tip of the capsule from the right atrial wall. The capsule can then be manipulated into the inferior vena cava.

LOADING AND INSERTION OF THE MU FILTER THROUGH THE JUGULAR VEIN

The stylet pin vise is retracted 5–6 cm away from the Luer–Lok hub and retightened, and the stylet is

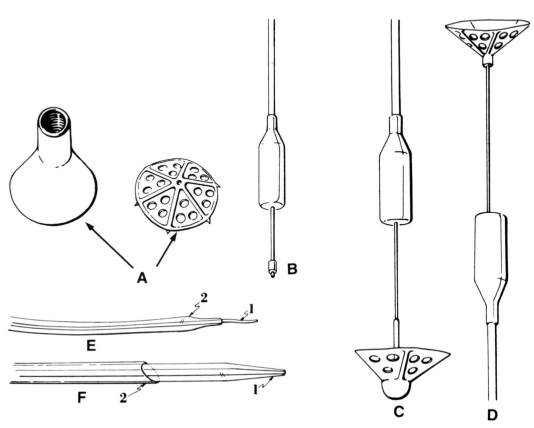

Fig. 22–3   Mobin-Uddin filter. A. Filter and loading cone for femoral introduction. B. Introducer capsule with stylet. C. Filter mounted on stylet for transjugular approach. D. Filter mounted on stylet for transfemoral introduction. E. 8F (1) and 24F (2) Teflon dilators. F. 24F dilator (1) with Teflon sleeve (2) for percutaneous introduction through either transjugular or transfemoral approach.

advanced until the pin vise is flush with the hub. The protruding stylet tip is then screwed onto the receiving end of the filter. The stylet is turned counterclockwise one-half turn to facilitate detachment of the filter and to ensure that the threads are not stripped.

Before collapsing the filter, the operator lubricates the inner surface of the loading cone and the filter adequately with either K–Y Jelly (Johnson & Johnson) or Lubafax (Burroughs–Wellcome). The filter should be loaded into the capsule gently, without damaging the spokes or the Silastic web. With an assistant holding the stylet catheter along with the mounted filter, the operator aligns the loading cone axially and, by gentle thrusts, collapses the filter. The carrier capsule is advanced by the assistant onto the loading cone, and the operator pulls the stylet backwards, thereby loading the filter. The previously retracted pin vise is loosened, moved forward until it is flush with the Luer–Lok, and retightened. This final step prevents accidental premature ejection of the filter. The loaded carrier catheter is advanced through the venotomy under fluoroscopic guidance across the right atrium into the inferior vena cava.

This filter device should always be placed below the renal veins, the level of which is determined from the inferior venacavogram as previously described. The carrier catheter is advanced distally into the lower inferior vena cava or, preferably, into the iliac veins to prevent accidental ejection of the filter into a vertically oriented renal vein. The applicator catheter is then retracted until the proximal end is at the level of the more inferior renal vein. The stylet pin vise is loosened, moved 2–3 cm away from the Luer–Lok, and retightened. The applicator catheter is held firmly by the assistant or the operator, and the filter is ejected by pushing the stylet pin vise. The springing of the filter is watched under fluoroscopy, and the filter is secured to the inferior vena caval wall by gently tugging on the stylet several times. After the filter firmly engages the wall, constant traction is applied to the stylet while it is turned counterclockwise to detach the filter. If accidental premature ejection occurs, the filter can be advanced inferior to the renal veins with the still engaged stylet.[40] The carrier catheter and the capsule are removed, and the venotomy incision is closed.

If the clinical situation permits, anticoagulants can be resumed in 12 hr[5] and continued for 3–6 months to diminish thrombus formation on the filter. However, in most cases, the filters are placed in lieu of anticoagulation, so that combined treatment with the filter and anticoagulants is not practical.

PERCUTANEOUS INTRODUCTION OF THE MU FILTER THROUGH THE FEMORAL VEIN

A method was proposed by Knight, Rizk, and Amplatz for introducing the umbrella filter percutaneously by the femoral route.[25,45,46] When the internal jugular vein cannot be approached because of infection, trauma, abscess secondary to surgical resection, congenital hypoplasia, or recent thrombosis of the superior vena cava, the femoral approach is an effective alternate route.

The antegrade approach from the femoral vein is accomplished by modifying the commercially available filter set as follows:

1. The cylindrical end of the loading cone is opened (Fig. 22–3A).
2. The central hole in the umbrella is extended through and through.
3. The stylet tip is shortened (Fig. 22–3B).

These three modifications allow mounting and loading of the capsule in a retrograde fashion (Fig. 22–3C).

In 1978, a warning was published in a bulletin from American Edwards Laboratories against inserting the MU filter from the femoral approach, with the contention that the filter could not be secured properly if ejected in the inverted position.[47] Several published and unpublished cases belie this claim.[25,45,46]

To insert the MU filter via the femoral vein, an inferior venacavogram is obtained by introducing the catheter through the femoral vein by the Seldinger technique. The presence or absence of thrombi in the femoral and iliac veins and the lower inferior vena cava is ascertained; if thrombi are found, this approach is not appropriate, because the introduction of dilators and catheters can dislodge the clots.

The filter is mounted on the carrier catheter as follows:

1. The open loading cone is held upright (so the flared end points upward).
2. A small amount of lubricant is applied to the inside of the cone and to the capsule and the modified filter.
3. The modified filter with its through-and-through hole in the center of the hub is placed on top of the flared end of the loading cone.
4. The shortened stylet is introduced through the narrow end of the cone and screwed onto the filter by clockwise rotation.
5. After the stylet is tightened, it is rotated counterclockwise one-half turn so the filter can be disengaged more easily after it is securely placed.
6. The stylet is pulled backward so that the filter collapses as it traverses the narrow segment of the cone. As it is collapsing, the filter is gently withdrawn into the capsule while central axial pressure is maintained.

With this technique, the filter nicely forces itself into the capsule. One should make sure the spokes are not protruding beyond the capsule edge.

Through the angiographic catheter used for the inferior venacavogram, a guidewire is introduced up to the junction of the inferior vena cava and the right atrium. Over the guidewire, a long 8F Teflon dilator is introduced. Over the dilator, the puncture site and femoral artery are sequentially dilated to 24F (Fig. 22–3E) after the skin and subcutaneous tissues have been anesthetized liberally. (The subcutaneous planes are spread apart with a hemostat to facilitate anesthetic injection.)

After dilatation to 24F is completed, the working sheath that comes with the filter set is advanced into the low inferior vena cava (Fig. 22–3F). One should make sure the tip of the working sheath reaches the lower inferior vena cava; otherwise, the filter capsule is difficult to advance. If the working sheath provided does not reach far enough, one of the longer commercially available working sheaths is used. During placement of the filter, hemostasis is achieved by placing a rubber stopper on the working sheath. Through the working sheath, the carrier capsule is advanced until it is below the renal veins (Fig. 22–4), and the stylet is advanced to release the filter, as in the conventional jugular approach. The filter is secured to the inferior vena caval wall by tugging on the catheter, and the stylet is released by counterclockwise rotation.

Hemostasis is secured by manual compression at the femoral puncture site for 5–10 min, and a pressure bandage is applied. Placing the patient in a slight Trendelenburg position lowers the femoral vein pressure to 0 so that effective hemostasis is secured rapidly.

Kimray–Greenfield Filter

This filter is a cone-shaped stainless-steel device with six limbs, each with a terminal recurved hook that assures fixation to the inferior vena caval wall (Fig. 22–5). The KG filter measures 45 mm from apex to base, with a maximum span at its base of 30 mm.

The principal advantage of this filter is that, even with 80% of the cone filled with clot, the cross-sectional area is reduced by only 64%.[10,13,48] By design, a properly positioned filter should trap emboli >3–4.5 mm. However, if

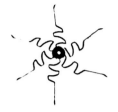
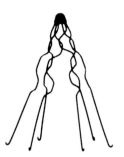

Fig. 22–5   Greenfield filter: Top and frontal views.

the central axis of the filter is tilted out of alignment with the axis of the inferior vena cava, larger clots can bypass the filter through the wider spaces between the limbs (Fig. 22–6). Because of its cone shape, the filter preserves laminar peripheral flow of blood around the entrapped clots, and this continuous flow permits lysis of the entrapped clots and so prevents complete occlusion of

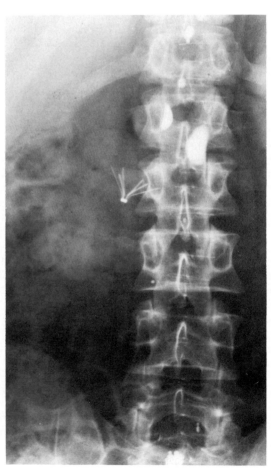

Fig. 22–4   Mobin-Uddin filter placed below renal veins. Observe tilting due to discrepancy between diameters of inferior vena cava and filter.

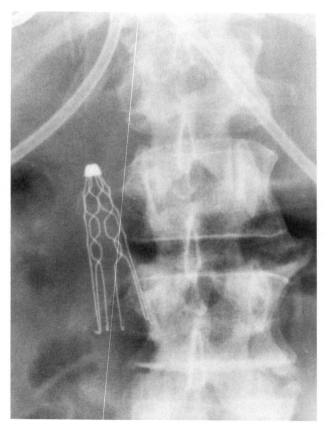

Fig. 22–6   Spot film of abdomen showing slightly tilted Greenfield filter within inferior vena cava.

the vena cava. The reported 95%–98% patency rate of the inferior vena cava in patients with the KG filter[12,14] has been attributed to this cone-shaped design that allows central retention of clots while maintaining the circumferential laminar blood flow.[10]

Because of their high patency rates, the KG filter and some of the newer designs such as the Amplatz–Lund, Günther, and bird's nest are best suited for placement above the renal veins when an infrarenal position is not possible or when suprarenal filtration is desirable. Such placements were carried out in 11 patients below the eustachian valve without any serious sequelae.[49] Suprarenal placement is desirable when the source of emboli is the renal veins, ovarian veins functioning as collaterals after infrarenal caval ligation, or thrombi extending along the inferior vena cava up to and beyond the renal veins and when there are recurrent thrombi despite infrarenal caval ligation with adequate anticoagulation.[49] Suprarenal placement of the filter probably will be required in <20% of cases.[49]

The filter should be placed straight up without any tilting and should be parallel to the central axis of the inferior vena cava. In a deviated vena cava, the filter may look misaligned without affecting filtration, if in reality it is parallel to the lumen. A truly off-axis position may cause several undesired effects:

1. Passage of larger clots;
2. Propagation of clots trapped in the apex of the filter;
3. Penetration, with subsequent perforation, of the inferior vena caval wall because of undue pressure on one of the walls.

The patency rate of the KG filter surpasses that of the MU filter, because the former design allows circumferential flow past the device.[11–14,20] Stasis complications occur in 38% of patients with the KG filter, compared with 75% with MU filters. The lower rate of complications may be a consequence of caval patency.[20]

INTRODUCTION OF THE KG FILTER FROM THE JUGULAR VEIN THROUGH A VENOTOMY OR PERCUTANEOUSLY

Venacavography before filter placement is appropriate, because caval size and abnormalities, as well as extension of thrombi, should be evaluated to permit correct filter placement.

A right internal jugular vein approach is generally preferred, because of its straighter course and direct alignment in the vertical plane with the right atrium and the inferior vena cava, unless the vein is not accessible because of hematoma, infection, or thrombosis. The large carrier capsules of the KG and MU filters are difficult to advance through the left internal jugular and innominate vein into the superior vena cava and right atrium, and complications such as perforation or mediastinal hemorrhage have been reported with this approach.[50]

Introduction through a Surgical Venotomy

A horizontal incision is made above the clavicle, and the internal jugular vein is dissected out. After proper control of the vein has been gained, a small venotomy is created. Initially, routine dilatation of the junction of the internal jugular with the subclavian vein with a Fogarty balloon catheter was recommended, but this probably is not necessary in every case.[12] The use of guidewires makes for easier advancement of the carrier capsules through the eustachian valve.[51]

The guidewire and pusher stylet are retracted fully, and the guidewire lock hub is tightened, thereby keeping the guidewire in place. After full retraction of the pusher stylet, it is locked by tightening the stylet seal to prevent premature discharge of the filter (Fig. 22–7A).

With the help of the loading tool, the tip of the filter is advanced into the carrier capsule until the hooks are a few millimeters from the edge of the capsule (Fig. 22–7B). The hooks are then gathered with the concave end of the loading tool and advanced fully into the capsule (Fig. 22–7C). One must make sure that the "legs" of the filter are not crossed during loading (Fig. 22–7E); if they are crossed, all the steps will have to be repeated. Alternatively, a loading cone can be used to load the filter into the capsule (Fig. 22–7F). The cone is also used for loading of the filter into the modified capsule for femoral approach (Fig. 22–7G,H).

The present design has two sideholes, one for flushing or guidewire introduction, the other for flushing of the carrier capsule that houses the filter. Flushing of the capsule prevents clot formation between the legs and apex of the filter, which might prevent complete expansion of the filter. Incomplete expansion can result in a tilted position, with consequent poor filtration.[52]

If the carrier capsule cannot be advanced across the eustachian valve easily, insertion can be accomplished either by curving the stylet to redirect the capsule[33] or by advancing the capsule over a prepositioned guidewire. Advancement over a guidewire also prevents persistent entry of the carrier capsule into the hepatic or right renal vein. In another maneuver to solve this problem, the patient is placed in the left lateral decubitus position; its weight will then force the capsule into the more dependent position away from the vein orifices.[51,53] The capsule can then be advanced to the desired location. Dislodgment of the filter into the right renal vein can be prevented by initially advancing the carrier capsule distally into the iliac vein and subsequently pulling it back into the inferior vena cava to the desired site.[12]

The filter is released by withdrawing the capsule while holding the filter in place (Fig. 22–8) rather than by advancing the pusher stylet, because the latter maneuver may place the filter further inferiorly than desired. With capsule withdrawal, the apex of the filter is placed at the desired location, usually below the renal veins at the level of the metallic marker placed on the anterior abdominal wall as described earlier. Other radiologists prefer to leave a catheter in the lowermost renal vein to serve as a marker; it is removed along with the catheter assembly through the venotomy.[24,54]

Percutaneous Introduction

Percutaneous introduction is performed under fluoroscopy guidance and local anesthesia without venotomy.

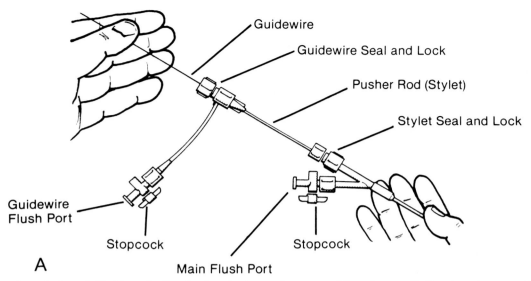

Fig. 22–7 Preparation of Greenfield filter. A. Proximal end of introducer catheter. B. Narrowed end of loading tool is used to advance filter into capsule until hooks are approximately 3–5 mm away from the capsule edge. C. Hooks are gathered with concave end of loading tool, which is then used to advance filter fully into the capsule. D. Cross-section of capsule with loaded Greenfield filter shows adequate position of struts. E. Crossing of struts within capsule will cause inadequate placement. F. Loading cone and tool being used to advance filter into capsule for jugular approach. G. Loading cone used to advance filter into capsule for femoral approach. H. Filter loaded into capsule modified for femoral approach. (Courtesy of Medi–Tech, Inc.)

Introduction can be accomplished only through the right internal jugular vein, because it involves the introduction of semirigid dilators and a 24F working sheath, and the tortuous course of the left internal jugular vein will not permit such manipulation without a high risk of perforation. The right internal jugular approach is preferred to the femoral approach because of the straighter venous course, which facilitates the passage of dilators and sheaths. Moreover, the filter will sit better within the lumen of the vena cava when introduced from above, thereby minimizing or avoiding off-axial seating and subsequent poor filtering.[24]

Filter insertion by the jugular vein approach. The patient is placed in the supine position with the head turned to the left side. The shoulders are elevated by placing a pillow between the scapulae posteriorly. The skin is infiltrated with local anesthetic approximately five fingerbreadths (10 cm) above the clavicle and lateral to the carotid artery.[55] The internal jugular vein is immediately posterior to the belly of the sternocleidomastoid muscle. The needle is directed toward the jugular notch at the medial end of the clavicle while the patient performs the Valsalva maneuver to distend the vein. The internal jugular vein is punctured high to avoid puncturing the apex of the lung and subsequent pneumothorax formation.

Following the puncture of the vein, a guidewire is passed through the needle and advanced into the inferior vena cava. Liberal amounts of lidocaine are then infiltrated into the subcutaneous tissues along the needle track. Over the guidewire, the 8F Teflon guiding catheter of the Amplatz coaxial dilator system is advanced into the infrarenal inferior vena cava (Fig. 22–9).[24,56] The subcutaneous tract is loosened with a hemostat, and the tract is dilated sequentially to 24F (Figs. 22–10 and 22–11). A 28F working sheath is then advanced over the 24F dilator into the superior vena cava.

Before the dilators and guidewire are removed from the sheath, the patient is instructed to hold his/her breath or to perform a Valsalva maneuver to increase the intrapulmonary pressure. A gush of blood will be noticed through the working sheath upon removal of the dilators. These measures are not required if the venous pressure is high secondary to pulmonary hypertension or if the patient is placed in the Trendelenburg position.

After removal of the dilators, the carrier capsule is immediately advanced through the working sheath (Figs. 22–12 and 22–13). If time elapses between dilator removal and carrier advancement, large amounts of air can be aspirated through the sheath, resulting in severe air embolism. As soon as the carrier capsule exits from the working sheath into the vein, the sheath is retracted (Fig. 22–14), and hemostasis is secured at the puncture site by manual compression over the catheter. While the assistant holds the puncture site, the catheter assembly is advanced under fluoroscopy into the infrarenal inferior vena cava, and the filter is released as discussed previously.

After filter placement, the catheter is removed, and the patient's upper body is elevated 20–30° above the horizontal level with a wedge. Because of negative pressure in the internal jugular vein, there is no oozing of blood at the puncture site. The incision is closed with No. 4 or No. 5 suture material. The patient's head is kept elevated for 1–2 hr.[24]

Filter insertion by the femoral vein approach. The femoral vein approach carries a risk of dislodgment of any iliac vein and lower inferior vena cava thrombi, so iliac and inferior vena cava venography should be performed first.

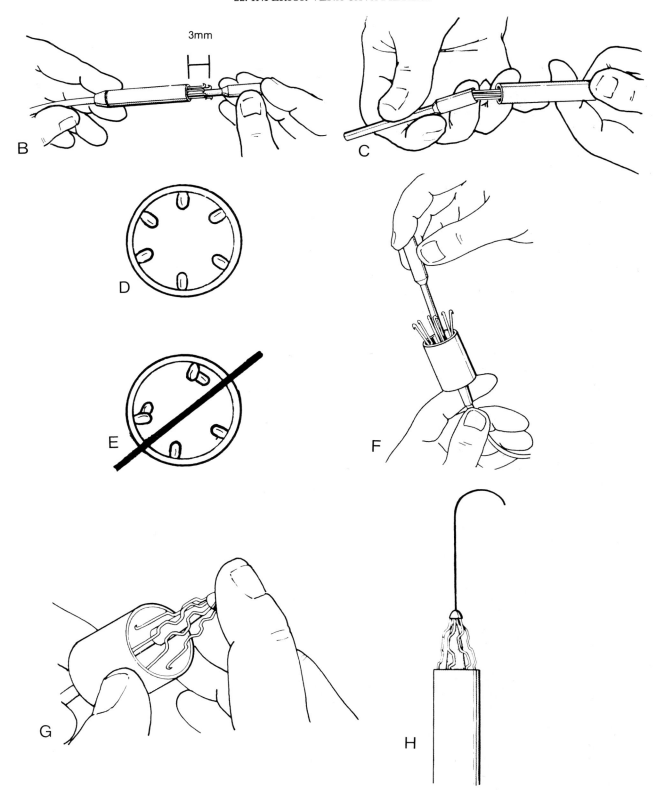

Fig. 22–7 B–H

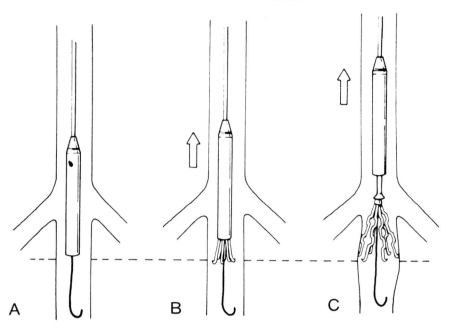

A   B   C

Fig. 22–8   Introduction of Greenfield filter. A. Most distal edge of introducer capsule has been placed at level where filter will be released. B. While stylet is held in place, capsule is pulled back. C. After capsule has been pulled back, Greenfield filter has re-expanded; legs are fixed to wall by gently pulling back on stylet. (Courtesy of Medi–Tech, Inc.)

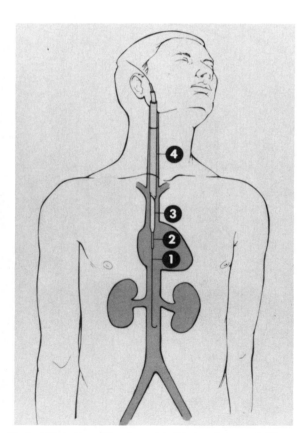

Fig. 22–9   Dilatation of jugular vein with Amplatz renal dilators and placement of Teflon sheath tip (4) within superior vena cava; 24F dilator (3); 8F dilator (2); guidewire (1). (Reproduced from Tadavarthy SM, Castañeda–Zuñiga WR, Salomonowitz E, et al: Kimray–Greenfield vena cava filter: percutaneous introduction. *Radiology* 1984;151:525–526.)

For femoral insertion, the carrier was redesigned by shortening the capsule (Fig. 22–15). The stylet over which the filter is mounted is tapered to admit a guidewire for easier manipulation of the catheter assembly. As in the jugular carrier, there are two sideholes, one to flush the guidewire and the other to flush the carrier capsule. The pusher stylet is advanced by unlocking the stylet seal, which is kept unlocked for loading the filter. The loading cone is placed over the carrier capsule, and the base of the filter is inserted slowly into the loader by gently pushing on the nose. The pusher stylet is then locked, so the loaded filter is not disturbed. Guidewire motion is checked, after unlocking the guidewire seal, by advancing the wire through the pusher stylet out through the nose of the filter.

For insertion via a femoral venotomy, the carrier capsule is advanced through the incision, and the catheter assembly is negotiated over the guidewire through the iliac system into the inferior vena cava (Fig. 22–16). During introduction, the guidewire and the main flush ports are flushed with heparinized saline to prevent clotting on the filter. When the desired position below the renal veins is reached, the shaft is held firmly, the pusher stylet is unlocked, and the filter is uncovered by withdrawing the capsule toward the groin. In this fashion, the filter is released from the tapered pusher. No further manipulation is attempted.

In most older patients, the carrier capsule, in spite of its redesign, is difficult to advance through the iliac system. The use of heavy-duty guidewires, such as the Lunderquist, the Lunderquist–Ring, or the Amplatz stiffening wire, is recommended. Usually, the carrier capsule is caught where the distal right iliac vein joins the inferior vena cava; at this site, the iliac artery crosses the iliac vein anteriorly and courses toward the right side of the pelvis.

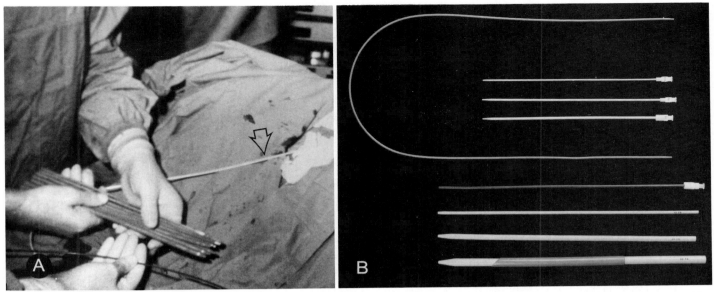

Fig. 22–10 Transjugular approach. A. Pigtail catheter passed through jugular puncture (arrow). Operator shows set of Amplatz renal dilators prior to dilatation. B. Amplatz dilator set with Teflon sheath over 24F dilator for percutaneous placement of Greenfield filter.

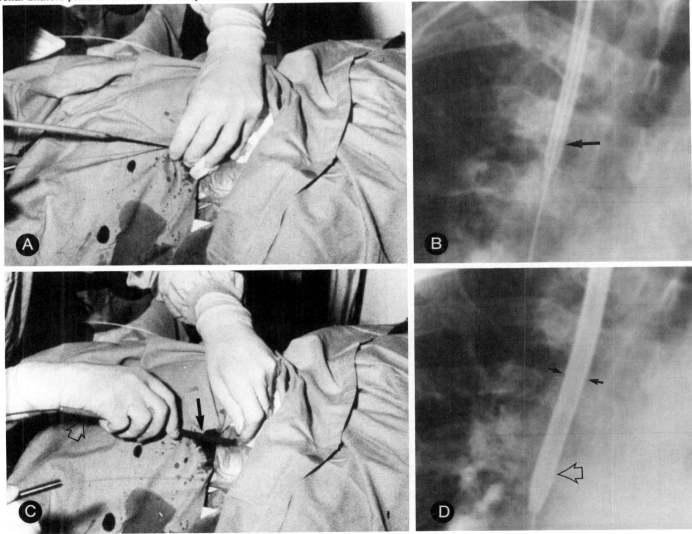

Fig. 22–11 Transjugular approach (continued). A. 20F dilator being advanced over guiding 8F catheter and guidewire. B. Spot film shows 20F dilator (arrow) with its tip within superior vena cava. C. Teflon sheath (arrow) being advanced over 24F dilator (open arrow) across puncture site. D. Spot film shows position of 24F dilator (open arrow) within superior vena cava during advancement of Teflon sheath, the edge of which is faintly visible (small arrows).

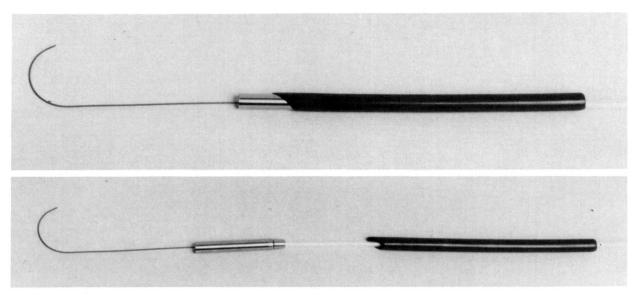

Fig. 22–12   Introducer catheter with capsule passed through Teflon sheath. Observe guidewire in lumen of introducer catheter.

Forceful advancement, even over the guidewire, is not advisable, because the iliac veins can be perforated easily.

To minimize problems in these older patients, the puncture site in the femoral vein is dilated to 24F with the coaxial dilator system, and a long Teflon sheath is advanced until its tip is located high in the distal iliac vein or in the lower inferior vena cava.[24] Through this working sheath, the carrier capsule can be advanced and the filter uncovered in the usual fashion. Simple manual pressure over the puncture site secures hemostasis, despite the large hole in the femoral vein, because of the low venous pressure.

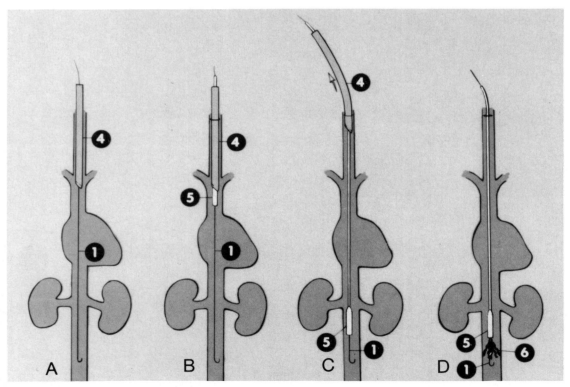

Fig. 22–13   Percutaneous introduction of Greenfield filter. A. Teflon sheath (4) in place with tip in superior vena cava. 1 = guidewire. B. Greenfield filter loaded in capsule (5) being introduced through Teflon sheath. C. Once capsule has been passed into superior vena cava, Teflon sheath is removed. D. Then, with manual compression of puncture site, Greenfield filter (6) is positioned below renal veins. (Reproduced from Tadavarthy SM, Castañeda–Zuñiga WR, Salomonowitz E, et al: Kimray–Greenfield vena cava filter: percutaneous introduction. *Radiology* 1984;151:525–526.)

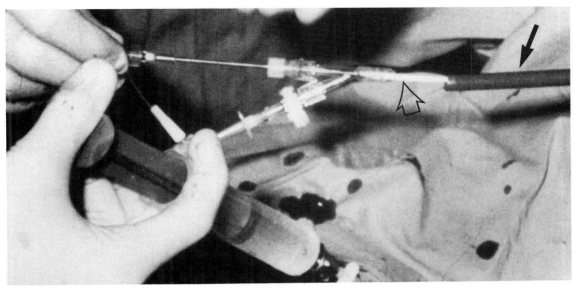

Fig. 22–14 After introduction of capsule, Teflon sheath has been pulled back (black arrow) over shaft of introducing catheter (open arrow). Contrast medium is being injected through sidearm fitting to verify position of capsule within inferior vena cava.

Hunter–Sessions Transvenous Balloon Occlusion

Hunter et al developed a balloon catheter for percutaneous inferior vena caval occlusion.[35,57–59] Excellent long-term results, with follow-up for as long as 13 years, have been reported.[57]

The shaft of the catheter is 17F and 75 cm long. The balloon is attached to the catheter by a collar, so it can be detached easily. The balloon was devised with six principles in mind[35,57–59]:

1. Avoidance of vessel trauma. The balloon has no hooks or pins to traumatize or penetrate the vena caval wall. Therefore, retroperitoneal hemorrhage and trauma to nearby organs such as the ureter and duodenum are avoided, as is migration of the device into the peritoneum.

2. Facilitation of radiologic studies. Venograms can be obtained by instilling contrast medium through the catheter shaft, and this facilitates the positioning of the balloon. Postocclusion venography is also advised to confirm proper positioning.

3. Avoidance of general anesthesia and laparotomy. Bal-

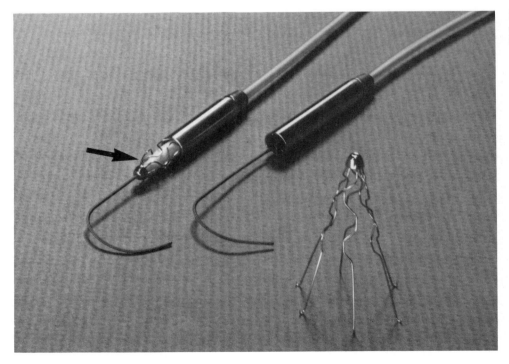

Fig. 22–15 Greenfield filter loaded in capsule for transfemoral placement (arrow).

loon occlusion of the inferior vena cava can be accomplished under local anesthesia through a jugular venotomy.

4. Precise fit of the device to the blood vessel. The balloon can be inflated with contrast medium so that it adapts to the dimensions of the inferior vena cava. The balloon usually remains inflated for 1–2 years.

5. Ability to use anticoagulants safely. Balloon occlusion of the inferior vena cava permits simultaneous administration of anticoagulants. Because the balloon does not penetrate the vessel wall, there is no risk of retroperitoneal hemorrhage. The combination of balloon occlusion and anticoagulants expedites clot resolution in the legs, thereby minimizing stasis sequelae.

6. Avoidance of thrombosis. Complete occlusion of the inferior vena cava is required to prevent recurrent pulmonary emboli, and this can be accomplished without laparotomy by the balloon technique. The transluminal filters are foreign bodies within a slow-flow venous system and thus may trigger clot formation with subsequent thrombosis.

Balloon occlusion usually is well tolerated even by very sick patients. No periprocedural deaths have been reported. In about 5% of cases, however, acute balloon occlusion is not well tolerated and causes hypovolemia and shock, which may create problems in patients with minimal cardiopulmonary reserve.[35] Hypotension is treated by deflation of the balloon, administration of fluids, and reinflation of the device.[35]

The balloon is placed through a venotomy under fluoroscopy guidance and inflated with 25% Hypaque (average volume: 17 ml).[35] Fluoroscopy and traction on the balloon assure correct position. The balloon gradually deflates, but within about 2 years, the inferior vena cava fibroses around the deflated balloon, and permanent complete occlusion is achieved.

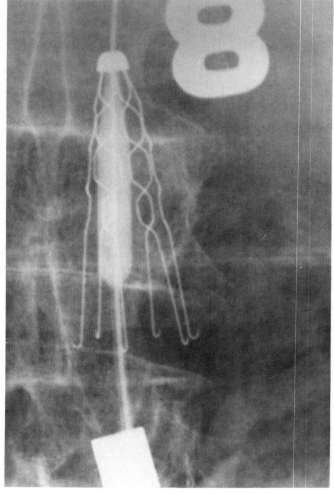

Fig. 22–16   Filter being positioned in inferior vena cava through femoral approach.

GENERAL CONSIDERATIONS IN THE DESIGN OF NEWER FILTERS

The authors' *in vitro* testing showed that the available filters have certain limitations and drawbacks. For example, filtration with the KG device is highly dependent on filter position. If the filter is off center, it does not filter some of the caval flow adequately and so may allow larger clots to pass.[32] *In vitro*, the KG filter is gravity dependent. Clots pass along the dependent part of the model vena cava, especially if the filter is not aligned with the vessel axis. Moreover, whereas the KG filter offers minimal resistance to the flow of blood so that the clotting tendencies in the inferior vena cava are low, the design of the MU filter offers higher resistance that may ultimately lead to thrombosis of the inferior vena cava.

Because of the shortcomings of the available occlusion devices, newer designs for caval filters have been developed. The ideal filter would have these characteristics:

1. It would be insertable through 8F–14F angiography catheters that can be introduced by the Seldinger technique through the femoral or jugular veins.[26,27,32]

Catheters and capsules of this size avoid the complications of air embolism.[32]

2. It would not migrate or damage the surrounding tissues.

3. If the filter is not in the correct position after release, it would be possible to make adjustments until the correct position is achieved.

4. The device would be removable percutaneously so that it could be inserted for prophylaxis and removed after the crisis to avoid the long-term complications of occlusion of the inferior vena cava.

5. Its material would be biocompatible, stress resistant, and nonthrombogenic.[26,27,32]

6. It would trap small emboli while maintaining the physiologic flow in the inferior vena cava.

These features are desirable to prevent complications such as thrombosis, leg edema, and stasis.

Several newer designs, such as the Nitinol,[26,27] bird's nest,[28–30] Lund–Amplatz retrievable,[32] and helix[31] filters are undergoing experimental and clinical evaluation. Some of these filters are promising to satisfy some or all of the above criteria.

Lund–Amplatz Filter

A newer design and material were chosen for this filter. It is shaped in the form of an umbrella ("spider" design) and is made from MP35 alloy (35% nickel, 35% cobalt, 20% chromium, and 10% molybdenum),[32] which is a biocompatible, corrosion-resistant material with higher fatigue resistance. It also is used in the production of endocardial pacer wires.[60]

The spider filter has a central stem that has a retrieval hook at one end and an attachment for a threaded cable wire at the other (Fig. 22–17A,B). Fixation of the filter is accomplished by pointed wires that pierce the caval wall; wire loops prevent the prongs from penetrating the wall

more than 2 mm (Fig. 22–17C). The filter is attached to a threaded guidewire and inserted through a 14F catheter. The prongs are compressed during passage through the catheter (Fig. 22–18A) and spring open (Fig. 22–18B) when extruded in the infrarenal vena cava. The filter is secured by gently pulling back (in the transjugular approach) or gently pushing forward (in the transfemoral approach) on the wire to engage the prongs firmly in the caval wall. The threaded guide is subsequently unscrewed, and all introducing catheters are removed.

Percutaneous retrieval is accomplished through the femoral vein. The hook on the caudal end of the filter is engaged by a snare (Fig. 22–19A–C), and the filter is held securely in position while the 14F removing Teflon sheath is advanced over it. The sheath compresses the prongs, freeing them from the wall of the vena cava (Fig. 22–20). Once the filter is completely inside the sheath, the sheath and filter are removed through the femoral vein as a sin-

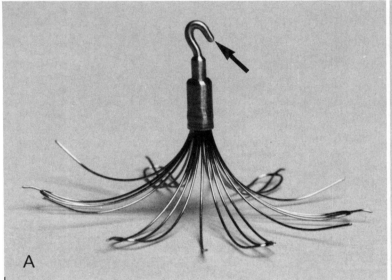

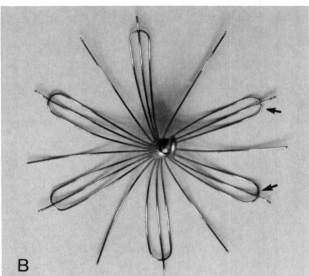

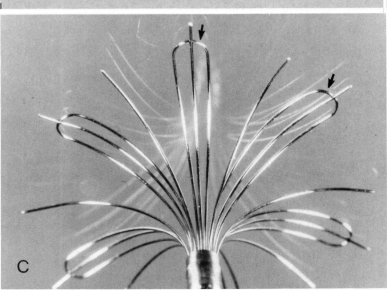

Fig. 22–17 Lund–Amplatz retrievable filter. A. Profile; observe hook for retrieval (arrow). B. Filter seen from top to show spaces between legs as well as stoppers (arrows) that restrict penetration of vena caval wall. C. Closeup view shows stoppers to better advantage (arrows) as well as decreasing size of spaces toward center of filter. (Reproduced from Lund G, Castañeda W, Amplatz, K: Retrievable vena caval filter percutaneously introduced. *Radiology* 155(3):831, 1985.)

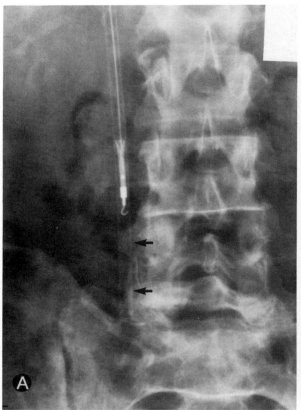
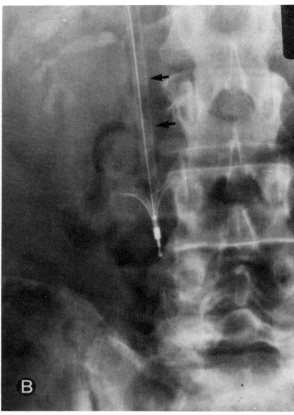

Fig. 22–18 Introduction of Lund–Amplatz filter. A. Long Teflon sleeve (arrows) has been advanced to level of right common iliac vein.

B. After placement of filter at desired level, Teflon sheath (arrows) is gently pulled back until filter is released.

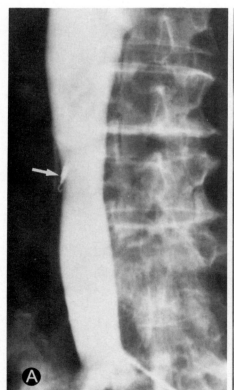
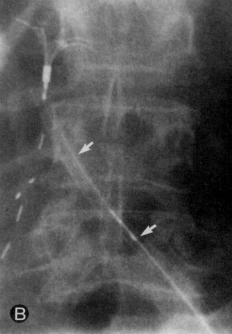
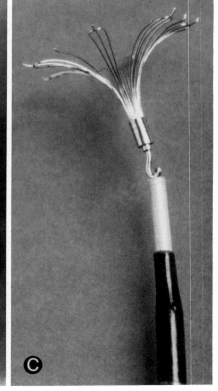

Fig. 22–19 Removal of Lund–Amplatz filter. A. Inferior venacavogram performed through left femoral vein shows tilting of filter (arrow) within vessel lumen. Hook appears to be embedded in caval wall, but this proved to be an artifact due to layering of contrast medium. B. Teflon sheath (arrows) has been advanced to a position distal to hook, and a snare has trapped hook. Teflon sheath is slowly advanced over filter to close legs. C. Snare and catheter for percutaneous retrieval of Lund–Amplatz filter.

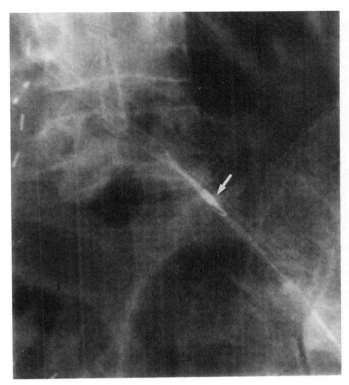

Fig. 22–20 Filter (arrow) has been disengaged from caval wall and is withdrawn slowly through Teflon sheath.

gle unit. The filter should not be pulled back into the sheath, because this would cause extensive laceration of the caval wall.

The present design of this filter is effective not only in trapping all the small clots but also in maintaining the normal flow in the inferior vena cava (Fig. 22–21). As was proved in the authors' *in vitro* experiments, the filter is not gravity dependent. After uneventful testing in dogs, the filter has been placed in patients with good results and without serious sequelae. In dogs, retrieval with the snare 2–3 weeks after placement was successful in most

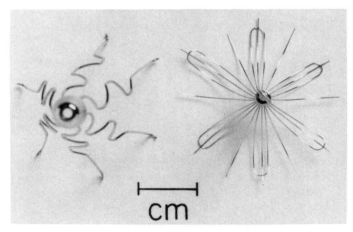

Fig. 22–21 View from above of Greenfield and Lund–Amplatz filters showing slightly smaller spaces between struts of Lund–Amplatz filter.

cases. Successful retrieval has been achieved recently in human beings.

Basket (Günther) Filter

This filter consists of two segments, the proximal in the shape of a basket and the distal composed of anchoring limbs.[61] The tips of the limbs form tiny balls, limiting penetration of the vessel wall. The two segments of the filter are constructed from 12 single pieces of 0.2-mm-diameter stainless-steel wires with no soldering, thereby avoiding breakage points between the segments. The total filter length is 7.5 cm, the diameter of the basket is 2.5 cm, and the anchoring limbs encompass a circle of 3.0 cm (Fig. 22–22). By virtue of its design, the basket traps emboli at three levels: the distal end outside the basket, inside the basket, and between the anchoring limbs and the basket.

In vitro and *in vivo* (canine) testing proved that the Günther filter captures tiny (15 × 2 × 2-mm) emboli. The filter also effectively maintained its position. Unlike the KG filter,[61] it stayed parallel to the central axis of the inferior vena cava without tilting, because of the presence of the proximal basket and of the distal anchoring segments. Filter position was stable, without migration, and only a 5-mm Hg gradient was noted across the filter after the capture of several clots. On postmortem examination of the dogs, the inferior vena cava demonstrated tiny nodular fibrotic changes, indicating a mild inflammatory reaction.

The method of introduction is simple. The filter is first inserted into a loading cartridge and then advanced with a guidewire through a 10F catheter from either the femoral or the jugular approach (Fig. 22–15). The device can be retrieved within 1–2 weeks without undue damage to the vessel wall. To date, the filter has been successful in three patients.[61] Long-term follow-up is needed to document the clinical effectiveness and complications.

Bird's Nest Filter

The bird's nest filter is composed of four 25-cm-long stainless-steel wires 0.18 mm in diameter with two short angled hooks at each end for venous fixation (Fig. 22–23).[28] It is shaped into a nonmatching mesh with gaps no larger than 3–4 mm (Fig. 22–24) and effectively traps emboli as small as 1–2 mm.[30]

The filter is designed to be introduced percutaneously by the Seldinger technique through an 8F catheter, thereby eliminating the venotomy and the need for bulkier capsules.[28,29] The wire mesh is loaded into an 8F Teflon catheter and introduced through a femoral or jugular sheath. The filter is positioned in the infrarenal vena cava with a detachable wire pusher (Fig. 22–25).[28,29] During advancement, the filter resumes its configuration and fixes to the vessel wall (Fig. 22–26).[28,29] The wire pusher is detached, and the Teflon catheter and sheath are removed together.

The patency rate of the inferior vena cava is expected to be as high as with the KG filters.[28] However, no long-term studies comparing the bird's nest with other filters in a large group of patients are available.

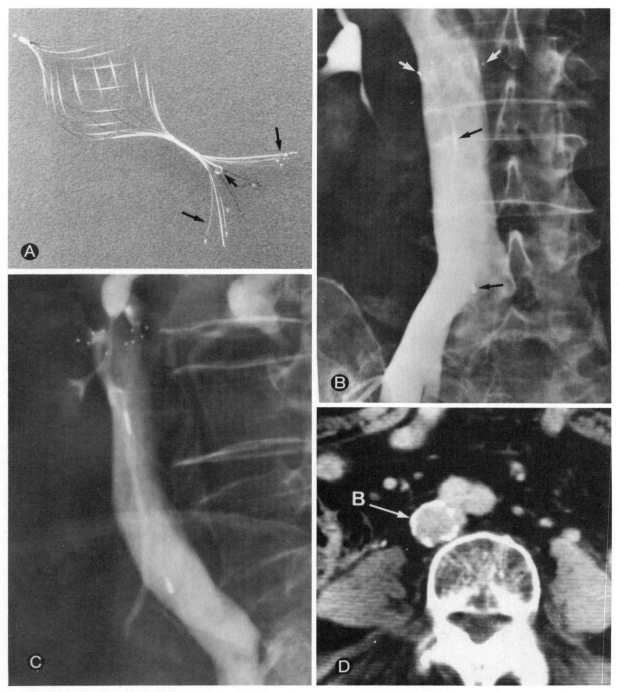

Fig. 22–22 Günther filter. A. Observe basket-like configuration of filter with a spider (long arrows) attached to one of its ends for fixation to caval wall. A hook is also placed in center of spider for percutaneous introduction and removal (short arrow). B. Inferior venacavogram in anteroposterior projection shows filter low in vessel (black arrows). Fixation hooks pierce wall of vein (white arrows). C. Lateral projection of inferior venacavogram shows filter centered in lumen. D. CT scan shows basket wires in filter midsection (B) braced against venous wall. (Reproduced from Günther RW et al: Basket filter for prevention of pulmonary embolism. *Semin Intervent Radiol* 1986;3:220–226.)

Nitinol Filters

Nitinol is a unique alloy of nickel and titanium that has a thermal-dependent memory.[26,27] The design of the filter is embodied in the wire at the time of annealing at high temperature[26,27]; by cooling, the wire can be made pliable and straight. In this condition, the Nitinol wire can be introduced through 8F catheters by the Seldinger technique.[27]

PALESTRANT FILTER

Palestrant et al recently designed a Nitinol inferior vena caval filter and tested it *in vitro*.[26] The filter has two

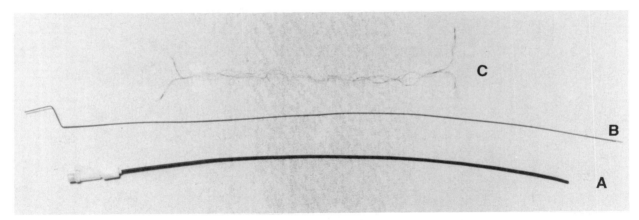

Fig. 22–23 Unassembled set of Gianturco bird's nest filter showing introducing catheter (A), fixation stylet (B), and filter (C).

components, one a filter mesh and the other a component with six anchoring limbs, which have terminal hooks that penetrate the vena caval wall up to 1 mm, thus securing the device (Figs. 22–27 and 22–28). The filter limbs span as much as 32 mm, and the filter mesh spans up to 25 mm with nonoverlapping loops formed by a set of seven wires. The design allows the filter to be centered in the inferior vena cava lumen; the anchoring limbs and filter mesh can capture all emboli >5 mm.[26] During *in vitro* testing, the filter was highly effective, allowing only 3% of short small

emboli to escape capture.[26] The gradient across the filter after clot capture was no greater than 5 cm H_2O.[26]

CRAGG FILTER

Cragg et al recently developed a simple spiral Nitinol filter that can remove clots very effectively without restricting the flow of blood (Fig. 22–29).[27] The spiral design has several advantages:

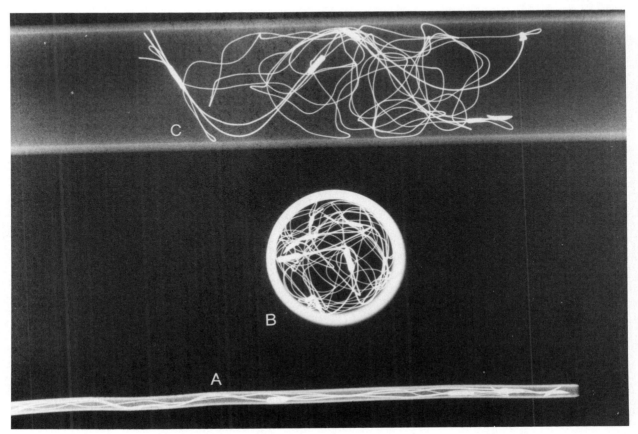

Fig. 22–24 Radiographs of bird's nest filter within introducer catheter (A) and cross-sectional (B) and longitudinal (C) views of filter within inferior vena caval model illustrate mesh formed by the wires, which helps prevent migration of embolus.

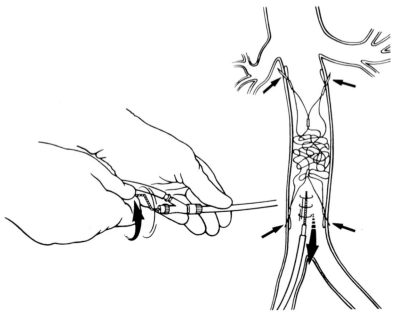

Fig. 22–25 Placement of bird's nest filter below renal veins. Proximal and distal fixation points (arrows) have been anchored to caval wall, and stylet has been removed by gentle unscrewing. (Courtesy of Cook, Inc.)

1. It can be introduced through 8F angiographic catheters.
2. It can be repositioned easily.
3. It allows easier adjustments in size by tightening or loosening the spiral, allowing the filter to be effective in many sizes of vena cava.
4. The loop maintains proper orientation of the filter in the caval lumen.
5. It is less thrombogenic because of its smaller amount of wire.[27]
6. As with the KG filter, the apex of the Cragg filter is oriented superiorly and the spiral distends the inferior vena caval wall (Fig. 22–30). The entrapped emboli at the apex of the spiral sieve therefore occlude less of the lumen, maintaining para-axial flow.

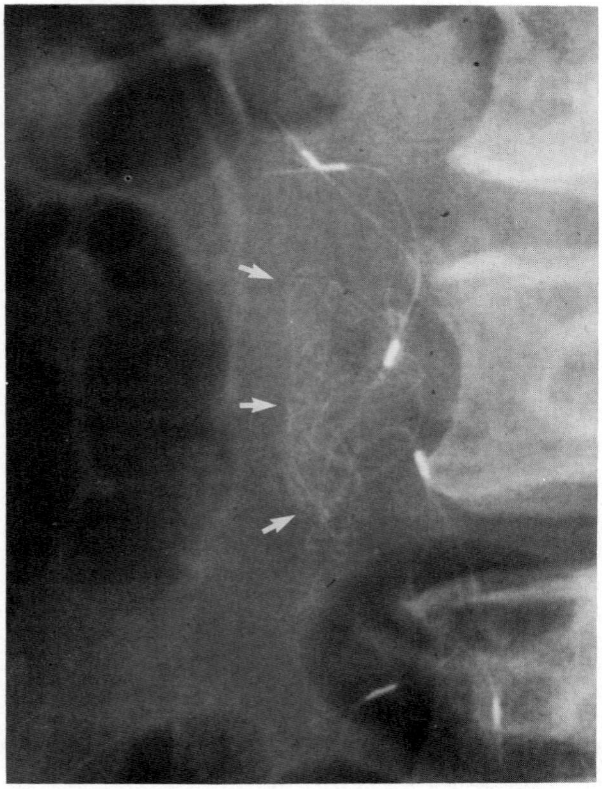

Fig. 22–26 Lateral view of abdomen showing bird's nest filter positioned in inferior vena cava (arrows).

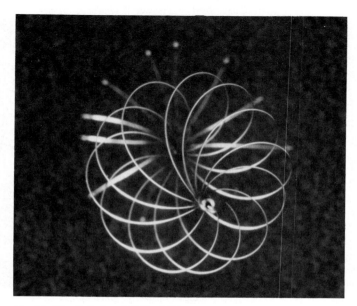

Fig. 22–27 Palestrant Nitinol filter.

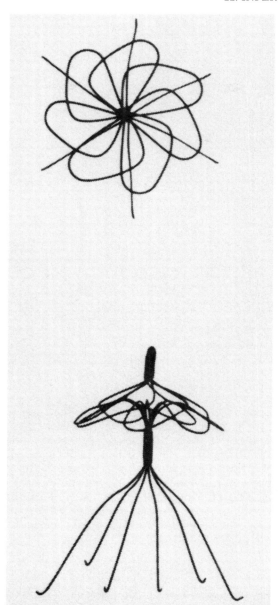

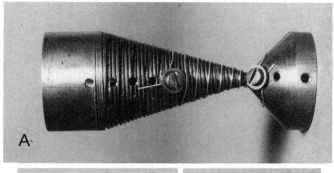

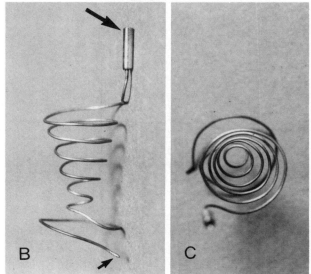

Fig. 22–29 Cragg filter. A. Nitinol wire is tightly wound around cone-shaped stainless-steel barrel for thermal shaping. Lateral (B) and frontal (C) views of filter show its cone-shaped configuration with distal prong (small arrow) for fixation and proximal screw-carrying capsule for introduction and release (large arrow). (Reproduced from Cragg A, Lund G, Salomonowitz E, et al: A new percutaneous vena cava filter. *AJR* 1983;141:601–604.)

Fig. 22–28 Cross-section and longitudinal views of Palestrant filter. (Reproduced from Palestrant AM, Prince M, Simon M: Comparative *in vitro* evaluation of the Nitinol inferior vena cava filter. *Radiology* 1982;145:351–355.)

COMPLICATIONS OF INTRALUMINAL FILTER DEVICES

Misplacement

Misplacement of the filter is one of the most common complications, although the frequency decreases with experience. Routine preoperative venography and labeling of renal vein position with metallic markers minimize the frequency of misplacement.

Misplacement of filters most often involves the right side of the heart, the right renal vein, and the iliac veins. The right renal vein can easily be involved if the kidney is ptotic or if the renal vein is vertical and parallel to the inferior vena cava. Initial advancement of the filter capsule into the iliac vein under fluoroscopy guidance, before

final ejection at the infrarenal position, minimizes the incidence of accidental misplacement into the hepatic, iliac, or renal veins.

Inadvertent placement of MU filters into the right renal vein has been reported[2,37,41] and can be corrected by operative removal and repair of the vein.[62] Misplacement into the right iliac vein[2] and perforation of the hepatic vein with filter extrusion into the retroperitoneal space also have been reported. Other, rare, sites of misplacement include the right atrium, right ventricle, and suprarenal inferior vena cava.[63] Persistent entry of the capsule into the right renal vein can be prevented by blocking this

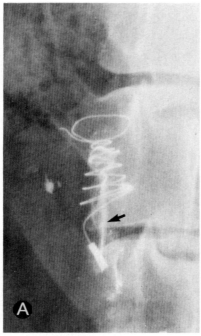
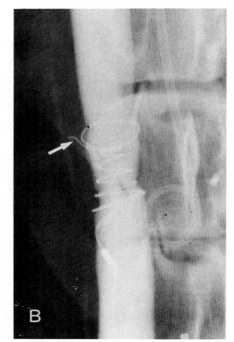

Fig. 22–30   Experimental use of Cragg filter. A. Spot film shows filter of proper size placed within inferior vena cava of dog after injection of radiopaque autologous clot (arrow). B. Superior venacavogram 6 weeks after placement shows patent caval lumen with some filling defects within filter representing trapped embolus. Distal prong has perforated venous wall (arrow).

vein with a Fogarty balloon catheter advanced through the venotomy.[64] Accidental placement of MU filters in the suprarenal inferior vena cava can be corrected by careful advancement of the filter downward by the carrier capsule.[2]

Migration

This complication can happen if there is a mismatch between the diameter of the filter device and the inferior vena cava (Fig. 22–22A). The size of the inferior vena cava can be assessed easily from an inferior venacavogram and is not related to the age, sex, body habitus, or weight of the patient. The width of the inferior vena cava in normal adults is usually between 15 and 28 mm. Megacava may occur in persons with chronic pulmonary hypertension, congestive heart failure, or tricuspid insufficiency and, rarely, as a congenital anomaly. Filters also can migrate if their limbs are not properly engaged in the caval wall prior to release.

Fig. 22–31   Chest radiograph showing migrating Mobin–Uddin filter lodged in right pulmonary artery (arrows).

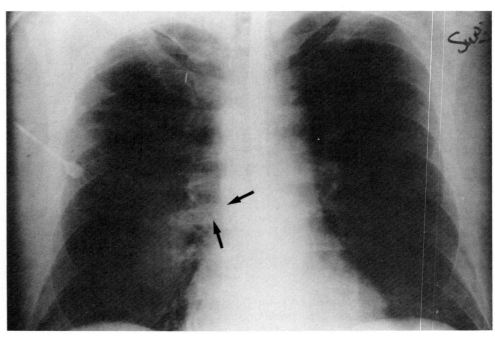

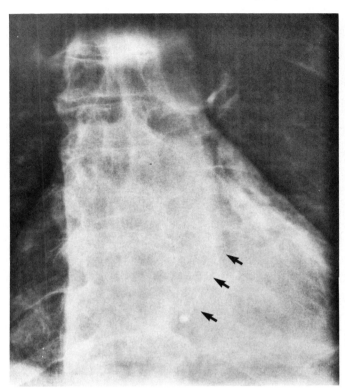

Fig. 22–32 Closeup of heart shows Greenfield filter that has migrated into right ventricle (arrows).

With the 23-mm MU filter, migration was reported in 22 patients (0.9%) of a large series and was fatal in 14 (0.6%).[11,42] With the newer design of 28-mm MU filters, the migration incidence has been decreased to 0.4% in a series of 300,333 patients.[65] The 2-mm (extended length) prongs from the 28-mm filter ensure secure seating of the device in the infrarenal inferior vena cava in most patients.

Migration of the MU filter to the right atrium or ventricle or to the pulmonary artery has been reported (Fig. 22–31).[63,66,67] Although less common, migration also has been reported with the KG filter (Fig. 22–32).[68]

Other complications reported with this type of filter include locking of the struts, which results in incomplete, asymmetrical opening of the filter,[69] perforation of the inferior vena cava,[70–72] misplacement,[71,73–75] distal migration,[76] and premature ejection into the right atrium.[69,70,73]

References

1. Dalen JE, Alpert JS: Natural history of pulmonary embolism. *Progr Cardiovasc Dis* 1975;17:259
2. Mobin–Uddin K, Utley JR, Bryant LR: The inferior vena cava umbrella filter. *Progr Cardiovasc Dis* 1975;17:391
3. Ochsner A, Ochsner JL, Sanders HS: Prevention of pulmonary embolism by caval ligation. *Ann Surg* 1970;171:923
4. Spencer FC, Quattlebaum JK, Quattlebaum JK Jr, Sharp EH, Jude JR: Plication of the inferior vena cava for pulmonary embolism. *Ann Surg* 1962;155:827
5. Sensenig DM, Achar BG, Serlin O: Plication of the inferior vena cava with staples. *Am J Surg* 1965;109:679
6. Moretz WH, Still MJ Jr, Griffin LH, Jennings WD, Wray CH: Partial occlusion of the inferior vena cava with a smooth Teflon clip: analysis of long-term results. *Surgery* 1972;71:710
7. Miles RM, Chappell F, Renner O: A partially occluding vena caval clip for the prevention of pulmonary embolism. *Am Surg* 1964;30:40
8. Adams JT, Deweese JA: Partial interruption of the inferior vena cava with a new plastic clip. *Surg Gynecol Obstet* 1966;123:1087
9. Deweese JA, Hunter JR: Vena cava filter for the prevention of pulmonary embolism: five years' clinical experience. *Arch Surg* 1963;86:852
10. Schroeder TM, Elkins RC, Greenfield LJ: Entrapment of sized emboli by the KMA-Greenfield intracaval filter. *Surgery* 1978;83:435
11. Cimochowski GE, Evans RH, Zarins CK, Lu C–T, DeMeester TR: Greenfield filter versus Mobin–Uddin umbrella: the continuing quest for the ideal method of vena caval interruption. *J Thorac Cardiovasc Surg* 1980;79:358
12. Gomez GA, Curler BS, Wheeler HB: Transvenous interruption of the inferior vena cava. *Surgery* 1983;93:612
13. Greenfield LF, McCurdy JR, Brown PP: A new intracava filter permitting continued flow and resolution of emboli. *Surgery* 1973;73:599
14. Greenfield LF: Current indications for and results of Greenfield filter placement. *J Vasc Surg* 1984;1:502
15. Eichelter P, Schenk WG Jr: Prophylaxis of pulmonary embolism: a new experimental approach with initial results. *Arch Surg* 1968;97:348
16. Moser KM, Harsany PG, Harvey–Smith W, Durante P, Gursan M: Reversible interruption of inferior vena cava by means of a balloon catheter: preliminary report. *J Thorac Cardiovasc Surg* 1971;62:205
17. Pate JW, Melvin D, Cheek RC: A new form of vena caval interruption. *Ann Surg* 1969;169:873
18. Hunter JA, Sessions R, Buenger R: Experimental balloon obstruction of the inferior vena cava. *Ann Surg* 1970;171:315
19. Mobin–Uddin K, McLean R, Bolooki H, Jude JR: Caval interruption for prevention of pulmonary embolism: long-term results of a new method. *Arch Surg* 1969;99:711
20. Wingerd M, Bernhard VM, Maddison F, Towne JB: Comparison of caval filters in the management of venous thromboembolism. *Arch Surg* 1978;113:1264
21. Bernstein E: The place of venous interruption in the treatment of pulmonary thromboembolism, in Moser K, Stein M (eds): *Pulmonary Thromboembolism*. Chicago, Year Book Medical Publishers, 1973, p 312
22. Rizk GK, Amplatz K: A percutaneous method of introducing the caval umbrella. *AJR* 1973;117:903.
23. Knight L, Amplatz K, Nicoloff DM: Alternate method for introduction of IVC filters. *Surg Gynecol Obstet* 1974;138:763.
24. Tadavarthy SM, Castañeda–Zuñiga WR, Salomonowitz E, et al: Kimray–Greenfield vena cava filter: percutaneous introduction. *Radiology* 1984;151:525
25. Formanek A, Castañeda WR, Knight L, Amplatz K: Three year experience with percutaneous introduction of inferior vena cava filter. *Rev Interam Radiol* 1977;2:171
26. Palestrant AM, Prince M, Simon M: Comparative in vitro evaluation of the Nitinol inferior vena cava filter. *Radiology* 1982;145:351
27. Cragg A, Lund G, Salomonowitz E, et al: A new percutaneous vena cava filter. *AJR* 1983;141:601
28. Roehm JO Jr: The bird's nest filter: a new percutaneous transcatheter inferior vena cava filter. *J Vasc Surg* 1984;1:498
29. Roehm JO Jr, Gianturco C, Barth MH, Wright KC: Percutaneous transcatheter filter for the inferior vena cava: a new device for treatment of patients with pulmonary embolism. *Radiology* 1984;150:255
30. Gianturco C, Anderson JH, Wallace S: A new vena cava filter: experimental animal evaluation. *Radiology* 1980;137:835

31. Maass D, Demierre D, Wallsten H, Senning A: The helix filter: a new vena caval filter for the prevention of pulmonary embolism. *J Cardiovasc Surg (Torino)* 1985;26:116

32. Lund G, Rysavy JA, Salomonowitz E, et al: A new caval filter for percutaneous placement and retrieval: experimental study. *Radiology* 1984;152:369

33. Gray RK, Buckberg GD, Grollman JH Jr: The importance of inferior vena cavography in placement of the Mobin–Uddin vena caval filter. *Radiology* 1973;106:277

34. Ferris EJ: The inferior vena cava, in Abrams H (ed): *Abrams Angiography*, ed 3. Boston, Little, Brown, p 939

35. Stansel MC: Vena cava interruption: three points of view. *Contemp Surg* 1982;20:63

36. Santos GH, Lansman S: Prevention of pulmonary embolism with use of Mobin–Uddin filter. *NY State J Med* 1982;82:185

37. Mobin–Uddin K: Invited commentary. *World J Surg* 1978;2:55

38. Greenfield LJ, Scher LA, Elkins RC: KMA–Greenfield filter placement for chronic pulmonary hypertension. *Ann Surg* 1979;189:560

39. Peyton JW, Hylemon MB, Greenfield LJ, Crute SL, Sugerman HJ, Quershi GD: Comparison of Greenfield filter and vena caval ligation for experimental septic thromboembolism. *Surgery* 1983;93:533

40. Mobin–Uddin K, Callarda M, Bolooko M, Rubinson R, Michie D, Jude JR: Transvenous caval interruption with umbrella filters. *N Engl J Med* 1972;286:255

41. Mensoian JO, LoGerfo FW, Weitzman AF, Ezpeleta M, Sequeira JC: Clinical experience with the Mobin–Uddin vena cava umbrella filter. *Arch Surg* 1980;115:1179

42. McIntyre AB, McCready RA, Hyde GL, Mattingly W: A ten year follow-up study of the Mobin-Uddin filter for vena cava interruption. *Surg Gynecol Obstet* 1984;158:513

43. Schlosser V, Spillner G, Kaiser W: Prevention of pulmonary embolism by inferior vena cava filters: results in 62 cases. *World J Surg* 1977;1:113

44. Wingerd M, Bernhard VM, Maddison F, Towne JB: Comparison of caval filters in the management of venous thromboembolism. *Arch Surg* 1978;113:1264

45. Knight L, Amplatz K, Nicoloff DM: Alternate method for introduction of IVC filters. *Surg Gynecol Obstet* 1974;138:763

46. Rizk GK, Amplatz K: A percutaneous method of introducing the caval umbrella. *AJR* 1973;117:903

47. Greenfield LJ, Crute SL: Retrieval of the Greenfield vena caval filter. *Surgery* 1980;88:719

48. Stewart JR, Greenfield LJ: Transvenous vena caval filtration and pulmonary embolectomy. *Surg Clin North Am* 1982;62:411

49. Orsini RA, Jarrell BE: Suprarenal placement of vena caval filters: indications, techniques, and results. *J Vasc Surg* 1984;1:124

50. Novelline RA: Practical points on transvenous insertion of inferior vena cava filters. *CardioVasc Intervent Radiol* 1980;3:319

51. Greenfield LJ, Stewart JR, Crute S: Improved technique for insertion of Greenfield vena caval filter. *Surg Gynecol Obstet* 1983;156:217

52. Leiter B, Sequeira J, Weitzman R, Menzoian J: A complication following Kimray–Greenfield filter insertion. *CardioVasc Intervent Radiol* 1981;4:215

53. Menzoian JO, Logerfo FW, Doyle JE, Weitzman AF, Sequeira JC: Technical modifications in the placement of inferior vena caval filter devices. *Am J Surg* 1981;142:216

54. Sequeira JC, Sacks BA, Tata J, Simon M: A safe technique for introduction of the Kimray–Greenfield filter. *Radiology* 1979;133:799

55. Gonzalez R, Narayan P, Castañeda–Zuñiga WR, Amplatz K: Transvenous embolization of the internal spermatic veins for the treatment of varicocele scroti. *Urol Clin North Am* 1982;9:17

56. Rusnak B, Castañeda–Zuñiga WR, Kotula F, Herrera M, Amplatz K: An improved dilator system for percutaneous nephrostomies. *Radiology* 1982;144:174

57. Hunter JA, DeLaria GA: Hunter vena cava balloon: rationale and results. *J Vasc Surg* 1984;1:491

58. Hunter JA, Dye WS, Javid H, Najafi H, Golding MD, Serry C: Permanent transvenous balloon occlusion of the inferior vena cava: experience with 60 patients. *Ann Surg* 1977;186:491

59. Stiegel D, Duesman JF: Experience with the Hunter–Sessions inferior vena cava balloon occluder. *Arch Surg* 1979;114:746

60. Williams DF: Implantable prostheses. *Phys Med Biol* 1980;25:611

61. Günther RW, Schild M, Fries A, Storkel S: Vena caval filter to prevent pulmonary embolism: experimental study. *Radiology* 1985;156:315

62. Fee HJ, McAvoy JH, O'Connell TX: Treatment and prevention of Mobin–Uddin umbrella misplacement. *Arch Surg* 1978;113:331

63. Isch JH, Shumacker HB Jr: Embolization of caval umbrella: discussion and report of successful removal from the right ventricle. *J Thorac Cardiovasc Surg* 1976;72:256

64. Edoga JK, Widmann WD: Avoiding renal vein entry when implanting the Mobin–Uddin vena cava umbrella filter. *Arch Surg* 1979;144:752

65. Mobin–Uddin K: Vena cava interruption: three points of view. *Contemp Surg* 1982;20:43

66. Nevin WS: Migration of vena cava filter. *JAMA* 1972;222:88

67. Flores L, Caldera F, Lotlikar U, et al: Arterial thromboembolism: a complication after insertion of Mobin–Uddin vena cava filter. *NY State J Med* 1982;82:1588

68. Castañeda F, Herrera M, Cragg AH, et al: Migration of a Kimray–Greenfield filter to the right ventricle. *Radiology* 1983;149:690

69. Leiter B, Sequeira J, Weitzman AF, Menzoian J: A complication following Kimray–Greenfield filter insertion. *CardioVasc Intervent Radiol* 1981;4:215

70. Simon M, Palestrant AM: Transvenous devices for the management of pulmonary embolism. *CardioVasc Intervent Radiol* 1980;3:308

71. Sequeira JC, Sacks BA, Tata J, Simon M: A safe technique for introduction of the Kimray–Greenfield filter. *Radiology* 1979;133:799

72. Phillips MR, Widrich WC, Johnson WC: Perforation of the inferior vena cava by the Kimray–Greenfield filter. *Surgery* 1980;87:233

73. Greenfield LJ, Crute SL: Retrieval of the Greenfield vena caval filter. *Surgery* 1980;88:719

74. Akins CW, Thurer RL, Waltman AC, Margolies MN, Schneider RC: A misplaced caval filter: its removal from the heart without cardiopulmonary bypass. *Arch Surg* 1980;115:1133

75. Allen MA, Cisterninos J, Otteseno E, Queral L, Dagher F: The Kimray–Greenfield filter: a case of unusual misplacement. *CardioVasc Intervent Radiol* 1982;5:82

76. Berland LL, Maddison FE, Bernhard VM: Radiologic follow-up of vena cava filter devices. *AJR* 1980;134:1047

23

Percutaneous Uroradiologic Techniques

S. MURTHY TADAVARTHY, M.D., CAROL C. COLEMAN, M.D., DAVID W. HUNTER, M.D., TONY P. SMITH, M.D., MICHAEL D. DARCY, M.D., ANDREW H. CRAGG, M.D., GUNNAR LUND, M.D., MORTEZA K. ELYADERANI, M.D., WON J. LEE, M.D., FLAVIO CASTAÑEDA, M.D., ERICH K. SALOMONOWITZ, M.D., JANIS GISSEL LETOURNEAU, M.D., PRATAP K. REDDY, M.D., JOHN C. HULBERT, M.D., PAUL H. LANGE, M.D., CHRISTOPH L. ZOLLIKOFER, M.D., KURT AMPLATZ, M.D., AND WILFRIDO R. CASTAÑEDA-ZUÑIGA, M.D., M.Sc.,

Percutaneous nephrostomy has come a long way since its original description 30 years ago by Goodwin et al.[1] First, it has virtually replaced surgical nephrostomy for the relief of supravesical obstruction because it is easier and has far lower morbidity and mortality rates.[2,3] Second, it now is often a prelude to rapid tract dilatation to gain access to the urinary tract for such interventional procedures as stricture dilatation, stenting of ureteral fistulae, biopsies of the renal pelvis and ureter, stone removal, intrarenal operations, and local infusion of drugs. The overall success rate for tract establishment is 95%–98%.[2-6] The rate is somewhat lower (85%–90%) when there is a nondilated renal pelvis or staghorn stone.[7]

RENAL ANATOMY

Position

The human kidneys are retroperitoneal organs lying on each side of the vertebral column between the 12th thoracic and the 2nd to the 3rd lumbar vertebrae. The renal axis parallels the psoas muscle approximately 13° from the midline and the lordotic curvature of the lumbar spine. Consequently, the upper pole is more posteriorly located than the lower (Figs. 23–1 and 23–2). In addition, because the kidneys rest over the psoas muscle edge, the lateral margin of the kidney is more posteriorly positioned than the medial edge, placing the medially positioned renal hilum more anteriorly. In a cross-section of the abdomen at this level, the kidney is tilted about 30° posterior to the coronal plane of the body (Fig. 23–3).

Retroperitoneal Relations

The retroperitoneal space is demarcated anteriorly by the posterior parietal peritoneum and posteriorly by the fascia transversalis. It extends from the pelvic brim inferiorly to the diaphragm superiorly. Several structures are found within the retroperitoneum, including (1) the adrenal glands, kidneys, and ureter; (2) the descending, transverse, and ascending portions of the duodenum and the pancreas; (3) the great vessels and their principal branches; and (4) the ascending and descending colon. The extraperitoneal space is distinctly outlined by fascial planes. Meyers described three individual extraperitoneal compartments: the anterior pararenal space, containing the ascending and descending colon, the duodenum, and the pancreas; the perirenal space, containing the adrenal glands, kidneys, and proximal ureters; and the posterior pararenal space, occupied by fat (Fig. 23–4).[8] Each space can produce characteristic radiographic findings when it is occupied by abnormal collections of fluid or gas.[9]

The surface of the kidney is covered by a fibrous nonadherent capsule. The organ is surrounded by the perirenal fat, which extends into the renal sinus. The fat is enclosed by the posterior and anterior layers of the renal fascia (Gerota's fascia). Laterally, the two layers of this fascia fuse behind the ascending and descending colon to form the lateroconal fascia (Fig. 23–5). Medially, the posterior fascial layer fuses with the psoas or quadratus lumborum fascia. The anterior renal fascia blends into the dense connective tissue surrounding the aorta and inferior vena cava in the root of the mesentery as well as behind the pancreas and doudenum. Inferiorly, Gerota's fascia fuses loosely around the ureter. Superiorly, the two layers fuse firmly to the diaphragmatic fascia above the adrenal glands.[9] These relations are particularly important in the evaluation of perinephric and paranephric fluid collections.

The musculature posterior and medial to the kidney consists of the erector spinae muscle, occupying the vertebrocostal groove of the back, and the quadratus lumborum muscle, adjacent to the posterior paranephric space. Posterolaterally are the latissimus dorsi, posterior inferior serratus, external oblique, internal oblique, and transversus abdominis muscles and their related fasciae (Fig. 23–6). The thoracolumbar fascia and the renal capsule commonly resist the puncturing needle or dilating catheter during percutaneous nephrostomies and tract dilations.

Renal Axis
13° 13°
FINCH '85
AFTER BRÖDEL

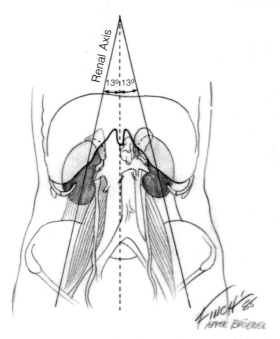

Fig. 23–1 The kidneys lie along course of psoas muscles, which tilt their axes approximately 13° from the vertical, placing upper pole more medially than lower pole.

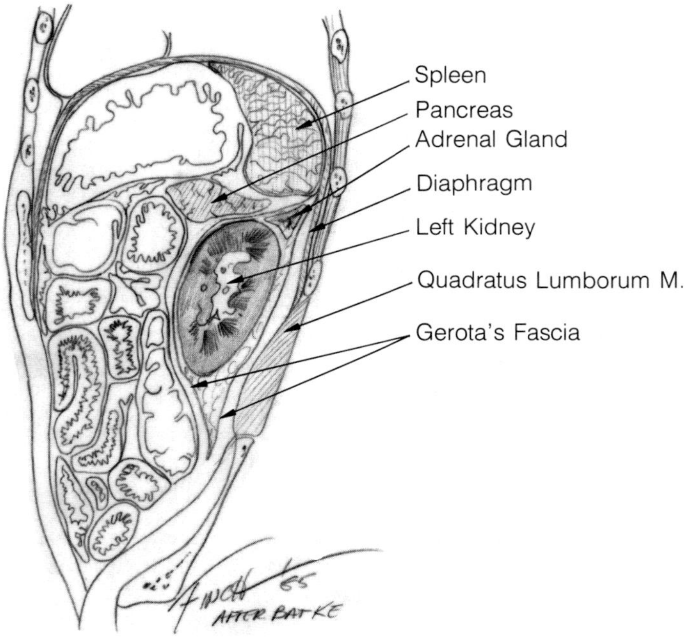

Spleen
Pancreas
Adrenal Gland
Diaphragm
Left Kidney
Quadratus Lumborum M.
Gerota's Fascia
FINCH '85
AFTER BATKE

Fig. 23–2 Left sagittal section of abdomen; kidneys lie next to psoas muscles anteroposteriorly and follow lordotic curvature of spine. Consequently, the upper poles are located more posteriorly than the lower poles.

Relations to the Pleura and Ribs

Posteriorly, the 12th rib crosses the kidney at a 45° angle (Fig. 23–7). On the left, the lower half of the kidney usually extends below the pleural reflection, whereas on the right, about two-thirds of the kidney is located below this reflection (Fig. 23–7). These relations are important when considering supracostal or infracostal approaches to the collecting system.

The posterior reflection of the parietal pleura is along a horizontal line starting at the level of the lateral surface of the 12th thoracic vertebra at the same level as, or slightly below, the origin of the 12th rib. It passes obliquely downward and laterally (Fig. 23–7).[10] At the level of the posterior axillary line, it lies below the level of the 10th rib. The 12th rib crosses the pleural reflection 4 cm from the rib's proximal edge; therefore, the distal portion of the rib lies below it.

Because of these anatomic relations, the two principal problems associated with supracostal punctures are pneumothorax and hydrothorax. The posterior recesses of the pleural space are occupied by the lung margin during deep inhalation (Fig. 23–8). During exhalation, the lung recess migrates superiorly, leaving the costophrenic angle empty. Consequently, when planning supracostal punctures, usually of the central or upper pole calices, lat-

POSTERIOR
FINCH '85
ANTERIOR

Fig. 23–3 Cross-section of the abdomen at the level of the kidneys; renal axis is tilted 30° posterior to coronal plane of body.

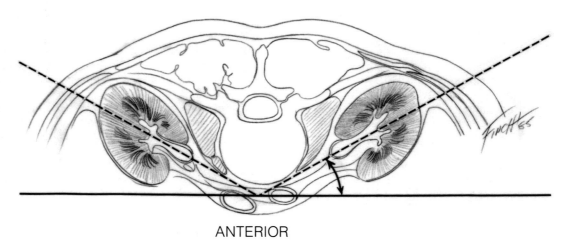

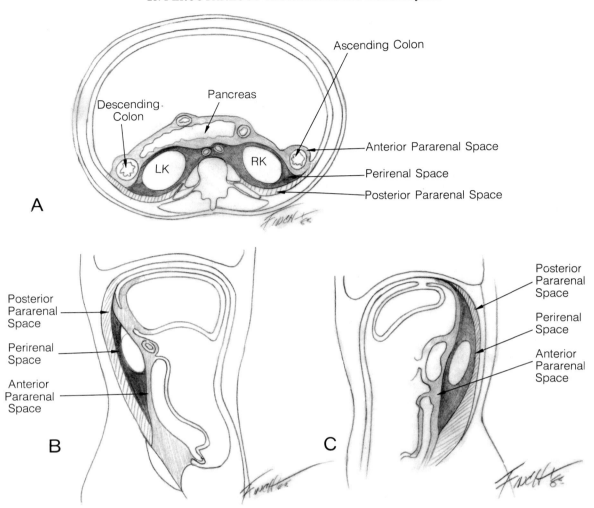

Fig. 23–4   Cross-section at the level of kidneys (A) and right sagittal (B) and left sagittal (C) views of kidney. Contents of anterior pararenal space include the ascending and descending colon, the duodenal loop, and the pancreas. Perirenal space contains the adrenal glands, kidneys, and proximal ureters. Posterior pararenal space contains only fat. LK = left kidney; RK = right kidney.

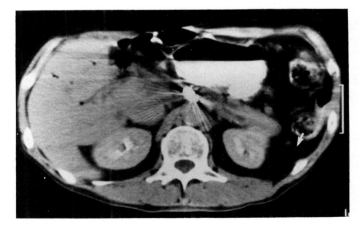

Fig. 23–5   CT scan at level of kidneys; lateral renal fascia (arrow) blends with peritoneal reflection to form paracolic gutter.

eral fluoroscopy should be used to determine the relation of the lung to the 11th and 12th ribs and to the chosen entry point to avoid lung puncture with subsequent pneumothorax development. The hydrothorax in supracostal punctures comes from dissection of irrigation fluid along the nephrostomy tract into the pleural space.

Additional problems, particularly common with intercostal punctures, are pain, caused by rubbing of the sheath or nephrostomy tube against the inferior costal margin, causing irritation of the intercostal nerve and periosteum, or significant bleeding, caused by laceration of the intercostal vessels. Therefore, in intercostal approaches, the best site for puncture is between the 11th and 12th ribs or at least 1 cm below the 12th rib. This subject is considered in more detail later in this chapter.

Relations to Adjacent Organs and Structures

The anatomic structures important in renal stone removal, in addition to the diaphragm and pleura, are the liver, spleen, and the splenic and hepatic flexures of the colon. Any of these can be perforated by the needle and dilators.

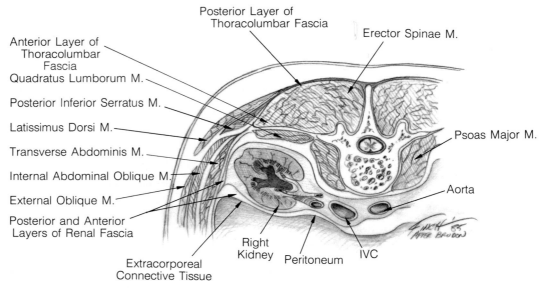

Fig. 23-6   Relations of paraspinal muscles to the kidney. IVC = inferior vena cava.

High in the abdomen (near the upper pole of the kidney), the liver and spleen are quite medial (Fig. 23-9). In more caudal punctures, the liver and spleen are more laterally placed, and the right and left portions of the colon begin to appear in the picture (Fig. 23-10). Because of these relations, the authors have found that puncturing just off the lateral border of the paraspinal muscles provides a consistently safe route into the renal collecting system by an infracostal route (Fig. 23-11). In the supracostal route, the puncture site is selected more medially, through the paraspinal muscle, to avoid injury of the spleen in particular (Fig. 23-11B). In the patient with hepatosplenomegaly, in patients with an atypical location

of bowel loops visible on the plain film of the abdomen, or in the emaciated patient (in whom the colon can be in an abnormally posterior position), a CT or ultrasound examination should be performed to determine the relation between the kidney and these organs before the percutaneous nephrostomy is performed (Fig. 23-12).

Lobar Anatomy

Embryologically, most fetal kidneys have 14 lobes, seven anterior and seven posterior. Deep surface clefts delineate the margins of the lobes. Caliceal development at this time corresponds to the pattern of lobar clefts:

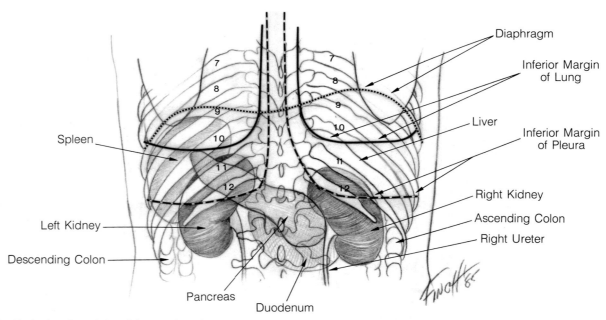

Fig. 23-7   Posterior view of the abdomen. One-third to one-half of kidneys is covered by the ribs and, therefore, by the pleura. Inferior posterior pleural reflection runs along horizontal line from 12th rib medially and passes slightly obliquely downward as it goes laterally. At axillary line, it is positioned under the 10th rib. Medially, pleura can be below the 12th rib.

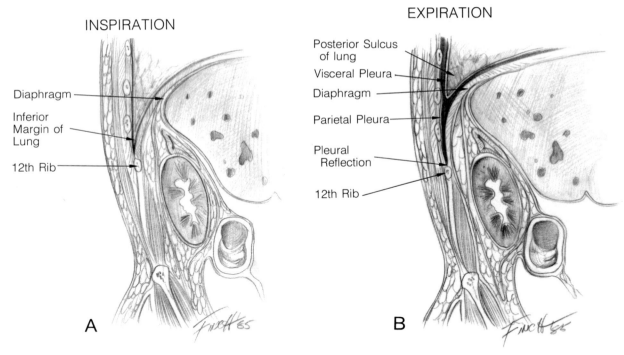

Fig. 23–8 Movement of the lungs with breathing. A. Lung fills posterior pleural recess; theoretically, puncture over 12th rib could cause pneumothorax. B. Lateral view of lower chest and upper abdomen during exhalation. Posterior sulcus of lung is well above 12th rib in most patients. Therefore, when planning a supracostal puncture, it is important to perform fluoroscopy of the lung in the lateral position to determine the depth of inhalation or exhalation at which puncture of the lung can best be avoided.

each lobe has one calix, one papilla, and surrounding cortex on its base (centrilobar cortex) and sides (septal cortex). After the 28th week of gestation, various degrees of assimilation of the independent lobes occur; and reduction in the number of calices, papillae, and surface lobar clefts follows. There is a greater degree of fusion of the calices than papillae by the time of birth. In the adult kidney, there are an average of 8.7 calices and 10.7 papillae.[10,11] The process of fusion results in a compound calix, usually in the upper and lower lobes, into which two, three, or more papillae drain. The calix therefore loses its one-to-one relation with an individual lobe and may drain several adjacent lobes.

Another possible result of fusion is the disappearance of the septal cortex. When the fusion is complete, the septal cortex is completely lost, and the medullary portions of adjacent lobes abut each other directly. When lobar fusion does not occur, the septal cortex fuses with the

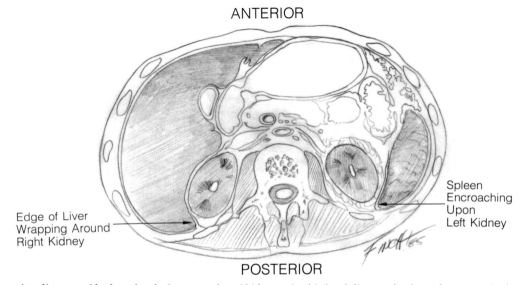

Fig. 23–9 Cross-section diagram of body at level of upper poles of kidneys. At this level, liver and spleen abut posterior lateral margin of the kidneys, leaving only a small space for entrance of puncturing needle.

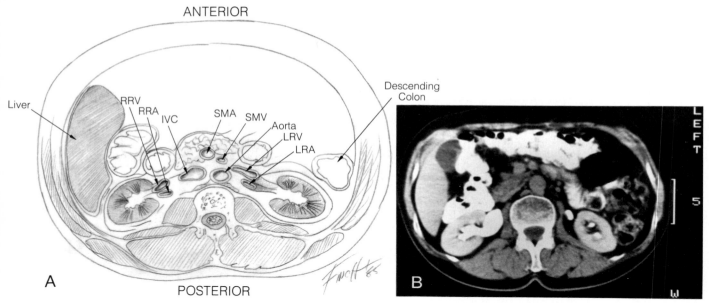

Fig. 23–10   Cross-sectional views at level of lower pole of kidneys. A. Diagram. On the left, this section is below tip of the spleen; descending colon is seen, although it is not encroaching on the kidney. On the right, liver has receded laterally, providing more room for more lateral puncture if needed. RRV = right renal view; RRA = right renal artery; IVC = inferior vena cava; SMA = superior mesenteric artery; SMV = superior mesenteric vein; LRV = left renal vein; LRA = left renal artery. B. CT cut; colon may be positioned posteriorly and medially, conpromising pathway for safe puncture.

adjacent septal cortex (septa of Bertin). Therefore, the relation of a single calix to a single papilla is preserved. Fusion between the anterior and posterior lobes in the interpolar region is rare, so in the midregion of the kidney, single calices are frequently found. In the upper and lower poles, there is usually fusion of anterior lobes to posterior lobes, with compound calices and papillae being common. Intermediate degrees of fusion also occur, in which case the septal cortex persists between the lobes to various depths.[11–15]

Offsetting the lobar pattern is the hilus, opening on the anterior surface of the kidney near its medial border. The effect is that, relative to the main renal coronal plane, the longitudinal plane between the two groups of lobes is on the posterolateral surface of the kidney. This places the anterior papillae more laterally and the posterior papillae

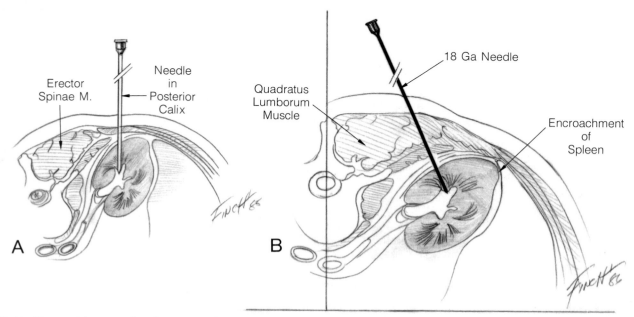

Fig. 23–11   Route of infracostal and supracostal punctures. Common skin entry site for puncturing needle is adjacent to lateral edge of paraspinal muscles; exact site will be influenced by relative position of underlying calices. B. For upper pole puncture of left kidney, a more medial entry site is selected through paraspinal muscle to avoid splenic injuries.

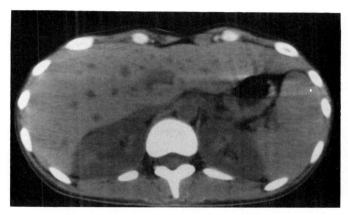

Fig. 23–12 CT scan through middle of kidney. Liver and spleen encroach on kidneys to variable degree. The only way to verify the presence of organs in the preselected needle path is by performing a CT or ultrasound examination before percutaneous puncture.

more medially relative to one another. This is more common in the midpolar region. Compound calices tend to be more in the midline of the kidney, without anterior and posterior positioning.

The posterior angulation of the kidney parallel to the psoas muscle accentuates the lateral position of any anterior calix and the medial position of any posterior calix (Fig. 23–13). The result is that the posterior calices are seen en face or end on and the anterior calices are seen tangentially (Fig. 23–14). The central calices generally are paired and arranged in two rows on either side of a line that divides the kidney longitudinally into anterior and posterior halves. The anterior calices are irregularly arranged about 70° anterior to the frontal plane of the kidney.[14,15] The posterior calices are more regular in position and lie about 20° posterior to the frontal plane (Fig. 23–13). However, there is great variability in the positioning of the calices, and occasionally just the opposite occurs (Fig. 23–15).[15] Therefore, before puncturing a

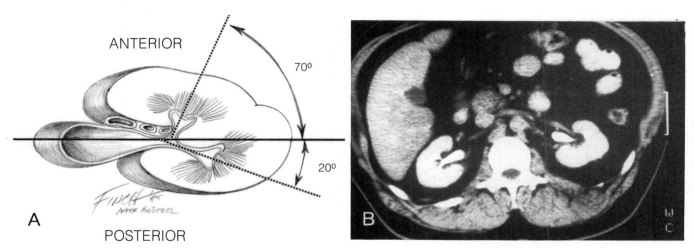

Fig. 23–13 Brödel type of kidney. A. Typically, in these kidneys posterior calix is located 20° behind sagittal plane and anterior calix 70° in front. B. CT scan at level of kidneys shows typical Brödel kidney on right.

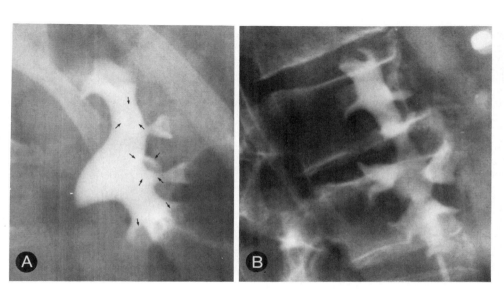

Fig. 23–14 A. IVU shows posterior calices on end (arrows) and anterior calices tangentially. B. Lateral film of retrograde pyelogram.

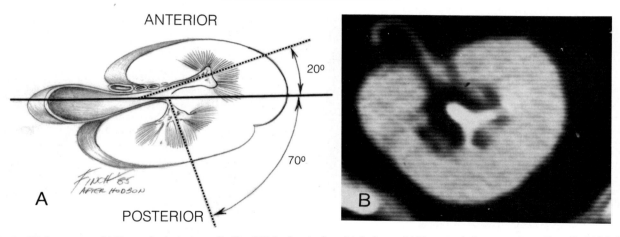

ANTERIOR

20°

70°

A

POSTERIOR

Fig. 23–15   Hudson type of kidney. A. Anterior calix lies 20° in front of sagittal plane of kidney and the posterior calices lie 70° behind. B. CT scan of Hudson's kidney.

calix, one should use lateral fluoroscopy or oblique views from an intravenous urogram or retrograde pyelogram to determine which calix or calices are posterior and which are anterior.

Arterial Anatomy

Brödel was the first to recognize the segmental distribution of the renal artery.[16] However, it was Graves, in 1954, whose excellent work described the constant distribution of intrarenal arteries which usually divides the renal parenchyma into specific anatomic segments.[17,18]

The main renal artery divides into anterior and posterior branches (Fig. 23–16). The anterior division is the direct continuation of the main renal artery and divides into three or four branches, whereas the posterior division continues without significant branching. From the two main divisions, there are five constant arterial segments (Fig. 23–17). There are four anterior segmental arteries— apical, upper, middle, and lower—and one posterior segmental artery.[19] These segmental arteries are end arteries that do not intercommunicate. The segmental arteries

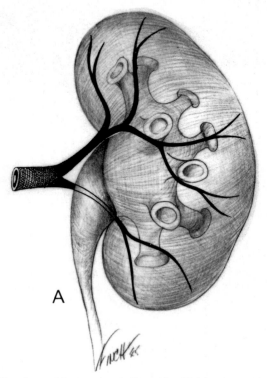

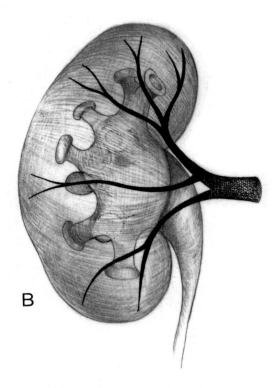

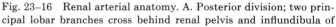

Fig. 23–16   Renal arterial anatomy. A. Posterior division; two principal lobar branches cross behind renal pelvis and infundibula of upper and lower caliceal groups. B. Anterior division supplies several lobar branches, which cross in front of renal pelvis and infundibula.

PLANE OF ARTERIAL DIVISION

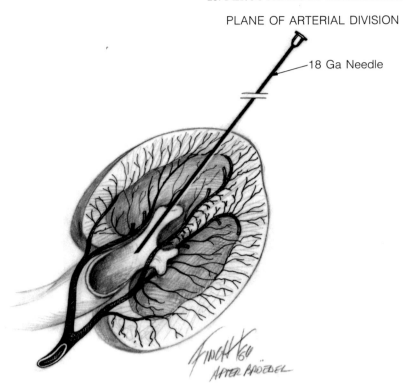

—18 Ga Needle

FINCH '61
AFTER BRÖDEL

Fig. 23–17 Cross-section of kidney showing relations of anterior and posterior divisions of renal artery to renal pelvis and infundibula. Plane of arterial division is the least vascular area of the kidney and is usually the place where nephrostomy punctures should be performed to avoid damage to large vascular structures.

divide into 8–12 interlobar arteries, which become arcuate arteries, generally upon entering the renal parenchyma at the corticomedullary junction. They are usually paired, one to each adjacent papilla. Therefore, each papilla is supplied by at least two interlobar arteries. The arcuates run in the corticomedullary junction, giving off perpendicular interlobular arteries supplying the cortex.[20–22]

The anterior segmental arteries supply the anterior and posterior surface of the anterior row of calices. They extend onto the posterior renal surface and provide the vascular supply to the anterior surface of the posterior row of calices.[14,18,22] The posterior segmental artery crosses the posterior aspect of the upper renal pelvis or proximal upper infundibulum and supplies the posterior aspect of the posterior row of calices.

The size of the posterior segmental artery is highly variable. In more than 50% of human kidneys, it is confined to the middle or upper half of the posterior renal surface without extending to the midcoronal plane or convex lateral border. In these kidneys, the posterior segmental artery vascularizes only the posterior parenchyma of the posterior row of calices. In 30% of the population, the posterior segmental artery reaches the lateral border of the kidney or beyond to meet the adjacent anterior segmental artery in the midcoronal plane. Here, the posterior segmental artery carries more of the vascular supply of the posterior row of calices. Only rarely does the posterior segmental artery supply the entire anterior surface of the posterior row of calices.[18]

It is obviously important that any puncture and subsequent tract dilation avoid transection of any large artery. The principal segmental arteries lie relatively deep within the kidney, running close to the infundibula within the hilar area. By the time their branches have reached the more peripheral level of the calices, they have become considerably smaller (Fig. 23–17). Once the corticomedullary junction has been reached (beyond the territory of the central collecting system), the vessels are small. Therefore, the puncture site should be chosen as far peripherally as possible. Ideally, the needle should enter the calix end on rather than side on, avoiding the interlobar arteries, which can cross the infundibula.

Positioning of the Patient: Overview

Generally, because of the smaller vessels involved, a posterior calix is entered end on. In order to do this, the affected side of the patient is raised from the table top. For example, in the patient with the kidney posteriorly obliqued 30° and the posterior calix angled 20° posterior to the frontal plane of the kidney, the affected side would have to be raised 30°–40° to see the posterior calix on end (Fig. 23–18). This angle will differ from patient to patient and can be determined fluoroscopically.

Selection of an appropriate skin entrance site is important because of the contiguous organs that could be punctured. The safest route is just adjacent to the paraspinal muscles; if one goes too far laterally, the liver, spleen, or colon could be punctured.

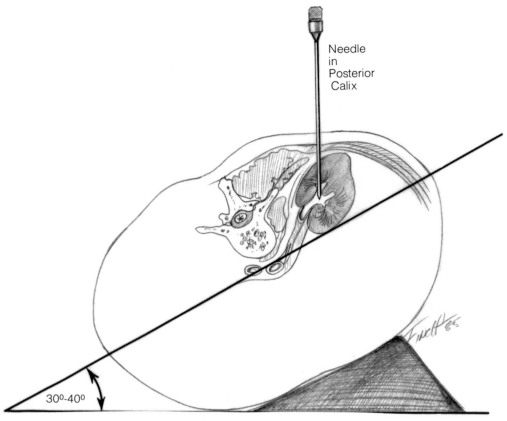

Fig. 23–18 To puncture posterior calix end-on, usually affected side of the patient is raised approximately 30°–40°. Alternatively, fluoroscope can be moved to line up calix with puncturing needle.

NEPHROSTOMY DRAINAGE

Catheters and Stents for Urinary Drainage

With the aid of cross-sectional imaging and fluoroscopy, catheters can easily be introduced into or near the renal pelvis for drainage of various fluid collections such as urinomas, seromas, lymphoceles, hematomas, and abscesses. Despite the attention paid to percutaneous nephrostomy as merely the first step in interventional uroradiologic techniques, simple urinary drainage remains a common indication. Nephrostomy drainage will not divert all the urine, and so will not be adequate by itself in conditions such as ureterocutaneous fistulae, but it can be invaluable—even lifesaving—in relieving renal obstruction.

The newer technical achievements in percutaneous nephrostomy drainage were made possible by:

1. The experience gained with interventions in cyst punctures and transcutaneous biopsies in and around the kidney;
2. The design of fascial, coaxial, and balloon dilators that make it possible to dilate a tract to as much as 30F within 15–30 min;
3. Development of trocar–cannula systems for single-step placement of nephrostomy catheters; and
4. Development of catheters of different sizes, shapes, and lengths made from materials such as polyethylene, silicone, Teflon, and combinations of plastic polymers

to achieve the stiffness necessary for introduction into the renal pelvis or ureters.

EXTERNAL DRAINAGE CATHETERS

Pigtail Catheter

This is an angiographic style catheter ranging in size from 5F–10F. (For drainage purposes, manufactured nephrostomy pigtail or polyethylene catheters are used in order to be able to create sideholes along the shaft, a step that obviously is not possible with wire-mesh torque control pigtail catheters.) The pigtail configuration of the distal end (Fig. 23–19A) reduces the likelihood of accidental dislodgment,[23] which gives this design an advantage over a straight catheter. However, the retaining capacity of the pigtail is definitely inferior to that of other self-retaining configurations, such as the Cope loop and Malecot and balloon catheters. Nonetheless, the configuration of the pigtail prevents the collapse of the renal pelvis, thereby allowing free drainage of urine. The authors commonly use these catheters for temporary drainage prior to introducing a Silastic internal–external or internal stent. A recent modification has added a Cope type of retention system to a classic pigtail catheter (Tegtmeyer catheter; Medi-Tech, Inc., Watertown, MA) (Fig. 23–19B).

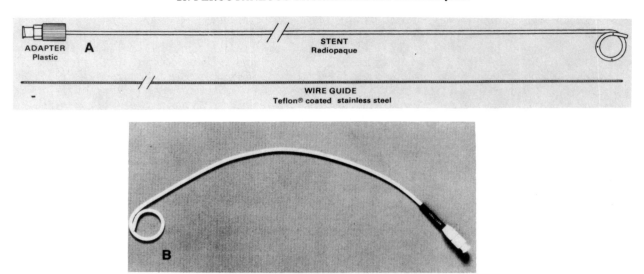

Fig. 23–19 Pigtail catheters. A. Polyethylene catheter with sideholes only in loop. (Courtesy of Cook Urological, Inc.) B. BUD Percuflex catheter. (Courtesy of Medi-Tech, Inc.)

The chief disadvantages of pigtail catheters are their stiffness, which makes them uncomfortable for long-term use; the lack of self-retention capabilities; their small size, which does not tamponade a larger nephrostomy tract such as that present after stone removal; and their small sideholes, which are easily clogged by clot and do not allow passage of debris.

Hawkins Accordion Catheter

This is a 5F–6F Teflon catheter with excellent self-retention capabilities and probably the best long-term patency rate because of the low encrustation coefficient of Teflon.[24] It can be inserted in one step when it is mounted on a long (20-inch) Chiba needle (see descrip-

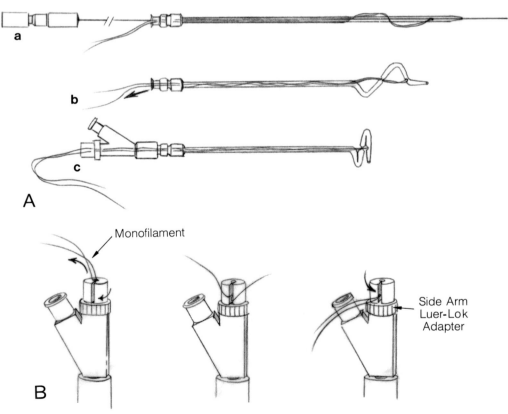

Fig. 23–20 Hawkins one-stick accordion catheter set. A. Diagram: a. 6F accordion Teflon catheter mounted over long Chiba needle. b. After needle is removed, pulling back on monofilament starts to reshape "accordion." c. Accordion has been completely reshaped and monofilament has been secured with Luer-Lok adapter. B. Close-up view of sidearm Luer-Lok adapter used to fix monofilament in accordion catheter. Sidearm is used for flushing or drainage.

tion of Hawkins one-step technique in puncture section), or it can be passed over a guidewire in the same fashion as any other angiographic catheter (Fig. 23–20). This catheter is now available from Cook, Inc. For exchange purposes, the monofilament thread is released, and a wire is passed through the lumen, gently straightening the accordion loops. Once the wire reaches the renal pelvis, the catheter is exchanged for a new one of equal dimensions. Because of the stiffness of Teflon, it is almost impossible to pull this catheter out when it is properly looped within the collecting system.

Cope Loop

This catheter is commonly used in interventional radiology, its distinct advantage being its self-retaining capacity.[25] The Cope loop has a monofilament string passed through its proximal end and the lumen and brought out through a proximal hole. The distal end of the string is attached to the tip of the catheter. Therefore, when the operator pulls on the proximal end, a loop is created. The configuration is maintained by tying the string to the proximal end of the catheter just below the hub and covering it with a rubber sleeve (Fig. 23–21). The size of the Cope loop may make reshaping difficult in a nondilated renal pelvis, although an experienced operator usually can reshape the loop even in a small collecting

system. Commercially, Cope loops, made from C-Flex, are available in 8F–14F diameters in different lengths for use as external or combined external–internal stents.

Occasionally, the encrustation of urinary salts on the string creates difficulties at the time of exchange or removal of this catheter, preventing the loop from being straightened with a guidewire. In such a case, the catheter hub and thread are cut off, a sheath introducer is passed over the catheter to the loop, and the catheter is pulled back forcefully against the advancing edge of the sheath; this usually straightens the loop (Fig. 23–22).[26] The catheter is then removed through the sheath, and a guidewire is passed into the renal pelvis for catheter replacement.

Because of the softness and high coefficient of friction of C-Flex, insertion of these catheters will be simplified by using either an introducer sheath or a cannula stiffener that fits a 0.038-inch wire and is flexible enough to follow gentle curves along the tract. Alternatively, the cannula can be curved before introduction to facilitate passage.

A modified form of this catheter (Cook, Inc.) is longer and has sideholes along its shaft to allow it to be used as an internal–external drainage stent with the loop in the bladder or the renal pelvis (Fig. 23–23A). The loop also has been modified for retrograde placement in patients with urinary diversions. This modification is necessary to eliminate the overlapping tip, and sideholes are made

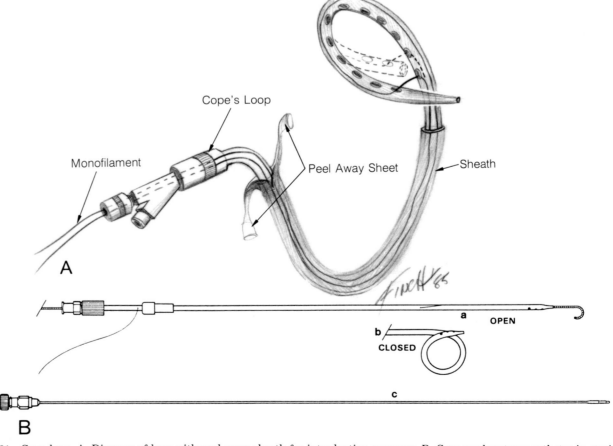

Fig. 23–21   Cope loop. A. Diagram of loop with peel-away sheath for introduction purposes. B. Cope nephrostomy catheter in straightened (a) and closed (b) positions. C. Introduction stiffening cannula.

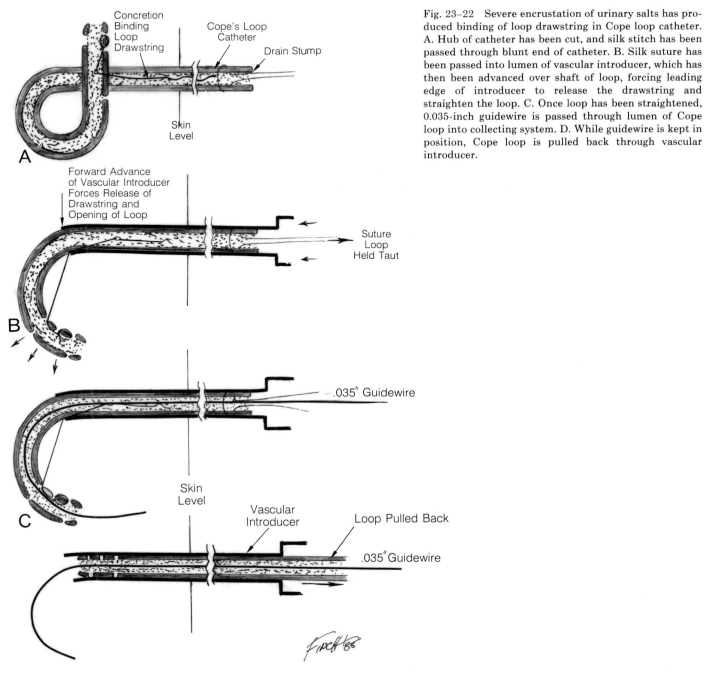

Fig. 23–22   Severe encrustation of urinary salts has produced binding of loop drawstring in Cope loop catheter. A. Hub of catheter has been cut, and silk stitch has been passed through blunt end of catheter. B. Silk suture has been passed into lumen of vascular introducer, which has then been advanced over shaft of loop, forcing leading edge of introducer to release the drawstring and straighten the loop. C. Once loop has been straightened, 0.035-inch guidewire is passed through lumen of Cope loop into collecting system. D. While guidewire is kept in position, Cope loop is pulled back through vascular introducer.

only within the catheter loop, because sideholes within the bowel will allow mucus to get into the catheter, which commonly results in obstruction and infection (Fig. 23–23B,C).

Stamey Suprapubic Malecot Catheter

In its 14F version modified for nephrostomy use, the Stamey catheter is packaged with a Teflonized internal stiffener that fits over a 0.038-inch guidewire (Fig. 23–24).[27] During stent insertion, the introducer—created from the original Stamey trocar by removal of the cutting edge to prevent puncture of the renal pelvis—holds the wings of the Malecot tip flat against the catheter shaft.

The Malecot tip minimizes accidental dislodgment, and the larger lumen is effective in draining not only urine but also pus and blood.

The chief disadvantage of this catheter is its stiffness, which makes it uncomfortable for the patient to lie supine. The stiff wings also irritate the collecting system to such an extent that, in a few instances, granulation tissue has grown into the wings, necessitating operative removal.

Amplatz Dual-Stiffness Malecot (Stamey) Catheter

This is a C-Flex larger lumen, 14F catheter with a Malecot tip at its distal end, giving it excellent retention

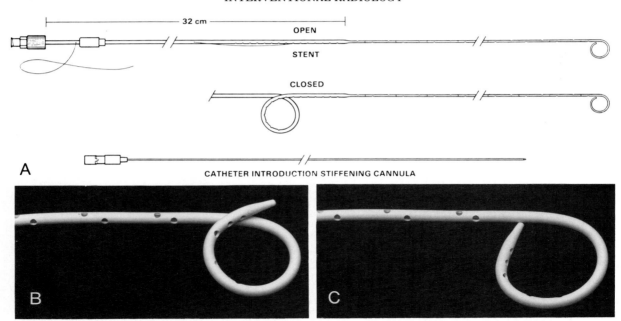

Fig. 23–23   Cope loops. A. Cope nephroureterostomy stent; loop is formed within renal pelvis to secure catheter in place; long ureteral stent ends in pigtail. Traditional (B) and modified (C) Cope loop for retrograde insertion in patients with ileal loops. Change in loop configuration avoids damage by catheter tip.

properties (Fig. 23–25). It drains not only clear fluid but also thick purulent or serosanguineous collections.

The catheter has a unique design. The distal segment is stiff, thereby preserving the retention capacity of the mushroom tip. This segment is joined to a longer, soft, flexible shaft that is well tolerated and accepted by patients for long-term drainage. Thus, the chief limitation of other Malecot designs —stiffness—has been eliminated by joining two plastics of different rigidities.[28] The Malecot wings are straightened with a flexible introducer, the combination being advanced over the guidewire into the renal pelvis.

Castañeda Malecot Catheter

This stent, manufactured by Medi-Tech, Inc., is made of Percuflex in 8F and 10.3F sizes. A stainless-steel spiral has been added to strengthen the Malecot wings and so improve the self-retention capabilities. No increase in the incidence of encrustation by urinary salts has been found as a result of the spiral. This design has one of the widest internal lumens relative to the outer diameter of all the catheters available. It comes in two lengths: 35 cm, for external drainage, and 55 cm, for internal–external drainage with the Malecot tip in the renal pelvis and a gentle curve with several sideholes in the bladder (Fig. 23–26A,B). Additional sideholes can easily be made with a paper punch. (One should practice before using these punches on actual catheters, because an error can cut out almost the entire circumference of the catheter.) The chief disadvantage of this catheter is its softness, which, although desirable for patient comfort, creates a need for an internal stiffener for introduction and removal. The stiffener is also needed to straighten the wings of the Malecot for introduction and removal. A straight universal drainage catheter made of C-Flex is available for internal–external drainage (Fig. 23–26C). Sideholes can be punched with a paper punch.

Argyle Ingram Trocar Catheter

This is a self-retaining, trilumen, polyvinyl chloride catheter available in 12F and 16F sizes (Sherwood Medical Industries) (Fig. 23–27). It was designed to prevent accidental dislodgment, and the presence of an inflatable balloon at its distal end is a unique feature. The 16F catheter has an inner lumen of 3.9 mm with an end hole of 2.5 mm and three sideholes, each measuring 3.2 mm × 5 mm, for effective drainage.[29] There are three lumens: one for balloon inflation, the second for irrigation, and the third (smaller than in other catheters) for drainage. Introduction of this soft catheter is facilitated by overdilation of the nephrostomy tract so that buckling is avoided. Also, during introduction, the catheter is stiffened with a translumbar aortography needle guide, by immersion in ice-cold sterile water,[29] or by introduction of an 11F dilator (into the 16F catheter) or a 7F dilator (into the 12F catheter).[29] The combination of dilator and catheter fits snugly over a 0.038-inch guidewire and can easily be advanced past the fascia into the renal pelvis.

The disadvantages of this catheter are, first, the many steps involved in its introduction. Second, the balloon has a tendency to rupture, even when underinflated.[18] Other problems are spontaneous balloon deflation and the reverse: the fact that sometimes the balloon does not deflate, making catheter removal difficult.[29]

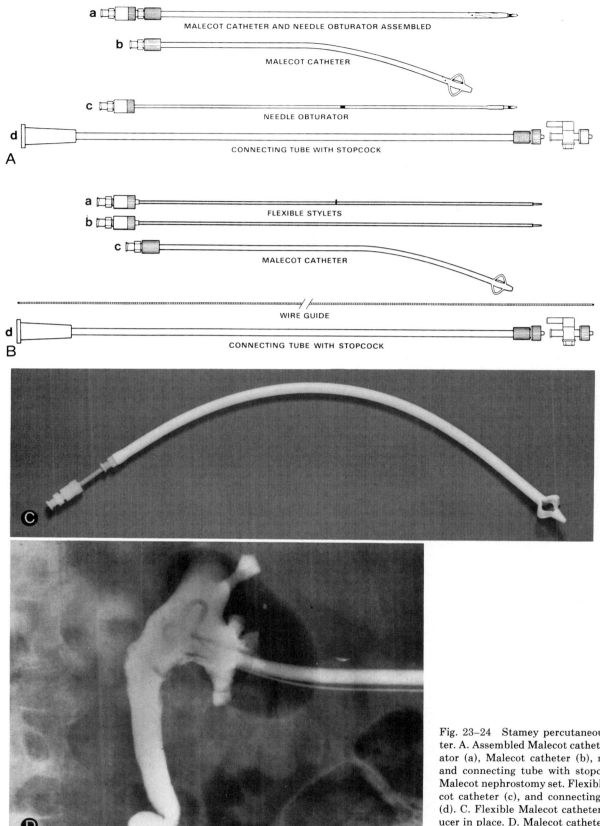

a MALECOT CATHETER AND NEEDLE OBTURATOR ASSEMBLED

b MALECOT CATHETER

c NEEDLE OBTURATOR

d CONNECTING TUBE WITH STOPCOCK

A

a
b FLEXIBLE STYLETS

c MALECOT CATHETER

WIRE GUIDE

d CONNECTING TUBE WITH STOPCOCK

B

C

D

Fig. 23–24 Stamey percutaneous suprapubic catheter. A. Assembled Malecot catheter with needle obturator (a), Malecot catheter (b), needle obturator (c), and connecting tube with stopcock (d). B. Flexible Malecot nephrostomy set. Flexible stylets (a,b), Malecot catheter (c), and connecting tube with stopcock (d). C. Flexible Malecot catheter with Teflon introducer in place. D. Malecot catheter within renal pelvis in patient with pyonephrosis. (Courtesy of Cook Urological.)

Fig. 23–25 Amplatz dual-stiffness Malecot catheter. A. Junction of stiffer Malecot front end (arrow) with softer shaft. B. Dual-stiffness catheter is advanced over 0.035-inch Bentson guidewire into collecting system without much difficulty.

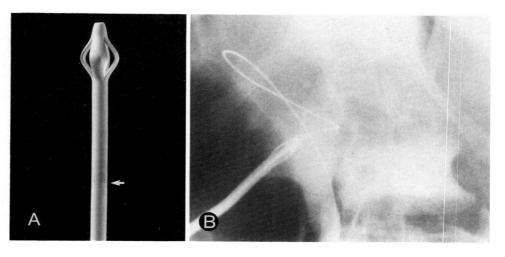

Councill Catheter

This is a self-retaining (balloon) rubber catheter in 8F–12F sizes with an end hole and two sideholes near the tip (Fig. 23–28). Because of its lower coefficient of friction, its slightly lower profile balloon, and its greater stiffness in comparison with a Foley catheter, a Councill catheter can be passed either directly over a guidewire or mounted on a stiffening angiographic catheter–dilator. The self-retention capabilities are excellent because of the balloon, making these catheters suitable for long-term drainage. The disadvantage of retention balloons is that less room is available in the renal pelvis for drainage. Generally, Councill catheters are used either in cases in which other self-retaining catheters (Cope loop, Malecot) keep falling out or after nephrostolithotomy, for tract tamponade and drainage.

Foley Catheter

This is a Silastic tube, 8F–30F in size, with no end hole and two sideholes near the tip. An end hole must be made for percutaneous introduction (Figs. 23–29 and 23–30). A metal introducer is available (Cook, Inc.) to facilitate percutaneous passage (Fig. 23–31),[30] which otherwise is extremely difficult because of the high coefficient of friction and the softness of Silastic (see section on introduction techniques). Foley catheters are used either for long-term nephrostomy drainage or following nephrostolithotomy for tract tamponade and drainage.

INTERNAL DRAINAGE WITH EXTERIORIZED CATHETERS

Amplatz Tapered Stent

This C-Flex stent is a 24F catheter that tapers to 8F for the intraureteral segment (Fig. 23–32).[31] Sideholes are present at the distal end and where the 24F portion tapers. Because of the high coefficient of friction and the softness of C-Flex, an internal Teflon stiffener that fits over a 0.038-inch wire is needed for introduction. The length of the ureteral segment can be trimmed to fit special anatomic needs, the undesired length being cut off

with scissors. A taper is then formed by pulling on the catheter tip while it is being held in steam. This catheter is ideal for use after difficult or traumatic nephrostolithotomies, particularly after manipulation in, or perforation of, the ureter and ensures that the catheter remains in the collecting system.

Smith Malecot/Ureteral Stent

This C-Flex catheter is 24F with a Malecot tip for self-retention and drainage and a long ureteral segment (Fig. 23–33). Like the Amplatz tapered catheter, the Smith stent is useful after nephrostolithotomy for tract tamponade, drainage, and ureteral stenting.

Smith Universal Stent

This is an 8F, 90-cm-long catheter made from silicone rubber (Heyer–Schulte, Cook Urological). It is frequently inserted for ureteral stenting during open surgical procedures such as pyeloplasty or ureterointestinal anastomoses and also is used in several endourologic procedures.[32] Its softer material is less irritating to the mucosa of the ureter and bladder, avoiding painful spasms and pressure feelings. The ureteral portion is cut off at the level appropriate for the particular patient, so one need not stock several lengths of catheters. The stent is provided with sideholes in a central 2.5-cm segment that is labeled on both sides with radiopaque markers (Fig. 23–34). From the nephrostogram, utilizing the endoruler or bent wire technique, the length of the ureter is measured. A similar length of catheter beginning at the segment of the sideholes plus an additional 1–2 cm is preserved, the remaining length being eliminated with scissors. At the distal end of the stent, several sideholes are made with an 18-gauge blunt needle or with a hole punch. The catheter can then be pulled through the renal pelvis and the ureter utilizing a pull-through (antegrade–retrograde) technique or be passed through a peel-away sheath.[33] The distal end rests against the bladder mucosa, and the proximal sideholes are in the renal pelvis.

Later exchanges of the catheter can be accomplished by advancing the guidewire from the proximal, exteriorized end of the stent. This end is fitted with a Luer-Lok

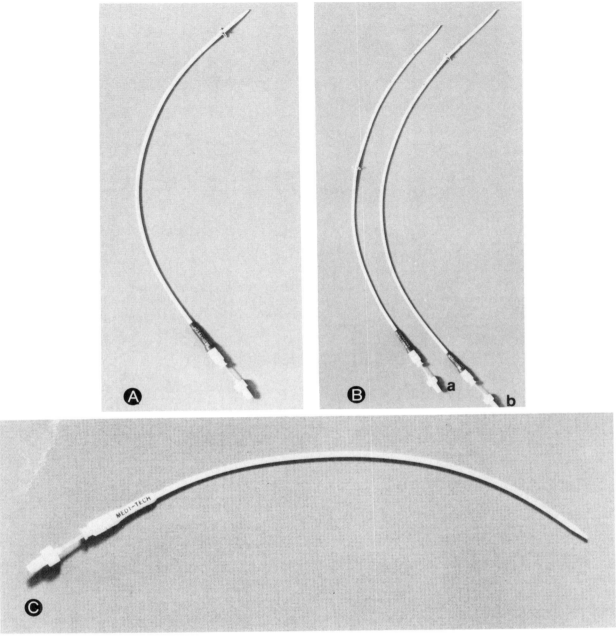

Fig. 23–26 Castañeda Malecot catheter. A. Catheter has short tip for external drainage. B. Various designs. a. Malecot placed in middle of shaft for internal drainage; Malecot is placed in renal pelvis and sideholes are placed in distal ureter and bladder. b. Modified for external–internal drainage; Malecot is placed in baldder with sideholes in renal pelvis. (Courtesy of Medi-Tech, Inc.) C. Universal straight drainage catheter with internal stiffener for introduction purposes. (Courtesy of Medi-Tech, Inc.)

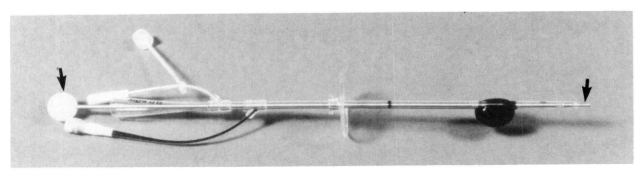

Fig. 23–27 Argyle triluminal catheter; balloon has been inflated with dye to show it to better advantage. Trocar (arrows) of catheter system is placed within central lumen for trocar introduction technique.

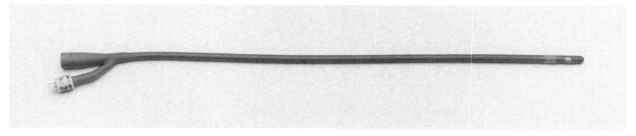

Fig. 23–28   Councill catheter.

and can be plugged to convert the patient entirely to internal drainage. A blocked universal stent can sometimes be reopened by reaming it with a guidewire or by flushing.

Looped Universal Stent (Coil)

This is a Silastic 8F stent (Medical Engineering Corp., Bardex) with three or four loops in its central segment where sideholes are located (Fig. 23–35). There are no radiopaque markers to show their position. These catheters have a small internal lumen and a high friction coefficient that makes it necessary either to place them intraoperatively or to use a pull-through technique. The friction problem has been reduced by the use of a hydrophilic compound in the surface of the Bardex catheter which makes it slippery. The large loop size often interferes with reformation in small collecting systems.

INTERNAL URETERAL STENTS

The ideal ureteral stent has features that keep it properly positioned in the ureter and is radiopaque to facilitate accurate placement. It is well tolerated and thus more likely to be made of silicone rubber than of the stiffer polyethylene. It is easy to insert by either endourologic or cystoscopic methods, and it resists encrustation by urinary crystalloids.

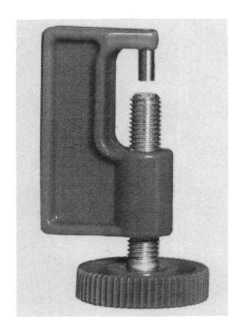

Fig. 23–29   Hole punch for perforating end holes in the tip of Foley catheters. (Courtesy of Cook Urological.)

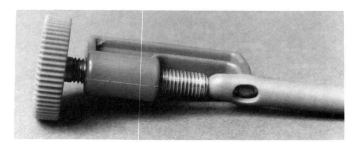

Fig. 23–30   Foley catheter with hole punch putting end hole in tip.

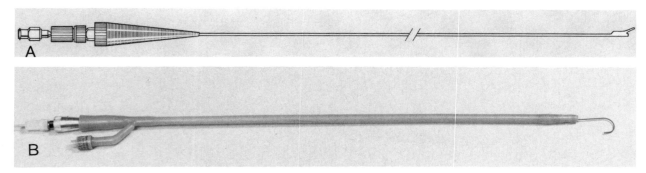

Fig. 23–31   Use of Foley introducer. A. Introducer. B. Foley catheter mounted over introducer with guidewire passed through introducer tip.

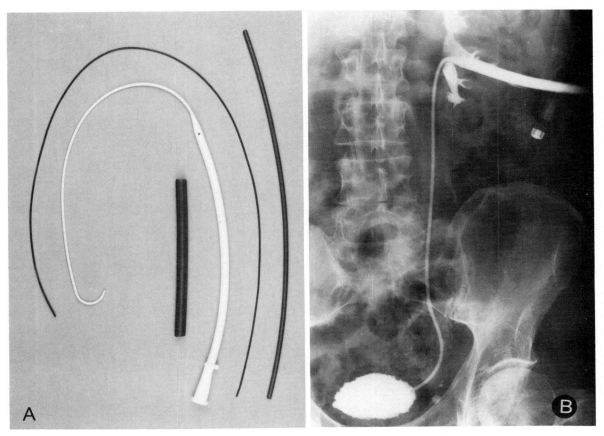

Fig. 23–32 Amplatz tapered pyeloureteral stent. A. Stent has 24F shaft for tract tamponade and 8F ureteral stent. B. Nephrostogram through stent.

Double-pigtail stents have many of these features. Unlike their single-pigtail predecessors, which are given to upward migration and to trigonal irritation,[34] double-pigtail stents are stabilized by retention curls in both the renal pelvis and the bladder, and the inward curl of the intravesical end minimizes bladder irritation.[34–36] These stents can be inserted endourologically, endoscopically, or intraoperatively.[35]

One caution is particularly important in using double-pigtail stents: there is a fine line between one that is too short, which may pull up into the ureter or damage the renal pelvis, and one that is too long, which may irritate the bladder mucosa. Accurate measurement of ureteral length and appropriate correction for radiologic magnification are mandatory.

Polyethylene Double-Pigtail Stent

These are available commercially in diameters of 5F–8F and in lengths of 8–30 cm (Cook Urological; Vance Products) (Fig. 23–36).

Polyethylene is a tasteless, odorless, thermoplastic resin with a molecular weight of 18,000.[37] It is inert and so causes minimal tissue reaction. It is also flexible, resilient, and nonwettable. The nonclotting properties diminish the tendency of catheters to become blocked by blood clots, exudates, or urinary salts.[37] However, polyethylene, like silicone, is not immune to encrustation, and deposition of crystalloids is common in patients with infected urine.[38,39]

Polyethylene stents can be introduced percutaneously without transurethral assistance. The manufacturer's set contains the stent, a guidewire, and a graduated pusher to advance the stent into place. These stents can also be introduced in retrograde fashion through a cystoscope; this procedure is facilitated by advancing the catheter over a guidewire that has already negotiated the ureteral orifice. Antegrade percutaneous insertion is successful in most cases in which retrograde passage proves impossible.[38]

Polyethylene catheters have higher flow rates than similar sizes of silicone Surgitech double-J or Heyer–Schulte Gibbons catheters.[38] Also, the stiffer nature of polyethylene is an attractive feature and is advantageous for percutaneous insertion. Its radiopacity also facilitates stent recognition under fluoroscopy.

It has been said that polyethylene catheters occlude early because of their high encrustation rate, but this has not been proved.[39] However, due to the higher encrustation, long-term indwelling catheters may become stiff and brittle, and some spontaneous fractures have been observed.[40]

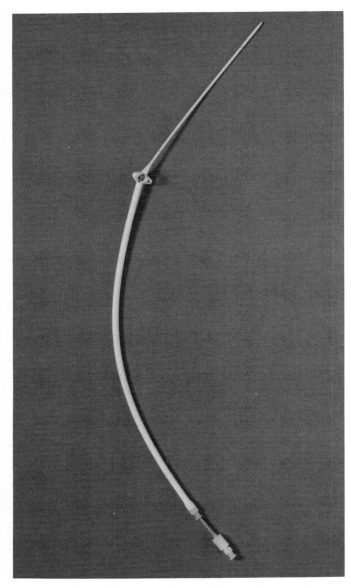

Fig. 23–33 Smith Malecot catheter with tapered ureteral stent. (Courtesy of Cook, Inc.)

Fig. 23–35 Looped Silastic universal stent; length of proximal and distal loops make this internal stent fit all lengths of pelvicaliceal systems.

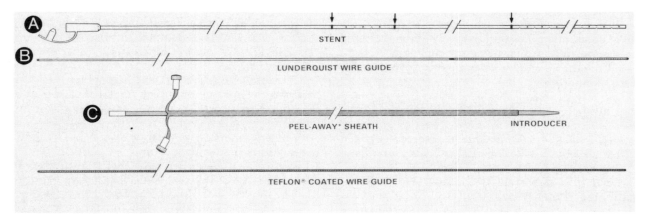

Fig. 23–34 A. Smith universal ureteral stent set. Silastic stent with sideholes in its midsegment and two radiopaque markers (arrows). Additional sideholes are placed in distal segment, with radiopaque marker showing their proximal extension. B. Lunderquist wire guide. C. Peel-away sheath introducer. (Courtesy of Cook Urological.)

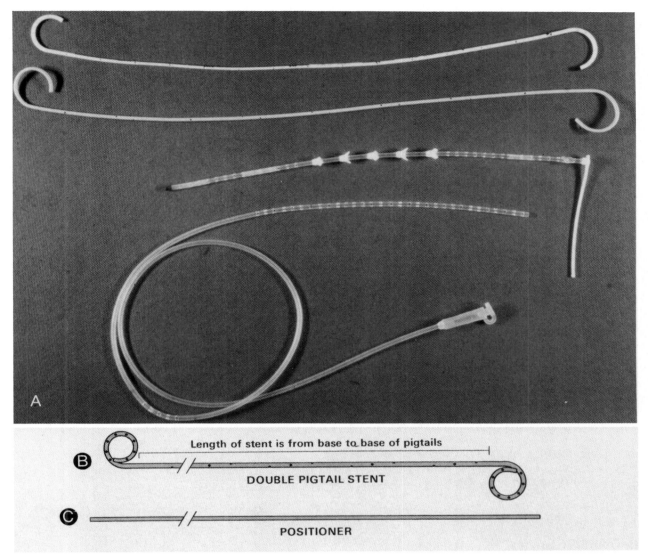

Fig. 23–36 A. Silastic double-pigtail stent. B. Gibbons stent. C. Universal stent. D. Polyurethane antegrade stent set consisting of a 6F double-pigtail stent, which comes in different lengths. E. 6F radiopaque polypropylene stent positioner. (Courtesy of Cook, Inc.)

Silicone Rubber (Silastic) Stents

Some urologists and radiologists prefer silicone to polyethylene catheters because of the spasm, irritation, and pain often associated with the use of the latter. Silicone rubber is a polymer of silicone, oxygen, and organic groups and is a flexible, inert, nonwettable material with a low encrustation coefficient that can be made as rigid as desired.[41–43] It is chemically stable in the body with little change due to temperature[43] and resists deposition of calcareous material, thereby increasing its patency compared to other catheters. Silicone rubber elicits minimal tissue reaction, and its softness and pliability eliminate irritation of the renal pelvis and bladder.[41]

Silicone rubber was first utilized as a urinary stent by Zimskind et al.[41] Later, various catheter insertion techniques were reported by other authors.[44–46] These catheters have remained indwelling with no problems for as long as 4 years,[47,48] although microscopic hematuria or pyuria is encountered occasionally.[49] Initially, silicone

rubber catheters were used as open-ended tubes with no provisions to prevent expulsion or migration. Later, Gibbons et al fabricated silicone rubber catheters with dentate barbs and a flange to prevent upward or downward migration,[46] and Finney designed a double-J silicone rubber catheter for easier insertion and to prevent migration.[47,50] The barbs of the Gibbons stent make its outer diameter 11F compared with a 7F inner lumen, and at times this design causes difficulties in placement.[48,49] Smith et al describe a pull-through technique to facilitate stent insertion.[51–53]

The encrustation rate is kept low by having the patient take plenty of oral fluids and a low-calcium diet and by preventing or treating infection. Female patients are often given low-dose prophylactic antibiotics.[47] In encrusted catheters, the inner lumen and the proximal and the distal ends are covered with urinary salts, whereas the segment that resides in the ureter is clean due to the peristaltic activity.[47]

The double-J catheters are available in 6F, 7F, and

8.5F diameters with lengths of 16, 26, 28, and 30 cm. The length of the stent is the length of its shaft: the J's are not included in the measurement. A self-retention J is molded at each end, with the two J's pointing in opposite directions, such that the proximal one hooks onto a lower calix or the renal pelvis and the lower one coils in the bladder.[50] Double-J stents can be placed endoscopically by advancing them with a pusher over a guidewire lubricated with mineral oil to minimize resistance. The catheter, guidewire, pusher, and mineral oil are available in a kit form (Medical Engineering Corp.).[47,50] The stents can also be placed during an open operation through the cut ends of the ureter utilizing a stylet.[47] Percutaneous placement is possible with slightly stiffer catheters made of modified soft silicone elastomers.

Silicone Rubber Double-J Stent

This stent comes in 6F–8F sizes, commonly with two lengths, 26 and 28 cm. The stent modified for percutaneous insertion (Medical Engineering Corp.) has two end holes and a tapered tip to facilitate introduction. Silicone rubber catheters are barely radiopaque and have a high friction coefficient. For easier recognition under fluoroscopy, Medical Engineering Corporation recently introduced a radiopaque version. To overcome the problem of friction, sterile mineral oil is applied liberally both inside and outside the catheter to facilitate passage over Teflon-coated guidewires. The commercially available set has a pusher, guidewire, and mineral oil. Silicone rubber catheters are often said to have higher patency rates because of their lesser encrustation; however, there are no data to support this claim. The principal advantage of silicone rubber is its softness, which avoids the pain and frequency of urination provoked by the stiffer polyethylene catheters.

C-Flex Double-J Stent

This catheter (Cook, Inc.), designed by Amplatz, has a lower friction coefficient and larger internal diameter than the 8F Silastic double-J stent. The stent is therefore easier to introduce while probably remaining patent for the same length of time.[54] An internal stiffener and a pusher are provided with the manufacturer's set (Fig. 23–37). These stents need further clinical evaluation, because they are the newest of the ureteral stents. Physically, C-Flex material is easier to introduce than polyethylene and, biologically, behaves much like silicone rubber.

Gibbons Ureteral Stent

The efficacy of silicone rubber for indwelling ureteral stents has been demonstrated repeatedly,[32,39,41,44–46] but the homemade catheters of this material were fraught with problems, such as migration, expulsion, and collapse.[48,49] Many of these problems were overcome by the stents designed by R.P. Gibbons.

The currently available Gibbons stent has a collar with a retrieval tail at the distal end to prevent upward migration. The catheter has a radiopaque tip, and its entire length resists radial compression by virtue of the incor-

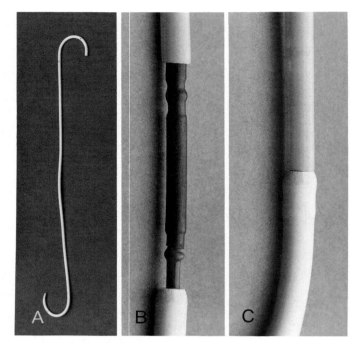

Fig. 23–37   Percuflex antegrade stent (A); black internal stiffener with retention beads and both stent and pusher advanced over (B); stent and pusher have been secured over the retention beads.

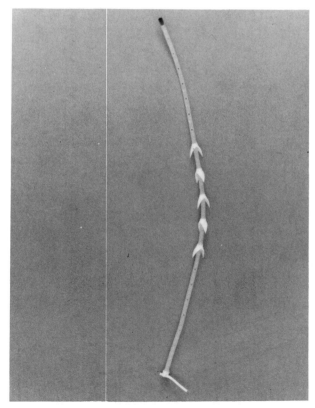

Fig. 23–38   Silastic ureteral Gibbon's stent.

poration of a spring coil into the wall. Radiopaque dentate protrusions (barbs) are present in the middle third of the stent; these protrusions rest on the obstructive site, preventing distal migration. However, the stent may migrate inferiorly if the dentate protrusions are below the site of stricture or obstruction.[49] Use of this stent is not advisable in patients with ureteral fistulae, because of the possible protrusion of the dentate wings through the openings. These stents are available in 7F and 9F sizes with a length of 15 or 23 cm (Fig. 23–36 and 23–38).

Even with the improved design, the Gibbons stent occasionally migrates upward. In this situation, a Fogarty balloon catheter can be introduced into the distal end, and, by gentle traction, the stent can be repositioned.[55] Alternatively, alligator forceps can be used under fluoroscopic control to grasp the retrieval tail.[56]

The other mechanical problems of indwelling stents, such as hematuria, infection, and reflux, are observed to a minor degree.[49] The extent of encrustation can be reduced by a high fluid intake.

The Gibbons stent is usually inserted retrograde using a cystoscope or a 24F panendoscope. At times, the stent is difficult to insert; in these cases Gibbons et al recommend softening the stricture by advancing a 4F catheter and leaving it for 4–5 days before stent insertion.[48,49]

An innovative technique has been described by Smith et al for introducing a Gibbons stent with the aid of a percutaneous nephrostomy (Fig. 23–39).[51,52] A 0.038-inch guidewire and angiographic catheter are advanced through the tract into the bladder. The guidewire is extracted from the bladder with the cystoscope in the usual fashion. Alternatively, when instruments cannot be advanced through the urethra, an end hole Foley catheter is inserted into the bladder, and a basket or snare is introduced through it to capture the wire and pull it out through the urethra (Fig. 23–40).[57] The distal end of the angiographic catheter is cut off, and a 10F filiform follower is screwed into the catheter. A 260-cm-long, 0.038-inch guidewire is passed retrograde through the sidehole of the angiographic catheter until it exits through the proximal end at the flank, where it is held with a hemostat. The ureteral end of the guidewire is threaded through the sidehole of the filiform follower and is subsequently passed through the lumen of a Gibbons catheter. An 8F angiographic catheter is inserted over the distal end of the guidewire and held with a second hemostat. By holding the guidewire taut at both ends, a mechanical advantage is gained, and the Gibbons stent can be pulled into the ureter until its distal end rests against the ureteral orifice in the bladder lumen. The angiographic catheter, the filiform follower, and the guidewire are pulled out through the nephrostomy tract, and the distally placed angiographic catheter is pulled out from the urethral end. Essentially the same steps are followed to insert a Gibbons stent in patients with ileal conduits,[53] the only difference being that the guidewire is brought out through the ileostomy stoma rather than through the urethra.

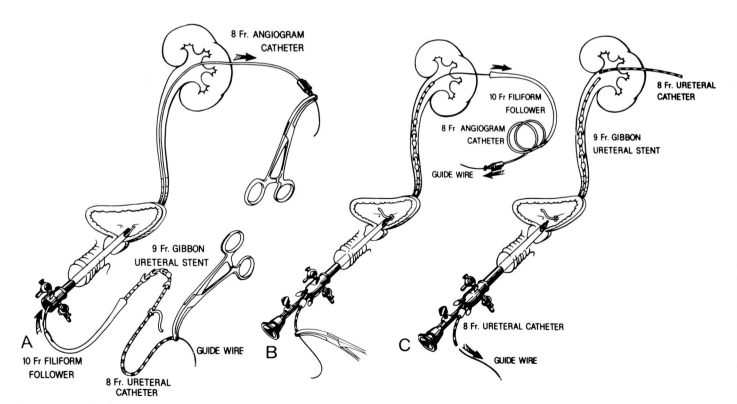

Fig. 23–39 Combined percutaneous–cystoscopic technique for placement of Gibbons ureteral stent. A. Cystoscope has been passed into bladder to withdraw angiographic catheter placed antegrade. To the end of the angiographic catheteter, 10F filiform and 9F Gibbons ureteral stent have been attached. B. By gently pulling back on angiographic catheter, Gibbons stent has been positioned. C. Gibbons stent has been detached from guidewire and angiographic catheter, which has been left in renal pelvis for temporary external drainage, and the rest of the instruments and wires are being removed from the urethra. (Reproduced from Smith AD, Lange PH, Miller RP, et al: Introduction of the Gibbons ureteral stent facilitated by antecedent percutaneous nephrostomy. *J Urol* 1978;120:543.)

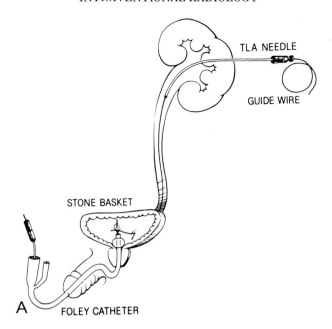

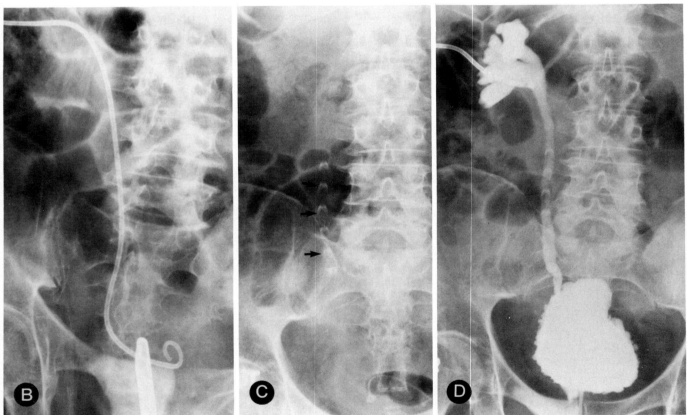

Fig. 23–40 Pull-through technique. A. Noncystoscopic technique for withdrawal of guidewire from bladder. Through Foley catheter with end hole, Dormia basket has been passed into bladder. Guidewire has been advanced antegrade from percutaneous tract and manipulated into basket, which is then closed and removed through urethra. B. External–internal drainage catheter has been passed through obstruction in distal ureter, placing tip within baldder. Cystoscope has been passed into bladder to extract angiographic catheter. C. Using the pull-through technique, Gibbons stent has been pulled into ureter (arrows). D. Nephrostogram through temporary external drainage catheter reveals widely patent Gibbons stent with free flow of contrast medium into bladder.

Guidewires

Many types of angiographic guidewires are available for use in urointerventional procedures. Of these, the authors have found the following most useful:

0.035-inch floppy-tip Bentson (Cook, Inc.);
0.038-inch wide-J (Cook);
Lunderquist (0.038-inch; Cook; Surgimed);
Lunderquist–Ring torque control (0.038-inch; Cook);
"Coat-hanger" (0.018-inch Cook);
"Rocket" (0.018-inch Hawkins–NASA);
Wire stiffeners (Dotter cannula);
Amplatz stiffening (0.035- and 0.038-inch; Cook).

FLOPPY-TIP (BENTSON) WIRE

This Teflonized wire (TSFB; Cook) is valuable in negotiating dilated, tortuous ureters with minimal trauma, particularly in the hands of less experienced operators. It is also helpful in collecting systems filled with staghorn calculi. A word of caution: when this is used as the primary or sole wire, the entire floppy segment should be coiled within the renal pelvis or advanced down the ureter before one attempts to pass dilators or catheters over it, because if part of the floppy segment is outside the collecting system, the wire can easily be dislodged during the passage of a dilator or catheter, causing loss of the tract and necessitating a new puncture.

TEFLONIZED J-WIRE

Until the recently developed Amplatz stiffening wire took over, this wire was the primary working wire for nephrostolithotomy. There is no advantage to a tight-J over a wide-J.

LUNDERQUIST WIRE

This 0.038-inch wire comes either Teflonized (Surgimed) or in stainless steel (Cook). This is an extraordinarily strong wire with a short (2–3 cm) floppy leading segment and a stiff stainless-steel shaft. It is useful in passing drainage catheters, dilators, or stents in patients with fibrotic stenoses along the urinary tract or in the retroperitoneum, as from previous surgery. The weak point of this wire is the junction of the stiff and floppy segments, where the wire may bend and, occasionally, break. If positioned near a curve in the urinary tract, this joint can bend sharply, producing a rigid, sharp point that can easily perforate the collecting system.

LUNDERQUIST–RING TORQUE CONTROL WIRE

This 0.038-inch stainless-steel wire (Cook) has a short floppy tip that, because of its method of construction (soldering the spring coil to the central stiff core), can be rotated for manipulation around corners. The stiffness of this wire also facilitates the passage of catheters through fibrotic tracts.

COAT-HANGER WIRE

This 0.018-inch wire has a semirigid stainless-steel shaft and a short flexible tip (Cook). It is passed through a 22-gauge Chiba needle in Cope's one-step nephrostomy technique.

ROCKET WIRE

The special alloy of this wire, made by the National Aeronautics and Space Administration (NASA) and used by Hawkins and collaborators, creates a strong wire available in 0.018 inch and larger sizes. This wire is ideal for one-step manipulations, because it has a short flexible tip but a stiff shaft that facilitates catheter placement or dilation through fibrotic tracts.[58] The wire is not yet commercially available but can be obtained from I.F. Hawkins (Gainesville, FL).

WIRE STIFFENERS (DOTTER CANNULA)

Dotter described the use of this semiflexible stainless-steel cannula for stiffening polyvinyl chloride angioplasty balloon catheters. It also can be used inside nephrostomy drainage catheters to support the guidewire, particularly in obese patients, in whom kinking of the wire in the perinephric tissues is common, or in patients with postoperative perirenal fibrosis.

A metal cannula introducer was designed by Cope for the introduction of Silastic Foley catheters.[30] In addition to providing added stiffness by stretching the catheter, it decreases its outer diameter.

AMPLATZ STIFFENING WIRE

This wire has a stiff shaft and a floppy tip that comes in short (2-cm) and long (8-cm) versions.[59] The two principal differences between this wire and the other stiff wires, such as the Lunderquist, are that it is Teflon coated and that the junction of the stiff and floppy portions is "graduated." This less abrupt change makes it easier for this wire to pass around tight corners and eliminates worries about the stiff portion perforating the collecting system. This combination of characteristics makes the Amplatz wire ideal for most urointerventional procedures.

Dilators

Several dilator sets are available to enlarge the percutaneous tract either for drainage catheter placement or for nephrostolithotomy:

Angiographic Teflon (6F–24F);
Fascial (8F–36F; Cook Urological);
Teflon coaxial (8F–18F; Cook Urological);
8F tapered-tip coaxial Amplatz dilators (8F–34F; Cook; Vantec; Medi-Tech);
Amplatz 6/10 or 6/12 long tapered Teflon;
Metal;
Balloon.

Fig. 23–41 Angiographic Teflon dilators tapered to fit 0.038-inch guidewire.

ANGIOGRAPHIC TEFLON DILATORS

These dilators come in French sizes of 6 to 24 (Fig. 23–41). Because of their rigidity, they can be used to dilate tracts in scarred postoperative flanks. Each dilator is tapered to fit a 0.038-inch guidewire. They are not truly radiopaque and so can be difficult to control fluoroscopically.

FASCIAL DILATORS

These radiopaque, semirigid polyurethane dilators come in 8F–36F sizes and have a tip tapered to fit a 0.038-inch guidewire (Fig. 23–42). They are used for tract dilation for nephrostolithotomy and are passed individually over the guidewire.[60,61] A working cannula is provided with the 24F dilator.

TEFLON COAXIAL DILATORS

As in Dotter's original design, these radiopaque Teflon dilators (8F–18F) telescope together so that the 10F dilator passes over the 8F, which is tapered to a 0.038-inch guidewire (Fig. 23–43).[62] The 12F, 14F, and 16F dilators taper to 10F and the 18F tapers to 12F. The Teflon construction of these dilators provides them with strength and a low friction coefficient, which makes them useful for dilating fibrotic perinephric tissues. Coaxial dilators are also used as a stiffening bridge in the ureter (see section on ureteral catheterization).

AMPLATZ TAPERED-TIP COAXIAL DILATORS

These radiopaque, semirigid polyurethane dilators come in 8F–34F sizes, all of which are tapered to the 8F Teflon guiding dilator.[61,63] Teflon working sheaths of 28F, 30F, 32F, and 34F outer diameters are provided that fit snugly over the 24F, 26F, 28F, and 30F dilators, respectively; these sheaths are used as instrument conduits during manipulations for nephrostolithotomy (Fig. 23–44). The main advantage of this system is that dilation of the tract is not done over a guidewire but rather over the guidewire–8F guiding dilator assembly, providing added safety.

AMPLATZ 6/10 AND 6/12 LONG TAPERED TEFLON DILATORS

These two coaxial systems include dilators whose largest outer diameters are either 6F and 10F or 6F and 12F (Fig. 23–45). The 6F leading dilator passes over a 0.038-inch guidewire. Both systems have a long, gradual taper to their largest external diameter. This taper, plus the coaxial design, makes them ideal for dilating tight, rigid stenoses, especially in the ureter.

METAL DILATORS

Stainless-steel dilators in 8F–24F (Wolf) and 8F–26F (Storz) are available as sets for dilation of percutaneous tracts for nephrostolithotomy. Each set starts with a long

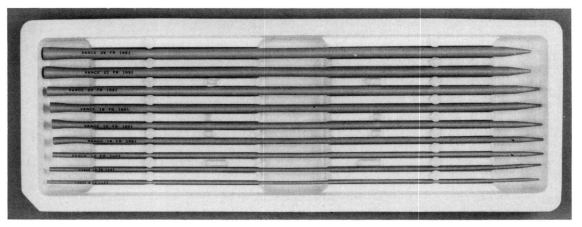

Fig. 23–42   Fascial dilators from 8F–24F with tip tapered to fit 0.038-inch guidewire.

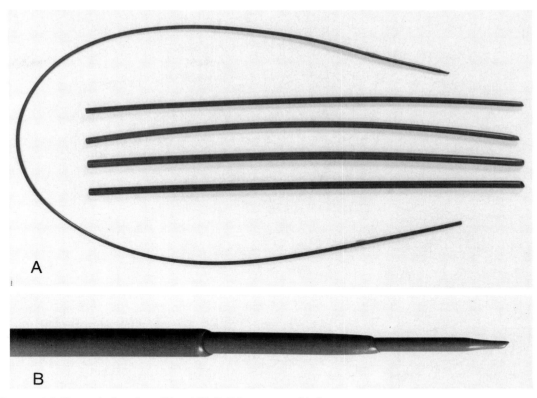

Fig. 23–43 Teflon coaxial dilator. A. Sets from 8F to 18F. B. Dilators assembled.

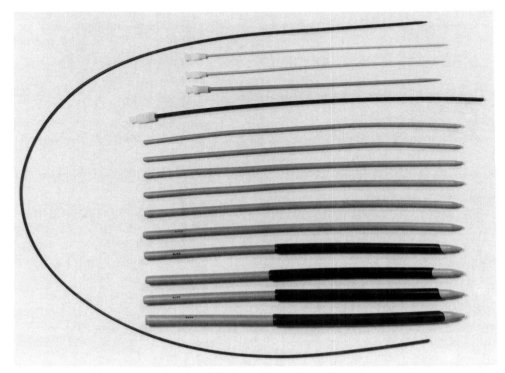

Fig. 23–44 Amplatz renal dilators with tips tapered to fit 8F Teflon guiding dilator. Note Teflon working sheaths above 24F, 26F, 28F, and 30F dilators.

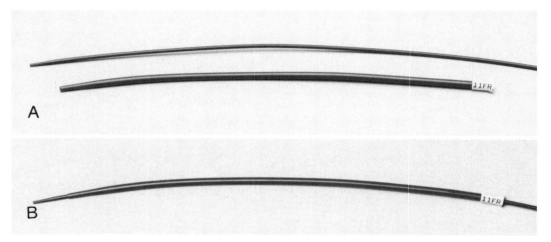

Fig. 23–45   6F/11F Teflon stricture dilator set. A. Parts of system. B. Assembled dilator.

8F cannula with a 0.038-inch lumen and a bead-like stopper in front that controls the forward motion of subsequent dilators (Fig. 23–46). The main advantages of metal dilators are rigidity, which makes them useful for dilation of the most resistant fibrotic perinephric tissues, and the fact that they can be resterilized and reused almost *ad infinitum.* However, their stiffness is also their main disadvantage, because an inexperienced operator can easily perforate the collecting system or tear renal parenchyma with them.

BALLOON DILATORS

Modified angioplasty balloons can be used for dilation of nephrostomy tracts. The balloon should be 8–15 cm long and able to withstand 10–15 atm of pressure,

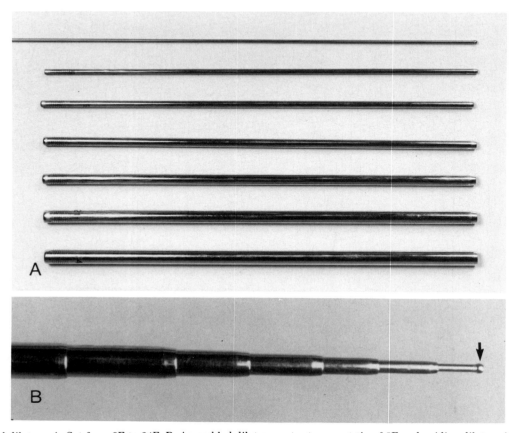

Fig. 23–46   Metal dilators. A. Set from 8F to 24F. B. Assembled dilators; note stopper at tip of 8F and guiding dilators (arrow).

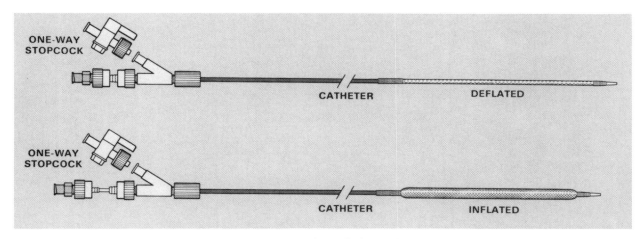

Fig. 23–47 Cook enforcer catheter dilator. A. Catheter with balloon deflated; observe low profile of balloon. B. Catheter with balloon inflated. (Courtesy of Cook, Inc.)

although in the typical case only 6–10 atm are needed. The diameter of the balloon is chosen to suit the type and size of the tract (Fig. 23–47).[60,61,64]

Needle Systems

Although almost any type of needle can be used for urointerventional procedures, the following are the most popular:

Chiba (skinny)(22–23-gauge);
Baltaxe–Mitty–Pollack;
Sheathed (translumbar aortogram, MEC, Hawkins);
Nonsheathed 18-gauge;
Trocar.

CHIBA (SKINNY) NEEDLE

These 22- or 23-gauge needles (Fig. 23–48A) are used either for the initial (localization) puncture, in patients with dilated, obstructed, or otherwise nonopacified collecting systems, or for the definitive puncture with the Cope and Hawkins one-step techniques.

BALTAXE–MITTY–POLLACK NEEDLE

This set consists of a fine needle over which an 18-gauge cannula is fitted (Fig. 23–49). A marker on the shaft of the 22-gauge needle signals the position of the cannula.[65]

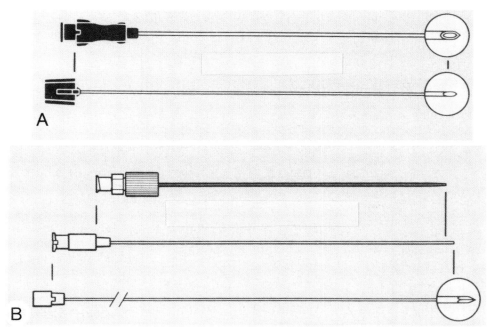

Fig. 23–48 Nephrostomy needles. A. 22-gauge Chiba needle with beveled tip. B. Sheathed 18-gauge needle with diamond tip. (Courtesy of Cook Urological.)

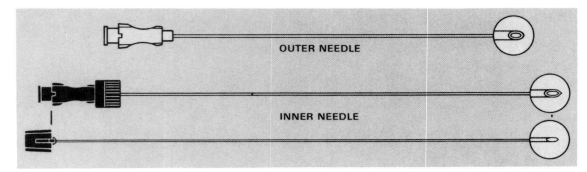

Fig. 23-49 Baltaxe–Mitty–Pollack needle consisting of inner needle with 22-gauge, 22.5-cm stylet; outer needle is 18-gauge and 4 cm long. (Courtesy of Cook Urological.)

SHEATHED NEEDLES

Hawkins Needle

The Hawkins needle is a 20-gauge, 20-inch-long needle with an "accordion" catheter mounted on its shaft (Fig. 23-50). A 0.018-inch coat-hanger wire or a 0.018-inch rocket wire is passed through the needle into the collecting system for catheter introduction.[24]

Translumbar Aortography (Amplatz TLA) Needle

This 18-gauge needle with either a diamond or a beveled tip comes with a snugly fitted Teflon sheath. A 0.038-inch guidewire fits through this needle.

MEC Needle

The needle–sheath assembly of this design has three components snugly fit over each other. It is 24 cm long and is used for the one-step method of nephrostomy catheter placement. The innermost component is a 22-gauge Chiba needle, over which a 19-gauge metal cannula fits snugly. A Teflon sheath with a hub is the outermost component (Fig. 23-51). The collecting system is punctured with the Chiba needle. Following aspiration of urine, the metal cannula and the Teflon sheath are advanced coaxially over the needle. As soon as the tips of the outer needle and the Teflon sheath reach the renal pelvis, the Chiba needle and the cannula are removed. The Teflon sheath then functions as a conduit for guidewire advancement and manipulations in the renal pelvis or the ureter.

NONSHEATHED NEEDLES

Diamond-Tip Needles

These 18-gauge needles are provided with all nephrostomy sets (Fig. 23-48B). They fit a 0.018-inch guidewire or 3F catheter.

Trocar Needle

A technique using a trocar needle for puncture of the collecting system was described by Newhouse and Pfister.[66] In this technique, the drainage catheter is passed into the collecting system through the outer cannula of the trocar after removal of the central stylet.

INDICATIONS FOR PERCUTANEOUS NEPHROSTOMY PUNCTURE

Percutaneous nephrostomy is indicated in the presence of urinary obstruction of benign or malignant origin. It also is part of many diagnostic and therapeutic maneuvers. A list of these indications is followed by a discussion of each.

1. Obstruction with dilatation or azotemia:
   a. Blood clots;
   b. Operative ligation or transection of the ureter;
   c. Trauma (external);
   d. Postpyeloplasty complications;
   e. Stone;
   f. Fungus infection;
   g. Retroperitoneal fibrosis;
   h. Postradiation fibrosis;
   i. Inflammatory and other fluid collections, such as pyonephrosis, perinephric abscess, urinoma, seroma, and lymphocele;
   j. Malignancy;

2. Ureteral stricture or fistula as a prelude to stent insertion;
3. For urodynamic studies;
4. Prior to stone removal, either mechanically, utilizing lithotripsy, forceps, or flushing, or by chemical dissolution with various solvents (chemolysis);
5. Nephroscopy to obtain biopsy material from or to resect a renal pelvic or ureteral tumor;
6. Foreign body removal;
7. Allograft evaluation and management;
8. Infusion of solvents and drugs;
9. Access for intrarenal surgery.

Benign Obstruction

Occlusion by blood clots necessitating percutaneous decompression is usually a complication of operation (pyeloplasty, ureteral reimplantation) or of renal biopsy.

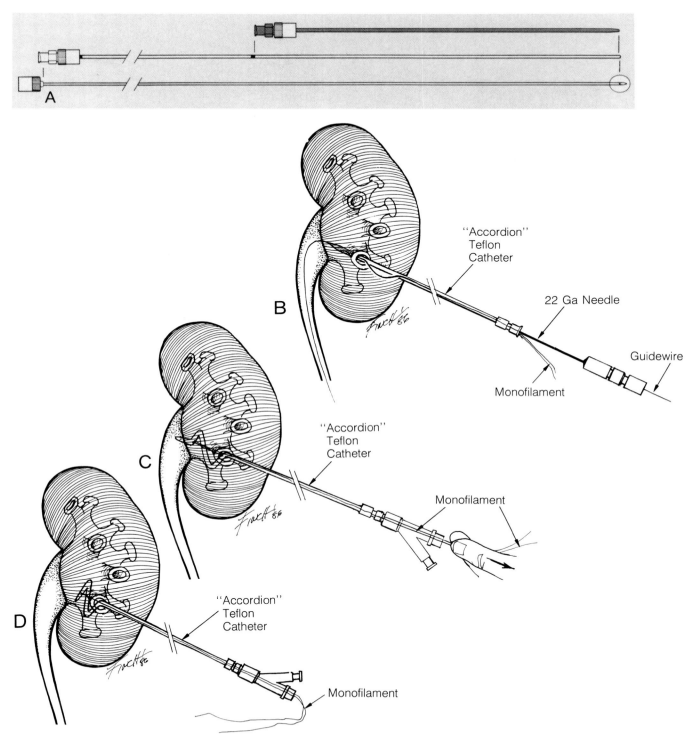

Fig. 23–50 Hawkins one-stick needle set. A. Components. Technique for drainage procedures; B. 21-gauge needle has entered posterior calix and coat-hanger guidewire has been passed through needle. 6F accordion catheter has been advanced over needle cannula and guidewire, which are held in position. C. After removing guidewire and needle the accordion catheter is reshaped. D. Accordion catheter in place.

In contrast, bleeding from benign conditions, such as arteriovenous malformations and trauma, or from malignant tumors usually does not necessitate percutaneous decompression, because such bleeding usually subsides spontaneously without clotting. Further, because malignant tumors are usually treated surgically or by arterial embolization rather than by percutaneous means, nephrostomy puncture is not needed.

External trauma is an uncommon indication for percutaneous decompression, with the immediate indication being either obstruction by blood clots or a urinary leak from a disrupted collecting system.

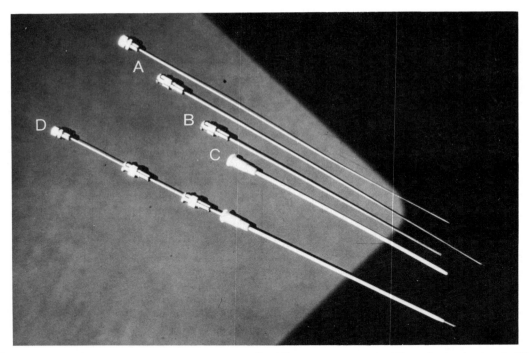

Fig. 23–51   MEC one-stick needle set consisting of 22-gauge needle (A), 18-gauge cannula (B), and plastic sheath (C). D. Assembled components.

Postoperative obstruction may necessitate decompression either as a temporary measure until edema subsides or for long-term management for failed plastic procedures in the renal pelvis, ureter, or ureterovesical junction.[67–70]

Percutaneous decompression has become the procedure of choice for the management of urinary stones causing symptoms of acute obstruction, such as pain, infection, and dysuria. After resolution of the symptoms and control of infection, the tract is dilated and the stones removed,[70–73] or, less often, extracorporeal shockwave lithotripsy (ESWL) is performed. This will be reviewed at length in the section on nephrostolithotomy.

Fungus infection with formation of fungus balls is an uncommon cause of acute urinary obstruction. Temporary percutaneous decompression may be necessary, particularly in patients with compromised renal function, such as the immunosuppressed recipient of a renal or bone marrow transplant. In these patients, a percutaneous nephrostomy catheter provides not only a means to decompress the obstructed collecting system, but also a route for infusion of antifungal drugs.[67,74,75]

Retroperitoneal fibrosis has been a difficult therapeutic problem. The prevailing treatment is still surgical, because recent attempts at percutaneous management, including decompression and dilation of obstructed ureteral segments, has proved unsuccessful in the long term.[66,67] However, percutaneous decompression is an efficient way to preserve renal function and stabilize the patient preoperatively.

After irradiation of the retroperitoneum or pelvis, the ureter can become obstructed by fibrosis. Percutaneous decompression and balloon dilation have been useful in the management of this complication.[70]

Infection, especially severe infection (pyonephrosis), is one of the principal indications for percutaneous decompression, and in these patients, the technique can be lifesaving.[2,3,66,71,73,76–79] Minimal manipulation is recommended in order to reduce the passage of bacteria into the blood. Initially, a one-step procedure (as with the Pfister, Medi-Tech, or Hawkins kits) can be used, although the catheter is small. As soon as possible after the patient is stable, a larger drainage catheter, such as the dual-stiffness Stamey, should be inserted to drain viscous debris.

Malignant Obstructions

Obstruction by genitourinary or any other malignancy causing uropathy and azotemia may be one of the leading indications for either percutaneous or surgical nephrostomy.[67,80–82] Percutaneous nephrostomy is now preferred as a faster, safer method of draining the obstructed kidney in critically ill cancer patients. This technique relieves the obstruction, purchasing time for effective chemotherapeutic agents or radiation to be administered for control or cure of the cancer. Also, in the presence of inoperable malignancies, a nephrostomy can be used to establish internal drainage by the insertion of a double-J stent.[38] Re-establishment of drainage reverses the azotemia and, sometimes, any associated hypertension[82] and may prolong the patient's life a few months to a year.[80,82]

One should proceed with nephrostomy in the cancer patient only after extensive discussion with oncologists, urologists, the patient's family, and, most importantly, the patient. It is seldom if ever appropriate to relieve urinary obstruction in a patient with severe pain for whom no appropriate anticancer treatment is available.[81,82]

Ureteral Strictures or Fistulae

In these cases, nephrostomy is a prelude to other interventional procedures within the ureter. Strictures might be the result of accidental ureteral ligation during pelvic surgery of idiopathic retroperitoneal or radiation fibrosis, of trauma, or of malignancy. Fistulae are commonly associated with strictures.

The management of ureteral strictures and fistulae is complex. Retrograde insertion of catheters is not possible in many patients, in which case percutaneous nephrostomy followed by the insertion of some type of stent markedly improves the patient's condition without open operation, which carries high morbidity and mortality rates.

Urodynamic Studies

Dilation of the ureters is not necessarily associated with obstruction or reflux. The anatomic significance of a dilated collecting system and ureter can be evaluated by performing what is now known as a Whitaker test.[83-87] Various conditions, such as neurogenic bladder, asymptomatic hydronephrosis, megaureters associated with reflux or obstruction, pelviureteral strictures, and apparently failed pyeloplasty, can be evaluated by this test from a physiologic point of view to determine if urodynamically significant obstruction is present, although in rare cases the test does not give clear-cut answers.[87] To reduce the frequency of this problem, Pfister, Newhouse, and their colleagues measure the pressure in the urinary bladder as well as in the renal pelvis, on the theory that the pressure differential obtained by subtracting the renal pelvic pressure from the intravesical measurement may be more meaningful than the intrapelvic pressure alone.[87] This pressure differential measurement eliminates the influence of external pressure, such as abdominal wall tension, that can increase the renal pelvic pressure. A pressure differential of about 10 cm H_2O at a perfusion rate of 10 ml/min with the bladder empty is abnormal.[86]

The Whitaker test is performed by introducing two needles percutaneously into the renal pelvis; one needle is utilized for perfusion, the other for measurement. The intrapelvic pressure can also be measured through a previously inserted nephrostomy catheter. The intravesical pressure is measured with a 5F pediatric feeding tube inserted transurethrally. The pressures are measured with a water manometer with its zero point level with the tip of the needles in the renal pelvis.

Stone Removal

Percutaneous nephrostomy is the initial step to obtain access to the renal pelvis for extraction of pelvic and proximal ureteral stones. Although this approach, called nephrostolithotomy or nephrolithotomy, is less widely practiced since the licensing of the ESWL machine,[88,89] it remains useful both in cities where ESWL is not available and in patients with obstruction or staghorn stones; there is low morbidity with rapid convalescence in most patients.[7,72,90-101] Some medical centers are even doing nephrostolithotomy on an outpatient basis.[102]

Endoscopic Exploration

Rigid and flexible fiberoptic nephroscopes are utilized for direct inspection, to perform biopsies of suspected lesions, and, increasingly, to resect renal pelvic tumors from patients who are not suitable candidates for open operation.[103,104] These instruments are introduced through 24F–30F nephrostomy tracts that have been created percutaneously.

Foreign Body Removal

Many broken or blocked stents that cannot be removed or replaced over a guidewire by the conventional transcystoscopic method can be retrieved via percutaneous nephrostomy tracts with the aid of different types of forceps and baskets.[105] Fragments of broken stone baskets have also been removed this way.

Allograft Evaluation and Management

After renal transplantation, such urologic complications as urine leak and ureteral obstruction occur in 10% of patients.[106] Conventional endoscopic retrograde catheter insertion may not be possible in all cases, and the fear of introducing sepsis with this approach is a real concern. Percutaneous nephrostomy is technically feasible without traversing the peritoneum and is the fastest method of establishing the diagnosis and managing the critically ill patient.[106-108] The dense, fibrous shell around the transplanted kidney, along with the abdominal wall, effectively closes the tract, preventing sequelae.

Infusion of Solvents and Drugs

Chemotherapeutic agents can be introduced through nephrostomy catheters for local treatment of unresectable malignant tumors, including those in a solitary kidney, or for adjunctive treatment after percutaneous resection. Also, upper tract candidiasis can be managed through percutaneous nephrostomy catheters in patients in whom catheters are difficult to insert retrograde. This approach reduces the side effects of these toxic drugs. Local treatment of the renal pelvis and ureter with amphotericin B has been successful in the management of upper tract candidiasis in an insulin-dependent patient with malignant obstruction.[75]

The placement of large catheters in the kidney via the nephrostomy tract has also facilitated the infusion of various solvents to dissolve renal pelvic stones.[109-112] Usually, two catheters are necessary, one for infusion of the solvent and the other for drainage. Alternatively, a patent ureter or ureteral stent can function as a drainage conduit, allowing rapid flow of solvent without causing undue pressure in the renal pelvis. Struvite, uric acid, and cystine calculi are dissolved with this approach. The potential complications of hypermagnesemia (with some solvents) and obstruction should be watched for during the infusion.

Chemolysis via a percutaneous approach is practical in patients with recurrent calculi, contraindications to open operation, and residual stones or dust following percutaneous extraction. The drawbacks of longer treatment and hospitalization time as well as the advent of ESWL have eliminated the use of this method as primary therapy.

Intrarenal Surgery

As uroradiology practitioners became more comfortable working via a percutaneous nephrostomy tract, they began adapting transurethral surgical procedures to the upper urinary tract. In addition to the resection of tumors, mentioned earlier, intrarenal procedures now in use include relief of stenotic infundibula, ablation of caliceal diverticula, and relief of ureteropelvic junction stenoses.[113-117]

CONTRAINDICATIONS TO NEPHROSTOMY PUNCTURE

The only true and absolute contraindication to percutaneous nephrostomy is the presence of bleeding diathesis that would make the puncture unacceptably risky. However, coagulation disorders can usually be corrected by the administration of fresh-frozen plasma, platelets, or specific blood components.

Sepsis is only a relative contraindication, because, as remarked earlier, percutaneous decompression may be lifesaving in the presence of pyonephrosis with urosepsis. However, in most cases, percutaneous puncture can wait for sepsis control.

Another relative contraindication is the presence of cancer. If the patient's quality of life is severely impaired and all avenues of cancer treatment have been exhausted, it is doubtful that relief of obstruction is appropriate.[81,82]

EVALUATION AND MANAGEMENT OF PATIENTS FOR PERCUTANEOUS NEPHROSTOMY

A clinical history and physical examination should be obtained in all cases. The necessary laboratory tests are:

Coagulation profile;
Complete blood count;
Creatinine and blood urea nitrogen (BUN) measurements;
Urinalysis;
Urine culture.

The radiologic examinations needed are:

Intravenous urogram (IVU);
Ultrasound scan;
Computed axial tomography (CT) scan;
Chest radiograph.

Preoperative Preparation

An adequate intravenous line should be started for administration of analgesics, sedatives, antibiotics, and fluids. The patient with pyonephrosis is given appropriate antibiotics as determined by the results of urine and blood cultures, whereas the patient undergoing decompression or stone removal is given broad-spectrum antibiotics until the last nephrostomy tube is taken out.[72]

Coagulation abnormalities are corrected with fresh-frozen platelets or specific coagulation factors before any percutaneous manipulation is done.

Although premedication is generally selected according to personal preferences, several analgesic–sedative–amnesic combinations are popular to decrease anxiety (meperidine or secobarbital with hydroxyzine pamoate). These drugs are usually started at the time the patient is called to the angiography suite. Atropine is used by some investigators to decrease both secretions and the incidence of vasovagal reactions.

Intraoperative Care

Vital signs (pulse, blood pressure, breathing) are monitored continuously by either a circulating nurse or an anesthetist. Electrocardiographic (ECG) monitoring is recommended, particularly in the following circumstances:

Elderly patients, in whom respiratory depression can accompany use of analgesics or sedatives;
Difficult manipulations where deep sedation and analgesia are needed—for example, stone manipulation under local anesthesia;
The septic patient;
The high-risk postoperative patient in need of a decompression procedure. In the patient housed in an intensive care unit, it is particularly useful to have either a circulating nurse or a nurse anesthetist to control all the intravenous, pressure, and respiratory lines.

Most urointerventional procedures can be performed under local anesthesia with the help of sedatives and analgesics. Several combinations have proven safe for intraoperative control of pain, such as diazepam with butorphanol tartrate, meperidine hydrochloride, morphine, or fentanyl. Of these, diazepam with butorphanol has proved safest for use in the absence of direct monitoring by the anesthesiology department.

PUNCTURE TECHNIQUE

Imaging

ULTRASOUND

The guidance system used to direct the needle for puncture of the pelvicaliceal system varies from institution to institution. In the past, most punctures were made under fluoroscopy utilizing the bony landmarks.[2] However, several authors have stressed the value of ultrasonographic guidance when puncturing the pelvicaliceal system with a 22- or 18-gauge needle.[118-125] Certainly its value in pregnant patients, in whom radiation exposure is thereby avoided, is indisputable.[3] Ultrasound also is useful in patients with renal failure, in whom iodinated contrast material does not opacify the collecting system, and in diabetic patients, in whom contrast material is hazardous to renal function.[120-123] Finally, ultrasound is the preferred method in the patient with an obstructed, poorly functioning kidney. It not only depicts collecting system dimensions and anatomy accurately but also shows the depth of the kidney below the skin and provides an excellent image of the perirenal space. The number of punctures required to enter the renal pelvis is definitely reduced with ultrasonography compared with fluoroscopy.[122] Therefore, the morbidity and the risk of significant damage to the kidney are reduced or eliminated. An initial puncture with ultrasonography to opacify the collecting system, with the final placement of the catheter under fluoroscopy, seems to be the accepted procedure now.

The right kidney is scanned through the sonic window of the liver (Figs. 23–52 and 23–53). Longitudinal (Fig. 23–52) and transverse views (Fig. 23–53) are obtained with the patient supine and in deep suspended inhalation. The left kidney is examined with the patient in a left anterior oblique or right decubitus position. This method provides a coronal section of the kidney (Fig. 23–54). Longitudinal and transverse views are obtained (Fig. 23–54).

Modern ultrasound scanners assess renal anatomy very accurately. Recall and compare anatomic details of a 19th-century drawing of a kidney (Fig. 23–55) with modern ultrasound pictures as in Figures 23–52 through 23–54. Sonographically, the parenchymal structure of a kidney is less echodense than the liver (Fig. 23–52). Within the parenchyma, renal pyramids are less echodense than renal cortex. The renal sinus encompasses the collecting system, vessels, fibrotic tissue, and fat and is strongly echogenic. There is only a little free fluid present in the normal collecting systems except during pregnancy.

Several techniques have been described. One uses ultrasound for locating and determining the depth of the collecting system. A mark is made on the skin at the best site for the needle puncture, and the depth is noted. After the field has been prepared and draped, the needle is introduced in the direction and to the depth determined by the ultrasound study. Another technique uses a special A-mode biopsy transducer, which was the first system to provide a method for puncturing the collecting system under ultrasound.[3,119] A special sterilizable transducer with a central hole for needle introduction allows imaging of the needle tip as a spike within the collecting system.[119] The depth of the collecting system can be marked on the needle. This technique has been abandoned for real-time methods.

Real-time ultrasound equipment has two distinct advantages over B-mode scanners. First, a faster live image is obtained; second, many of the new units are portable.[121,125] The actual insertion of the needle is monitored continuously, two-dimensional imaging of the renal pelvis ensuring safe placement (Figs. 23–56 and 23–57).[123] The newer generation real-time transducers are more

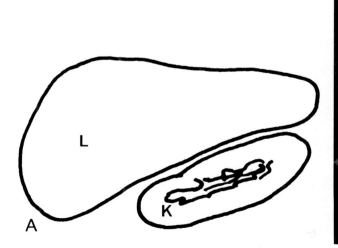
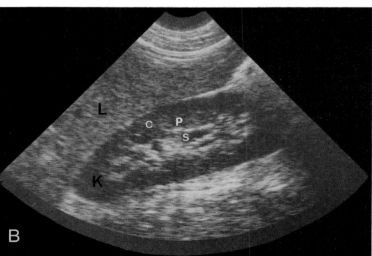

Fig. 23–52   Anatomy for ultrasound-guided puncture. A. Longitudinal liver–kidney view with right lobe of liver (L) serving as sonic window for kidney (K). B. Normal right kidney in supine longitudinal sonogram: L = liver; K = kidney; S = sinus echoes encompassing collecting system, vessels, fat, and connective tissue; P = pyramid; C = renal cortex.

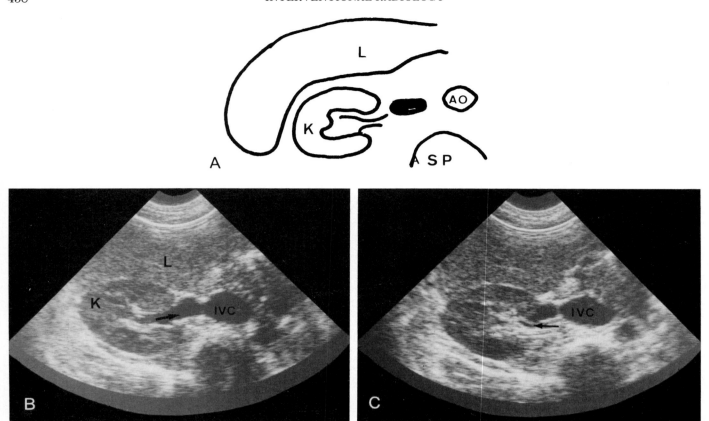

Fig. 23–53 Anatomy for ultrasound-guided puncture. A. Transverse liver–kidney view. L = liver; K = kidney; AO = aorta; SP = spine. B. Normal right kidney in supine transverse sonogram: L = liver; K = kidney. Arrow indicates blood flow in right renal vein joining inferior vena cava (IVC). C. One centimeter caudally; arrow indicates right renal artery crossing under inferior vena cava (IVC).

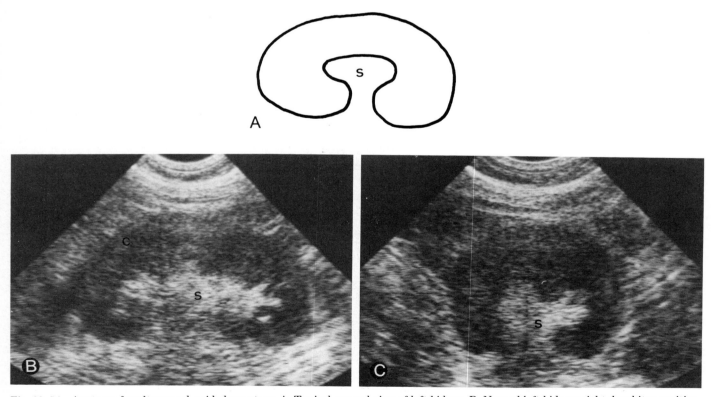

Fig. 23–54 Anatomy for ultrasound-guided puncture. A. Typical coronal view of left kidney. B. Normal left kidney; right decubitus position, coronal view. S = renal sinus. C. Transverse section of B. C = cortex; S = renal sinus.

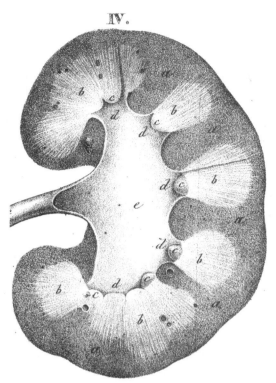

Fig. 23–55 A 19th-century graphic (artist unkown) demonstrating renal cortex (a), renal pyramids (b), tips of pyramids (c) and inside collecting system (d and e).

practical, because the targeted calix can be entered precisely.[3]

One technique for real-time ultrasound guidance uses a sidearm attachment for the transducer (Fig. 23–58) that allows imaging of the needle as it advances on an oblique pathway and enters the collecting system, which is kept in the center of the field. Another technique uses a linear array real-time transducer with a removable central crystal (Fig. 23–59) that allows continuous observation of the

needle tip within the target area (Figs. 23–56B and 23–57B). A sterilizable funnel-shaped attachment is used to fit the needle through the special transducer so the entire transducer need not be sterilized.

A practical, easier approach was suggested by Dubuisson et al.[124] The real-time transducer is placed in a sterile glove, and images are obtained in several planes. The needle is then advanced in an oblique pathway intersecting the path of the sound beam (Fig. 23–60). This method obviates sterilization of the transducer.

Ultrasound does have some limitations. For example, it can give a false-positive diagnosis of pyelocaliectasis, particularly in renal allograft recipients with full bladders. Second, the image of the collecting system anatomy is frequently inadequate for a precise caliceal puncture, as is needed for nephrostolithotomy.

COMPUTED TOMOGRAPHY

Computed tomography best demonstrates the transverse anatomy of the renal pelvis and calices, as well as the relation of the kidney to nearby organs and viscera. Although CT can be used to guide needle insertion, this approach is expensive and time consuming and generally has no advantages over ultrasound. Further, the patient must be transferred to the fluoroscopy unit for the final placement of the catheter, and this, too, is time consuming and may cause accidental withdrawal of guidewires or needle sheaths.

Antegrade pyelography of the nonfunctioning kidney can be guided by the anatomic information obtained from the cross-sectional images of CT scans (Figs. 23–61 and 23–62).[6] In patients with severe kyphoscoliosis, the cross-sectional anatomy observed on CT is invaluable in guiding needles and catheters.[126] Computed tomography also is valuable for nephrostomies as a prelude to stone removal in patients with congenital anomalies, such as horseshoe kidney. In these cases, exquisite anatomic detail and the relations of the pelvicaliceal system to the surrounding hollow and solid viscera are clearly depicted.

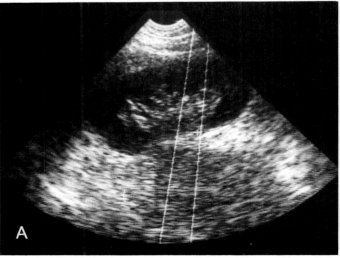
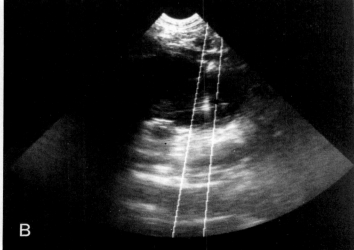

Fig. 23–56 Nephrostomy puncture under real-time ultrasound. A. Puncture calipers indicate needle path. Maximum depth of puncture is measured by white cross. B. Puncture. Echogenic needle (arrow) is seen within parenchyma.

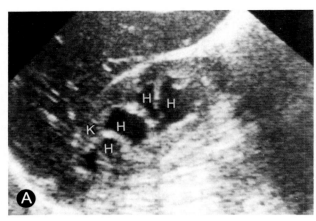

Fig. 23–57 Hydronephrotic right kidney (K) on supine longitudinal sonogram. Note distended collecting system (H). B. Ultrasonically guided needle puncture of hydronephrotic system (H); needle tip (arrow) is seen entering fluid.

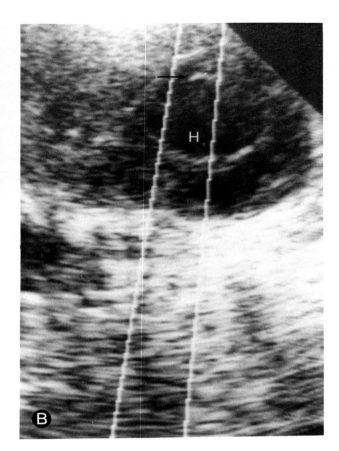

SECTOR TRANSDUCER

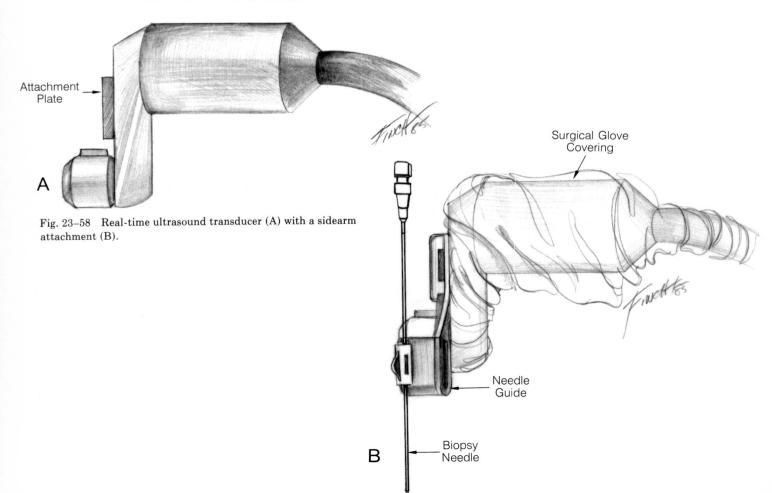

Fig. 23–58 Real-time ultrasound transducer (A) with a sidearm attachment (B).

TOP VIEW

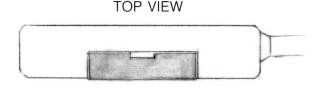

FRONT VIEW

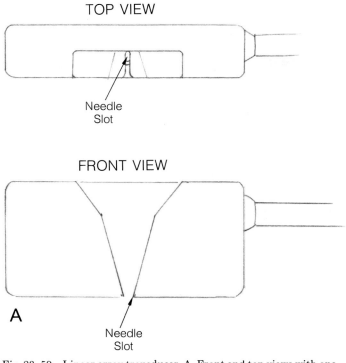

Needle
Slot

FRONT VIEW

Needle
Slot

A

Insert

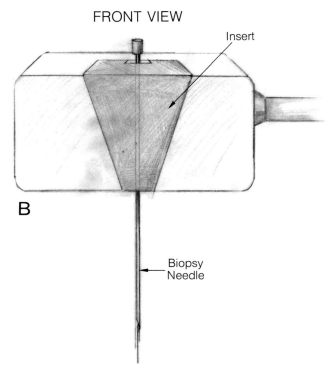

B

Biopsy
Needle

Fig. 23–59   Linear array transducer. A. Front and top views with one crystal removed in center, where adapter can be placed to guide introduction of needle under direct real-time imaging. B. Top view with insert in place and front view with insert assembled and needle going through insert.

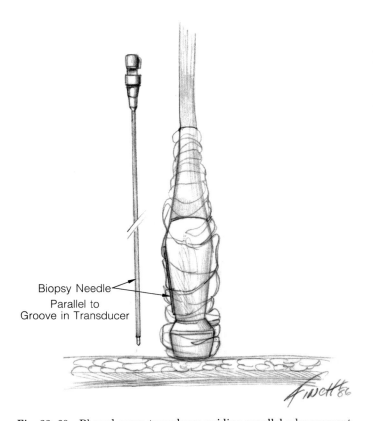

Biopsy Needle
Parallel to
Groove in Transducer

Fig. 23–60   Phased array transducer guiding parallel advancement of needle.

BLIND PUNCTURE

If ultrasound is not available and the collecting system is not opacified by the intravenous administration of contrast medium, a blind puncture of the collecting system is usually successful. A previous IVU or a recent plain film of the abdomen can be used to locate the kidney margins. The relative position of the renal pelvis is then related to bony landmarks: the thoracic and lumbar spine, vertebral bodies, and 12th rib (Fig. 23–63A). A direct puncture into the area where the renal pelvis is expected is done under fluoroscopic control following these landmarks. The skinny (22- or 23-gauge) needle usually enters the collecting system in one or two passes, particularly if the system is dilated. Once the collecting system has been opacified through the skinny needle with contrast medium, CO_2, or both (Fig. 23–63B), a second puncture is made into a posterior calix, either with another Chiba needle (for the Cope or Hawkins one-step technique) or with an 18-gauge needle (for the two-step technique).

Approach Selection

GENERAL CONSIDERATIONS

To select the approach for a percutaneous nephrostomy, one must take several points into consideration.

Fig. 23–61 CT scan through upper renal pole shows intimate relations between superolateral margins of kidney and liver on the right side and spleen on the left side. Also note relations of upper pole to diaphragm and pleural space.

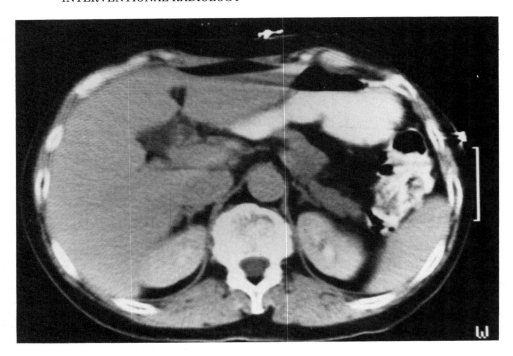

CT SCAN

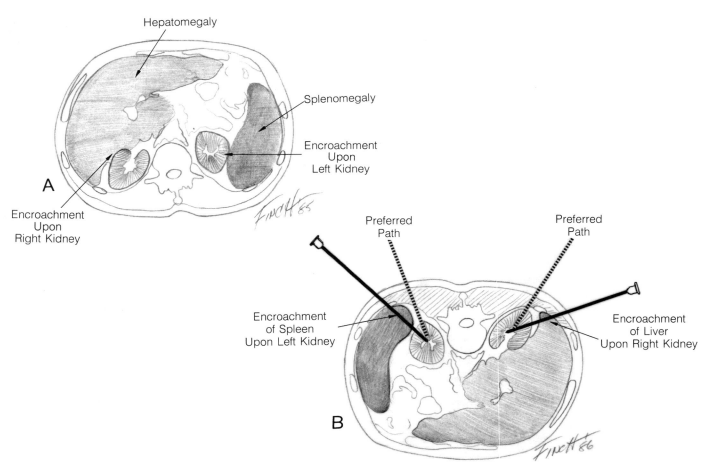

Fig. 23–62 Alteration of needle path in patient with hepatosplenomegaly. A. Encroachment of liver and spleen on right and left kidneys, respectively, in patient with hepatosplenomegaly. B. Need to change path of percutaneous tract from posterior axillary line to more medial position to avoid puncutures of liver or spleen in patient with hepatosplenomegaly or in patients in whom upper pole puncture is desirable.

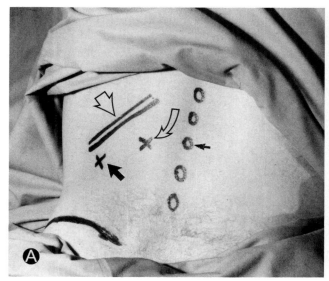

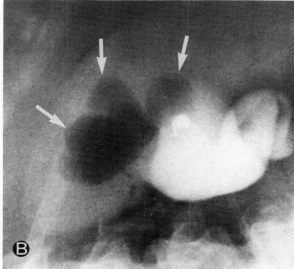

Fig. 23–63 Technique of blind puncture. A. Bone landmarks for blind punctures of pelvicaliceal system: 12th rib (open arrow); spinous process (short black arrow); medially placed cross marks entry site of Chiba needle (curved open arrow); laterally placed cross (large black arrow) marks entry of 18-gauge needle. B. Puncture of renal pelvis using Chiba needle with aid of double contrast to demonstrate posterior calices (arrows).

First, the renal pelvis should not be punctured directly, either from a posterior or an oblique approach, because of the higher incidence of vascular complications[127,128] caused by the position of the branches of the renal artery supplying the posterior division of the kidney behind the renal pelvis and the proximal segments of the upper and middle infundibula (Fig. 23–64).[14,129] A puncture into this area thus can cause an arterial laceration (Fig. 23–65) that will necessitate selective arterial embolization (the treatment of choice) or surgery (see section on complications). Instead, the puncture should be performed through the posterolateral margin of the kidney on Brödel's avascular line (Fig. 23–66). Puncture through this area theoretically avoids damage to any branch of the renal artery.[14,130,131] Entry of the renal pelvis through the posterolateral aspect of the kidney also purchases long length, thereby minimizing accidental dislodgment. The tract through the renal parenchyma avoids or minimizes the urine leakage compared with direct entry to the renal pelvis, wherein lack of supporting structures favors urinoma formation. Catheters leaving the posterolateral aspect of the flank allow the patient to rest comfortably on his or her back without fear of kinking or accidental guidewire or catheter dislodgment.

A second consideration of puncture site selection is that, because of the oblique orientation of the coronal plane of the kidney with respect to the transverse plane of the body (Fig. 23–67), the area of the kidney where the puncture should be performed is generally projected just off the paravertebral muscles when the patient is in a prone oblique position (Fig. 23–67). A more lateral puncture increases the risk of puncturing the liver, spleen, or colon (Figs. 23–67 through 23–69); this complication has been reported with the wider use of the percutaneous approach to the kidney not only for drainage but also for stone removal. Perforation of the colon is a particular risk in the patient who has had a partial ileal bypass operation or who has minimal fat in the retroperitoneal area, because in such cases, the different organs and viscera shift posteriorly (Fig. 23–70). One way to decrease these complications is to obtain two or three CT or ultrasound cuts through the kidney routinely, although if care is used, this is probably not necessary. Most investigators just try to stay as close as possible, or even medial to, the lateral edge of the paravertebral muscles (Fig. 23–63).

A posterior calix of the lower or middle caliceal group is usually selected for drainage purposes. The needle

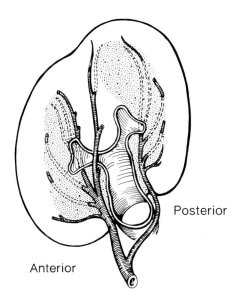

Fig. 23–64 Direct relations of renal artery branches with renal pelvis and infundibula. Ideal entry site is through a posterior calix to avoid injury to major vessels.

Posterior

Anterior

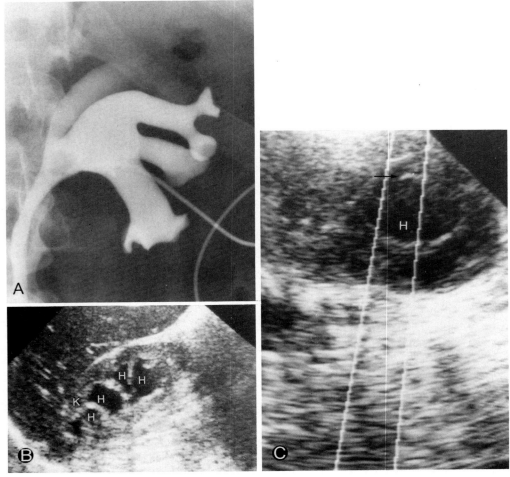

Fig. 23–65 Avoiding arterial lacerations. A. IVU after successful puncture. Note entry site medial on infundibulum. B. Medially placed puncture caused laceration of lobar artery. Note extensive extravasation of contrast medium (arrows). C. Balloon inflated at site of arterial laceration stops bleeding.

Fig. 23–66 Cross-section of kidney showing needle pathway through Brödel's avascular line.

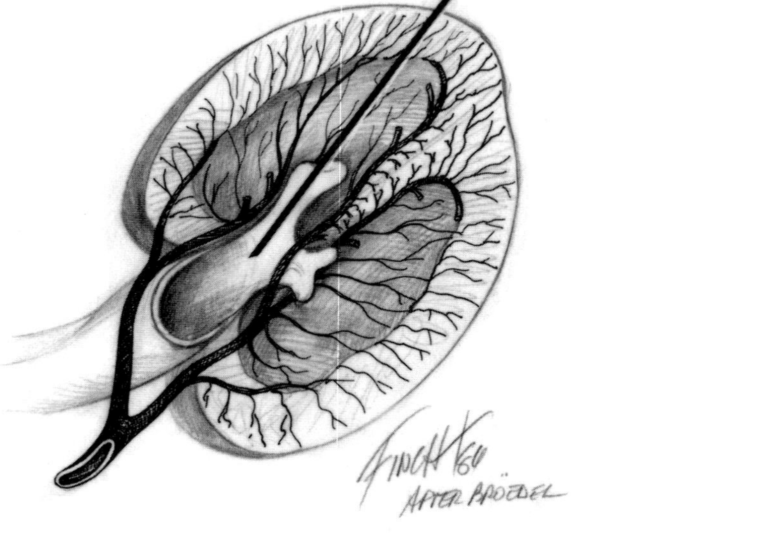

PLANE OF ARTERIAL DIVISION

18 Ga Needle

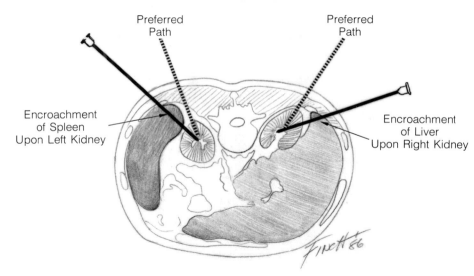

Preferred Path

Preferred Path

Encroachment of Spleen Upon Left Kidney

Encroachment of Liver Upon Right Kidney

Fig. 23–67 Modification in technique required to create percutaneous tract into kidney safely in patient with splenomegaly or in whom upper pole puncture is desirable. More medial tract is required for the 18-gauge needle to avoid injury to spleen that would occur if positional landmarks are not used.

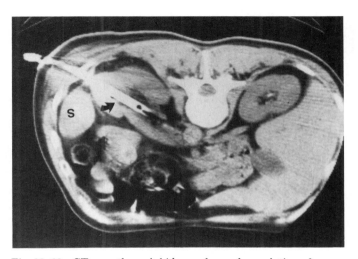

Fig. 23–68 CT scan through kidneys shows close relation of percutaneous tract to spleen in patient in whom posterior calix in lower pole was punctured using the inside-out technique. S = spleen. Foley catheter in tract (curved arrow).

puncture is placed either through the calix itself (Fig. 23–71A) or at the junction of the calix with the infundibulum (Fig. 23–71B).[57]

For drainage, the authors keep the puncture site below the 12th rib, because this is generally below the pleural reflection. However, when the nephrostomy tract is to be used for nephrostolithotomy or internal stent placement, a puncture above the 12th rib is acceptable and often preferred.

For circle loop nephrostomy drainage, two punctures are needed, one in the lower pole and the other in the upper pole.[132] The upper puncture is occasionally above the 12th rib.

SUPINE OBLIQUE APPROACH

Fernström and Andersson performed nephrostomies with the patient in the supine oblique position solely to enter the renal pelvis through the lateral aspect of the cortex.[128] This approach was proposed because of the

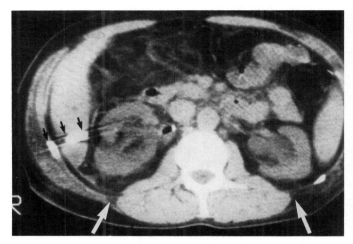

Fig. 23–69 Percutaneous tract created with inside-out nephrostomy technique traverses liver at level of posterior axillary line (black arrows). A more medially placed tract (white arrows) just off the paravertebral muscles would have been safe.

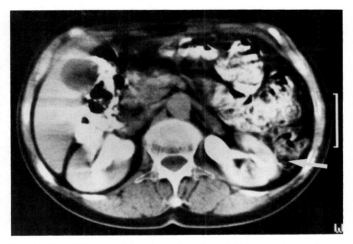

Fig. 23–70 CT scan through midsection of kidneys shows abnormally posteriorly positioned splenic flexure–descending colon (arrow) near lateral margin of left kidney. Puncture through an anterior calix could easily perforate colon.

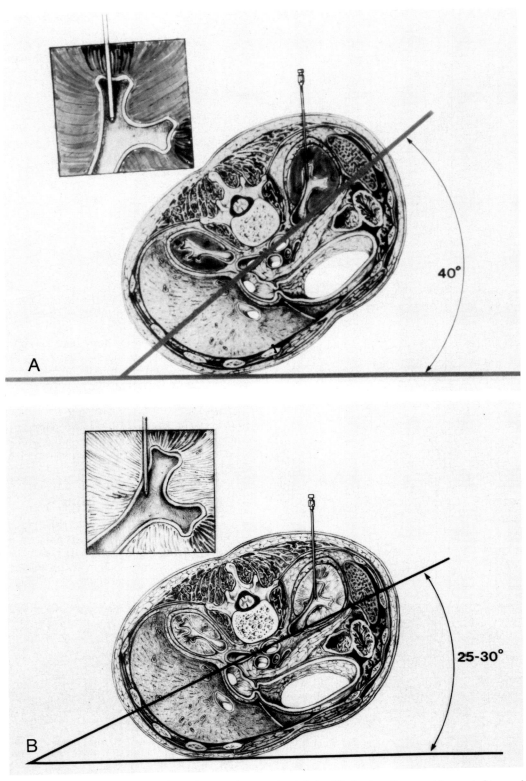

Fig. 23–71 Punctures for drainage. A. Puncture through posterior calix provides direct access to renal pelvis. B. Puncture through cal-iceal–infundibular junction must be angled toward pelvis to provide direct access to renal pelvis.

realization that posterior punctures lead to direct entry of the renal pelvis, risking damage to the renal pedicle. The puncture is made under fluoroscopy from the posterior axillary line while the patient lies supine rotated 25° to the opposite side (Fig. 23–71). The needle is aimed toward the renal pelvis and is tilted 10° to the anterior abdominal wall. Sudden flow of urine with slow withdrawal of the needle indicates correct positioning of the needle tip in the renal pelvis, which is verified by contrast injection. The potential for entry into the peritoneum or the viscera is certainly high compared to the posterolateral prone approach. Entry into the peritoneum is signaled by pain, and withdrawal of the needle is recommended.

The supine oblique position is also utilized in performing nephrostomies with ultrasonography at the bedside in seriously ill patients who cannot be transported to the radiology suite.[125] In this refined method of real-time ultrasonography guidance, the organs between the puncture site and the renal pelvis are clearly identified, and the needle is monitored until it enters the collecting system. Supine oblique entry may be the only possible approach in seriously ill patients maintained with life-supporting equipment such as respirators, who cannot be rotated to the conventional prone oblique position.[77]

Definitive Puncture

Several techniques have been described for making the definitive puncture:

Single stick:
    Cope technique;
    Hawkins technique;
    MEC technique;
    Pfister trocar–cannula technique;
Double-stick technique;
Inside-out retrograde technique.

SINGLE-STICK METHODS

The single-stick techniques have in common the use of a single needle puncture of the collecting system, through which opacification of the pelvicaliceal system and placement of a drainage catheter can be performed.

Cope Technique

Cope described insertion of a drainage catheter using a single puncture with a 23-gauge skinny needle (Fig. 23–72).[133] After opacification of the collecting system, if the needle entry site proves appropriate, a 0.018-inch coat-

hanger wire is passed through the needle into the collecting system, and the needle is removed (Fig. 23–73). A 6.3F Teflon dilator, tapered to the wire and having a sharp bend 2 cm behind the tip and a hole into the medial side of the bend, is mounted on a stiffening metal cannula. The two are then advanced over the guidewire until the tip of the dilator is within the collecting system, taking care not to perforate the opposite wall of the renal pelvis. The metal cannula is removed, which allows gentle manipulation of the dilator tip into a more desirable position within the renal pelvis. The wire is then exchanged for a 0.038-inch Teflon-coated tight (3-mm) J-wire. Because of the position of the sidehole in the angled portion of the dilator and the fact that the distal end of the dilator is tapered to 0.018 inch, the curved 0.038-inch wire will always exit through the sidehole. The wire is advanced within the collecting system before the Teflon dilator is removed. Dilation of the tract and placement of a drainage catheter can then be performed over the 0.038-inch wire.

Hawkins Technique

Hawkins described a simpler single-stick technique and designed a kit consisting of a 20-inch-long, 20-gauge needle over which a 6F Teflon accordion drainage catheter is tightly fitted.[24] A 0.018-inch coat-hanger wire or rocket wire is used for catheter placement (Fig. 23–74). The initial puncture is done with the skinny needle using either ultrasound or fluoroscopic guidance after intravenous administration of contrast medium. If needle position is appropriate, the guidewire is passed through the needle until it has coiled within the renal pelvis. While the needle hub and wire are held with one hand to prevent forward movement, the Teflon drainage catheter is gently advanced with the other hand over the needle–wire combination until enough catheter is within the collecting system. The needle and wire are removed, and, by pulling on the monofilament string, the loops of the accordion catheter are pulled together. This maneuver, although easy in a dilated renal pelvis, can be difficult in a less dilated collecting system.

The greatest disadvantage of this technique lies in the use of the long skinny needle, which is cumbersome. Hawkins recommends holding the needle with both

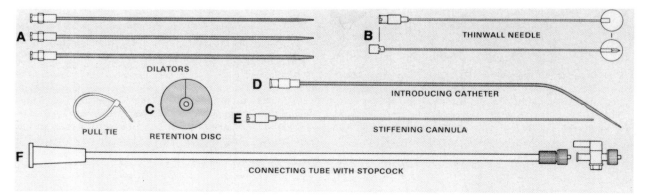

Fig. 23–72 Cope's one-stick nephrostomy set. A. 6F, 7F, and 8F Teflon dilators. B. 18-gauge diamond-tip dilators. C. Retention disk. D. Introducing catheter. E. Stiffening cannula. F. Connecting tube with stopcock. (Courtesy of Cook, Inc.)

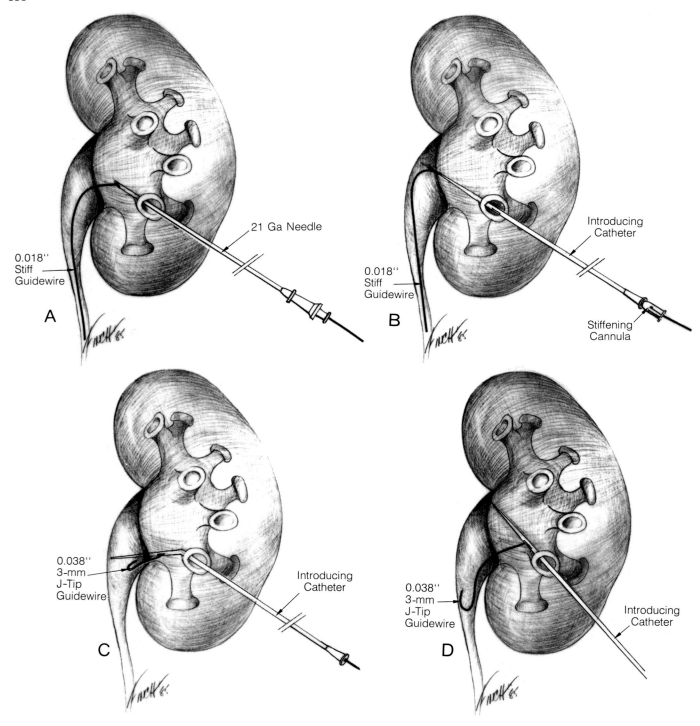

Fig. 23–73 Cope single-stick technique. A. 21-gauge needle has been placed into posterior calix and 0.018-inch coat-hanger guidewire has been passed and manipulated into ureter. B. After removal of needle cannula, introducing catheter with stiffening cannula has been passed over guidewire. C. Guidewire has been removed and 0.038-inch J-tip guidewire has been passed; this wire has exited through sidehole at bend in introducing catheter. D. Introducer catheter is being removed while wire is kept in place. E. Close-up of distal end of introducer catheter: a. Oval sidehole at bend; note smooth tapering of introducer tip to fit over 0.018-inch guidewire. The 19-gauge steel cannula fits within introducer catheter, providing added stiffness and straightening during introduction. b. Tight-J 0.038-inch guidewire exits through sidehole regularly, because distal lumen is smaller than diameter of guidewire.

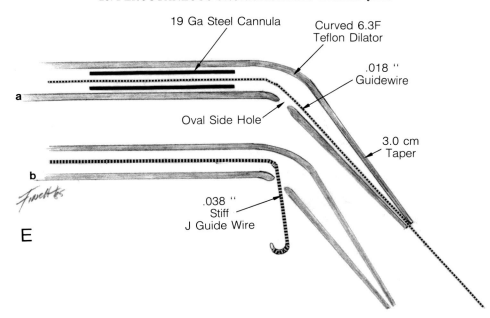

hands, one at the tip and the other 6–8 inches behind, leaving the rest of the needle hanging loose.

MEC Technique

A simplified version of the Hawkins kit was developed by MEC. It consists of a 22-gauge, 25-cm-long needle, a 19-gauge stiffening cannula, and a 6F plastic sheath. No wire is provided. The needle, cannula, and sheath are assembled, and the collecting system is punctured under ultrasound or fluoroscopy. Only the needle enters the renal parenchyma and collecting system (Fig. 23–75A). The position of the needle tip within the collecting sys-

tem is proved by the aspiration of urine. Dilute contrast medium can be injected to opacify and distend the collecting system further. While the needle is held in place with one hand, the cannula and sheath are advanced until the tip of the cannula is seen within the collecting system (Fig. 23–75B). At this point, the forward motion of the cannula is stopped while the sheath is advanced over the cannula and needle until the sheath passes a mark on the surface of the cannula (Fig. 23–75C). (The mark is needed because the sheath is only barely radiopaque.) Once the position of the sheath is considered adequate, the needle and cannula are removed. A 0.038-inch guidewire can be used to position the sheath more advantageously.

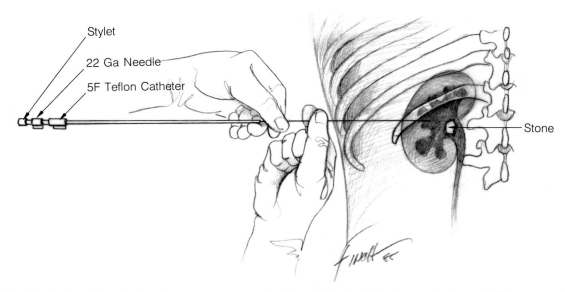

Fig. 23–74 Hawkins single-stick technique for percutaneous nephrostomy. Using both hands, proximal part of 22-gauge needle is carefully advanced through posterior calix into collecting system.

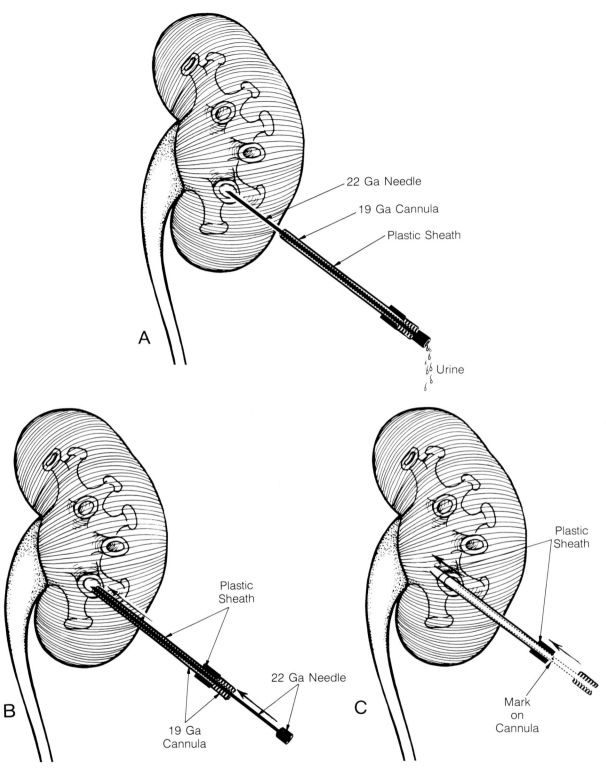

Fig. 23–75   MEC needle one-stick technique. A. 22-gauge part of needle has been passed into posterior calix in lower pole of kidney; 19-gauge cannula and plastic sheath are seen outside renal capsule. Urine leaks back through lumen of 22-gauge needle. B. While 22-gauge needle is held in place, 19-gauge cannula and plastic sheath are synchronously advanced into collecting system. C. After removal of 22-gauge needle and verification of position of 19-gauge plastic sheath within collecting system, the 19-gauge cannula is held in position while advancing plastic sheath to mark on the cannula; this means that tip of plastic sheath is within collecting system.

The disadvantages of this technique are:

Lack of an 0.018-inch wire for sheath guidance; a coat-hanger wire (Cook, Inc.) can be used to solve this problem;

The fact that the sheath has only an end hole and no self-retention features. In general, it has to be replaced by a conventional drainage catheter.

A similar kit has been described by Baltaxe, Mitty and Pollack.[65]

Trocar–Cannula Technique

In the original description of percutaneous nephrostomy by Goodwin et al, a trocar–cannula system was used to insert polyethylene tubes through a hollow cannula.[1] Later, Pfister and his colleagues refined the technique,[66,71,134] and the equipment is now available commercially. Initially, a 10F metal cannula fitted with a pencil point stylet was used; lately, the metal cannula has been replaced with a peel-away Teflon outer sheath.[33] The trocar has a sidehole proximal to its sharp tip, so as soon as the trocar–cannula assembly enters the renal pelvis, urine emerges spontaneously through the hollow trocar.

As an initial step, the pelvicaliceal system is opacified by injecting contrast medium with a 22-gauge Chiba needle. The desired calix is punctured under fluoroscopy. The assembly is advanced as a single unit under intermittent fluoroscopy (Fig. 23–76), maintaining its direction toward the target by gentle short thrusts. As soon as urine emerges, the trocar is removed, an 8F–12F Silastic catheter is introduced, and a longer segment of catheter is coiled in the renal pelvis to prevent dislodgment. The cannula is removed by sliding it back over the Silastic catheter.

The two principal advantages of the trocar–cannula system are:

Faster placement of drainage catheters, achieved by avoiding the intermediate steps such as dilating the nephrostomy tract. The risks of guidewire kinking and loss of the tract are thereby eliminated; and

Usage of soft Silastic catheters, which have the desirable properties of low encrustation with urinary salts, higher urine flow rates, and efficient drainage of debris and purulent material.[71]

The trocar–cannula puncture technique is not as popular as placement of catheters with the Seldinger technique, maybe because of radiologists' familiarity with the latter. The courage needed to introduce a trocar–cannula without a guidewire thus is often absent in radiologists trained in the United States. Also, puncture of the nondilated collecting system is somewhat difficult with the trocar–cannula technique.

DOUBLE-STICK TECHNIQUES

Two punctures are commonly used in obstructed, poorly functioning kidneys. The first (localization puncture[7]) is made into the renal pelvis with a 22- or 23-

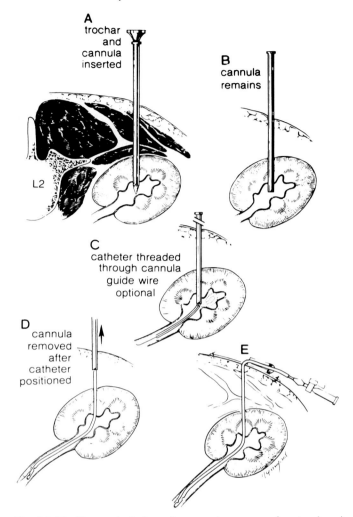

Fig. 23–76 Trocar technique for percutaneous nephrostomies. A. Metal trocar and cannula have been inserted; tips lie within collecting system. B. Trocar has been removed, leaving cannula in place. C. Drainage catheter has been threaded through cannula with or without a guidewire. D. Cannula is being removed, leaving catheter in position. E. After removal of cannula, catheter is secured to the skin and connected to drainage bag. (Reproduced from Newhouse JH, Pfister RC: Percutaneous catheterization of the kidney and perinephric space: trocar technique. *Urol Radiol* 1981;2:157.)

gauge needle under either ultrasonic or fluoroscopic guidance. Contrast medium, CO_2, or both are injected, and the definitive puncture of a calix with an 18-gauge needle is then performed with a high degree of accuracy on the first pass.[57,71,76,126]

Inside-Out Technique

It is easier to establish a tract in retrograde fashion than by conventional percutaneous nephrostomy in the nondilated collecting system. A technique for retrograde percutaneous nephrostomy, described by Hawkins et al, utilizes the experience and principles of transvenous liver biopsies.[135,136] In this system, a 9F catheter is advanced into a posterior calix via a cystoscope. Therefore, two people are usually involved: one, usually the urologist, handles the cystoscope, while a radiologist familiar with percutaneous catheter–guidewire techniques handles the other equipment.

A complete set of equipment for this technique (Fig. 23–77) consists of:

1. A 5F–9F coaxial catheter system. The 9F Teflon catheter is 90 cm long with a 3-cm-long curved tip. The inner (5F) catheter is 3 cm longer than the outer catheter and has a J configuration at its distal tip to prevent trauma to the calices by the larger catheter;
2. A 110-cm-long, 20- or 21-gauge needle with a 93-cm-long 5F Teflon-sheathed Seldinger catheter;
3. Two 50-cm-long, 0.02-inch rocket wires.

With the patient under adequate regional anesthesia, a cystoscope is used to gain access to the bladder, and the coaxial 5F–9F catheter combination is negotiated through the ureter under fluoroscopic guidance (Fig. 23–78A). In tortuous ureters, torque control guidewires are used so the coaxial system does not perforate the ureter. The 9F catheter is placed in the appropriate calix, and its position is verified by injecting contrast medium (Fig. 23–78B). The inner, 5F catheter is removed by loosening the Tuohy–Borst adapter on the 9F catheter. The 100-cm needle, covered by the 93-cm 5F Teflon sheath, is introduced into the lumen of the 9F catheter.

While the operator maintains the posteriorly directed position of the guiding catheter, the needle is advanced until it reaches the skin, which is tented (Fig. 23–78C). The skin is incised with a blade to allow the needle to exit. Liberal use of 1% lidocaine precedes passage of the needle out through the skin.

Occasionally, in postoperative kidneys, the 21-gauge needle will not penetrate the fibrotic tissues. In these cases, a 0.02-inch sharp rocket wire is advanced through

the 21-gauge needle; it commonly penetrates the kidney and skin easily.

The 100-cm rocket wire is pulled through the skin so that it extends from the urethra through the kidney and beyond the skin. This wire is used for subsequent dilation of the nephrostomy tract (Fig. 23–78D).

After penetration of the skin, the 5F sheathing catheter and needle are removed. A standard 0.038-inch guidewire is introduced through the 9F catheter, and the 9F catheter and cystoscope are removed. Over the 0.038-inch guidewire, a balloon or angiographic catheter is advanced into the renal pelvis for subsequent intervention.

Occasionally, the needle will find a rib in its path. To get around the rib, the needle is pulled back 2 or 3 cm, and the patient is asked to inhale or exhale deeply. The needle can then be advanced without resistance because of the change in kidney position in relation to the ribs (Fig. 23–79).

The advantages of creating a nephrostomy tract by retrograde puncture are:

1. Dilation of the tract is easier and safer, becasue the wire passes from the urethra through the kidney and skin, even in obese patients with a scarred kidney;
2. The exiting of the wire through a posterior calix reduces the risk of trauma to renal hilar vessels in comparison with percutaneous puncture.

The chief disadvantage of this technique is that the natural tract of the needle points more laterally than is desirable, usually toward the posterior axillary line. This produces a longer tract and increases the risk of perforating adjacent organs (Figs. 23–80 through 23–82). The more lateral orientation can be explained by the oblique position of the kidney within the body and by the orientation of calices, as seen on transverse tomography (Fig.

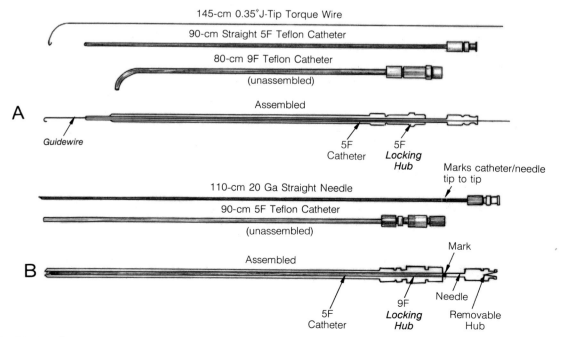

Fig. 23–77 Hawkins inside-out nephrostomy set.

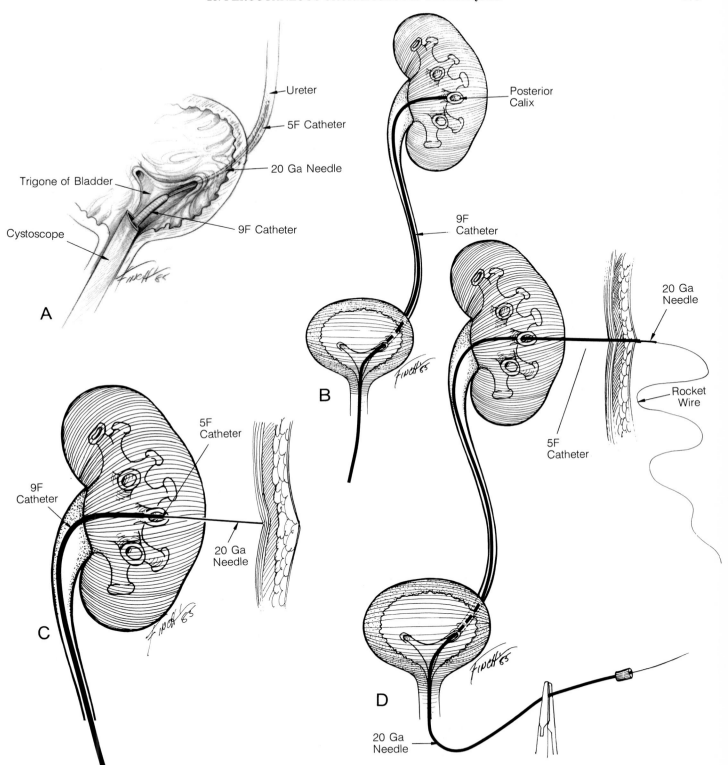

Fig. 23–78 Diagrams illustrating inside-out nephrostomy technique. A. Through cystoscope, ureteral orifice has been catheterized, and 5F catheter has been advanced into ureter. Over 5F catheter, 9F Teflon guiding catheter is being advanced. B. Cystoscope has been removed, leaving 9F catheter with its tip in a posterior calix in lower pole of kidney. C. Through 9F catheter, 5F catheter–20-gauge needle assembly hs been advanced. Once tip of 5F catheter reaches tip of 9F guiding catheter, they are both held in position, and 20-gauge needle is thrust forward until it tents the skin. D. After cutting of the skin, needle has been pulled through, and rocket wire has been passed through needle to provide safe pull-through system. 5F catheter has been advanced over needle–rocket wire assembly.

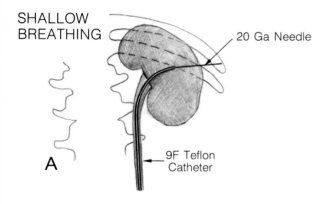

SHALLOW
BREATHING

20 Ga Needle

9F Teflon
Catheter

A

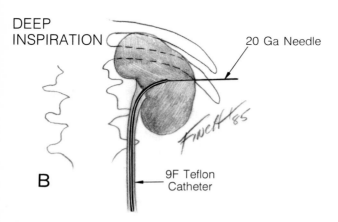

DEEP
INSPIRATION

20 Ga Needle

9F Teflon
Catheter

B

Fig. 23-79 Avoiding the ribs during retrograde nephrostomy puncture. A. During normal shallow breathing, forward advancement of 20-gauge needle has been stopped by a rib. B. By withdrawing the needle slightly and changing the degree of lung inflation, path of needle has been cleared for percutaneous exit.

23–83). Furthermore, the position of the calices is variable; some calices point straight posteriorly, whereas others point directly laterally, causing the needle to exit in the midaxillary line (Fig. 23–84). This obviously cannot be predicted from the analysis of the IVU, so it probably is advisable to obtain two or three CT cuts before the procedure to study the anatomy. One can try to avoid this lateral orientation of the tract by placing a radiopaque marker at the desired skin exit point and then trying to direct the needle toward this marker. This sometimes takes more than one needle passage. Another disadvantage of this technique is encountered when the coaxial catheter–needle system punctures an anterior calix, because the needle might exit anterolaterally, risking puncture of the liver or spleen.

All in all, the authors believe that, although the retrograde technique has some advantages, namely creation of a straight tract and a through-and-through guidewire, which makes dilation of the tract and the placement of a nephrostomy catheter safe and fast, the disadvantages of the lateral and superior orientation of the tract, the inability to select a specific calix in some cases, and the need for cystoscopy outweigh the advantages. This is particularly true in preparation for nephrostolithotomy, where a short tract into a specific calix is needed.

FLUOROSCOPIC PUNCTURE TECHNIQUES

Two techniques are used for the puncture of the renal collecting system: the straight-on-target approach or down-the-barrel technique.

In the straight-on technique, the selected calix is placed in the center of the x-ray field to avoid parallactic shift. After a small skin incision has been made with a

Fig. 23–80 Puncture of adjacent organs during retrograde nephrostomy puncture. A. CT scan through mid area of kidney shows extremely laterally placed nephrostomy path that passes through liver (arrows). Note tip of Foley catheter within renal pelvis (open arrow).

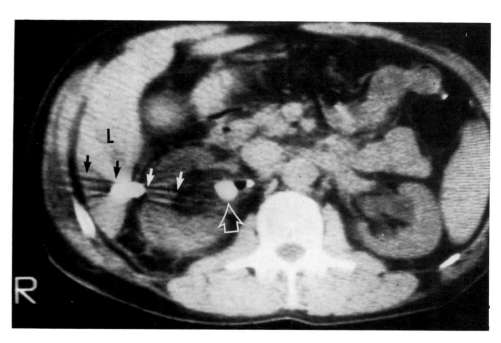

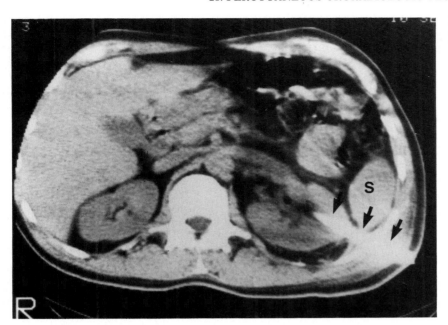

Fig. 23–81 CT scan through mid area of kidney shows extremely lateral nephrostomy tract dangerously close to tip of spleen (S).

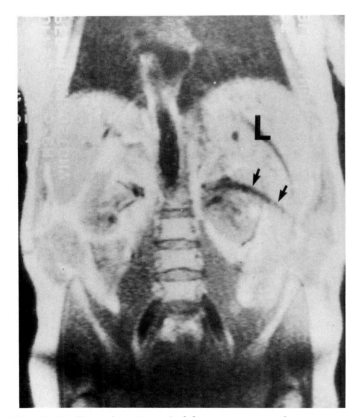

Fig. 23–82 Coronal section of abdomen on magnetic resonance imaging shows path of percutaneous tract through mid area of kidney (arrows), which in this projection seems to be through liver (L). By CT, tract did not pass through liver but was dangerously close to it.

blade, the diamond-tip needle (Fig. 23–85), held by a radiolucent plastic handle (Fig. 23–86),[137] is advanced directly into the target under continuous fluoroscopic monitoring (Fig. 23–87). The diamond-tip needle is preferred to the beveled-tip design because it pursues a straighter course, without swaying to one side or the other as beveled-tip needles commonly do.[129] The needle can be angled in almost any direction if a C- or U-arm unit is used; with such equipment, the needle is always advanced in the direction of the x-ray beam, so the diamond tip should be seen as a dot through its radiolucent hub under fluoroscopy.[129]

The advantage of this straight-on approach is that anyone with any degree of expertise can reach the targeted calix without undue complications. Penetration of the calix or infundibulum can be judged by the observation on the fluoroscopy monitor of indentation of contrast medium by the needle tip, as well as by the tactile sensation of "giving" as soon as the needle reaches the collecting system. The position of the needle is confirmed by aspirating urine, followed by contrast injection. Biplane or oblique C-arm fluoroscopy is better than single-plane fluoroscopy, because the position of the tip of the needle can be confirmed with ease in two planes without aspirating the urine or turning the patient (Figs. 23–88A and 23–89).

When only a conventional fluoroscope is available, a straight-on approach is frequently impossible if the patient cannot be rotated or if cephalad or caudad angulation is required, inasmuch as the area of interest would be directly in the path of the primary x-ray beam. This can be avoided by creating an oblique tract. For this purpose, the patient is arranged in the prone decubitus position. After opacification of the collecting system, the desired site of entry is selected under fluoroscopy. A skin entry site is prepared just off the paravertebral muscles and under the 12th rib. The needle is then advanced

Fig. 23–83   Variability in anatomic relations of calices and central axis of kidney. A. Posterior calices point almost straight posteriorly and anterior calices point in more lateroposterior direction (arrows) than in normal Brödel kidney.

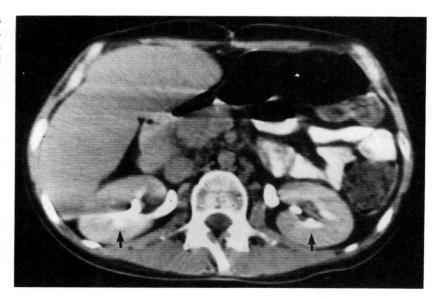

Fig. 23–84   Both posterior and anterior calices point posteriorly (arrows).

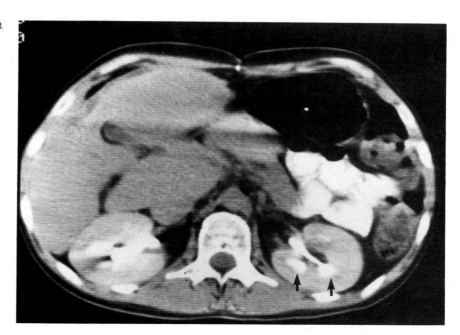

toward the target area, which is kept in the center of the x-ray field. By rotating the patient or moving the table at intervals during needle advancement, the direction of the needle path is corrected. Once the needle is in the target, the patient is rotated so that the collecting system is inside the x-ray field, while the puncture site at the skin is outside, minimizing radiation exposure to the operator's hands.

A simpler way of accomplishing the same objective is to place the patient under fluoroscopy in the prone oblique decubitus position with the side of interest elevated. A target area is selected, and the needle is advanced in straight-on fashion into the collecting system (Fig. 23–90A). Once the target area has been reached, the patient is rearranged in the prone decubitus position, which will place the puncture site outside the x-ray field (Fig. 23–90B).

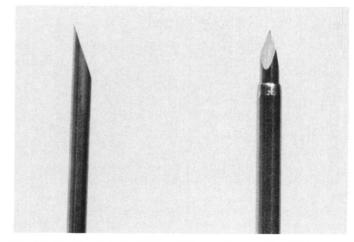

Fig. 23–85   Beveled-tip (left) and diamond-tip needles (right).

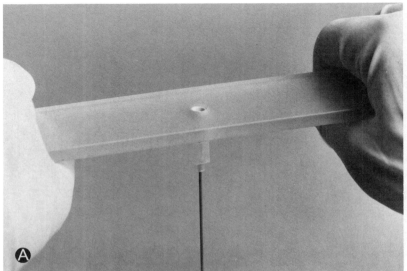

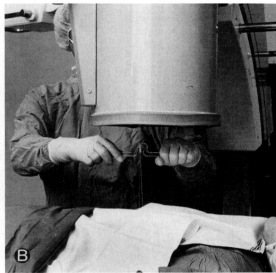

Fig. 23–86 Plastic handle with 18-gauge needle in central opening. A. Observe position of operator's hands holding handle away from primary x-ray beam. B. Use of plastic handle under multidirectional fluoroscopy. Note hands away from primary x-ray beam during advancement of needle under continuous fluoroscopy.

CATHETER PLACEMENT TECHNIQUE FOR EXTERNAL DRAINAGE

Once a 0.038-inch guidewire is in the collecting system, the tract is enlarged to the desired diameter with angiographic Teflon dilators. The authors usually overdilate by 2F to facilitate passage of the drainage catheter. After removal of the last dilator, the drainage catheter is inserted, and the wire is removed. Contrast medium is injected to verify the proper positioning of the sideholes within the collecting system, and the catheter is secured to the skin with suture and tape.

Pigtail Catheters

If a pigtail catheter is to be introduced, it is simply advanced over the guidewire under fluoroscopic control until the pigtail loop is seen within the collecting system. The wire is removed, and the position of the loop and sideholes within the collecting system is checked fluoroscopically by the fast injection of 2–3 ml of contrast medium. All the sideholes should lie within the collecting system; otherwise, bleeding through the catheter can be a problem, and the catheter may become blocked by clots.

Hawkins Catheter

The Hawkins accordion catheter is placed in one step, guided by the needle cannula and coat-hanger wire.

Cope Loop

For insertion of the Cope loop, the 8F–10F catheter with the stiffening cannula is advanced over the guidewire until the desired length of catheter is seen within the collecting system. Making a gentle curve in the cannula can help to direct the catheter tip. One should be careful not to perforate the wall of the pelvis, particularly a small intrarenal pelvis, with the tip of the catheter–stiffener combination. Once the guidewire and cannula have been removed, by simultaneously pulling the silk thread and rotating the catheter, the operator can easily reshape the loop.

The USCI Cope loop, the peel-away introducer sheath,

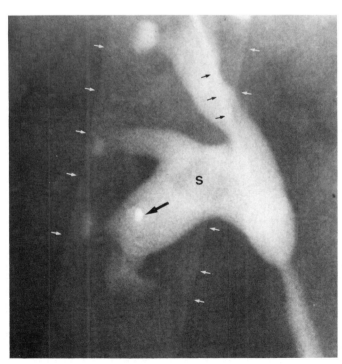

Fig. 23–87 Spot film showing down-the-barrel puncture of lower pole posterior calix. Needle is seen as dot (arrow); stone (S) is faintly visible within renal pelvis. Ureteral catheter with tip in upper pole (small black arrows) was inserted retrograde before procedure. Plastic handle is barely visible (small white arrows).

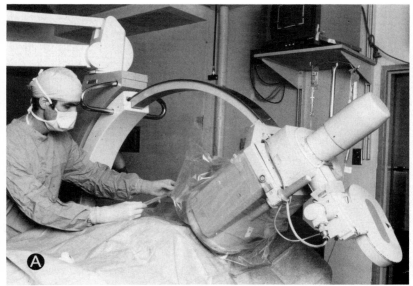

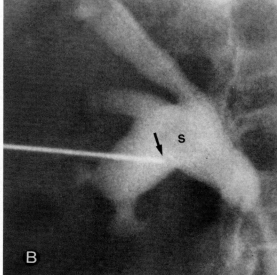

Fig. 23–88   Value of lateral fluoroscopic imaging. A. Lateral view of kidney under continuous fluoroscopy facilitates access to operating field. B. Spot film taken during lateral fluoroscopy shows entry of needle tip (arrow) through caliceal–infundibular junction, avoiding perforation of distal wall of infundibulum. S = stone.

and its dilator are first positioned inside the collecting system. The dilator is then removed, leaving the sheath and guidewire in place. The blunt-ended drainage catheter is inserted through the sheath into the collecting system, where the tip is advanced, the guidewire removed, and the loop reshaped and fixed. After demonstrating adequate placement of the loop by contrast injection, the sheath is peeled away.

In some patients, urinary salt encrustation on the

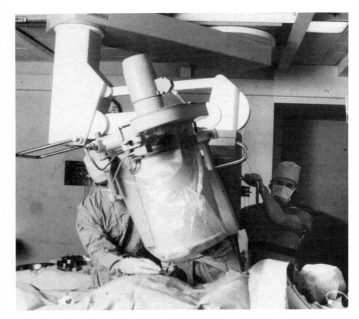

Fig. 23–89   Multidirectional fluoroscopy with cephalad angulation of percutaneous puncture provides straighter tract along central axis of infundibulum.

monofilament thread blocks urine flow and prevents the release of the loop for exchange purposes. In these cases, a smaller (0.035-, 0.025-, 0.018-inch) wire can usually be passed through the lumen after cutting the catheter. A peel-away sheath (Fig. 23–91) or a 10F or 14F coaxial Teflon dilator is advanced into the collecting system over the catheter–wire combination until it reaches the loop (Fig. 23–92). The catheter is yanked back into the sheath or dilator, forcing the loop open (Fig. 23–92), and slowly removed by advancing the sheath and dilator slightly into the collecting system. A new drainage catheter can then be inserted through the sheath or dilator.

Malecot Catheter

Because of the softness of the C-Flex material of the Medi-Tech and Cook Malecot drainage catheters, a stiffener is needed for introduction and to straighten the wings of the catheter. For exchange purposes, a straight-end guidewire is passed through the end hole; if the wire does not pass spontaneously, the stiffener is inserted through the catheter up to the wings, and the catheter is gently pulled back over the stiffener, closing the wings by pushing the stiffener against the tip of the catheter.

With the Medi-Tech catheter, this process is slightly complicated by the presence of the spring-coil thrillium lock inside the Malecot. One should be careful not to push too hard, since this may fracture or loosen the spring–plastic bond. When this accident occurs, it usually happens at only one point, so the catheter can be removed after passage of a wire into the collecting system.

Once the Malecot wings have been straightened by the stiffener, passage of a wire through the end hole is easy. If these maneuvers fail, the wire is passed through the Malecot openings until at least 10 cm are coiled in the

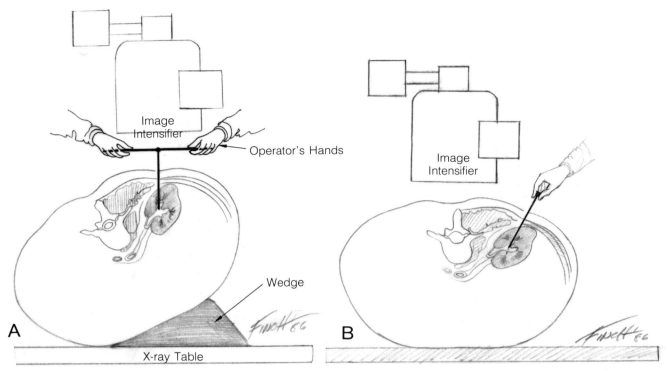

Fig. 23–90 DIagram illustrating puncture of collecting system using conventional fluoroscopic equipment. A. Down-the-barrel puncture is performed with patient rotated approximately 25°–35° in prone decubitus position with side of interest elevated with wedge. B. After needle has been placed within collecting system wedge is removed, and patient can be moved to flat prone decubitus position, which helps to keep operator's hands away from primary x-ray beam.

collecting system, and the catheter is gently pulled back under fluoroscopic control (Fig. 23–93).

The polyethylene Malecot catheter is stiff and therefore usually easy to introduce.

Argyle Catheter

The Argyle three-lumen catheter can be inserted in a single step with the help of the accompanying trocar needle. However, this is not an easy task due to the high friction coefficient of the catheter material. A preferred method of introduction is by puncturing the collecting system with an 18-gauge needle and dilating the tract 2F larger than the catheter, which can then be advanced easily over the guidewire. Because of its two functional lumens, this catheter can be used for drainage of pyonephrosis.

Councill Catheter

The Councill catheter, being slightly stiffer than the Foley catheter, can be introduced fairly easily over a guidewire. For introduction in fresh tracts, dilation 2F larger than the catheter is recommended. An internal stiffener (5F–8F angiographic catheter) is used to decrease the bluntness of the Councill catheter tip and increase stiffness (Fig. 23–94).

Foley Catheter

Several techniques have been recommended for introducing Foley catheters, which are soft and have a high friction coefficient. One method involves making an end hole and freezing the catheter to increase its stiffness. Another involves making an end hole and stiffening the catheter with a dilator or angiographic catheter.

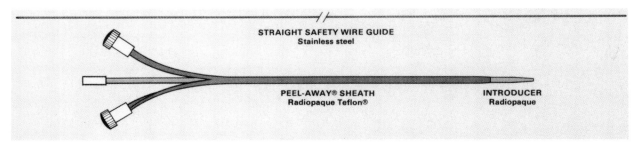

Fig. 23–91 Peel-away introducer set for the introduction of Silastic stents.

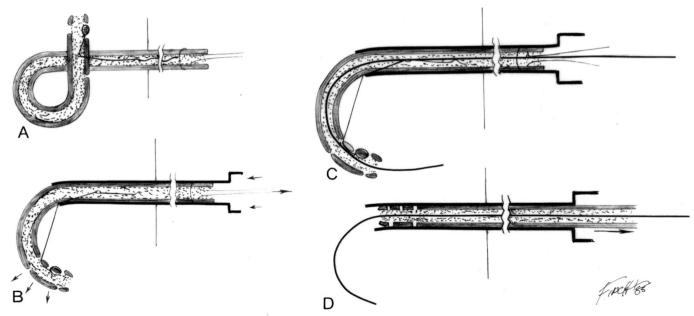

Fig. 23–92 Diagram illustrating removal of stuck Cope loop. A. Severe encrustation of urinary salts has produced binding of loop drawstring in Cope loop. Hub of catheter has been cut, and silk stitch has been passed through blunt end of catheter. B. Silk suture has been passed into lumen of vascular introducer, which has then been advanced over shaft of Cope loop, forcing leading edge of introducer to release drawstring and straighten loop. C. Once loop has been straightened, 0.035-inch guidewire has been passed through lumen of loop into collecting sytem. D. While guidewire is kept in position, Cope loop is pulled back through introducer.

The Cope Foley introducer is an ingenious device that stretches the rubber material of the catheter over a stiff metal, thus decreasing the diameter and increasing the stiffness. A thin slit, not an end hole, is cut in the tip of the catheter, and the cannula–catheter assembly is inserted over the guidewire into the collecting system (Fig. 23–95). The tract needs to be dilated only to the size of the catheter. Once the balloon is inflated to assure its position within the collecting system, the cannula is removed and contrast medium is injected.

When using large-bore drainage catheters, one should make sure, first, that the catheter tip is not within the

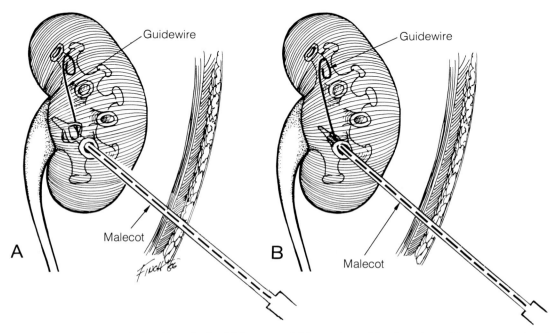

Fig. 23–93 Diagram illustrating removal of malfunctioning Malecot catheter. A. Guidewire has been passed, exiting through openings of Malecot tip, and has been looped into upper pole calix. B. With guidewire held in place, Malecot catheter is pulled back.

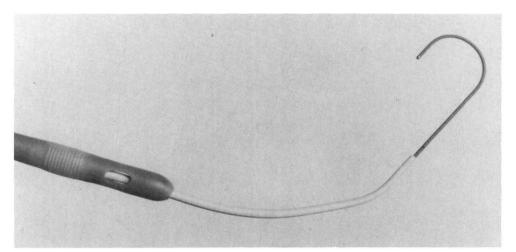

Fig. 23–94 Councill catheter with angiographic torque control catheter passed through it over guidewire.

proximal ureter or ureteropelvic junction, because it may induce local irritation with subsequent stricture formation, and, second, that the tip is not pressing on the renal pelvic wall, because this frequently causes pain, nausea, and vomiting.

For exchange of these large-bore catheters, a guidewire is passed, ideally through the end hole. If the wire passes through a sidehole, enough wire (8–10 cm) should be coiled within the collecting system to prevent dislodgment during catheter removal (Fig. 23–96).

Occasionally, the balloon of a Councill or Foley catheter will not deflate, particularly when filled with contrast medium. In such a case, the balloon can be punctured percutaneously with a 20- or 22-gauge needle under fluoroscopic control (Fig. 23–97). This is preferable to pulling the inflated balloon forcefully through the tract.

Circle Tube (U-Loop) Nephrostomy Catheter

Patients who require long-term external drainage are best managed by creating circle tube nephrostomy drainage. Long-term external drainage is fraught with complications, such as obstruction, tube dislodgment, and hemorrhage. Thus, since its inception in the 1950's and 1960's, surgically created circle tube nephrostomies have become popular as a way to reduce the frequency of those problems.[138-143] Silicone rubber catheters are preferred because of their resistance to encrustation and because they remain soft and pliable even after long usage, and so are comfortable for the patient.

Smith et al proposed an innovative technique to establish circle tube nephrostomy drainage in patients who already have a single nephrostomy tract created either

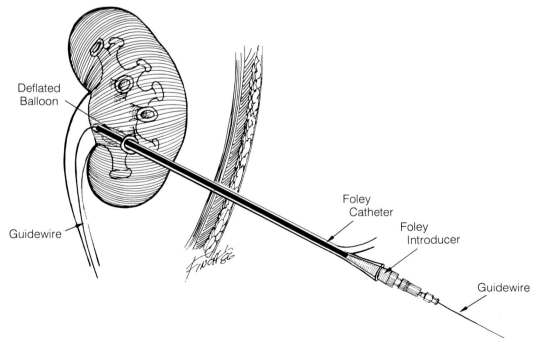

Fig. 23–95 Diagram illustrating placement of Foley nephrostomy catheter with aid of Foley introducer.

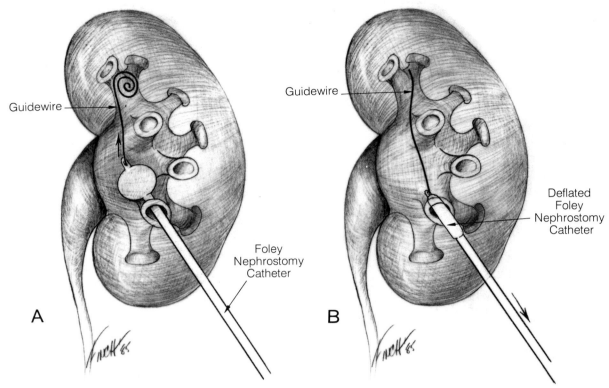

Fig. 23-96   Diagram illustrating removal of Foley catheter placed surgically. A. In the absence of end hole in Foley catheter, guidewire has been manipulated through sideholes and looped into upper pole

calix. B. After deflation of balloon, Foley catheter is pulled back while guidewire is kept in place.

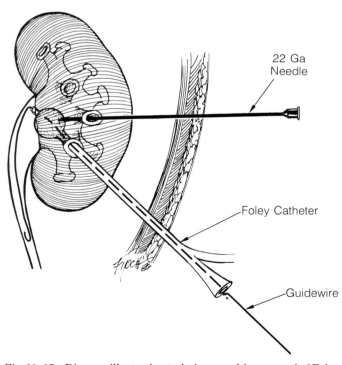

Fig. 23-97   Diagram illustrating technique used for removal of Foley balloon catheter when balloon cannot be deflated because of drying and consolidation of contrast medium used to fill it. A 22-gauge Chiba needle is placed percutaneously to puncture balloon, which can then be withdrawn over guidewire.

percutaneously or surgically.[132,144] The principal indications are:

Poor surgical risks that preclude radical surgery;
Unresectable carcinoma in patients who are uncooperative or incapable of taking care of single-tube nephrostomies.

The principal advantages of circle tube nephrostomy drainage are:

1. Avoidance of bleeding from the chronic irritation by single nephrostomy catheters;
2. The higher patency rate of the Silastic tubes used because of their lower encrustation;
3. Greater comfort, because the tubes are softer;
4. Avoidance of accidental loss of the catheter;
5. Easy exchange of the catheter by connecting it to an adapter attached to a new tube that is pulled into place over a guidewire;
6. Excellent drainage, even in patients with a small renal pelvis.

Technique

To place a circle tube requires two nephrostomy tracts. Ideally, they should go through posterior calices in the upper and lower poles, because it is advisable to have considerable renal parenchyma between the tracts. However, if an upper pole approach would require a puncture above the 12th rib, a posterior calix of the middle group can be

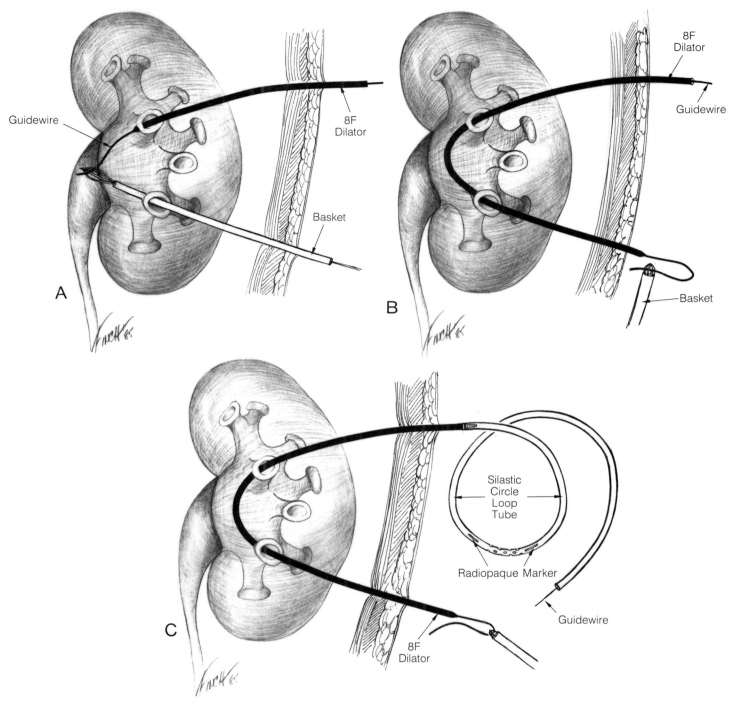

Fig. 23–98 Placement of circle loop nephrostomy. A. Two separate percutaneous nephrostomy tracts have been placed; one through an upper pole and one through a lower pole calix. Both tracts have been dilated to 8F; through one tract, basket has been introduced to trap guidewire passed through second tract. B. Basket and trapped guidewire have been pulled back, creating through-and-through guidewire path. The 8F Teflon dilator has been advanced to dilate tract.

C. Bifunnel plastic adapter (arrow) has been attached to ends of Teflon dilator and Silastic circle loop tubes. D. By pulling forward on Teflon dilator, Silastic circle loop nephrostomy tube has been positioned with sideholes within renal pelvis. Observe position of radiopaque markers within collecting system. A T-connector has been used to connect both limbs of circle loop nephrostomy tube to drainage bag.

used for the upper tract. Through one of the tracts, a stone basket or snare loop is introduced to trap a guidewire introduced through the opposite tract (Fig. 23–98A). Frequently, it is easier to snare the wire down the ureter than it is to trap it within the dilated renal pelvis. Once

the wire is snared, it is extracted gently through one tract (forceful extraction is to be avoided, because the wire might cut the intervening renal parenchyma) while being advanced through the other.

Once the trail is established with the guidewire

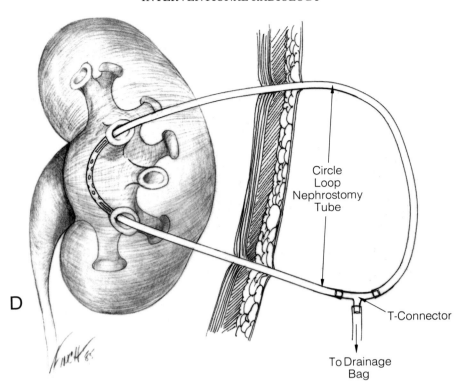

Fig. 23–98D

between the upper and lower puncture sites, the tract can be dilated in one of three ways (Fig. 23–98B). First, for small tracts, the coaxial Amplatz renal dilators or the Vance tapered-tip dilators that fit snugly over the 0.038-inch guidewire can be utilized without kinking the guidewire. Second, the tract can be dilated with balloon catheters. Third, a filiform follower can be attached to an angiographic catheter by passing the distal end of the guidewire through a sidehole immediately in front of the distal end of the angiographic catheter and threading it back through the lumen of the filiform catheter. The tract is then dilated with a succession of filiform followers of gradually increasing size.

After the desired dilation is achieved, an angiographic "guiding" catheter or dilator the same size as the circle nephrostomy tube is inserted over the through-and-through guidewire and passed through both tracts. A plastic bifunnel adaptor is connected flush to the end of both the Silastic tube and the guiding catheter dilator (Fig. 23–98C). The assembled system can be pulled and pushed through under fluoroscopic control until the radiopaque markers that outline the sideholes of the circle tube lie within the collecting system (Fig. 23–98D). The wire and angiographic catheter or dilator are then removed. After clamping of one end of the Silastic tube, contrast medium is injected to assess the position of the sideholes, which can be adjusted by pulling on either end of the loop. If the position is satisfactory, both ends are hooked to a Y connector, which is connected to the drainage bag. Both arms of the Silastic loop can then be stitched to the skin to prevent migration.

Cooperative patients with a long-term loop learn to adjust it when they sense either the discomfort or the urine leak that occurs when the sideholes are misplaced, partially blocking and distending the renal pelvis. The loop can easily be replaced by attaching a bifunnel connector between one arm of the old and new loops and pulling the latter into position. The tubes are usually changed once every 3–6 months. The same technique can be used for patients with obstructed ureterostomies (Fig. 23–99).

EMERGENCY BEDSIDE PERCUTANEOUS NEPHROSTOMY

Portable real-time sonography plays an important role in critically ill patients who cannot be transported to the radiology department.[125] In emergencies, percutaneous nephrostomy is performed mostly for drainage of urinary obstruction or pyonephrosis.

Preoperative and Intraoperative Care

The procedure, possible complications, and risks are explained to the patient's family. Bleeding factors and times are evaluated and any abnormalities corrected. Sedation is administered as needed, depending on the condition of the patient.

Technique

The first step is a diagnostic screening. After thorough examination, the patient is positioned to allow the nephrostomy needle to enter through the posterolateral margin of the kidney. The kidney is evaluated again and

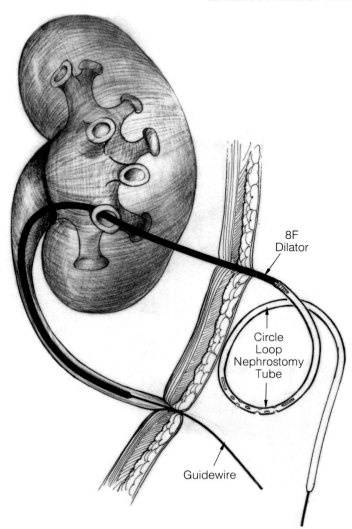

a puncture site is selected (Fig. 23–100). The entry site is scrubbed and draped.

After administration of local anesthetic, the needle is advanced into the pelvicaliceal system under ultrasonic guidance (Fig. 23–101) until urine can be aspirated.[3,76,125] After successful puncture of the collecting system, urine is aspirated, and samples are sent for cytology, Gram stain, and culture. Ideally, a one-stick Hawkins set is used for the initial puncture, because the accordion drainage catheter can immediately be advanced into the collecting system under either ultrasonic guidance or portable fluoroscopy.[24] An 18-gauge needle can be inserted along the 22-gauge needle at the same angle and to the same depth.[2,3] The exchange for the 18-gauge needle should be performed under portable fluoroscopic control. A few milliliters of contrast medium are instilled into the collecting system through the 22-gauge needle and the further steps observed with the portable C-arm fluoroscope.

When the patient is in the decubitus position, contrast medium tends to accumulate in the renal pelvis or proximal ureter, and the posterior calices—the site of entry for the nephrostomy needle—will not be opacified.[3] The entire procedure can be markedly facilitated by the introduction of CO_2 into the renal pelvis, because it will float into the posterior calices.

Only guidewires with long floppy tips should be used during bedside nephrostomies to minimize the chances of perforation. The advancement of the guidewire should be

←

Fig. 23–99   Use of circle loop nephrostomy technique in patient with cutaneous ureterostomy. Over guidewire manipulated across stricture at level of anastomosis with help of angiographic catheter, an 8F dilator has been passed. To the end of the 8F dilator, bifunnel pastic adapter has been attached to pull circle loop nephrostomy tube into position.

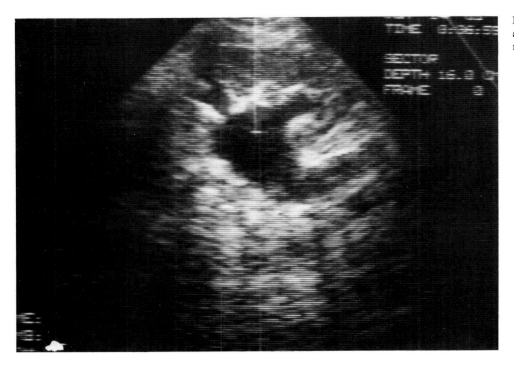

Fig. 23–100   Longitudinal sonogram along posterior axillary line shows marked hydronephrosis.

Fig. 23–101 Longitudinal sonogram shows position of needle tip within renal pelvis (arrow).

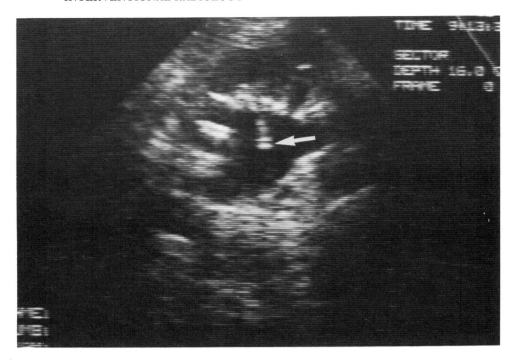

observed adequately (Figs. 23–102 and 23–103). At the end of the procedure, the drainage system is fixed to the skin, and a scout film is obtained for documentation after contrast medium has been administered through the catheter.

PERCUTANEOUS NEPHROSTOMY IN CHILDREN

Percutaneous nephrostomy is performed in infants for diagnostic and temporizing purposes.[4,145] Diagnostic antegrade urography provides clear definition of the anatomy and, in association with dynamic studies (Whitaker test), permits better evaluation of the anatomic and physiologic problems than do static radiographic studies. Ultrasound is preferred to delineate the collecting system, inasmuch as it entails no radiation exposure and because renal function commonly has deteriorated to the extent that opacification of the dilated collecting system by iodinated contrast medium is poor at best. Ultrasound will image poorly functioning kidneys clearly.

Fig. 23–102 Transverse sonogram at level of renal pelvis showing guidewire introduced through needle into renal pelvis (arrows).

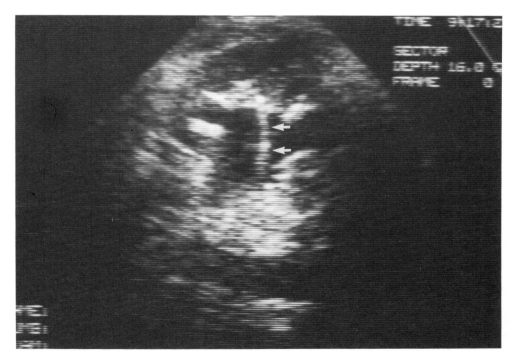

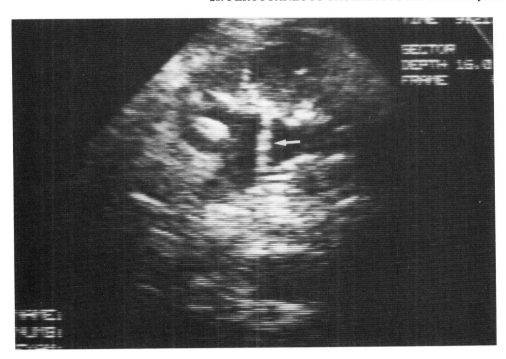

Fig. 23–103 Transverse sonogram showing position of pigtail catheter within renal renal pelvis (arrow).

Technique and Indications

The technique for placement of nephrostomy tubes is similar to that used in adults, with these differences:

The kidneys of infants and young children lie lower than in adults;

The soft tissues in the renal fossa are less developed than in adults; therefore, the kidneys are closer to the skin;

Commonly, because of the nature of the disease process with long-standing obstruction, less renal parenchyma is available, so its contribution to tract formation is slight;

Heavy sedation or general anesthesia is required because of the lack of cooperation from these patients;

The use of a small needle and tubing (e.g., 5F) is necessary to minimize renal damage and the risk of vascular injury. The 5F Hawkins accordion catheter is a good system, because the puncture is done with a 22-gauge needle. Over this needle the 5F Teflon catheter is advanced into the collecting system, providing a reliable, self-retaining drainage tube. The retention capability is a particularly desirable feature in children.

Common indications are posterior urethral valves, congenital hydronephrosis and megaureter, postoperative strictures, pyonephrosis, obstructed allografts, fistulae (post-traumatic or postoperative), and renal calculi.

Functional Studies

Pressure–flow measurement as a diagnostic urodynamic study was first described by Backlund and Renterskold in 1969 and popularized by Whitaker and Pfister.[83–87] Antegrade evaluation of obstruction of the upper urinary tract requires a simple set-up, namely a pump to deliver a given flow rate and a pressure transducer or a water manometer. A Foley catheter is placed in the bladder for vesical pressure recording, and a 22-gauge needle or small angiographic catheter is placed in the renal pelvis. The needle or catheter is connected through a three-way stopcock to a water manometer and to the infusion pump. Alternatively, two needles can be placed in the renal pelvis, one connected to the infusion pump, which delivers normal saline or dilute contrast medium at a selected rate, and the second to a pressure transducer.[87] Simultaneously, the pressure in the bladder is recorded via the Foley catheter. The bladder pressure is then subtracted from the pelvic pressure, and in this way the pressure required to propel fluid accross the ureteropelvic junction at a given flow rate is determined. Whitaker recommends perfusion at 10 ml/min and regards a pressure gradient of <12 cm H_2O across the ureterovesical or ureteropelvic junction as normal. Values of 13–22 cm H_2O suggest mild obstruction, and pressure gradients >22 cm H_2O indicate severe obstruction.

Discussion

Infants and young children with severe hydronephrosis and megaureter pose a difficult therapeutic problem. Various approaches have been proposed, such as cutaneous ureterostomy and primary ureteral repair, in which the ureter is tapered and reimplanted and continuous antibacterial suppression is instituted. However, these dilated ureters often drain compromised kidneys, and the child frequently presents with sepsis or uremia.

Drainage of an infected obstructed megaureter in a sick baby is best achieved by nephrostomy, which, if done percutaneously, obviates cutaneous ureterostomy and general anesthesia. This is desirable because fixation of the ureter and possible compromise of the ureteral blood supply during cutaneous ureterostomy render subsequent reconstruction awkward and unnecessarily delay the definitive repair of the megaureter. Indeed, Gonzalez and Sheldon, who have treated several newborn infants who had septic obstruction, recently changed their recommendations of immediate open operation[146] to percutaneous nephrostomy.[147] Although noting that open operation does permit biopsy of grossly abnormal areas of the kidney, those authors remark that the safety of multiple percutaneous skinny-needle biopsies and the availability of urine from the nephrostomy tract for analysis make open biopsy seem less necessary.

The antegrade pyelogram and the Whitaker test have an important place in clinical practice, and percutaneous nephrostomy has distinct advantages over open nephrostomy or cutaneous ureterostomy, particularly in the very sick infant and younger child.

PERCUTANEOUS NEPHROSTOMY IN THE RENAL ALLOGRAFT

Introduction

Urologic complications occur in approximately 10% of all renal allograft recipients.[148] Most of these complications involve either a urine leak, which usually occurs in the early postoperative period (within a month) or ureteric obstruction, which can occur either early or late (*i.e.,* >6 months postoperatively). A precise anatomic and physiologic diagnosis should be made quickly to permit prompt surgical correction if necessary. Percutaneous antegrade pyelograms and placement of percutaneous nephrostomy drainage catheters are rapid and accurate ways to make a diagnosis and initiate therapy. The most common presenting symptoms are elevation of the creatinine level and pain over the allograft.

Indications

Prior to 1977, urologic complications occured in 8%–13% of those renal allograft recipients who had a Starzl or Politano–Leadbetter submucosal tunnel ureteroneocystostomy (Fig. 23–104) or a variation. Other types of urinary tract anastomoses had even less favorable results. In the last several years, increasing experience with improved surgical and immunologic techniques has lowered the rate of urologic complications to 1%–5%.[148] Most urologic complications involve either leaks, which occur in the early postoperative period (*i.e.,* within 1 month), or ureteral obstruction, which occurs both early and late (*i.e.,* >6 months postoperatively). Urologic complications are associated overall with a two- to three-fold increase in morbidity and mortality,[149–151] and those that occur within 2 or 3 weeks after surgery have an even higher risk of fatal outcome or loss of the allograft.[150–152] Therefore, it is imperative that a diagnosis be made quickly and appropriate treatment be instituted. Percutaneous procedures are playing an increasing part in this management.

Obstruction. The important and often difficult distinction to be made in a patient presenting with worsen-

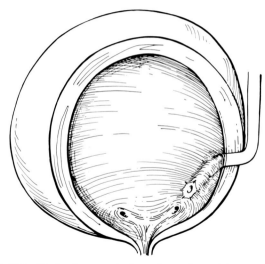

Fig. 23–104 Ureteral neocystostomy is performed low on posterolateral aspect of bladder wall as close as possible to the relatively immobile trigone. Ureter passes obliquely through muscular part of bladder wall and then in short submucosal tunnel to its orifice. (Reproduced from Hunter DW, Castañeda–Zuñiga WR, Coleman CC, Herrera M, Amplatz K: Percutaneous techniques in the management of urological complications in renal transplant patients. *Radiology* 1983;148:407 with permission of the Radiological Society of North America.)

ing allograft function, especially in the late postoperative period, is between rejection and obstruction.[150] Obstruction is primarily due to surgical problems, not immunologic ones.[153] This view is supported by the finding that the rate of obstruction in patients requiring reimplantation of the native ureter, primarily for reflux, is 4%,[154] *i.e.,* approximately the same as that in allograft recipients. The most common site of obstruction is the ureterovesical junction.[148,150] A large number of causes have been found, including kinks; fibrosis following inflammation, rejection, or ischemia; calculi or clots; extrinsic compression by fluid collections, including lymphocele, hematoma, urinoma, and abscess; tumor; and edematous allografts; ischemia; and functional obstruction secondary to bladder distention.[149]

Several authors offer suggestions on which test to order to diagnose obstruction. These include a renogram, IVU, cystogram, and cystoscopy with retrograde pyelography, in that order.[152,155,156] All authors recommend making an accurate diagnosis rapidly, because morbidity and mortality increase markedly if treatment is delayed, and reoperation is difficult even under favorable circumstances. Reimplantation is often impossible, necessitating a salvage procedure such as pyeloureterostomy or pyelovesical anastomosis.[150,155]

Urine leak. Most urine leaks occur at the ureteroneocystostomy, at the cystostomy through which the ureteroneocystostomy was created,[149–151,153,157] or at the renal pelvis and ureter. The usual cause of a urine leak from the renal pelvis or ureter is ischemia, most likely due to excessive dissection of the donor kidney that compromises blood supply from the small peripelvic or periureteric vessels.[151,158–160] In those leaks appearing >4 weeks postoperatively, ischemia may be secondary to rejection.[150,155] Leaks usually occur in the first 2 or 3 postoperative weeks[150,153,160] and almost invariably in the first 5–6 weeks.[152,161] Rarely, urine leaks occur as late as the tenth week.

Urine leaks are supposedly more common in allografts from living related donors,[155] but in the present authors' series there was no significant difference in the incidence between living related and cadaver allografts. Leaks are more common in diabetic patients[157]; two of the authors' patients with urine leaks had juvenile onset diabetes. Urine leaks are more common in patients who, instead of the Politano–Leadbetter ureteroneocystostomy, have a ureteroureterostomy, pyeloureterostomy, or extravesical anastomosis.[152,155,162] They also are more common after operation for obstruction.[150]

The recommended approach to the diagnosis and treatment of urine leaks varies widely. Rapid diagnosis and early correction are generally believed to be important, because delay in treatment increases the morbidity and mortality.[151,152,163,164] Nonetheless, several investigators recommend waiting for a few days after the diagnosis of a urine leak or fistula to see if it will close spontaneously.[152,155,165] One report said that 12 of 14 urinary fistulae closed without operation,[165] whereas another asserted that none closed without treatment.[151] The mortality rate from untreated urinary fistulae is as high as 50%,[153] and even with adequate treatment it is approximately 33%.[150,152]

Radiologic Diagnosis

The approach to the radiologic evaluation of the allograft recipient with a suspected urologic complication begins with ultrasound and a renogram. Ultrasound can detect small abnormal fluid collections that may be an early sign of a leak and is a sensitive indicator of hydronephrosis or hydroureter, which suggests obstruction but can be due to other causes, especially rejection.[159,166,167] Some investigators suggest that the renogram is insensitive (a high false-negative rate), anatomically inaccurate, and nonspecific.[155–168] However, in the authors' series, the renogram was a good indicator of allograft viability, and a persistent abnormal collection of activity was a reliable sign of a leak and urinoma. In addition, concomitant vascular flow studies and diuresis excretion studies can help in evaluating the vascular supply and may allow one to differentiate rejection from obstruction. However, even with the additional refinement of diuresis, a renogram may miss a partial but significant obstruction and is usually unable to define or locate the cause.

In the present authors' experience, as well as in that of others, the allograft renal pelvis is often prominent on ultrasound even without obstruction, especially in the early post-transplantation period. Furthermore, the level of the obstruction is often difficult to locate. On the other hand, the pelvicaliceal system may not be dilated, and can be compressed, in the presence of fibrotic changes in the transplanted kidney (Fig. 23–105). In these cases, the ultrasound study will be negative in spite of marked obstruction at the ureteral level. To improve its accuracy in obstruction, a functional ultrasonic evaluation can be performed by obtaining scans first with an empty bladder and then, after a few hours without voiding, with a full

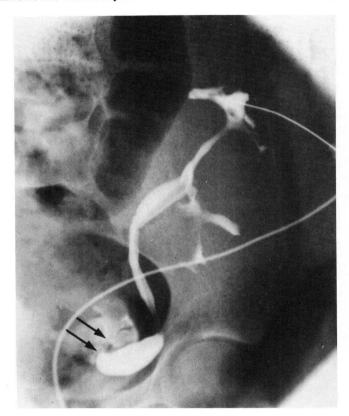

Fig. 23–105 Antegrade pyelography in patient with interstitial fibrosis of allograft kidney and elevated serum creatinine levels for 2 years. In spite of high-grade stenosis of intramural distal ureter, there is no dilatation of pelvicaliceal system. Note dilated aperistaltic distal ureter (arrows). (Reproduced from Zollikofer C, Hunter DW, Castañeda–Zuñiga WR, et al: *RöFo* 1985;42:193.)

bladder. Theoretically, the degree of dilatation of the collecting system should not change, or change only minimally, in cases with a fixed organic obstruction but should increase significantly as the bladder fills in cases of functional obstruction (Fig. 23–106). Differentiation between functional and organic obstruction caused by bladder distention is still not possible, however.

A cystogram is done next, especially if a bladder leak is suspected.

The surgical literature suggests cystoscopy and retrograde studies as the next step. Retrograde studies are accurate when successful, but they carry an increased risk of infection, and the ureteroneocystostomy is often difficult to locate and cannulate.[155,160,169] In the authors' experience, attempts at retrograde studies failed in >50% of cases. Further, a retrograde study done without fluoroscopy may not image the ureter or a point of extravasation optimally, and it may be impossible to get contrast above a tight stenosis to evaluate the proximal collecting system.[166]

Instead of cystography, the authors recommend a percutaneous antegrade pyelogram. When performed with a skinny needle, there are few or no complications,[166,169–171] and because the allograft kidney is denervated, there is little or no pain. The test is particularly good in patients with poor renal function, in whom an IVU or renogram will be inadequate. The site of a urine leak can be deter-

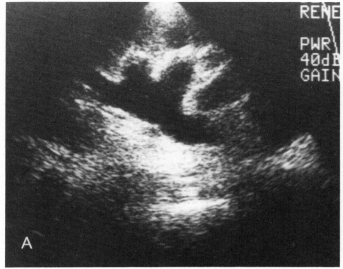

Fig. 23–106   Longitudinal sonogram over transplanted kidney shows collecting system of normal dimensions, indicating that marked dila- tation of renal pelvis and calices is related to compression of ureter by distended bladder.

mined accurately, as can the location and extent of any fistulous tracts or urinomas. Stenoses and the proximal end of any obstruction can be clearly seen. An antegrade pyelogram through the skinny needle, possibly combined with a Whitaker test for objective physiologic evaluation of obstruction, may be the only test necessary. This was true in 30% of the authors' patients, who, on the basis of the antegrade pyelogram, either did not require or were unsuitable candidates for percutaneous catheter drainage.

In some cases, contrast medium may be instilled into the bladder through a Foley catheter and the collecting system opacified by reflux into the allograft ureter. This method should be used only when a previous cystogram has demonstrated low-pressure reflux without extrava- sation and when there is no urinary infection.

Catheter Insertion

The approach to the allograft kidney for placement of a nephrostomy catheter depends on the surgical anatomy. In the usual situation, the kidney is in an extraperitoneal location with the renal pelvis on the posteromedial sur- face. In these cases, an anterolateral approach to the col- lecting system should be used which avoids overlying bowel, traverses as much renal parenchyma as possible, and enters through an anterolateral calix or infundibu- lum (Fig. 23–107). If the nephrostogram reveals a prob-

Fig. 23–107 Schematic drawing of anatomic relations of transplanted kid- ney and its orientation in its extraper- itoneal pelvic position. Anterolateral approach with needle avoids peritoneal cavity and overlying bowel and tra- verses maximum amount of renal parenchyma before entering collecting system. IVC = inferior vena cava. (Reproduced from Hunter DW, Casta- ñeda–Zuñiga WR, Coleman CC, Her- rera M, Amplatz K: Percutaneous tech- niques in the management of urological complications in renal transplant patients. *Radiology* 1983;148:407 with permission of the Radiological Society of North America.)

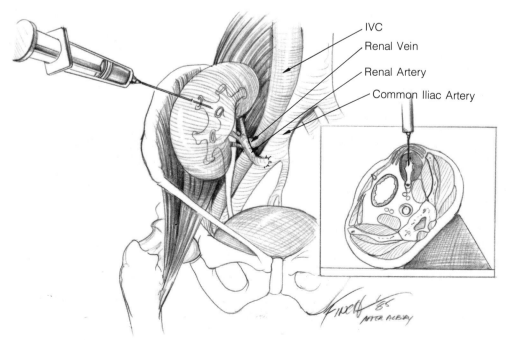

IVC
Renal Vein
Renal Artery
Common Iliac Artery

lem that will require imminent surgical correction, the drainage tube is usually left in the renal pelvis. Otherwise, it may be advanced to the bladder to permit internal drainage with normal urination.

Perioperative care. Prophylactic broad-spectrum antibiotics (ampicillin and gentamicin) are begun just prior to the invasive studies or nephrostomy and continued for as long as a drainage catheter is in place. Coagulation factors and times should be normal if possible.

Guidance methods. The method used to image the collecting system depends on the clinical situation. In most cases, elevated creatinine levels and depressed renal function preclude the use of intravenous contrast medium. In most of the authors' cases, the collecting system could be entered on the first or second pass with a 22-gauge needle under ultrasound guidance (Fig. 23–108). In other cases, the location of the collecting system on the skin is marked, and a puncture is made in the direction and to the depth determined by ultrasound or CT in the angiographic suite (Fig. 23–109). After adequate opacification of the collecting system, the percutaneous nephrostomy is created under fluoroscopic guidance. Multidirectional fluoroscopy with a rotational fluoroscope (C-arm or U-arm) is of great advantage in selecting the best approach.

Urodynamic Studies for Evaluation of Obstruction

To assess the functional significance of a stenosis, or to determine if hydronephrosis is due to partial obstruction, a Whitaker test can be done.[167,170–172] The test can diagnose obstruction even if it is associated with reflux. It has been used to document functional ureterovesical-junction obstruction in children with ureteroneocystostomies and to differentiate functional ureterovesical obstruction from a noncompliant detrusor.[173] In addition, studies of ureteral peristalsis by means of cine ureterography or

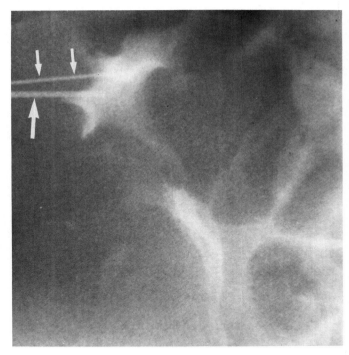

Fig. 23–108 Spot film showing position of 22-gauge Chiba needle used for initial puncture under ultrasound guidance (small arrows) and the position of 18-gauge needle (large arrow) placed in tandem fashion for definitive puncture or for drainage catheter placement.

rapid (6 frames/sec) filming with a 100-mm camera may give additional information, especially in equivocal cases.

Technique of the Whitaker test in allograft kidney. The authors performed the Whitaker test according to his methods and those described by Pfister and Newhouse.[170] Figure 23–110 shows the equipment used. Antegrade ureteral perfusion is performed using a 22-gauge Chiba needle or through a percutaneous nephros-

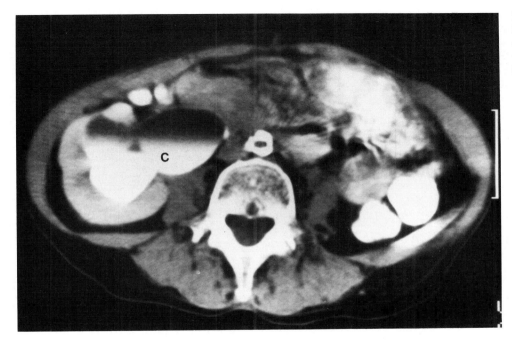

Fig. 23–109 CT scan through allograft kidney illustrates problems imposed by specific gravity of contrast medium (c) within collecting system; lighter urine floats on top.

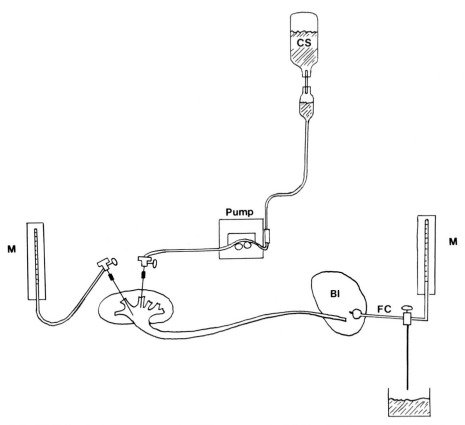

Fig. 23–110   Set-up used for Whitaker test. From reservoir, 20%–30% contrast medium (CS) is pumped through 22-gauge Chiba needle into collecting system. Simultaneously, pressure in renal pelvis is registered through second Chiba needle in collecting system. Pressure in baldder (Bl) is measured via Foley catheter (FC). For pressure measurements, two simple water manometers (M) are sufficient. A three-way stopcock allows emptying and retrograde filling of urinary bladder.

tomy tube. When the needle is used, the authors recommend the double-needle technique, using one needle for perfusion and one for measuring pressures in the renal pelvis. This technique is especially helpful in cases with little or no dilation of the pelvicaliceal system. The first needle, which is placed under ultrasonic or fluoroscopic control, may show free flow for perfusion but may not allow aspiration and pressure reading if its tip is against the pelvic wall. However, by dilating the pelvicaliceal system by the injection of contrast medium, a second needle can be placed selectively in a calix or infundibulum, which will best guarantee free backflow for pressure measurement. This technique offers the advantage of simultaneous perfusion and pressure readings. In the authors' experience, there has been no increase in morbidity or rate of bleeding in conjunction with inserting two skinny needles into the pelvicaliceal system. Pressures in the urinary bladder are usually recorded using a Foley catheter. Ureteral perfusion is regulated by a pump capable of delivering flow rates of as much as 15–20 ml/min.

The perfusion studies are started at a flow rate of 2–5 ml/min. If no significant pressure increase occurs at low flow rates, the rate is increased in increments of 5 ml/min every 5–10 min to a maximum of 15–20 ml/min. To allow observation of flow fluoroscopically, a 20%–30% contrast solution is used. For pressure measurements, simple water manometers are sufficient. Perfusion is usually started with the bladder empty. If no significant pressure gradient or an equivocal pressure gradient is found, the test is repeated with the bladder full to rule out functional obstruction. According to Mayo and Pfister and their coworkers, a pressure gradient between the pelvicaliceal system and the bladder of >20 cm H_2O at a flow rate of 10 ml/min is definitely abnormal; gradients below 15 cm H_2O are normal, and those between 15 and 20 cm H_2O are equivocal.[170,173] In the authors' hands, the combined use of antegrade pyelography and the Whitaker test in renal allografts definitely clarified the differential diagnosis between rejection and obstruction in >80% of cases, and in about 45%, the initial clinical diagnosis was corrected.

Evaluation of Ureteral Peristalsis

In native kidneys, peristaltic waves normally occur 2–6 times per minute. The rate of ureteral contraction depends on the amount of urine production; at low flow rates (<0.2 ml/min), the rate drops to 2 or 3 per minute, whereas at high flow rates (3–5 ml/min or more), the rate may increase to 12 per minute. At extremely high flow rates, such as the 10 ml/min used in perfusion studies, a continuous column of fluid forms in the ureter. Mechanical stretch, such as that by urine or a fluid bolus, may initiate peristalsis. In addition, peristalsis is influenced by

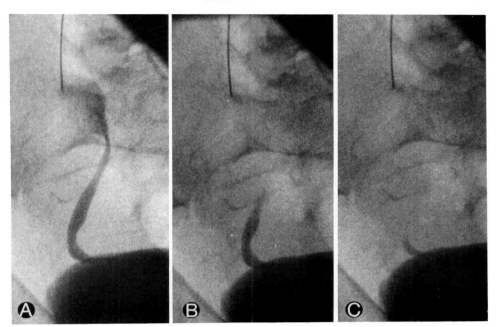

Fig. 23–111 Cine sequence of antegrade pyelogram in patient without obstruction. Note normal peristaltic wave, with rapid and complete emptying of renal pelvis and ureter after injection of single bolus of contrast medium.

the intrapelvic pressure. In partial obstruction with an increase in basal pelvic pressure, the frequency of contraction increases and, depending on the severity of obstruction, there may be retrograde spread of activity or discoordination and a decrease in the amplitude of the contractile pressure waves, rendering urine transport inefficient. With dilation of the ureter in severe stenosis, peristaltic waves are completely lost.

According to the literature, ureteral peristalsis is seen in 84%–90% of renal transplant recipients with stable renal function on standard excretory urography. Much as in the normal kidney, peristalsis in an allograft may be changed or lost due to obstruction and infection. In addition, rejection, periureteral fibrosis, surgical trauma, and compromise of the blood supply may inhibit peristalsis.

In the authors' experience, peristalsis is best studied during perfusion studies at low flow rates or with short manual injections of contrast medium at the time of antegrade pyelography (Fig. 23–111). For documentation, cine ureterography or a series of rapid spot films (100-mm camera, 6 films/sec) is best. In all cases of proved obstruction in the authors' series, ureteral peristalsis was abnormal or absent. With obstruction at the ureterovesical junction, at least the distal part and often the entire ureter was aperistaltic (Fig. 23–112). When the obstruction was in the mid or distal ureter, peristalsis was sometimes seen distal to the stenotic area or a proximal retrograde contracting wave could be demonstrated. Patients with normal reaction of renal function after operation or long-term stenting for obstruction regained normal peristalsis (Figs. 23–113 and 23–114). In contrast, abnormal or absent peristalsis was seen in only 4 of 10 patients with acute rejection.

Discussion

Urodynamic studies. Antegrade pyelography combined with urodynamic studies locates exactly and

defines clearly the site and significance of an obstruction. The diagnostic yield of the studies is significantly greater than that of conventional studies. Although invasive, antegrade pyelography carries a low risk when done with a thin needle. If obstruction cannot be excluded clinically

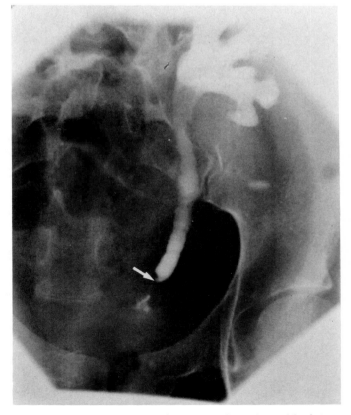

Fig. 23–112 Percutaneous nephrostogram in patient with obstruction at ureterovesical junction (arrow) and positive Whitaker test. Collecting system as well as ureter is dilated. There is no peristalsis.

Fig. 23–113 Antegrade pyelograms in 14-year-old girl with increased serum creatinine (280 μmol/liter) 3 months after transplantation. A. Prevesical ureteral kinking with obstruction (arrow); note comparatively high site of ureteroneocystostomy. Dilated, aperistaltic ureter proximal to kink, with some peristalsis in prevesical ureter distal to the kinking (B).

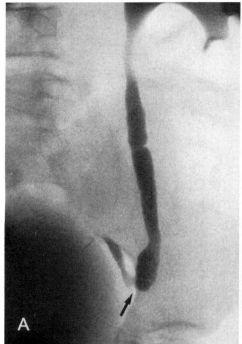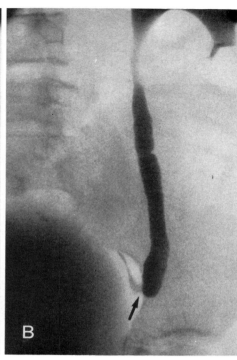

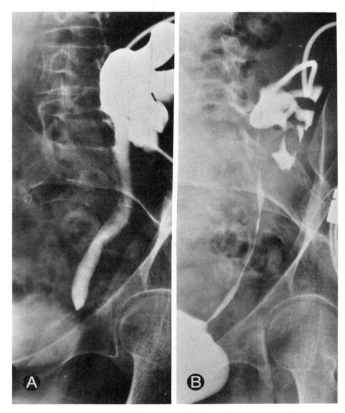

Fig. 23–114 Percutaneous nephrostomy was performed in patient with obstruction at ureterovesical junction 3 weeks post-transplantation. A. Hydronephrosis with dilated and noncontracting ureter proximal to obstruction. B. Nephrostogram 10 days after ureteroneocystostomy shows collecting system and ureter of normal caliber and normal peristalsis.

or by conventional studies (ultrasound, IVU), a fine-needle antegrade pyelogram should be done. To further assess the functional significance of a stenosis, the Whitaker test is the method of choice, and significant obstruction can be assumed if a pressure gradient of >20 cm H_2O between the renal pelvis and the bladder is shown. During these studies, ureteral peristalsis should be closely watched and perhaps recorded on video tape, cine film, or rapid spot-film sequences, especially if there is a question of stenosis in the presence of a normal or equivocal Whitaker test.

As Coolsart et al state, a low pressure gradient does not necessarily exclude an obstruction.[174] Under normal conditions, ureteral contractile pressures exceeds the intravesical pressure, so the urine passes into the bladder. A dilated, poorly contractile ureter thus must have an increased baseline internal pressure to overcome the intravesical pressure. In other words, the adynamic ureter probably represents a relative obstruction to urine flow, thereby compromising renal function in spite of the absence of proof of organic obstruction on the antegrade pyelogram. This theory was substantiated by one of the authors' cases, in which stenting of an adynamic ureter (with a normal Whitaker test) for 1 month led to recovery of normal renal function and ureteral peristalsis (Fig. 23–115). Lack of peristalsis with dilation in this patient was probably due to recurrent urinary infections, which subsequently were treated with adequate antibiotics.

Therefore, patients with adynamic ureters but without a pathologic gradient must be evaluated for other causes of aperistalsis such as infection or rejection. As demonstrated, these patients may benefit from temporary stenting to relieve the relative obstruction, allowing the ureter to regain its normal peristaltic activity. In contrast, in the

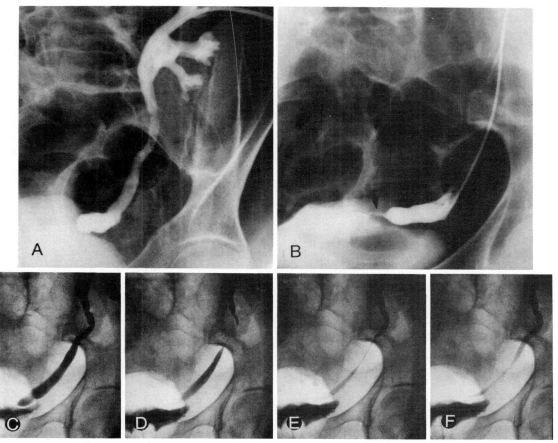

Fig. 23–115 Percutaneous nephrostomy and subsequent stenting in patient with recurrent pyelonephritis and elevated serum creatinine 3 weeks after transplantation. Whitaker test was negative. A. Nephrostogram shows pelvicaliceal system within normal limits but dilated, noncontracting ureter. B. Oblique view shows intramural part of ureter to be patent and of normal caliber (arrow). C–F. Cine nephrostogram after 1 month of ureteral stenting shows well-contracting ureter with normal antegrade peristalsis.

authors' experience, a nondilated ureter with normal peristalsis virtually excludes significant obstruction; in none of their cases was obstruction with normal peristalsis ever substantiated in the clinical follow-up. In addition, almost all patients with normal renal function following operation or stenting for obstruction regained normal ureteral tone and peristalsis within days or a few weeks.

As stated above, the absence of ureteral peristalsis may also mean rejection. The rate of pathologic peristalsis in this condition may vary considerably, ranging from 36% in the authors' case material to 75% in the series reported by Newhouse et al.[175] Therefore, rejection has to be considered in the absence of a negative or equivocal Whitaker test. Renal biopsy and the reaction of the serum creatinine level to percutaneous drainage or to appropriate treatment for rejection will eventually reveal the diagnosis.

An increase in intravesical pressure or kinking of the ureter with bladder filling also can act as an obstruction. Therefore, it is important that pressure measurements be performed with the bladder filled to various degrees. In one of the authors' patients, a stenosis of the ureterovesical junction was significant only with the bladder full (Fig. 23–116). Ureteral peristalsis also disappeared completely when the bladder was full (Fig. 23–117). In another patient, intermittent hydronephrosis of unknown etiology was a recurring problem. A 5F catheter was placed percutaneously into the renal pelvis. With the bladder emptied through a Foley catheter, there was unobstructed flow of contrast medium into the bladder, whereas with the bladder filled with sterile water, the flow of contrast medium into the bladder stopped. The bladder was re-emptied, and a guidewire and catheter were advanced without difficulty into the bladder. When the bladder was refilled with sterile water, the angle at which the catheter and guidewire entered the bladder, and, by extrapolation, the angle at which the intramural portion of the ureter was bent, became acute (Fig. 23–118).

The few references to functional ureterovesical junction obstruction secondary to bladder distention suggest that the pathologic mechanism is, as in this case, an implantation site located too high on the very mobile, muscular portion of the bladder wall. Percutaneous antegrade techniques appear to be the only way to make this diagnosis definitely and, in particular, to differentiate this entity from other functional causes of obstruction such as a noncompliant bladder or a hypoperistaltic ureter, which may be due to episodes or ureteric rejection or ischemia.

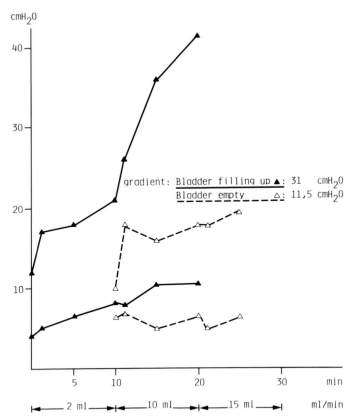

Fig. 23–116 Whitaker test in patient with elevated serum creatinine (200 μmol/liter) 4 months after transplantation. Gradient is normal with bladder empty. Note increasing gradient with progressive filling of bladder. At operation, distal ureter was found to be necrotic.

Percutaneous Therapy

Nephrostomy drainage. On the basis of the antegrade pyelogram or Whitaker test performed through a Chiba needle, the decision is made whether to place a nephrostomy drainage catheter. The indications for a catheter include obstruction, if it has resulted in decreased renal function (increased creatinine), symptoms (pain, fever, oliguria, or anuria), or urinary infection; and a urinary leak.

In patients with a urinary leak, the drainage catheter is commonly left in the renal pelvis in an attempt to divert urine from the site of the leak and either allow it to close or to stabilize the patient's clinical status for surgery. A stent across the site of the leak is theoretically desirable,[143,145] but it can be associated with complications such as false passage at a site of ureteral necrosis or rupture.

In cases of ureteral obstruction by clot (Fig. 23–119), the catheter can be advanced to the bladder to remove the obstruction physically; alternatively, clots can be aspirated through the catheter or flushed down into the bladder (Fig. 23–120). Catheters can also be used to straighten a ureteral kink (Fig. 23–120) and to allow internal drainage both for the psychologic benefit of normal urination and to decrease the risk of infection. To prevent recurrent blockage, large (10F–12F) drainage catheters should be used (Figs. 23–121 and 23–122).

In organic obstruction, the advantage of installing a percutaneous nephrostomy is two-fold: first, to provide rapid decompression and to allow recovery of renal function before corrective operation is performed, and second, to assess the potential for recovery of renal function; *i.e.*, the rate and amount of decrease in serum creatinine levels are important prognostic parameters. Other factors that seem to influence the outcome are the duration and severity of impairment of renal function before drainage, the interval since transplantation, and the extent of interstitial fibrosis as determined by renal biopsy. In the authors' experience, patients with recent anuria or oliguria who were admitted within 1 month after transplantation did significantly better than those admitted later. Furthermore, patients with a definite fall in serum creatinine levels and no interstitial fibrosis had the best results, with normal renal function postoperatively. Normalization of serum creatinine during nephrostomy drainage or postoperatively was always associated with long-term graft survival. In contrast, patients presenting >1 month postoperatively, with high creatinine levels (>250 μmol/liter) and with persistent or rising serum creatinine levels during percutaneous drainage always have lost graft function in spite of surgery. These patients also showed definite interstitial fibrosis on renal biopsy.

A third indication for nephrostomy drainage in the differential diagnosis of obstruction and rejection is when a nonperistaltic dilated ureter is not accompanied by a definite obstruction on antegrade pyelography or by a pathologic Whitaker test. As discussed previously, rejection and infection may cause abnormal or absent peristalsis. In such cases, percutaneous drainage is very helpful, because decompresssion of the collecting system usually leads to recovery of ureteral peristalsis. Furthermore, the reaction of the serum creatinine level and peristaltic activity after clamping of the drainage tube and treatment of rejection or infection will provide enough evidence to rule out functional obstruction.

Balloon dilation for obstruction. Ureteral strictures secondary to periureteral fibrosis, anastomotic fibrotic strictures, and ischemic strictures can be dilated (Fig. 23–123). Diffuse strictures secondary to rejection or necrosis cannot be dilated. The authors routinely create nephrostomy tracts through an anterior calix of the upper pole in allografts to facilitate the passage of guidewires, catheters, and balloon dilators into the ureter.

A high-pressure angioplasty balloon 6–8mm in diameter is chosen. Commonly, 0.038-inch guidewires are adequate to pass the balloon catheter across the stricture; occasionally, a Lunderquist wire is required, particularly in severe strictures involving a long segment. Predilation to 10F with Teflon dilators facilitates the passage of the balloon. After dilation, an external–internal stent is left for drainage; it may be replaced with a large (12F–14F) double-J stent as soon as the urine is bloodless to minimize the chances of infection in these immunosuppressed patients. The stent should stay in place for 3–4 months to increase the chances of long-term success. A combined internal–external stent has the advantage of permitting a two-step pull-back to the renal pelvis prior to final removal and allows observation of the dilation results by

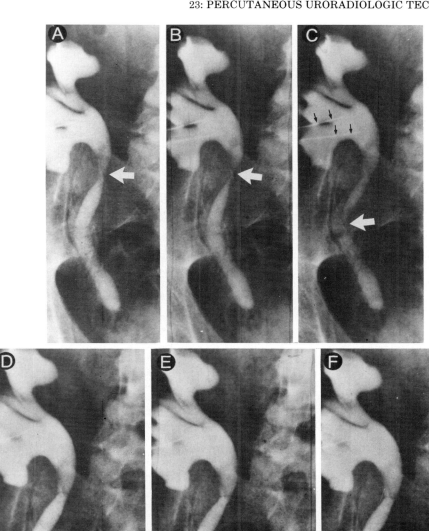

Fig. 23–117 Antegrade pyelography of patient in Figure 23–116. A–C. Spot film sequence taken with bladder empty. Pelvicaliceal system and ureter are dilated. However, peristaltic wave can be seen starting at ureterovesical junction and propagating antegrade (large white arrows). There is high-grade stenosis of prevesical ureter (short white arrow). Note two Chiba needles in place for Whitaker test (small black arrows). D–F. Spot film sequence with bladder filled. There is progressive dilatation of collecting system and ureter. No peristaltic activity is apparent. A markedly dilated aperistaltic prevesical ureter is seen (long white arrows). Narrow distal ureter (short white arrows).

following the serum creatinine levels with the catheter clamped. If necessary, the obstruction can be easily redilated and restented. This option is relinquished, in favor of the potential advantage of a decreased risk of infection and better patient tolerance, by stenting with a double-J catheter. Follow-up of these patients is by determination of creatinine levels. A retrograde cystogram can be performed to evaluate the patency of the stent if there is any suggestion of obstruction. The stent is removed via a cystoscope.

Sometimes, sophisticated methods must be applied to treat a recurrent stenotic anastomosis, as shown in Figures 23–124 through 23–126. A combined approach by the urologist and interventional radiologist finally stabi-

lized one patient's condition after three previous operations for anastomotic strictures.

Complications

Antibiotic coverage is provided for all diagnostic and therapeutic interventional procedures and as long as a drainage catheter is in place, because these immunocompromised patients are subject to severe opportunistic infections. In the authors' material, two of three patients suffered intercurrent urinary infections when antibiotic therapy was temporarily stopped.

In the authors' experience with >50 patients, no severe complications directly related to the percutaneous punc-

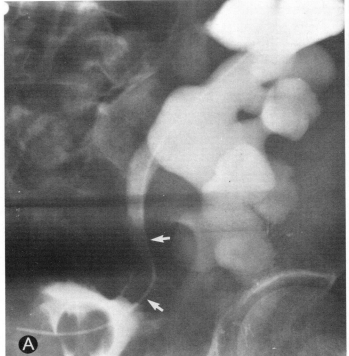

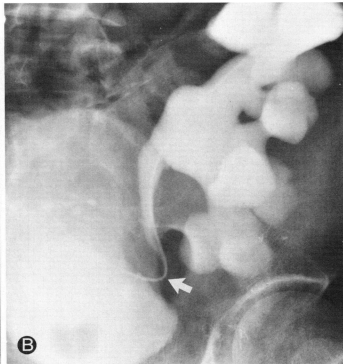

Fig. 23–118 Renal allograft recipient with recurrent anuric episodes and elevated creatinine. A. Antegrade pyelogram shows marked dilatation of pelvicaliceal system and ureter with apparent narrowing of distal ureter. Guidewire has been passed into the bladder (arrows). B. Distention of bladder with contrast medium produces marked angulation of distal ureter, manifested by kinking of guidewire (arrow). C. Further distention of bladder accentuates kinking of distal ureter (arrow), which causes functional obstruction.

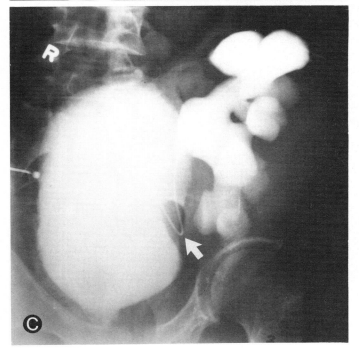

ture or to the placement of a nephrostomy tube occurred. Hematuria usually subsides within 24–48 hr. In patients with bleeding and obstruction of the pelvicaliceal system secondary to renal biopsy or coagulopathy, large-bore (10F–12F) stents should be used to prevent obstruction by clots (Figs. 23–119 and 23–120).

As long as there is no obstruction to antegrade urine flow, the nephrostomy tract will usually close within 1–3 days after removal of the catheter. Occasionally, in patients who are being treated for rejection, prolonged urinary leakage follows removal of the nephrostomy catheter. In these patients, the drainage catheter should be left in place until rejection has been controlled and the corticosteroid dose has been reduced. In one patient, the tract had to be plugged with Gelfoam to stop the leakage of urine.

Irritability and spasm of the ureter when it is entered by a guidewire and catheter through the ureterovesical

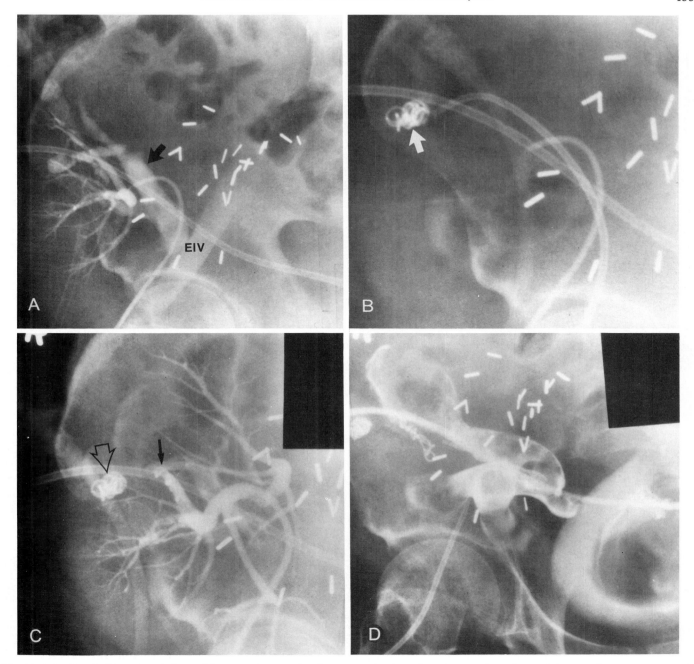

Fig. 23-119 Renal allograft recipient with severe hematuria after renal biopsy. Selective renal arteriogram shows extensive arteriovenous shunting through fistula created by biopsy needle. Renal vein (black arrow); external iliac vein (EIV). B. Because of difficult arterial anatomy in this patient and the desire to preserve as much renal parenchyma as possible, attempt was made to close fistula by placing GWC coils from venous side (arrow); coils were partially successful in controlling fistula. C. Persistent hematuria led to selective cathe- terization of renal artery branch supplying arteriovenous communi- cation; GWC coils were placed (black arrow). Note no forward flow across fistula. Open arrow points to GWC coils in venous side. D. Because of acute urinary retention, percutaneous nephrostomy was created. Note large clots within pelvicaliceal system, causing obstruc- tion. E. Nephrostogram performed 48 hr later shows that clots have been flushed out of pelvicaliceal system into bladder. Note coils within arterial (open arrow) and venous sides (short white arrow).

junction can induce acute edema. A two-step pull-back of the drainage tube to the renal pelvis is recommended prior to final removal of a catheter that has been placed into the bladder for internal drainage. Functional ure- teral patency should be documented with pyelogram and, if necessary, with a Whitaker test prior to final removal.

Conclusions

If obstruction cannot be definitely excluded on the basis of clinical findings and conventional diagnostic methods, antegrade pyelography and the Whitaker test are fast and accurate means of diagnosing the location

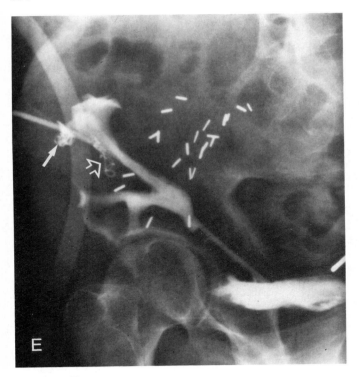

Fig. 23–119E

and significance of urinary obstruction in the renal allo-graft. Ureteral obstruction must be sought and treated aggressively, especially in the early post-transplantation period. In patients with persistent or rising levels of serum creatinine (>250 μmol/liter) during percutaneous drainage, especially if the patient presented in the inter-mediate or late post-transplantation period, treatment of ureteral obstruction does not halt graft failure.

For the initial treatment of obstruction, a percutaneous nephrostomy should be performed for rapid decompres-sion. Continuous urinary drainage by nephrostomy is a good method for assessing the potential functional recov-ery of the graft, so operation can be delayed until recov-ery of renal function has been demonstrated. In some cases, i.e., prolonged postoperative edema of the uretero-vesical junction, further treatment after stenting may not be necessary at all.

The dynamics of ureteral peristalsis are important to observe, especially in patients with a negative or equivo-cal Whitaker test in combination with aperistalsis and dilation of the ureter. In these patients, percutaneous drainage is indicated as a first step in order to evaluate further other causes of an adynamic ureter, such as rejec-tion or infection.

In certain cases, particularly in patients with recurrent anastomotic strictures, dilation with angioplasty balloons

Fig. 23–120 Flushing of clot. A. Nephrostogram after percutaneous nephrostomy shows large amount of clot in pelvis and ureter with obstruction of flow to bladder. B. After decompression and flushing, collecting system appears clear.

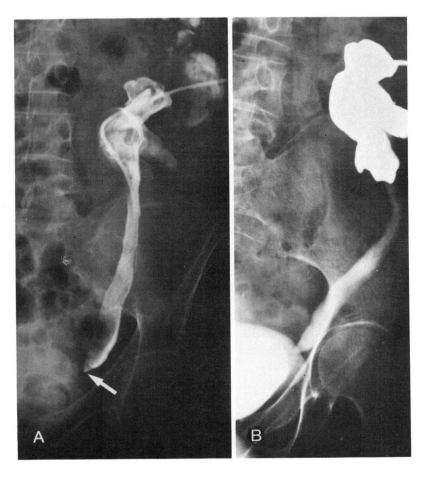

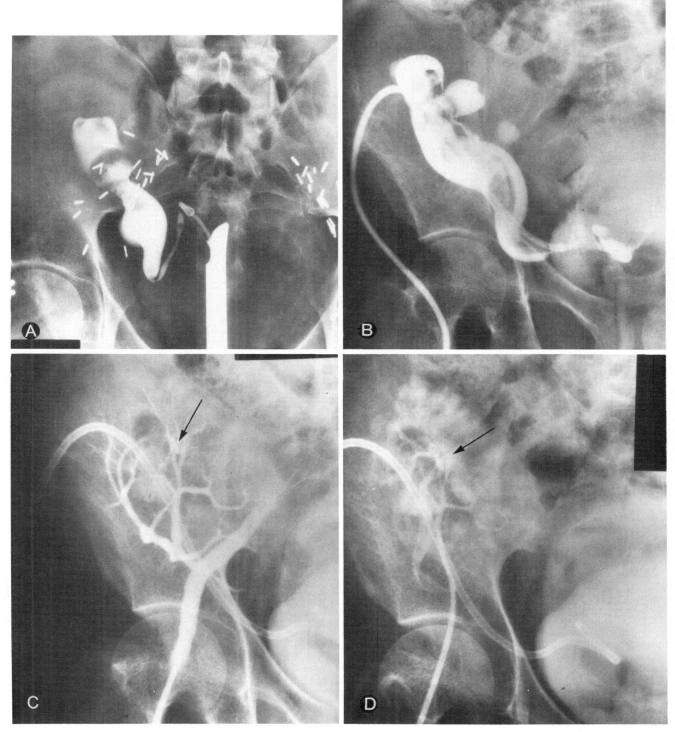

Fig. 23–121   Renal allograft recipient presenting with acute urinary retention by clots after renal biopsy. A. Retrograde pyelogram shows marked kinking of midureter and large number of clots within renal pelvis. Attempts to catheterize ureter retrograde were unsuccessful. B. Nephrostogram performed after percutaneous placement of drainage catheter shows large amount of clot within renal pelvis and calices. C. Because of persistent hematuria, arteriogram was performed which revealed extravasation of contrast medium from branch in upper pole of kidney (arrow). D. Late phase of arteriogram shows pooling of contrast medium in area of extravasation (arrow). E. Repeat renal arteriogram after embolization of bleeding site with two pieces of Gelfoam shows complete obstruction with no further extravasation.

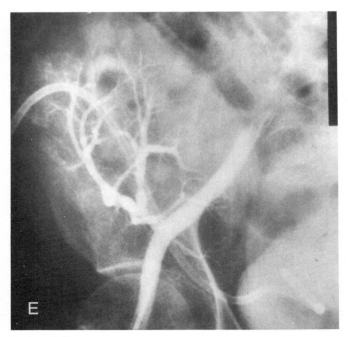

Fig. 23–121E

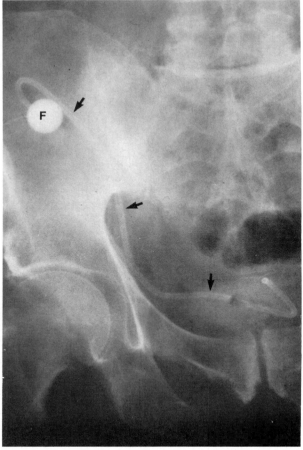

Fig. 23–122 Double-J stent has been placed for internal drainage (arrows). Foley catheter (F) is seen with its tip within renal pelvis for external temporary drainage.

followed by long-term stenting is a valid alternative to operation.

Urinary leaks or fistulae should be treated early with percutaneous nephrostomy to stabilize the patient's condition or for diversion of urine flow to allow the leak to close.

Securing the Catheter to the Skin

Stitching the catheter (Chinese finger trap) to the skin has proved reliable.[176] In the long term, however, sutures tend to cut through the skin or to be accidentally cut off during cleansing. Taping the catheter to the skin offers fair security for the short term if the skin is dry and tincture of benzoin is used. The adhesive properties are lost, however, in the presence of urine leakage or bleeding, both of which are common after a percutaneous nephrostomy. In addition, nurses' habits of removing unclean dressings and tapes become a problem because frequently, one will find a nice clean wound with a partially pulled-out untaped catheter. Nurses must be properly instructed about appropriate care of patients with taped catheters.

Molnar disks and derivatives of different shapes and sizes are currently available from several manufacturers (Fig. 23–127). This probably is one of the best ways to secure a drainage catheter long term,[177,178] although it has the disadvantage that secretions tend to collect under the disk where it is difficult to clean. The authors designed a variant of the Molnar disk that consists of two concentric metal rings joined by three arms (Fig. 23–128). The catheter is passed through the central ring, to which it is stitched. A wide surface area allows easy cleaning of the puncture site, and its flat configuration makes it well tolerated.

Stoma adhesive is another excellent way of securing a long-term catheter, particularly one that is draining internally so that the puncture site is clean and dry.[178,179] A small central circular hole is made in the skin adhesive, which is then applied to the skin around the puncture site after the catheter has been pulled through. The catheter is then looped and covered by the second layer of adhesive (Fig. 23–129). The only disadvantage of adhesive is that it is difficult to care for. Special care has to be taken when removing the adhesive for periodic flushing and inspection. One method of taping the catheter leaves the end out for flushing.

Another catheter-securing technique uses a Tuohy–Borst adapter tightened around the catheter at the puncture site (Fig. 23–130). The adapter is then stitched to the skin. This technique has been more useful for biliary drainage procedures than for nephrostomy drainage, where the patient has to lie on the rigid device.

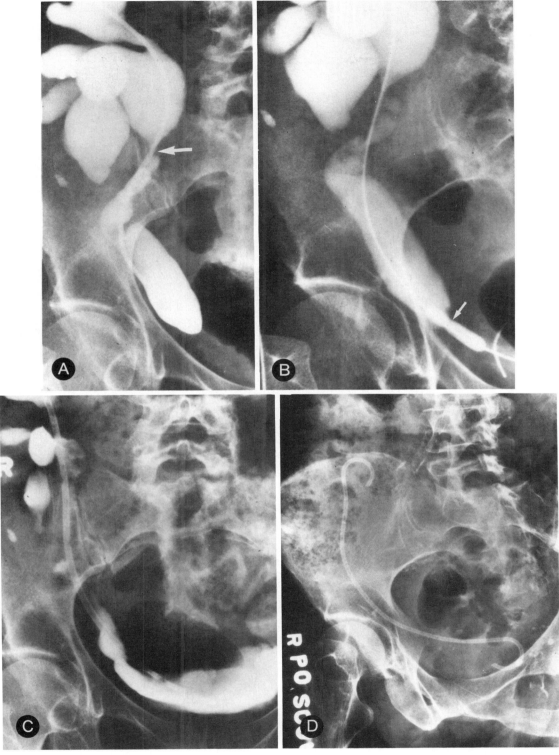

Fig. 23–123   Renal allograft recipient with deteriorated renal function and creatinine of 7.5 mg/dl. A. Nephrostogram shows complete obstruction of distal ureter proximal to ureteroneocystostomy. Also note narrowing of proximal ureter just beyond ureteropelvic junction (arrow) and marked dilatation of calices. B. After passage of guide-wire across area of obstruction in distal ureter, 6-mm angioplasty balloon catheter was passed across stricture and inflated for 15 min at 8 atm of pressure. Note small waist in balloon (arrow). C. Nephrostogram performed 2 days after dilatation of ureteral stricture shows adequate opening, with good decompression of pelvicaliceal system by 10F Malecot catheter. D. Malecot catheter has been replaced by 8F double-J Silastic stent for internal drainage.

Fig. 23–124 Fifty-eight-year-old patient. A. Film 10 days after second pyeloureterostomy for recurrent stricture at ureteropelvic junction. Patient had previous operation for stricture at ureterovesical junction. B. After removal of ureteral catheter, anuria developed. Percutaneous nephrostogram shows complete obstruction at ureteropelvic junction (arrow). Ureter could not be catheterized antegrade.

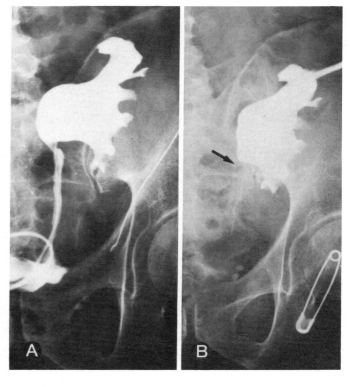

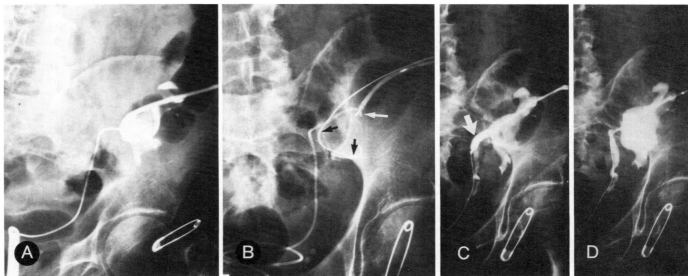

Fig. 23–125 Same patient as in Figure 23–124. A. Retrograde placement of ureteral catheter allowed crossing of stricture. B. Using alligator forceps (white arrow) passed through steerable catheter system, catheter could be snared and pulled out through nephrostomy tract. Note position of safety wire (black arrows). C. After introduction of guidewire through snared catheter, the latter was exchanged for 6-mm Grüntzig balloon catheter (arrow) and stenosis was dilated repeatedly. D. Immediately after dilatation, proximal ureter is patent; area of previous stenosis was stented with 12F polyurethane catheter.

DISLODGED NEPHROSTOMY DRAINAGE CATHETER

General Principles

Accidental dislodgment of a nephrostomy drainage catheter is a relative emergency, because the patient frequently has only one functioning kidney. Symptoms and a rise in serum creatinine concentration start soon after, because the ureter is obstructed and the nephrostomy tract usually closes within hours of tube loss. At present, with the innovative modern angiography techniques involving specialized torque control guidewires and different combinations of catheters, one can re-establish the nephrostomy tract with diligent probing under fluoroscopy.

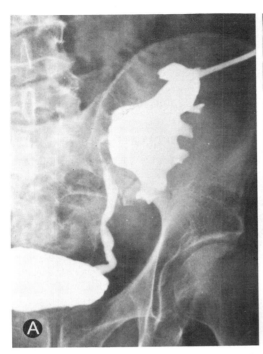

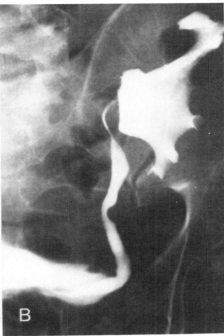

Fig. 23–126 Same patient as in Figures 23–124 and 23–125. A. After 2 months of stenting, nephrostogram shows patent but relatively narrow proximal ureter. Pigtail catheter was therefore left in renal pelvis. B. Nephrostogram 1 week later shows practically unchanged patent, somewhat narrow proximal ureter. However, there was good antegrade flow, so nephrostomy tube was removed. Patient did well and had normal urine output as of 2-year follow-up.

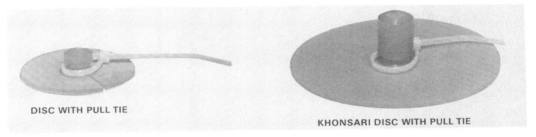

DISC WITH PULL TIE

KHONSARI DISC WITH PULL TIE

Fig. 23–127   Molnar disk with pull tie (A) and Khonsari disk with pull tie (B). (Courtesy of Cook Urological.)

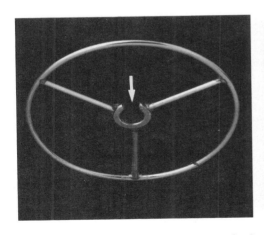

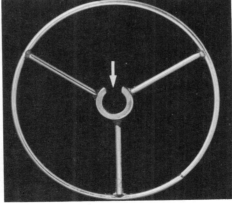

Fig. 23–128   Metallic retention device made of flat stainless-steel wire. Central opening is for catheter placement (arrow).

The sooner the patient reports to the hospital, the better. Immediate establishment of drainage of urine is crucial in patients who are infected.[180] Usually, the tract is patent for 6–8 hr in patients previously drained with 8.3F–10F nephrostomy catheters.[181]

Two cardinal rules should be remembered:

1. Do not attempt blind manipulations through a tract, regardless of how old and mature it is, because these tracts will be tortuous even if they were created straight, and once a false passage is created by blind manipulations, it becomes almost impossible to catheterize a tract. However, in patients with large tracts drained with Foley or other retention catheters, the tract will be mature, and one can easily introduce pediatric feeding tubes or small (5F) 45° angle soft polyethylene catheters with or without coaxial guidewire techniques.

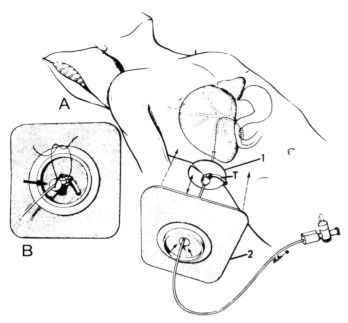

Fig. 23–129 A. Molnar disk has been tightened around drainage catheter at skin level; stoma adhesive patch is being advanced over catheter after cutting hole in its center (arrows) to fit center of Molnar disk through it. B. Close-up view of final arrangement showing the stoma adhesive attached to the skin and the Molnar disk (arrow) protruding through the center hole in the stoma adhesive patch. (Reproduced from Shoenfeld RB, Ring EJ, McLean GK, Freiman DB: Stabilization of percutaneous catheters. *AJR* 1982;138:972.)

2. Do not infiltrate the tract with local anesthetic before attempting to catheterize it, because injections can traumatize and obstruct it. It is preferable to administer sufficient sedation and analgesics to make the patient comfortable before manipulation. Once the tract is catheterized, local anesthetic can be given before any further manipulations are performed.

Technique

Infected patients should receive intravenous antibiotics prior to the manipulation to prevent septicemia. The patient is placed prone, and the side of interest is cleansed and draped. Under fluoroscopy, and, if possible, with digital road mapping or video recording, a "Christmas tree" adapter (Fig. 23–131) is inserted into the nephrostomy tract opening, and 50% contrast medium is instilled to opacify the tract (Fig. 23–132).[116] Still-framing on the video recorder is valuable to guide catheterization; if it is not available, a film of the abdomen or a good memory will have to suffice.

Once the tract is opacified, the Christmas tree adapter is removed, and a floppy-tip 0.035-inch guidewire (Cook, Inc.) is gently manipulated through the bends in the tract (Fig. 23–133A,B) with the help of a steerable multipurpose or cobra angiographic catheter until the wire reaches the collecting system (Fig. 23–133C), from which it must be manipulated down the ureter into the bladder if one plans internal drainage.

Another method of gaining access to the renal pelvis is the advancement of an 8F pediatric nasogastric tube with a soft tip in combination with a coaxial soft 0.038-inch

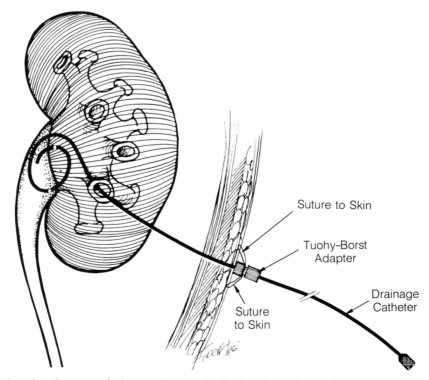

Suture to Skin

Tuohy–Borst Adapter

Drainage Catheter

Suture to Skin

Fig. 23–130 External fixation of nephrostomy drainage catheter using Tuohy–Borst adapter. Skin sutures are subsequently tightened around catheter, which is therefore fixed in this position.

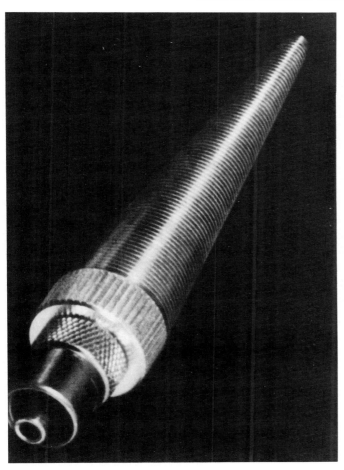

Fig. 23–131 Christmas tree adapter.

can be achieved by utilizing various guidewires and angiographic and balloon catheters under fluoroscopic control.[2,57,184–187] Antegrade stenting is successful in most cases where retrograde ureteral stents cannot be inserted by the conventional transcystoscopic method.[38,186] Recently developed smaller flexible nephroscopes and ureteroscopes have been utilized for inspection of the renal pelvis and ureter, to perform biopsies, and to remove stones and foreign bodies.[2,57,183,188–190] These percutaneous techniques have offered an alternative treatment for patients who are not suitable candidates for operation. In most cases, percutaneous ureteral procedures are convenient and safer than open surgical intervention and are now often the procedures of choice. Catheterization of the ureter by a percutaneous translumbar approach with subsequent placement of stents in cases of malignancy, fistulae, or strictures avoids the bothersome management of external nephrostomy catheters and collection bags. It also reduces the risk of urosepsis, a frequent problem in patients on long-term external drainage. The social and psychologic stigmata of carrying drainage bags are also avoided. Percutaneous placement of ureteral stents is the only logical alternative in patients with ileal conduits[40,191] and in patients in whom transcystoscopic insertion is not possible because of bladder tumor. Other extensive tumors preventing cystoscopic visibility of the ureteral orifices also necessitate percutaneous placement of the ureteral stent.

Following a discussion of stent insertion, the role of percutaneous ureteral manipulation will be discussed in detail in four pathologic conditions: fistulae, strictures, stones, and foreign bodies.

flexible guidewire that exits through the sidehole proximal to the distal end.[181] In this fashion, traumatization of the tract by the tip of the angiographic catheter is avoided.[182]

The third method of gaining access to the tract is utilization of a coaxial 5F 45° nonbraided catheter along with the soft, straight, flexible-tip guidewire.[180] The tract is probed with the catheter with or without advancing the tip of the wire, thereby avoiding traumatizing the tract.

As a final resort, a nonbraided angiographic catheter is used along with a Lunderquist torque control guidewire.[181]

If the patient is not seen until >72 hr after tube dislodgment, the tract is frequently closed, and attempts to reopen it rarely succeed. In these cases, and in those in which blind manipulations have created one or more false passages, creating a new nephrostomy tract will be faster and safer than manipulating a traumatized and possibly infected old one.

Interventions in the Ureter

Percutaneous nephrostomy is often a prelude to various interventions in the ureter. The first percutaneous ureteral catheterization was reported by Weiss et al for treatment of lithiasis.[183] Interventions within the ureter, such as negotiating strictures, obstructions, or fistulae,

Techniques for Internal Drainage with Exteriorized Catheter

TRAVERSING THE URETER

Once a guidewire has been placed in the collecting system, the tract is enlarged to 10F with Teflon dilators, and a second wire is introduced through a safety wire introducer (Cook, Inc.; Cook Urological). When the introducer is removed, two wires are in place: one is the safety wire, which is stitched to the skin, and the other is the working wire, which is used for the manipulations in the ureter.

Although a large variety of catheters and wires can be used to traverse the ureter, the two techniques the authors prefer are the following:

1. With the help of a torque control cobra (Cordis) or multipurpose (Cook, Inc.) catheter, a 0.038-inch floppy-tip wire is advanced into the ureter. By skillful, gentle manipulation, all the bends of tortuous, dilated ureters can be negotiated (Figs. 23–134 and 23–135).[57,189] Generally, once a guidewire has been passed into the bladder, the ureter can be straightened by applying gentle traction to the wire (Fig. 23–135D,E).

2. A slightly curved Lunderquist or a torque control Lunderquist–Ring wire is manipulated gently around the bends in the ureter and into the bladder. One should be careful not to apply too much axial pressure to the Lunderquist wire when advancing around curves, par-

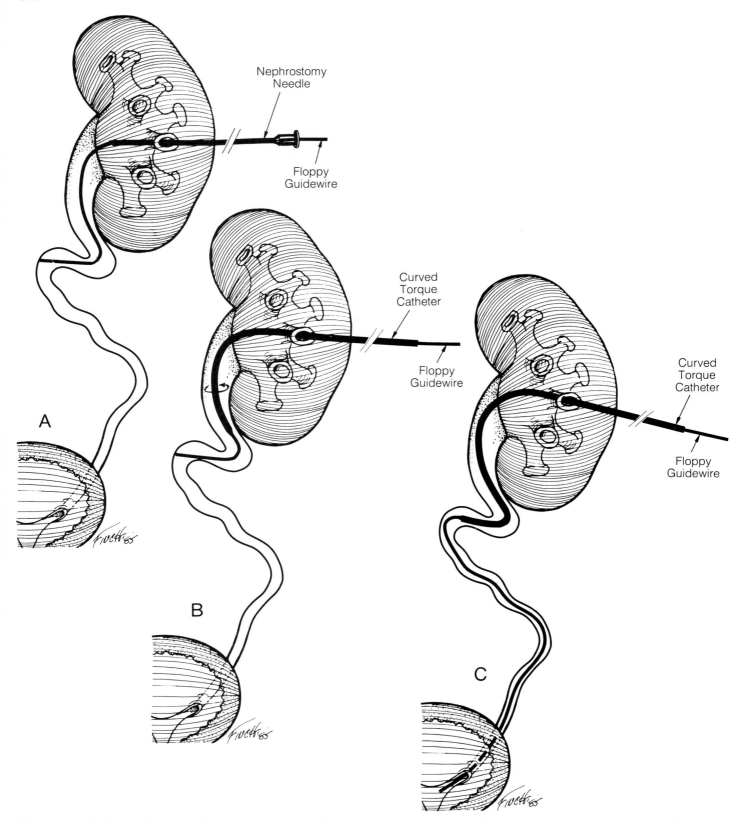

Nephrostomy Needle

Floppy Guidewire

Curved Torque Catheter

Floppy Guidewire

Curved Torque Catheter

Floppy Guidewire

A

B

C

Fig. 23–134 Technique for manipulations of catheters and wire through tortuous, dilated ureters, especially those with severe obstructions. A. Floppy guidewire has been passed through 18-gauge needle placed through posterior calix. B. After removal of needle, angiographic torque control catheter has been introduced over wire.

C. By gentle manipulation of angiographic catheter and guidewire, tortuous ureter has been negotiated, and tip of wire has been advanced into bladder. D. Angiographic catheter has been advanced over guidewire into bladder. E. By gentle traction on guidewire and catheter, ureter has been straightened.

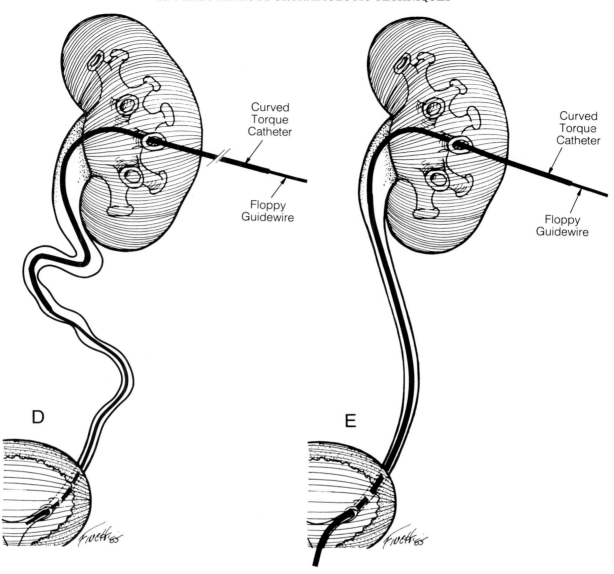

Fig. 23–134D,E

subsequent dilation and drainage catheter placement.[57,189] This maneuver requires heavy analgesia and sedation, and topical anesthetics are recommended for the urethra and bladder.

MEASUREMENT OF URETERAL LENGTH

For internal–external catheters, accurate placement of the sideholes in the collecting system is important and sometimes tricky. Determining the length of catheter between the bladder and the renal pelvis where sideholes should be is relatively easy if one of the following techniques is used:

1. Once the guidewire is in the bladder, an angiographic catheter is passed into the center of the bladder. The wire is then pulled back even with the tip of the catheter, and a clamp is placed on the wire at the skin (Fig. 23–139A). While this clamp is kept in place, the wire is pulled back until its tip is in the renal pelvis. A second clamp is then placed on the wire at skin level (Fig. 23–139B), and the wire is removed. The segment of wire between the clamps corresponds to the length of catheter needed between the bladder and renal pelvis (Fig. 23–139C).

2. A second simpler technique uses an endoruler, which consists of 0.038-inch Teflon tubing inside of which radiopaque markers are placed 1 cm apart (Fig. 23–140A).[192] Once an angiographic catheter is in the bladder, the guidewire is removed, and the endoruler is introduced in the same manner as any other guidewire. The exact distance from the bladder to the renal pelvis can then be directly measured on the fluoroscope screen or from a film of the abdomen (Fig. 23–140B). This measurement is transferred to the drainage catheter to determine where to make the sideholes.

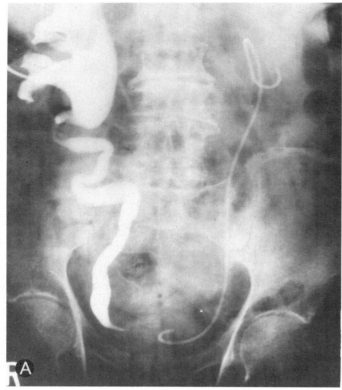

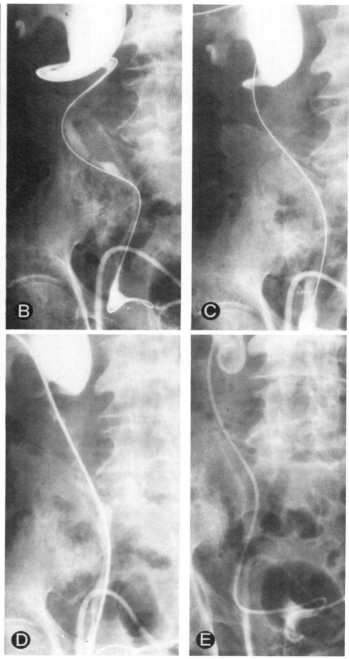

Fig. 23–135 Patient with obstruction of distal ureter by pelvic mass. A. Nephrostogram shows marked hydronephrosis and very dilated and tortuous right ureter. Double-J catheter had been placed previously in left pelvicaliceal system and ureter. B. With help of angiographic catheter, floppy-tip Bentson wire has been manipulated across all bends and curves in the ureter until its tip has reached bladder. C. By gentle pulling back on guidewire, tortuosity of ureter has been eliminated. D. Angiographic catheter has been advanced over guidewire, further straightening ureter. E. Double-J stent has been placed over guidewire.

Types of Catheters and Their Insertion

As has been mentioned, there are several drainage catheters that can be used to obtain internal drainage with an exteriorized catheter. They can be divided into three types, depending on the material they are made of (polyethylene,[37,38] C-Flex, and Silastic[39]), and into two types, depending on whether they have self-retaining features.

The most common stent is the angiographic pigtail catheter. Because of the need to create sideholes along the shaft, the pigtail should be made of polyethylene, not wire mesh. The limitations of pigtail catheters include their small inner diameter, their rapid encrustation that

necessitates frequent exchanges because of catheter plugging by urinary salts, and their poor retention capabilities.

Because of these problems, larger internal diameter catheters with lower encrustation rates and better self-retention capabilities have been developed. The most commonly used material is C-Flex, a soft polymer with a low encrustation rate. Because of the softness of the material, an inner stiffener is needed for introduction. In addition, the tract should be slightly (at least 2F) over-dilated. Catheters of this material come in three shapes: Malecot (Medi-Tech; Cook Urological), Cope loop (Cook, Inc.), and Amplatz funnel (Cook, Inc.).

The Medi-Tech Castañeda Malecot catheter comes in

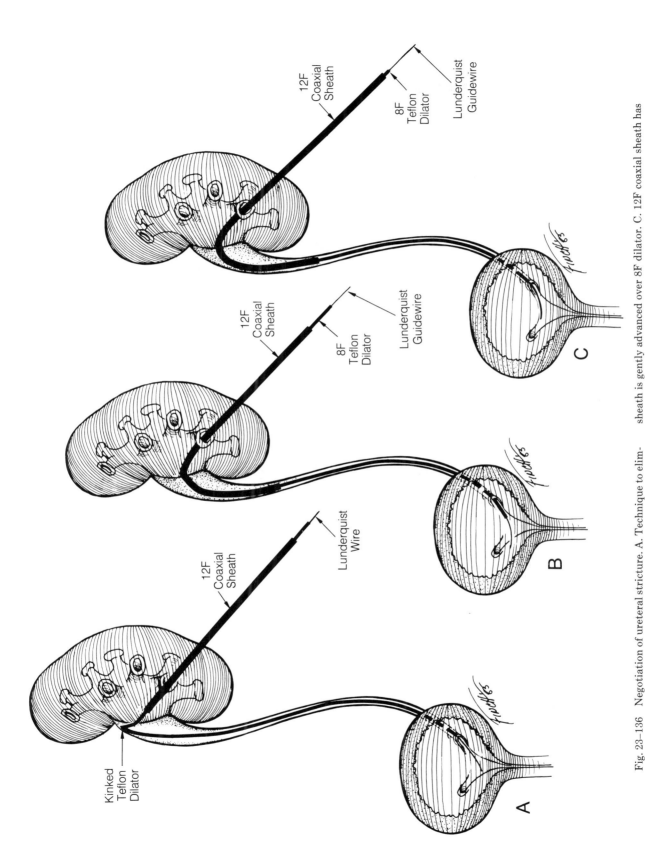

12F
Coaxial
Sheath

8F
Teflon
Dilator

Lunderquist Guidewire

12F
Coaxial
Sheath

8F
Teflon
Dilator

Lunderquist Guidewire

12F
Coaxial
Sheath

Lunderquist Wire

Kinked
Teflon
Dilator

A

B

C

Fig. 23–136 Negotiation of ureteral stricture. A. Technique to eliminate kinking and looping of wire within renal pelvis. B. To eliminate
kinking of Teflon dilator in dilated renal pelvis during attempts to
pass it over a guidewire across site of obstruction, 12F Teflon coaxial

sheath is gently advanced over 8F dilator. C. 12F coaxial sheath has
been advanced into proximal third of ureter, and 8F Teflon dilator
has been manipulated across stricture.

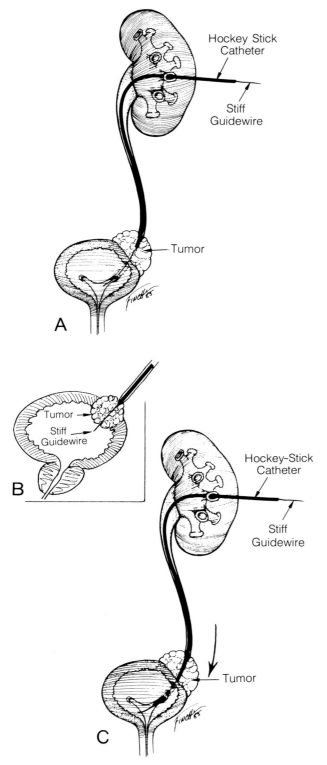

Fig. 23–137 Technique for bypassing complete obstruction of distal ureter by tumor mass. A. Hockey-stick catheter has been manipulated into distal ureter. After opacification of distal ureter and bladder with contrast medium, stiff guidewire is advanced through hockey-stick catheter. B. Close-up view of bladder in tangential projection during advancement of stiff guidewire through tumor mass into bladder. C. Catheter has been advanced over stiff guidewire into bladder.

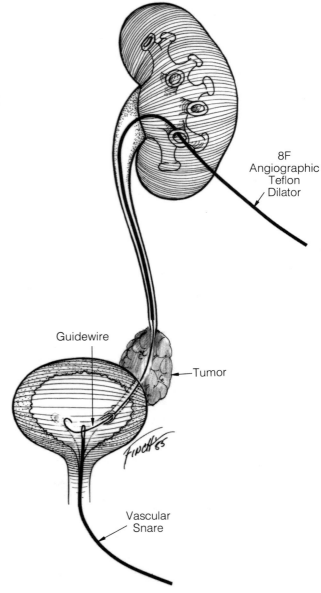

Fig. 23–138 Extraction of guidewire from bladder with vascular snare in a patient with large tumor causing marked obstruction of distal ureter that prevented advancement of dilators or catheters over wire.

8F and 10F sizes and has excellent drainage characteristics. No increased encrustation has been reported on the stainless-steel spiral used to reinforce the Malecot wings, but a recent version eliminates the steel spring. This change simplifies removal and manipulation, but the wings do not hold their shape as well.

The Smith Malecot (Cook Urological) and the Amplatz funnel designs are large-bore (24F) catheters that taper to an 8F long ureteral stent with distal sideholes only.[31] The chief use of these tubes is for tract tamponade and ureteral stenting after nephrostolithotomy, particularly when the ureter has been perforated or traumatized. The use of these tubes eliminates the need for a separate ureteral stent in addition to a nephrostomy tube. The length

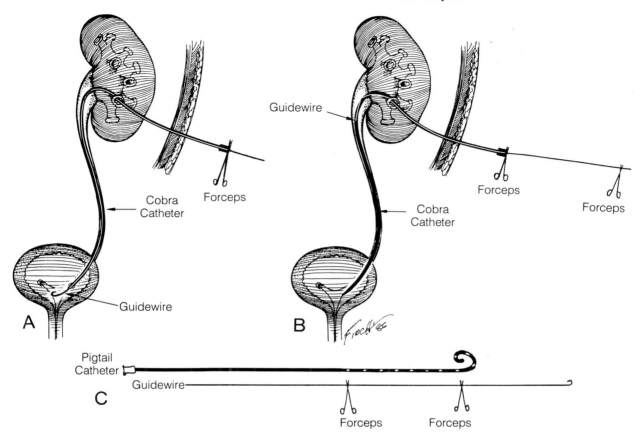

Fig. 23–139 Technique for measurement of distance from the ureterovesical junction to renal pelvis. A. Through angiographic catheter passed into bladder, guidewire has been introduced and passed beyond tip of angiographic catheter. Forceps have been applied to guidewire as it exits from hub of catheter. B. While angiographic catheter is kept in same position, guidewire has been pulled back until its tip lies within renal pelvis; at this point, second forceps have been applied over guidewire, which is then removed. C. Distance between forceps represents distance from bladder to renal pelvis; corresponding sideholes have been created in drainage catheter.

of the stent portion can be adapted easily to the individual needs of each patient by cutting off its tip. The presence of the stent segment also obviates a safety catheter. If the catheter is accidentally pulled back during patient activities or care of the wound, the stent is long enough so that the tube will not fall out into the perinephric tissues. The catheter can easily be readvanced under fluoroscopy with or without a guidewire to reposition the sideholes within the collecting system. In tubes without this feature, readvancement can be a problem, depending on the age of the tract.

The external drainage Cope loop (Cook, Inc.) has been modified for internal–external use by increasing the length. The loop is placed in the bladder. Sideholes are present on the shaft, 20 cm proximal to the loop for drainage of the collecting system. For retrograde placement in patients with an ileal diversion, the loop is modified by making its tip point directly against the shaft, decreasing mucosal trauma. Sideholes are present only on the loop to avoid the passage of mucus from the ileal conduit into the tube, which would rapidly occlude the lumen. The urine drains through the tube into the bag.

Silastic catheters have the best encrustation resistance and patency rate and are well tolerated by the patient. Their main disadvantage is a high friction coefficient,

which makes introduction difficult. Three techniques are used to overcome this problem:

1. One week before stent insertion, the nephrostomy tract is overdilated and stented 2F larger than the Silastic stent to be used. The stent usually can then be introduced directly over the guidewire.
2. A long peel-away sheath mounted on a dilator is passed through the tract into the bladder. The dilator is removed, leaving the guidewire and sheath in place. A mineral oil-lubricated stent can then be introduced easily through the sheath over the guidewire, because friction between the Silastic stent and the Mylar sheath is minimal. The inside of the stent is also lubricated to decrease the friction between the stent and the guidewire. Once the stent is in place, the guidewire is pulled back slowly and carefully, because it tends to bind at the curves. After the guidewire is out, the sheath can be peeled away. The stent can also be introduced through the sheath without a guidewire. When using the peel-away sheath technique, a calix is punctured that provides a direct path to the ureteropelvic junction. This often requires a middle or upper pole intercostal approach.
3. The catheter can also be pulled through the tract over

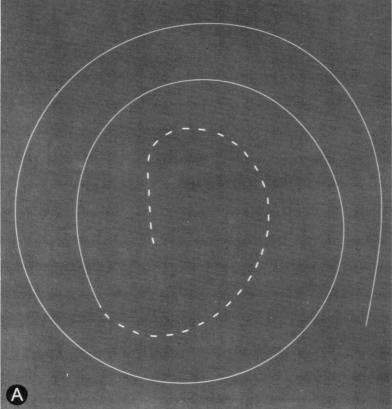

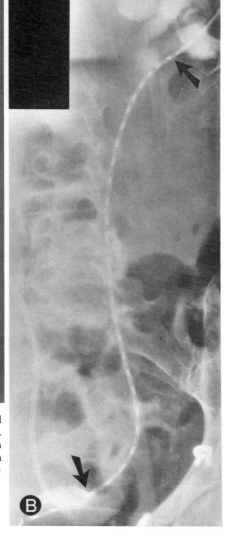

Fig. 23-140 Endoruler. A. Metalic markers spaced 1 cm apart with attached guidewire for easier introduction. Entire system is coated with Teflon tubing. B. Endoruler passed through angiographic catheter showing exact length from bladder (lower arrow) to renal pelvis (upper arrow). (Reproduced from Herrera M, et al: The Endocatheter ruler: a useful new device. *AJR* 1982;139:828-829. © by American Roentgen Ray Society, 1982.)

a through-and-through guidewire, an approach commonly used by urologists as a staged procedure.[32,57,189] In the first stage, an 8F angiographic or multipurpose catheter is passed through the percutaneous tract into the bladder. In the second stage, in the cystoscopy suite, the catheter is extracted endoscopically from the bladder (Fig. 23-141A). The renal or hub end of the catheter is cut off, and an exchange wire is passed through until it exits from both ends (Fig. 23-141B). A plastic bifunnel adapter is passed over the wire and connected to the renal end of the angiographic catheter, and the stent is advanced over the guidewire and connected to the plastic adapter. With the guidewire and both catheters held together as a unit, the urethral end of the angiographic catheter is slowly pulled out until the leading end of the Silastic catheter exits through the urethral meatus (Fig. 23-141C). The guidewire is removed, and the end of the Silastic catheter is cut off just distal to the sideholes. The catheter is then pulled back slowly until its radiopaque markers indicate that the proximal sideholes are within the renal pelvis (Fig. 23-141D). Excess distal catheter can

be pushed back into the bladder. Too much length in the bladder can be irritating, however, because it tends to slip into the urethra during urination, and the catheter may need to be trimmed transcystoscopically. These catheters are usually connected to external drainage for a few days, until the urine clears, and then are clamped externally to force internal drainage.

For exchange of long-term Silastic tubes, a lubricated guidewire is passed through the tube into the bladder. The tube is removed under fluoroscopic control, keeping the tip of the wire in the bladder, and a new tube is passed over the wire. Normally, due to softening or dilation of the obstruction, the new tube passes easily. If not, the wire can be retrieved endoscopically and the steps of the procedure repeated as just outlined.

Miller uses another technique to extract the wire from the bladder. A long floppy-tip wire is looped near the bladder neck in a distended bladder, and the patient is asked to void. The wire frequently will be voided together with the fluid (R.P. Miller, personal communication).

Smith described using a Foley catheter with the tip cut

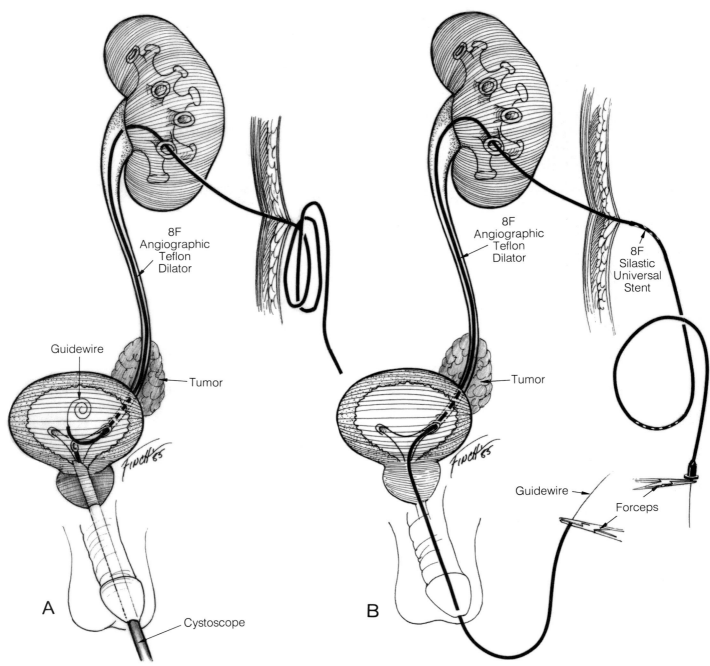

Fig. 23–141 Pull-through technique. A. Angiographic Teflon dilator has been passed over guidewire into bladder; with the help of cystoscope, catheter and guidewire are being extracted through urethra. B. 8F Silastic universal stent has been attached with bifunnel plastic adapter to end of 8F angiographic Teflon dilator. Forceps have been applied to both ends of guidewire to prevent it from moving. C. By gently pulling forward on Teflon dilator, stent has been pulled through until distal sideholes exit through urethra. Note sideholes for renal pelvis overlying midureter. D. After distal end of stent has been cut, stent is pulled back to position sideholes within bladder and renal pelvis.

off. Through this catheter, he passes a basket or snare to entrap the wire, which is then pulled out through the catheter.[57]

The pull-through technique can also be used for long-term stenting in patients with ileal loop urinary diversions. As with the modified Cope loop, the Silastic tube placed in an ileal conduit should have sideholes only in the renal pelvis and collecting bag to prevent plugging of the catheter by mucus from the intestinal segment.

Internal Stenting

TYPES AND INSERTION TECHNIQUES

Internal stents are divided into three groups according to the plastic they are made of: polyethylene, Silastic, and C-Flex. Polyethylene double-J catheters have the disadvantage of stiffness and a high encrustation rate (Fig. 23–142). Also, the change in the chemical and physical com-

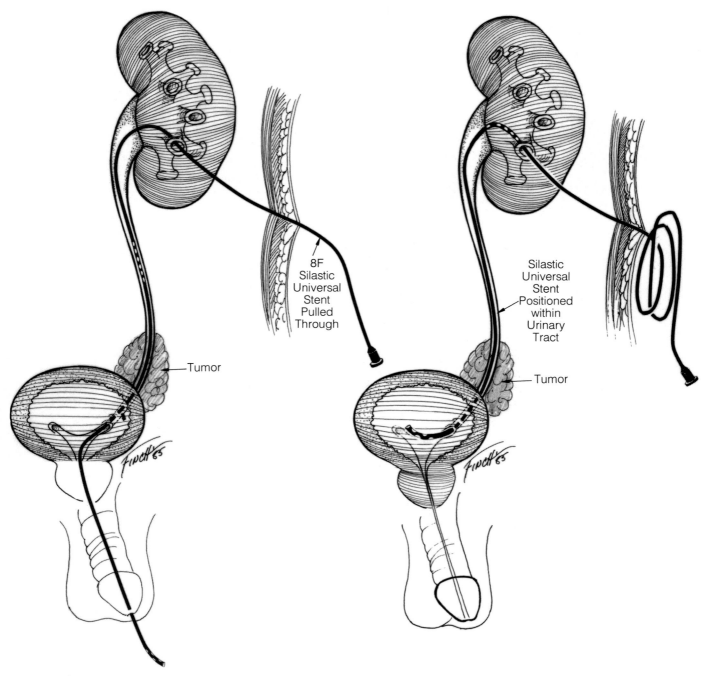

Fig. 23–141C,D

position of the plastic during long-term use may be so pronounced as to cause the stent to fracture. There is no difference between Silastic and polyethylene catheters in the efficiency of urine drainage or reactivity of the ureteral tissue, but longer patency has been claimed for Silastic. However, others have found no significant difference in the patency of the two types. Of all the double-J stents, the polyethylene ones are the easiest to place percutaneously; no prematuration or overdilation of the tract is needed.

There are three techniques for placement of internal stents. Polyethylene ureteral stents can be introduced without transurethral assistance following percutaneous nephrostomy. The tract is dilated to the stent size, and a guidewire is manipulated into the bladder with the help of an angiographic catheter. The distance from the bladder to the renal pelvis is determined as described earlier, and a stent of adequate length is chosen. Prior to introduction, a silk thread is passed through the last sidehole of the stent and withdrawn through the end hole (Fig. 23–143A). The stent is passed over the guidewire to the skin and advanced with the pusher, which has markers at 1-cm intervals to help determine when its tip has reached the renal pelvis. If the stent has been advanced too far, it

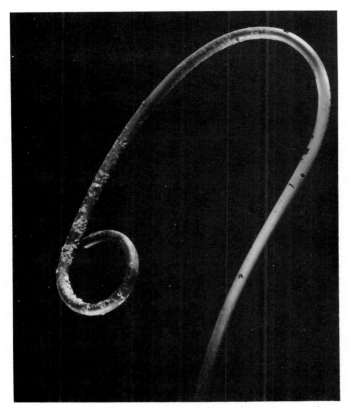

Fig. 23–142 Polyethylene double-J stent showing marked encrustation by urinary salts after 3 months.

can easily be pulled back into the renal pelvis by gently tugging on the silk thread. Once a good position has been reached (Fig. 23–143B), the pusher is used to hold the stent in place while the silk thread is removed. The guidewire is pulled back into the pusher (Fig. 23–143C). When the wire leaves the stent's lumen, the J will reform (Fig. 23–143D). The wire is then readvanced into the renal pelvis, and the pusher is removed. A 5F or 6F angiographic pigtail catheter is left in the renal pelvis open to external drainage for 24–36 hr until the urine clears (Figs. 23–143E and 23–144) to prevent blockage of the stent by the blood clots often present after the manipulation. When the urine is clear, a nephrostogram is performed to ensure that the stent is patent and that the collecting system is intact. The temporary external drainage tube can then be removed. Subsequently, patency of the stents can be checked by demonstrating reflux during cystography (Fig. 23–144C).

For introduction of Silastic stents, one of two techniques must be used:

Overdilation of tract (2F larger) with tract maturation for 1 week;
Passage of a Mylar sheath introducer.

For the first of these techniques, the ureter is catheterized, and the tract is dilated and stented with a catheter 2F larger than the stent of choice. One week later, the patient is brought back, and, after cleansing of the skin, an endoruler is passed through the drainage catheter to determine the distance from the bladder to

the renal pelvis. A Silastic stent of adequate length is prepared for introduction by passing a suture through the last sidehole and the end hole. The stent is then lubricated internally and externally with sterile mineral oil. A lubricated guidewire is introduced through the drainage catheter and passed into the baldder, and the drainage catheter is withdrawn over the guidewire. The stent is advanced over the guidewire until the skin level is reached, being careful to keep the suture threads untwisted. Further advancement of the stent is accomplished by the pusher. It is difficult to see the stent and pusher because both are barely radiopaque; moving the pusher back and forth is helpful. A more accurate way to gauge the position is to insert the pusher first so that the distance from the skin to the renal pelvis can be measured and marked on its outer surface. The position of the double-J stent can be adjusted by pulling on the suture threads or by pushing with the pusher. Once a satisfactory position has been obtained, the suture is pulled back while the stent is held in place with the pusher. While continuing to hold the stent in place, the guidewire is pulled back into the pusher. The double-J loops will then reform in the renal pelvis and bladder. The guidewire is advanced into the renal pelvis, and the pusher is exchanged for a temporary 5F–6F drainage catheter, which stays in place until the urine clears and is removed after a nephrostogram demonstrates the integrity of the collecting system and the patency of the stent.

Occasionally, there is a need to place an internal Silastic stent in one step. This can be done with the aid of the Mylar sheath introducer. First, a puncture is made through a posterior calix or infundibulum that provides a straight line approach to the ureteropelvic junction and ureter to decrease the friction within the sheath during introduction. This implies, in some cases, a puncture above the 12th rib. The ureter is catheterized, and the entire tract is dilated to the sheath size. The distance from the bladder to the renal pelvis is determined with an endoruler. The Mylar sheath, mounted on its dilator–introducer, is passed over the guidewire until its tip is in the bladder (Fig. 23–145A). The dilator is removed, leaving the sheath in place (Fig. 23–145B). A lubricated and suture-looped double-J Silastic stent is then advanced over the guidewire through the Mylar sheath with the help of a pusher until the ends of the pusher and stent are within the renal pelvis (Fig. 23–145B). While the stent is held with the pusher, the Mylar sheath is pulled away. The position of the stent is adjusted by gently pulling back on the suture or by advancing the pusher. Once satisfactory placement is obtained, the suture is removed, and a temporary external drainage catheter is placed as described.

The new Amplatz double-J catheter, made of C-Flex, can be introduced in one step, without the need for an introducer, because an internal stiffener is used (Fig. 23–146). The tract should be dilated to 2F larger than the stent. The same steps for stent positioning and wire removal are followed as for the other double-J stents, except that suture threads are not required. The catheter fits so snugly over the stiffener that it can be advanced or withdrawn at will until the desired position is reached.

Teflon coaxial dilators (Cook), the polyurethane ure-

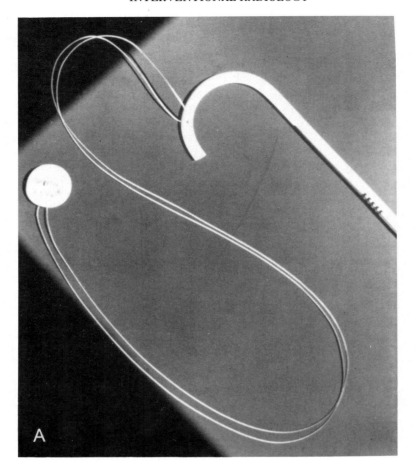

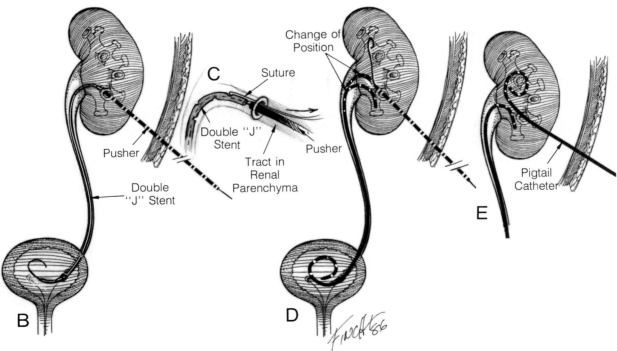

Fig. 23–143 Silastic double-J stent. A. Close-up view of proximal end of Silastic double-J stent with string passed through sidehole for repositioning purposes during introduction. B. Advancement of double-J stent over guidewire passed beyond site of obstruction. C. While end of stent is held in place with pusher, suture is pulled back. D. Stent has doubled back into lower pole infundibulum. E. Pusher has been replaced by pigtail catheter for temporary external drainage.

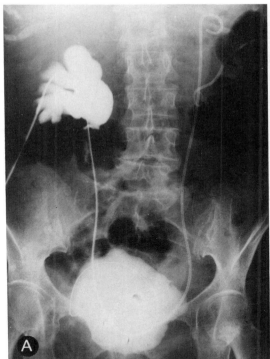

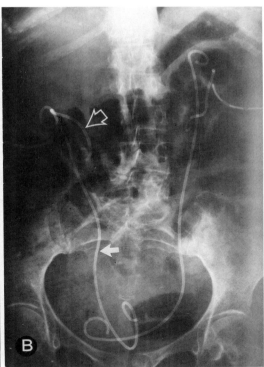

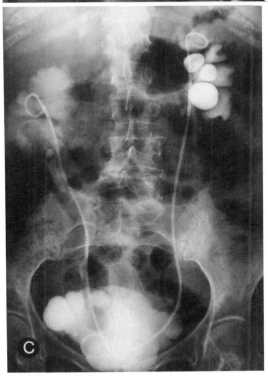

Fig. 23–144 Marked hydrohnephrosis of right kidney. A. Guidewire and angiographic catheter have been manipulated into bladder. Double-J stent has been previously placed in left pelvicaliceal system. B. Double-J stent has been passed over guidewire (white arrow), and pigtail catheter (open arrow) has been left for temporary external diversion in right kidney. C. Cystogram performed to assess patency of double-J stents shows free reflux of contrast medium from bladder into renal pelvis. In spite of patency of double-J stents, note marked hydronephrosis in both pelvicaliceal systems.

teral dilators (Cook Urological), or long (10-cm) 4- or 5-mm balloon dilators can be used to enlarge the tract and the obstruction.

THE OBSTRUCTED DOUBLE-J STENT

The duration of patency of double-J stents varies from 2 or 3 to 18–24 months. When an internal stent becomes obstructed, either by salt encrustation or blood clots, it must be replaced. This can be done using one of several techniques.

In one technique, the bladder end of the stent is grabbed through an endoscope and slowly pulled back until it exits through the urethra, and a guidewire is passed through it into the ureter and renal pelvis. The stent is then replaced with a new one under fluoroscopic

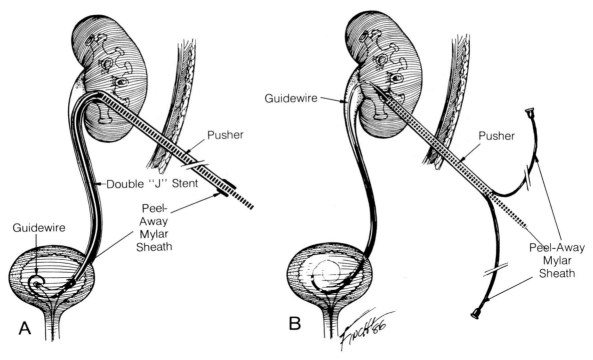

Fig. 23–145 Introduction of double-J stent through peel-away sheath. A. Through sheath beyond site of obstruction, double-J stent is being positioned with help of pusher. B. Mylar sheath is being peeled away while double-J stent is being positioned with help of pusher. B. Mylar sheath is being peeled away while double-J stent is kept in place with pusher.

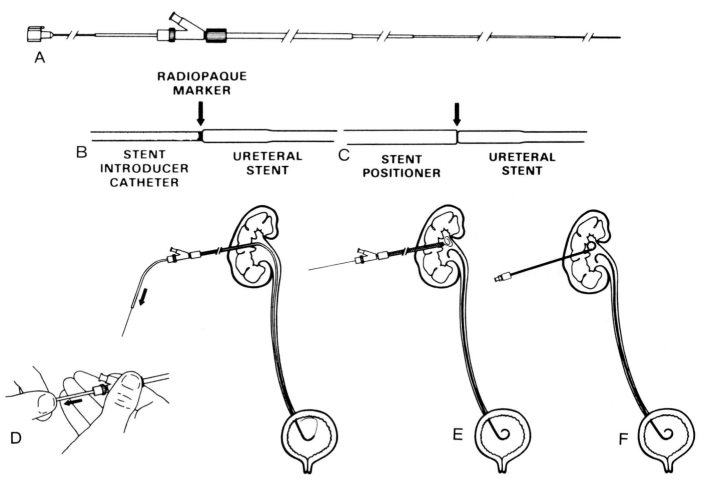

Fig. 23–146 Amplatz double-J stent set. A. Preassembled stent introducer. B. Assembled double-J stent and introducer. C. Stent positioner advanced over introducer until it meets end of double-J stent. D. After Tuohy–Borst adapter is loosened, stent introducer is pulled back while double-J stent is held in place with stent positioner. E. Double-J stent is held in place with positioner while guidewire is pulled back into renal pelvis. F. Pigtail catheter has been passed over the guidewire for temporary drainage. (Courtesy of Cook, Inc.)

control over the guidewire, the new stent being advanced deep into the renal pelvis until the distal end is in the bladder. While the stent is held in place with the pusher, the guidewire is pulled out. The position of the stent is adjusted cystoscopically if necessary by gently pulling it back with alligator forceps. Alternatively, the position of the double-J stent can be adjusted with the suture thread technique described for percutaneous introduction.

In a second technique, the bladder end of the obstructed double-J stent is trapped with a basket or snare loop introduced through a Councill catheter passed into the bladder for this purpose.[57] Once the stent is trapped, it is pulled back, together with the Councill catheter, until it exits through the urethra. The same steps described above are then followed for stent exchange and positioning.

In patients in whom endoscopy is contraindicated or too difficult, a third technique is used. A new percutaneous tract into the collecting system is created and dilated to 10F–16F,[39,193,194] and a second guidewire is passed into the renal pelvis. The renal end of the double-J stent is trapped under fluoroscopic control with a basket, snare loop, or alligator forceps (Fig. 23–147), and the stent is pulled out through the tract, being careful to keep the second (safety) wire in place. Once the stent exits through the skin, a lubricated guidewire is passed through it into the bladder. If this is not feasible, the stent is pulled out, and the second (safety) wire is manipulated down into the bladder with the help of an angiographic catheter. If the manipulation from the renal pel-

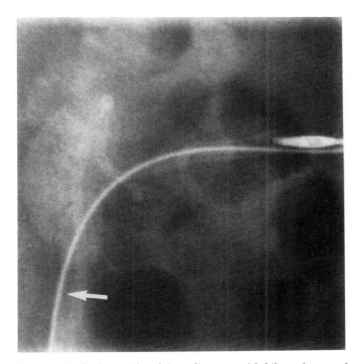

Fig. 23–147 Patient with pelvic malignancy with bilateral ureteral obstruction, treated by placing internal ureteral stent, presenting with rising creatinine. Cystogram revealed no evidence of reflux through stent, suggesting obstruction. Through percutaneous tract, alligator forceps have been used to grasp proximal end of double-J stent, which is gently pulled back through percutaneous tract. Note presence of safety wire in ureter (arrow).

vis into the ureter proves difficult, it pays to replace a safety wire in the renal pelvis, because occasionally during difficult manipulations the wire is dislodged from the collecting system, and reinsertion through a fresh tract is practically impossible. Once the wire has passed into the bladder, a new Silastic stent can be advanced over it. Because the obstruction is already dilated from the previous stent, the new stent usually slides in easily.

THE MIGRATING INTERNAL STENT

Occasionally, a double-J stent migrates either proximally or distally, impairing its function. If it migrates distally (Fig. 23–148), it can usually be replaced by one of the cystoscopic techniques described earlier. If it migrates proximally (Fig. 23–149) a new percutaneous nephrostomy must be created in order to extract and replace the stent.[195]

Management of Fistulae

Ureteral fistulae may result from pelvic neoplasm or from radical pelvic operations.[196,197] Other causes of dehiscence of the ureter with ultimate fistula formation are radiation injury, penetrating or missile trauma,[198] and injuries during transplantation.[199] In surgical or penetrating trauma, the fistulae are the result of direct transection or of ischemia from stripping of blood vessels or thrombosis.

Surgical repair of fistulae involves either anastomosing the viable ureter to other organs such as bowel or autotransplantation. An effective alternative is percutaneous placement of ureteral stents, which gives equally good results with much lower morbidity.[200,201] Frequently, retrograde catheterization is not possible in patients with complete severence or partial dehiscence. In these cases, antegrade passage of guidewires with subsequent placement of internal stents can be successful.[187,200,202]

TECHNIQUE OF CATHETERIZATION

For easier catheterization of the ureter, the nephrostomy puncture should be made as superiorly as possible, at least in the midsegment of the kidney.[189]

As emphasized by Coleman et al, negotiating the traumatized ureter is facilitated by knowing the location of the proximal and distal limits of the injury, which can be achieved with a nephrostogram and a retrograde ureterogram (Fig. 23–150).[189] Usually, utilizing a combination of a soft, straight, floppy-tip guidewire and a torque control catheter, one can probe the fistula and pass the wire into the distal ureter (Fig. 23–151). Once the guidewire crosses the fistula site, it is easier to advance an 8F or 10F catheter with sideholes placed proximally in the renal pelvis and distally in the bladder. There are no holes in the ureteral segment of the stent, thus maximizing drainage and avoiding soiling the fistula with urine.[189] The technique is extremely useful in the management of patients with fistulae in the recent postoperative period (Fig. 23–152) or critically ill patients (Fig. 23–153).

In cases in which only the wire can be advanced and kinking is noted at the time of catheter advancement, the

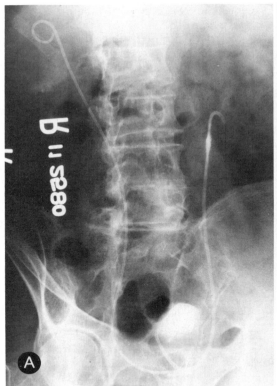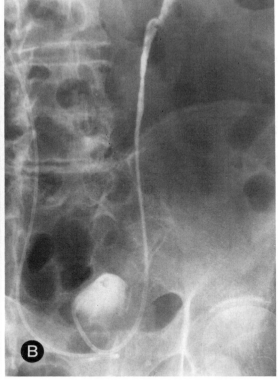

Fig. 23–148   Bilateral double-J stent placement in patient with pelvic malignancy. A. Observe very low position of left stent due to distal migration. B. Left antegrade pyelogram performed during crea-tion of new percutaneous tract for stent removal confirms low position of double-J stent.

guidewire is extracted through the urethra with either a cystoscope or a basket snare passed through a Foley catheter.[57] By holding the guide proximally at the lumbar level and distally at the urethra, fixation is achieved, and stenting is easily accomplished.[189]

EMBOLIZATION

Embolization has been performed to defunctionalize the kidney, achieving effective control of fistulae and avoiding open operation. An innovative technique of embolization, with butyl-2-cyanoacrylate, was reported by Günther et al to manage the complicated vesicovaginal or vesicocutaneous fistulae associated with pelvic malignancy.[203] Ureteral embolization, along with external drainage via a percutaneous nephrostomy, accomplishes the goal of managing the patient comfortably. Butyl-2-cyanoacrylate was chosen because of its efficacy in vascular occlusion. The results were not optimal, however, because the embolic material was partially or totally expelled by ureteral peristalsis, perhaps because of detachment of the glue secondary to regeneration of uroepithelium. A patent ureter results.[189,203]

An alternative technique of embolizing the ureter, with latex or detachable silicone rubber balloons, was proposed by the same authors.[204,205] Apparently, balloons do not dissolve in urine and are nonwettable, so ureteral recanalization is avoided. With this technique, temporary urinary diversion is achieved, and the ureter becomes amenable to surgical intervention if the balloon is removed.[204]

One should try initially to manage ureteral fistulae with a simple diversion nephrostomy and stent placement. The extreme approach of medical nephrectomy by renal embolization[206–208] is drastic and is undesirable in patients whose lesions are not cancerous.

OTHER TECHNIQUES

Another innovative technique, by Lund et al, occludes the ureter proximal to the fistula with rubber bands and clips similar to those used for ligating the fallopian tubes.[205] A percutaneous tract is created by direct puncture of the ureter proximal to the fistula (Fig. 23–154A) and the ureter is opacified through a puncture of the renal pelvis with a Chiba needle. The tract into the ureter is dilated to 26F (Fig. 23–154B). Over a 20F Teflon sheath, the rubber ring is introduced through the 26F working sheath. The ureter is trapped and mobilized with long forceps, a loop is pulled into the 20F tube, and the rubber ring is advanced onto the ureter with the outer Teflon sheath. This technique has been successful in dogs and in human patients.

Ureteral Stricture Dilation

Patients with strictures in the urinary tract have traditionally been managed operatively. Recently, however,

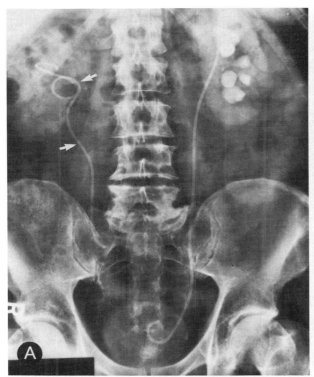

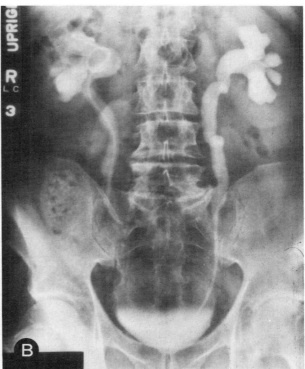

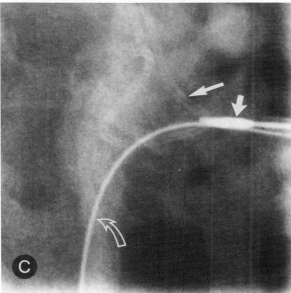

Fig. 23–149 Bilateral double-J stents placed for internal drainage in patient with pelvic malignancy. A. IVU shows adequate function of left double-J stent and proximal migration of right double-J (arrows). B. Late film of IVU shows adequate flow of contrast medium from left pelvicaliceal system into bladder through double-J stent and marked hydronephrosis of right pelvicaliceal system due to proximal migration of stent. C. Through percutaneous tract, stent (large arrow) has been grabbed with alligator forceps (short arrow) and is slowly pulled through tract. Safety wire is in ureter (open arrow).

attempts have been made at several institutions to dilate benign strictures percutaneously. Short-term results have been good. Dilation of malignant obstructions has generally failed, however, and these strictures are more common, generally as a result of primary cancer of the bladder, ureter, or renal pelvis or of secondary involvement by cancer in adjacent organs or lymph nodes.

Benign strictures have several causes, most of which are iatrogenic: trauma during major pelvic or retroperitoneal operation, previous ureteral surgery (reimplantation, lithotomy, ileal diversion, ureterostomy), or trauma during endourologic manipulations of instruments to remove stones. Other causes are retroperitoneal fibrosis, radiation, congenital narrowing, and infection.

The traditional nonoperative approach to the management of ureteral strictures was retrograde catheter dilation,[209] but the technique often failed because of inability to introduce larger catheters without undue trauma or perforation.[210] The recent availability of the Grüntzig balloon[211] overcomes this problem and permits dilation of strictures in the biliary tract and ureter.[212] Single case reports of ureteral dilation describe success,[213,214] and success also has been reported in 13 of 23 cases and in 6 of 7 cases.[189] These promising results have encouraged

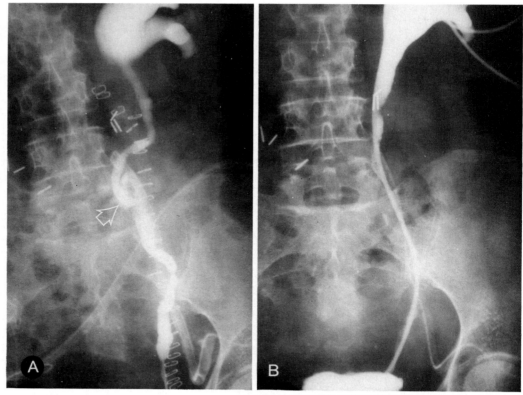

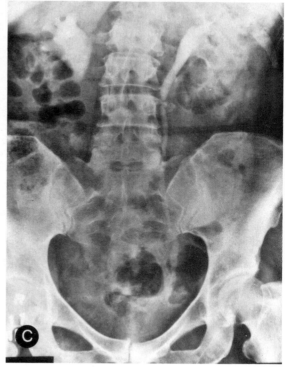

Fig. 23–150 Patient with partial intraoperative transection of ureter. A. Retrograde pyelogram shows opacification of distal ureter with extravasation of contrast medium at level of L5 (arrow). Attempts to catheterize ureter retrograde for placement of double-J stent were unsuccessful. B. Antegrade pyelogram performed after placement of drainage catheter shows adequate control of extravasation from site of partial transection. C. IVU performed 3 months after removal of external–internal drainage shows no evidence of extravasation and good decompression of both pelvicaliceal systems.

other investigators to research the pathophysiologic mechanisms that lead to strictures, decide upon the ideal type of balloon, and determine the number and duration of balloon inflations required for successful dilation.[215] Further studies are needed to determine the efficacy of the technique and the duration of postdilation stenting required to keep the ureter patent.

Patient Selection

The patients are evaluated by thorough physical examination and medical history in order to determine the severity and etiology of the stricture. The following laboratory examinations are usually ordered at the time of hospital admission:

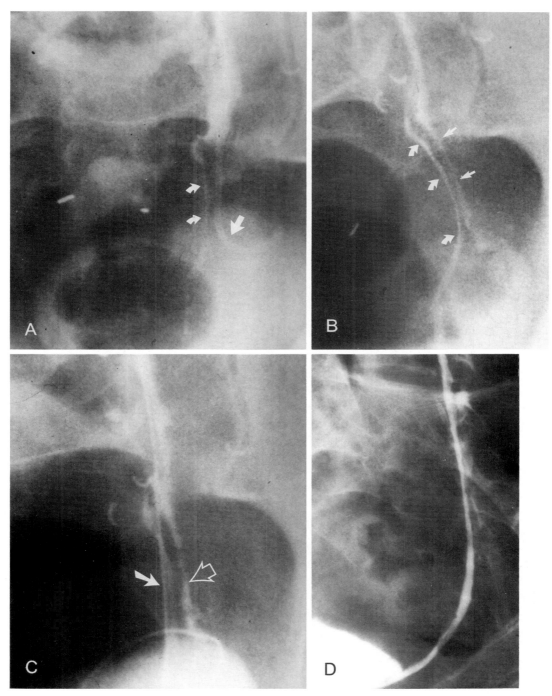

Fig. 23–151 Patient with partial transection of left ureter during radical pelvic surgery. Primary suture with double-J stent placement was attempted. Drainage of urine through Penrose drain indicated percutaneous management. A. Stenting of ureteral injury. Antegrade pyelogram reveals that distal end of double-J catheter (short arrow) is outside ureter. Distal ureter is faintly opacified; it is medially displaced (curved arrows) by urinoma. B. After removal of double-J stent thorugh percutaneous tract, angiographic torque control catheter has been advanced to level of ureteral tear. Contrast medium is seen extravasating (short white arrows) but contrast medium flows into distal ureter (curved arrows). C. Guidewire has been manipulated with the help of a torque control catheter into the distal ureter (white arrow), passing the tip of the wire to the bladder. Observe continuous extravasation of contrast medium (open arrow). D. Follow-up nephrostogram 2 months later before removal of stent shows intact ureteral walls.

Coagulation profile (prothrombin time, partial thromboplastin time, thrombin time, platelets); any coagulation abnormality is corrected before percutaneous manipulation is attempted;

Hemoglobin and hematocrit;
Blood urea nitrogen (BUN), creatinine;
Urine culture. (If infection is present, appropriate antibiotics are started).

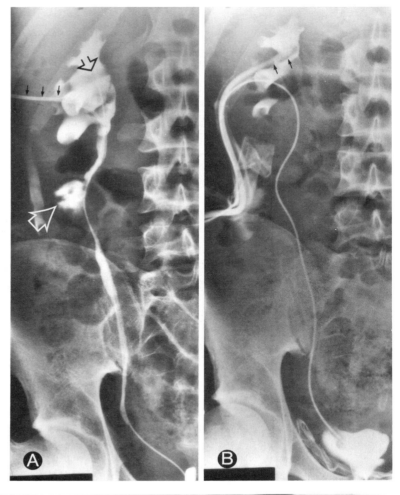

Fig. 23–152 Management of postoperative fistula. Retrograde pyelogram shows extravasation of contrast medium in upper third of right ureter (open white arrow) at site of ureterostomy for stone removal. An 8F catheter is seen within renal pelvis (small black arrows), as is large rubber tube (open black arrow). B. Nephrostogram after removal of ureteral catheter shows antegrade placement of 6F ureteral stent with its tip in bladder. Rubber tube is seen within renal pelvis (arrows).

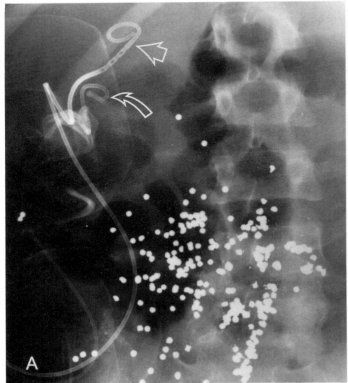

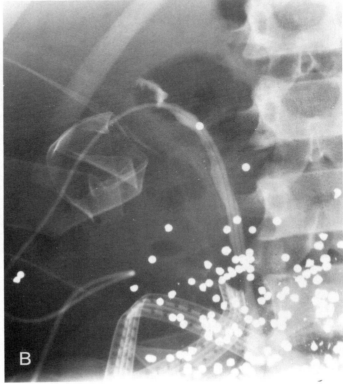

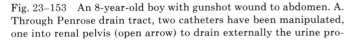

Fig. 23–153 An 8-year-old boy with gunshot wound to abdomen. A. Through Penrose drain tract, two catheters have been manipulated, one into renal pelvis (open arrow) to drain externally the urine produced by the kidney and a second into urinoma found around kidney by CT (curved arrow). B. Through Penrose drain tract, angiographic catheter has been manipulated into ureter.

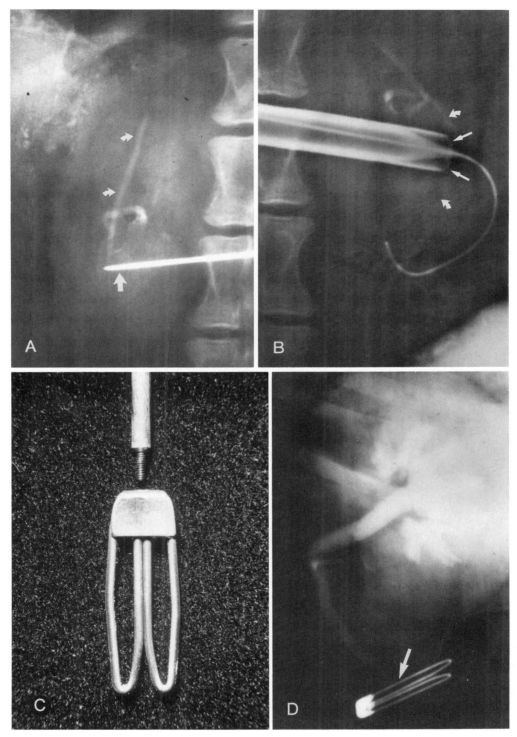

Fig. 23–154   Clip obstruction of ureter. A. IVU in mongrel dog shows adequate opacification of ureter (curved arrows). Large needle has been introduced percutaneously and advanced to level of ureter (short arrow). B. Through needle, guidewire has been advanced, and tract has been dilated to 24F. Teflon sheath (arrows) is being advanced over dilator. Observe medial displacement of ureter by sheath (curved arrows). C. Close-up view of metallic clip used to obstruct ureter. D. Flat view of abdomen after intravenous injection of contrast medium shows dilatation of proximal ureter and renal pelvis after obstruction of ureter with clip (arrow).

Various radiologic examinations are performed as appropriate to clarify the nature and severity of the stricture:

An IVU, to help define both the anatomy and the function of the kidney and ureter;

A "loopogram" in patients with ileal diversions; this usually is the best way to opacify the collecting system;

An antegrade pyelogram, when renal function is impaired by the obstruction, to demonstrated the anatomy;

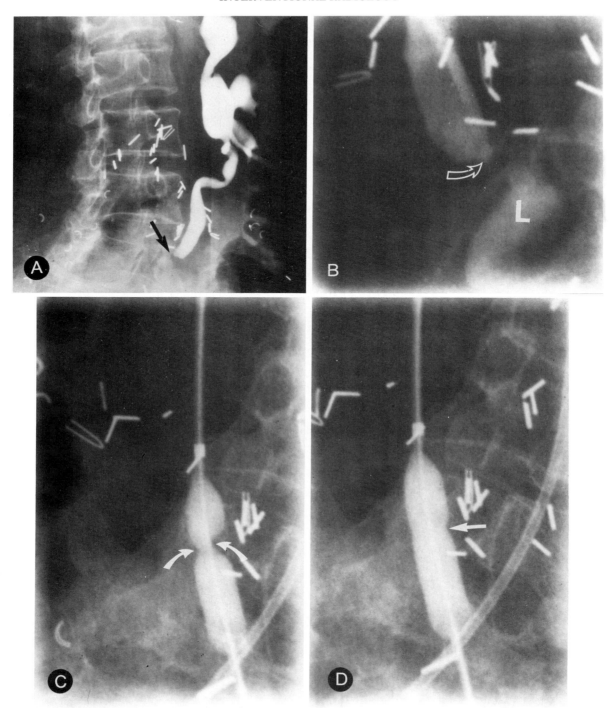

Fig. 23–155   Patient with ileal diversion presenting with rise in creatinine. A. Antegrade pyelogram shows dilatation of renal pelvis and calices from complete obstruction of distal ureter (arrow). B. Angiographic catheter has been advanced to obstruction (open arrow); contrast medium slowly opacifies loop (L). C. Guidewire has been passed through site of obstruction; over guidewire, 8-mm, 4-cm-long angioplasty balloon catheter has been inserted. Observe indentation in balloon at site of stricture (arrows). D. With increasing pressure in the balloon, indentation has almost completely disappeared (arrow). E. Flat plate of abdomen showing position of balloon across stricture during trial of long-term inflation. Note ileus presenting as a complication in this patient. F. Nephrostogram 3 months after dilatation and before stent removal shows adequate increase in diameter of ureter at site of balloon dilation (arrows).

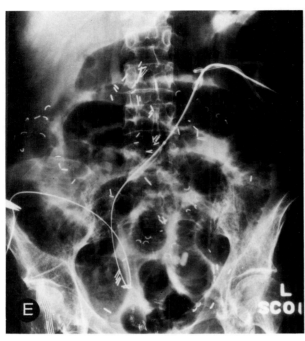
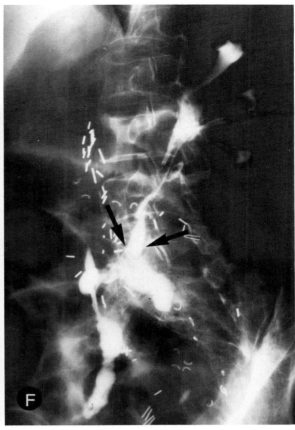

Fig. 23–155E,F

A Whitaker test if there is any question about whether an apparent stricture is functionally important. A pressure gradient between the renal pelvis and bladder of >20 cm H_2O is significant. The modification of the Whitaker test used in renal allograft recipients where the source of the obstruction is suspected of being a high implantation of the ureter in the bladder has already been discussed.

PREOPERATIVE PREPARATION AND INTRAOPERATIVE CARE

Before the procedure, similar steps are taken as for other urointerventional procedures, including making sure there is an adequate intravenous line for fluids, sedatives, and analgesics. Broad-spectrum antibiotics (gentamicin and ampicillin or an equivalent combination) are given either 6–8 hr prior to or immediately before the procedure, and the patient receives some preoperative sedation as described earlier. During the procedure, vital signs are monitored, and analgesics are given intravenously as needed.

TECHNIQUES

There are two principal steps: dilation and long-term stenting. Dilation of strictures can be performed with either semirigid or balloon dilators. Because of the easier passage of the latter, they are preferred in most cases, and

most strictures respond rapidly. However, some strictures will require a second balloon dilation or dilation overnight. The second balloon dilation, 1 or 2 days later, is often remarkably successful even when the first has seemingly had little or no effect. The new 6F/10F or 6F/12F Teflon, long-taper coaxial dilators developed by Amplatz are often successful when everything else has failed.

There are three approaches for dilating strictures with balloon catheters:

1. Short balloon inflation with short-term stenting;
2. Short balloon inflation with long-term stenting;
3. Long balloon inflation with long-term stenting.

Currently, the authors stent all dilated strictures, either for short periods, if the stenosis was less severe, or for longer periods, often coupled with later redilation, if it was more severe. Which of these approaches will prove best in the long term remains to be seen.

The optimal approach for ureteral dilation requires a tract through a posterior calix of the superior or, preferably, the middle caliceal group (Fig. 23–155A).[184,189,202] The ureter is catheterized with a cobra or multipurpose angiographic catheter. By gentle manipulation of the catheter and guidewire, the stricture is traversed, and the guidewire is advanced into the bladder or ileal loop (Fig. 23–155B). The angiographic catheter is removed, the nephrostomy tract is dilated to 10F, and a second wire is introduced. A 10-mm-diameter, 10-cm-long, high-pressure balloon catheter is passed over the stiffer wire until the balloon is traversing the stricture, and the balloon is inflated with an inflation device. A simple inflation device is necessary because repeated adjustments must be made by the nurses during the 10–12 hr that the balloon is inflated and deflated.[189] A pressure of 6–10 atm is usually sufficient, although occasionally pressures up to 15–20 atm are needed. Immediately after the start of balloon inflation, a "waist" is seen at the site of the stricture (Fig. 23–155C), which disappears as the pressure is raised (Fig. 23–155D).[213,214]

If a short inflation is planned, the balloon is deflated either after 10–15 min or when the waist disappears and is exchanged for an 8F–10F drainage catheter with sideholes proximal and distal to the dilated area.[210] The safety wire is pulled out.

If a long inflation is planned, the balloon is left in the stricture inflated at 4–6 atm (Fig. 23–155E). A drainage catheter is passed over the safety wire into the renal pelvis for external drainage while the balloon is in place.[189] Alternatively, a special balloon with sideholes proximal to the balloon can be used for dilation and drainage. Generally, the authors leave the balloon inflated for 30 min, alternating with 30 min of deflation for 12 hr. Once the sequence is completed, the balloon catheter is exchanged for a 10F internal–external stent, which is left in place for 3–4 months. At this time, the status of the dilated site is re-evaluated by contrast medium injection (Fig. 23–155F). If needed, redilation can be done at this time and followed by long-term stenting.[189] Repeated short inflations, every 2 or 3 days for as long as 10–15 days, seem to be safer and probably are more effective than long-term inflations.[210]

In some patients, the stricture is so hard that it does not stretch with balloon inflation. In such cases, the Teflon coaxial dilators and the new Teflon long-taper Amplatz coaxial dilators have proved useful.[69,189]

In some patients, it is possible to pass a wire through the stricture but not a dilator. In these cases, a through-and-through wire provides the only approach for successful dilation.

Discussion

Ureteral catheterization via the lumbar route is the natural extension of percutaneous nephrostomy.[184,185,215] Greater force can be exerted on the catheter to advance it through the stricture when proper puncture of either a superior or a middle calix is performed. The management of immediate postoperative complications, such as partial transection of the ureter, by percutaneous nephrostomy[187,200,202] led to trials of stenting and dilation of strictures with the newer balloon catheters.[189,209,210,214,216] The success in negotiating strictures with guidewires and arteriography catheters after failure by the retrograde cystoscopic approach revealed an additional advantage of the antegrade method. Another point in the favor of the new method was the experimental demonstration, in the dog model, that ureteral strictures can be dilated via the percutaneous route.[214] Balloon catheter dilation is preferred because it does not require creation of a large tract through the renal parenchyma, yet it achieves maximum dilation.

Balloon or coaxial dilation of malignant strictures should not be attempted for fear of ureteral rupture. In these cases, mere stenting with indwelling catheters maintains the natural conduit of urine between the kidneys and the bladder.

Which strictures will respond to dilation is difficult to predict, and the time required to dilate strictures is not well established, ranging from 30 sec to 16 hr of balloon inflation.[189,209,215,216] Banner et al reported favorable results in patients with "fresh" postoperative strictures and postulated that old ischemic, fibrotic strictures may not respond to dilation.[210] Those authors also predicted that the strictures that have resulted from fistulae, being densely fibrotic because of the urine leakage, may not respond to dilation. The desmoplastic reaction in retroperitoneal fibrosis may also prevent successful dilation of strictured ureters.[210] Other unfavorable types are:

1. Ureteroileostomy strictures following radical surgery for carcinoma of the cervix;
2. Strictures associated with fistulae following radical hysterectomy;
3. Postoperative pyeloplasty strictures of longer duration associated with urine leakage.

The strictures that respond favorably are:

1. Those following ureteroneocystostomy, ureteroileostomy, and ureterolithotomy[210];
2. Recent ureteropelvic strictures following pyeloplasty[217];
3. Those following accidental ligation of the ureter.[69]

Transient obstruction may develop secondary to ureteral edema in patients with indwelling stents.[218] Nephrostograms may reveal mucosal irregularities, "thumb-printing," or bullous edema secondary to the pressure effect of large catheters for long periods of time (Fig. 23–156). These changes may be related to hypersensitivity to catheter material with or without infection.[218] Such obstruction is treated simply by placing an external catheter for urinary drainage and usually clears within 5–8 days.

Further investigative human and animal work is needed to establish protocols for successful dilation of ureteral strictures of various etiologies.

Patient Follow-up

Microhematuria and pyuria are frequent after catheter placement. Infection is uncommon and usually easy to eradicate with appropriate antimicrobials. Vesicoureteral reflux is to be expected due to the presence of an open system (the stent) but may require higher than usual vesical pressure. Reflux should cause no problems unless there is a lower urinary tract infection. Urine cultures are obtained monthly, and infections are treated according to the antibiotic sensitivity results. Prophylactic antibiotics are recommended for females, for males with a history of urinary tract infection, or for anyone who develops an infection while a stent is indwelling.

Irritation of the bladder mucosa by the stent may cause symptoms, especially when a long segment of the stent protrudes into the bladder. Antispasmodics are useful to

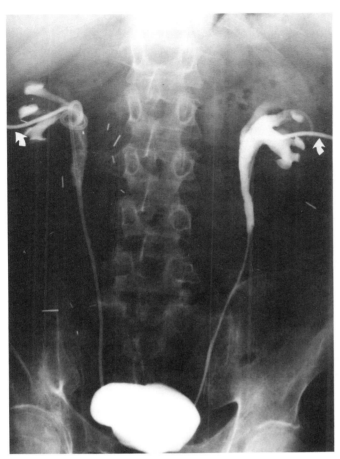

Fig. 23–156 Bilateral nephrostogram in patient with double-J stents placed bilaterally and with temporary external diversion (arrows). Note marked prominence of endothelium in both kidneys, predominantly on right side, suggestive of inflammatory changes secondary to catheter placement.

control these symptoms. If trigonal irrigation causes intractable symptoms, a polyethylene or C-Flex stent may have to be replaced by a softer Silastic stent.

Encrustation usually occurs with all of the available stents if they are left indwelling long enough. A diluted, acidic urine will delay the onset of this problem, so the patient should be instructed to maintain an intake of at least 2 liters of fluid daily. Prophylactic control with antimicrobials aimed specifically at urea-splitting organisms will also retard the onset and the progression of encrustation. There seems to be no difference in the encrustation rates of polyethylene and silicone stents, although there have been claims of a lower encrustation rate for silicone.

For follow-up purposes, the authors distinguish those patients with an externally accessible catheter from those with internal stents. Patients with external or internal–external catheters should be evaluated every 3 months if asymptomatic or any time there is a decrease in urinary output, creatinine elevation, hematuria, or leakage of urine or blood along the catheter. As a rule, the authors replace the catheters whenever an evaluation is required for any of these reasons and every 6 months otherwise.

Malfunction of an internal stent can be difficult to detect, especially if the other kidney is unobstructed and functioning. Subtle symptoms, such as back pain, malaise, dysuria, hematuria, frequency, and fever, must be asked about at each visit and their significance carefully explained to the patient so he or she can watch for problems at home. Decreased urine output and creatinine elevation are late signs and mandate an immediate radiologic evaluation.

Radiologic studies should be obtained as necessary to confirm or disprove obstruction. In the patient requiring long-term stent drainage, a baseline renogram and an ultrasound scan should be performed 4–6 weeks after stent placement for subsequent comparison in case problems arise. If the renogram or ultrasound scan confirms the presence of obstruction, a plain film of the abdomen should be obtained to assess stent position, because proximal or distal migration can be the cause of the obstructive symptoms (Figs. 23–147 through 23–149). If an internal stent has migrated or is obstructed, it must be replaced by one of the techniques described above. A cystogram is one of the best methods to diagnose stent obstruction (Fig. 23–144C).

Obstruction of an external–internal stent can be relieved either by simple irrigation of the stent or by passing a guidewire through the stent lumen. However, with internal stents, this problem becomes more difficult. Obstructed stents are commonly replaced endoscopically. This is easier in females due to the shorter urethra. In males, the stent usually is pulled out, and the ureter then has to be catheterized *de novo* endoscopically.

Complications and Management Problems during Short- and Long-Term Nephrostomy Drainage

Serious complications, such as hemorrhage in and around the kidney and exacerbation of infection or onset of new sepsis, occur in about 4%–5% of nephrostomies.[3,71] Other serious complications, such as pneumothorax, urine peritonitis, and retroperitoneal extravasation of urine with subsequent urinoma, are rare.[2] The deaths (0.2% incidence) have been caused by severe hemorrhage in all cases.[3] Several of these fatalities followed puncture as a last resort in patients with severe septic obstruction and known coagulation deficits. In contrast, the mortality rate of surgical nephrostomy is 6%–12%.[3,80]

Minor complications occur in 10% of nephrostomies and are hemorrhage, pain, and catheter malfunction.[2,3,71]

URINE LEAKAGE

Leakage of urine along the tract occurs for one of three reasons:

1. Catheter obstruction. In these cases, the catheter should be replaced by one of the same dimensions.
2. Catheter sidehole malpositioning. The catheter should either be repositioned or be replaced by one of the same caliber with fewer sideholes.
3. Tract larger than drainage catheter. The catheter must be replaced by a larger one.

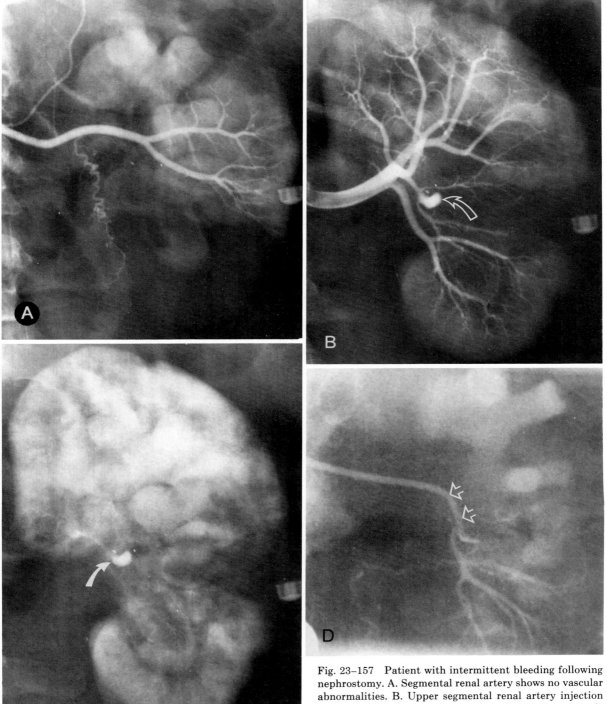

Fig. 23–157   Patient with intermittent bleeding following nephrostomy. A. Segmental renal artery shows no vascular abnormalities. B. Upper segmental renal artery injection reveals false aneurysm involving branch (open arrow). C. Nephrographic phase shows persistent opacification of false aneurysm (arrow) and dense parenchymal staining. D. Tip of catheter (arrows) has been selectively placed into false aneurysm to deposit two pieces of Gelfoam. E. Repeat segmental artery injection shows complete obliteration of false aneurysm (arrow) with preservation of remaining renal artery branches.

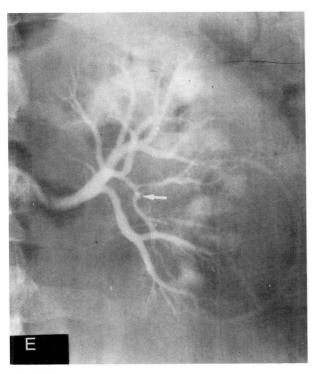

Fig. 23–157E

PAIN

Pain after nephrostomy catheter placement can have any of at least three causes:

1. Periosteal irritation when the puncture was done too close to a rib;
2. Intercostal nerve irritation when the puncture is placed too close to the lower costal margin. Both intercostal nerve and periosteal pain are best managed by an intercostal nerve block;
3. The catheter tip pushing against the renal pelvic wall. This is a problem particularly with large drainage catheters. It is managed by repositioning the catheter.

INFECTION

Infection is prevented by the administration of antibiotics (gentamicin–ampicillin or a similar combination) before, during, and 2 days after urointerventional procedures. In the long-term care of these patients, antibiotics are usually not needed prophylactically. The patients are instructed on how to take care of the nephrostomy site and how to irrigate the drainage catheter to minimize the risk of infection.

The infection can be exacerbated by percutaneous nephrostomies in patients with pyonephrosis. High-pressure injections and diagnostic nephrostograms should be avoided in order to prevent reflux of contaminated urine via the pyelovenous route into the systemic veins.[3,78]

Urine may be contaminated with other organisms if aseptic technique is not practiced for catheter placement or if the catheters are poorly handled during irrigation.

HEMORRHAGE

Bleeding can be either immediate or delayed. All patients have hematuria after the percutaneous nephrostomy puncture, but generally the urine clears within 24–36 hr, so this is not considered a complication.[3,71] If the urine does not clear but the amount of blood is not excessive, it is probably caused by the position of a sidehole or the catheter tip within the renal parenchyma. Repositioning of the catheter usually takes care of this problem. Catheter blockage secondary to clots from any bleeding should be prevented by frequent saline irrigation.[7] The rare case of a falling hematocrit without external bleeding is probably secondary to perirenal hemorrhage[7] and occurs in patients with coagulation defects.[78] In this situation, CT is extremely helpful.[219]

If the bleeding is severe, it is usually due to major vascular injury, either arterial laceration, with or without false aneurysm formation, or formation of an arteriovenous fistula.[131,219,220] In some patients, the bleeding can be arrested by inserting a larger nephrostomy tube to tamponade the tract. Ideally, this will be a self-retaining catheter. If the bleeding stops with this treatment, the catheter should stay in the tract for 2–4 weeks before any further manipulations are attempted. Severe bleeding that cannot be controlled by tamponade usually necessitates selective arteriography to locate the vascular injury followed by selective embolization (Fig. 23–157).

Renal vascular complications, such as arteriovenous fistulae and pseudoaneurysms, are more common in patients who undergo renal biopsies than in those who undergo percutaneous nephrostomy, perhaps because of the mechanical removal of a tissue core at the time of renal biopsy rather than the mere tissue displacement in nephostomies.[220]

The vascular complications of nephrostomy, are attributed to:

1. Use of larger (16-gauge) needles, which, unlike the smaller (20–22-gauge) needles, cause trauma[219];
2. Diabetes, hypertension, or other types of nephrosclerosis that impair the contractility of the vessel walls[221];
3. Direct trauma to branches of the renal artery around the renal pelvis, leading to significant bleeding because of the lack of supporting connective tissue and its tamponade effect[219];
4. Too early removal of the nephrostomy tube, before blood vessels injured during tract creation and dilation have sealed properly.[96]

Fortunately, the severe hemorrhage secondary to renal arteriovenous fistulae and pseudoaneurysms can be stopped by selective arteriography and embolization with Ivalon, Gelfoam, or steel coils.[219] This approach preserves most of the renal parenchyma without undue loss of renal function even in patients with a single kidney.

Perirenal hematomas can be found by CT examination in practically every patient following percutaneous manipulations (Fig. 23–158). These collections are asymptomatic and seldom require any therapy, resolving spontaneously without sequelae.

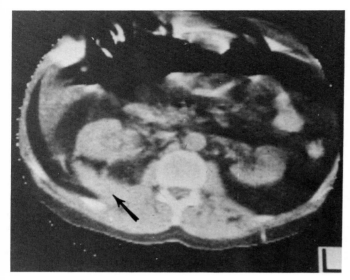

Fig. 23–158   CT scan at midsection of kidneys shows large perirenal hematoma around right kidney (arrow).

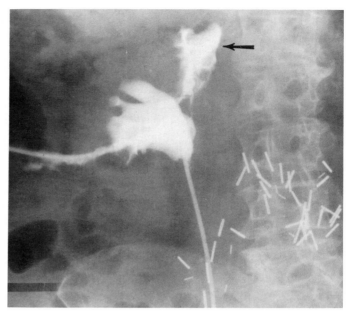

Fig. 23–159 Nephrostogram shows extravasation of contrast medium (black arrow) into perirenal space superiorly.

URINOMA

This is an uncommon complication that is usually secondary to severe lacerations of the renal pelvis (Figs. 23–159 and 23–160) or ureter during manipulation for stone removal. Urinomas also are seen in patients with collecting system tears associated with distal obstruction and continued normal renal function.[222] There are a few case reports of urinoma formation secondary to poor drainage by kinked or obstructed catheters.[223] Generally, these tears heal spontaneously with adequate drainage of the renal pelvis and ureter. If the collection is undrained, the urine can evoke a fibrotic reaction that forms a thick wall around the fluid collection, creating a fluctuant mass that displaces the kidney.

MECHANICAL PROBLEMS OF CATHETER MANAGEMENT

These problems include obstruction secondary to plugging of drainage holes either with debris or purulent material in pyonephrosis or by blood clots in severe hemorrhage. Obstruction can be prevented by using large-bore nephrostomy catheters to drain pus and by frequent saline flushes to dissolve clots.[2] Completely obstructed catheters can be replaced by introducing a Desilets–Hoffman sheath (Cook, Inc.) over the existing catheter. The plugged catheter is then replaced with a new one, thereby avoiding a new puncture.

Catheter dislodgment is a serious problem that should be minimized by proper securing methods such as Molnar disks and stoma adhesives instead of simple suturing, which tears through the skin, making the catheter easy to dislodge. The patient and the nursing staff should be trained in the proper handling of catheters. Slight catheter migration can cause urine leakage.

INTERVENTIONS IN THE URETHRA

Suprapubic cystostomy drainage has traditionally been used for emergency urinary decompression and commonly required a surgical procedure. With the advances in endourologic techniques, a different approach is available, not only for diagnostic but also for therapeutic purposes.

Technique of Suprapubic Cystography and Urethral Catheterization

With the patient supine on the x-ray table, the skin of the suprapubic area is cleansed and draped. The bladder is localized either after intravenous administration of contrast medium or, more commonly, under real-time ultrasound guidance. After administration of adequate sedation and local anesthesia, the bladder is entered with an 18-gauge needle in the midline just above the symphysis pubis at a caudad angle. After aspiration of urine, contrast medium is injected to opacify the bladder, a 0.038-inch J-tip guidewire is passed, and the needle is withdrawn. The tract is dilated until a 10F dilator is in place (Fig. 23–161A). At this point, a second guidewire is introduced. Over one of the guidewires, a 7F cobra or multipurpose angiographic catheter is introduced and manipulated into the bladder neck; and a 0.035-inch floppy-tip guidewire is carefully passed through the posterior urethra (Fig. 23–161B) until it exits through the urethral meatus. The angiographic catheter is then passed over the guidewire, through the urethra, and out the meatus (Fig. 23–161C).

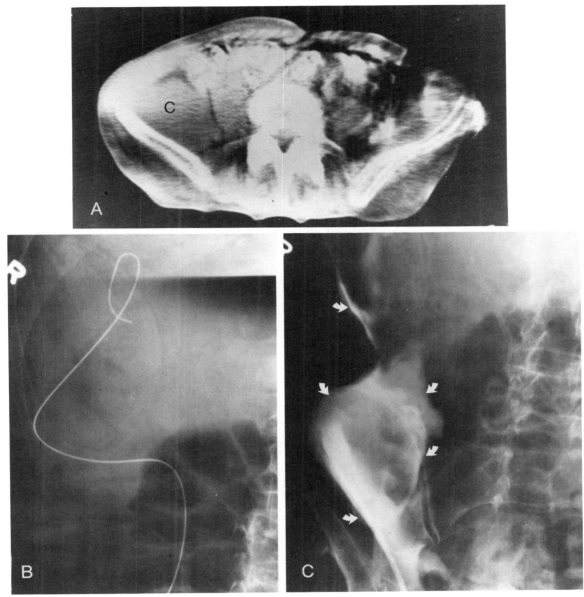

Fig. 23-160   Patient presenting with abdominal distention and pain after accidental removal of his nephrostomy tube. A. CT scan at level of pelvis shows large fluid collection (c) extending along paracolic gutter. B. After percutaneous puncture under fluoroscopy, guidewire has been passed through needle; it can be seen to extend high in paracolic gutter. C. Contrast medium injected through pigtail catheter is seen to outline right paracolic gutter (arrows).

After removal of the catheter, and depending on the problem present (obstruction or disruption), balloon dilators or semirigid urethral dilators are advanced over the guidewire to dilate the urethra. Once the dilation is completed, an end hole can be cut in a Foley catheter, which is then advanced into the bladder. The position of the catheter is verified by a cystogram performed while keeping the wire in place, passing it into the dye-injecting syringe. If the urethral catheter is in a good position, the wire is withdrawn into the bladder, and a catheter is placed through the percutaneous tract into the bladder.[224]

Percutaneous urethral catheterization is becoming more common as interventional endourologic procedures become more widely used. Antegrade catheterization has advantages over retrograde urethral catheterization, which is a blind procedure that usually provides only a temporary solution. Indications for retrograde catheterization include obstructing prostatic hyperplasia, postgonococcal strictures, obstructing urethral stones, and urethral trauma. The procedure itself, because of the traumatic, blind manipulation of the urethra, can cause severe inflammation in the urethral mucosa and periurethral tissue. Antegrade catheterization, on the other hand, provides a controlled, simplified approach to the urethra. In cases where attempts at retrograde catheterization are contraindicated—for example, in suspected urethral rupture—antegrade urethrography and catheterization have been successful, and surgical intervention has been avoided (Fig. 23-162).[225] Antegrade urethral

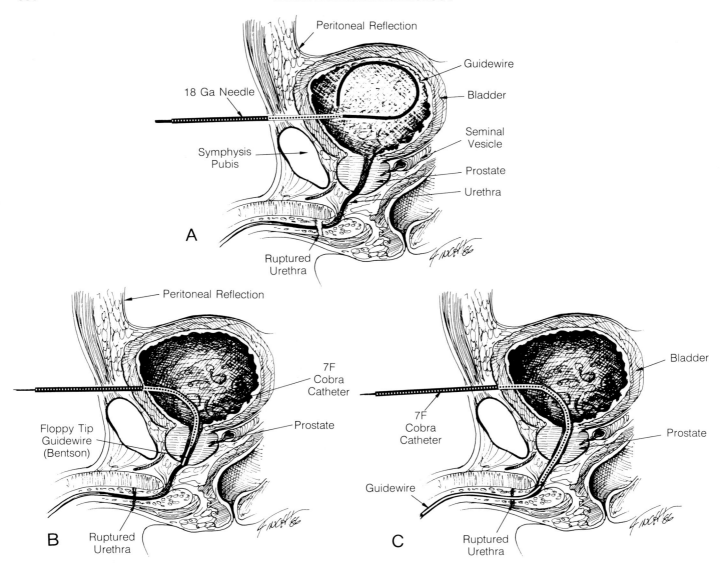

Fig. 23–161 Suprapubic antegrade catheterization of urethra in patient with trauma or severe strictures. A. Using suprapubic approach, 18-gauge needle was used to puncture bladder, and 0.038-inch guidewire was passed into bladder. Angiographic torque control catheter has been passed over guidewire after dilatation with Teflon dilators. B. Tip of angiographic catheter has been directed toward bladder neck, and guidewire has been manipulated down prostatic urethra. C. Guidewire has been manipulated with help of angiographic catheter across area of trauma in urethra until wire exits through meatus.

catheterization provides a means for imaging and stenting a severely traumatized urethra, permitting it to heal rapidly with minimal manipulation.

Other Urethral Procedures

As in so many other areas of interventional radiology, a basic technique—antegrade urethral catheterization—and appropriate instruments had no sooner appeared then ingenious practitioners thought of several new ways to combine them into nonoperative solutions to formerly surgical problems. Among these new techniques are antegrade recanalization of strictured or disrupted urethras,[226–228] percutaneous ablation of posterior urethral valves,[229,230] and relief of obstructive prostatic hyperplasia.[231–233] As these are predominantly techniques for the surgeon, they will not be discussed further here.

NEPHROSTOLITHOTOMY (NLT)

Historical Background

In 1946, Rupel and Brown reported removing renal calculi through surgically created nephrostomy tracts.[234]

Removal of stones through percutaneously created nephrostomy tracts was initially reported by Fernström and Johansson.[235] Thereafter, partly as the result of the

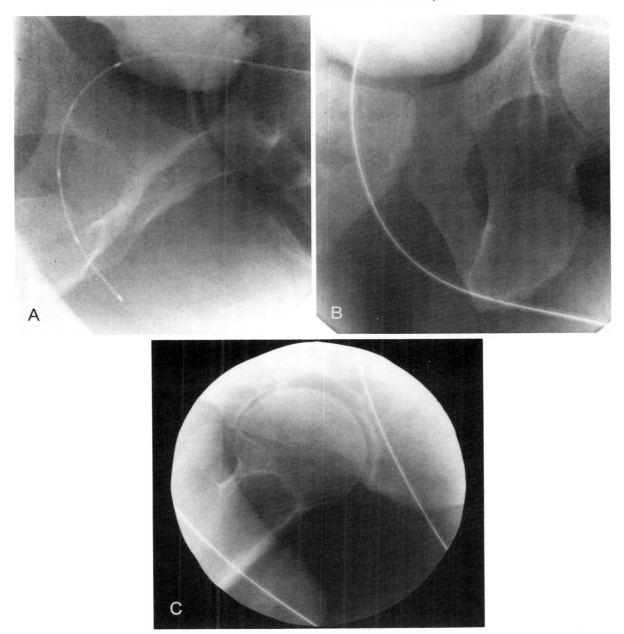

Fig. 23–162 Patient suffered rupture of urethra in motor vehicle accident. A. Through suprapubic puncture, Lunderquist–Ring torque guidewire has been manipulated through traumatized ure-thra. B. Anteroposterior projection showing passage of Teflon dilator over guidewire. C. Lateral projection showing guidewire and dilator at entry and exit point at urethral meatus.

development of new instruments and the refinement of old ones, NLT virtually replaced open stone operations, even for large stones; some series of 400 or more patients have been reported,[95,96,99] and no doubt there are others.

In 1978, Smith, then at the University of Minnesota, and his colleagues wrote the first report of the uroradiologic extraction of a ureteral calculus. This patient had an ileal loop.[236] Since that time, many hundreds of nephrostolithotomies have been performed at this institution. Close cooperation between the radiologists and urologists has been essential to the development of the new techniques for extraction of renal stones through a percutaneous tract. The knowledge of the interventional radiologist is necessary for the placement of the needle and

guidewires in the appropriate calix utilizing multidirectional fluoroscopy to obtain a three-dimensional image. Further, that person's knowledge of cardiovascular techniques for maneuvering the catheters and guidewires and for the passage of rigid or flexible dilators is needed. The urologist is the patient's primary physician and is practiced in the direct removal of the stones by endoscopic techniques, utilizing flexible and rigid nephroscopes and electrohydraulic or ultrasonic lithotriptors, or with various other instruments such as baskets.

The nephrostomy tract can be dilated within a few minutes to 30F with flexible dilators or balloons with subsequent placement of 30F Amplatz working sheaths. In cases in which stones are <1.5 cm and lie free in the renal pelvis, they can often be extracted in a single session, resulting in a shorter hospital stay. Even when more complex methods are needed, there is less postoperative morbidity than with open operation and almost no mortality. Patients can reassume normal activity sooner than after conventional surgical lithotomy even when staghorn stones are removed, because the convalescent period is only 3–10 days after discharge from the hospital.[7,90–92,97,98,100,101,237–243] The overall success rate for removal of renal pelvic stones is 96%–98%. The somewhat lower success rate (85%) for ureteral stones may be related to adherence or submucosal burying of these stones in the wall. In summary, NLT is a safe, cost-effective procedure with low morbidity and a low rate of stone recurrence. At the University of Minnesota, the authors became so confident of NLT that they removed a number of asymptomatic stones when there were social indications, such as inability to practice one's profession.

As rapidly as NLT has developed, however, extracorporeal shock wave lithotripsy (ESWL) has begun to curtail its use. Percutaneous techniques are now thought applicable principally where ESWL is not available, when ESWL has failed, and for particular types of stones, particularly those made of cystine, those trapped behind an obstruction, those that are radiolucent or infected, and those that fill most of the collecting system. Thus, despite the appeal of ESWL, percutaneous methods of stone removal are expected to continue to play an important part in the total stone removal effort.

Indications

Almost any retained urinary stone may be removed by NLT. In most patients, the stone should be the cause of symptoms, such as hematuria, pain, or infection, although stones are sometimes removed for "social" indications.

Contraindications

Nephrostolithotomy has two chief contraindications: infection and bleeding diathesis, although both of them can be considered relative. The treatment of choice for obstructed, infected uropathy is percutaneous decompression and specific antibiotic therapy, stone removal being performed in a subsequent step once the infection has been controlled. Bleeding diathesis also is a relative contraindication, because it can be corrected by the transfusion of fresh-frozen plasma, platelets, and specific blood products.

SOLITARY KIDNEY

A vascular injury from a nephrostomy tract in a solitary kidney is a serious complication, and radiologists hesitate to perform NLT in these cases.[244] However, a solitary kidney does not rule out NLT. Clayman and Castañeda–Zuñiga propose that stone extraction in these patients be performed in stages. On the first day, a nephrostomy catheter is placed; 2 or 3 days later, the tract is dilated to 24F, and the patient is sent home while the tract matures for 1 or 2 weeks; and the stone is

extracted in a final session.[245] The authors have extracted stones from patients with a solitary kidney without any serious complications. However, the radiology–urology team without extensive experience in NLT should consider solitary kidneys a contraindication to the procedure, because this method of treatment is still being evaluated in large medical centers.

UNUSUAL STONE CONFIGURATIONS AND ANOMALOUS RENAL ANATOMY

Staghorn calculi, particularly large ones with several branches, were once considered a contraindication to NLT because of the possibly higher incidence of complications. In the authors' experience, although the procedures are technically difficult, these patients have not had a higher incidence of bleeding.[246] The reason for this is unknown; the authors have speculated that the repeated infections that are common in these patients lead to urothelial or parenchymal hypervascularity or subtly alter the structure of the existing vessels. Comparisons of open and percutaneous procedures for removing staghorn calculi point clearly to the superiority of the latter, even though the hospitalization costs may be slightly higher.[97,98,100,102]

Multiple large caliceal stones together with difficult pelvicaliceal anatomy are a relative contraindication, because the removal of all the stones will require more than one percutaneous tract. However, experienced operators can remove even these stones.[247,248]

Vascular malformations of the kidney can be a contraindication, inasmuch as they would definitely increase the chances of bleeding.

IODINE ALLERGY

Opacification of the collecting system and localization of the stones within the renal pelvis or calices is crucial to successful NLT, because proper selection of the nephrostomy site and a precise puncture of an appropriate calix are required. In general, retrograde injection of iodinated contrast medium through ureteral catheters does not precipitate anaphylactic reactions in iodine-allergic persons, although contrast extravasation during nephrostomy puncture and stone manipulations or absorption of pyelovenous backflow from the distended renal pelvis may precipitate an anaphylactic reaction.

Because of these facts, previous mild allergic reactions such as hives are not considered to be contraindications to NLT. However, if an anaphylactic reaction is considered possible, prophylactic oral corticosteroids, antihistamines, and cimetidine can be administered 48–72 hr prior to the procedure. One hour before the procedure, an infusion of 1 g of hydrocortisone sodium succinate in 500 ml of dextrose in water is started at the rate of 200 mg of hydrocortisone per hour. The drip should be continued during and for 2–4 hr after the procedure. An anesthetist should be available for tracheal intubation in cases of severe laryngeal edema.

To avoid these serious complications, the authors have recently administered CO_2 through a ureteral catheter to

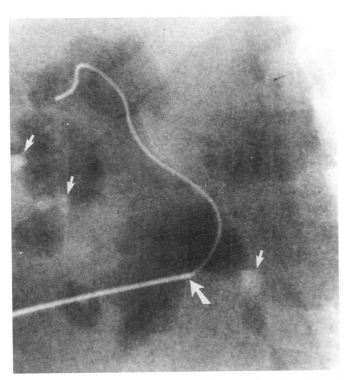

Fig. 23–163 Spot film taken after opacification of renal pelvis and calices with CO_2 injected through ureteral catheter. Note excellent demonstration of pelvicaliceal system and stones (small arrows) in patient with allergy to contrast medium. An 18-gauge needle (large arrow) has been placed through posterior lower calix; guidewire has been passed into upper pole.

guide the percutaneous procedure (Fig. 23–163). The dorsal calices of the collecting system are well delineated by this technique, and the puncture site is easily selected.[249,250]

OBESITY

Nephrostomy puncture and insertion of working sheaths are difficult or impossible in obese patients. Even when the procedure is possible, longer working sheaths may be needed to gain access to the renal pelvis; these are commercially available. Also, at times, fluoroscopy examination is difficult in the obese patient. Again, experienced operators are more likely to succeed in these patients, many of whom are *not* candidates for ESWL because the image intensifiers cannot be positioned for stone location and beam focusing.

Patient Evaluation

A thorough medical history and physical examination are performed before or at the time of admission, with particular emphasis on evidence of allergies to contrast medium, local anesthetic, or analgesics; infection (fever, urinary symptoms); and bleeding disorders or other medical problems such as cardiac or pulmonary disease that could complicate intraoperative or postoperative management.

LABORATORY STUDIES

The necessary laboratory studies are:

1. A complete blood count with hemoglobin and hematocrit, both as a baseline and to evaluate the differential leukocyte count for evidence of infection;
2. Blood typing and cross-matching of 2 units as a prophylactic measure. The authors make sure that at least 2 units are immediately available when difficulties are likely, such as in patients with a horseshoe kidney, staghorn calculus, or postoperative stone recurrence;
3. Urinalysis and culture, with sensitivity studies of any organisms so that infection can be treated with specific antibiotics;
4. BUN and creatinine to evaluate renal function.

RADIOLOGIC STUDIES

The appropriate radiologic studies include some or all of the following:

Unless a recent film is available, an IVU with at least one oblique film should be obtained to delineate the pelvicaliceal anatomy and to determine accurately the location of the stone (Fig. 23–164); the minimum recommended study for proper planning of the case is four films: prone and prone oblique (stone side elevated 30°–40°) views before and after injection of contrast medium.

Ultrasound seldom provides any useful information but is needed occasionally to direct the first puncture of a poorly functioning or totally obstructed kidney.

CT is used by some radiologists routinely prior to NLT to study the anatomy of the pelvicaliceal system (Fig. 23–165), because there is such great variability in the relation of the calices to the renal pelvis (Fig. 23–166).[15] The authors do not believe this is appropriate, because CT usually will not provide any information not available from a high-quality IVU and careful fluoroscopy at the time of puncture, especially if the latter is augmented with angled views (C-arm) or injection of contrast medium and CO_2. There are some situations, however, in which CT can provide invaluable information:

a. When there is a malrotated kidney, in which there may be profoundly distorted pelvicaliceal relations;
b. Where there is hepatosplenomegaly, so that it is critical to determine a safe pathway for the percutaneous tract to avoid splenic or hepatic injury (Figs. 23–167 and 23–168);
c. Patients who are emaciated, who have undergone ileal bypass or splenectomy, or in whom the plain films suggest that the colon is lodged next to the kidney in the usual path of the percutaneous tract (Fig. 23–169).

A retrograde pyelogram, done at the time of retrograde ureteral catheter placement, sometimes provides invaluable information about stone location and pelvicaliceal anatomy, particularly when steep oblique and lateral films are taken.

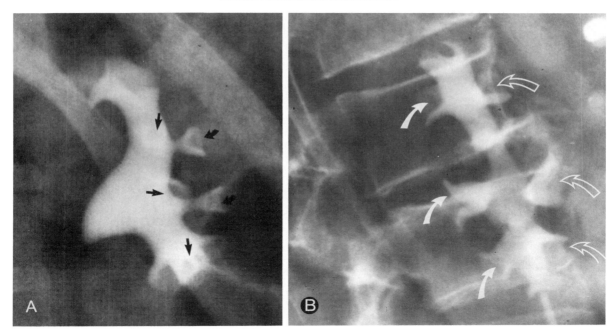

Fig. 23–164   Orientation of calices. A. Anteroposterior view of kidney showing typical on-end appearance of posterior calices (small arrows) and on-side projection of anterior calices (curved arrows). B. Lateral view of collecting system shows posterior calices pointing in a straight posterior direction (white arrows) and more anterior position of anterior calices (open arrows).

Preoperative Management

The patient is usually admitted to the hospital the evening before NLT. An anesthesiology consultation is obtained, because occasionally an emergency open operation is necessary. An intravenous line is secured, and the patient is hydrated to a positive fluid balance if the cardiac and renal status permit. Broad-spectrum antibiotics, such as gentamicin and ampicillin or a similar combination, are administered intravenously starting 12 hr before the procedure until 24–48 hr after the procedure. At least one antibiotic is continued orally until the last tube is removed from the percutaneous tract. The use of this strict antibiotic regimen probably is the reason that the authors have had no serious infections in their large series.

Intramuscular sedatives and analgesics are administered on call to help relax the patient.

Fig. 23–165   Tomographic section shows classic Brödel-type kidney on left.

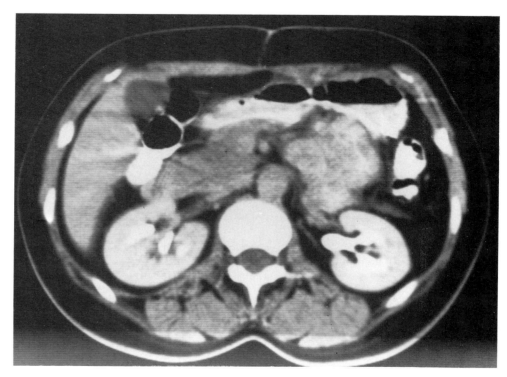

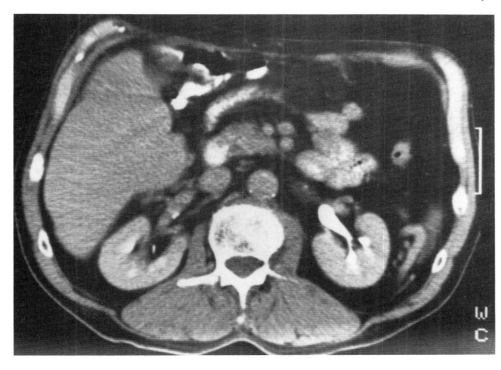

Fig. 23–166 Tomographic section shows classic Hudson-type kidney on left.

Intraoperative Care

The ECG and vital signs are monitored constantly during the procedure, either by the circulating nurse or, preferably, by a nurse anesthetist.

Several analgesics and sedatives can be used to control pain and anxiety. A combination of diazepam and morphine has proved the most useful and safe, particularly in older patients. The doses are tailored to the patient's needs. As discussed earlier, other drugs are meperidine (pethidine), fentanyl with or without droperidol, and intermittent nitrous oxide. Drugs are usually administered by the nurse anesthetist. Some operators prefer to use mild sedation supplemented by nitrous oxide administered by the patient according to need.[251]

Intravenous fluids and mannitol, or a diuretic such as furosemide, are used by some operators in the hope of decreasing the chances for pyelotubular reflux, which could cause infection.[194] Saltzman et al recently demonstrated that proper use of a working sheath during NLT,

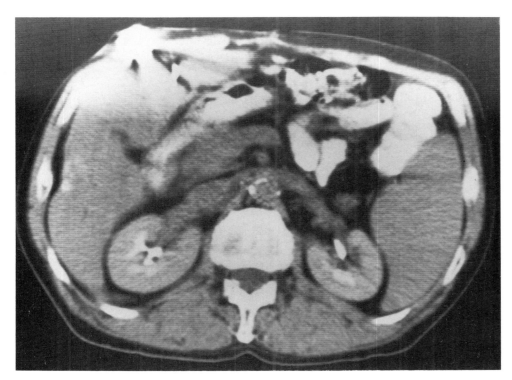

Fig. 23–167 Pronounced posterior extension of both liver and spleen is clearly seen in tomographic section through kidneys.

Fig. 23–168 Tomographic section through kidney shows nephrostomy tube (arrows) traversing liver parenchyma due to very lateral placement of percutaneous tract, which was created through an anterior calix using inside-out technique.

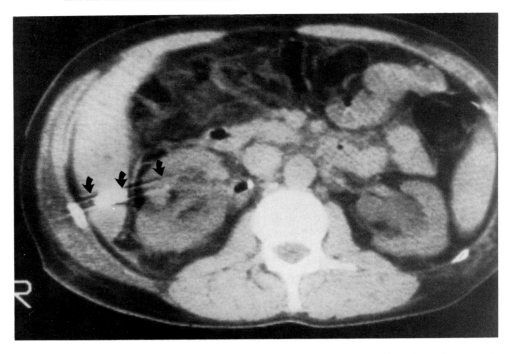

by keeping the renal pelvic pressure below 16 cm H_2O, also helps prevent backflow.[252]

Fluid replacement and blood transfusion are given as needed.

In the authors' institution, the whole NLT procedure is performed in one stage in a special procedures room in the operating suite using local anesthesia and intravenous sedation and analgesia. A long-acting local anesthetic (bupivacaine 0.24%) was used effectively for several years, but following reports of adverse reactions such as cardiac arrhythmias associated with large doses of this drug, the authors decreased the usual dosage and eventually replaced bupivacaine with short-acting local anesthetics such as 1% lidocaine. Patients in whom they might consider using general anesthesia are the very

infirm; those with respiratory function impairment, in whom sedatives and analgesics might compromise respiratory function; those who clearly psychologically will not tolerate being awake during the procedure; and those who have been heavy analgesic users and who will not tolerate any manipulations in spite of excessive doses of sedatives and analgesics.

Plans for NLT

ONE-SESSION REMOVAL

A one-session procedure consists of the initial nephrostomy puncture followed immediately by tract dilation and stone removal under either local or general anes-

Fig. 23–169 Tomographic section through kidney shows very posterior location of distal splenic flexure (C) in patient with minimal retroperitoneal fat.

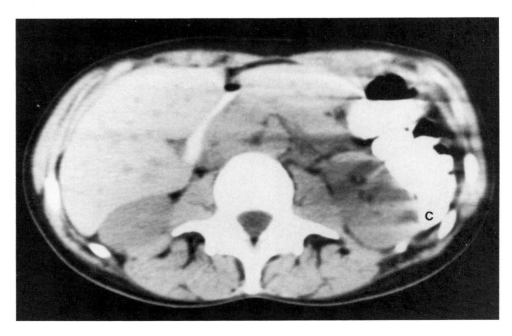

thesia, depending on the preference of the radiology–urology team and the institution. The initial nephrostomy is performed after opacification by contrast medium given intravenously, via a 22-gauge needle in the renal pelvis, or by retrograde infusion through a catheter placed endoscopically.

The one-stage removal is the most expeditious, and >90% of all stones have been extracted in this fashion at the University of Minnesota Hospitals. The entire procedure, including nephrostomy, tract dilation, and stone extraction, is performed in the radiology suite. The average procedure takes 2–3 hr; some departments may not be able to afford to spend so much time on one procedure. Another disadvantage is that most angiographic suites are not equipped to handle the large amount of irrigation fluid that is used during the endoscopic procedures.

Profuse bleeding that interferes with endoscopic visibility may be a significant drawback in the one-stage procedure, because the nephrostomy tract is fresh. In practice, the authors have not found this to be a serious problem; with a working sheath and adequate irrigation, extraction can be accomplished in a large percentage of cases.

TWO-STEP PROCEDURE

Two methods have evolved that differ in the time interval between the initial nephrostomy and the stone extraction.

Immediate Two-Step Procedure

The initial nephrostomy and tract dilation up to 24F are followed by nephrostomy catheter placement with or without ureteral catheter placement in the radiology department. The next day, or the same day in the afternoon, usually with general anesthesia, the stone is extracted in the operating room under fluoroscopic control. In certain institutions, only 8F–10F nephrostomy catheters, along with ureteral catheters, are initially placed; because tract dilation is painful without assisted local or general anesthesia, tract dilation with working sheath placement is performed in the operating room immediately before stone removal.

The immediate two-stage procedure requires a single hospital admission, and logistically, it works better in most institutions, because the initial nephrostomy puncture does not tie up the radiology suite for a long time. The immediate two-stage procedure minimizes the length of the hospital stay and the anesthesia requirements. The visibility problem of working through fresh, bleeding tracts may be encountered, just as in the one-stage procedure.

Delayed Two-Step Procedure

Nephrostomy tract creation and dilation to 24F–30F are followed by placement of an appropriate nephrostomy tube by the radiologist during the first hospital admission. The patient is then discharged home, to return in 5–7 days for the second stage, stone extrac-

tion.[245] This is the safest method, and radiologist–urologist teams who are learning NLT procedures should use this plan. The bleeding and clot problems do not exist, because the tract is mature, and at times a single stone can be extracted with endoscopy without fluoroscopy. This plan also is recommended for complicated cases, such as patients with multiple caliceal stones and stones within solitary or horseshoe kidneys. One drawback is that between the sessions, improper tube maintenance, tube dislodgment, or migration of stones to a different location in the collecting system may cause problems.

The NLT Procedure

The steps in stone removal are as follows. Each will be discussed in turn.

Retrograde ureteral catheter placement;
Approach selection;
Collecting system opacification;
Puncture;
Tract anesthetizing;
Calculus extraction;
Nephrostomy tube placement;
Nephrostomy tube securing.

RETROGRADE URETERAL CATHETER PLACEMENT

Although not universally accepted, this step provides invaluable help in several respects[72,91,239,253–258]:

1. Retrograde injection of contrast medium or CO_2 provides optimal opacification of the entire collecting system and distends the calices (Figs. 23–170 and 23–171). This combination of distention and opacification is indispensable for making accurate punctures.
2. In cases where distention of the collecting system is even more critical, such as in a patient with a small intrarenal pelvis or a bifid collecting system, or in a patient with a large staghorn calculus, the catheter, possibly with a balloon, can be used to occlude the ureteropelvic junction (UPJ) (Fig. 23–172) while fluid or gas distends the collecting system for easier guidewire and instrument insertion.
3. A ureteral catheter, even without a balloon, will usually obstruct the UPJ enough to prevent migration of calculous fragments down the ureter during lithotripsy and removal.[258,259]
4. When large perforations of the renal pelvis occur, the passage of a guidewire through the ureteral catheter into the renal pelvis, from which it can be percutaneously extracted, often provides the only way to get a stent or drainage catheter into the pelvis or ureter.
5. The catheter provides a way to opacify the collecting system with CO_2 in patients with a contrast allergy.[249,250]
6. In patients with impacted ureteral calculi, flushing through the catheter with CO_2 or diluted contrast medium is the fastest and easiest method to release the stone.[260,261] (See section on extraction techniques.)

Fig. 23–170 IVU showing good opacification of pelvicaliceal system and ureter in patient with ileal diversion. B. Loopogram in same patient produces much better opacification and distention of renal pelvis, infundibula, and calices.

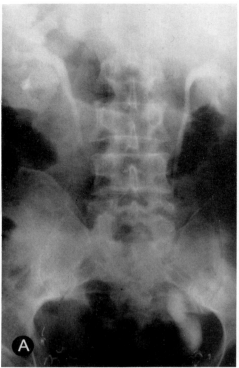
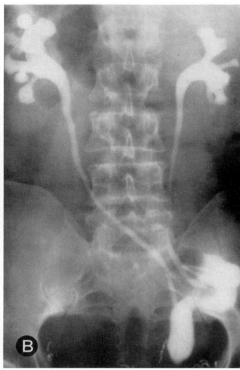

APPROACH SELECTION

Before attempting to puncture the collecting system, a recent IVU and the retrograde pyelograms made at the time of ureteral catheter placement must be studied to determine the collecting system anatomy and the location of all calculi. Steep oblique or lateral films are particularly helpful, not only to pinpoint stone location but also to search for anatomic variants. If there is evidence of malrotation of the kidney, a CT scan can provide more detailed information. In general, in cases of malrotation, the authors prefer to approach the collecting system through the upper caliceal group (see discussion below) (Fig. 23–173).[262]

Selection of the entry site into the collecting system is

probably the most important decision in the NLT procedure. A wrong choice can result in an extremely difficult procedure, perhaps requiring the creation of another percutaneous tract (Fig. 23–174),[129,262,263] or complete failure. If the initial puncture is not ideal (Fig. 23–175), it is better to stop, re-evaluate the situation, and start with a new puncture in a better position than to go ahead, dilate the tract, and then, after several frustrating hours, realize that it will be impossible to extract the calculus through it.

The following general guidelines have been useful in selecting the best approach:

Stay below the 12th rib if possible.

Puncture through the posterolateral edge of the par-

Fig. 23–171 A. IVU shows adequate opacification of pelvicaliceal system. Observe faint opacification of upper pole infundibulum (curved arrow) and small dimensions of central and lower pole infundibula. B. Retrograde opacification of pelvicaliceal system through ureteral catheter shows far better distention of infundibula and calices than after intravenous contrast injection.

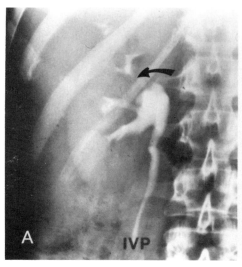
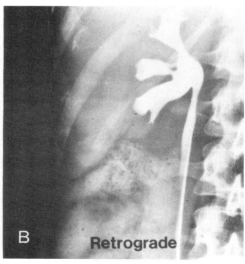

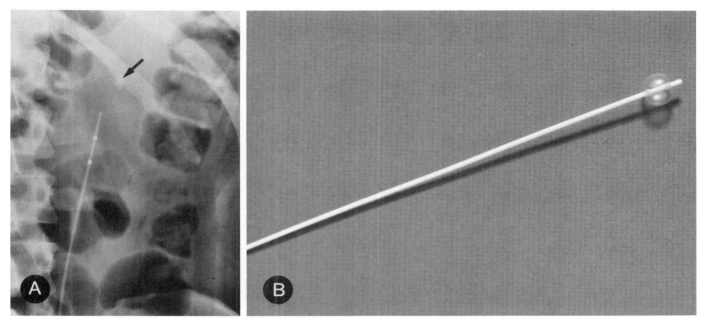

Fig. 23–172 Technique for distention of collecting system. A. Small angioplasty balloon catheter has been inserted retrograde to occlude UPJ in patient with calculus (arrow) in small intrarenal pelvis in order to distend pelvis to facilitate puncture and dilatation. B. Close-up view of occlusion balloon catheter.

avertebral muscles but avoid going too far laterally, especially if above the 12th rib, in order to avoid the colon, liver, and spleen.

For renal pelvic and ureteral calculi, puncture through a posterior calix.[72,99,129,239,262]

For caliceal calculi, puncture the affected calix at the medial edge of the calculus.[72,129,262]

The specific guidelines depend on renal anatomy, on calculus location and size, and on whether there are multiple or staghorn calculi.

Renal Pelvic Calculi

These are the simplest calculi to extract. They are approached through a posterior calix of the lower or mid-

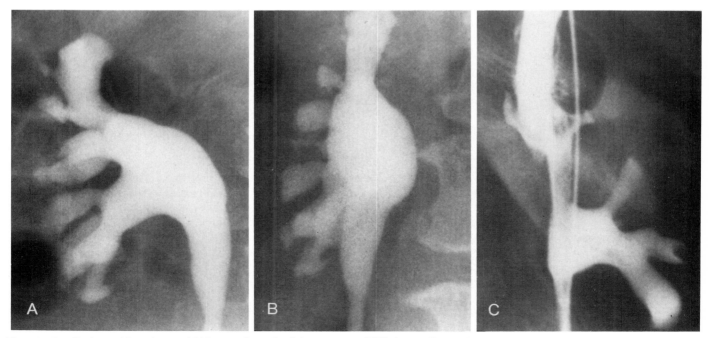

Fig. 23–173 Patient with malrotated kidney and renal pelvic stone. A. IVU shows abnormal radiographic pattern of anterior and posterior calices in anteroposterior projection. B. Lateral projection of IVU shows all of calices pointing anteriorly. C. Lateral projection during percutaneous puncture through upper pole calix.

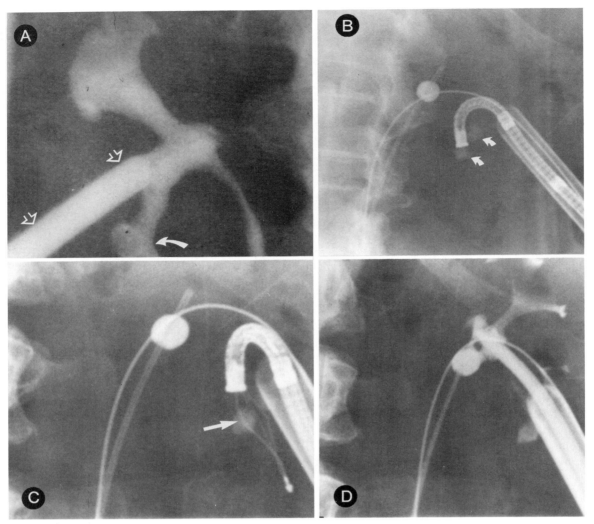

Fig. 23–174   Patient with two >4-mm calculi in posterior calix of lower pole of right kidney. A. Percutaneous tract was created in posterior calix adjacent to one where stones were lodged (curved arrow). Teflon sheath (open arrows) is seen within percutaneous tract with its tip within infundibulum. B. Flexible nephroscope has been introduced through Teflon sheath and manipulated into calix with calculi (arrows). Note presence of safety wire in ureter and occlusion balloon catheter blocking UPJ. C. Through flexible nephroscope, Dormia basket has been passed to capture stones. Note that front part of basket is way beyond stones (arrow), indicating that it is lodged within renal parenchyma, which inhibits its free expansion. D. After unsuccessful manipulations, Foley balloon catheter has been passed through Teflon sheath into renal pelvis.

dle groups with a puncture below the 12th rib (Fig. 23–176).[72,129,240,259,262,263]

Staghorn Calculi

Large, multiple, branched staghorn calculi usually require more than one puncture for complete removal. Puncture of the infundibulum of a posterior calix of the lower group usually provides access to most of the collecting system, not only for the flexible endoscopes, but also for the rigid instruments (Fig. 23–177). A second puncture (Fig. 23–178) or a Y tract (Figs. 23–179 and 23–180)[247] is commonly required for the removal of the remaining fragments, particularly those in posteriorly directed central calices. Residual fragments are best approached by an extended tract (Fig. 23–181) or a needle push technique (Fig. 23–182).

Small staghorn calculi are best approached with a direct puncture of the calix containing the largest branch, provided this is a posterior calix.[129,262] If the largest or sole branch is in an anterior calix, the best approach is either through the upper caliceal group or through an adjacent posterior calix, whichever affords a direct path through the renal pelvis to the stone.

Posterior Lower or Middle Caliceal Calculi

One or more calculi in a single posterior lower or middle calix are approached with a direct puncture of that calix (Figs. 23–183 and 23–184). If possible, the puncture is made on the medial edge of the stone to trap it and prevent migration.

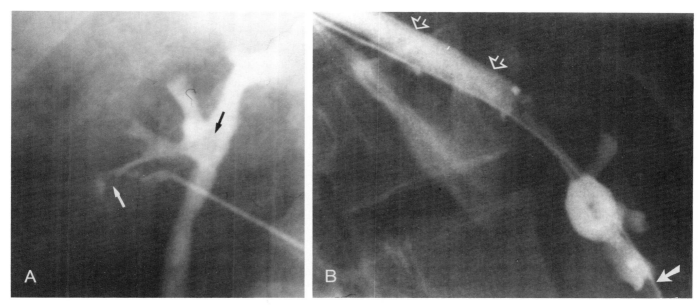

Fig. 23–175   Approach to stone in anterior calix. A. Lateral view of antegrade pyelogram after puncture of anterior calix with 18-gauge needle shows sharp angle between calix and renal pelvis. Observe calculus in anterior calix (white arrow) and larger one within renal pelvis (black arrow). B. Lateral projection shows relation of Teflon sheath (open arrows) and upper pole calix. Also note gentle angle between Teflon sheath, upper pole infundibulum, and renal pelvis. Safety wire in ureter (white arrow).

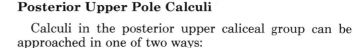

Fig. 23–176   Approach via posterior lower calix to free-floating stone in renal pelvis.

Posterior Upper Pole Calculi

Calculi in the posterior upper caliceal group can be approached in one of two ways:

1. For those <0.4 mm, a puncture below the 12th rib through a posterior calix of the lower or middle group provides easy, safe access for flexible, and sometimes rigid, endoscopes (Fig. 23–185) provided there is no infundibular stenosis.[72,129,262]
2. If there is infundibular stenosis, or if the calculus is >4 mm, a direct puncture of the affected calix above the 12th rib provides the best access (Figs. 23–186 and 23–187). After stone removal, the stenotic infundibulum can be dilated and stented.[129,262] Another approach is to insert a 16F flexible nephroscope through either a middle or a lower calix, aiming it toward the stenotic infundibulum. The stenosis is incised with a 5F cutting electrode, and the stone is extracted with 7F or 9F alligator forceps. In this fashion, Clayman et al removed stones from 10 patients whose stones were lodged in stenotic infundibula or in caliceal diverticula.[114] However, this method should not be attempted by neophytes, because extensive experience in handling the nephroscopes, as well as three-dimensional mental views of trapped stones in the stenotic infundibulum, are required.

Anterior Caliceal Calculi

These stones are approached either through a posterior calix or by direct puncture into the calix containing the stone (Fig. 23–188). The authors prefer the former method, because it is technically easier and carries less risk of bleeding. Choosing the correct posterior calix, so

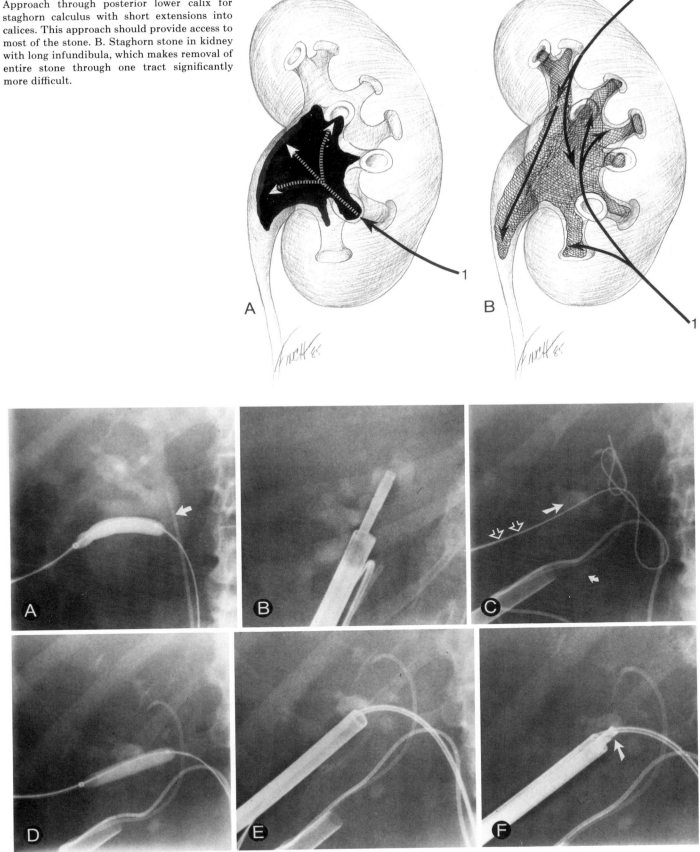

Fig. 23–177 Approach to staghorn stone. A. Approach through posterior lower calix for staghorn calculus with short extensions into calices. This approach should provide access to most of the stone. B. Staghorn stone in kidney with long infundibula, which makes removal of entire stone through one tract significantly more difficult.

Fig. 23–178 Patient with large staghorn calculus and long infundibula. A. Stone is seen to occupy most of renal pelvis, infundibula, and calices. Ureteral catheter with tip within renal pelvis (arrow). Percutaneous tract has been created, with wire passed down ureter; bal-

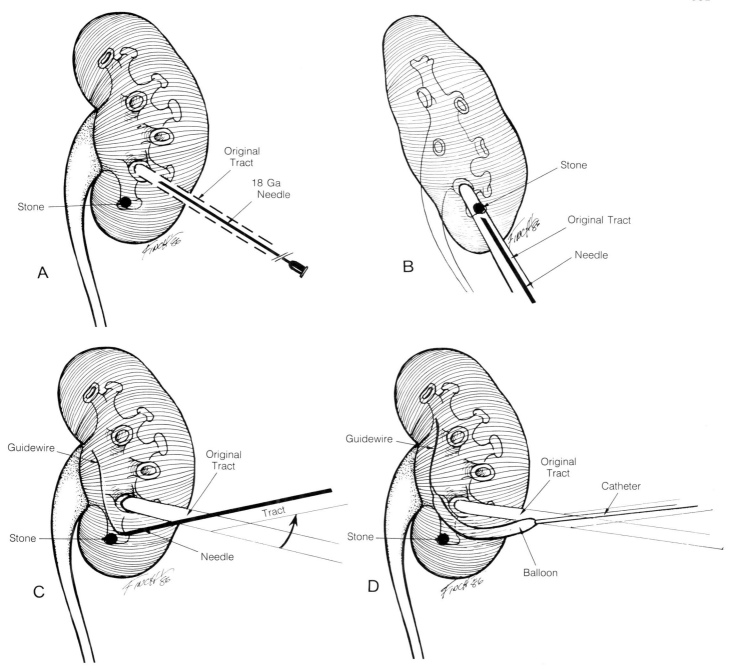

Fig. 23–179   Creation of Y tract. A. An 18-gauge needle has been passed through percutaneous tract until its tip lies at level of retained stone in adjacent calix. B. Lateral view. C-arm has been rotated until percutaneous tract overlaps adjacent calix containing stone. C. With caudal angulation, needle has been advanced into adjacent calix, and guidewire has been passed into renal pelvis. D. After exchange of needle for dilators, balloon has been passed to dilate new tract.

loon catheter is being used to dilate percutaneous tract. B. With help of ultrasonic lithotripter, most of calculus has been removed from renal pelvis and lower pole infundibulum; probe is seen fragmenting stone in upper pole infundibulum and calix. C. Most of stone has been removed through lower pole tract. Two fragments are seen, one in lower pole calix (small arrow) and one in central calix (large arrow). Guidewire is seen (open arrows) in a second percutaneous tract created directly onto stone fragment in posterior central calix.

D. Second percutaneous tract is being dilated with help of angioplasty balloon catheter. E. Teflon sheath has been placed in tract after completion of dilation. F. Ultrasonic lithotripter (arrow) is being used to fragment rest of stone. Observe two safety wires in ureter from upper tract, one catheter down ureter from upper tract, one catheter down ureter from lower tract, and second catheter into upper pole calix for irrigation.

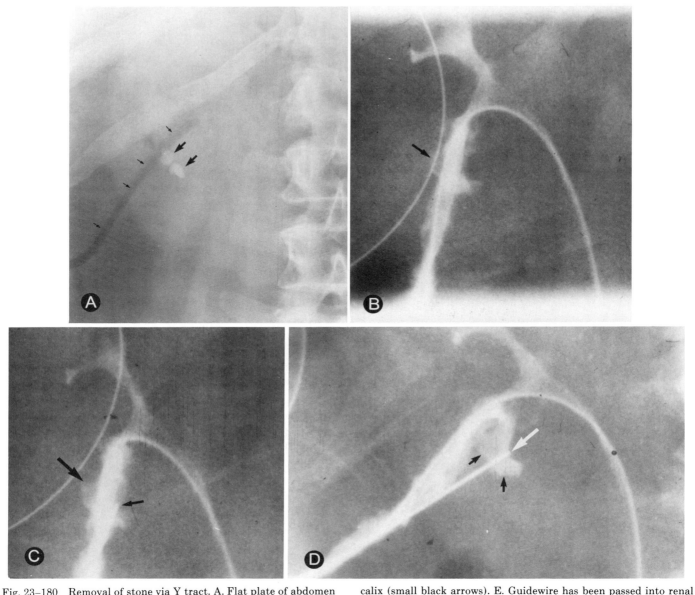

Fig. 23–180   Removal of stone via Y tract. A. Flat plate of abdomen shows Foley catheter (small arrows) within percutaneous tract with its tip at renal pelvis. Calculi are adjacent to percutanoeus tract (large arrows). B. Collecting system has been opacified with contrast medium, and wire has been passed down ureter. By rotation of either patient or image intensifier, percutaneous tract has been overlapped with adjacent calix, where calculi are lodged (arrow). C. An 18-gauge needle has been advanced through tract until its tip (small arrow) overlies most peripheral area of calculi (large arrow). D. After providing moderate degree of caudad angulation, needle has been advanced about 1.5 cm; at this point, either by rotation of patient or rotation of image intensifier, lateral fluoroscopic projection has been obtained to appreciate entrance of needle (white arrow) into adjacent calix (small black arrows). E. Guidewire has been passed into renal pelvis and, with the help of flexible nephroscope (arrow), guidewire is being pulled through original percutaneous tract. F. Wire is now seen to pass from original tract across newly created branch (small arrows), crossing infundibulum into renal pelvis and then out through original tract. G. Using angioplasty balloon catheter, Y tract is being dilated. Observe indentation in balloon at level of renal capsule (small arrow) and relation of retained calculus (large arrow) to leading edge of balloon. H. After dilation of tract, Teflon sheath (white arrow) has been advanced into calix for stone extraction. Observe safety wire in ureter (small black arrow), circle loop safety wire (large black arrow), and catheter with wire through Teflon sheath (open arrow).

that the path through the collecting system to the stone can be negotiated by the necessary instruments, often requires intensive analysis of the anatomy. For instance, many anterior lower pole caliceal stones have been removed through posterior upper pole caliceal punctures.

Multiple Caliceal Calculi

Small multiple caliceal calculi are best approached through a puncture of a posterior calix, either of the lower group or, as the authors prefer, of the upper group, because with the flexible endoscope the anterior calices

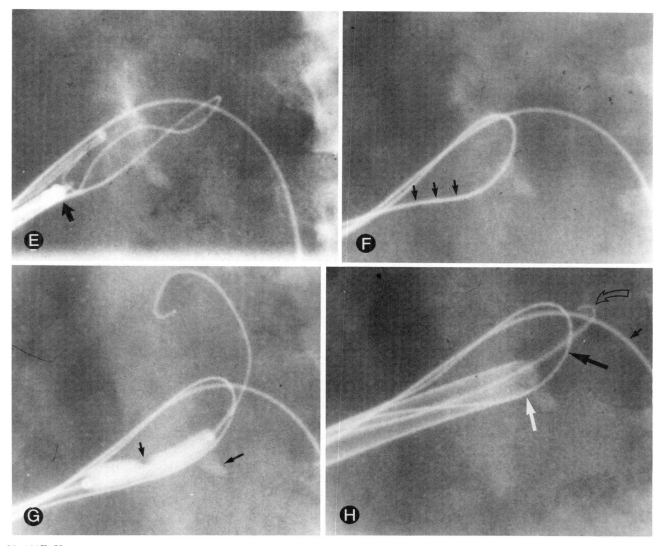

Fig. 23–180E–H

are more easily approached from the upper pole than from the lower. On occasion, an additional puncture, either a separate second one or a Y tract, is needed to extract all the calculi (Fig. 23–189).[129,262]

Multiple Calculi with Complex Location

For posterior caliceal calculi associated with a renal pelvic or ureteral calculus, a direct "trap" puncture of the calix containing the calculus allows easy removal of that stone and provides an adequate path to the renal pelvic or ureteral calculus (Figs. 23–190 through 23–193).

Anterior caliceal calculi associated with renal pelvic or ureteral calculi demand a more devious plan. Because of the sharp angle between the tract into the anterior calix and the infundibulum back toward the renal pelvis, manipulation of wires and catheters from the calix into the renal pelvis is exceptionally difficult, and the passage of large dilators or rigid instruments into the renal pelvis

is practically impossible.[262] For these reasons, the preferred approach is usually through a posterior calix of the upper group, because from this one site the pelvic, ureteral, and caliceal calculi often can all be reached (Figs. 23–194 and 23–195).[262]

Ureteral Calculi

Whether the stone is removed by retrograde flushing or by passage of instruments into the ureter, a caudally directed tract that points into the UPJ is preferred. This usually requires the puncture of a posterior calix in the middle or upper groups, which is often above the 12th rib (Fig. 23–196). Recently, as the authors have become more confident of the capabilities of the flush technique to get the stone completely out of the patient or at least out of the ureter into the renal pelvis, they have used a puncture below the 12th rib of a posterior calix of the middle or lower groups.[94,197]

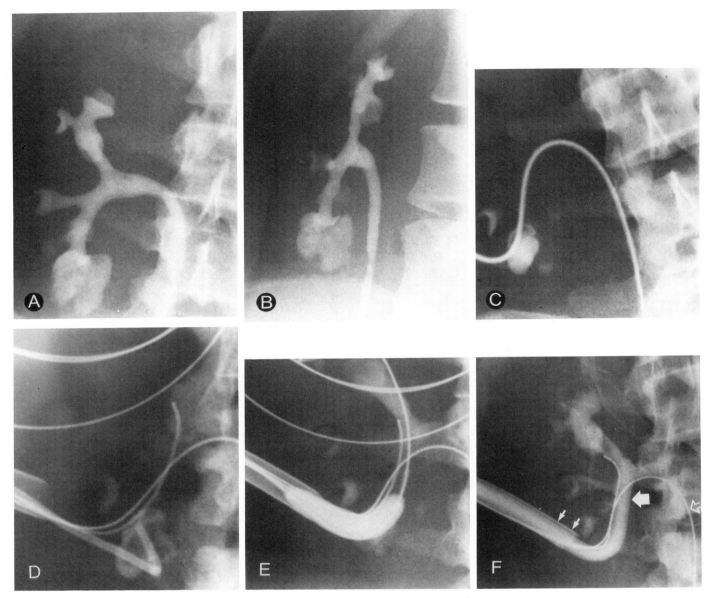

Fig. 23–181 Removal of stone from kidney with anomalous anatomy. A. IVU showing compound papilla with large calix in lower pole of right kidney containing multiple calculi. B. Steep oblique view of IVU shows to better advantage anatomy of large compound calix; filling defects represent calculi. C. Direct approach into most posterior part of calix led to realization that membranous partition separated this large compound calix into anterior and posterior divisions. Calculi in posterior division were removed easily, but attempts to pass flexible nephroscope into anterior division were unsuccessful. Observe tract created into posterior segment of large calix. Catheter and wire in ureter. D. Forward extension of tract was then accomplished by advancing needle through original tract to perforate membrane. Guidewire was passed through needle, and, after removal of needle, catheter has been passed into anterior division of this calix. Larger filling defect within calix represents blood clot. Observe safety wire in ureter; second wire has been passed into renal pelvis. E. Anterior extension of tract has been dilated with angioplasty balloon catheter. F. Rubber tube (large arrow) advanced through Teflon sheath (small arrows) into renal pelvis. Safety wire is in ureter (open arrow).

Diverticular Calculi

Depending on their location, above or below the 12th rib, diverticular stones are approached differently. If the diverticulum is below the 12th rib, a direct puncture of the diverticulum provides the fastest and surest access. After the calculi are removed, the stenotic neck can be dilated and stented. If the diverticulum is above the 12th rib, it can be approached either by a direct puncture over the 12th rib (Fig. 23–197) or by a subcostal puncture of a posterior calix. From this point, the diverticular neck must be reached, observed, catheterized, and dilated or incised under direct vision. The calculi are then extracted, and the neck is stented.[262] A significant problem can arise at any point with this latter approach. A frequent problem is seeing the diverticular opening

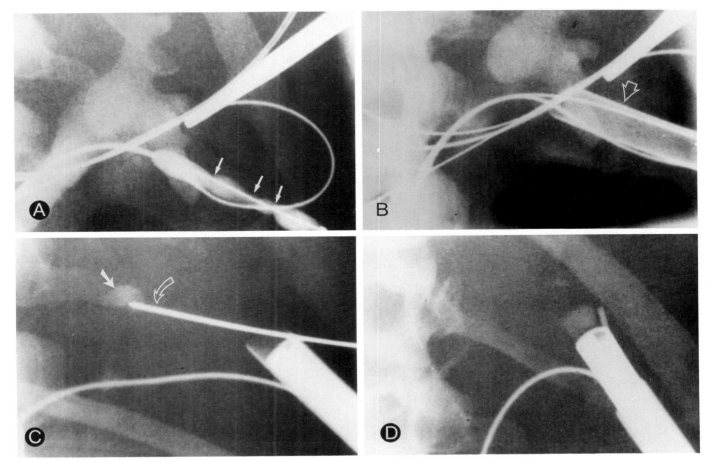

Fig. 23–182 Large staghorn calculus entirely filling renal pelvis, infundibula, and calices. A. Percutaneous tract has been created through posterior lower calix, and tract is being dilated with 10-cm-long, 10-mm-diameter balloon catheter. Observe multiple indentations in balloon (arrows) representing renal capsule and fasciae around kidney. Two wires are seen in ureter. B. Dilation of tract complete; Teflon sheath (arrow) has been placed for ultrasonic lithotripsy. C. Most of staghorn calculus has been removed. Fragment in posterior central calix remains beyond reach of rigid nephroscope because of sharp angle between infundibula where fragment is lodged and renal pelvis. Fragment is too large for removal with flexible nephroscope. An 18-gauge needle (open arrow) placed directly over fragment (white arrow) is being used to push it into renal pelvis, where it can be seen by endoscopist. D. After manipulation of stone fragment with needle push technique, endoscopic extraction is successful.

endoscopically. A helpful maneuver is puncture of the diverticulum with a 22- or 23-gauge needle and injection of CO_2 or other contrast agent such as methylene blue, which can be seen by the endoscopist as it bubbles through the diverticular neck.[249,250]

Calculi in a Horseshoe Kidney

Because of the extremely anterior position of the lower pole of the kidney in these patients, a puncture of the upper caliceal group provides the shortest tract possible from which almost any location can be reached (Fig. 23–198).[129,262] Stones, including staghorn calculi, have also been removed from pelvic and transplanted kidneys by abdominal transperitoneal puncture.[148,264,265] In a renal allograft draining into an ileal conduit, a stenotic infundibulum causing hydrocalix was dilated and stented after a staghorn stone was removed.[265]

COLLECTING SYSTEM OPACIFICATION

Although the collecting system can be adequately opacified by intravenous contrast medium, an accurate caliceal puncture is greatly facilitated by a distended, maximally opacified system created by direct infusion of radiopaque material. The method the authors have found best is retrograde infusion of contrast medium through the ureteral catheter (Fig. 23–199). The same result can frequently be obtained by puncturing the collecting system with a skinny needle either under ultrasound guidance or after the intravenous administration of contrast medium,[99,242,263] but this method is technically more difficult and more often creates extravasation that obscures the fluoroscopist's vision. With either method of opacification, if it is difficult to distinguish the anterior from the posterior calices, injecting 10–15 ml of CO_2 will make the distinction simple: the gas floats to the highest parts of the collecting system, which are the posterior calices in a

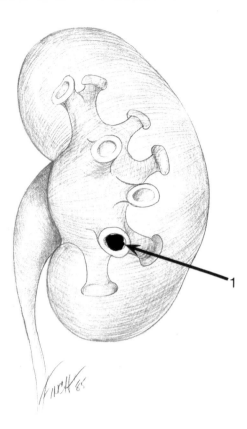

Fig. 23–183 Single stone in posterior calix; approach (1) is into calix containing stone.

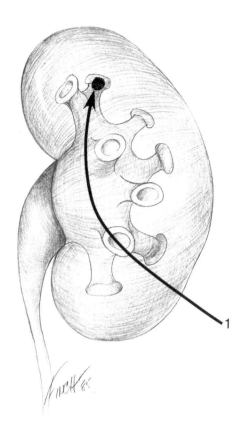

Fig. 23–185 Single small (2–3-mm) stone in upper pole calix; preferred approach (1) is through posterior lower calix if anatomy provides straight access into upper pole.

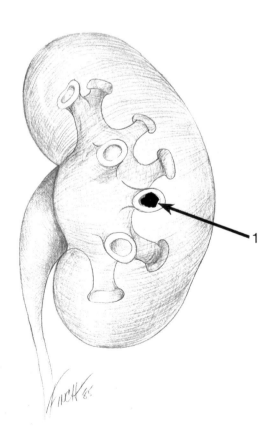

Fig. 23–184 Single stone in posterior central calix; approach (1) is directly into calix containing stone.

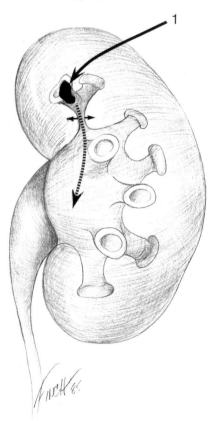

Fig. 23–186 Single stone in upper pole calix with infundibular stenosis (small black arrows); preferred approach (1) is directly into calix containing stone, with subsequent dilatation of infundibulum.

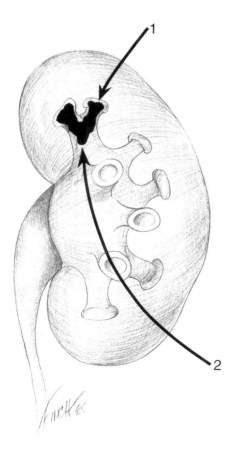

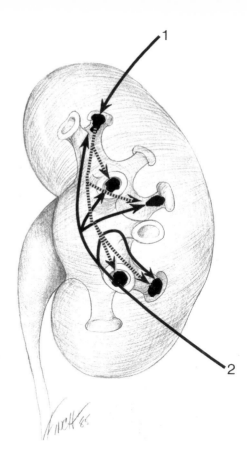

Fig. 23–187   Partial staghorn calculus in upper pole calix; preferred approach (1) is directly into calix containing the stone (S). Alternative approach (2) is through posterior lower calix if anatomy provides straight access into upper pole and if infundibula are short.

Fig. 23–189   Multiple caliceal stones; best approach is either from posterior lower calix (2) or from upper pole calix (1).

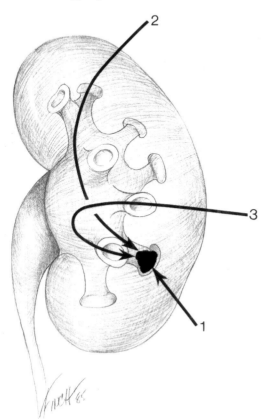

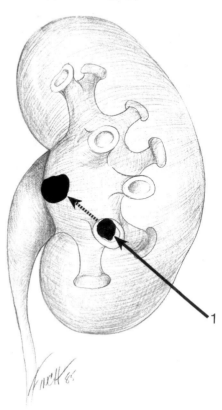

Fig. 23–188   Solitary stone in anterior calix; preferred approach (1) is directly into this calix, particularly if stone is >3 mm. Alternative approaches are from upper pole (2) or posterior central calix (3).

Fig. 23–190   Combination of stones, with one in posterior lower calix and additional one in renal pelvis; preferred approach (1) is directly into calix containing stone, through which both stones can be removed.

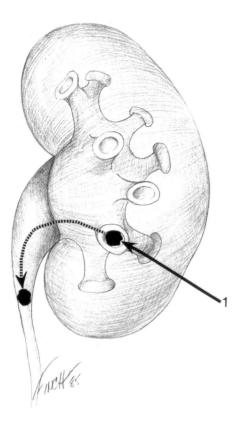

Fig. 23–191 Combination of stones in posterior calix and upper ureter; preferred approach (1) is through posterior calix containing stone.

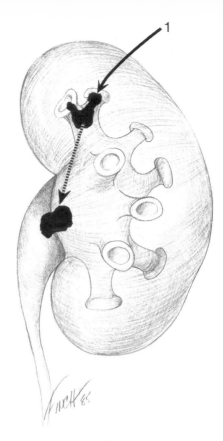

Fig. 23–193 Combination of partial staghorn stone in upper pole calix and free-floating stone in renal pelvis; preferred approach (1) is through upper pole calix, which facilitates removal of caliceal stone with excellent access to pelvic stone.

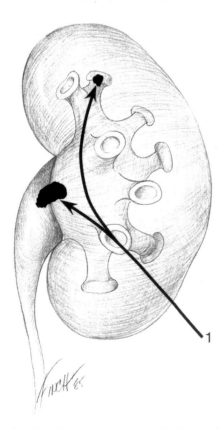

Fig. 23–192 Combination of stones in renal pelvis and upper pole calix; preferred approach (1) is through posterior lower calix, which provides easy access to both areas.

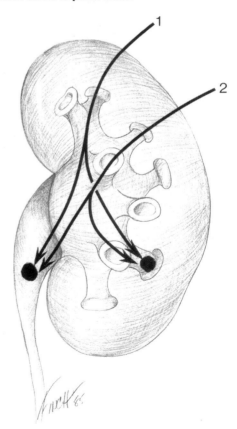

Fig. 23–194 Combination of anterior caliceal and UPJ stones; preferred approach (1) is through upper pole, which provides convenient access to both areas. Alternatively (2), posterior central calix can be used.

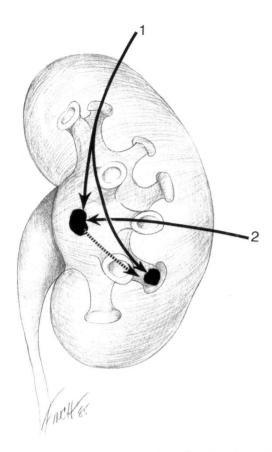

Fig. 23–195 Combination of anterior caliceal and renal pelvic stones; preferred approach (1) is through upper pole calix, which provides convenient access to both areas. Alternatively (2), posterior central calix can be used.

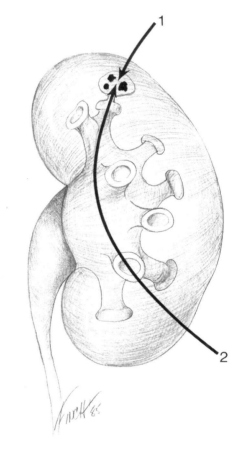

Fig. 23–197 Diverticulum with multiple retained stones in upper pole; best approach (1) is through direct puncture of diverticulum. Alternatively (2), posterior lower calix can be punctured, with subsequent catheterization of diverticular opening.

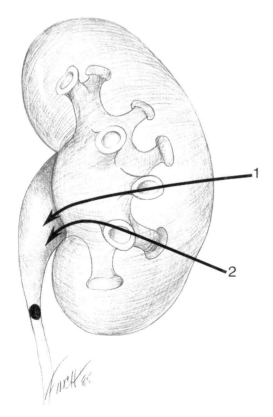

Fig. 23–196 Ureteral stone is best approached through posterior central (1) or lower (2) calix.

Fig. 23–198 Horseshoe kidney in anteroposterior and right posterior oblique views showing complex anatomy. Important anatomic point to remember is that only upper pole of kidney is in direct contact with posterior wall of abdomen. R12 = 12th rib; L2 = second lumbar vertebra.

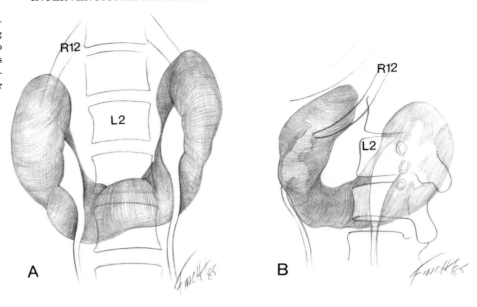

prone oblique-positioned patient (Figs. 23–200 and 23–201). In the patient with a history of allergy to contrast medium, CO_2 can be introduced through either the skinny needle or the ureteral catheter to opacify the collecting system before the definitive puncture is performed with the 18-gauge needle.[249,250]

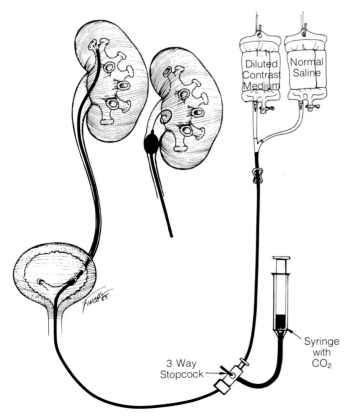

Fig. 23–199 Infusion system for injection of contrast medium or CO_2 through ureteral catheter.

Fluoroscopy *vs.* Ultrasound Guidance

Ultrasound guidance provides one of the best methods to puncture a dilated or poorly functioning collecting system, because location and depth can be determined accurately. However, ultrasound is not accurate enough to guide the definitive 18-gauge needle puncture of a specific calix. Rather, it is best confined to guiding the localization puncture with the skinny needle, especially in the patient with no or poor opacification of the collecting system after intravenous contrast medium or in whom a ureteral catheter could not or has not been placed. With an adequately opacified collecting system, fluoroscopy is the most accurate method of guidance.

Radiographic Equipment

Although NLT can be performed with a conventional fixed over-table image intensifier system, it is greatly facilitated by the use of multidirectional radiographic systems (C- or U-arm) or biplane fluoroscopy. The greatest advantages of multidirectional or biplane fluoroscopy over single-plane conventional fluoroscopy are the three-dimensional capability, which allows rapid and accurate determination of depth; the ability to get angled views (C- or U-arm), which allows cephalad or caudad punctures with the needle still seen as a "end-on dot" superimposed on the target calix; reduced radiation exposure to patient and operator; and easy maneuverability, which allows the operator to move the equipment out of the way in an emergency.[245] Multidirectional fluoroscopy has an advantage over biplane fluoroscopy in that it is commonly much less bulky.

PUNCTURE TECHNIQUE

General Considerations

The following guidelines will help to ensure a successful definitive puncture.

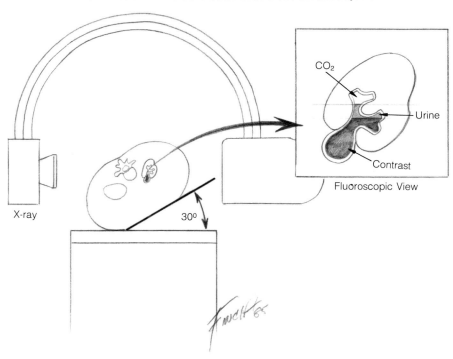

Fig. 23–200 Layering of contrast medium, urine, and CO_2 within collecting system in patient lying in prone oblique decubitus position as seen on cross-table fluoroscopy.

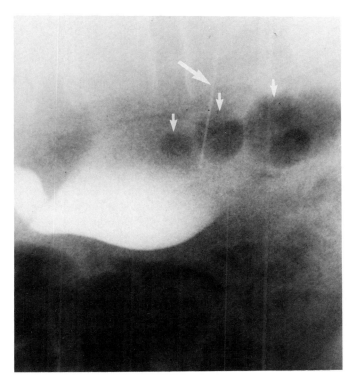

Fig. 23–201 Cross-table lateral view of kidney showing three different densities within collecting system: contrast medium lying in most dependent portion of kidney, partially opacified urine in intermediate position, and CO_2 outlining posterior calices (small arrows). Chiba needle is in renal pelvis (large arrow).

First, of the two types of 18-gauge needles available, bevel- and diamond-tipped (Fig. 23–202), the latter is preferred, because the design of the tip helps to direct the needle in a straight pathway.[245]

Second, a plastic handle (Fig. 23–203) is used to hold the needle, allowing a puncture under continuous fluoroscopic control while keeping the operator's hands away from the x-ray beam.[137]

Third, the puncture is performed during normal or quiet breathing by the patient. This is done to avoid cre-

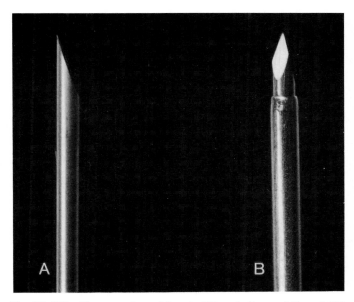

Fig. 23–202 Close-up view of bevel- (A) and diamond-tipped (B) needles.

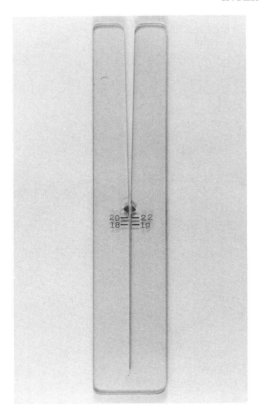

Fig. 23–203   Universal handle for manipulation of needles of different gauges.

ating a tract with sharp angulations, which can result if the puncture is performed during a deep inhalation or exhalation.

Fourth, if multidirectional fluoroscopy is available, the needle path should be slightly angulated in a direction parallel to the long axis of the infundibulum of the calix that is punctured. A straight-down puncture could result in a sharp angle between the entry site and the infundibulum.

Fifth, the puncture should be either through the calix itself or through the caliceal–infundibular junction (Fig. 23–204). A puncture of the more central portion of the infundibulum can result in a dangerous vascular injury, due to the close relation of the larger renal vessels to this part of the collecting system.

The different puncture techniques used, which depend on the relations of the entry site to the 12th rib, on whether an anterior or posterior calix is being punctured, or on whether the puncture is for a staghorn calculus, will be described.

Puncture above the 12th Rib

Anatomic considerations. Because the pleural reflection normally reaches the level of the 12th rib, every puncture above this rib should be considered to be transpleural. The lung, however, is usually not at the level of the 12th rib. During deep inhalation, it reaches down to the level of the 9th or 10th rib and during normal or shallow breathing, it is generally at the level of the 10th or 11th rib. Therefore, a puncture through the intercostal space between the 11th and 12th ribs will pass through the pleural reflection but not through the lung (Fig. 23–205). If the kidney is located high underneath the diaphragm, so that the lower pole lies beneath the 11th intercostal space, the costodiaphragmatic recess and pleural space are obliterated.[254] This anatomic safety feature may be one of the reasons why the incidence of pneumothorax is not higher than it is after punctures of the 11th intercostal space.

Two other anatomic features are important in these punctures. First, the posterior division of the renal artery gives a branch to the upper pole which crosses the midportion of the upper pole infundibulum. Thus, punctures of this infundibulum should be avoided, because they might injure this vessel.[14] Second, the spleen, liver, and colon can be contiguous with the lateral edge of, or even posterior to, the upper pole of the kidney. For this reason, upper pole punctures are commonly done in a more medial position than usual through the paravertebral muscle (Fig. 23–206).

Technique. When a puncture through the 11–12th intercostal space is planned, the entry site is selected with the patient in the prone oblique position and marked with a 25-gauge needle. The patient or the fluoroscope is then rotated so that fluoroscopy can be done tangential (usually nearly lateral) to the entry path. The position of the needle at the entry site is then observed in relation to the lung and kidney during normal, shallow breathing and during forced inhalation and exhalation. After the operator has confirmed that the lung will not be traversed by the puncture tract, the patient is replaced in the prone oblique position and prepared for the puncture. The patient is instructed to continue shallow breathing during the puncture.

The needle should be kept away from the lower margin of the 11th rib, where the intercostal nerves and vessels run. Pain can result either from nerve irritation (puncture too close to the 11th rib) or from periosteal injury (too close to the 11th or 12th rib). The large diameter of the nephrostomy tubes placed in the tract during and after the NLT procedure, as well as breathing motion, exacerbate the pain. Occasionally, an intercostal nerve block will be needed.

Another complication of intercostal punctures is hydrothorax, which is caused by leakage of irrigation fluid along the tract and into the pleural space. To avoid this, a Teflon sheath should be kept in the tract at all times with its tip inside the collecting system.[254,266] Thirty-eight per cent of patients with an intercostal puncture have small asymptomatic pleural effusions or plate-like atelectasis, which resolve spontaneously, and 8% have large hydrothoraces that require thoracocentesis.[254]

An NLT via an intercostal approach should be planned as a one-step procedure, because these tracts tend to become tortuous with time due to breathing motion. For the same reason, a balloon retention catheter (Foley, Councill) should be left in the tract, because other types of tubes are commonly dislodged by the breathing movements.[245,254]

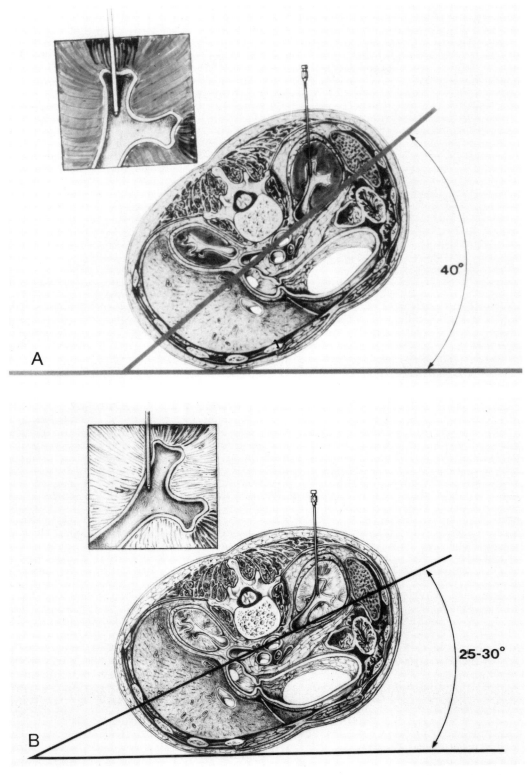

Fig. 23–204   Positions for particular punctures. A. Prone oblique position used for direct puncture through calix. B. Diagram showing patient in prone oblique decubitus position for puncture at junction of calix with infundibulum.

As a precaution, the lung is periodically checked by fluoroscopy during the procedure to look for early pneumothorax or hydrothorax. At the end of the procedure, inhalation and exhalation posteroanterior, and inhalation lateral chest radiographs are taken to look for pneumothorax and hydrothorax. Pneumothorax has not occurred in the authors' experience[254] but has been rather frequent in other series.[266]

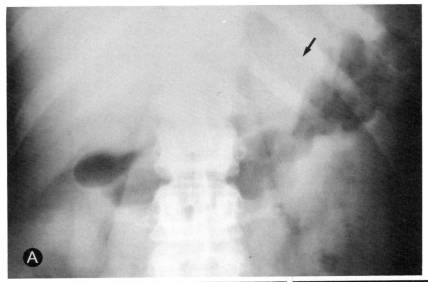

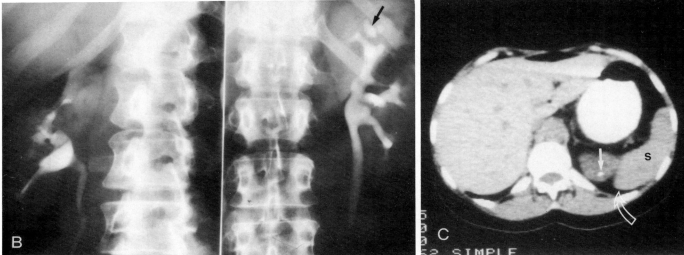

Fig. 23–205   Upper caliceal stone. A. Flat plate of abdomen shows small calcific density (arrow) in upper pole of left kidney above the 12th rib. B. IVU shows stone to be located within caliceal diverticulum (arrow) of upper pole calix. C. Tomographic section through upper pole of left kidney shows marked posterior extension (open arrow) of spleen (S). Note calcification in upper pole of kidney (small arrow).

Punctures under the 12th Rib

Posterior calix.   Posterior calices can frequently be identified by their end-on orientation. In some (Hodson) kidneys, however, the normal pattern is reversed.[15] Careful observation of steep oblique and lateral films from the IVU or retrograde pyelogram usually helps to differentiate the two sets of calices. If previous films are not helpful or not available, the pelvicaliceal system is studied under fluoroscopy. The injection of 10–15 ml of CO_2 is a helpful maneuver, because the gas will readily float toward the uppermost part of the collecting system (*i.e.,* the posterior calices).[249,250]

Once a posterior calix has been selected, the patient or the multidirectional fluoroscope is rotated until the calix is seen almost end-on. Excessive rotation laterally should be avoided; the skin entry site should not be past the lateral edge of the paravertebral muscles. More laterally placed entry sites could lead to splenic, hepatic, or colonic lacerations.

With the selected calix in the center of the x-ray field to avoid parallactic shifts, the needle in the plastic radiolucent handle is advanced forward for 8–10 cm.[7,253,267] The needle and hub should be seen as a dot (Fig. 23–207). After reaching this depth, or as soon as the needle tip is noted to move up and down with the kidney, either the patient (when using single-plane fluoroscopy) or the fluoroscope is rotated to obtain a lateral projection of the area (Fig. 23–208). End-on advancements and oblique or lateral depth checks are alternated until the needle tip enters the calix (Fig. 23–209). This method allows one to perform a one-wall puncture of the collecting system, thus avoiding the extravasation of contrast medium that interferes with observation during the initial maneuvers. Once the needle tip appears to lie within the collecting system, the trocar is removed; urine or froth of CO_2 and

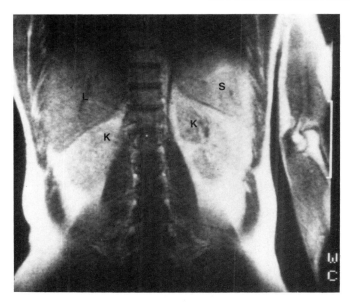

Fig. 23–206 Coronal section of body on magnetic resonance imaging shows relations of upper pole of left kidney (K) with spleen (S) and of upper pole of right kidney (K) with liver (L).

urine usually leaks out (Fig. 23–210). If it does not, a syringe with flexible connecting tubing (Argyle K50) is attached to the needle hub, and suction is applied while the needle tip position is adjusted. When urine is obtained, 10–15 ml of contrast medium are injected, further dilating the collecting system. A guidewire usually passes easily from a posterior calix into the renal pelvis (Fig. 23–209).

When a large calculus is lodged in the infundibulum or calix where the puncture was performed, passage of the wire into the renal pelvis is impossible. There are two techniques that can be used in these situations. First, if there is sufficient space behind the calculus, a floppy-tip 0.035-inch wire can be passed through the needle and 8–10 cm of it looped in the calix to ensure that all of the floppy segment is within the calix. Attempts to dilate over the floppy segment can result in loss of the wire position and tract. Newer guidewires, such as the Amplatz stiffening wire (Cook, Inc.) or a movable core wire, can also be effective in this situation.

Alternatively, if there is no space in either the calix or the infundibulum because of the calculus, the wire is advanced through the needle against the calculus. Upon exiting the needle tip, the wire will be within the collecting system, and as it is advanced, it will slip off the stone surface and perforate the wall of the calix or infundibulum, looping outside the collecting system in the renal parenchyma (Fig. 23–211). The tract can then be dilated

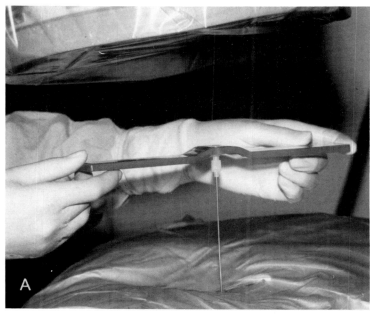

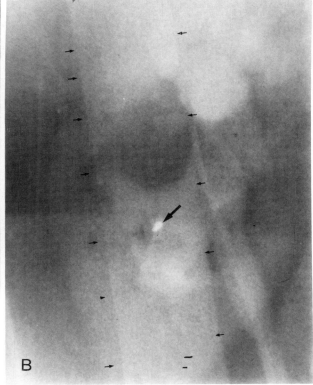

Fig. 23–207 "Down-the-barrel" puncture of collecting system. A. Anteroposterior plane position of needle held by plastic handle. B. Spot film on anteroposterior projection during advancement of needle under continuous fluoroscopy. Needle appears as a dot (large arrow) advancing toward infundibulum of lower pole calix. Plastic handle is faintly seen (small arrows). Note ureteral catheter with tip in upper pole calix.

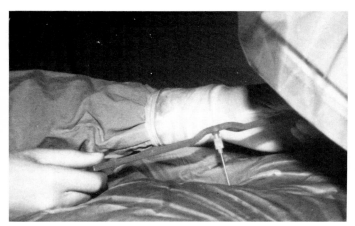

Fig. 23–208   After needle has been advanced for 7–8 cm, C-arm has been angled to provide lateral fluoroscopic image of kidney.

over this wire, being careful not to advance the dilator further after its tip strikes the calculus. Once the tract is dilated, the endoscopist can introduce the ultrasonic lithotripter to fragment the calculus, with care to keep the wire in place, because it is the only link with the collecting system. When enough of the calculus has been removed, a second wire usually can be passed under direct endoscopic vision into the renal pelvis and fluoro-

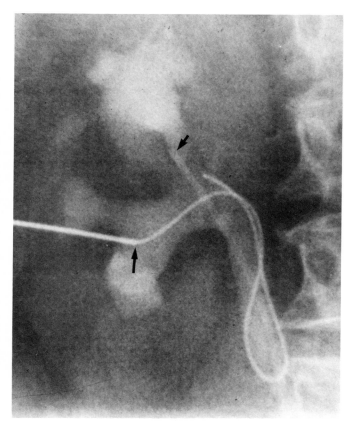

Fig. 23–209   Spot film taken during guidewire advancement shows tip of needle within infundibulum (lower arrow) and guidewire in upper third of ureter. Ureteral catheter has its tip in upper pole infundibulum (upper arrow).

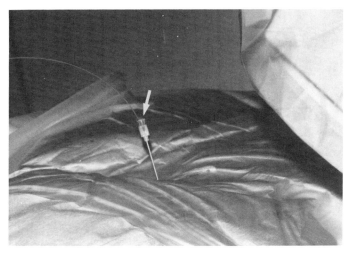

Fig. 23–210   With C-arm providing lateral fluoroscopy, guidewire has been advanced through 18-gauge needle into collecting system. Observe urine reflux through needle (arrow).

scopically manipulated into the ureter. The procedure then continues in the usual fashion. (See section on safety wire placement and tract dilation.)

Large staghorn calculi.   Large branched calculi are usually approached through a posterior lower pole calix,[72,129,246,262] although an upper caliceal puncture occasionally proves better, particularly when the branching involves primarily the anterior or upper calices.

Occlusion of the UPJ with a large-diameter (at least 8F) balloon or retrograde catheter is very helpful, because the collecting system can then be distended with contrast medium to facilitate the manipulation of wires, catheters, and dilators around the large calculus. This distention can be painful, and the patient should be adequately sedated.

The patient is positioned obliquely, and the needle in the handle is advanced until it reaches the calculus. It should be forcefully pushed against the calculi for another 1–2 mm[262] to assure that, upon removal of the trocar, the cannula will lie within the collecting system (Fig. 23–212). When the trocar tip initially hits the calculus, the cannula might be outside the collecting system if the calculus fills the infundibulum and calix (Fig. 23–213). If the cannula is advanced against the calculus, retrograde leakage of urine will not occur when the trocar is removed. A syringe with connecting tubing is attached to the needle hub, and a small amount of dilute contrast medium is injected; commonly, it will flow around the calculus, outlining the calix and infundibulum. A guidewire can then be advanced through the needle. A floppy 0.035-inch wire will usually slip alongside the calculus and into the renal pelvis. If the wire cannot be passed into the renal pelvis, it is looped inside or outside the calix or infundibulum as discussed in the previous section.

Anterior calix.   Although a posterior caliceal approach is often simpler, a solitary calculus in an anterior calix can be removed by the creation of a tract directly into that calix. The same puncture technique is followed as for posterior calices except that the patient is

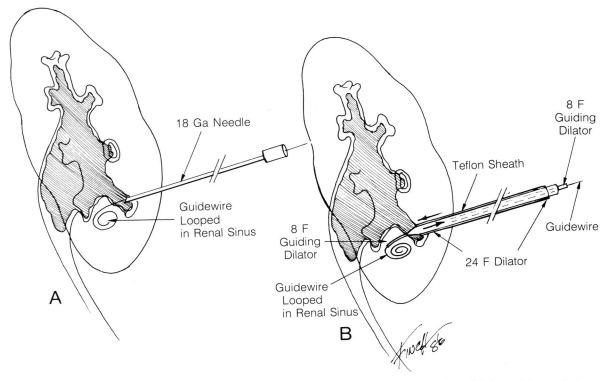

Fig. 23-211 Alternative technique used in patients with large branched calculi that do not allow passage of guidewire into renal pelvis. A. Needle has been placed through infundibular–caliceal junction and is pointing against opposite wall of infundibulum. Guidewire has perforated wall and is looped in renal sinus. B. During dilatation, dilators are advanced carefully until their tips meet opposite infundibular wall; this leaves sheath barely within collecting system after its advancement over dilator.

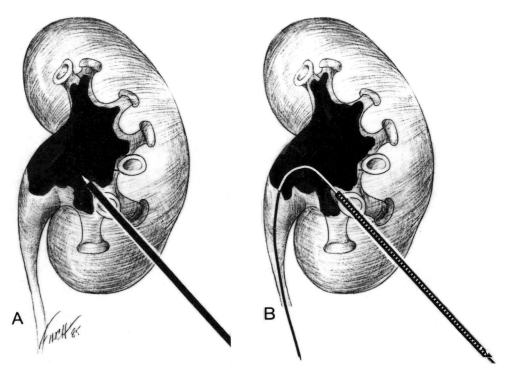

Fig. 23-212 Correct technique for needle puncture in patient with large staghorn calculus. A. Through posterior lower calix, needle has been advanced and pushed into calculus to ensure that cannula of needle is within collecting system. B. After removal of stylet, cannula tip is within collecting system and guidewire can be manipulated into renal pelvis.

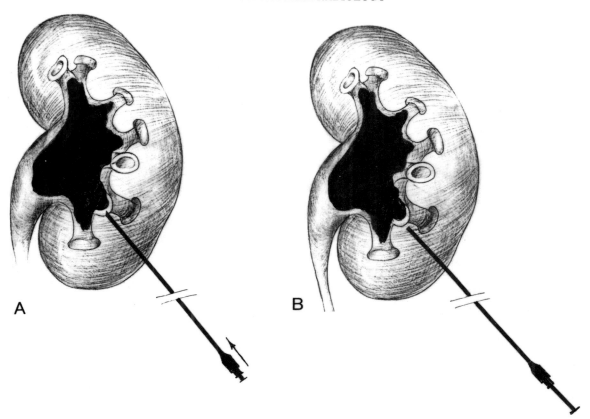

Fig. 23–213   Incorrect positioning of 18-gauge needle. A. Needle has been advanced until its tip hits stone. B. Upon removal of stylet, cannula of needle is seen to lie outside collecting system.

arranged in a steeper prone oblique position to bring the anterior calix into profile. However, if the caliceal pattern is such that the anterior calix is seen end-on in the usual prone oblique position (Hodson-type kidney), cephalad or caudad angulation alone can be used, because there usually will be no overlap with the posterior calices.

In the most common pelvicaliceal pattern, the calix is approached in profile, and, because of the sharp angle between the tract and the infundibulum going back to the renal pelvis, passing a guidewire into the renal pelvis is difficult.[262] Two techniques can be used. First, after the position of the needle tip within the calix has been verified, a 0.035-inch floppy-tip wire is passed through the cannula. If the wire does not pass spontaneously into the renal pelvis the needle can be tilted so that it points more toward the pelvis. The wire will then frequently find its way into the renal pelvis (Fig. 23–214).[129] Second, if the wire advances toward the calix rather than the pelvis, it is looped within the calix (Fig. 23–215A). The tract is carefully dilated, and a 7F, cobra, or multipurpose torque control catheter is advanced over the wire until its tip lies within the calix or infundibulum (Fig. 23–215B). The catheter tip is rotated until it points more toward the renal pelvis, and the wire is carefully withdrawn inside the catheter and then readvanced in the new direction (Fig. 23–215C).

Dilating a tract to an anterior calix is one instance where a balloon dilator definitely should be used, because semirigid or rigid dilators will not follow the wire around the sharp angle toward the renal pelvis. In addition, semi-

rigid dilators tend to push and rotate the kidney away from the patient's back, which elongates and curves the tract. To avoid this, the dilators should be used gently with a predominantly rotating, not pushing, motion; and only the tip of the dilator should enter the calix. These precautions will also help to minimize bleeding and per-

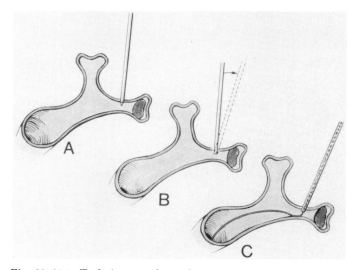

Fig. 23–214   Technique used to advance guidewire from anterior calix into renal pelvis. A. Because of relation between advancing needle and wall of infundibulum, guidewire has a tendency to go peripherally into papilla rather than into renal pelvis. B. Needle is tilted toward renal pelvis. C. Guidewire is advanced into renal pelvis.

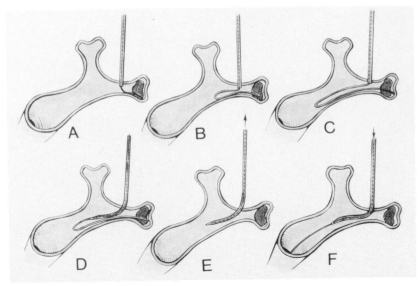

Fig. 23–215 Passage of guidewire into renal pelvis. A–C. Floppy 0.035-inch guidewire has been advanced into papilla, where it bounces back and loops into renal pelvis. D. After exchange of needle cannula for torque control angiographic catheter, tip of catheter has been advanced over guidewire in the direction of renal pelvis. E. Guidewire has been withdrawn into catheter and subsequently advanced (F) in the direction of renal pelvis through angiographic catheter.

foration, which are a greater hazard with this longer tract through the parenchyma.

Tract Anesthesia

If an extensive procedure is planned, a long-acting local anesthetic, such as 0.25% bupivacaine (Marcaine) can be used, because its effects will last for 3–4 hr.[72,245,262] However, this anesthetic has been associated with several adverse reactions, especially when used in large doses, and is therefore not currently used at the authors' institution. For most cases, they now use 1% lidocaine (Xylocaine). Its duration of action can be extended by using the form with epinephrine. Care must be taken to avoid large intravascular injections. Only rarely is general or spinal anesthesia necessary.

The skin entry site and subcutaneous tissues are infiltrated widely with 10–15 ml of lidocaine using 25- and 21-gauge needles. A 1–1.5-cm-long skin incision is made with a No. 11 surgical blade. A 6-inch 22-gauge needle is then advanced under fluoroscopic control along the planned tract to a point just outside the collecting system, and lidocaine is liberally deposited in the tract as the needle is slowly withdrawn (total dose: 10–15 ml). Once the tract is well anesthetized, the puncture of the selected calix is performed with an 18-gauge needle, and a guidewire is passed into the renal pelvis.

If anesthesia of the tract is inadequate, there are several methods to reinfiltrate it from the renal casule to the subcutaneous tissues. First, a Tuohy–Borst adapter with a sidearm can be passed over the wire and connected to the cannula's hub. The adapter is then tightened around the wire, and local anesthetic is injected through the sidearm into the tract. The disadvantage of this method is that it is time consuming and awkward to loosen and tighten the adapter every time the needle is pulled back

another small step along the wire to infiltrate a different area.

A second technique uses a short catheter with multiple sideholes (Fig. 23–216). A Tuohy–Borst adapter is attached to the catheter, and both are advanced over the wire until the tip of the catheter reaches the renal capsule. After tightening of the adapter on the wire, local anesthetic is infiltrated along the entire tract.[61]

The simplest technique is to use the 6-inch 22-gauge needle again to infiltrate the tract alongside the guidewire (Fig. 23–217).

TRACT DILATION EQUIPMENT

The several available dilator systems have been discussed at length earlier in this chapter. Emphasis will now be put on the indications, advantages, and disadvantages of each system.

Balloons

Balloon catheters are the primary dilators for NLT. High-pressure balloons 10–15 cm long and 8–12 mm in diameter (Fig. 23–218) are now commercially available (Cook, Inc.; Surgimed; USCI; Medi-Tech). Some balloons are a woven nylon coaxial design (Fig. 23–219), whereas others are of the more traditional wrap-around design and light-weight plastic materials. Either design can be used to dilate a percutaneous tract, and most will accept a back-loaded dilator and sheath (Fig. 23–220). If the tract is to be dilated under local anesthesia, balloon dilators are definitely preferred, because the inflation of the balloon is much less painful than repeated passes with sequentially larger semirigid dilators. Balloon dilators are also preferred in the dilation of difficult tracts such as intercostal, Y, and anterior caliceal ones and those where

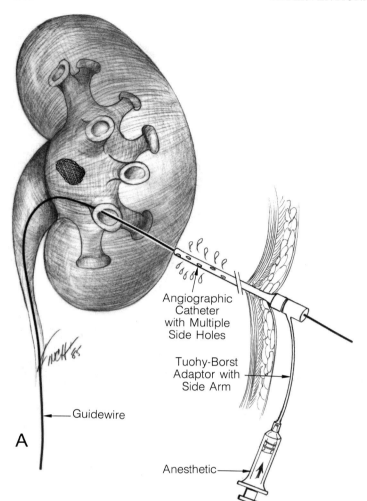

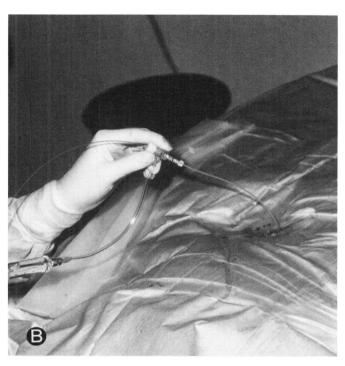

Fig. 23–216 Infiltration of percutaneous tract with local anesthetic using catheter with multiple sideholes and Tuohy–Borst adapter with sidearm. A. By tightening Tuohy–Borst adapter over guidewire, anesthetic can be injected into tract. B. Infiltration of percutaneous tract using catheter with multiple sideholes and Tuohy–Borst adapter passed over guidewire.

the guidewire is in an unstable position or outside the collecting system.

Another advantage of balloons is speed, because one inflation of an 8- or 12-mm diameter, 10-cm-long balloon, for 20–30 sec at a pressure of 12–15 atm dilates an entire tract to 24F or 36F, respectively. In addition, balloon dilation is less traumatic than use of semirigid dilators, so there is less bleeding. This is important for one-stage procedures when endoscopy is planned.

Balloon dilators do have some minor disadvantages. They increase the cost of the procedure, because they are expensive and are not reusable. Also, balloons usually are unable to dilate tracts in scarred postoperative flanks even with 12 atm of pressure. Further, an interesting problem can result if a balloon ruptures transversely. If the distal end blows out like a parachute, it can be impossible to remove. In this situation, the catheter hub is cut off, and a 10F or 12F blunt-ended Teflon dilator (Cook, Inc.) is advanced over the catheter shaft until it reaches the "parachute" site. The catheter is then forcefully pulled back into the dilator while the guidewire is kept in place (Fig. 23–221).

Semirigid Dilators

Semirigid dilators are classified into several types depending on their primary use and their method of introduction:

1. 0.038-inch tapered tip:
   a. Fascial (Cook Urological);
   b. Vessel (Cook, Inc.);
2. 8F tapered tip:
   a. Biliary coaxial (Cook, Inc.);
   b. Renal Amplatz (Cook, Inc.; Cook Urological; Van-Tech).

0.038-inch tapered-tip dilators. Both systems are tapered at the tip to fit a 0.038-inch guidewire and come in sizes increasing in 2F steps. The vessel dilators range from 8F–24F and the fascial dilators from 8F–36F. The principal difference between the systems is their relative stiffness. The vessel dilators, being made of Teflon, are significantly stiffer and are therefore used almost exclusively for dilation of scarred, fibrous tracts. Another difference is that a working cannula (Rutner

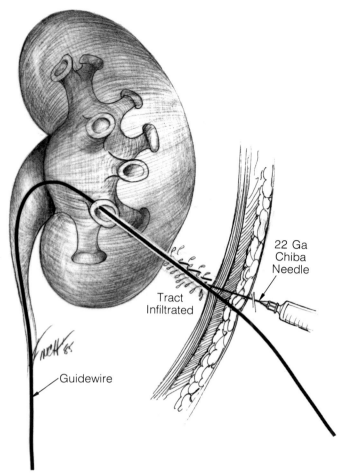

Fig. 23–217 Infiltration of percutaneous tract with anesthetic using 22-gauge Chiba needle alongside guidewire originally passed through 18-gauge needle into pelvicaliceal system. Multiple passes of Chiba needle ensure adequate infiltration around guidewire.

cannula; Cook Urological) is available for introduction over the 24F fascial dilator (Fig. 23–222).

8F tapered-tip dilators. Both systems of this type are introduced coaxially over a guiding 8F Teflon dilator, which is passed over the working wire and remains in

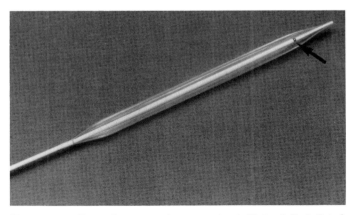

Fig. 23–218 Grüntzig-type nephrostomy tract dilator fully inflated to its 10-mm diameter. Balloon length is 15 cm. Observe radiopaque marker (arrow) indicating beginning of balloon.

place during the entire dilation (Fig. 23–223). The advantage these systems have over the 0.038-inch tapered-tip dilators is that the large dilators are not introduced over a guidewire but rather over the significantly stiffer combination of a guidewire and 8F Teflon dilator. As a result, they are guided much more reliably into the collecting system, so guidewire kinking in the tract, which can cause perforations, bleeding, and loss of the tract, is much less common.

The biliary coaxial dilators are seldom used for tract dilation because of their size (18F maximum diameter). The Amplatz renal dilators come in 10F–30F sizes with Teflon working sheaths for the 24F, 26F, 28F, and 30F dilators. Larger dilators with sheaths, and sheaths for smaller dilators, can be special ordered.[61,63,72,253,257,258,267]

DILATION TECHNIQUES

Introducing the Safety Wire

The manipulations required to remove a urinary calculus are frequently difficult and extensive, and it is not unusual for the working sheath and instruments to get dislodged so that the operator loses the tract into the collecting system or creates false tracts that make re-entry difficult or impossible. For these reasons, it became obvious early in the authors' experience that they needed an extra wire in the tract to be assured of expeditious access to the collecting system at all times.

Two systems for introduction of this extra ("safety") wire are available. The first comes as a part of the Amplatz renal dilator set (Cook, Inc.; Van-Tech) (Fig. 23–224A–C). The 8F Teflon guiding dilator is advanced over a wire into the collecting system and followed by a thin-walled 10F introducer passed coaxially. The 8F dilator is then removed, keeping the original guidewire in place. A second guidewire is introduced into the collecting system through the 10F introducer, which is then removed (Fig. 23–224D). One of the two wires (usually the less stiff one) is then properly positioned in a secure place, such as the ureter or a remote calix.

The second method is to use the commercially available safety wire introducer set (Cook Urological). This set consists of a 12F sheath with a central stiffener tapered to fit a 0.038-inch guidewire (Fig. 23–225). The two parts are introduced together over the initial wire into the collecting system (Fig. 23–226A), and the stiffener is removed, leaving the wire in place (Fig. 23–226B). A second wire is passed through the lumen of the sheath, which is then removed (Fig. 23–226C,D).

Because most guidewires are Teflonized, they are slippery and tend to pull out through the stitches that are fixing them to the skin. For this reason, a 5F polyethylene catheter is passed over the safety wire; tying the stitch to the plastic makes the safety wire much more secure.

Except in cases of ureteral stones, both the safety and the working wires should be advanced into the mid or distal third of the ureter. Sometimes, the initial wire will advance spontaneously into the ureter; if not, it can be placed there with the help of a torque control angiographic catheter. This manuever can be done either

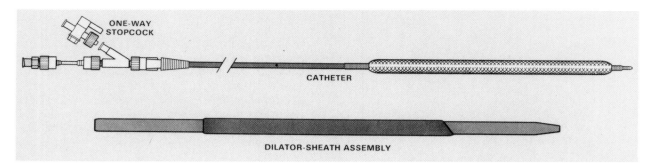

Fig. 23–219 Dilator sheath assembly and Cook enforcer balloon. Observe that tip of dilator is tapered down to size of shaft of balloon catheter on which it will be back-loaded for advancement immediately after balloon dilatation of tract. (Courtesy of Cook, Inc.)

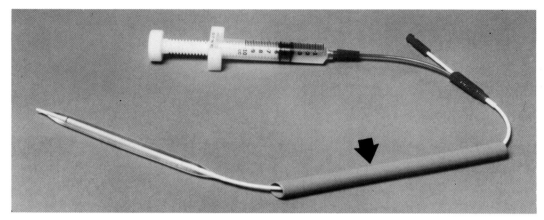

Fig. 23–220 Tract-Master one-step tract dilatation system with sheath. Observe that 10-mm diameter, 15-cm-long balloon has been assembled with 30F (lumen) Teflon sheath (arrow). Sheath can be advanced easily over fully inflated balloon into renal pelvis.

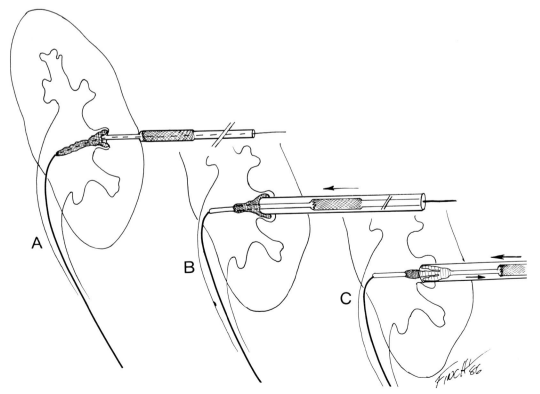

Fig. 23–221 Technique used for removal of parachuting, transversely broken Grüntzig-type dilating balloon. A. Attempts to remove balloon produced parachuting. B. Teflon sheath has been advanced over shaft of catheter until it meets edges of broken balloon. C. Balloon has been pulled into dilator.

572

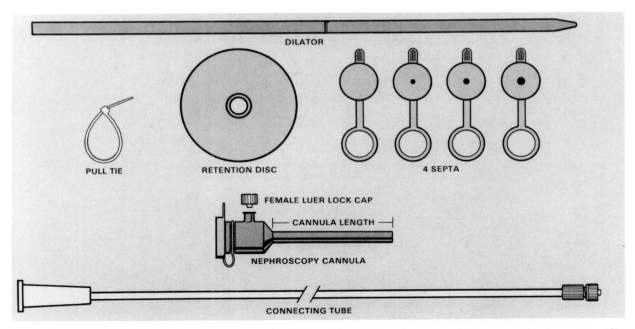

Fig. 23–222 Nephroscopy cannula set consisting of cannula with 24F lumen and several silicone septa for introduction of endoscopic instruments. Molnar retention disk is provided for fixation to skin.

Note side port on cannula for connection to suction. (Courtesy of Cook Urological.)

before or after the second wire has been added. When there is an impacted stone at the UPJ or in the proximal ureter, the wires cannot be advanced down the ureter. In these cases, or in cases of ureteral stones (where the wires become a hindrance if they are in the ureter), the wires should be looped in a remote calix (Fig. 23–227). At least 8–10 cm of wire should be looped to prevent accidental dislodgment.

Dilating with Balloons

A 10F dilator is passed over the working wire to enlarge the tract enough to facilitate balloon introduction. The

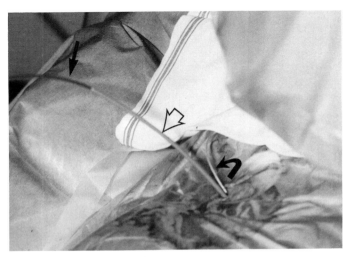

Fig. 23–223 Dilatation of percutaneous tract using Amplatz renal dilators. Note that individual dilators (open arrow) are passed over 8F Teflon guiding dilator (large arrow). Safety guidewire is to the side (curved arrow).

balloon catheter is advanced over the wire until the most distal radiopaque marker is within the collecting system. In most cases, the tip of the balloon is passed into the renal pelvis, which means that the infundibulum is also dilated; this is particularly helpful if the plan calls for the sheath or a large rigid instrument to pass through the infundibulum. For direct approaches to anterior caliceal stones, and in cases with an obstructed infundibulum such as those with a staghorn stone, the balloon dilates only up to the calix.

A pressure gauge (Fig. 23–228) is attached to an inflation device (Fig. 23–229), which is then connected to the balloon catheter. The balloon is inflated with dilute contrast medium to a pressure of 12–14 atm. Initially, a waist is seen in the balloon at the level of the renal capsule, the posterior perirenal fascia, and the subcutaneous tissue (Fig. 23–230A). By maintaining or slowly raising the pressure, these deformities generally can be made to disappear in 20–30 sec (Fig. 23–230B),[64] although on occasion, long use of very high pressures (17–20 atm) is required. When the waist is gone, the balloon is deflated and removed, and either the sheath of the ultrasonic lithotripter (Fig. 23–231) or the working Teflon sheath and its dilator are passed into the collecting system (Fig. 23–232).

A variation of this technique involves a Teflon working sheath with or without a dilator back-loaded on the balloon catheter. Once the tract is dilated, either the back-loaded sheath is passed over the inflated balloon or the balloon is deflated and the back-loaded dilator and sheath are advanced over the shaft of the balloon catheter. The balloon catheter and dilator are then removed, leaving the Teflon sheath and wire in place. The minor advantage of this system is that it saves one step.[61,64,72,240,258,268]

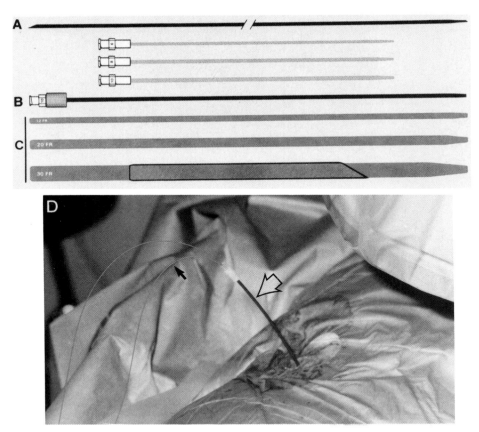

Fig. 23–224   Top: Partial set of Amplatz renal dilators showing 8F guiding dilator (A); 10F blunt-ended Teflon dilator, which doubles as safety wire introducer (B); and 12F, 20F, and 30F dilators (C). Teflon sheath is mounted over 30F dilator. (Courtesy of Cook, Inc.) Bottom (D): 10F Teflon dilator (open arrow) of Amplatz set being used to pass two guidewires (small arrows) into collecting system.

Dilating with Semirigid Dilators

0.038-inch tapered-tip dilators.   Each individual dilator is introduced over the working wire under continuous fluoroscopic control until its tip is in the collecting system. No attempt should be made to advance the tip to the UPJ, because the stiff dilator might bend the wire and perforate the renal pelvis. Care should be taken at the level of the renal capsule and fascia, because trying to advance the dilator through this site of higher resistance may, if the dilator is at all off line, cause kinking or buckling of the wire. Trying to advance a semirigid dilator past a kink in the wire is almost always unsuccessful and frequently results in the wire being dislodged and that tract being lost. If a kink occurs, it is probably wise to exchange the wire for a stiffer one (Lunderquist, Lunderquist–Ring, Amplatz stiffening). Such precautions are usually used from the outset in patients who have had renal surgery. On the other hand, in a patient with a soft back, an experienced operator might choose to dilate in 4F steps (examples in references 3 and 28) rather than in 2F steps.

Tapered-tip dilators.   Of the two systems, only the Amplatz renal dilators or their equivalent are used for NLT. The 8F Teflon guiding dilator is passed over the working wire and remains in place until the final dilator

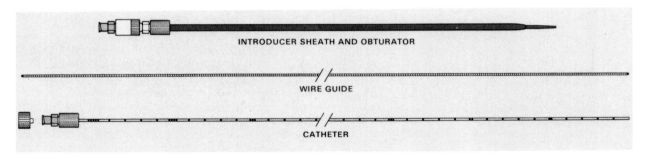

Fig. 23–225   Safety wire introducer set consisting of 12F radiopaque polyethylene introducer sheath (22 cm long) with radiopaque polyethylene obturator. (Courtesy of Cook Urological.)

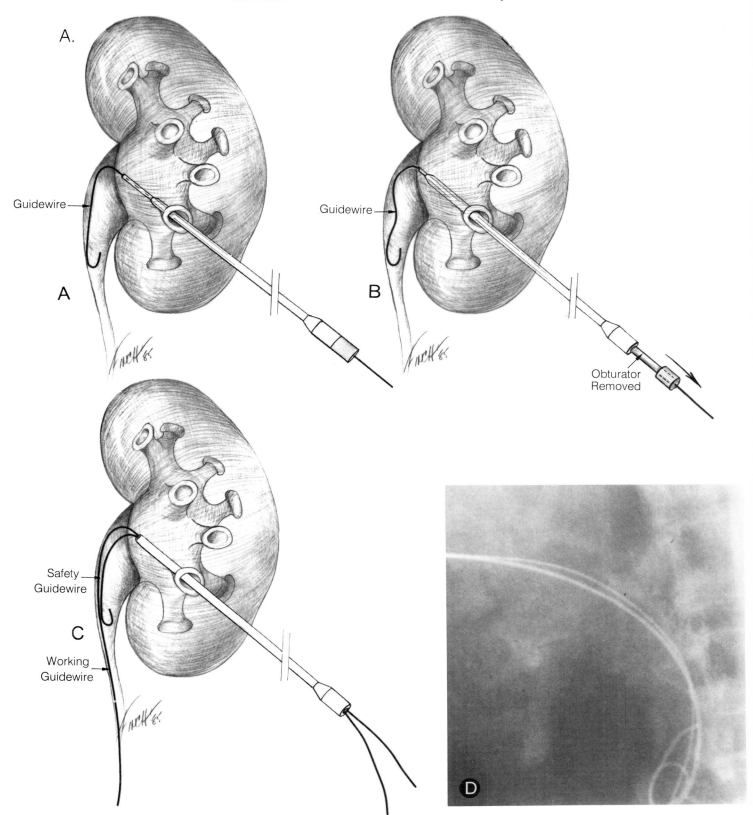

Fig. 23–226 Use of safety wire introducer. A. Over initial wire passed through 18-gauge needle, safety wire introducer has been advanced until its tip lies well within collecting system. B. While guidewire is kept in place, obturator is removed. C. Second guidewire has been passed through safety wire introducer, which is then removed. D. Spot film showing position of both guidewires in upper ureter through safety wire introducer.

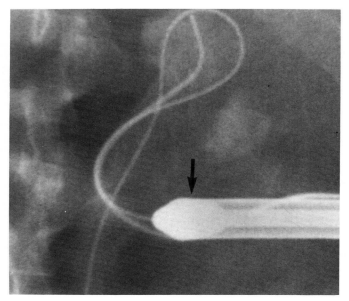

Fig. 23–227 Nephroscope with its obturator (arrow) advanced directly through tract over wire.

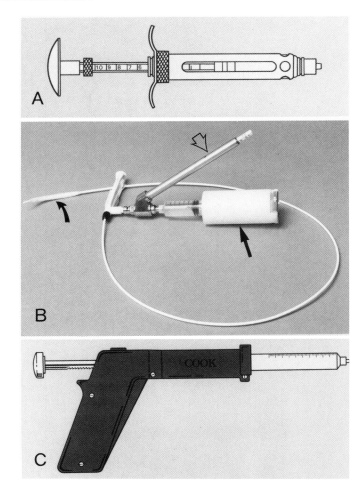

Fig. 23–229 Inflation devices. A. Syringe for manual inflation of high-pressure balloons. (Courtesy of Cook, Inc.) B. Helic injector for high-pressure balloons (black arrow); pressure gauge (open arrow); Olbert balloon (curved arrow). C. Inflation pistol with standard 10-ml disposable syringe. (Courtesy of Cook, Inc.)

and Teflon sheath have been introduced. The dilators are used in steps of 2F or 4F, depending on the operator's experience. With tension kept on the 8F dilator, each larger dilator is carefully advanced under fluoroscopic control until its tip is at the desired depth in the collecting system (Fig. 23–233). With these systems, there is less chance of bending the guidewire–Teflon dilator assembly at the perirenal level, although this can be done. Therefore, if the larger dilator is not passing easily, a brief fluoroscopic check at an angle that allows one to see "down the barrel" of the dilator may help to realign the dilator and guidewire before a kink occurs. Once the desired French size for the tract is reached, commonly 24F–30F,

a Teflon working sheath or metal lithotripter sheath is passed over the dilator into the collecting system (Fig. 23–234A). The tip of the sheath should not be advanced past the "shoulder" area of the dilator (Fig. 23–234B,C), because the tip will then no longer be in contact with the dilator and may cause significant tissue damage and bleeding.

Dilating with metal dilators. Metal dilators are made by two companies, Wolf and Storz, and have a coaxial telescope design; they are manufactured in French sizes of 8 to 24 (Wolf) and 8 to 28 (Storz). Each set consists of a leading 40-cm-long, 8F cannula that fits over a 0.038-inch guidewire and has a round or pyramidal stopper on the leading end that prevents the next larger dilator from advancing past the leader and causing a perforation (Fig. 23–235). The set consists of several dilators, each 3F larger than the prior size. The bleeding is minimal because of the telescopic nature of the system. Dilation is straight, so this system should not be used in curved tracts, because the dilator cannot follow the guidewire without kinking or bending it. The front end of the larger dilators is open, whereas the back end is closed

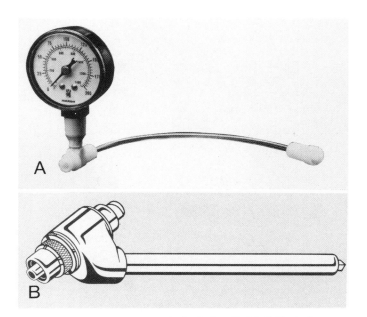

Fig. 23–228 Pressure gauges. A. Cook, Inc. B. Medi-Tech, Inc.

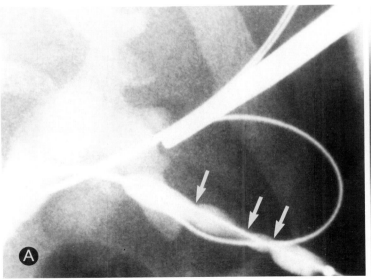
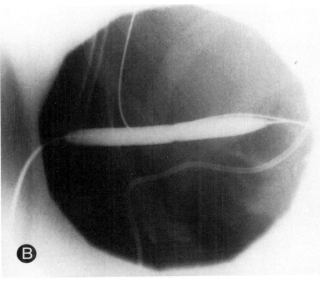

Fig. 23–230 Dilatation with balloons. A. Inflated in percutaneous tract; note indentation at level of renal capsule and perirenal fasciae (arrows). B. After increase in intraballoon pressure, indentation has disappeared, and balloon is fully inflated.

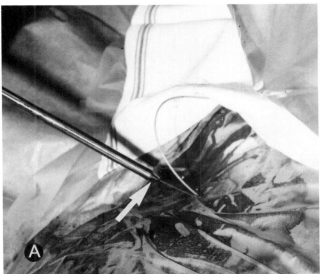
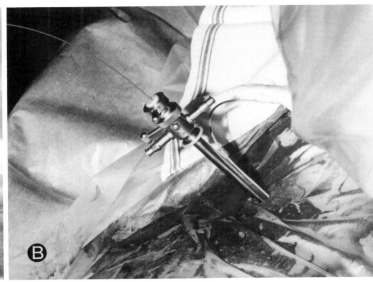

Fig. 23–231 Insertion of working sheath. A. Metallic sheath of ultrasonic lithotripter with its open-ended obturator is being advanced over working wire. B. Under fluoroscopic control, tip of obturator has been passed into renal pelvis over guidewire.

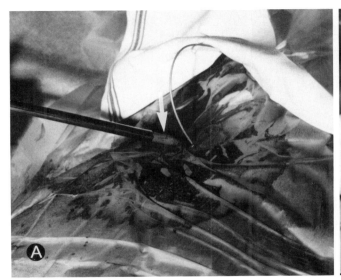
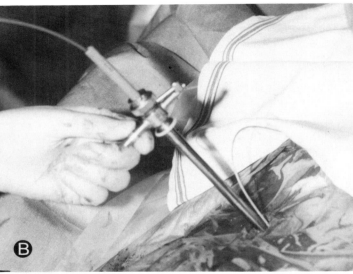

Fig. 23–232 Insertion of working sheath.. A. Metal sheath of ultrasonic lithotripter is advanced into collecting system over 24F Amplatz renal dilator (white arrow). B. Under fluoroscopic control, sheath has been advanced into renal pelvis over Amplatz renal dilator.

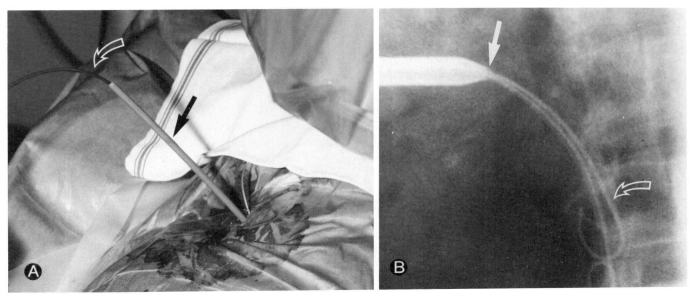

Fig. 23–233 Dilation with Amplatz system. A. 18F (arrow) Amplatz renal dilator has been advanced under fluoroscopic control over 8F Teflon guiding dilator (open arrow). B. Spot film taken during advancement of 18-gauge Amplatz renal dilator showing relation of tip of dilator to UPJ (white arrow) and safety wire (open arrow).

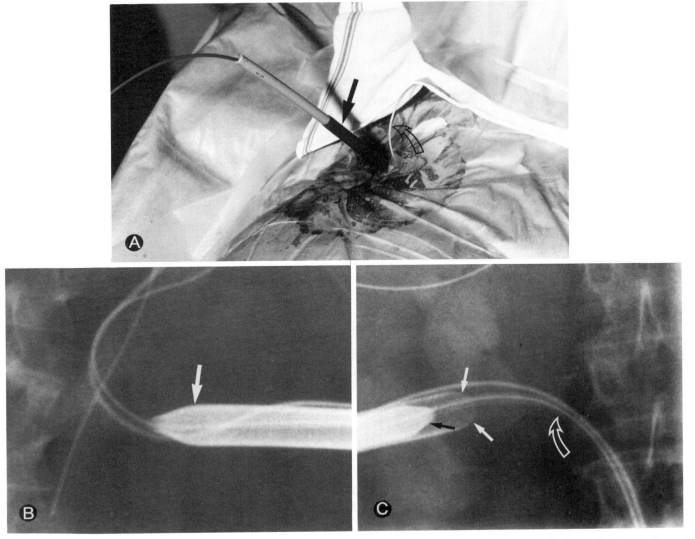

Fig. 23–234 Insertion of working sheath. A. 28F Amplatz renal dilator has been passed under fluoroscopic control over 8F guiding dilator, and Teflon sheath has been advanced into collecting system (black arrow). Note safety guidewire (open arrow). B. Two guidewires have been advanced through percutaneous tract and looped in upper pole calix. Over working wire, 24F dilator has been advanced into collecting system (arrow). C. 24F dilator (black arrow) is removed over 8F guiding dilator (open arrow) leaving Teflon sheath (white arrows) within collecting system.

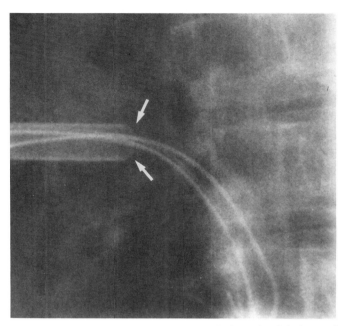

Fig. 23-235 Teflon sheath is seen at level of renal pelvis (arrows). Two guidewires are within proximal ureter.

with a central 8F hole for the leading cannula. The closed back end stops each dilator at the end of the dilators already in place.

The 8F leading cannula is passed under fluoroscopic control over the working wire until its tip lies at the desired point inside the collecting system. Each successive dilator is then advanced coaxially over the previous one until it reaches the stopper (Fig. 23-236). The key to successful dilation lies in holding the leading cannula steady to avoid perforations of the collecting system. Once the dilation is completed, the sheath of the ultrasonic lithotripter is introduced over the last dilator. At the University of Minnesota Hospitals, metal dilators are not routinely used despite their effectiveness because of the ease with which they can perforate the renal pelvis. A fascial inciser has been recently developed for the percutaneous incision of fasciae or scar tissue over the guidewire (Fig. 23-237).

WORKING SHEATHS

A working sheath or cannula is needed when performing NLT in one stage or by the immediate two-stage method. A sheath is also required whenever work is done

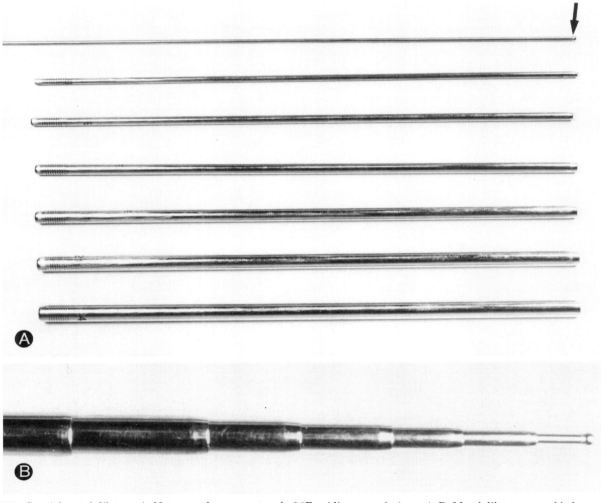

Fig. 23-236 Coaxial metal dilators. A. Note round stopper at end of 8F guiding cannula (arrow). B. Metal dilators assembled.

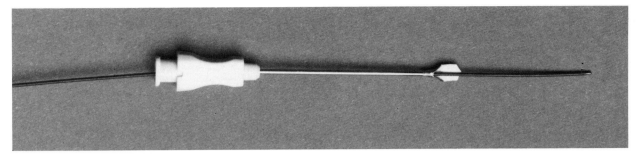

Fig. 23-237   Fascial blade advanced over guidewire.

through a tract above the 12th rib regardless of its age or maturity. A sheath is used for several purposes:

It tamponades the tract, which invariably bleeds, particularly in the kidney, after dilation, especially with semirigid dilators. Tamponading the tract minimizes blood loss and improves endoscopic visibility.

It permits removal and reintroduction of instruments, gently facilitating exchange if one instrument is not working well and allowing the endoscopist to move in and out of the collecting system quickly and easily when removing clots or small stone fragments with a grasper.

It prevents seepage of large amounts of irrigation fluid into the retroperitoneal space or, after supracostal or 11th intercostal punctures, into the pleural space.[254]

Its routine use keeps the intrarenal pressure low during stone extraction or nephroscopy and minimizes perforations of the renal pelvis.[252] To achieve this effect, the sheath should be 2F–4F larger than the nephroscope to allow free retrograde flow of the fluid.

It allows easy introduction into the renal pelvis of 20F–22F Foley or Councill catheters with a Cope intro-ducer. After tube placement, the working sheath is slipped back and then removed by cutting it lengthwise.

There are three types of working sheaths:

1. Teflon sheaths. The standard sizes have 28F, 30F, 32F, and 34F outer diameters with inner diameters 4F smaller. These sheaths are faintly radiopaque and have a blunt and a beveled end. The blunt end can be used for endoscopy in small areas where a bevel may not fit, whereas the beveled end is particularly well suited for flushing techniques because the bevel can be directed toward the calculi for more efficient irrigation and aspiration.

   Teflon sheaths are introduced over the corresponding dilator (i.e., a 24F dilator for a 28F internal diameter sheath). The dilator is advanced until its shoulder is at the point within the collecting system where the sheath tip should lie. The dilator is held in position, and the sheath is gently advanced over it until the tip is at the shoulder of the dilator (Fig. 23–238A). The dilator and the 8F Teflon guiding catheter are then

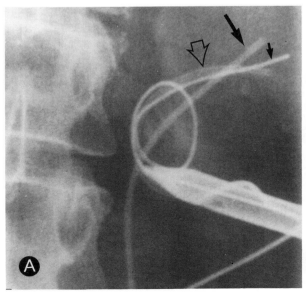
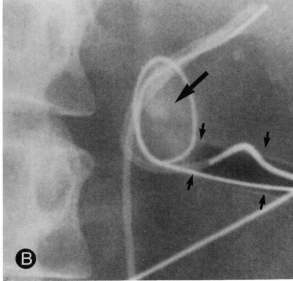

Fig. 23-238   Approach to free-floating renal pelvic stone. A. Percutaneous tract through posterior lower pole calix has been dilated to 24F. Note presence of safety wire (small black arrow), 8F dilator (open arrow), and uretral catheter (large black arrow). B. Teflon sheath has been placed within collecting system (small black arrows). Note stone within renal pelvis (large arrow).

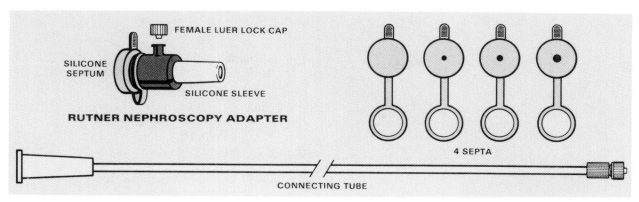

Fig. 23–239 Rutner nephroscopy adapter used in conjunction with renal dilating sheath to control fluid flow and to provide access for endoscopes. Silicone sleeve slides over end of Teflon sheath. Forceps are provided for introduction of different sized instruments. (Courtesy of Cook Urological.)

removed (Fig. 23–238B). The wire is usually left in place to give the endoscopist a visual guide into the pelvis. This implies that a sheath which is slightly larger than the instruments should be used. Having the wire as a guide is often valuable, and the wire, if not dislodged, can be used at the end of the procedure to guide the drainage catheter.

If the sheath is too long for the instruments, or if it sticks out so far above the skin that it gets in the way of the endoscopist, it can be cut off with scissors. The sheath can even be cut flush with the skin; but if this is done, a double stitch should be passed through the side of the sheath to keep control of it, because otherwise it may slip under the skin during manipulations.

The only minor disadvantage of Teflon sheaths is the lack of control over irrigating fluids, which flow freely from the outer end and necessitate a watertight draping system. A silicone nephroscopy adapter has been described for use with the Amplatz Teflon sheath, to control irrigating fluids during endoscopic manipulations (Fig. 23–239).

2. Rutner cannula (Cook Urological). This plastic molded working cannula is 28F with an inner diameter of 24F.[61] It has a side port for suction and a rubber seal to prevent backflow of fluid around the instruments. The Rutner cannula is introduced over the corresponding dilator (Fig. 23–240). Its two chief disadvantages are the thickness of its wall, which produces a blunt advancing edge during introduction, and the fact that only one size is available.

3. Ultrasonic lithotripter cannula. This cannula is a tight-fitting metal sleeve through which the ultrasonic lithotripter is inserted. When the lithotripter is fully inserted, it can be locked into place. Excess irrigation fluid must be aspirated either through a side port or through the ultrasonic wand. The cannula can be inserted either mounted on the appropriate semirigid dilator, with passage over the guidewire–8F dilator combination, or attached to the blunt-tipped metal obturator that comes as part of the set with passage directly over the guidewire. The blunt metal obturator-over-guidewire system has proved both more difficult to use and more likely to kink the wire.

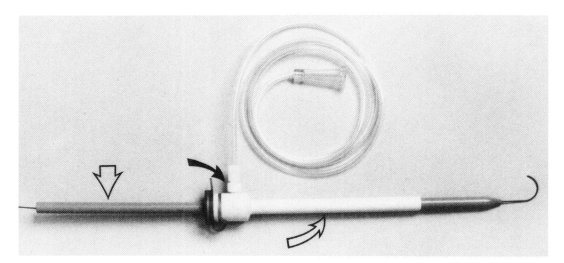

Fig. 23–240 Rutner cannula (curved open arrow) introduced over 24F dilator (short open arrow). Black arrow points to side post. (Courtesy of Cook Urological.)

EXTRACTION TECHNIQUES

The techniques for percutaneous removal of calculi can be divided for descriptive purposes into two groups, fluoroscopic and endoscopic, depending on the primary guidance method used to control the instruments used. Plainly speaking, however, fluoroscopy is used in both methods, because it facilitates spatial orientation during the performance of endoscopy. Both the fluoroscopic and the endoscopic techniques can be further subdivided into two large groups:

1. Fluoroscopic techniques:
   a. Flushing;
   b. Grasping;
2. Endoscopic techniques:
   a. Grasping;
   b. Fragmentation.

Fluoroscopic Techniques

Flushing for renal pelvic and caliceal calculi. Flushing is the simplest and least traumatic of all the extraction techniques. It is particularly useful in the removal of multiple small calculi or of fragments from ultrasonic or electrohydraulic lithotripsy.[258,267] The following technical tips will help to make flushing successful:

1. The lumen of the Teflon sheath should be larger than the calculi.
2. The UPJ should be blocked with either a large catheter or a balloon catheter to prevent migration of calculi down the ureter.[258] (This is probably not so important when irrigating through a ureteral catheter.)
3. Irrigation should be performed with a power injector at a flow rate of 10–15 ml/sec with dilute contrast medium under fluoroscopic control.
4. If perforation of the collecting system has occurred during the dilation maneuvers, flushing techniques should not be used, because they could cause severe extravasation.
5. Suction should be applied to the end of the Teflon sheath during the irrigation but should be gentle to avoid collapsing the collecting system against the sheath (Fig. 23–241).

Depending on the set-up used, the flushing techniques can be divided into two groups: indirect and direct.

Indirect methods. For these methods, a Teflon sheath is inserted alongside the safety wire, which is passed down the ureter, with its bevel inside the collecting system pointing in the direction of the calculus.[253] A flexible plastic tube is connected to the sheath, and suction is applied with a catheter-tipped syringe. A second catheter is placed for irrigation. Several arrangements of second catheters have been used:

1. Retrograde ureteral balloon catheter with an end hole only (Berman or Medi-Tech occlusion balloon catheter) (Fig. 23–242)[258];
2. Antegrade balloon catheter with sideholes proximal to the balloon and no end hole (Berman or Swan–Ganz catheter) (Fig. 23–243). Placement of this type of balloon catheter alongside the sheath into the UPJ can be difficult;
3. Retrograde balloon occlusion of the UPJ with a Berman or Medi-Tech occlusion balloon, with an additional catheter for irrigation purposes. Both of these catheters must be passed alongside the sheath (Fig. 23–244).
4. For removal of small stones or fragments, the irrigation catheter can be passed through the sheath and positioned adjacent to the calculi or fragments (Fig. 23–245).

Direct method. This method is particularly useful for stones lodged in an infundibulum or calix remote from the puncture site. A large-caliber (24F or 26F) red rubber (Robinson) catheter is modified by cutting the tip at an

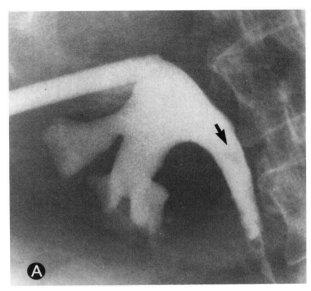
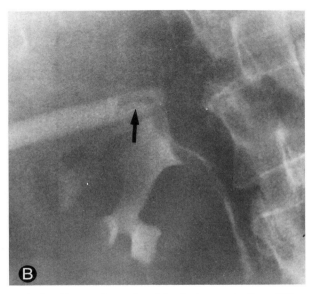

Fig. 23–241 Flushing (A) and aspiration (B) through Teflon sheath in patient with free-floating stone in renal pelvis (small arrow). Note marked collapse of renal pelvis during aspiration; filling defect within Teflon sheath represents clot and stone (arrow).

angle to create a wide, slanted opening. This tube is then passed through the Teflon sheath over a previously positioned angiographic catheter (Fig. 23–246A) into the infundibulum or calix where the calculus is lodged (Fig. 23–246B).[258] The angiographic catheter is removed, and the slanted opening of the tube is rotated until it lies in direct contact with the calculus. Forceful aspiration generally pulls the calculus against the tube opening (Fig. 23–246C), although in most cases, alternating irrigation and suction must be applied before this happens. Once the calculus has been trapped, the suction is maintained while slowly withdrawing the rubber tube. It may be possible to remove the calculus through the sheath, but usually, it gets loose in the renal pelvis, from which it can be removed easily by some other technique.

Ureteral calculus extraction. The standard treatment of upper ureteral calculi has been surgical removal through a ureterostomy via a flank or dorsal lumbotomy incision, because retrograde endoscopic basketing, so often effective in the lower ureter, is associated with trauma and sometimes avulsion in the upper ureter. Fortunately, the recent, rapidly evolving, methods of extracting pelvicaliceal stones through percutaneous nephrostomy tracts have been extended to the ureter,[72,91,236,240,258,269–273] and the ureterorenoscope has extended the endoscopist's reach from below. Open operations are seldom performed now for ureteral stones without some other indication, such as a need for plastic repair. The 94% success rate of percutaneous extraction of upper ureteral calculi remains higher than that of ureteroscopic techniques at present. Moreover, specially experienced urologists are needed to perform the latter

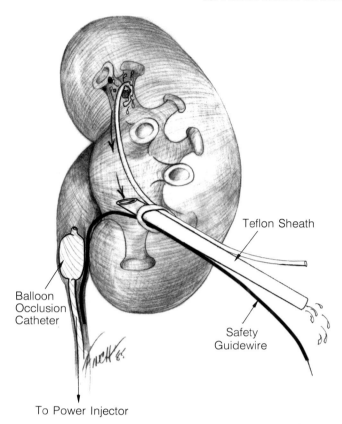

Fig. 23–242 Irrigation through occlusion balloon catheter placed retrograde at level of UPJ. Irrigating fluid and stones exit through Teflon sheath. Safety wire has been placed alongside Teflon sheath in percutaneous tract.

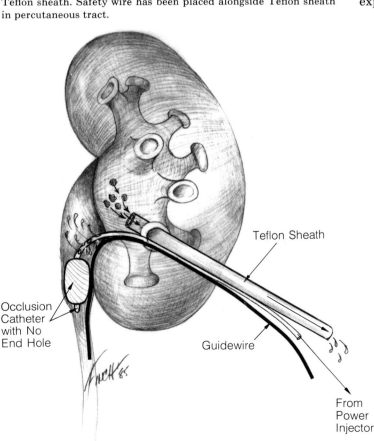

Fig. 23–243 Flushing technique using occlusion balloon catheter with no end hole and with proximal sideholes; guidewire is placed alongside Teflon sheath and balloon catheter. Irrigating fluids and stones exit through Teflon sheath.

Fig. 23–244 Flushing technique using angiographic
catheter placed near stones to maximize effect of irrigation in patient with caliceal stones. Observe placement of irrigating catheter and safety wire alongside
Teflon sheath within percutaneous tract. Balloon
occlusion catheter has been placed retrograde to block
UPJ.

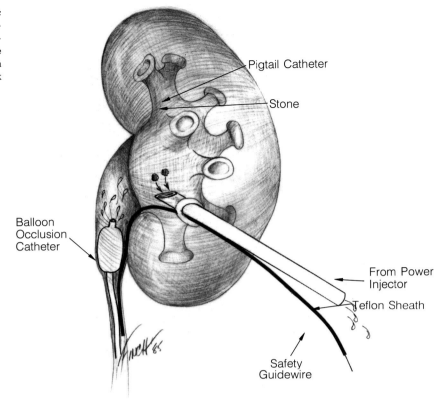

Fig. 23–245 Flushing technique using catheter passed
through Teflon sheath in patient with small stone fragments
within renal pelvis. Occlusion balloon catheter blocking UPJ
was inserted retrograde.

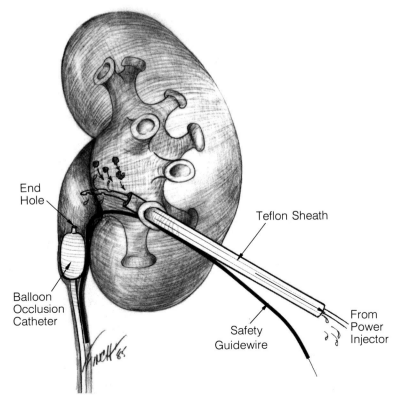

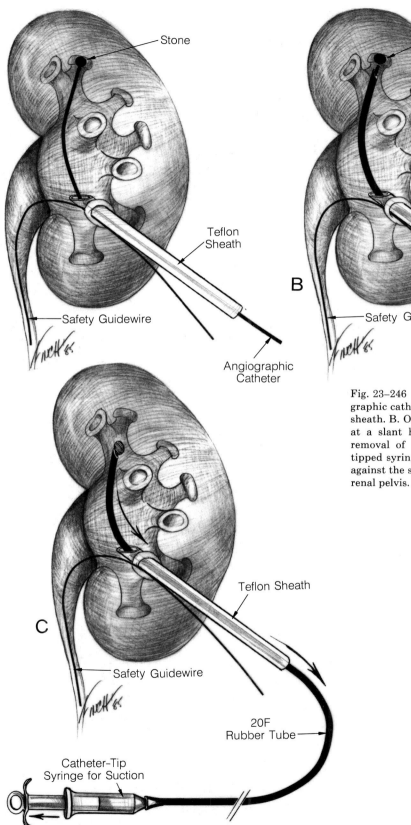

Fig. 23–246 Suction technique for removing caliceal stones. A. Angiographic catheter has been passed into calix containing stone via Teflon sheath. B. Over angiographic catheter, 20F rubber tube with its tip cut at a slant has been advanced into stone-containing calix. C. After removal of angiographic catheter, suction is applied with catheter-tipped syringe to end of rubber tube, whose tip must be applied right against the stone; suction causes stone to be pulled by rubber tube into renal pelvis.

procedure, which now is limited to large medical centers. Thus, the percutaneous method seems superior to the endoscopic approach. As pointed out by Narayan and Smith,[269] it is easier to bypass a stone or obstruction with a guidewire or catheter from above than it is retrograde from below, because the proximal ureter supports the catheter and guidewire. This fact may account for some of the difficulties of ureteroscopic stone removal.

The frustrating ureteral spasm and the inability of stone baskets to open fully in nondilated ureters are the primary technical reasons for the lower success rate of removal of ureteral, in comparison to pelvicaliceal, stones. However, the development of new basket designs,[72,272,274,275] of balloon catheters for both blocking and flushing, and of innovative techniques such as flushing with either CO_2 or dilute contrast medium through a catheter inserted retrograde[276] have improved the success rate of ureteral stone extraction. Nonetheless, some of the larger, irregularly shaped stones cannot be flushed up or snared with baskets from above; this may reflect entrapment or embedding of the stones within edematous ureteral mucosa.[58]

Flushing methods.   Flushing has been the most useful and least traumatic technique for the extraction of ureteral calculi and is the primary reason that the authors' success rate with ureteral calculi has recently increased to 100%. Flushing is done through a ureteral catheter inserted retrograde with its tip positioned below the stone. The flushing agents used are CO_2 or dilute contrast medium. The following technical tips will help to make flushing in the ureter successful and safe:

1. A Teflon sheath with an inner diameter larger than the stone should be placed in the collecting system before any flushing takes place, because flushing with contrast medium without the sheath to act as a vent can cause severe extravasation into the renal sinus.
2. It is helpful to choose an entry site that provides direct access to the UPJ, because, if the flushing method fails, other manipulations will be needed. This usually requires a caudal approach through a middle or upper pole calix. Flushing is also facilitated if the tip of the Teflon sheath is located near the UPJ.
3. A 7F or 8F open-ended catheter with no sideholes is placed cystoscopically in the ureter with its tip immediately below the calculus (Fig. 23–247A,B). An end hole balloon catheter is particularly useful in two situations:
   a. When the catheter tip cannot be placed next to the calculus;
   b. When the calculus is lodged in the distal third of the ureter, because in these cases there is a tendency for the flushing agent to drain into the bladder and for the catheter to recoil back into the bladder as the flushing solution is injected.
4. Each time the calculus moves, the catheter should be advanced over a guidewire until it is once more immediately below the calculus.
5. Manipulation or placement of wires or catheters in the ureter above the calculus should be avoided, because they can impede the flushing effort either indirectly, by causing increased mucosal edema or perforations, or directly, by their mechanical presence. Instead, the working and safety wires should be parked in some remote calix.
6. Ureteral spasms can be minimized by:
   a. Intravenous administration of glucagon and sedatives;
   b. Local instillation of 10 ml of 1% lidocaine into the ureter proximal to the stone.[273]
7. CO_2 flushing is tried first, because it has usually been both safer and more effective.

For the CO_2 flushing method, once the Teflon sheath with attached suction tubing and safety wire have been properly positioned, a 60-ml syringe loaded with CO_2 is connected directly to the ureteral catheter hub. The gas is forcefully injected as fast as possible with both hands. Under fluoroscopy, the sudden marked increase in the diameter of the ureter produced by the high-speed bubble of gas can easily be detected. As the ureteral size changes, the calculus usually appears to be "rattling" about freely inside the ureter. If this type of motion is seen, then usually on a subsequent injection (the authors have done as many as eight) the stone will suddenly get completely free and be carried into the renal pelvis or even out through the sheath. It seems to be helpful to fill the ureter with a few milliliters of saline before injecting the gas, because the bubbles and turbulence created by the gas in the liquid help to free the stone.[276] If the stone does not appear to be moving even after four or five injections, CO_2 will usually fail.

This method is safe and has never caused significant extravasation even when perforations were present. Further, any slight extravasation that does occur clears rapidly. Not only does CO_2 not obscure the stone, it actually highlights it, making verification of position and motion simple.[276]

For flushing with dilute contrast medium, the standard 60% contrast medium is diluted with normal saline to a concentration of 10%–20%. It is delivered with a power injector connected by high-pressure angiographic tubing to the hub of the ureteral catheter. For the first injection, a flow rate of 10–15 ml/sec is used under fluoroscopic control.[253,258,267,276] Both short bursts and a continuous injection for 2–3 sec have been successful. Here, as in the CO_2 technique, the keys to success are using a large enough catheter, positioning the ureteral catheter tip next to the stone, and ensuring predominantly retrograde flow toward the renal pelvis. (If antegrade flow into the bladder predominates, exchanging the ureteral catheter for a balloon catheter might provide the needed ureteral occlusion.) If the first injection is not successful, the flow rate is raised by 5 ml/sec on each subsequent injection until a maximum flow rate of 25 ml/sec is reached.

Commonly, when irrigating with diluted contrast medium, the calculi spontaneously exit through the Teflon sheath (Fig. 23–247C,D), particularly if suction is applied. After the tubing and syringe have been filled with the aspirated fluid and debris, the tubing is clamped near the sheath end and removed from the sheath. The clamp is removed over a filter or gauze so that the fluid can be checked for stones.

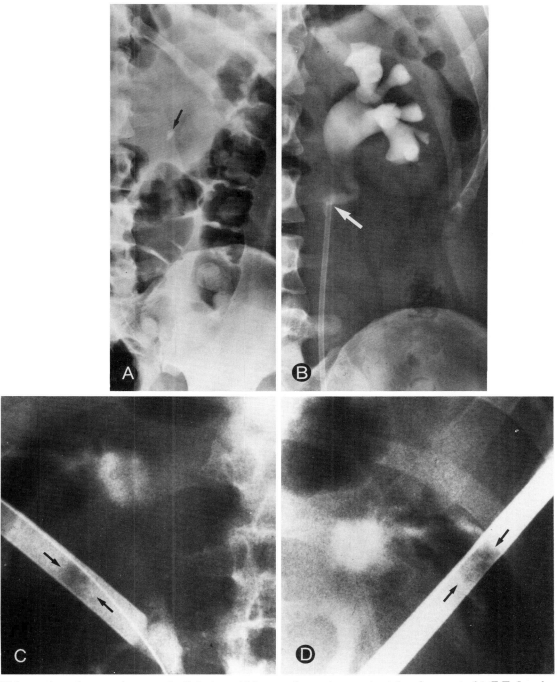

Fig. 23-247 Disimpaction of ureteral stone. A. Calculus within upper third of left ureter (arrow). B. Ureteral catheter (arrow) has been placed retrograde immediately underneath stone. Contrast medium delineates collecting system. C. After creation and dilatation of percutaneous tract for placement of 24F Teflon sheath, stone has been disimpacted from ureter and is seen within sheath (black arrows). D. Stone is seem migrating outward within sheath (arrows).

Some precautions must be observed when using dilute contrast medium for flushing:

1. Do not flush if a significant perforation of, and extravasation from, the collecting system occurred during tract creation.
2. Flush under fluoroscopic control.
3. Do not flush with nonopaque fluid unless flushing with dilute contrast has shown that there is no significant extravasation and has caused severe problems in seeing the stone.

Other methods. Retrograde passage of ureteral catheters may displace the stone if it is not impacted in the ureteral wall.

Balloon catheters (4 mm in diameter, 2 cm long, 5F shaft) can be advanced through the working sheath and carefully manipulated beyond the stone with a 0.038-inch guidewire. The balloon is then fully inflated immediately below the stone. Careful traction may dislodge the stone into the proximal ureter or renal pelvis (Fig. 23–248). At times, ureteral stones can be displaced downward with balloon catheters either in patients with intact bladders[272] or in those with ileal conduits.

Multiple ureteral stones can be extracted through a nephrostomy tract. The ureter is catheterized, and a guidewire is advanced past the stone into the bladder. The guidewire is removed, and a Dormia basket is tied to the end of the angiographic catheter until both ends of the guidewire are secured, one at the flank, the other at the urethra.[182,203] By pulling back on the angiographic catheter, the basket is manipulated to the level of the most distal stone. The wires of the basket are kept fully open by simultaneous pressure applied to both the angiographic and basket catheters until the stone has been entrapped. The basket is allowed to close, and the stone is extracted. The same maneuver is repeated to extract the other stones. A stent is placed over the guidewire

after the removal of the basket and angiographic catheter (Fig. 23–249). A variation of this technique uses a special basket with two long arms (Fig. 23–250).

If the manipulation under fluoroscopy fails, UPJ stones can sometimes be removed with flexible alligator or 3-pronged rigid forceps introduced through a nephroscope and carefully manipulated under direct vision.

The 7F Rutner's catheter has a helical stone basket distally and a 6-mm dilating balloon proximally (Fig. 23–251).[210] If the catheter is advanced in antegrade fashion, the ureter distal to the stone is dilated (Fig. 23–252A–C); this allows expansion of the basket in the ureter and increases the chances of snaring the stone.

Grasping techniques. These techniques can be divided into subgroups according to the instrument used: baskets, flexible forceps, and rigid forceps. These techniques are indicated in the percutaneous extraction of radiopaque calculi up to 1.5 cm in size. A tract of at least 28F is required. For baskets and flexible forceps, a Teflon sheath is used; rigid forceps are passed directly through the tract without a sheath.

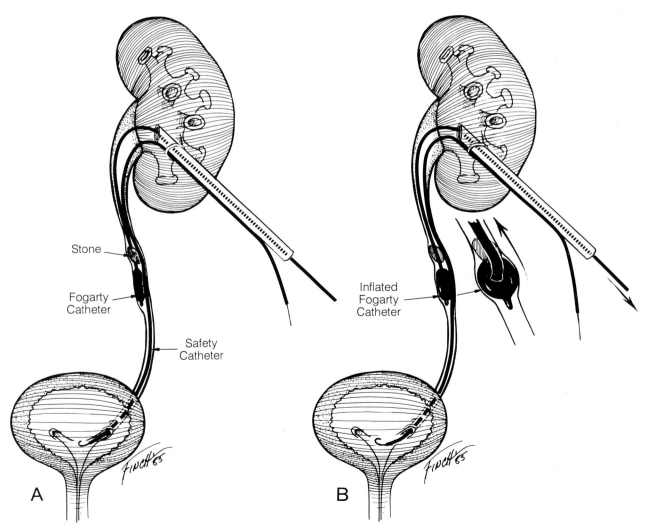

A

B

Fig. 23–248 Stone extraction from ureter with Fogarty balloon catheter. A. Catheter has been manipulated beyond stone. Note presence of safety catheter alongside Teflon sheath with its tip in bladder. B. Balloon has been inflated and is slowly withdrawn, pulling stone back into renal pelvis.

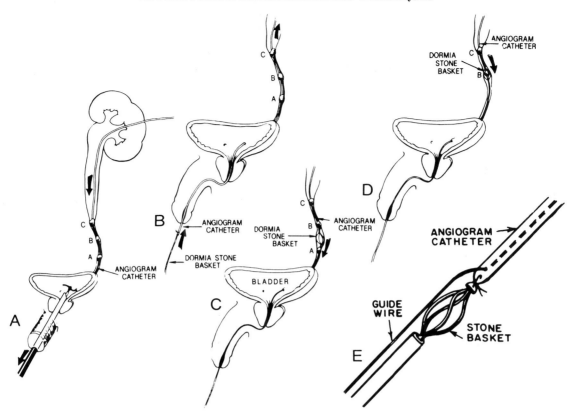

Fig. 23–249 Combined percutaneous and cystoscopic manipulation of multiple ureteral stones. A. Endoscope is used to extract tip of guidewire introduced antegrade through percutaneous tract. Observe presence of three stones in distal ureter (A,B,C). B. Over exteriorized guidewire, angiographic catheter has been advanced, and proximal end of Dormia basket has been attached to its end; basket is then slowly and gently pulled back through urethra and bladder. C. Basket has been positioned just proximal to most distal ureteral stone. D. After extraction of first stone, basket has been repositioned and second stone has been captured. E. Close-up view of assembled angiographic catheter with stone basket. Observe wire extended through sidehole of catheter and running along basket sheath for safety purposes. (Reproduced from Smith AD, Lange PH, Reinke DB, et al: Extraction of ureteral calculi from patients with ileal loops: a new technique. *J Urol* 1978;120:623.)

Baskets. Several designs and sizes of baskets are available:

1. Pfister–Schwartz type with a 3-, 4-, 6-, and 8-wire helicoidal pattern and a long floppy filiform tip (Fig. 23–253A);
2. Dormia, with a 3- and 4-helicoidal wire pattern without a floppy tip and with a detachable introducing sheath (Fig. 23–253B);
3. Universal basket with a 3-, 4-, and 6-wire helicoidal pattern, a floppy tip, and a detachable introducing sheath (Fig. 23–253C);
4. Hawkins basket, with a 4-wire pattern in either an 8F or a 10F Teflon sheath (Fig. 23–254);
5. Segura basket made of flat wire and with a blunt end (Fig. 23–255);
6. Rutner basket with a 7F angioplasty balloon and a 3- or 4-wire helicoidal basket.

The size of the basket needed depends on the size of the calculus except when using a Hawkins basket, where the size of the basket can be changed as needed by advancing or retracting the Teflon sheath (Fig. 23–256).[209]

The value of baskets for caliceal or infundibular calculi is limited, because the small dimensions of these structures generally do not allow complete opening of the basket and because the basket tip can easily perforate the calix[207] except with the Segura or the Hawkins basket that can be safely advanced, due to their blunt end. In addition the Hawkins basket shaft can be preshaped to facilitate entrance into a calix (Fig. 23–257).

The Burhenne's handle (Medi-Tech) and steerable catheters can be used to guide the baskets into the calices or the proximal ureter (Fig. 23–258).[202]

In the renal pelvis, there is ample space for manipulation and opening of the basket. The Hawkins basket is slightly more versatile than the others.[170] The length of the basket can be easily changed, the basket can be safely pushed against the renal pelvic wall to force the wires open, the strength of the 4-wire shaft and Teflon sheath allow the basket to be easily rotated, and the sheath can be preshaped to facilitate reaching stones in distant parts of the renal collecting system or proximal ureter.[209]

Baskets with a long filiform tip are preferred for manipulations in the ureter for two reasons. First, the long floppy segment is kept beyond the calculus during manipulation of the basket, which allows the basket to be drawn up and down past the stone without losing its position.[207] Second, the floppy tip is less traumatic than the end of the nonfiliform tip baskets. Baskets with a detach-

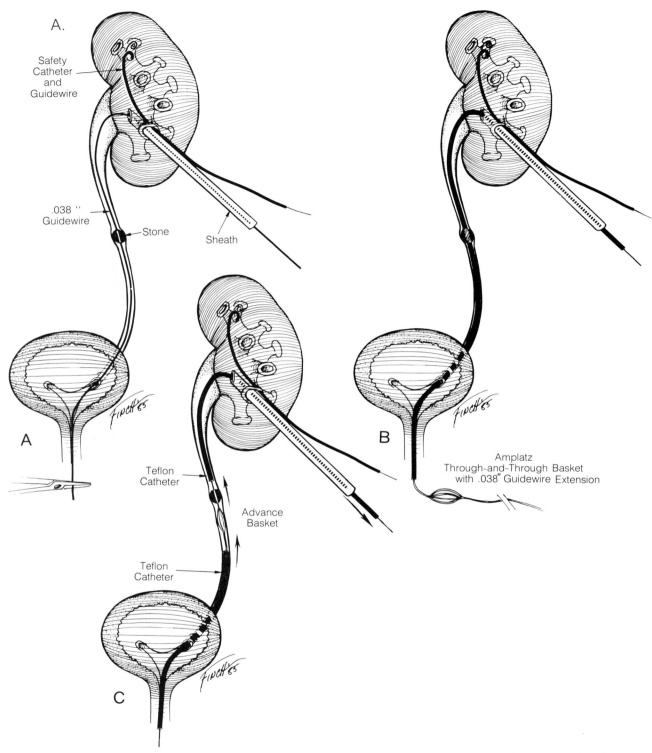

Fig. 23–250 Use of Amplatz through-and-through basket. A. Through Teflon sheath, guidewire has been manipulated into bladder, from which it was extracted with cystoscope. B. Teflon catheter has been passed over guidewire, which has been replaced by through-and-through basket with its two wire extensions. C. Basket has been pulled through Teflon sheath to level of stone in midureter; Teflon catheter has been pulled back proximal to the basket, and second Teflon catheter has been advanced distal to basket. D. By pushing both Teflon catheters against the basket, it is forced to open, and stone is captured. E. Combination of Teflon catheters and basket is withdrawn through collecting system into Teflon sheath. F. Continuous Amplatz helical stone extractor set consisting of continuous constructed stainless-steel helical stone extractor, 158 cm long, with two 5F radiopaque sheaths and two pin vise handles. (Courtesy of Cook Urological.)

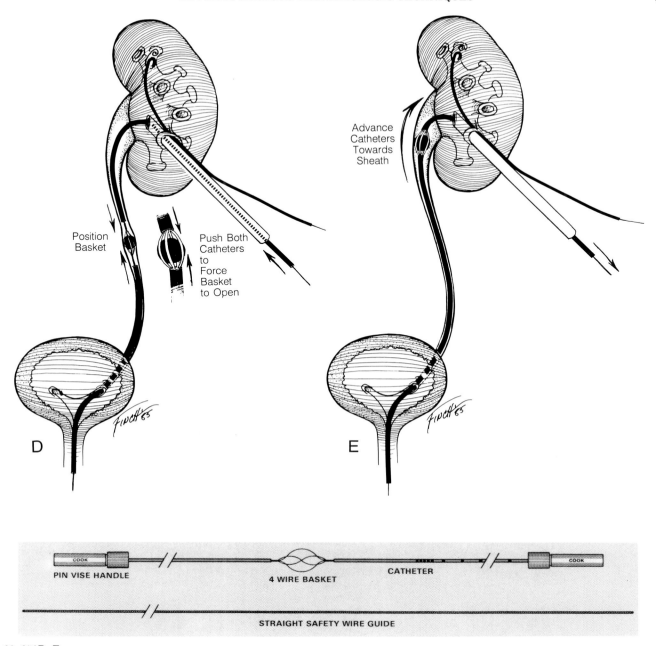

Position Basket

Push Both Catheters to Force Basket to Open

Advance Catheters Towards Sheath

D

E

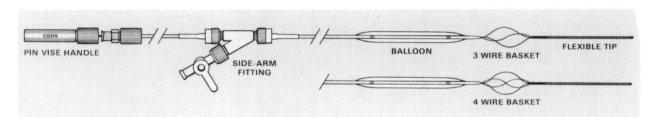

Fig. 23–250D–F

PIN VISE HANDLE   4 WIRE BASKET   CATHETER   COOK

STRAIGHT SAFETY WIRE GUIDE

PIN VISE HANDLE   SIDE-ARM FITTING   BALLOON   3 WIRE BASKET   FLEXIBLE TIP

4 WIRE BASKET

Fig. 23–251 Rutner balloon dilatation helical stone extractor set consisiting of 7F radiopaque polyethylene balloon catheter with 4-cm-long balloon (6-mm inflated diameter) and stainless-steel helical basket with 5-cm flexible tip matched to balloon catheter. Both 3- and 4-wire baskets are available. (Courtesy of Cook Urological.)

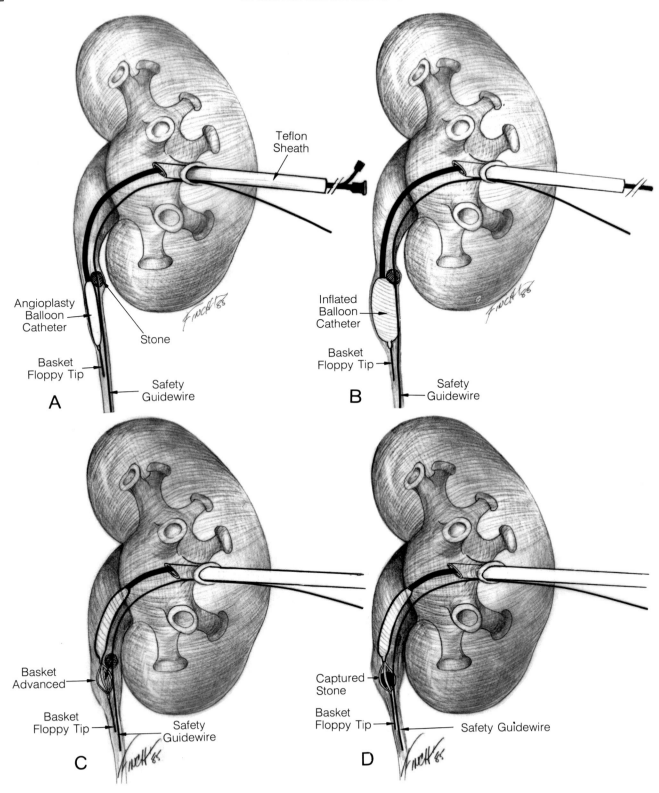

Fig. 23–252   Use of Rutner balloon dilatation helical stone extractor. A. Angioplasty balloon has been manipulated beyond ureteral stone. Note safety wire. B. Balloon has been inflated below stone to dilate ureter and facilitate extraction maneuvers. C. After deflation of balloon, basket has been advanced beyond tip of catheter. D. Stone has been captured by basket within dilated segment of ureter.

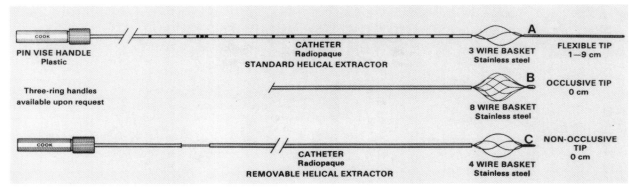

Fig. 23–253   Stone basket designs. A. Pfister–Schwartz basket with flexible tip. B. Dormia basket. C. Removable sheath helical extractor.

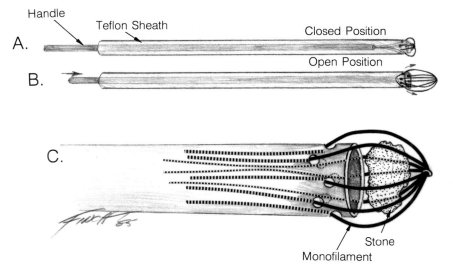

Fig. 23–254   Hawkins stone basket in closed (A) and open (B) positions. C. Hawkins monofilament basket with trapped stone. D. Hawkins wire basket.

able sheath (universal) are also useful in the ureter. The ureter is first catheterized with an angiographic catheter to pass a wire beyond the stone. Over this wire, the basket's sheath is passed. The wire is removed and the basket is passed through the sheath. The baskets with a nondetachable sheath (Pfister–Schwartz) are passed either through a Burhenne handle or a nontapered catheter.

Baskets are often unsuccessful and frustrating to use in the ureter. Space for complete basket opening is restricted due in part to the normally small ureteric dimensions and to the further decrease in dimensions by the urothelial edema caused by the calculus. Indeed, the edematous mucosal folds can entrap the stone, making it impossible to reach it with a basket. Manipulations in the ureter increase the amount of edema significantly and should be minimized.

Rutner described another type of basket mounted on an angiographic balloon catheter for retrograde use; this design is supposed to decrease trauma to the distal ureter.[210] The balloon is used to dilate the ureter distal to the calculus either before or after trapping the stone.

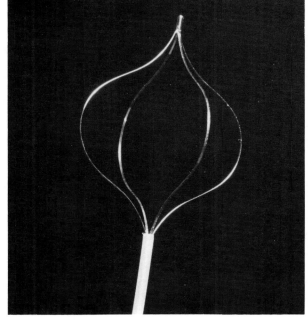

Fig. 23–255   Segura basket made of 4 flat wires with blunt end.

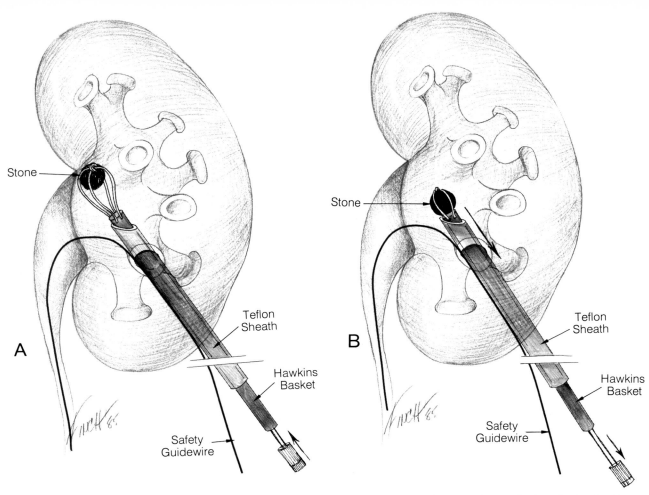

Fig. 23–256   Use of Hawkins basket. A. Hawkins basket has been introduced through Teflon sheath, and basket has been enlarged to capture stone. B. By retracting guidewires, basket has been closed; captured stone is pulled out through Teflon sheath.

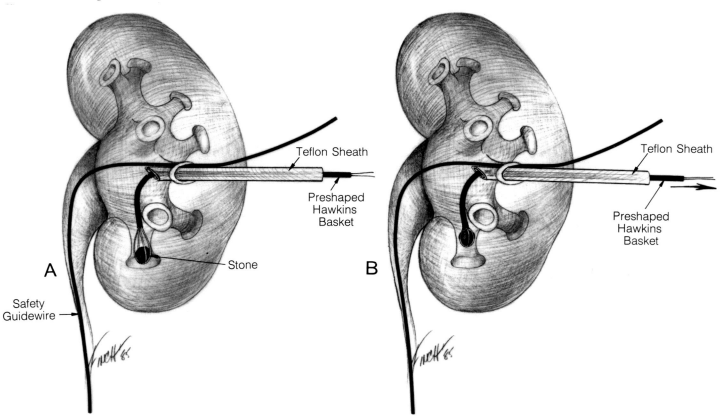

Fig. 23–257   Modification of Hawkins basket for removal of caliceal stones. A. Preshaped Hawkins basket has been passed into anterior lower pole calix containing stone, and basket has been enlarged. B. Captured stone is slowly removed through Teflon sheath.

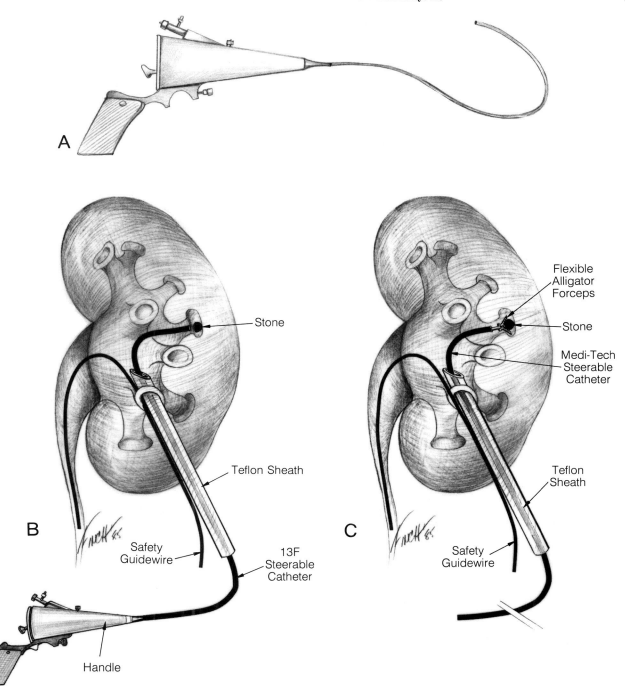

Fig. 23–258 A. Steerable catheter system (Medi-Tech). B. Use of system in patient with caliceal stones. A 13F steerable catheter has been manipulated into calix with stone. C. Alligator forceps have been passed to grasp stone.

Recently, the authors have begun using an angiographic 2-wire snare for stones in tight places. It has been remarkably successful for stones in calices, infundibuli, and the ureter. Although they expected the stone to slip out of the snare, once pulled against the end of the nephroscope or catheter (Fig.23–259), it usually does not move. The softer, floppier snare is much easier to work around the edge of a stone than is a basket. Perforation has not occurred.

Flexible forceps. There are two types of flexible forceps used under fluoroscopic control: 3- or 4-pronged types (Fig. 23–260A) and the 7F alligator type (Fig. 23–260B). Flexible forceps should be used only for radiopaque calculi and when multidirectional fluoroscopy is available. The forceps are usually introduced through a 13F Burhenne catheter (Fig. 23–258C).

The 3- and 4-pronged forceps are limited by the small pulling force they can exert without loosing their grip on

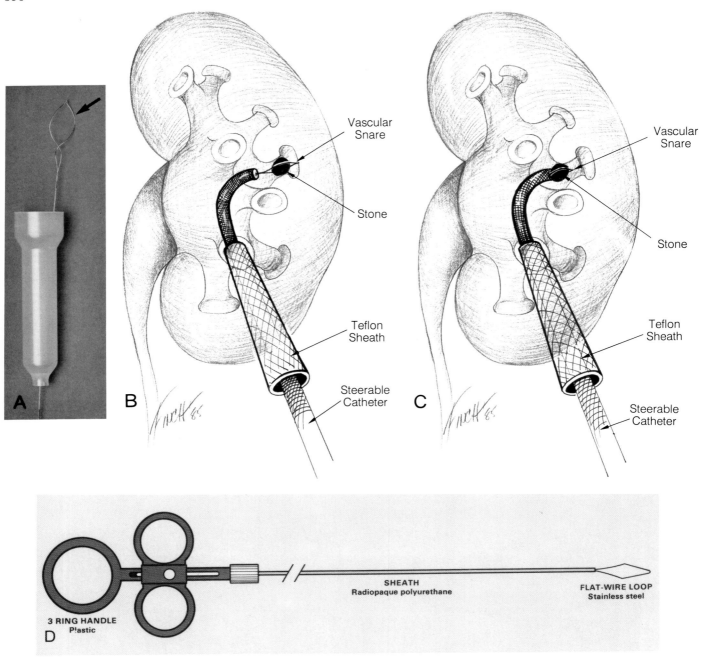

Fig. 23–259   A. Vascular snare (arrow). B. Capture of caliceal stone with vascular snare introduced through steerable catheter. Snare has been gently manipulated around stone. C. Snare has been closed to trap stone, which is then gently pulled from calix into renal pelvis and Teflon sheath. D. Loop retriever used for removal of stones from ureter or renal pelvis, as well as for removal of foreign bodies. (Courtesy of Cook Urological.)

the calculus. They are useful mainly for rough-surfaced, small (2–3-mm) calculi. Their principal disadvantage is that the small curved "claws" or "hooks" of the grasping element can easily grasp and tear the collecting system wall. Also, once the wall has been grasped, there is no way to loosen the tissue from the hooks. What little fluoroscopic use these forceps have seen has not been notably successful, and they probably should be used only under direct vision.

The 7F flexible alligator forceps provide a firmer grip on calculi, and the jaws can be rotated to find a better

grasping point. If tissue is also grasped, it can easily be released. These forceps need a 13F Burhenne steerable catheter for introduction and guidance.

Rigid forceps.   Three types of rigid forceps can be used for percutaneous calculus removal:

1. Randall's forceps (Fig. 23–261A) open with a scissors motion (Fig. 23–262A). A groove (Fig. 23–263A) must be made in the tip for introduction over a guidewire (Fig. 23–264A).[58,74,128,167,168,170,194,207]
2. Mazzariello–Caprini forceps (Fig. 23–261B) open by

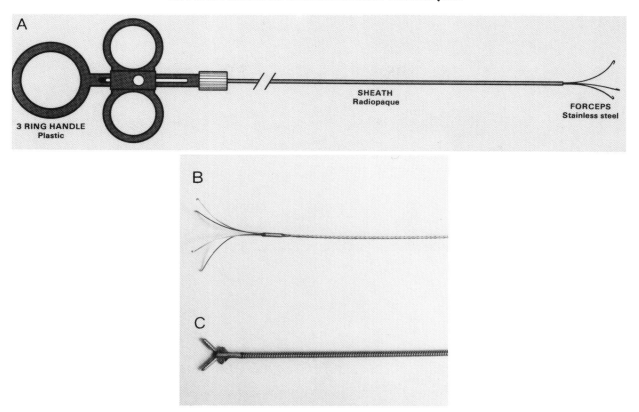

Fig. 23–260   Forceps designs. A. 3-prong grasping forceps. (Courtesy of Cook Urological.) B. 4-prong grasping forceps. C. 7F alligator forceps.

rotating along the axis (Fig. 23–262B) so the transverse diameter does not increase. A long groove down the entire distal shaft (Fig. 23–263B) is necessary for introduction over a guidewire (Fig. 23–264B).[58,74,128,167,194,207,213]

3. Laryngeal biopsy forceps come in two shapes that have either a direct or a side bite.

The Randall's and the Mazzariello–Caprini forceps are introduced directly through the tract, whereas the laryngeal biopsy forceps must be introduced through a Teflon sheath.

Several precautions should be observed. Unskilled operators should not use rigid forceps, because the collection system can be severely damaged. Multidirectional

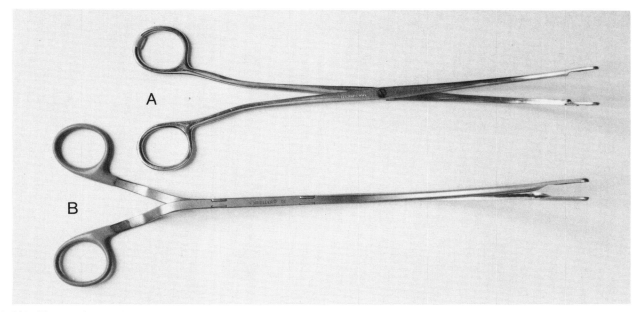

Fig. 23–261   Forceps designs (continued). A. Randall forceps. B. Mazzariello–Caprini forceps.

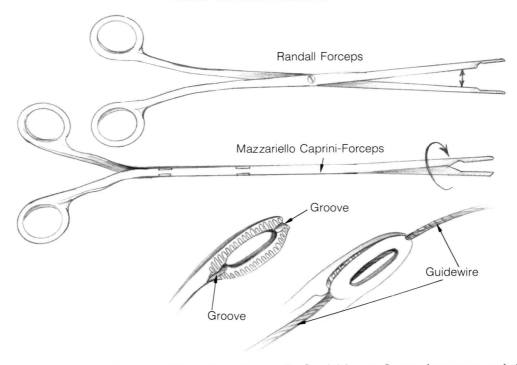

Fig. 23–262   Difference in mechanism of opening of Randall and Mazzariello–Caprini forceps. Inserts show groove made in Randall forceps and fitting of forceps over wire for introduction.

fluoroscopy is mandatory to facilitate manipulation and minimize trauma. Calculi should be smaller than 1.5 cm and preferably located in the renal pelvis, although calculi in calices can also be extracted in this way (Fig. 23–265). Adequate sedation of the patient is critical, because these maneuvers are usually painful.

After dilation of the percutaneous tract, the location of the stone is re-evaluated in several planes. The safety

wire should be in the distal ureter, and one or two working wires should be available in the collecting system adjacent to the stone, because on occasion more than one introduction of the forceps will be needed. The Randall's

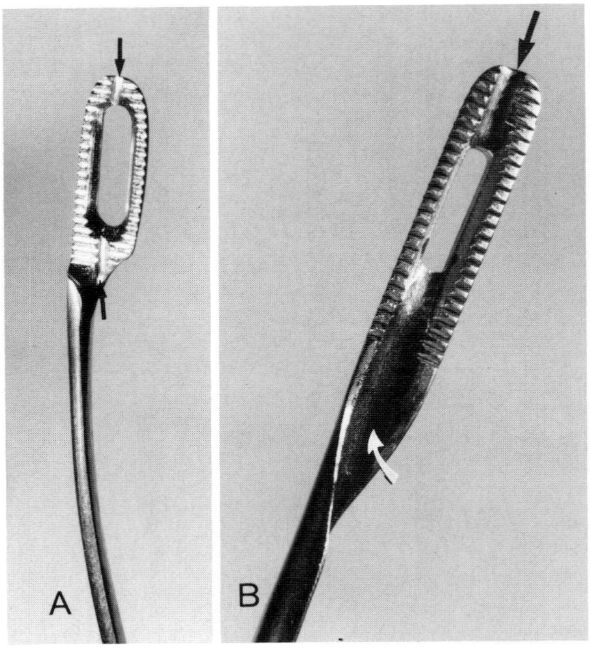

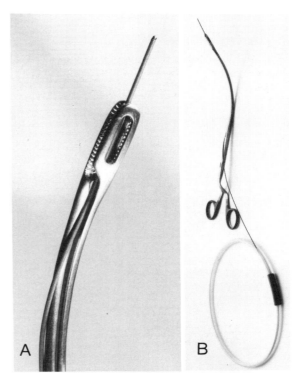

Fig. 23–263   A. Groove made in Randall forceps (arrow). B. Mazzariello–Caprini forceps with groove made in grasping element.

Fig. 23–264   Passage of modified forceps. A. Grooved Randall forceps being advanced over guidewire. B. Mazzariello–Caprini forceps with wire in groove.

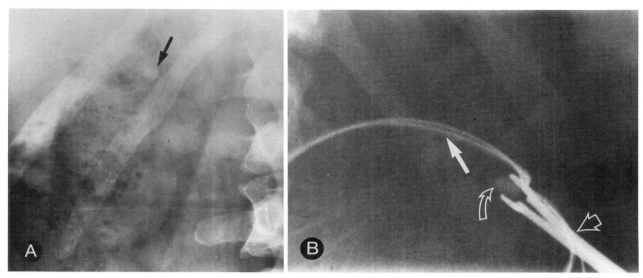

Fig. 23–265 Use of Randall forceps. A. Flat plate of abdomen showing calcific density overlying upper pole of right kidney above level of 12th rib (arrow). B. Two wires have been passed through percutaneous tract (white arrow). Randall forceps (open arrow) have been advanced over one wire and are seen grasping stone (curved arrow) in upper pole calix.

or Mazzariello–Caprini forceps are mounted on the working wire (Fig. 23–266A) and, while holding tension on the wire, the forceps are advanced under continuous fluoroscopy until they reach the vicinity of the calculus (Fig. 23–267A–C). The position of the forceps adjacent to or in contact with the calculus is then verified in two planes 90° apart (Figs. 23–266B,C and 23–267D,E) either with multidirectional fluoroscopy or by rotating the patient. The position of the forceps can be adjusted by moving them back and forth over the guidewire. Once the correct position is reached, the wire is released. (Opening and rotating the jaws or gently shaking the wire is usually sufficient, although occasionally, the wire must be pulled back, particularly with the Mazzariello–Caprini forceps.[213]) With the wire out of the way, the closed forceps are gently manipulated to "tap" the stone. Multidirectional fluoroscopy is used liberally to assess progress. Only when the stone can be "felt" with the forceps are the jaws opened.

The opened jaws are not used to "bite" at the stone; instead, they are gently rotated around the stone until the stone "falls" between the jaws. Only then are the jaws closed. With the stone thus firmly in the center of the "spoon" of the graspers, loss of the stone into the urinary tract is essentially impossible. A good grasp of the stone is definitely needed before starting to pull it back through the tract (Fig. 23–267F), because there are several naturally narrower areas where it might get dislodged from the forceps. During the pullback, the position of the safety wire should be carefully maintained, because profuse bleeding is not unusual in these acutely dilated tracts after rigid forceps manipulation. Not uncommonly a combination of techniques is necessary; fragmentation and grasping are used to speed the extraction process of large hard stones (Fig. 23–268).

Nasopharyngeal forceps. Of the two types available, the direct-biting forceps are the most useful. They are introduced through the Teflon sheath, because they cannot be grooved for introduction over a wire (Fig. 23–269A–C). Smaller calculi (4–5 mm) are easily grasped if they are directly in the path of the sheath (Fig. 23–269D).[91,267] The jaws open without a corresponding increase in shaft diameter. With the side-bite forceps, one can grasp stones that are not in a direct path with the nephrostomy tract.

Nephrostolithotomy in Renal Allografts

Renal transplantation has become routine in the management of end-stage renal disease. Newer and more effective immunosuppressive drugs have lowered the incidence of rejection, thus prolonging the life of the allograft; and improved technical expertise has decreased the incidence of vascular and urologic complications.[278] Nonetheless, many complications occur, an increasing number of which are amenable to interventional radiology techniques, as discussed earlier in this chapter.

The formation of calculi is one of the least common of the urologic complications of renal transplantation, 78 cases having been reported.[279–285] However, it remains an important cause of deterioration of renal function and can cause symptoms and signs that may be mistaken for an episode of rejection. The most common etiology appears to be hypercalcemia due to hyperparathyroidism as a result of adenoma or hyperplasia of the gland.[282–288] However, other causes, such as renal tubular acidosis and hyperoxaluria, have been described. A special group of patients, those who have allografts draining into an ileal loop, are particularly prone to the formation of kidney stones as a result of recurrent infection.[283]

These calculi often have been removed by traditional techniques such as open operation (for stones in the renal pelvis) and endoscopic retrograde manipulation (for stones in the lower part of the allograft ureter). Nonoperative management has been preferable provided there are no complications because of the increased risk of

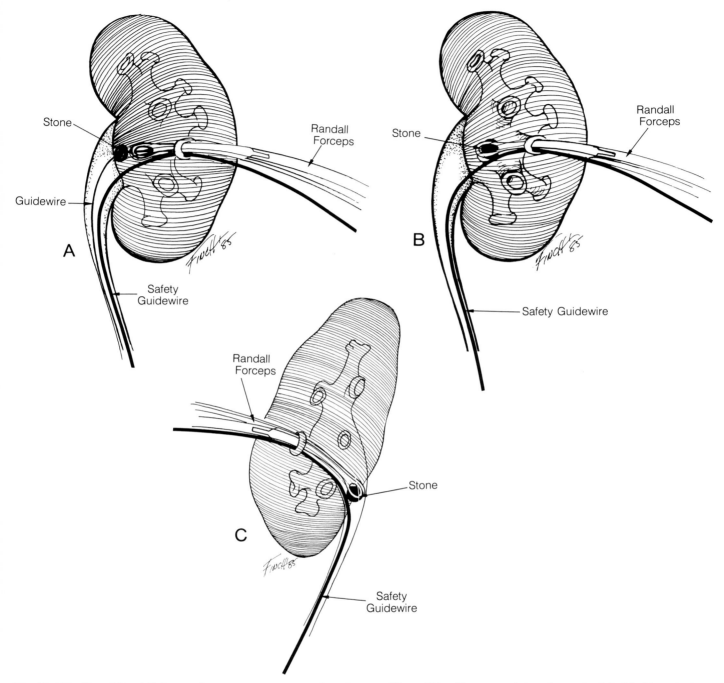

Fig. 23–266   Use of Randall forceps for percutaneous extraction of stones from renal pelvis. A. Forceps have been advanced over working wire into renal pelvis near stone. Note presence of safety wire with its tip in ureter. B. Posteroanterior diagram showing relative positions of tip of forceps and stone in renal pelvis. Working wire has been removed. C. Lateral diagram showing direct relation of tip of forceps to stone.

Fig. 23–267   Patient with large staghorn calculus that was almost completely removed through tract in upper pole of kidney. Retained fragment within posterior lower pole calix could not be reached. A. Second puncture was created into calix containing fragment (large black arrow); two wires have been passed into renal pelvis (small black arrow). Over one guidewire, Randall forceps are being advanced (open arrow). B. Randall forceps at level of renal capsule (open arrow). White arrow points to stone. C. Forceps are seen in more proximal position relative to stone (arrow). D. In anteroposterior projection, forceps are seen close to stone. E. Steep oblique projection shows direct relation of tip of forceps to stone. Forceps have been opened to grasp fragment (arrow). F. Spot film during removal of stone (arrow) to percutaneous tract.

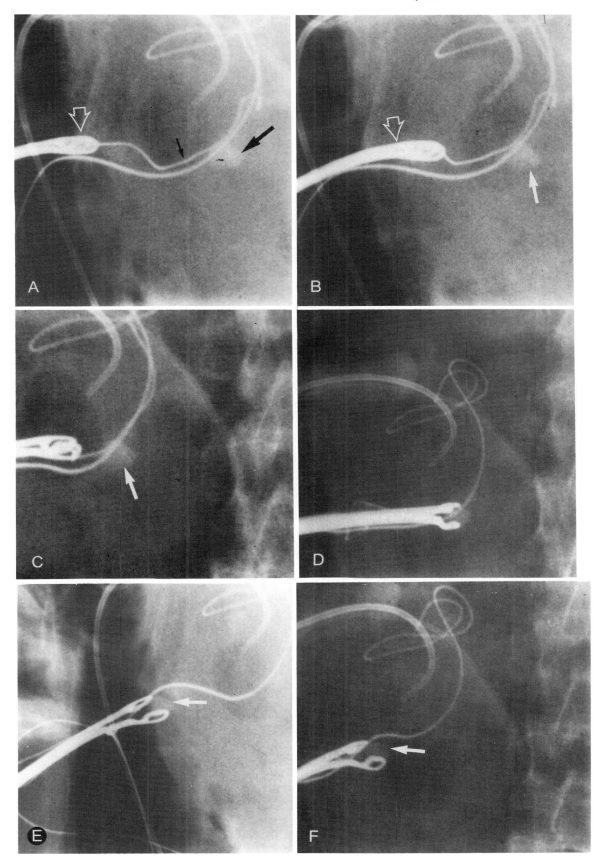

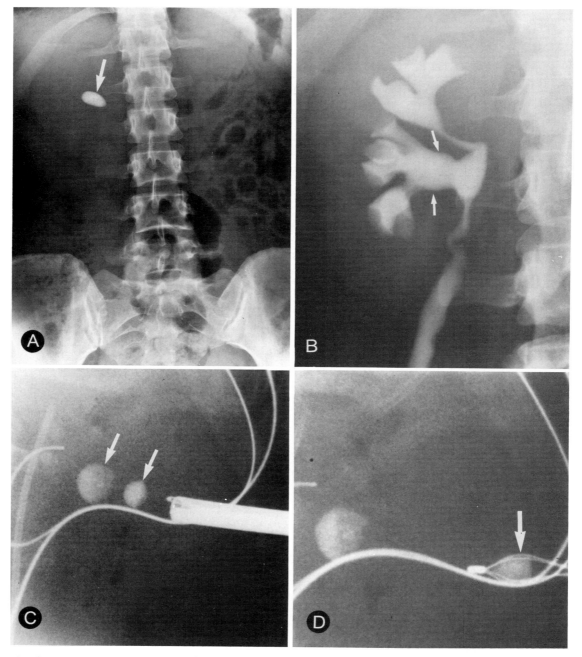

Fig. 23–268 Combination of fragmentation and grasping techniques. A. Large, highly calcified oval stone in right renal pelvis (arrow). B. Bifid renal pelvis with stone lodged in lower chamber (arrows). C. Stone has been fragmented (arrows) with help of ultrasonic lithotripter. Attempts to remove stone under direct vision were unsuccessful. D. Using basket, smaller of the fragments has been pulled out through percutaneous tract (arrow). E. Using Randall forceps, largest fragment has been tilted and extracted through percutaneous tract (arrow).

infection and impairment of wound healing in the immunosuppressed patient.

The percutaneous antegrade techniques described here can be adapted to the removal of calculi from allograft kidneys. The special technical considerations are as follows:

The pelvic location of the allograft necessitates a puncture in the anterior abdominal wall.

The superficial position of the allograft facilitates the puncture into the collecting system.

Perirenal inflammation tends to encase the kidney and restrict its mobility, an important factor when using rigid instruments to reach different areas of the kidney.

The insertion of a large nephrostomy tube after each procedure allows the development of a mature tract (this seems to be unaffected by immunosuppressive

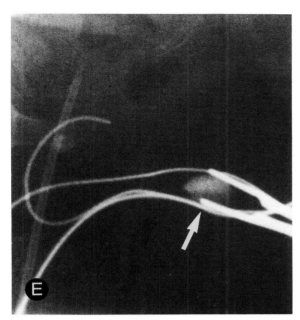

Fig. 23–268E

therapy), which can be used to reinspect the collecting system for residual stone fragments on an outpatient basis.

Other endourologic maneuvers can also be performed through the percutaneous tract. In one case, suture material was removed from within the collecting system. In another case, dilation of a stenotic infundibulum with an angioplasty balloon permitted access to a previously unsuspected stone after a tract had been created into a different part of the kidney to remove a large stone.

Stones ≤1 cm in diameter can be removed intact (Fig. 23–259); larger stones are broken up by ultrasonic lithotripsy and the fragments are aspirated simultaneously through the ultrasonic probe.

Flexible nephroscopy allows inspection of the entire collecting system. The nephroscope can even be passed down the ureter into the bladder or, as has been described in one case, into an ileal loop. Stone baskets or small grasping forceps may be passed through this flexible instrument to remove smaller stones.

Nephrostolithotomy in Pediatric Calculous Disease

Urinary calculi in children are rare in industrialized countries; <1% of the urinary calculi in the United States occur in the pediatric population.[281–291] However, in many parts of the world, including the Middle East, India, and Southeast Asia, there is a significant incidence of urinary calculi in children.[292–296]

In the United States, those stones that do occur in children tend to be the result of metabolic disorders such as hyperparathyroidism, renal tubular acidosis, hyperoxaluria, or diseases that result in hyperuricemia, such as leukemia. Children subject to recurrent urinary tract infections are also at risk, this being particularly important in those patients with neurovesical dysfunction due to conditions such as myelomeningocele or sacral agenesis.

The techniques the authors use for these patients involve puncture of the collecting system with a 19-gauge diamond-tip needle. Once access has been established, the tract is gently dilated to 12F so that a second guidewire can be passed into the ureter. Over the second guidewire, the tract is dilated with balloon dilators or with the Amplatz rigid dilators until a 24F–30F tract is established, depending on stone size. A Teflon sheath is then inserted into the renal pelvis. In children, these procedures are carried out under general anesthesia.[94]

Traditionally, treatment for children with urinary calculi consisted of endoscopic manipulation with a stone basket for stones in the lower third of the ureter, whereas open procedures, such as ureterolithotomy, pyelolithotomy, and nephrolithotomy, were performed for stones located higher in the ureter or in the renal pelvis and calices. There was understandable reluctance on the part of the pediatrician to subject a child to a major surgical procedure for the removal of calculi unless the symptoms were significant. More appealing options are now available, such as percutaneous techniques and extracorporeal shock wave lithotripsy. The authors' initial experience with NLT in children included six patients. The procedure was successful in all cases, with an average hospital stay of 4.5 days and no complications. There is some concern about the long-term effects of nephrostomy tracts. In adults, such tracts in the kidney produce little long-term renal damage.[297–299] Whether the same benign consequences will obtain in children, with their smaller and still growing kidneys, remains to be seen. However, the authors feel confident at present that NLT can be performed in children 8 years of age and older. They are somewhat concerned about establishing tracts of 24F in younger patients because their kidneys are so small and mobile. However, instruments and sheaths of finer caliber will likely become available in the near future for dealing with stones in the younger patients. Extracorporeal lithotripsy may also prove satisfactory.

Nephrostomy Tube Placement

After an uneventful extraction is completed or the procedure is stopped, a drainage catheter equal to or slightly smaller than the tract must be introduced to tamponade the tract, as well as to drain the urine externally. The fastest method is to introduce a drainage catheter through the Teflon sheath (Fig. 23–270A), which is subsequently pulled back over the catheter (Fig. 23–270B,C). If a balloon (Foley, Councill) catheter is introduced, the sheath will have to be cut with scissors in order to remove it from the catheter.

Ideally, a self-retaining catheter (Foley, Councill, Malecot) should be placed (Fig. 23–271), particularly in obese patients (Fig. 23–262), in cases of supracostal punctures or caliceal diverticula (Fig. 23–272), or in patients in whom significant bleeding occurred during manipulations. A self-retaining tamponade catheter has been

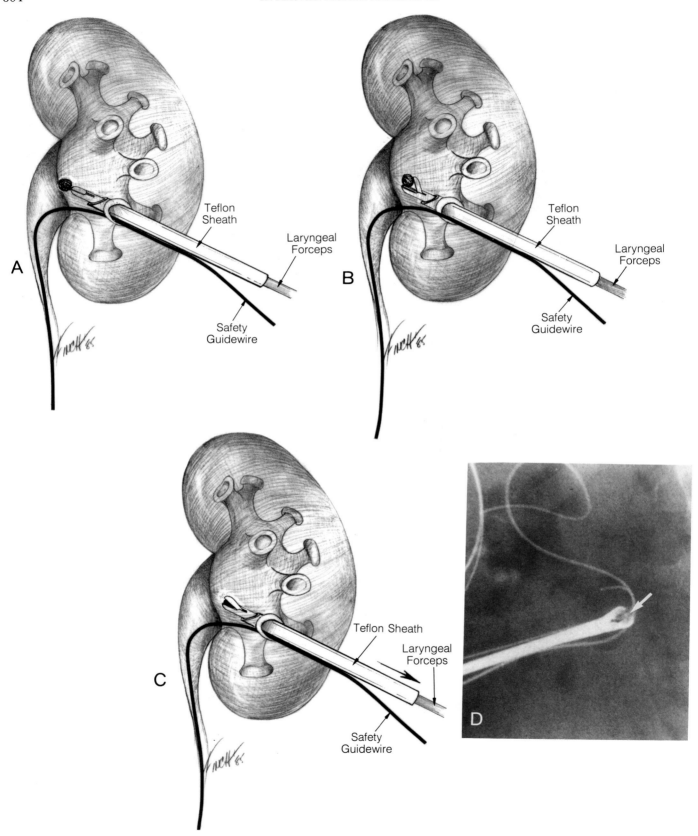

Fig. 23–269 Technique of stone removal using laryngeal forceps. A. Straight-bite forceps have been passed through Teflon sheath until it lies next to stone. B. Forceps have been opened, and stone has been captured by the arms. C. Captured stone is slowly pulled out through sheath. D. Spot film during stone extraction with laryngeal biopsy forceps shows stone trapped by arms (arrow).

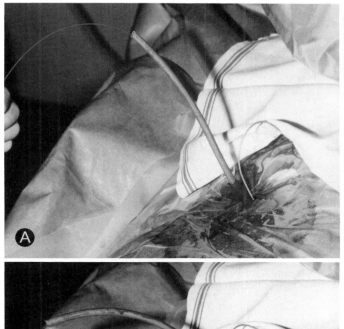

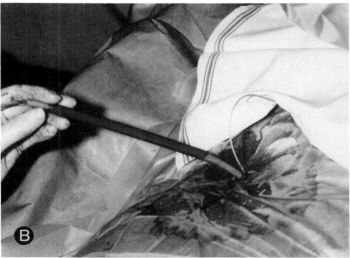

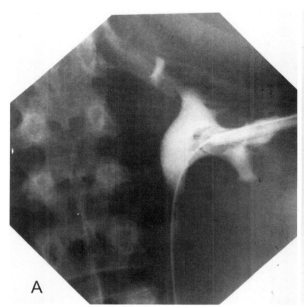

Fig. 23–270 Insertion of drainage tube. A. Straight 22F rubber tube with end hole has been passed over guidewire through Teflon sheath into collecting system. B. Sheath has been pulled back over 22F rubber tube. C. Sheath has been removed, leaving 20F rubber tube within collecting system. Note safety wire beside rubber tube.

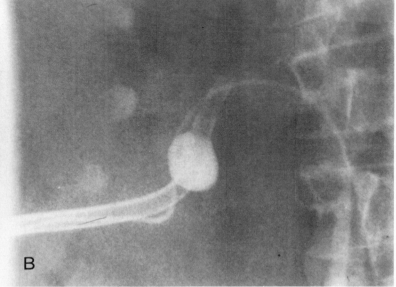

Fig. 23–271 Placement of retention catheter. A. Foley catheter placed through percutaneous tract with balloon inflated in renal pelvis. Safety wire in ureter. B. Spot film showing ideal position of catheter tip away from renal pelvic wall and pointing toward upper pole infundibulum. Safety catheter is in ureter.

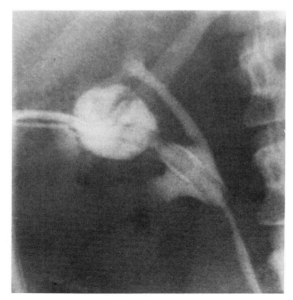

Fig. 23–272 Argyle catheter placed through neck of caliceal diverticulum after stone removal and dilatation of neck with angioplasty balloon catheter. Observe contrast medium partially filling balloon.

developed for use after NLT (Fig. 23–273). In patients with double punctures, either individual drainage catheters (Fig. 23–274) or a circle nephrostomy tube can be placed. In Y tracts, only one tube is required.

Complications of Nephrostolithotomy

As with all invasive procedures, there are certain risks associated with NLT. A few complications are inherent in the use of percutaneous nephrostomy techniques, such as puncture of the kidney, passage of guidewires into the ureter, and dilation of the tract. The use of a nephroscope, ultrasonic lithotripter, and various stone extraction forceps and baskets may produce significant injury to the upper urinary tract. The authors' experience, involving >1200 patients, clearly shows that the complication rates associated with percutaneous extraction of renal and upper ureteral stones depend on the complexity of the stone, the renal anatomy, and the skill of the operator. A small (<1 cm) floating stone in the renal pelvis is the easiest to remove, and no specific complication should occur. In the authors' series, most complications occurred with impacted caliceal and ureteropelvic junction stones, multiple stones, and staghorn calculi requiring extensive manipulations. Embedded ureteral stones were the chief cause of complications such as ureteral avulsion, perforation, and stricture.

The most common complication of this procedure was bleeding necessitating transfusion (11%). Other complications of ultrasonic lithotripsy include incomplete stone disintegration with small fragments remaining in the kidney (4%), displacement of stone fragments (1%), and pneumothorax or hydrothorax (3%). Transient pleural effusion was commonly observed after puncture above the 12th rib. Nephroduodenal fistula was seen in one patient. Some other well-documented complications of nephrostolithotomy include infection, urinoma, injury to

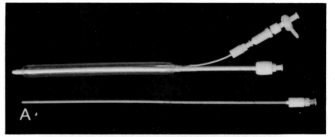

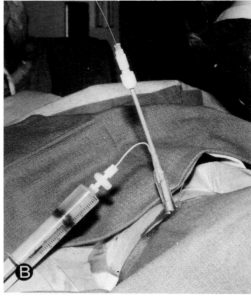

Fig. 23–273 Kaye tamponade catheter. A. Catheter (top) and stiffener (bottom). B. Balloon catheter inflated in percutaneous tract.

adjacent organs, avulsion of the ureter, stone fragment displacement, renal infarction, ileus, and atelectasis/pneumonia. Theoretical complications include hyponatremia and irrigation fluid ascites. The overall complication rate of nephrostolithotomy is low (4%–8%) in the literature, with a mortality rate estimated at 0.2%.

MORTALITY

Obviously, death is the single most important complication. Pulmonary embolism, myocardial infarction, and irrigation fluid intoxication have been responsible for deaths. There has been one death directly related to NLT in an obese, elderly, diabetic patient who had bilateral staghorn calculi. After the second session for removal of residual calculi, this patient suffered a myocardial infarction.[99] The relative risk factors for patients undergoing NLT include hypertension, diabetes mellitus, infected stone, and advanced age.

COMPLICATIONS

Complications can be divided into two groups: periprocedural and delayed. The 5.1% rate of the former, which include bleeding, pulmonary emboli, urinary extravasation, pulmonary problems, and myocardial infarction, is low when compared to the 14%–45% complication rate

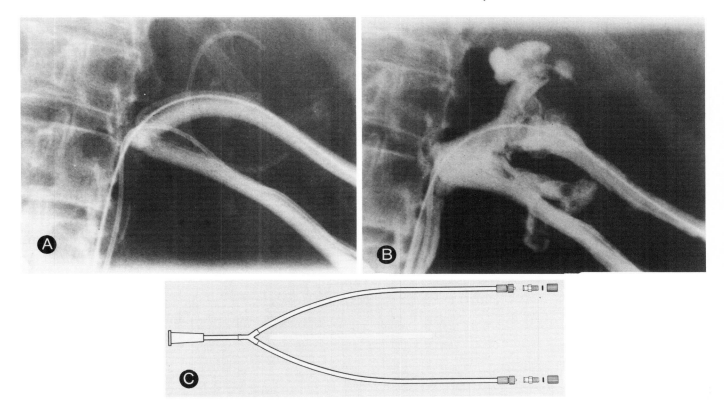

Fig. 23–274 Placement of drainage tubes in patient with double punctures. A. Two percutaneous tracts after removal of large staghorn calculus. Note safety wire alongside each catheter. Additional catheter has its tip in upper pole calix. B. Nephrostogram performed through one of drainage catheters shows multiple filling defects within collecting system, representing stone fragments and clots. There is no evidence of extravasation of contrast medium. C. Plastic flexible Y connector for patients with either circle loop nephrostomies or two percutaneous tracts.

produced by the open surgical method.[91] A delayed complication rate of 30% has been reported after open operation (reviewed in reference 7).

Periprocedural Complications

The following problems have been reported during or immediately after NLT:

1. Hemorrhage;
2. Perforation–avulsion of the renal pelvis or ureter;
3. Urinoma;
4. Retroperitoneal hematoma;
5. Hematuria;
6. Infection;
7. Fever;
8. Contrast medium reaction;
9. UPJ obstruction;
10. Hydrothorax or pneumothorax;
11. Nephrostomy tube dislodgment;
12. Loss of nephrostomy tract;
13. Failure to reach or retrieve the stone;
14. Residual stones;
15. Equipment failure;
16. Foreign body;
17. Electrolyte imbalance.

The management of the most significant of these will be discussed.

Perforation of the renal pelvis or proximal ureter. Perforations of the renal pelvis can occur when the needle passes through the anterior wall at the time of initial nephrostomy. This technical problem is avoidable if the operator watches the needle advancement step by step under multidirectional fluoroscopy. Perforations occur predominantly in small renal pelves (Fig. 23–275), bifid collecting systems, and renal pelves filled with calculi so that there is no room for manipulations (Fig. 23–276). Also, perforations are more common when the nephrostomy tract is dilated with metal or semirigid dilators and less common with balloon dilatation.[130] Undue force on the medial or anterior wall of the renal pelvis may tear the collecting system. The advancement of dilators over a coaxial catheter or a guidewire, along with distention of the renal pelvis with saline or contrast medium through a ureteral catheter, lessens the chance of perforations.[130]

At the time of renal stone removal, perforations of the renal pelvis impair visibility of the area of interest due to the contrast extravasation. If it becomes impossible to locate the instruments or the stone, the procedure should be postponed, leaving a safety catheter in the ureter and a Malecot or balloon catheter in the renal pelvis for drainage. Usually, tears in the renal pelvis heal within 48–72 hr[258,268]; this can be verified with a nephrostogram.

If there is a discrepancy of ≥1 liter between the input and the output of the irrigant at the time of nephroscopy,

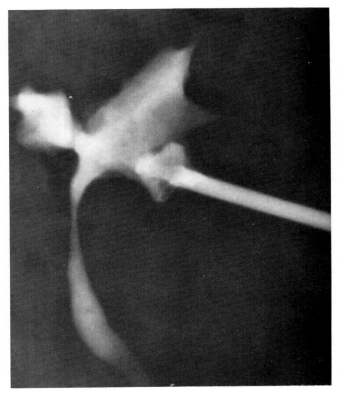

Fig. 23–275 Nephrostogram following percutaneous stone extraction shows perforation of renal pelvic wall by stiff Malecot nephrostomy tube. No intervention was necessary other than repositioning of tube.

a tear in the renal pelvis should be suspected and the procedure terminated.

Extraction of stones from the proximal ureter with baskets or graspers can result in avulsion. Perforation leads to periluminal positioning of the instruments and perhaps of stones. Thus, it is crucial to check the position of baskets with biplane fluoroscopy or under direct vision before they are opened.[130]

Withdrawal of graspers or baskets can entrap the ureteral wall, perhaps avulsing it. The presence of a safety guidewire or catheter in the ureter helps in dealing with these problems; a catheter with multiple sideholes can be placed over the guidewire to stent the ureter until the perforation heals. Concomitant external drainage of the renal pelvis is required (Fig. 23–277). Perforation of the ureter may result in migration of renal pelvic or proximal ureteral stones into the retroperitoneal tissues; such displacement appears to cause no problems if the stones are free of infection, and no further treatment may be required.

Urinoma. A urinoma may result from a tear in the renal pelvis associated with ureteral obstruction or poor drainage from an improperly positioned nephrostomy catheter. In the latter instance, the distal holes of the tube are outside the kidney in the perinephric space and the proximal holes are within the renal pelvis, draining the urine into the retroperitoneum. Unrecognized large urine collections in the retroperitoneal space can displace

the kidney and, by their mass effect, cause secondary hydronephrosis.

In NLT procedures, 24F–30F tracts are created. In cases complicated by perforations of the renal pelvis, placement of a smaller (8F–10F) nephrostomy catheter allows backflow of urine along the nephrostomy tract, the result being urinoma formation. In these cases, the tract should be tamponaded with a 20F–24F balloon catheter. The 24F funnel catheter described by Amplatz (Cook, Inc.) is ideal in this situation. It consists of a 24F proximal shaft with multiple sideholes that tapers to a long 8F stent. The sideholes are placed within the renal pelvis and the 8F segment in the ureter with the tip in the bladder.

Urinomas are easily identified with cross-sectional imaging techniques, such as ultrasonography or CT. These fluid collections can easily be drained under fluoroscopic guidance, following their opacification, with pigtail, Malecot, or VanSonnenberg catheters.[130]

Infection with or without abscess or pyonephrosis. At the University of Minnesota, routine prophylactic antibiotics are administered before, during, and after the procedure until the last tube comes out of the patient. This regimen has drastically reduced infection rates, although one case of perirenal abscess was encountered among the first 600 cases.[237] Patients with known urosepsis are treated with parenteral antibiotics for 48–72 hr prior to the procedure and then with oral antibiotics for several days after stone extraction.[130]

The extraction procedure is terminated in patients with infected stones whenever inadvertent perforations are detected during the puncture or dilation.[130] This prevents the passage of infected urine and irrigant into the perinephric space. Perinephric abscess may thereby be avoided.

The obstructed infected collecting system results in pyonephrosis. Extraction procedures should not be contemplated until the infected urine is drained by a percutaneous nephrostomy and the infection is brought under control with parenteral antibiotics. Even slight manipulations such as nephrostograms may result in frank systemic urosepsis, so manipulations must be minimized.

Postlithotomy pyonephrosis can develop in infected patients if the collecting system is obstructed with blood clots or if no effective external drainage system is in place.

The rate of bacteriuria during hospitalization has been <2%, and the condition has occurred in 7%–14% of patients after stone extraction.[130]

Chest complications, such as pneumothorax and hydrothorax. Nephrostomies below the 12th rib are associated with a 1% rate of pleuropulmonary complications. At the University of Minnesota Hospitals, 60 patients have undergone stone extraction through the 11th intercostal space, and 9 of these had various degrees of pleural fluid accumulation. In six, the accumulation was minimal. Two patients had moderate collections, and only one required thoracocentesis and chest tube placement. In this patient, 1500 ml of blood-stained fluid were drained without sequelae (Fig. 23–278). No cases of pneumothorax have been encountered.

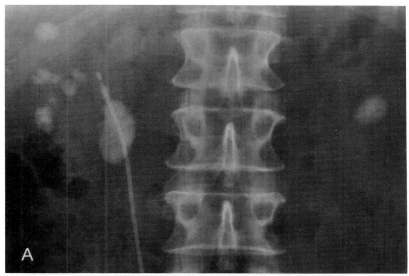

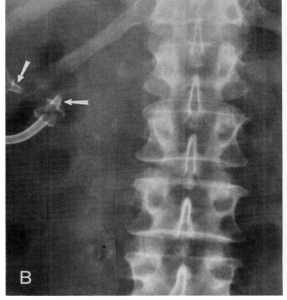

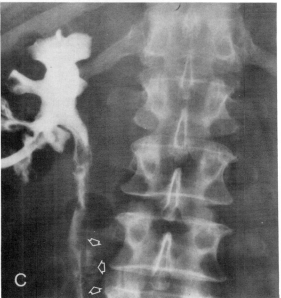

Fig. 23–276 Loss of stone fragments from urinary tract. A. Plain film of abdomen shows multiple caliceal stones and large pelvic stone. Ureteral catheter is in place. B. Plain film after percutaneous stone extraction including ultrasonic lithotripsy shows multiple residual fragments. Two nephrostomy tubes are in place (arrows). B. Nephrostogram shows fragments to be outside ureter in retroperitoneum (open arrows). Filling defects in collecting system and upper ureter represent clotted blood.

With the patient in the prone position, the posterior costodiaphragmatic recess usually extends to the level of the 12th rib. Therefore, at the time of the initial nephrostomy tube placement, careful observation is needed to avoid puncturing the lung.

As pointed out by Young et al, in patients with higher than usual kidneys, the posterior costodiaphragmatic recesses are obliterated.[255] In this institution, routine use of 30F Amplatz working sheaths has prevented the leakage of air and fluid into the pleural space even in these patients.[254] In the patient who required thoracentesis, the stone extraction had been carried out without a working sheath.

Ureteropelvic-junction obstruction. This type of acute obstruction may result from hemorrhage secondary to instrumentation and manipulations at the time of lithotripsy (Fig. 23–279). Also, mechanical trauma and edematous reaction of the mucosa secondary to basket or grasper manipulation may result in obstruction. When obstruction is discovered, the drainage catheter is kept open with no irrigations. Vigorous diuresis is produced by the administration of fluid at 100–200 ml/hr along with the administration of 6 g of mannitol or 10–20 mg of furosemide (Lasix) to help decrease clot formation within the collecting system.[245] Usually, within 1–2 days, the blood clots are lysed by the urokinase in the urine, and external drainage of blood-tinged urine is observed.

Nephrostomy tube dislodgment. Nephrostomy tubes that were placed through the intercostal space (Fig. 23–280) in a small renal pelvis and in obese patients are

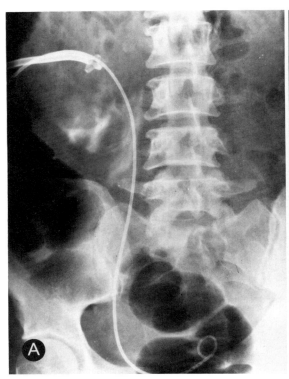

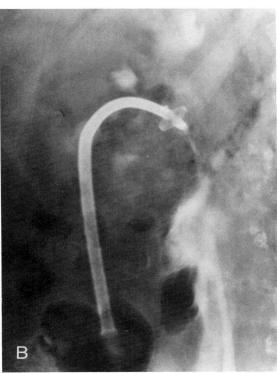

Fig. 23-277 Ureteral perforation during stone removal. A. 7F angiogram catheter passed into bladder after first-stage percutaneous nephrostomy; 14F Malecot nephrostomy tube in place for drainage. Extravasated contrast medium in perinephric space is result of leakage during tract dilatation. B. At completion of basket removal of upper ureteral stone, nephrostogram demonstrates extravasation from proximal ureter. Patient had uneventful recovery.

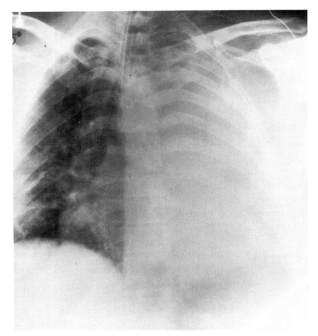

Fig. 23-278 Large hydrothorax following puncture above 12th rib.

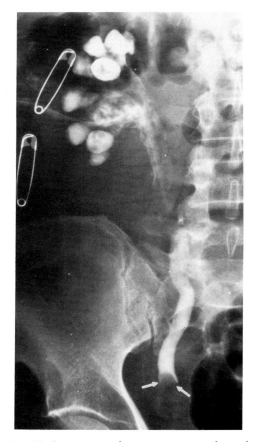

Fig. 23-279 Nephrostogram demonstrates complete obstruction (arrows). Following balloon dilatation, ureter was stented.

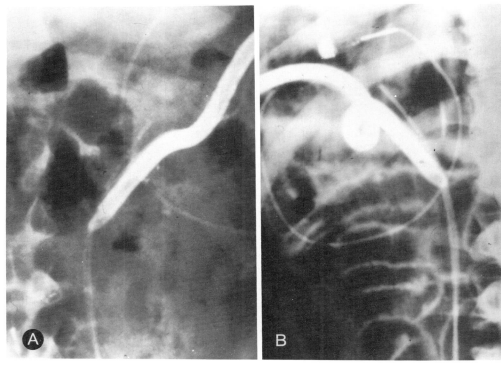

Fig. 23–280 A. Straight 24F rubber tube placed with tip in renal pelvis following supercostal puncture for percutaneous stone removal. Observe tip of ureteral catheter within upper pole. B. Flat plate of abdomen taken 3 hr after manipulation because of pain shows kinking of catheter at level of intercostal space due to breathing motion.

more easily dislodged.[130] In the supracostal approach, the excursions of breathing and the movements of the diaphragm are transmitted to the drainage catheter, which is therefore prone to dislodgment. In obese patients, even though a longer (15–20 cm) tube is utilized, only a small distal segment is within the renal pelvis, and it can easily be pulled out by excessive movements and the shifting of abdominal panniculus (Fig. 23–281).[245]

To reduce the risk of tube loss in these situations, the safest measure is the placement of a retention tube, such as the Foley or the Councill catheter. If a smaller nephrostomy tube is desired, a Malecot catheter or a

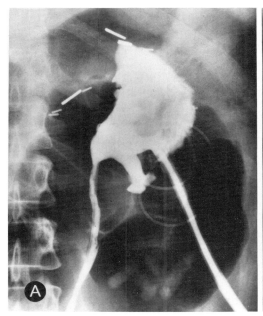

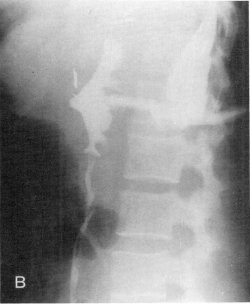

Fig. 23–281 A. Nephrostogram in anteroposterior projection shows extravasation of contrast medium. B. Lateral projection shows extravasation to be in subcutaneous tissues as result of positioning of sideholes within tract. Note indentation of renal pelvis by tip of catheters.

Cope loop can be placed. The newer 24F Amplatz funnel catheter and the Smith–Malecot ureteral stent are ideally suited for this situation, because the long 8F ureteral component secures the position of the 24F proximal segment in the renal pelvis and nephrostomy tract. The techniques for "recapture" of a lost nephrostomy tract were discussed earlier.

Retained stones. Retained stones are a frustrating problem seen in 4%–35% of patients who undergo NLT. The higher incidences usually are seen in patients treated by lithotripsy for staghorn or other large stones.

Residual stone fragments should be searched for by tomography without contrast medium after completion of the NLT. If fragments are found, they usually should be removed by flexible or rigid nephroscopy through the initial nephrostomy tract, although tiny fragments may be left to pass spontaneously. Stones that can be dissolved chemically may be subjected to chemolysis, thereby avoiding further instrumentation. Some operators regularly use chemolysis as an adjunct to primary nephrostolithotomy.[92]

Stone recurrence. The rate of recurrent stones is in the range of 7%–8% at 1 year in patients who underwent fragmentation extraction, as opposed to 10%–15% following open surgery. If the stone was removed whole, without fragmentation, an incidence of 2% at 1 year has been described.

Any residual fragments left at the time of the initial NLT might grow into larger fragments, so every effort should be made to remove them with flexible or rigid nephroscopes or by flushing.

Hemorrhage. Bleeding is a frequent problem in NLT procedures and ranges in severity from the slight bleeding nearly always observed after nephrostomy puncture and tract dilatation to life-threatening blood loss.

Transient hematuria that does not require transfusion is common for 12–24 hr after puncture or NLT. Slow oozing of blood with a drop in the hematocrit is conservatively treated with bed rest, sedation, and transfusion. This form of bleeding may be encountered in 4%–10% of NLT cases.

Severe bleeding may manifest either acutely or after a delay. Acute severe bleeding is secondary to transection of segmental arteries and calls for termination of the procedure. A fascial dilator as big as the nephrostomy tract, usually 24F–30F, or a 10-cm-long, 10-mm-diameter angioplasty balloon catheter is inserted over the guidewire into the tract until the tip is within the renal pelvis, and the balloon is inflated. This maneuver commonly controls the bleeding within 20–30 min, at which time the balloon or fascial dilators are replaced by a retention balloon catheter such as the Foley or Councill with a diameter equal to that of the dilated tract. The patient is observed for 24 hr in the hospital, and the stone extraction is postponed for 2 weeks to allow the development of a mature fibrous tract into the collecting system.

If no hemostasis is achieved by the initial inflation of the balloon within the tract, the patient is transferred to the angiography suite and turned into a supine position. A selective renal angiogram is performed to identify the site of bleeding. During the selective injection into the renal artery, the balloon should be deflated, because otherwise it will inhibit extravasation through the site of arterial injury (Fig. 23–282A,B). The injury is usually identified by selective renal artery injection and is usually a laceration of a lower branch, a false aneurysm, or an arteriovenous fistula. The affected renal artery branch is subsequently embolized with Gelfoam or Gianturco coils, depending on the antomy (Fig. 23–283). If embolization fails, surgical intervention may lead to partial or total nephrectomy.

At times, after successful extraction of stones, a slow, continuous venous ooze with large blood clots in the renal pelvis is noted. This problem is easily managed by the placement of a Foley or Councill catheter and inflating the balloon within the renal pelvis; this maneuver tamponades the renal parenchyma. The catheter should not be irrigated for 12–24 hr.

Delayed bleeding can occur (in <1% of patients) at the time of nephrostomy tube removal or a few weeks later secondary to pseudoaneurysm or arteriovenous malformation.

Vascular complications are encountered frequently when the tract is not properly placed anatomically. The main renal artery divides into a single dorsal and four anterior segmental arteries. The single dorsal segmental artery crosses the infundibulum of the upper pole calix; the other four segmental arteries pass anterior to the renal pelvis.

The puncture should be made into Brödel's avascular area, which is 1–2 cm behind the lateral convex border of the kidney. The needle should be aimed toward the middle or inferior dorsal calix or its junction with the infundibulum. Through-and-through punctures of the renal pelvis may traumatize the anterior segmental arteries and veins and should be avoided.

Nephrostomies in subcostal positions may traumatize the intercostal vessels, and tube placement may erode them, with subsequent pseudoaneurysm formation.[254]

Delayed Complications

Strictures may result from mechanical trauma, including avulsion or perforation, during stone removal (Fig. 23–284).[130,215,258] Many of these strictures can be dilated with a 6–8-mm angioplasty balloon catheter. Afterward, the ureter should be stented for 3–4 months to keep the area open. A nephrostogram should be performed to check ureteral patency before the stent is removed. Strictures at the ureteropelvic junction have been managed by percutaneous incision with a cold knife urethrotome (endopyelotomy) and long-term stenting.[116]

One year after lithotripsy, 7%–8% of patients have recurrent stones, whereas after intact removal, the recurrence rate is 2%.[91,245] The higher rate in patients whose stones were fragmented emphasizes the importance of extracting all the pieces. After open stone operations, the 1-year recurrence rate is 10%–15% (reviewed in reference 91).

Delayed bleeding at the time of nephrostomy tube removal occurs in <1% of patients and can be alarming. Therefore, some operators insert a guidewire before the tube is removed to permit expeditious insertion of a balloon catheter to tamponade the tract.[131] Later bleeding

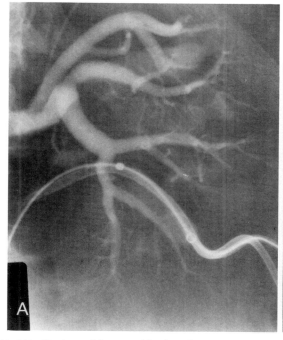

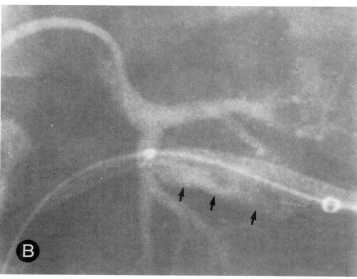

Fig. 23–282 Patient with severe bleeding during dilatation of tract. A. Selective renal arteriogram with dilatation balloon inflated in tract shows no evidence of extravasation. B. Repeat arteriogram after balloon deflation shows extensive extravasation of contrast medium from lobar branch adjacent to balloon (arrows).

secondary to pseudoaneurysms or arteriovenous malformations occurs in 0.6%–1% of patients and is managed by arteriography and embolization.[130,131,300,301] Perirenal hematomas can be detected by CT imaging following NLT (Fig. 23–285).

Colonic perforation. Colonic perforations have been reported with a low frequeny and appear to be most common in patients with little fat in the retroperitoneum, because in those patients the colon tends to have a more posterior location. Most of the patients had an uneventful

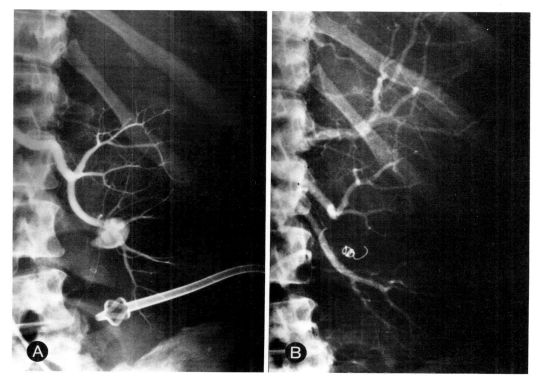

Fig. 23–283 Embolization of pseudoaneurysm. A. Selective renal angiogram demonstrates large pseudoaneurysm. B. Flush aortogram after successful embolization. Note obliteration of false aneurysm. Unfortunately the entire lobar branch has occluded.

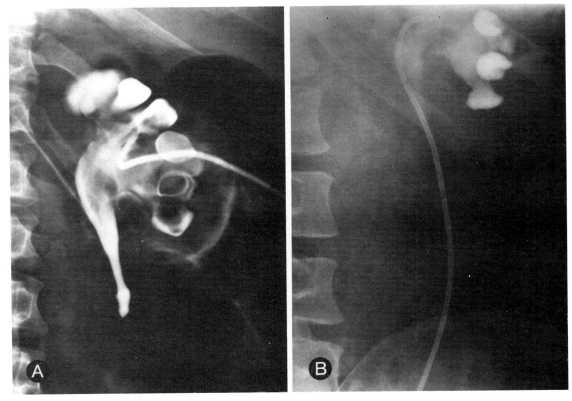

Fig. 23–284   Late stricture. A. Nephrostogram after removal of embedded upper ureteral stone under direct vision shows complete obstruction by stricture. B. Following balloon dilatation, ureter was stented.

recovery with conservative management (intravenous alimentation, antibiotic therapy, and local care) (Fig. 23–286).

Discussion

Initially, it was felt that NLT was ideal only for patients too sick to undergo open surgical procedures for stone removal. Since then, the remarkable success rates

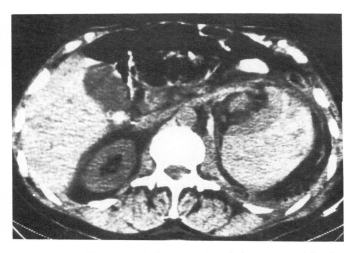

Fig. 23–285   CT scan of large perirenal hematoma following nephrostolithotomy.

(96%–98% for stone extraction from the renal pelvis) have changed the initial philosophy. At present, in most institutions, NLT has replaced the conventional operations, becoming the primary method of treatment in the absence of ESWL. Even staghorn calculi can be extracted by the percutaneous approach, although this may require several sessions and be a frustrating experience for a less experienced team of urologists and radiologists.

Especially in staghorn stones, there is little or no difference in the length and cost of the hospital stay. However, NLT has a striking advantage over the surgical method of stone removal in the length of convalescence, the reduction in morbidity, and the virtual absence of mortality. Patients are able to return to normal activities within 2–5 days after hospital discharge, in contrast to the 6–8 weeks needed after open operation.

A great concern existed initially over whether significant renal damage was produced by the percutaneous procedures. In a series of 82 patients followed for 12–43 months (mean 22 months) after the procedure, Marberger et al found no evidence of arteriovenous fistulae and minimal scars without any deterioration of renal function.[297] Also, Mayo et al performed differential renal function studies by calculating the creatinine clearance with radionuclides 2–3 months after percutaneous stone removal. In patients with normal renal function preoperatively, no functional loss was observed. Indeed, there was significant improvement in patients with preoperatively impaired renal function secondary to infected

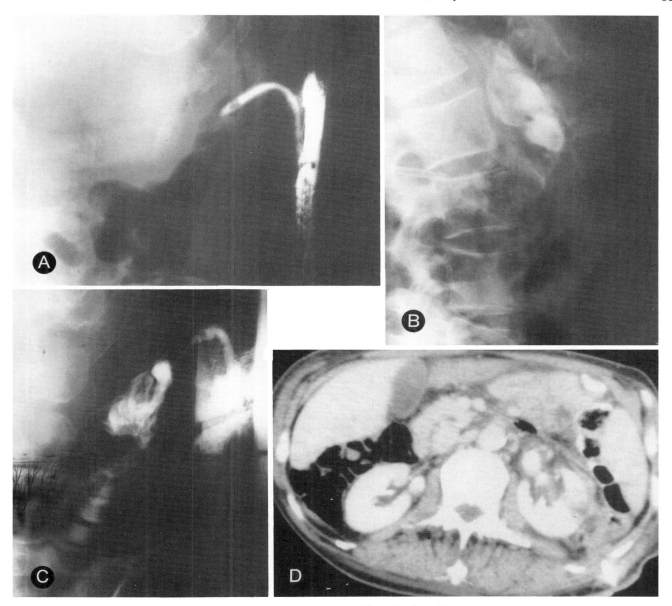

Fig. 23–286 Inadvertent perforation of colon during nephrostolith-otomy. Gas was seen coming out through Teflon sheath during manipulations. After removal of stone, Foley catheter was left within colon and was subsequently exchanged for catheters of smaller dimensions. Patient had uneventful recovery with no evidence of sepsis. A. Spot film showing tip of Foley catheter within splenic flexure of colon. B. Lateral view of abdomen showing extremely posterior position of colon. Observe tip of catheter. C. Injection of contrast medium after withdrawal of Foley catheter from tract opacifies splenic flexure of colon and tract; no evidence of communication with renal collecting system is noted. D. CT scan at level of lower pole of kidneys shows extremely posterior location of colon at this level and loss of fascial planes behind left kidney with area of low density in renal parenchyma.

stones.[298] Early radionuclide studies at the authors' institution likewise showed no loss of function.

The key to a successful extraction procedure is the close cooperation and exchange of ideas between the radiologists and the urologists. The urologists by training are capable of utilizing flexible and rigid nephroscopes and applying electrohydraulic or ultrasonic lithotripsy to fragment stones. The radiologist is responsible for radiation protection, including instructing the staff in how to minimize radiation dose; for formulating a three-dimen-

sional picture of the location of the stone in the renal pelvis; for deciding, together with the urologist, the best approach to each case; and for establishing the percutaneous tract with subsequent placement of a working sheath. These initial steps are the key to the success or failure of the entire procedure.

Until considerable experience has been gained by the team, complicated cases, such as staghorn calculi in solitary kidneys, caliceal stones, and stones in horseshoe or ectopic pelvic kidneys, should not be pursued.

References

1. Goodwin WE, Casey WC, Woolf W: Percutaneous trocar (needle) nephrostomy in hydronephrosis. *JAMA* 1955;157:891

2. Stables DP, Ginsberg NJ, Johnson ML: Percutaneous nephrostomy: a series and review of the literature. *AJR* 1978;130:75

3. Stables DP: Percutaneous nephrostomy: techniques, indications, and results. *Urol Clin North Am* 1982;9:15

4. Babcock JR Jr, Shkolnik A, Cook WA: Ultrasound guided percutaneous nephrostomy in the pediatric patient. *J Urol* 1979;121:327

5. Link D, Leff RG, Hildel J, et al: The use of percutaneous nephrostomy in 42 patients. *J Urol* 1979;122:9

6. Haaga JR, Zelch MG, Alfidid RJ, et al: CT guided antegrade pyelography and percutaneous nephrostomy. *AJR* 1977;128:621

7. Castañeda–Zuñiga WR, Clayman R, Smith A, et al: Nephrostolithotomy: percutaneous techniques for urinary calculus removal. *AJR* 1982;139:721

8. Meyers M: The extraperitoneal spaces: normal and pathologic anatomy, in *Dynamic Radiology of the Abdomen: Normal and Pathologic Anatomy.* New York, Springer Verlag, 1976, p 113

9. McVay C: Abdominal cavity and contents, in *Surgical Anatomy,* ed 6. Philadelphia, WB Saunders, 1984, p 585

10. Davidson AJ: Renal anatomy, in *Radiologic Diagnosis of Renal Parenchymal Disease.* Philadelphia, WB Saunders, 1977, p 17

11. Hodson J: The lobar structure of the kidney. *Br J Urol* 1972;44:246

12. Hodson JC: The renal parenchyma and its blood supply. *Curr Prob Diagn Radiol* 1978;7:1

13. Spirnak JP, Resnick MI: Anatrophic nephrolithotomy. *Urol Clin North Am* 1983;10:665

14. Kaye KW, Goldberg ME: Applied anatomy of the kidney and ureter. *Urol Clin North Am* 1982;9:3

15. Kaye KW, Reinke DB: Detailed calyceal anatomy for endourology. *J Urol* 1984;132:1085

16. Brödel M: The intrinsic blood vessels of the kidney and their significance in nephrostomy. *Johns Hopkins Hosp Bull* 1901;12:10

17. Graves FT: The anatomy of the intrarenal arteries and its application to segmental resections of the kidneys. *Br J Surg* 1954;42:132

18. Graves FT: The vascular anatomy and the principles of intrarenal access, in Wickham JEA (ed): *Intra-Renal Surgery.* Edinburgh, Churchill Livingstone, 1984, p 1

19. Resnick MI, Parker MD: Intrarenal anatomy, in *Surgical Anatomy of the Kidney.* Mount Kisco, NY, Futura, 1982, p 17

20. Boyce WH: Anatropic nephrotomy, in *Surgical Anatomy of the Kidney.* Mount Kisco, NY, Futura, 1982, p 154

21. Sykes D: The correlation between renal vascularization and lobulation of the kidney. *Br J Urol* 1964;36:549

22. Graves FT: *The Arterial Anatomy of the Kidney: The Basis of Surgical Technique.* Bristol, Wright, 1971

23. Elyaderani MK, Durn JS, Gabriele OF: Percutaneous nephrostomy utilizing a pigtail catheter: a new technique. *Radiology* 1979;132:250

24. Hawkins IF: Single-step placement of a self-retaining "accordion" catheter. *Semin Intervent Radiol* 1984;1:15

25. Cope C: Improved anchoring of nephrostomy catheters: loop technique. *AJR* 1980;135:402

26. Cope C: Replacement of obstructed loop and pigtail nephrostomy and biliary drains. *AJR* 1982;139:1022

27. Smith AD, Castañeda–Zuñiga WR, Tadavarthy SM, Amplatz K: A modified Stamey catheter kit for long-term percutaneous nephrostomy drainage. *Radiology* 1981;139:230

28. Tadavarthy SM, Coleman CC, Hunter DW, Castañeda–Zuñiga WR, Amplatz K: Dual stiffness Malecot (Stamey) catheter. *Radiology* 1984;152:225

29. Gerber WL: Use of the Argyle catheter for nephrostomy drainage. *Urol Clin North Am* 1982;9:61

30. Cope C: New Foley catheter introducer for percutaneous nephrostomy. *Urology* 1981;17:606

31. Cardella JF, Castañeda–Zuñiga WR, Hunter DW, Young AT, Amplatz K: A new pyeloureteral drainage catheter. *Radiology* 1985;155:527

32. Smith AD: The universal ureteral stent. *Urol Clin North Am* 1982;9:103

33. Rich M, Smith AD: Applications of the peel-away introducer sheath. *J Urol* 1987;137:452

34. Oswalt GC, Bueschen AJ, Lloyd LK: Upward migration of indwelling ureteral stents. *J Urol* 1979;122:249

35. Mardis HK, Hepperlen TW, Kammandel H: Double pigtail ureteral stent. *Urology* 1979;14:23

36. Camacho MF, Pereiras R, Carrion H, et al: Double-ended pigtail ureteral stent: useful modifications to single end ureteral stent. *Urology* 1979;13:516

37. Brown JP, Harrison JH: The efficacy of plastic ureteral and urethral catheters for constant drainage. *J Urol* 1951;66:85

38. Mardis HK, Kroeger RM, Hepperlen TW, et al: Polyethylene double-pigtail ureteral stents. *Urol Clin North Am* 1982;9:95

39. Lieberman RP: Percutaneous placement and removal of silicone rubber ureteral stents. *Semin Intervent Radiol* 1984;1:19

40. Pollack HM, Banner MP: Percutaneous nephrostomy and related pyeloureteral manipulative techniques. *Urol Radiol* 1981;2:127

41. Zimskind PD, Fetter TR, Wilderson JL: Clinical use of long-term indwelling silicone rubber ureteral splints inserted cystoscopically. *J Urol* 1967;97:840

42. Davis DM: Use of silicone rubber in urology. *J Urol* 1967;97:845

43. Mullison EG: Silicones as artificial internal tissue and organ substitutes. *Ann NY Acad Sci* 1964;120:540

44. Marmar JL: The management of ureteral obstruction with silicone rubber splint catheters. *J Urol* 1970;104:386

45. Orikasa S, Tsuji I, Siba T, Ohashi N: A new technique for transurethral insertion of a silicone rubber tube into an obstructed ureter. *J Urol* 1973;110:184

46. Gibbons RP, Mason JT, Correa RJ Jr: Experience with indwelling silicone rubber ureteral catheters. *J Urol* 1974;111:594

47. Finney RP: Double-J and diversion stents. *Urol Clin North Am* 1982;9:89

48. Gibbons RP, Correa RJ Jr, Cummings KB, et al: Experience with indwelling ureteral stent catheter. *J Urol* 1976;115:22

49. Gibbons RP: Gibbons ureteral stents. *Urol Clin North Am* 1982;9:85

50. Finney RP: Experience with new double-J ureteral catheter stent. *J Urol* 1978;120:678

51. Smith AD, Lange PH, Miller RP, et al: Introduction of the Gibbons ureteral stent facilitated by antecedent percutaneous nephrostomy. *J Urol* 1978;120:543

52. Smith AD, Miller RP, Reinke DB, et al: Insertion of Gibbons ureteral stents using endourologic techniques. *Urology* 1979;14:330

53. Smith AD, Lange PH, Miller RP, et al: Percutaneous dilation of ureteroileal strictures and insertion of Gibbons ureteral stents. *Urology* 1979;13:24

54. Cardella JF, Castañeda–Zuñiga WR, Hunter DW, Young AT, Amplatz K: Long term ureteral stenting: techniques and effectiveness. *Radiology* 1986;161:313

55. Niendorf DC, Kahmi B: Retrieval of indwelling ureteral stent utilizing Fogarty catheter. *Urology* 1975;6:662

56. Smith AD, Hekmet K: Retrieval of Gibbons ureteral stents under fluoroscopic control (letter). *J Urol* 1979;12:133

57. Miller RP, Reinke DB, Clayman RV, Lange PH: Percutaneous approach to the ureter. *Urol Clin North Am* 1982;9:31

58. Hawkins IF Jr: Retrograde nephrostomy tract creation. *Semin Intervent Radiol* 1984;1:9

59. Cardella JF, Kotula F, Hunter DW, et al: The super stiff–floppy guidewire. *Radiology* 1985;156:837

60. LeRoy AJ, May GR, Segura JW, Patterson DE, McGough PF: Rapid dilation of percutaneous nephrostomy tracts. *AJR* 1984;142:355

61. Coleman CC, Kimura Y, Castañeda–Zuñiga WR, et al: Dilatation of nephrostomy tracts for percutaneous renal stone removal. *Semin Intervent Radiol* 1984;1:50

62. Ben WJ, Smith SL, Calonje MA: T-tube dilation for removal of large biliary stones. *Radiology* 1975;115:485

63. Rusnak B, Castañeda–Zuñiga WR, Kotula F, Herrera M, Amplatz K: An improved dilator system for percutaneous nephrostomies. *Radiology* 1982;144:174

64. Clayman RV, Castañeda–Zuñiga WR, Hunter DW, et al: Rapid balloon dilation of nephrostomy track for nephrostolithotomy. *Radiology* 1983;147:884

65. Baltaxe HA, Mitty HA, Pollack HM: Multipurpose coaxial needle used for percutaneous nephrostomy. *Radiology* 1984;153:229

66. Newhouse JH, Pfister RC: Percutaneous catheterization of the kidney and perinephric space: trocar technique. *Urol Radiol* 1981;2:157

67. Lang EK, Price ET: Redefinitions of indications for percutaneous nephrostomy. *Radiology* 1983;147:419

68. Coleman CC, Kimura Y, Lange PH, et al: Percutaneous nephrostomy: indications, contraindications, preparation, and complications. *Semin Intervent Radiol* 1984;1:38

69. Kaplan JO, Winslow OP Jr, Sneider SE, et al: Dilatation of a surgically ligated ureter through a percutaneous nephrostomy. *AJR* 1982;139:188

70. Ekelund L, Karp W, Klefsgard O, et al: Percutaneous nephrostomy—indications and technical considerations. *Urol Radiol* 1980;1:227

71. Pfister RC, Newhouse JH: Interventional percutaneous pyeloureteral techniques II: percutaneous nephrostomy and other procedures. *Radiol Clin North Am* 1979;17:351

72. Clayman RV, Castañeda–Zuñiga WR: Nephrolithotomy: percutaneous removal of renal calculi. *Urol Radiol* 1984;6:95

73. Barbaric ZL: Percutaneous nephrostomy for urinary tract obstruction. *AJR* 1984;143:803

74. Dembner AG, Pfister AC: Fungal infection of the urinary tract: demonstration by antegrade pyelography and drainage by percutaneous nephrostomy. *AJR* 1977;129:415

75. Mazer MJ, Bartone FF: Percutaneous antegrade diagnosis and management of candidiasis of the upper urinary tract. *Urol Clin North Am* 1982;9:157

76. Saxon HM: Percutaneous nephrostomy—technique. *Urol Radiol* 1981;2:131

77. Barbaric ZL, Wood BP: Emergency percutaneous nephropyelostomy: experience with 34 patients and review of the literature. *AJR* 1977;128:453

78. Yoder IC, Lindfors KK, Pfister RC: Diagnosis and treatment of pyonephrosis. *Radiol Clin North Am* 1984;2:407

79. Barbaric ZL, Davis RS, Frank IN, et al: Percutaneous nephropyelostomy in the management of acute pyelohydronephrosis. *Radiology* 1976;118:567

80. Holden S, McPhee M, Grabstald H: The rationale of urinary diversion in cancer patients. *J Urol* 1979;121:19

81. Ortlip SA, Fraley EE: Indications for palliative urinary diversion in patients with cancer. *Urol Clin North Am* 1982;9:79

82. McNamara TE, Butkus DE: Nephrostomy in patients with ureteral obstruction secondary to nonurologic malignancy. *Arch Intern Med* 1980;140:494

83. Whitaker RH: Methods of assessing obstruction in dilated ureters. *Br J Urol* 1979;45:15

84. Whitaker RH: An evaluation of 170 diagnostic pressure flow studies of the upper urinary tract. *J Urol* 1979;121:602

85. Pfister RC, Newhouse JH: Interventional percutaneous pyeloureteral techniques: antegrade pyelography and ureteral perfusion. *Radiol Clin North Am* 1979;17:341

86. Newhouse JH, Pfister RC, Hendren WH, et al: The Whitaker test after pyeloplasty: establishment of normal ureteral perfusion pressures. *AJR* 1981;137:223

87. Pfister RC, Newhouse JH, Hendren WH: Percutaneous pyeloureteral urodynamics. *Urol Clin North Am* 1982;9:41

88. Bush WH, Gibbons RP, Lewis GP, Brannen GZ: Impact of extracorporeal shock wave lithotripsy on percutaneous stone proceduures. *AJR* 1986;147:89

89. Charig CR, Webb DR, Payne SR, Wickham JEA: Comparison of treatment of renal calculi by open surgery, percutaneous nephrolithotomy, and extracorporeal shockwave lithotripsy. *Br Med J* 1986;292:897

90. Segura JW, Patterson DE, LeRoy AJ, McGough PF, Barrett DM: Percutaneous removal of kidney stones: preliminary report. *Mayo Clin Proc* 1982;57:615

91. Clayman RV, Surya V, Miller RP, et al: Percutaneous nephrolithotomy: extraction of renal and ureteral calculi from 100 patients. *J Urol* 1984;131:868

92. White EC, Smith AD: Percutaneous stone extraction from 200 patients. *J Urol* 1984;132:437

93. Woodside JR, Stevens GF, Stark GL, Borden TA, Ball WS: Percutaneous stone removal in children. *J Urol* 1985;134:1166

94. Hulbert JC, Reddy PK, Gonzalez R, et al: Percutaneous nephrolithotomy: an alternative approach to the management of pediatric calculus disease. *Pediatrics* 1985;76:610

95. Reddy PK, Hulbert JC, Lange PH, et al: Percutaneous removal of renal and ureteral calculi: experience with 400 cases. *J Urol* 1985;134:662

96. Segura JW, Patterson DE, LeRoy AJ, et al: Percutaneous removal of kidney stones: review of 1,000 cases. *J Urol* 1985;134:1077

97. Adams GW, Oke EJ, Dunnick NR, Carson CC: Percutaneous lithotripsy of staghorn calculi. *AJR* 1985;145:803

98. Kerlan RK Jr, Kahn RK, Laberge JM, Pogany AC, Ring EJ: Percutaneous removal of renal staghorn calculi. *AJR* 1985;145:797

99. Lee WJ, Smith AD, Cubelli V, Vernance FM: Percutaneous nephrolithotomy: analysis of 500 consecutive cases. *Urol Radiol* 1986;8:61

100. Snyder JA, Smith AD: Staghorn calculi: percutaneous extraction versus anatrophic nephrolithotomy. *J Urol* 1986;136:351

101. Kahnoski RJ, Lingeman JE, Coury TA, Steele RE, Mosbaugh PG: Combined percutaneous and extracorporeal shock wave lithotripsy for staghorn calculi: an alternative to anatrophic nephrolithotomy. *J Urol* 1986;135:679

102. Preminger GM, Clayman RV, Curry T, Redman HC, Peters PC: Outpatient percutaneous nephrolithotomy. *J Urol* 1986;136:355

103. Streem SB, Pontes JE: Percutaneous management of upper tract transitional cell carcinoma. *J Urol* 1986;135:773

104. Smith AD, Orihuela E, Crowley AR: Percutaneous management of renal pelvic tumors: a treatment option in selected cases. *J Urol* 1987;137:852

105. Smith AD: Retrieval of ureteral stents. *Urol Clin North Am* 1982;9:109

106. Hunter DW, Castañeda–Zuñiga WR, Coleman CC, Herrera M, Amplatz K: Percutaneous techniques in the management of urological complications in renal transplant patients. *Radiology* 1983;148:407

107. Barbaric ZL, Thomson KR: Percutaneous nephropyelostomy in the management of obstructed renal transplants. *Radiology* 1978;126:639

108. Glass NR, Crummy AB, Fischer R, et al: Management of ure-

teral obstruction after transplantation by percutaneous ante-grade pyelography and pyeloureterostomy. *Urology* 1982;20:15

109. Dretler SP, Pfister RC, Newhouse JM: Renal-stone dissolution via percutaneous nephrostomy. *N Engl J Med* 1979;300:307

110. Newhouse JH, Pfister RC: Therapy for renal calculi via percutaneous nephrostomy: dissolution and extraction. *Urol Radiol* 1981;2:165

111. Smith AD, Lange PH, Miller PH, et al: Dissolution of cystine calculi by irrigation with acetylcysteine through percutaneous nephrostomy. *Urology* 1979;13:422

112. Sheldon CA, Smith AD: Chemolysis of calculi. *Urol Clin North Am* 1982;9:121

113. Wickham JEA, Keller MJ: Percutaneous pyelolysis. *Eur Urol* 1983;9:122

114. Clayman RV, Hunter DW, Surya V, Castañeda–Zuñiga WR, Amplatz K, Lange PH: Percutaneous intrarenal electrosurgery. *J Urol* 1984;131:867

115. Cardella JR, Hunter DW, Castañeda–Zuñiga WR, et al: Electrolysis for recanalization of urinary collecting system obstructions: a percutaneous approach. *Radiology* 1985;155:87

116. Badlani GH, Eshghi M, Smith AD: Percutaneous surgery for ureteropelvic junction obstruction (endopyelotomy): technique and early results. *J Urol* 1986;135:26

117. Smith AD, Badlani GH: Percutaneous endopyelopyelotomy: endourological management of a bifid pelvis with ureteropelvic junction obstruction. *J Urol* 1985;134:327

118. Pederson JF: Percutaneous nephrostomy guided by ultrasound. *J Urol* 1974;112:157

119. Pedersen JF, Cowan DF, Kristensen JH, et al: Ultrasonically guided percutaneous nephrostomy. *Radiology* 1976;119:429

120. Stables DP, Johnson ML: Percutaneous nephrostomy: the role of ultrasound. *Clin Diag Ultrasound* 1979;2:73

121. Baron RL, Lee JKT, McClennan BL, et al: Percutaneous nephrostomy using real-time sonographic guidance. *AJR* 1981;136:1018

122. Zegel HG, Pollack HM, Banner MP, et al: Percutaneous nephrostomy: comparison of sonographic and fluoroscopic guidance. *AJR* 1981;137:925

123. Heckemann R, Meyer–Scwickerath M, Hezel J, et al: Percutaneous nephropyelostomy under continuous real-time ultrasound guidance. *Urol Radiol* 1981;3:171

124. Dubuisson RL, Eichelberger RP, Jones TB: A simple modification of real-time sector sonography to monitor percutaneous nephrostomy. *Radiology* 1983;146:232

125. Elyaderani MK: Technique of bedside percutaneous nephrostomy under real-time ultrasonographic guidance. *Semin Intervent Radiol* 1984;1:5

126. Reznek RH, Talner LB: Percutaneous nephrostomy (abstract). *Radiol Clin North Am* 1984;22:393

127. Cope C: Single stick percutaneous nephrostomy. *Semin Intervent Radiol* 1984;1:1

128. Fernström I, Andersson L: Percutaneous puncture nephrostomy, in Andersson L (ed): *Handbuch der Urologie, V/1 Supplement: Diagnostic Radiology*. Berlin, Springer–Verlag, 1977, p 129

129. Coleman CC, Castañeda–Zuñiga WR, Kimura Y, et al: A systematic approach to puncture-site selection for percutaneous urinary tract stone removal. *Semin Intervent Radiol* 1984;1:42

130. Coleman CC, Kimura Y, Reddy P, et al: Complications of nephrostolithotomy. *Semin Intervent Radiol* 1984;1:70

131. Clayman RV, Surya V, Hunter DW, et al: Renal vascular complications associated with the percutaneous removal of renal calculi. *J Urol* 1984;132:228

132. Reddy P, Smith AD: Circle tube nephrostomy and nephroureterostomy. *Urol Clin North Am* 1982;9:69

133. Cope C: Conversion from small (0.018") to large (0.038") guidewires in percutaneous drainage procedures. *AJR* 1982;138:170

134. Pfister RC, Newhouse JH: Percutaneous nephrostomy: types of catheters for drainage, occlusion, and dilation, and fiberoptics for endoscopy, in Anthanasoulis CA, et al (eds): *Interventional Radiology*. Philadelphia, WB Saunders, 1982, p 1025

135. Hawkins IF Jr, Hunter P, Leal G, et al: Retrograde nephrostomy for stone removal combined cystoscopic/percutaneous technique. *AJR* 1984;143:299

136. Hawkins IF Jr: Retrograde nephrostomy tract creation. *Semin Intervent Radiol* 1984;1:9

137. Rusnak B, Castañeda–Zuñiga WR, Kotula F, Herrera M, Amplatz K: Radiolucent handle for percutaneous punctures under continuous fluoroscopic monitoring. *Radiology* 1981;141:538

138. Weyrauch HM, Rous SN: U-tube nephrostomy. *J Urol* 1967;97:225

139. Comarr AE: The improved U-tube catheter. *J Urol* 1964;92:78

140. Comarr AE: Experience with the U-tube for renal drainage among patients with spinal cord injury. *J Urol* 1966;95:741

141. Lunglmayr C, Pecherstorfer M: Long term drainage of the kidney by U-tube pyelonephrostomy. *Br J Urol* 1969;41:394

142. Binder C, Gonick P, Ciaverra V: Experience with Silastic U-tube nephrostomy. *J Urol* 1971;106:499

143. Brantley RG, Shirley SW: U-tube nephrostomy: an aid in the postoperative removal of retained renal stones. *J Urol* 1974;111:7

144. Smith AD, Lange PH, Miller RP, et al: Percutaneous U-loop nephrostomy. *J Urol* 1979;121:355

145. Stanley P, Bear JW, Reid BS: Percutaneous nephrostomy in infants and children. *AJR* 1983;141:473

146. Sheldon CA, Gonzalez R, Mauer SM, et al: Obstructive uropathy, renal failure, and sepsis in the neonate—a surgical emergency. *Urology* 1980;16:457

147. Gonzalez R, Sheldon CA: Septic obstruction and uremia in the newborn. *Urol Clin North Am* 1982;9:297

148. Hunter DW, Castañeda–Zuñiga WR, Salomonowitz EK, Lund G, Cragg AH: Percutaneous nephrostomy in the renal transplant recipient, in Smith AD, Castañeda–Zuñiga WR, Bronson JG (eds): *Endourology: Principles and Practice*. New York, Thieme, 1986, p 56

149. Malsk GH, Urkling ST, Daouk AA, et al: Urological complications of renal transplantation. *J Urol* 1973;109:173

150. Mandy AR, Podestra ML, Bewick M, et al: The urological complications of 1000 renal transplants. *Br J Urol* 1981;53:397

151. Palmer JM, Chatterjie SN: Urologic complications in renal transplantation. *Surg Clin North Am* 1978;58:305

152. Starzl TE, Groth CH, Putnam CW, et al: Urological complications in 216 human recipients of renal transplants. *Ann Surg* 1970;172:1

153. Becker JA, Kutcher R: Urologic complications of renal transplantation. *Semin Roentgenol* 1978;13:341

154. Marshal S, Guthrie T, Jeffs R, et al: Ureterovesicoplasty: selection of patients: incidence and avoidance of complications: a review of 3,527 cases. *J Urol* 1977;118:829

155. Ehrlick R, Smith R: Surgical complications of renal transplantation. *Urology* 1977;10(suppl):43

156. Weil R, Simmons RL, Tallent MB, et al: Prevention of urological complications after kidney transplantation. *Ann Surg* 1971;174:154

157. Simmons RL, Kjellstrand CM, Kyriakides GK, et al: Surgical aspects of transplantation in diabetic patients. *Kidney Int* 1974;1(suppl):129

158. Barry JM, Lawson RK, Strong D, et al: Urologic complication in 173 kidney transplants. *J Urol* 1974;112:567

159. Hackemann R, Hartmann EG, Eicksonburg HU: Combined ultrasound-radiographic detection of ureteral obstruction in renal transplants. *Urol Radiol* 1979;1:233

160. Cayne SS, Walsh JW, Tisnado J, et al: Surgically correctable

renal transplant complications: an integrated clinical and radiologic approach. *AJR* 1981;136:113

161. Salvatierra O, Olcott C, Amend WJ, et al: Urological complications of renal transplantation can be prevented or controlled. *J Urol* 1977;117:421

162. Mekta SN, Kennedy JA, Laughridge WGG, et al: Urological complications in 119 consecutive renal transplants. *Br J Urol* 1979;51:184

163. Colfry AJ, Schlegel JU, Lindsey ES, et al: Urological complications in renal transplantation. *J Urol* 1974;112:56

164. Bewick M, Collins REC, Saxon HM, et al: The surgery and problems of the ureter in human renal transplantation. *Br J Urol* 1974;46:493

165. Pastershank KP, Ty M: Urologic complications in renal transplantation. *J Can Assoc Radiol* 1978;29:34

166. Lieberman RP, Crummy AB, Glass NR, et al: Fine needle antegrade pyelography in the renal transplant. *J Urol* 1981;126:155

167. Mitchell A, Fellows GJ, Wright FW, et al: Hydronephrosis in a transplant kidney: the use of pressure-flow studies to exclude ureteric obstruction. *Transplantation* 1981;32:152

168. La Masters D, Katzberg RW, Confer DJ, et al: Ureteropelvic fibrosis in renal transplantations: radiographic manifestations. *AJR* 1980;135:79

169. Turner AG, Howlatt KA, Eban R, et al: The role of antegrade pyelography in the transplant kidney. *J Urol* 1980;123:812

170. Pfister RC, Newhouse JH: Interventional percutaneous pyelouretered techniques: antegrade pyelography and ureteral perfusion. *Radiol Clin North Am* 1979;17:341

171. Babaric ZL, Thompson KR: Percutaneous nephropyelostomy in the management of obstructed renal transplants. *Radiology* 1978;125:639

172. Shiff M, Rosenfield AT, McGuire EJ: The use of percutaneous antegrade renal perfusion in kidney transplant recipients. *J Urol* 1979;122:246

173. Mayo M, Ansell J: The effect of bladder function on the dynamics of the ureterovesical junction. *J Urol* 1980;123:229

174. Coolsaet BLRA, Griffiths DJ Jr, van Mastrigt R, et al: Urodynamic investigation of the wide ureter. *J Urol* 1980;124:666

175. Newhouse JH, Pfister RC, Hendren WH: The Whitaker test after pyeloplasty: establishment of normal ureteral perfusion pressures. *AJR* 1981;137:223

176. Pfister RC, Newhouse JH, Hendren WH: Percutaneous pyeloureteral urodynamics. *Urol Clin North Am* 1982;9:41

177. Molnar W, Stockum AE: Transhepatic dilation of choledochoenterostomy strictures. *Radiology* 1978;129:59

178. Bron KM: The non-suture skin fixation of drainage catheters. *AJR* 1982;139:404

179. Shoenfeld RB, Ring EJ, McLean GK, Freiman DB: Stabilization of percutaneous catheters. *AJR* 1982;138:972

180. Miller RP, Reinke DB, Clayman RV, et al: Reestablishment of a nephrostomy tract. *Urol Clin North Am* 1982;9:75

181. Pollack HM, Banner MP: Replacing blocked or dislodged percutaneous nephrostomy and ureteral stent catheters. *Radiology* 1982;145:203

182. Gordon RL, Oleaga JA, Ring EJ, et al: Replacing the "fallen out" catheter. *Radiology* 1980;134:537

183. Weiss EQ, Leyva A, Hernandez A: Treatment of lithiasis by the forced injection of liquid and ureteral catheterization by the translumbar route. *Int Surg* 1976;61:419

184. Elyaderani MK, Gabriele OF, Kandzari SJ, Belis JA: Percutaneous nephrostomy and antegrade ureteral stent insertion. *Urology* 1982;20:650

185. Mazer MJ, LeVeen RF, Call JE, et al: Permanent percutaneous antegrade ureteral stent placement without transurethral assistance. *Urology* 1979;14:413

186. Bigongiari LR: The Seldinger approach to percutaneous nephrostomy and ureteral stent placement. *Urol Radiol* 1981;2:141

187. Lang EK: Diagnosis and management of ureteral fistulas by percutaneous nephrostomy and antegrade stent catheter. *Radiology* 1981;138:311

188. Pollack HM, Banner MP: Work in progress: percutaneous fiberoptic endoscopy of the upper urinary tract. *Radiology* 1982;145:651

189. Coleman CC, Kimura Y, Castañeda-Zuñiga WR, et al: Interventional techniques in the ureter. *Semin Intervent Radiol* 1984;1:24

190. Lang EK, Alexander R, Barnett T, Palomar J, Hamway S: Brush biopsy of pyelocalyceal lesions via a percutaneous translumbar approach. *Radiology* 1978;129:623

191. Rosen RJ, McLean GK, Frieman DB, et al: Obstructed ureteroileal conduits: antegrade catheter drainage. *AJR* 1980;135:1201

192. Herrera M, Beawerman S, Castañeda-Zuñiga WR, Kotula F, Amplatz K: The Endocatheter ruler: a useful device. *AJR* 1982;139:828

193. Boren SR, Dotter CT, McKinney M, Rosen J: Percutaneous removal of ureteral stents. *Radiology* 1984;152:230

194. Zegel HG, Teplick SK, Khanna OM: Removal of a dislodged ureteral stent through a percutaneous nephrostomy. *AJR* 1981;137:629

195. Elyaderani MK, Kandzari SJ: Ureteral stent insertion and brush biopsy, in *Invasive Uroradiology*. Lexington, MA, Collamore Press, 1984, p 55

196. Guerriero WG: Gynecologic injuries to the ureter, bladder, and urethra, in Raz S (ed): *Female Urology*. Philadelphia, WB Saunders, 1983, p 357

197. St Martin EC, Trichel BE, Campbell JH, Locke CM: Ureteral injuries in gynecologic surgery. *J Urol* 1953;70:51

198. Rohner TJ Jr: Delayed ureteral fistula from high velocity missiles: report of 3 cases. *J Urol* 1971;105:63

199. Schiff M Jr, McGuire EJ, Weiss RM, Lytton B: Management of urinary fistulas after transplantation. *J Urol* 1976;115:251

200. Lang EK, Lanasa JA, Garrett J, et al: The management of urinary fistulas and strictures with percutaneous ureteral stent catheters. *J Urol* 1979;122:736

201. Goldin AR: Percutaneous ureteral splinting. *Urology* 1977;10:165

202. Bigongiari LR, Lee KR, Moffet RE, et al: Percutaneous ureteral stent placement for stricture management and internal urinary drainage. *AJR* 1979;133:865

203. Günther R, Marberger M, Klose K: Transrenal ureteral embolization. *Radiology* 1979;132:317

204. Günther R, Klose K, Alken P: Transrenal ureteral occlusion with a detachable balloon. *Radiology* 1982;142:521

205. Lund A, Rysavy JA, Hunter DW, Castañeda-Zuñiga WR, Amplatz K: Percutaneous occlusion of the ureter: a new approach for relief of urinary tract fistulae. *Semin Intervent Radiol* 1984;1:92

206. Nadalini VF, Bruttini M, Piccardo M, et al: Angiographic nephrectomy as a nonsurgical treatment of ureteral fistulas. *Urol Radiol* 1981;2:249

207. May ARL, North EA, Nash AG: Renal embolisation for urinary fistula caused by irreparable ureteric injury. *Br Med J* 1981;283:1086

208. Abaskaron M, Peterson GH: Embolization of kidney: treatment for laceration of ureter producing intractable urinary ascites. *Urology* 1984;23:299

209. Witherington R, Shelor WC: Treatment of postoperative ureteral stricture by catheter dilation: a forgotten procedure. *Urology* 1980;16:592

210. Banner MP, Pollack HM, Ring EJ, Wein AJ: Catheter dilation of benign ureteral strictures. *Radiology* 1983;147:427

211. Grüntzig A, Kumpe DA: Technique of percutaneous transluminal angioplasty with the Grüntzig balloon catheter. *AJR* 1979;132:547

212. Russinovich NAE, Lloyd LK, Griggs WP, Jander HP: Balloon dilation of urethral strictures. *Urol Radiol* 1980;2:33

213. Dixon GD, Moore DJ, Stockton R: Successful dilation of ureteroileal anastomotic stenosis using Grüntzig catheter. *Urology* 1982;19:555

214. Pingoud EG, Bagley DH, Zeman RK, Glancy KE, Pais OS: Percutaneous antegrade bilateral ureteral dilation and stent placement for internal drainage. *Radiology* 1980;134:780

215. Barbaric ZL, Gothlin JH, Davis RS: Transluminal dilation and stent placement in obstructed ureters in dogs through the use of percutaneous nephrostomy. *Invest Radiol* 1977;12:534

216. Elyaderani MK, Belis JA, Kandzari SJ, et al: Facilitation of difficult percutaneous ureteral stent insertion. *J Urol* 1982;128:1173

217. Kadir S, White RI, Engel R: Balloon dilation of a ureteropelvic junction obstruction. *Radiology* 1983;147:429

218. Levine RS, Pollack HM, Banner MP: Transient ureteral obstruction after ureteral stenting. *AJR* 1982;138:323

219. Cope C, Zeit RM: Pseudoaneurysms after nephrostomy. *AJR* 1982;139:255

220. Gavant ML, Gold RE, Church JC: Delayed rupture of renal pseudoaneurysms: complications of percutaneous nephrostomy. *AJR* 1982;138:948

221. Boiysen E, Kohler R: Renal arteriovenous fistulae. *Acta Radiol (Stockh)* 1962;57:433

222. McInerney D, Jones A, Roylance J: Urinoma. *Clin Radiol* 1977;28:345

223. Portela LA, Patel SK, Callahan DH: Pararenal pseudocyst (urinoma) as complication of percutaneous nephrostomy. *Urology* 1979;13:570

224. Schwartz BA, Wise HA II: Endourologic techniques for the bladder and urethra. *Urol Clin North Am* 1982;9:165

225. Lee WJ, Greenbaum R, Susl R, Khashu B, Smith AD: Percutaneous antegrade urethral catheterization of the traumatized urethra. *Radiology* 1984;141:251

226. Hare WSC, McOmish D, Nunn IN: Percutaneous transvesical antegrade passage of urethral strictures. *Urol Radiol* 1981;3:107

227. Gonzalez R, Chiou RK, Hekmat K, Fraley EE: Endoscopic reestablishment of urethral continuity after traumatic disruption of the membranous urethra. *J Urol* 1983;130:785

228. Chiou RK, Gonzalez R: Endoscopic treatment of complete urethral disruption using this trocar. *Urology* 1985;25:47

229. Zaontz MR, Gibbons MD: An antegrade technique for ablation of posterior urethral valves. *J Urol* 1984;132:982

230. Zaontz MR, Firlit CF: Percutaneous antegrade ablation of posterior urethral valves in premature or underweight term neonates: an alternative to primary vesicostomy. *J Urol* 1985;134:139

231. Burhenne HJ, Chisholm RJ, Quenville NF: Prostatic hyperplasia: radiological intervention. *Radiology* 1984;152:655

232. Quinn SF, Dyer R, Smathers R, et al: Balloon dilatation of the prostatic urethra. *Radiology* 1985;156:57

233. Castañeda F, Reddy P, Wasserman N, et al: Retrograde transurethral dilatation of the prostate in humans: work in progress. *Radiology* 1987;163:645

234. Rupel E, Brown R: Nephroscopy with removal of stone following nephrostomy for obstructive calculus anuria. *J Urol* 1946;46:177

235. Fernström I, Johansson B: Percutaneous pyelolithotomy: a new extraction technique. *Scand J Urol Nephrol* 1976;10:257

236. Smith AD, Lange PH, Reinke DB, et al: Extraction of ureteral calculi from patients with ileal loops: a new technique. *J Urol* 1978;120:623

237. Clayman RV: Nephrolithotomy (nephrostolithotomy): concepts and rationale. *Semin Intervent Radiol* 1984;1:75

238. Preminger GM, Clayman RV, Hardeman SW, Franklin J, Curry T, Peters PC: Percutaneous nephrostolithotomy vs open surgery for renal calculi: a comparative study. *JAMA* 1985;254:1054

239. Pollack HM, Banner MP: Percutaneous extraction of upper urinary tract calculi. *Urol Radiol* 1984;6:124

240. Wickham JEA, Kellet NJ: Percutaneous nephrolithotomy. *Br Med J* 1981;283:1571

241. Banner MP, Pollack HM: Percutaneous extraction of renal and ureteral calculi. *Radiology* 1982;144:753

242. Dunnick NR, Carson CC III, Moore AV, et al: Percutaneous approach to nephrolithiasis. *AJR* 1985;144:451

243. Wickham JAE, Kellet MJ, Miller RA: Elective percutaneous nephrolithotomy in 50 patients: an analysis of the techniques, results, and complications. *J Urol* 1983;129:904

244. Letourneau J, Lange PH, Kimuri Y, Castañeda F, Castañeda-Zuñiga WR: Nephrostolithotomy: the percutaneous approach to kidney stones, in Elyaderani MK, Kandzari SJ, Castañeda WR, Lange PH (eds): *Invasive Uroradiology*. Lexington, DC Heath and Co, 1984, p 97

245. Clayman RV, Castañeda-Zuñiga WR: *Techniques in Endourology: A Guide to the Percutaneous Removal of Renal and Ureteral Calculi*. Minneapolis, EndoPress, 1984

246. Clayman RV, Surya V, Miller RP, et al: Percutaneous nephrolithotomy: an approach to branched and staghorn renal calculi. *JAMA* 1983;250:73

247. Lange PH, Reddy PK, Hulbert JC, et al: Percutaneous removal of caliceal and other "inaccessible" stones: instruments and techniques. *J Urol* 1984;132:439

248. Reddy PK, Lange PH, Hulbert JC, et al: Percutaneous removal of caliceal and other "inaccessible" stones: results. *J Urol* 1984;132:443

249. Salomonowitz E, Castañeda-Zuñiga WR, Lange PH, et al: Percutaneous renal stone removal: use of carbon dioxide as contrast medium. *Radiology* 1984;150:833

250. Hunter DW, Young A, Castañeda-Zuñiga WR, et al: Carbon dioxide as a lighter than urine contrast medium for percutaneous nephrostomy. *Radiology* 1984;152:211

251. Katzen BT, Edwards KC: Nitrous oxide analgesia for interventional radiology. *AJR* 1983;140:145

252. Saltzman B, Khasidy LR, Smith AD: Elevated renal pelvic pressures during percutaneous renal procedures: reduction by use of working sheath. *Urology* 1987;30:472

253. Amplatz K, Castañeda-Zuñiga WR, Clayman R, et al: Percutaneous stone removal. *Appl Radiol* 1983;12:31

254. Lee WJ, Lom G, Smith AD, et al: Percutaneous extraction of renal stones: experience in 100 patients. *AJR* 1985;144:457

255. Young AT, Hunter DW, Castañeda-Zuñiga WR, et al: Percutaneous extraction of urinary calculi: use of the intercostal approach. *Radiology* 1985;154:633

256. Segura JW, Patterson DE, LeRoy J, May GR: Percutaneous lithotripsy. *J Urol* 1983;130:1051

257. Bush WH, Brannen GE, Burnett LL, Wales GR: Ultrasonic renal lithotripsy. *Radiology* 1984;152:387

258. Kerlan RK, Kahn I, Ring EJ: Percutaneous renal and ureteral stone removal. *Urol Radiol* 1984;6:113

259. Smith AD, Lange PH, Reinke DB: Extraction of ureteral calculi from patients with ileal loop: a new technique. *J Urol* 1978;120:623

260. Young AT, Castañeda-Zuñiga WR, Hunter DW, et al: The CO_2 flush: a new technique for percutaneous extraction of ureteral calculi. *Radiology* 1985;154:828

261. Hulbert JC, Reddy PK, Lange PH, et al: Percutaneous management of ureteral calculi facilitated by retrograde flushing with carbon dioxide or diluted radiopaque dye. *J Urol* 1985;134:29

262. Coleman CC, Castañeda-Zuñiga WR, Miller R, et al: A logical approach to renal stone removal. *AJR* 1984;143:609

263. LeRoy AJ, May GR, Bender CE, et al: Percutaneous nephrostomy for stone removal. *Radiology* 1984;151:607

264. Eshghi AM, Roth J, Smith AD: Percutaneous transperitoneal approach to a pelvic kidney for endourologic removal of staghorn calculi. *J Urol* 1985;134:525

265. Eshghi M, Smith AD: Endourologic approach to a transplant kidney. *Urology* 1986;28:504

266. Picus D, Weyman PJ, Clayman RV, McCleenan BL: Intercostal-

space nephrostomy for percutaneous stone removal. *AJR* 1986;147:393

267. Castañeda–Zuñiga WR, Miller RP, Amplatz K: Percutaneous removal of kidney stones. *Urol Clin North Am* 1982;9:113

268. LeRoy AJ, Segura JW: Percutaneous ultrasonic lithotripsy. *Urol Radiol* 1984;6:88

269. Narayan P, Smith AD: Percutaneous nephrostomy as an adjunct in the management of ureteral calculi. *Urol Clin North Am* 1982;9:137

270. LeRoy AJ, Williams MJ, Bender CE, et al: Percutaneous removal of small ureteral calculi. *AJR* 1985;145:109

271. Bush WH, Brannen GE, Lewis GP, Burnett LL: Upper ureteral calculi extraction via percutaneous nephrostomy. *AJR* 1984;144:795

272. Twomey BP, Wilkins RA: Ureteric stone displacement using a new technique. *Radiology* 1983;146:832

273. Coleman CC, Kimura Y, Castañeda F, et al: Fluoroscopically guided techniques for renal and ureteral stone removal. *Semin Intervent Radiol* 1984;1:63

274. Hawkins IF: New monofilament and soft wire basket. *Semin Intervent Radiol* 1984;1:60

275. Rutner AB: Balloon dilation of lower ureter to facilitate cystoscopic extraction of large ureteral calculi. *Urology* 1983;21:226

276. Young AT, Castañeda WR, Hunter DW, et al: Carbon dioxide as a lighter than air contrast medium for percutaneous nephrostomy. *Radiology* 1984;152:211

277. Clayman RV, Surya V, Castañeda–Zuñiga WR, et al: Percutaneous nephrostolithotomy with Mazzariello–Caprini forceps. *J Urol* 1983;129:1213

278. Williams G, Birch AG, Wilson RE: Urological complications of renal transplantation. *Br J Urol* 1970;42:21

279. Loughlin KR, Tilney NL, Richie JP: Urologic complications in 718 renal transplant patients. *Surgery* 1984;95:297

280. Schweiler RT, Bartus SA, Gradon RJ, Berlin BB: Pyelolithotomy of a renal transplant. *J Urol* 1977;117:665

281. Fisher ME, Haaga JR, Persky L: Renal stone extraction through a percutaneous nephrostomy in a renal transplant patient. *Radiology* 1982;144:95

282. Brien G, Scholz D, Oesterwitz H: Urolithiasis after kidney transplantation: clinical and mineralogical aspects. *Urol Res* 1980;8:211

283. Narayana AS, Loening S, Culp DA: Kidney stones and renal transplantation. *Urology* 1978;12:61

284. Rattazzi LC, Simmons RL, Markland C: Calculi complicating renal transplantation into ileal conduits. *Urology* 1975;5:29

285. Rosenberg JC, Arnstein AR, Ing TS: Calculi complicating a renal transplant. *Am J Surg* 1975;129:326

286. Motayne GG, Jindal SL, Irvine AH, Abele RP: Calculus formation in renal transplant patients. *J Urol* 1984;132:448

287. Christensen MS, Nielsen HE, Torring S: Hypercalcaemia and parathyroid function after renal transplantation. *Acta Med Scand* 1977;201:35

288. Lerut J, Lerut T, Growes JA, Michelson P: Donor graft lithiasis—unusual complication of renal transplantation. *Urology* 1979;14:627

289. Malek RS, Kelalis PP: Pediatric nephrolithiasis. *J Urol* 1975;113:545

290. Bennett AH, Colodny AH: Urinary tract calculi in children. *J Urol* 1973;109:318

291. Bass HN, Emanuel B: Nephrolithiasis in children. *J Urol* 1966;95:749

292. Loutfi A, Abdel HG, Francis M, et al: Study of urinary tract calculi in Egyptian children. *J Egypt Med Assoc* 1972;55:805

293. McCarrison R: Causation of stone in India. *Br Med J* 1931;1:1009

294. Gershoft SN, Pren EH, Chondraparoud A: Urinary stones in Thailand. *J Urol* 1963;90:285

295. Westermeyer JJ: Urinary calculi in Laos. *JAMA* 1971;217:82

296. Thalut K, Rijal A, Brockis JG, et al: The endemic bladder stones of Indonesia—epidemiology and clinical features. *Br J Urol* 1976;48:617

297. Marberger M, Stackl W, Hruby W, Kroiss A: Late sequelae of ultrasonic lithotripsy of renal calculi. *J Urol* 1985;133:170

298. Mayo ME, Krieger JN, Rudd TG: Effect of percutaneous nephrostolithotomy on renal function. *J Urol* 1985;133:167

299. Eshghi M, Schiff RG, Smith AD: Absence of permanent morphologic and functional changes after percutaneous renal stone removal: prospective quantitative study in patients with unscarred, unobstructed kidneys. *AJR* 1986;147:283

300. Cope C, Zeit RM: Pseudoaneurysms after nephrostomy. *AJR* 1982;139:255

301. Gavant ML, Gold RE, Church JC: Delayed rupture of renal pseudoaneurysms: complication of percutaneous nephrostomy. *AJR* 1982;138:948

24

Retrograde Transurethral Prostatic Dilatation with Balloon Catheter

FLAVIO CASTAÑEDA, M.D., PRATAP K. REDDY, M.D., JOHN C. HULBERT, M.D., BERT W. LARSON, M.D., DAVID W. HUNTER, M.D., JANIS GISSEL LETOURNEAU, M.D., KURT AMPLATZ, M.D., AND WILFRIDO R. CASTAÑEDA-ZUÑIGA, M.D., M.Sc.

The prostate is one of the largest glands in the human body, the physiologic function of which remains unknown. Granted, the prostate supplies a large number of components to the ejaculate; their biologic function is essentially unknown. There has been no shortage of speculation on these matters but little compelling evidence.

Despite this gap in our knowledge, it is clear that the growth and function of the prostate depend primarily on androgenic stimulation. In the normal male, the principal circulating androgen is testosterone, which is almost exclusively (>95%) of testicular origin. Under physiologic conditions, the Leydig cells of the testis are the main source of androgens.[1] Other endocrine and growth factors intervene in regulating the growth of the prostate gland, but their role is minimal in comparison with testicular androgens.

The prolonged androgenic stimulation of the prostate throughout the prime reproductive years takes its toll in middle-aged and senior men. The incidence of significant benign prostatic hyperplasia (BPH) in men older than 50 exceeds 80%.[2] Recent statistics reveal that a 50-year-old man has a 20%–25% chance of undergoing a prostatectomy during his lifetime,[3] and a much larger number will suffer intermittent or chronic pain and disability.

Thus, BPH is a serious health problem. The most recent data reveal that 297,000 prostatectomies were performed in 1978 in the USA alone,[4] and it is estimated that 500,000 prostatectomies are now being performed per year in this country. Approximately 44% of these patients present to the clinician in acute urinary retention, and 54% present initially with prostatism. Of the latter, 7% will experience acute urinary retention during the next 5 years.[5]

This common male ailment has been afflicting humanity for centuries. Knowledge of micturition problems dates as far back as the 15th century B.C., having been described in Egyptian papyruses discovered at Luxor in 1856.[6] Thus, it is not surprising that several techniques have been devised throughout the centuries to alleviate obstructive urinary symptoms and their consequences. Some techniques were as radical as castration,[7] whereas others were recommendations of a leisurely life, perhaps of golf and frequent vacations. Dilatation also has been practiced for centuries with the aid of bougies made of all sorts of materials, but it was not until 1844 that L.A. Mercier from France[8] designed a metal dilator specifically for this purpose (Fig. 24–1). Mercier postulated that the mechanism by which obstruction was relieved was stretching of the muscular sphincter at the bladder neck. It is likely that his dilator also stretched the surgical and external prostatic capsules.

In 1910, E. Hollingsworth, during the performance of a suprapublic prostatectomy and because of problems in obtaining good anesthesia, attempted to dilate the prostatic urethra by inserting his index finger through the bladder neck.[9] His results were so gratifying, not only in relieving voiding symptoms, but also in the absence of some of the complications of prostatectomy such as impotence, that he employed this procedure routinely from then on. In 1938, Otto Frank from St. Franziskus Hospital in Flensburg, Germany, reported a large series of patients treated by digital disruption of the prostate.[10] This technique still involved surgery, but it was much less extensive. In 1910, F. Kraemer of Frankfurt was utilizing retrograde transurethral dilatation with dilators as large as 2 cm in diameter.[11]

It was not until the late 1940s that dilatation techniques became widely used throughout Europe and Russia as a consequence of the modifications of the Mercier dilator made by Werner Deisting.[12] The Deisting dilator consisted of a 24F shaft made of two angled dilator branches that remain parallel as they spread apart (Fig. 24–2). Gradual rotation of the wheel with parallel ventrodorsal displacement of the branches caused blunt disruption of the adenoma at the anterior and posterior commissures (Fig. 24–3). The procedure was performed under local anesthesia. Rectal examination was used to evaluate the relation of the dilator to the external sphincter, ensuring that this structure was not injured (Fig. 24–4). The dilatation was carried out in small increments. The noted optimum dilatation ranged from 4–8 cm (Fig. 24–4) with the maximum dilatation being determined by three factors: (1) a distinct increase in the resistance in the screw mechanism; (2) the patient's urgent desire to void; and (3) the maximum desired opening of the blades, as recorded on the measuring rod of the instrument. Once

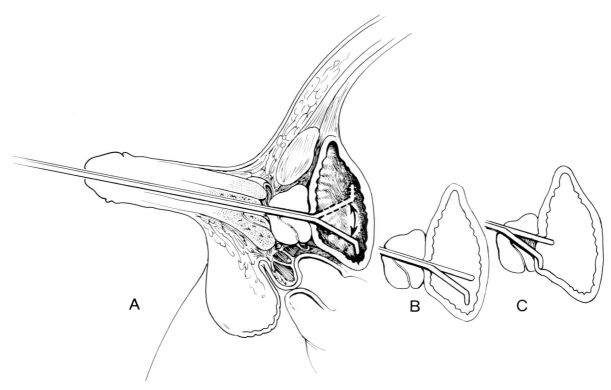

Fig. 24-1 Mercier's urethral dilator. A. Dilator has been rotated from its introduction position (dotted lines) to dilating position. B. Arms of dilator have been opened. C. Dilator has been pulled back slowly to dilate bladder neck and prostatic urethra.

the maximum dilatation was achieved, the dilator was left in place for various lengths of time to exhaust the elasticity of the prostatic capsule (Fig. 24-5).

In Deisting's original work, he reported on 324 patients, followed for 8 years. The immediate success rate was 95.3%, with the failures being due to middle lobe hyperplasia or bladder atony. The long-term failure rates were 1.7%, 5.4%, and 15.2% at 3, 5, and 8 years, respectively, with return of symptoms or postvoiding residual urine being considered a failure or recurrence. The method was found to be easy and to have few complica-

tions, the most frequent of which were epididymitis and prostatovesiculitis. The former was noted in approximately 35% of patients but was not encountered if vasectomy preceded the dilatation. Prostatovesiculitis was seen in 60% of the cases and attributed to the free communication between urethra, prostatic ducts, and seminal vesicles brought about by the tearing caused by the dilatation and permitting the ready spread of infected material to and from these organs. In most instances, the inflammation did not produce clinical symptoms, probably owing to the good drainage from the prostatic ducts

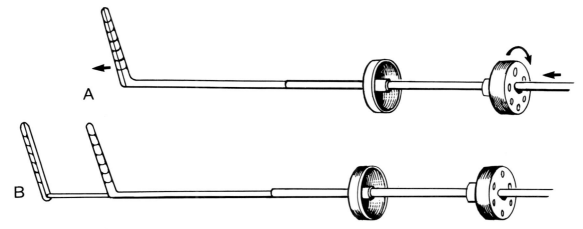

Fig. 24-2 Deisting's prostatic dilator. A. 24F dilator with two-angle dilating branches in closed position. B. By gradual rotation of the wheel with parallel displacement of branches in the ventrodorsal direction, two-angle dilating branches have spread apart.

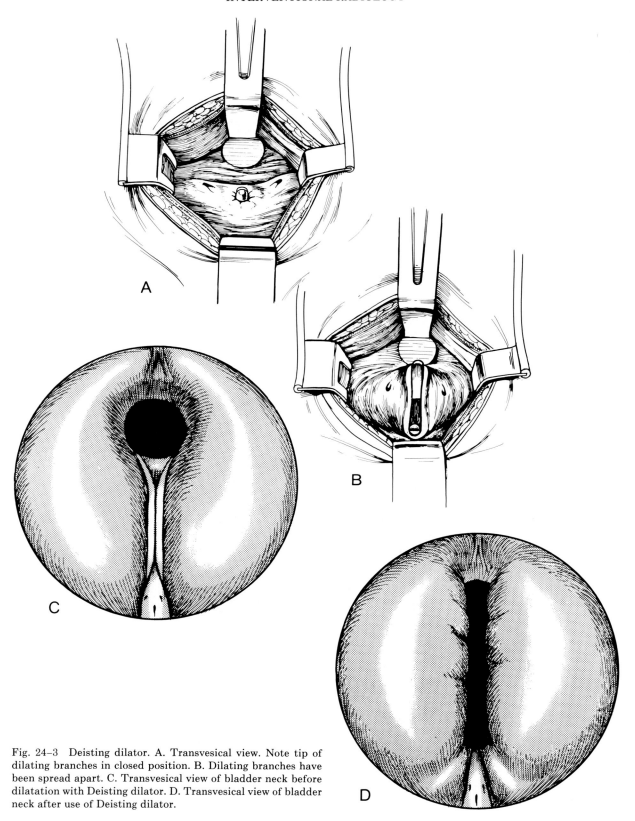

Fig. 24–3 Deisting dilator. A. Transvesical view. Note tip of
dilating branches in closed position. B. Dilating branches have
been spread apart. C. Transvesical view of bladder neck before
dilatation with Deisting dilator. D. Transvesical view of bladder
neck after use of Deisting dilator.

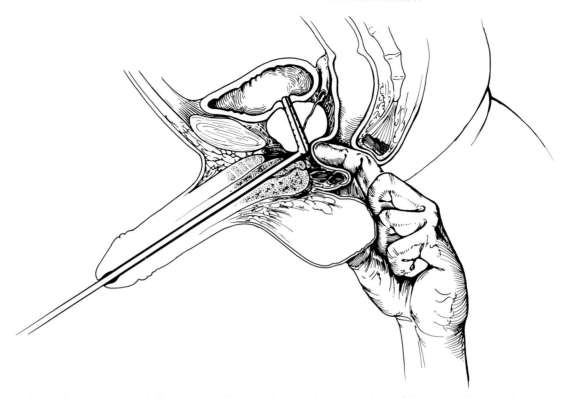

Fig. 24–4   Through rectal examination, relation between dilator and external sphincter is carefully assessed before dilatation.

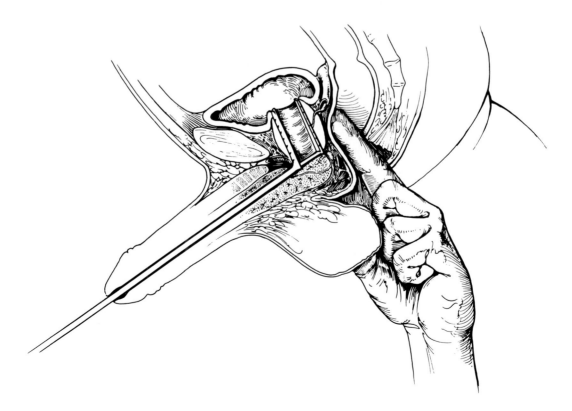

Fig. 24–5   Effects of dilatation on prostate are assessed by transrectal examination.

and vesicles. Approximately 4% of patients developed urethral strictures, most occurring in the external urethral orifice. Several reports of large series of patients followed, with similar results.[12-17]

The current treatment for BPH is either open or transurethral resection of the prostate (TURP). The latter, when properly done, is relatively safe but does have a low rate of morbidity and mortality. Many costs are involved, including surgeon and anesthetist fees, operating room and anesthesia time, hospitalization, and pharmacy charges, amounting to around $10,000 in 1987.

It is surprising that, with the excellent previous results of prostatic dilatation by mechanical means, and in spite of significant advances in interventional radiology and balloon catheter technology, balloon dilatation techniques had not been used to treat this extremely common ailment. The authors decided to try the method in an animal model.

EXPERIMENTAL WORK

A pilot study was undertaken in dogs to evaluate the feasibility of retrograde transurethral dilatation of the prostate by balloon catheters, with the realization that the dog is not the optimal model for BPH because the mechanism of obstruction is different than that in men.[18] That is, canine BPH is characterized by diffuse epithelial or glandular proliferation throughout the prostate[19] (Fig. 24–6), whereas human BPH arises specifically within the periurethral tissue and is characterized primarily by stromal hyperplasia.[20] Nonetheless, the dog is the only readily available animal known to develop BPH, and despite the histologic differences, there are sufficient similarities between the two species to regard the canine condition as a useful model.

The animal study consisted of two phases. In the first phase, the authors tried to find the optimal balloon size and duration of inflation for long-lasting results. In the second phase, the technique was used to evaulate the

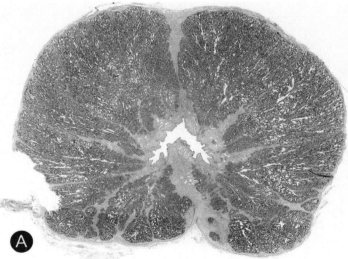

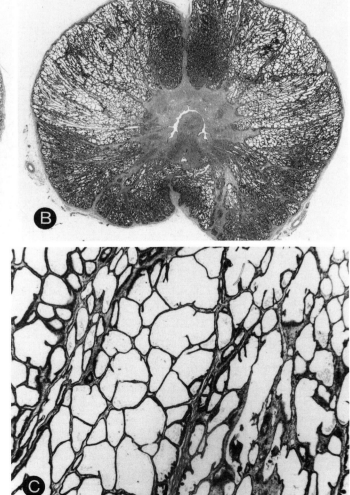

Fig. 24–6 Histopathology of canine BPH. A. Cross-section through prostate of young normal dog. B. Cross-section through prostate of older dog with BPH; note diffuse epithelial and glandular proliferation. C. Cross-section of dilated glands at higher magnification. Original magnification × 100.

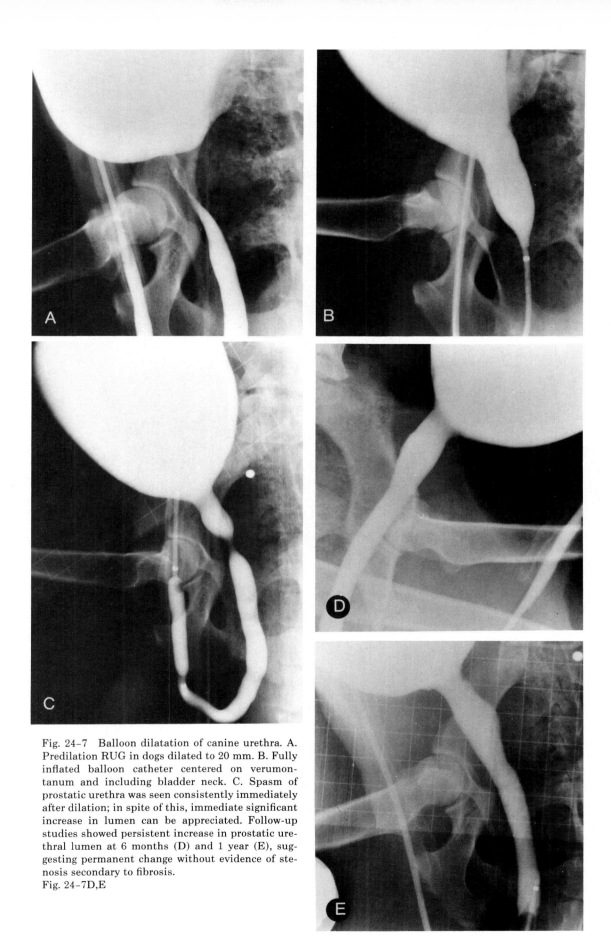

Fig. 24–7 Balloon dilatation of canine urethra. A.
Predilation RUG in dogs dilated to 20 mm. B. Fully
inflated balloon catheter centered on verumon-
tanum and including bladder neck. C. Spasm of
prostatic urethra was seen consistently immediately
after dilation; in spite of this, immediate significant
increase in lumen can be appreciated. Follow-up
studies showed persistent increase in prostatic urethral lumen at 6 months (D) and 1 year (E), suggesting permanent change without evidence of stenosis secondary to fibrosis.
Fig. 24–7D,E

acute, subacute, and long-term effects on the urethra and prostate. A total of 28 dogs was used: 18 for the first phase and 10 for the second. The results were evaluated by an initial retrograde urethrogram (RUG) and by follow-up studies immediately; at 2, 4, 8, 12, 16, 20, and 24 weeks; at 6 months; and at 1 year. Histologic sections were studied immediately after dilatation and at 2 weeks, 3 and 6 months, and 1 year. For the first phase, balloon diameters of 8, 10, 15, and 22 mm were tested, with periods of dilatation ranging from 3–10 min. For the second phase, all dogs were dilated to 20 mm for 10 min.

The study showed that no significant dilatation could be obtained with a balloon ≤15 mm in diameter and that any dilatation obtained with these smaller balloons

tended to decrease to baseline levels with time. On the other hand, with the use of balloons of 20 mm inflated for 10 min, the effects on the prostatic urethra were significant and long-lasting, with no decrease in the postdilation urethral diameters for as long as 14 months. The prostatic urethral diameters ranged from 2.5–4.1 mm before dilatation and from 16.5–18.0 mm afterward (Fig. 24–7).

Histologic study showed partially denuded urothelium with mild subepithelial congestion and minimal focal hemorrhage immediately after dilation (Fig. 24–8). These changes were largely repaired by 2 weeks. No other changes were noted histologically that could be attributed to the procedure.

These results were very encouraging and suggested

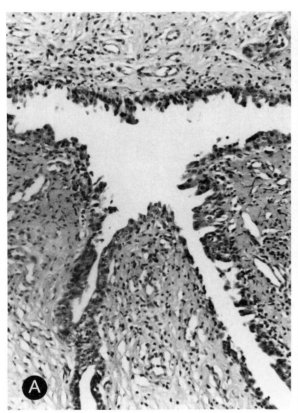

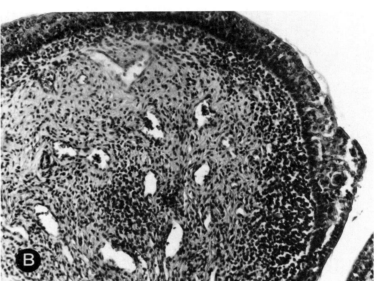

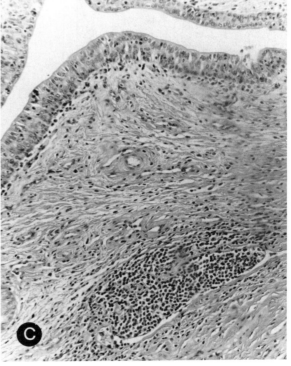

Fig. 24–8 Histologic changes after dilatation of canine urethra. A. Prostatic urethra immediately postdilatation, showing denuded epithelium with acute and chronic inflammatory changes in the adjacent gland. Hematoxylin and eosin, original magnification ×120. B. Prostatic urethra 2 weeks postdilatation; acute and chronic inflammatory infiltrates in urethra, with some polymorphonuclear neutrophils (PMNs) and lymphocytes. Atrophic glands in areas of inflammation with PMNs and histiocytes in inflamed ducts and glands. C. Prostatic parenchyma 6 months postdilatation, showing stromal proliferation, glandular atrophy, and chronic inflammation typical of BPH. Hematoxylin and eosin; original magnification × 48. Histologic study shows mature glands with patchy hyperplasia and atrophy. Urethral epithelium was intact.

that clinical human trials were warranted,[18] especially because dilatation techniques had been successful prior to the TURP era. This study also served to develop a balloon dilatation technique that could be used in humans and to determine the optimal balloon size and duration of inflation for adequate long-term results.

HUMAN EXPERIENCE

Materials and Methods

Patients were considered eligible for the procedure if they had BPH and were candidates for TURP to relieve the obstructive symptoms. Symptoms referable to BPH had been present for an average of 1.5 years and consisted of hesitancy, urgency, frequency, dribbling, and nocturia. Each patient was evaluated by cystoscopy, uroflow studies (UF), residual urine volume (RUV), voiding cystourethrogram (VCUG), RUG, rectal ultrasound (US), and magnetic resonance imaging (MRI) prior to the procedure. The VCUG, RUG, US, and MRI were repeated immediately after the procedure and again at 2 weeks and 3, 5, and 12 months; they will be repeated again at 2 years.

The procedure is performed with topical anesthesia using 2% viscous lidocaine applied liberally within the urethra. An intravenous line is placed for administration of any needed sedative or emergency drugs. Prophylactic antibiotics are given beginning 1 day before the procedure and continuing for 7 days. The penis is prepared and draped as it is for a surgical procedure. An interventional radiologist and a urologist participate jointly in the procedure. All maneuvers are conducted under fluoroscopic guidance to ensure proper positioning of the urethroplasty catheter. Immediately prior to dilatation, RUG is performed (Fig. 24–9) through a 14F Foley catheter, with the minimally inflated balloon occluding the external meatus to define precisely the location of the external sphincter. The level of the sphincter is marked with a 25-gauge needle on the skin or a surgical clamp securely in place on the drapes.

A 16F Councill catheter is advanced into the bladder, a 0.025-inch Amplatz stiffening guidewire is advanced through the catheter, and the catheter is removed. A 25-mm urethroplasty balloon (Fig. 24–10) of appropriate length is placed in the prostatic urethra above the external sphincter (Fig. 24–11) under fluoroscopic control. If there is concern about the position of the external sphincter, the balloon can be inflated to a low pressure and its position verified by rectal palpation or by injection of contrast medium alongside the balloon through an 8F feeding tube (Fig. 24–12). The balloon pressure is then increased to 6 atm, where it is maintained for 10 min (Fig. 24–13). Upward adjustment of the pressure is often needed, because the compliance of the prostate and its capsule decreases in response to the balloon, allowing the balloon to expand. Because of the sensory innervation of the prostatic capsule, mild pain is common, but at the time of balloon inflation, the predominant symptom is a strong urge to void caused by distention of the internal sphincter.

The urethroplasty catheter is subsequently removed, leaving the guidewire in place. Through a Councill catheter placed alongside the guidewire, an RUG is obtained (Fig. 24–14A). After the bladder is distended with contrast medium, the catheter is removed, and a VCUG is obtained on the table (Fig. 24–14B). Further dilatation is performed if needed. A 16F Councill catheter is then advanced over the guidewire and left in the bladder for approximately 24 hr.

Results

Significant increases in the diameter of the prostatic urethra were demonstrated by the radiographic studies, and reduction in symptoms and improvement in UF results were also seen in each patient (Fig. 24–15). The increased urethral caliber has persisted without significant modification throughout the follow-up period of as long as 18 months at the time of this writing. The MRI and ultrasound studies have shown no evidence of intraprostatic or periprostatic hematomas (Fig. 24–16). Three patients reported minor residual postmicturition dribbling. The symptoms were unrelieved in two patients in whom there was cystoscopic evidence of middle lobe hyperplasia, but there was significant reduction in the volume of residual urine (Fig. 24–17). Transient hema-

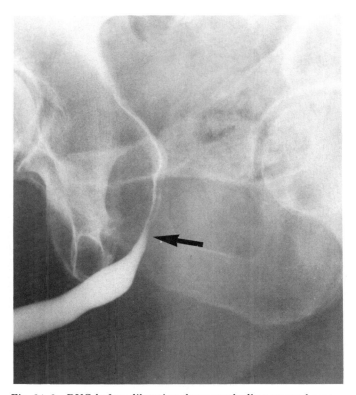

Fig. 24–9 RUG before dilatation shows markedly narrowed prostatic urethra and level of external sphincter (arrow).

Fig. 24–10 Urethroplasty balloon catheter fully inflated to 25 mm.

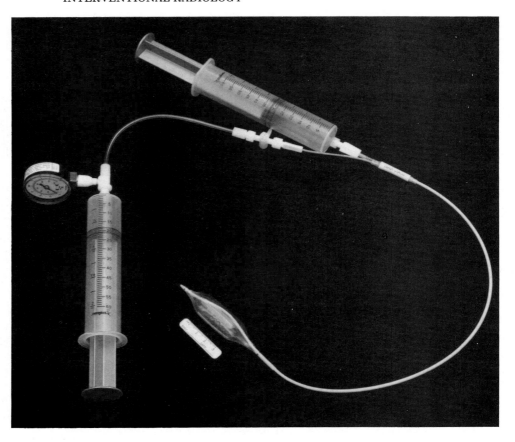

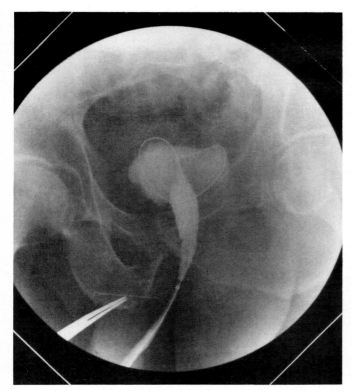

Fig. 24–11 Urethroplasty balloon has been partially inflated at low pressure, verifying its position above external sphincter, which is marked by needle placed on skin under fluoroscopic guidance at the time of RUG. Clamp is placed at same level.

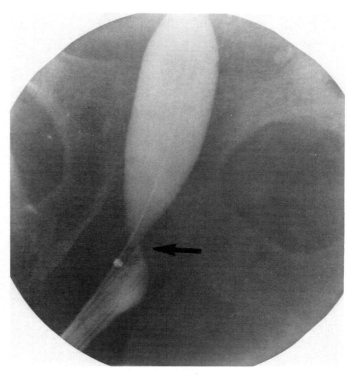

Fig. 24–12 After full inflation of balloon, contrast medium has been injected through 8F feeding tube to verify its placement above external sphincter (arrow).

turia occurred in every patient; it usually ceased within 4–12 hr. Every patient also experienced mild to moderate dysuria, which abated in 48–72 hr.

Complications

No complications have been seen other than mild transient hematuria. The potential for postprocedure incontinence is always there, which is why extreme care must be taken to avoid dilating the external sphincter. This did not occur in any patients in this series. Sepsis and hemorrhage are potential complications, but they are minimized by using strict aseptic techniques, preprocedural urine culture, and periprocedural antibiotic coverage. Hemorrhage is a possibility but should be preventable through correction of any hematologic abnormalities.

Contraindications

The contraindications to retrograde transurethral prostatic urethroplasty by balloon catheter are few. Predominant hyperplasia of the middle prostatic lobe has not responded well in the authors' experience; the same problem was also noted with the Deisting technique. The authors think a hyperplastic median lobe produces a large intravesical component that mimics a flap-like valve. The lobe is displaced cephalad and posteriorly by balloon inflation but falls back to its original position with balloon deflation (Fig. 24-18A,B). Such patients are therefore poor candidates for balloon dilatation (Fig. 24-18C,D). A careful evaluation of the intravenous urogram, RUG, VCUG, rectal ultrasound, MRI, and cystoscopy

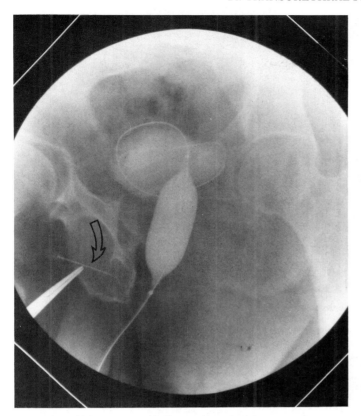

Fig. 24–13   Oblique view of balloon fully inflated in prostatic urethra. Note wire within bladder and needle marking location of the external sphincter (arrow).

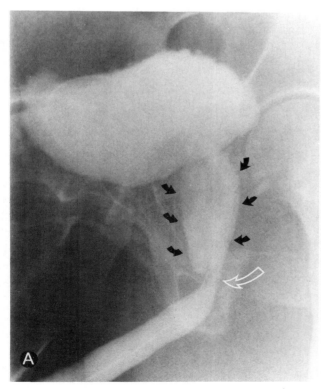

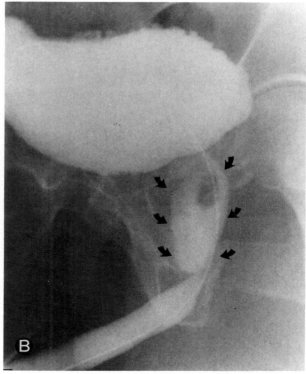

Fig. 24–14   Results of dilatation. A. RUG immediately after dilatation of prostatic urethra (curved arrows) shows preservation of external sphincter (open arrow). B. VCUG immediately after dilatation confirms marked widening of prostatic urethra (curved arrows).

tation confirms marked widening of prostatic urethra (curved arrows).

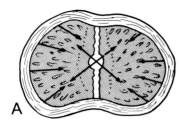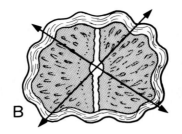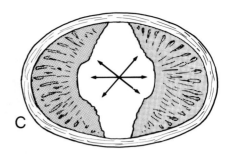

Fig. 24–19 Action of mechanical dilators. A. Transvesical digital technique disrupts adenoma but preserves elasticity of prostatic capsule, which will yield only moderately to increased intravesical pressure. B. Deisting technique displaces adenoma but also overstretches the capsule and exhausts its elasticity. C. With increase in intravesical pressure, prostatic capsule yields to accommodate urine flow, with marked widening of prostatic urethra.

CONCLUSIONS

Traditionally, TURP has mortality rates of 1.3%–3.2%[21–24] and a signifcant morbidity, especially in less fit patients. For example, patients with a serum creatinine of $\geq$1.5 mg/dl have a 6-fold increase in morbidity and mortality.[25] Increased morbidity and mortality are also seen in patients with prostates >60 g.[23,24] Other factors that increase morbidity and mortality are obesity, venous insufficiency, chronic obstructive pulmonary disease, cardiovascular disease, and chronic illnesses such as diabetes mellitus. Acute complications include priapism, extravasation of urine, urinary retention, incontinence, epi-

didymitis,[22] and hemorrhage due either to the procedure or to postoperative coagulopathy. Long-term complications include retrograde ejaculation in 40%–50%, impotence in as many as 40%,[21,26] urethral stricture in 6%,[27] incontinence in 4%–5%, and epididymitis in 2.3%.[23] In addition, obstruction recurs in 3.9% because of the continued growth of adenomatous tissue.[23]

Dilatation techniques were widely used in the past, with excellent results. With the current technologic and imaging methods, the time had come to try prostate dilatation using the new, relatively atraumatic balloons. In

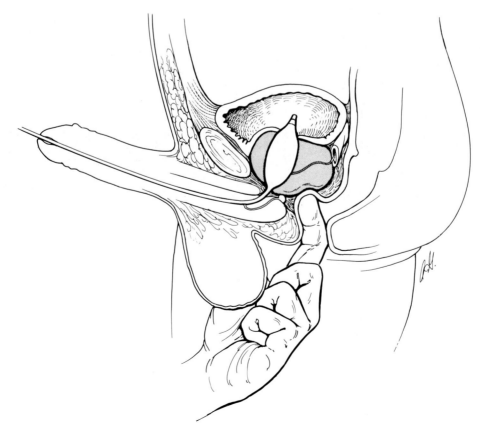

Fig. 24–20 Palpation to prevent damage to external sphincter during balloon inflation.

the authors' series, the presence of urgency or pain during balloon inflation was used as an indicator of adequate balloon size, because as previously reported by Deisting, pain results from the distention of the nerve fibers in the prostatic capsule and of the internal sphincter[12] (Fig. 24–19). Extreme care should be taken to avoid dilating the external sphincter, inasmuch as injury to this structure could cause urinary incontinence. This risk is minimized by performing an RUG prior to prostatic dilatation or by palpating the balloon transrectally during the initial inflation (Fig. 24–20). Once the RUG has been performed with the patient in an oblique position, he must remain still so that the fluoroscopic landmarks will not change. All catheter manipulations after dilatation should be done over the guidewire to avoid injuring the already traumatized urethra. Dilatation of the prostatic urethra must include the bladder neck where BPH causes functional obstruction. If necessary, short balloons can be inflated a second time at a slightly higher level to ensure the dilatation of this area.

Hematuria and dysuria are presumed to arise from tears in the urethra and underlying tissues. However, these complications have never been of importance or concern to either the patient or the clinician.

These patients are being closely monitored with VCUG, RUG, UF, and MRI. If the current record of safety and efficacy holds, however, simple symptomatic follow-up may prove adequate for most patients. The relatively short-term results in human volunteers are encouraging, and the authors are hopeful about the long-term results in view of the results obtained in earlier clinical studies with rigid dilators and in their animal study using balloon catheters.

The increasing life expectancy of the male population magnifies the importance of BPH as a clinical problem. The technique described significantly decreases medical costs, because it can be done as an outpatient procedure under local anesthesia with minimal morbidity and no mortality. The procedure can be performed on almost any patient regardless of his medical condition. Because of these minimal risks, the procedure could be performed as frequently as necessary. Additionally, the risks associated with TURP are avoided. This procedure is therefore attractive in a cost-conscious medical economy such as ours.

References

1. Horton RJ: Androgen hormones and prehormones in young and elderly men, in Grayhack JT, Wilson JD, Scherbenske MJ (eds): *Benign Prostatic Hyperplasia: Proceedings of a Workshop Sponsored by Kidney Disease and Urology Program of NIAMDD.* Washington DC, US Government Printing Office, 1976, p 183

2. Coordinating Committee (National Institutes of Health): Lower urinary tract diseases: obstruction, in *Research Needs in Nephrology*, volume I. DHEW Publication No. (NIH) 78-1481. Washington DC, US Government Printing Office, 1978, p 19

3. Birkhoff JD: Natural history of benign prostatic hypertrophy, in Hinman F Jr (ed): *Benign Prostatic Hypertrophy*. New York, Springer–Verlag, 1983, p 7

4. Vital and Health Statistics: *Utilization of Short Stay in Hospitals*, series 13, No. 46. DHEW Publication No. (PHS) 80-1797. Washington DC, US Government Printing Office, 1980

5. Craigen AA, Hickling JB, Saunders CRG, Carpenter RG: Natural history of prostatic obstruction. *J R Coll Gen Practitioners* 1969;18:226–232

6. Hinman F Jr (ed): *Benign Prostatic Hypertrophy*. New York, Springer–Verlag, 1983, p 5

7. Cabot W: The question of castration for enlarged prostate. *Ann Surg Phila* 1968;165:438

8. Mercier F: *Recherches sur les Valvules du Col de la Vessie.* Paris, 1850

9. Hollingsworth E: Dilatation of the prostatic urethra for relief of symptoms of prostatic enlargement. *Ann Surg* 1910;51:597–599

10. Frank O: Die Sprengung des Prostataringes. *Münch Med Wochenschr* 1938;21:777–782

11. Kraemer F: Ein Beitrag zur Behandlung der Prostata-Hypertrophie durch Prostatadehnung. *Dtsch Med Wochenschr* 1910;36:757–758

12. Deisting W: Transurethral dilatation of the prostate: a new method in the treatment of prostatic hypertrophy. *Urol Int* 1956;2:158–171

13. Oravisto KJ: Indications for Deisting's prostatic dilatation in the treatment of prostatic hypertrophy. *Urol Int* 1961;11:202–206

14. Backman KA: Dilatation of the prostate according to Deisting: results of follow-up one and two years after the operation. *Acta Chir Scand* 1963;126:266–274

15. Aalkjaer V: Transurethral resection/prostatectomy versus dilatation treatment in hypertrophy of the prostate II: a comparison of late results. *Urol Int* 1965;20:17–22

16. Sandberg I, Sandstrom B: Dilatation according to Deisting for prostatic hyperplasia. *Scand J Urol Nephrol* 1967;1:224–226

17. Aboulker P: La divulsion de la prostate: d'apres 218 observations personelles. *J Urol Nephrol* 1964;70:337–364

18. Castañeda F, Lund G, Larson BW, et al: Experimental dilatation of prostatic urethra in dogs. Presented at the Annual Meeting, Radiological Society of North America, Chicago, IL, 1986

19. Huggins C: The etiology of benign prostatic hypertrophy. *Bull NY Acad Med* 1947;23:696–704

20. McNeal JE: Origin and evolution of benign prostatic enlargement. *Invest Urol* 1978;15:340–345

21. Melchoir J, Valk WL, Foret JO, Mebust WK: Transurethral prostatectomy: computerized analysis of 2223 consecutive cases. *J Urol* 1974;112:634–642

22. Ashley JSA, Howlett A, Morris JN: Case–fatality of hyperplasia of the prostate in two teaching and three regional board hospitals. *Lancet* 1971;2:1308–1311

23. Melchoir J, Valk WL, Foret JO, Mebust WK: Transurethral prostatectomy in the azotemic patient. *J Urol* 1974;112:643–646

24. Mebust WK, Valk WL: Transurethral prostatectomy, in Hinman F Jr (ed): *Benign Prostatic Hypertrophy*. New York, Springer–Verlag, 1983, pp 829–846

25. Lentz HC, Jr, Mebust WK, Foret JO, Melchoir J: Urethral strictures following transurethral prostatectomy: review of 2223 resections. *J Urol* 1977;117:194–196

26. Blandy JP: *Transurethral Resection*, ed. 2. London, Pitman, Tunbridge Wells, 1978

27. Holtgreive HL, Valk WL: Late results of transurethral prostatectomy. *J Urol* 1964;92:51–55

25

Percutaneous Thermal Occlusion of the Ureter

PRATAP K. REDDY, M.D., AND WILFRIDO R. CASTAÑEDA–ZUÑIGA, M.D., M.Sc.

Occlusion of the ureter is a procedure that is seldom considered. Patients with ureteral pathology usually undergo a reconstructive operation or perhaps a simple nephrectomy if the contralateral renal unit is normal. However, urologists are now frequently faced with patients who need some form of urinary reconstruction or diversion but who are too sick to undergo any operation or whose life expectancy is so short that surgery is best avoided. This scenario includes terminally ill cancer patients who have lower urinary tract fistulae from cancer and radiation therapy. These fistulae could be from either the distal ureter or bladder to the vagina, rectum, or skin. Vesicovaginal fistulae are more frequent than the other types. In these patients, management of the fistula becomes a distressing problem for both the patient and the nursing home staff in hospital-confined patients. External collection devices are either impractical because of the location of the fistula or simply do not stay in place long enough because of the urine seepage. Percutaneous nephrostomy drainage is an ideal urinary diversion in these patients, but it has been the authors' experience that nephrostomy drainage in itself does not totally divert the urine, so some still passes down the ureter to the fistula. If the ureter could be occluded by a simple nonsurgical technique, all urine could be diverted through the nephrostomy tube, thereby keeping the fistula site dry. Other indications for ureteral occlusion with nephrostomy drainage include advanced inoperable bladder cancer with hematuria, dysuria, and urgency and terminal metastatic prostatic cancer with urinary frequency, urgency, or incontinence from previous local radiation or locally invasive cancer. Most of these patients have long-standing disease causing ureteral obstruction and may have only one functioning kidney. Occlusion of the ureter with nephrostomy drainage appears to be the least invasive procedure, with no morbidity and good patient acceptance. If patients have two functioning kidneys, bilateral nephrostomy drainage with either separate drainage bags or a single bag with a Y connector and occlusion of both ureters may be necessary.

TECHNIQUES

Percutaneous nephrostomy is performed via a central or upper pole calix under local anesthesia, and drainage is instituted through a 20F nephrostomy tube placed into the renal pelvis.[1] Nephrostomy drainage is tried for 1 week to see if it diverts all the urine. If significant quantities of urine still pass down the ureter, then thermal occlusion of the ureter is performed.

The nephrostomy tract is infiltrated with 0.5% bupivacaine. Supplemental intravenous analgesics or sedatives also are used. The tract needs no further dilatation. The procedure can be performed through either the mature tract or an Amplatz sheath. A 16F flexible choledochonephroscope is passed through the nephrostomy tract to examine the proximal ureter. If the ureteropelvic junction is narrow, it can be balloon dilated to accommodate the flexible nephroscope. A 4F electrode passed through the flexible nephroscope is used to fulgurate the ureteral mucosa (Fig. 25–1). A 2-cm segment of the proximal ureteral mucosa is coagulated in a concentric manner starting distally and working one's way upward. The reddish ureteral mucosa can be seen to whiten and narrow the lumen. The average time needed for fulguration is 15 min.

Following fulguration, a nephrostogram can be performed by injecting contrast medium through the flexible nephroscope (Fig. 25–1C). The nephroscope is withdrawn, and a 20F nephrostomy tube is placed in the renal pelvis for drainage. These patients usually do not require analgesics during the postoperative period.

COMPLICATIONS

The potential complications of percutaneous nephrostomy are reviewed elsewhere (Chapter 23 and reference 2) and will not be considered here. Thermal occlusion of the ureter could cause urinary extravasation, but this has not occurred in the authors' experience.

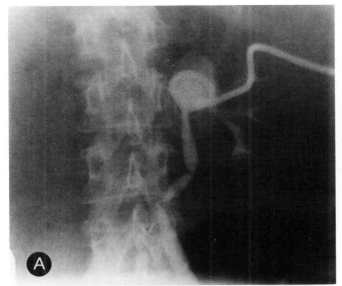

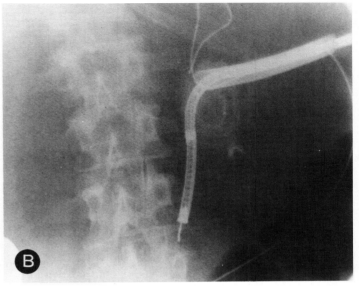

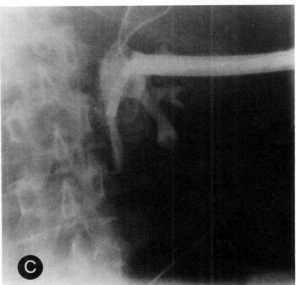

Fig. 25–1 Percutaneous thermal occlusion of right ureter. Patient is in prone position. A. Nephrostogram shows free flow of contrast medium down ureter. B. Nephrostomy tube was replaced with Amplatz sheath, and flexible nephroscope was passed through sheath into proximal ureter. Thermal occluson was performed with 4F electrode, seen here exiting from tip of nephroscope. C. Postprocedure nephrostogram performed through flexible nephroscope shows occlusion of ureter and no extravasation.

CONTRAINDICATIONS

A dilated ureter may be a relative contraindication. The authors have not had occasion to do this procedure on a dilated ureter.

Because this procedure is irreversible, it should be considered only for patients who are not operative candidates or who have a short life expectancy.

DISCUSSION

Several techniques for the nonsurgical occlusion of the ureter have been tried. Tissue adhesive (butyl-2-cyanoacrylate) has been used to occlude the lumen but has been of only temporary help because of recanalization or expulsion of the substance.[3] Ureteral occlusion with detachable balloons has had good short-term results,[4] but in the authors' experience, both balloons and coils tend to migrate. Nylon plugs to occlude the ureter, along with injection of sclerosing agents into the wall, have been tried with fairly good results.[5] However, this appears to

be a technically tedious procedure with complications including migration of the plugs and pyelonephritis. The authors have occluded the ureter in the retroperitoneum in dogs by a percutaneous approach[7]; clinical trials are being conducted. However, there is a potential for ureteral necrosis at the site of clipping.

Thermal occlusion of the ureter, on the other hand, is a fairly simple procedure. There have been no complications. Also, the authors believe that occlusion is best performed in the proximal part of the ureter, because occluding the ureter lower down by any technique leaves a stagnant column of urine that is a potential source of infection.

The authors' experience with thermal occlusion of the ureter has been successful in all cases, but more extensive experience is necessary to see if this is a suitable technique for some cases of ureteral pathology.

References

1. Castañeda–Zuñiga WR, Miller RP, Amplatz K: Percutaneous removal of kidney stones. *Urol Clin North Am* 1982;9:113
2. Coleman CC, Kimura Y, Reddy P, et al: Complications of nephrostolithotomy. *Semin Intervent Radiol* 1984;1:70
3. Günther R, Marberger M, Klose K: Transrenal ureteral embolization. *Radiology* 1979;132:317
4. Günther R, Klose K, Alken P: Transrenal ureteral occlusion with a detachable balloon. *Radiology* 1982;142:521
5. Kinn AC, Ohlsen H, Brehmer–Andersson A, Brundin J: Therapeutic ureteral occlusion in advanced pelvic malignant tumors. *J Urol* 1985;135:29
6. Reddy PK: Percutaneous ureteral fulguration (PUF): a nonsurgical technique for ureteral occlusion. *J Urol* 1987;138:724
7. Lund G, Rysavy JR, Hunter DW, Castañeda–Zuñiga WR, Amplatz K: Percutaneous occlusion of the ureter: a new approach for relief of urinary tract fistulae. *Semin Intervent Radiol* 1984;1:92

26

Endoscopy of the Upper Urinary Tract: An Interspecialty Common Ground

RALPH V. CLAYMAN, M.D., AND PETER BUB, M.D.

Rapid advances in fluoroscopic imaging techniques and in methods for dilating percutaneously established nephrostomy tracts have made it possible to create tracts suitable for the passage of a variety of rigid and flexible endoscopic equipment. Accordingly, the entire intrarenal collecting system and ureters can now be viewed using a percutaneous route. In the following discussion, instruments, techniques, indications, and interspecialty interactions of nephroscopy are addressed.

INSTRUMENTATION

Instruments for rigid nephroscopy were first developed in 1948 by Trattner,[1] who designed a straight pyeloscope for intraoperative use. This instrument was later modified by Leadbetter, who placed a 90° angle in its distal limb, thereby improving its maneuverability.[2] The first purposely built percutaneous nephroscopes were developed in 1970 by Alken for stone removal.[3] These nephroscopes had a sidearm 5° viewing system that resulted in a large, unobstructed central channel, which was necessary to accommodate the rigid ultrasound probes used to fragment renal calculi. Recently, Miller and Wickham designed a nephroscope with a 30° sidearm viewing system and a 30° lens system (Fig. 26–1).[4] The traditional cystoscopes (*e.g.*, the 20F or 24F McCarthy or the smaller pediatric panendoscopes) also may be used to perform nephroscopy. Although these familiar endoscopes will not accommodate an ultrasonic probe, they can be used with all the other types of stone removal equipment, including the electrohydraulic lithotripter. A comparison of the various rigid instruments designed for nephroscopy is provided in Table 26–1.

Flexible fiberoptic nephroscopy was first performed in a retrograde manner in 1964, when Marshall used a fiberoptic ureteroscope to examine a stone-containing renal pelvis intraoperatively.[5] In 1979, a 16F 13-cm-long flexible fiberoptic nephroscope was marketed by American Cystoscope Makers, Inc. for intraoperative use; again, the collecting system was viewed in a retrograde fashion. Antegrade percutaneous nephroscopy was first reported in 1975 by Harris and associates, who used a flexible bronchoscope to locate and remove a renal calculus through a surgically established nephrostomy tract.[6] More recently, 15F choledochoscopes have been adopted for use via the nephrostomy tract, although it has been only during the last few years that these instruments have actually been *adapted* for nephroscopy. Changes were essential because the angulation and size of the renal infundibula are anatomically unique, necessitating development of flexible endoscopes with as much as an 83° angle of view in water and with deflection capabilities of 180° in either direction.

In general, the flexible nephroscopes are 15F in diameter and have a working length of 30–37 cm. They usually are constructed with two fiberoptic light bundles, a solitary fiberoptic image bundle, and a 2-mm working port (Table 26–1 and Fig. 26–2). Flexion capabilities vary from 160°–180° in any one direction, and the angle of view in water varies from 51°–83°. All of these newer instruments are completely sealed, allowing sterilization by immersion.

PATIENT PREPARATION

Before percutaneous nephrostomy, it is of great value to obtain contrast-filled renal radiographs in the lateral, oblique, and anteroposterior positions, because these films allow the urologist and radiologist to delineate accurately the relations of the planned nephrostomy tract to the renal pelvis, calices, ureter, and calculi. The time spent in determining the optimal route to the area of pathology will save considerable time during the actual procedure and enhance the chances of a successful outcome.

In general, patient preparation for nephroscopy is simple.[7] Routine studies include a blood cell count, serum electrolyte measurements, a chest radiograph, and an electrocardiogram (if the patient is older than 40 years). A urine culture is obtained; in all cases, it is better to proceed only when the urine is sterile. If the urine is infected,

639

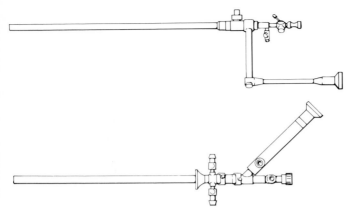

Fig. 26–1 Rigid nephroscopes. Top: Alken and Marberger-type rigid nephroscope with a 90° offset viewing system. Bottom: Wickham–Miller-type nephroscope with a 30° offset viewing system. Note that in both models the central channel is straight to allow passage of rigid ultrasonic probe used for renal stone disintegration.

appropriate antibiotics should be administered before nephroscopy. If the urine cannot be sterilized after 48–72 hr, nephroscopy can be performed under continued antibiotic coverage. If the urine culture is sterile, prophylactic parenteral antibiotics (usually a penicillin derivative and an aminoglycoside) are administered immediately before and for 24 hr after nephroscopy.

If a nephroscopy tube has been in place for longer than 3–5 days, the nephrostomy tract is usually well established, in which case the procedure may be done under assisted local anesthesia. However, if nephroscopy is planned at the time of the establishment of the nephrostomy tract, an epidural, spinal, or general anesthetic is recommended. Also, it is helpful to have the patient's blood typed, although a cross-match is done only if a lengthy or difficult procedure is expected.

Diuretics are used to establish a brisk flow of urine before and during nephroscopy. Usually, 6–12 g of mannitol or 10–20 mg of furosemide are administered intravenously along with 250–500 ml of intravenous fluid over a 30–60-min period. By increasing the urine output, the problems associated with intrapelvic blood clot formation and pyelotubular backflow may be decreased. In this regard, it is important that, prior to nephroscopy, all patients have an indwelling urethral catheter placed.

The draping procedure is extremely important in order to protect the fluoroscopy table. If the sheath of the nephroscope is inserted directly into the nephrostomy tract (i.e., closed system), then the draping procedure can be simplified, because there should be no outflow of irrigant onto the table. Most of the nephroscopes are designed for continuous flow. However, if the sheath of the nephroscope is passed through a wide-lumen Amplatz working sheath (i.e., open system), then the irrigant from the nephroscope will flow from the working sheath and must be collected. In this case, the working sheath serves as a conduit to the kidney. An advantage of such an open system is that intrapelvic pressure always remains low, because it cannot exceed the 20-cm length of the working sheath. With an open system, a cranial incise drape is helpful, as it contains a reservoir to collect the effluent. More recently, a nephroscopy drape (Surgikos; Arlington, TX) has been developed that includes a reservoir for collecting the fluid as well as a drain for emptying the reservoir. In addition, it contains a series of parallel perforated ridges in which the urologic and radiologic equipment used during the procedure can be stabilized.

ADDITIONAL MATERIALS FOR NEPHROSCOPY

It is necessary to have a light source that is compatible with the endoscope. In many situations, the type of rigid endoscope is different from the brand of flexible endoscope, so two light sources may be necessary.

Irrigation fluid for the endoscope should be warmed to 37°C. This solution should always be of a physiologic nature, preferably normal saline or Ringer's lactate; water, glycine, or sorbitol should be used only during intrarenal electrosurgery. A ⅙ or ⅒ normal saline solution should be used only during electrohydraulic lithotripsy. Use of these hypotonic solutions other than when indicated exposes the patient to a risk of water intoxication, hemolysis, and hyponatremia secondary to intraperitoneal/retroperitoneal extravasation or pyelovenous backflow. In order to decrease the chances of this problem, the irrigant is usually kept at a height of ≤40 cm. Also, an open system is recommended. If a closed system is used, a balance sheet for irrigant input and outflow is necessary. A discrepancy of >1 liter is a direct indication to conclude the procedure promptly.

Table 26–1
Instruments for Percutaneous Nephroscopy

	Rigid			Flexible		
Company	ACMI	Storz	Wolf	ACMI	Olympus	Pentax
Model no.	ARN-19	27092A	8962.31	APN-37	CHF-P10	FCN-15H
Outer diameter	24F	20F	24.5F	15F	15F	15F
Field of view (water)	58°	85°	60°	51°	64°	83°
Working length (cm)	19	18.5	19.5	37	33	30
Working port (mm)	4	5	4	1.8	2	2
Flexibility (up/down°)				180/180°	160/130°	160/130°
Immersible?	Yes	Yes	Yes	Yes	Yes	Yes

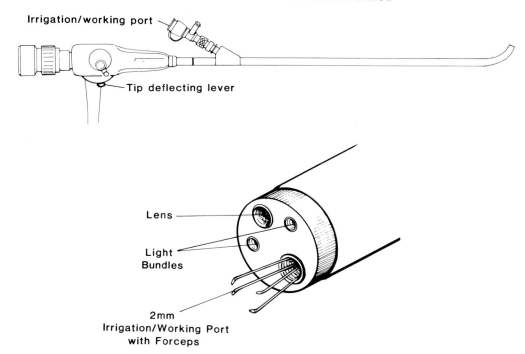

Fig. 26–2 Flexible nephroscope. Top: Deflecting lever is moved slightly forward, deflecting tip of instrument upward. Bottom: Irrigant and instruments must pass through the same channel; flow of irrigant is markedly decreased when an instrument is in the working port.

TECHNICAL ASPECTS OF NEPHROSCOPY

Prior to rigid or flexible nephroscopy, establishment of a "safety guidewire" and a "safety guidewire catheter" is advisable. This can be done by placing a 0.038-inch (3F) guidewire through the nephrostomy tract and, preferably, down the ureter and covering this with a 5F angiographic catheter. The latter is much easier to see during nephroscopy than is the wire and also can be more easily secured to the skin with a 2-0 silk suture. The safety wire system precludes loss of contact with the collecting system during the procedure. In addition, at the end of the procedure, the 5F angiographic catheter and guidewire provide ready access to the collecting system for passage of an end-hole nephrostomy (i.e., 20F or 22F Councill) catheter.

Rigid Nephroscopy: Techniques

When performing rigid nephroscopy through an open system, it is important to realize that the distal end of the Amplatz working sheath may not be in the collecting system.[7] This occurs when the nephrostomy tract misses the renal parenchyma and traverses only the renal pelvis, when the renal parenchyma is markedly thinned, or when the sheath has not been advanced far enough into the system. In the first two circumstances, the anterior and posterior walls of the collecting system may be pushed against each other during dilation. In this circumstance, the sheath may appear fluoroscopically to be deep enough in the collecting system yet still reside in the retroperitoneum. When the endoscopist approaches the distal opening of the sheath, red or fatty tissue may be observed (Fig. 26–3). When this occurs, it is helpful to locate the safety wire catheter as it passes beyond the distal end of the sheath. The tip of the rigid nephroscope (20F or 24F McCarthy) can then be guided along the safety wire catheter until the intrarenal collecting system is gained. The urothelium of the normal intrarenal collecting system has a smooth white background with an overlying fine vascular pattern.

Four situations can cause marked consternation during rigid nephroscopy (Fig. 26–4). First, when the tip of the endoscope or the working sheath abuts the urothelium, a "white-out" occurs. This can be resolved by retracting the endoscope or working sheath 1–2 cm. Indeed, it is always best, upon first gaining entry into the collecting system, to pull the working sheath back until its distal opening lies at the entry of the nephrostomy tract into the collecting system, where the smooth white urothelium is replaced by the markedly irregular or fatty tissue of the renal capsule or calix. A second problem is that of a "red-out," which is due to blood clots that have accumulated during placement of the nephrostomy tube. They need to be removed by flushing, suction, or endoscopic grasping. A third problem, which can follow perforation of the renal collecting system by a dilator, is the appearance of perirenal fat alone (i.e., a "yellow-out"). Finally, in a patient with a history of renal surgery, the maneuverability of the rigid nephroscope is severely limited, and in these cases, excessive or forceful manipulation may cause a significant laceration of the renal parenchyma and attendant hemorrhage.

Flexible Nephroscopy: Techniques

There are certain features common to all of the flexible nephroscopes. A focusing wheel is always present at the

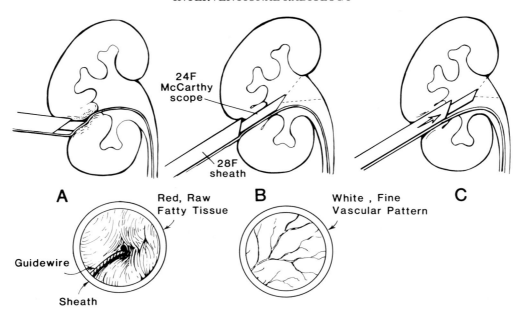

Fig. 26–3 Rigid nephroscopy: entering the collecting system. A. Amplatz working sheath lies just outside collecting system. Red and fatty tissue are seen by the endoscopist, indicating improper position of sheath. B. Beveled-tip McCarthy panendoscope is used to follow safety guidewire visually into the collecting system. The urothelium has a fine vascular pattern overlying a white background. In this case, an open system (*i.e.*, Amplatz working sheath) is being used. Note position of safety guidewire alongside working sheath. C. Upon entering the collecting system, working sheath is advanced over McCarthy panendoscope. For this maneuver to be successful, nephroscope must fit snugly into working sheath.

distal end of the handle; this should be adjusted by the examiner before nephroscopy. For orientation, there is always a field marker, usually at the 12 o'clock position (*i.e.*, when the examiner holds the endoscope as if it were a bottle of beverage, with the thumb resting on the deflection lever and the fingers grasping the handle, the field marker appears at 12 o'clock). The field marker often shows the direction of maximal tip deflection.

Nephroscopy is accomplished by moving the thumb in conjunction with the wrist. The deflection lever, which is controlled by the thumb, can move the tip of the instrument through an arc of 220–360°. The wrist can be used to rotate the nephroscope in order to direct the deflection mechanism along any desired plane of the collecting system.

The following sequence is one tested method for examining the intrarenal collecting system with a flexible nephroscope.[7] Upon entering the kidney, the safety guidewire catheter is followed to the ureteropelvic junction and into the ureter, which appears as an endless tunnel. After it enters the ureter, the flexible nephroscope is pulled slowly backward. As the renal pelvis is entered, its spaciousness is immediately appreciated, and the safety guidewire catheter, rather than being close to the wall of the collecting system, now appears to be suspended within the renal pelvis. Next, the upper and lower pole

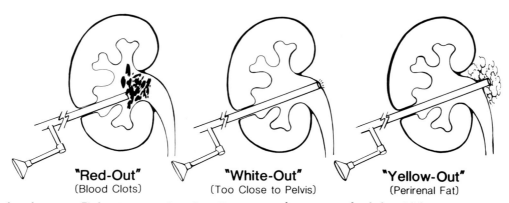

Fig. 26–4 Colors of nephroscopy. Red-out occurs when the collecting system is filled with blood clots or during active bleeding. In the former situation, clots must be cleared using suction or grasping forceps; in the latter situation, a large (22F–24F) nephrostomy tube should be placed and the procedure terminated. White-out occurs when nephroscope is applied against the urothelium. In this case, nephroscope need only be withdrawn 1 cm to gain proper view of collecting system. Yellow-out occurs when tip of nephroscope is within retroperitoneal fatty tissue. This means either that the endoscope is short of collecting system and in the tract or that renal pelvis has been perforated and nephroscope has exited the collecting system. In both situations, the nephroscope must be repositioned.

infundibula are identified. The infundibulum to the lower pole calices is nearest the ureteropelvic junction. The conical configuration of the pelvis begins to flatten as it flows into the lower pole infundibulum. This effacement of the pelvis, or "valley," occurs as the renal pelvis blends into the anterior wall of the lower pole infundibulum (Fig. 26–5A). If the nephroscope is pulled further backward, the posterior wall of the lower infundibulum comes into view as a "ridge" (Fig. 26–5B). Indeed, this ridge of tissue may actually snap across the tip of the nephroscope as the instrument is withdrawn, thereby obscuring the operator's view and resulting in a white-out. After identification of the ridge to the lower pole infundibulum, the nephroscope is turned so that the field marker points to the ridge. The nephroscope is then advanced just beyond the ridge, and its tip is deflected maximally. This results in a curling of the tip over the ridge and up into the calices of the lower pole.

The upper pole infundibulum lies approximately 180°

opposite the opening to the lower pole infundibulum. After examination of the lower pole calices, the nephroscope is withdrawn to the ostium of the lower pole infundibulum and rotated 180°, and the medial wall of the pelvis is followed until the upper pole infundibulum is gained. Again, the concept of a valley and a ridge applies.

After identification of both polar calices, the anterior and posterior middle region infundibula are sought. These may be difficult to identify, because they are usually at a sharp angle to a lower polar nephrostomy tract. Under these circumstances, the injection of contrast medium through the flexible nephroscope and guidance of the nephroscope under fluoroscopic control may be helpful. The most difficult calix to enter via a lower polar nephrostomy is the middle posterior calix, because entry requires the instrument to make a sharp U-shaped bend. In essence, then, the examiner is looking backward at himself as he tries to direct the tip of the endoscope into the posterior middle infundibulum.

INDICATIONS AND INSTRUMENTS FOR NEPHROSCOPY

Rigid nephroscopy is most often used to remove renal and upper ureteral calculi.[8] Calculi ≤1.5 cm radiographically can be removed intact with a rigid nephroscope. For this purpose, the following graspers are recommended: 7F alligator graspers for calculi ≤7 mm in diameter; 10F ureteral dilating and stone-grasping forceps (Olympus; New Hyde Park, NY) for calculi ≤10 mm in diameter; and the 26F optical kidney stone grasper (Storz; Culver City, CA) for calculi 1.0–1.5 cm in diameter. Calculi >1.5 cm can

most easily be dealt with by either ultrasonic or electrohydraulic lithotripter probes, both of which can be passed through the central channel of the rigid nephroscope.

In addition, rigid nephroscopy with a direct vision urethrotome is helpful in the percutaneous treatment of ureteropelvic junction stenosis. This procedure, termed pyelolysis or endopyelotomy, involves cutting the stenotic area under direct vision with a cold knife.[9,10] An indwelling ureteral stent is usually left for 4–6 weeks. This tech-

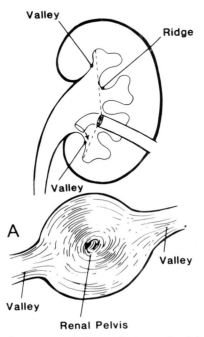

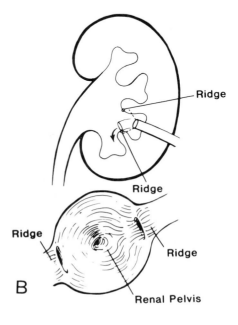

Fig. 26–5 Flexible nephroscopy techniques. A. As renal pelvis flattens toward lower pole infundibulum, a valley is formed. Similar furrow can be seen as pelvis flows into upper pole infundibulum. If tip of the flexible nephroscope is "walked" along valley, the calices will be seen. B. Posterior walls of upper and lower pole infundibula form a ridge, which is more prominent than the valley. To gain access to the calices, tip of nephroscope must be made to curl over the ridge.

nique is reportedly successful in at least 80% of patients with either primary or secondary ureteropelvic junction stenosis.

The flexible nephroscope is most useful as a diagnostic modality, because it can be maneuvered into 90% or more of the renal calices (Fig. 26–6). It is helpful in diagnosing the presence of a foreign body, ureteropelvic junction obstruction, arteriovenous malformations, leukoplakia, and many other diseases affecting the renal collecting system. Also, it has been effective in identifying the site of bleeding in patients with intermittent unilateral gross hematuria.[7]

In contrast, therapeutic flexible nephroscopy presents the endoscopist with a significant challenge.[8,11] The instruments available for use through the flexible nephroscope include stone baskets, alligator and biopsy forceps, 5F electrohydraulic lithotripter probes, a 4F electrosurgical unit, and a variety of 3- and 4-prong graspers. The grasping and basket instruments can be used to retrieve renal calculi, and the electrohydraulic lithotripter can be used to destroy larger calculi lying remote from the nephrostomy tract. The electrosurgical unit is helpful in either fulgurating a site of bleeding or cutting a stenotic infundibulum to allow access to the caliceal system. However, there are significant problems with instrumentation through the flexible nephroscope, including impaired flow of irrigant and decreased tip deflection (Table 26–2). Effective maneuvers to overcome problems of flow include placing the irrigant in a blood pressure cuff or blood pump to pressurize the flow (150 mm Hg), attaching a 50-ml syringe in line with the irrigant port so the

examiner can deliver a forceful jet of fluid during manipulation, and placement of a 5F angiographic catheter into the stone-containing calix alongside the flexible nephroscope and instilling irrigant through the catheter. This method provides a clear field of view and also helps flush the stone toward the flexible nephroscope, thereby facilitating removal.

The passage of stiff 5F biopsy forceps through the nephroscope significantly decreases tip deflection; an average of 20–30° of deflection is lost. Hence, a nephroscope with 160° of flexion will make only a 120–130° bend with the biopsy forceps in place. This problem can be partially alleviated by using finer grasping instruments such as a 3- or 4-prong grasper (see below).

The two most effective instruments for grasping calculi with a flexible nephroscope are the 4-prong grasper with a retractable sheath (ACMI; Stamford, CT) and a "W" grasper (Millrose; Mentor, OH). The former consists of four very fine wires, the tips of which are shaped into prongs (Fig. 26–7). The prongs are extended by retracting the sheath, so the closed instrument can be placed directly on a stone and the prongs opened without disturbing the position of the stone. This is most helpful, because it is difficult to see all four prongs through any of the available nephroscopes; whereas if the probe is flush on the stone, then seeing that at least two of the prongs have passed over one surface of the stone suggests that the other two, unseen, prongs have traversed the other side of the stone (providing the stone's diameter is <1.0 cm). The sheath is then advanced over the extended prongs, thereby closing them around the stone. The other

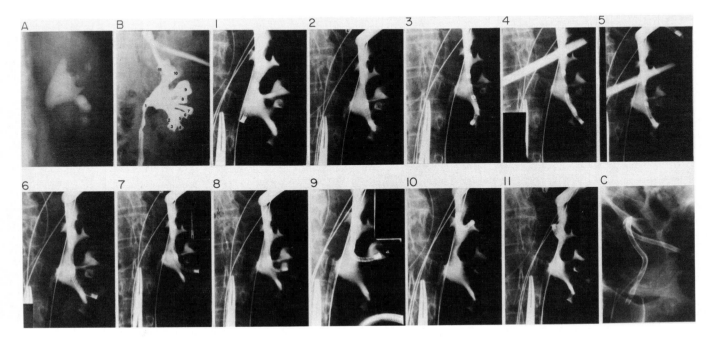

Fig. 26–6 Flexible nephroscopy: caliceal examination. A. Plain radiograph of abdomen reveals staghorn calculus with four branches. B. An intercostal (ribs 11 and 12) puncture is made into upper pole of collecting system. This permits the endoscopist to use the normal axis of the kidney to help guide the nephroscope and provides direct access to the renal pelvis and, at times, to the lower pole. The calices and ureter are numbered and correspond to the numbered (1–11) panels. Bulk of stone has been removed through upper pole nephros-

tomy. Flexible nephroscope is being used to examinne all calices for any stone remnants. By injecting dilute contrast medium through nephroscope, endoscopy and fluoroscopy can be used in combination to access all calices. C. Stone has been completely removed; Councill catheter is in place as nephrostomy tube. Note presence of antegrade ureteral catheter and retrograde ureteral occlusion balloon catheter. The latter is inflated during stone destruction to prevent migration of stone debris into ureter.

Table 26–2
Effect of Instruments on Irrigant Flow Rates in Flexible Nephroscope[a]

	ml/min
Unoccupied channel (gravity flow 65 cm)	52
Unoccupied channel	178
3F instrument	130
4F instrument	89
5F instrument	21
6F instrument	13

[a]Unless otherwise specified, all values were obtained with the irrigant pressurized to 150 mm Hg.

advantage of these grasping forceps is that the fine wires minimize loss of tip deflection of the nephroscope.

A second useful grasping instrument is the W or 3-nail grasper (Fig. 26–8). It is much stiffer and more durable than the 4-prong grasper. It is best used in the removal of impacted ureteral calculi. This instrument has a W jaw that is made of spring metal housed within a metal cylindrical sheath. Thus, when the outer restraining sheath is withdrawn, the jaws of the forceps spring open. This is a stiff instrument and must never be forcibly introduced through the working channel, because this may damage the channel. Likewise, passage of the W grasper significantly limits the range of tip deflection of the nephroscope.

The flexible nephroscope can also be used with a 4F electrosurgical probe (Greenwald Inc.; Lake Staton, IN) to incise stenotic infundibula in order to reach caliceal calculi, as well as to fulgurate an intrarenal site of bleeding, such as an arteriovenous malformation. Likewise, the electrosurgical unit can be used to incise the neck of a caliceal diverticulum and thus marsupialize the diverticulum into the renal pelvis, thereby effectively draining it.

Finally, there have been reports of using rigid and flexible nephroscopes to treat low-grade transitional cell cancer of the renal pelvis in high-risk patients or in patients with a solitary kidney. In these patients, the only alternatives would have been nephrectomy and dialysis or no treatment at all. Early reports of this method have been favorable, in that it has reduced the hospital stay and the immediate patient expense. Long-term follow-up data are not available. It must be stressed that the application of this procedure to patients with two kidneys is highly controversial. Currently, the recommended treatment for transitional cell carcinoma of the renal pelvis in a healthy patient with two kidneys remains nephroureterectomy with excision of a cuff of bladder to ensure removal of the possibly tumor-bearing ureteral tunnel and meatus.

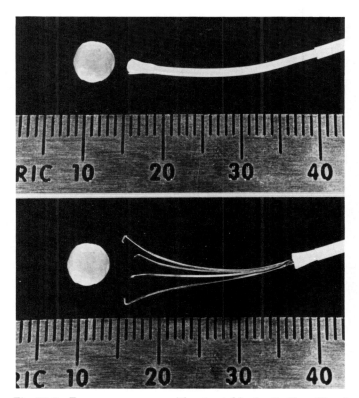

Fig. 26–7 Four-prong grasper with retractable sheath. Top: Closed grasper next to calculus; outer sheath is 5F. Bottom: Sheath is retracted, allowing prongs to spring open. Note that opening of prongs has not advanced them and that stone is still in its originial position. These forceps are quite pliable and result in only a slight decrease in nephroscope tip deflection. They are ideal for grasping caliceal calculi.

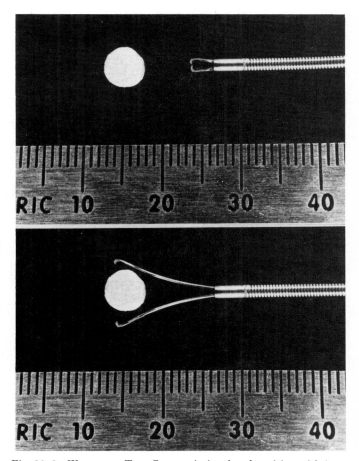

Fig. 26–8 W grasper. Top: Grasper in its closed position with jaws approximated. Bottom: Sheath remains fixed as jaws are advanced. Jaws are positioned so they actually pass over and a bit beyond stone; as they are retracted, they catch on stone and fix it firmly. These graspers are quite stiff and significantly reduce nephroscope tip deflection; however, they are stronger than any other grasper that can be passed through the flexible nephroscope. These forceps are best suited for retrieving impacted ureteral calculi.

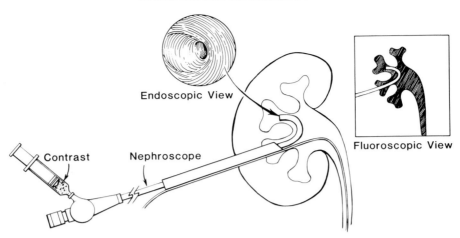

Fig. 26–9 Endofluoroscopy. By injecting dilute contrast medium through the nephroscope, the endoscopist can better understand the position of the endoscope in relation to the rest of the collecting system. Note, again, use of an open system and a safety guidewire catheter down ureter.

ENDOFLUOROSCOPY

The combination of nephroscopy and fluoroscopy (*i.e.*, endofluoroscopy) can be valuable in several situations: guidance of the nephroscope to a stone-containing calix, placement of a needle guide for subsequent electrosurgery to enter a stenotic calix, retrieval of a ureteral guidewire to permit establishment of a "through-and-through" drainage system, and creation of additional nephrostomy tracts. The fluoroscope displays the entire contrast-filled intrarenal collecting system, whereas the nephroscope provides only a direct view of a specific area of the system (Fig. 26–9). Therefore, it is often helpful to inject dilute contrast medium through the working port of the nephroscope with a 50-ml syringe and use the nephroscope fluoroscopically as though it were a steerable catheter. Indeed, in many situations, the radiologist may guide the nephroscope fluoroscopically to the affected calix so the urologist can proceed with stone removal. With practice, almost any calix, unless it is serviced by a stenotic infundibulum, can be entered using fluoroscopy and injection of contrast medium to help guide the nephroscope. However, it must be remembered that excessive exposure of the flexible nephroscope to ionizing radiation may damage fiber bundles, resulting in a yellowing of the transmitted light.

The infundibulum to a calix may be completely stenosed, thereby precluding access. Under these circumstances, it is helpful first to pass a sheathed needle through the stone-containing calix and into the renal pelvis. The endoscopist can then identify the sheathed needle and use an electrosurgical probe to cut along it and enter the calix. Note that when using electrosurgery along a nephrostomy needle, a sheath should be passed over the needle so the electric current is not transmitted along the needle shaft. Also, the patient must be properly grounded, and the irrigant must be changed from saline to sorbitol or glycine. Water should never be used as the irrigant. As an alternative to cutting to free the stone, a nephrostomy needle can be placed right behind the stone and used to push the stone into the neck of the infundibulum, where it can at times be seen and grasped by the nephroscopist. This method may avert the creation of additional nephrostomy tracts. In addition, the mere placement of a nephrostomy needle in a calix serviced by a stenotic infundibulum can also be helpful. A small amount of air or CO_2 can be injected through the needle, and the nephroscopist can follow the bubbles to the neck of the infundibulum.

Endofluoroscopy is also helpful in establishing a through-and-through guidewire system (Fig. 26–10). During nephroscopy, an exchange guidewire can be passed through an open-ended ureteral catheter under fluoroscopic control. Once the wire exits the catheter, it

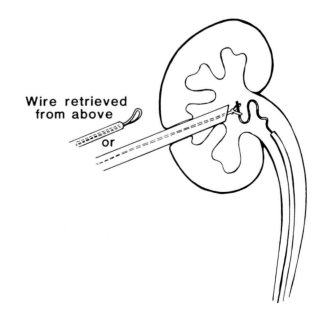

Fig. 26–10 Establishment of through-and-through guidewire. Under fluoroscopic guidance, exchange guidewire is passed through ureteral catheter until it is seen by endoscopist. Wire is then grasped with forceps and withdrawn through nephrostomy tract, thereby providing control over entire ipsilateral collecting system from flank to urethral meatus.

can be seen directly by the endoscopist, who can grasp it and pull it out through the nephrostomy tract. This wire now establishes complete control over the ipsilateral renal unit from the nephrostomy site in the skin to the urethral meatus. This is most valuable when an extensive perforation of the renal pelvis has occurred. With a through-and-through wire, proper placement of a draining ureteral stent and a nephrostomy tube within the collecting system is assured.

Finally, additional nephrostomy tubes can be quickly placed using endofluoroscopy. In patients with staghorn calculi, two or more nephrostomy tracts often are needed to reach all branches of the stone. In this situation, the flexible nephroscope is introduced through the initial nephrostomy tract and maneuvered until the stone in the affected calix is identified (Fig. 26–11). The radiologist then passes a nephrostomy needle so it enters the collecting system directly in front of the tip of the nephroscope (*i.e.,* "stick the 'scope"). The endoscopist actually sees the needle as it enters the collecting system, thereby preventing an anterior false passage. A 5F loop retrieval catheter (*i.e.,* snare) can be passed through the flexible nephroscope and used to encircle the tip of the needle. When a guidewire is passed through the metal sheath of

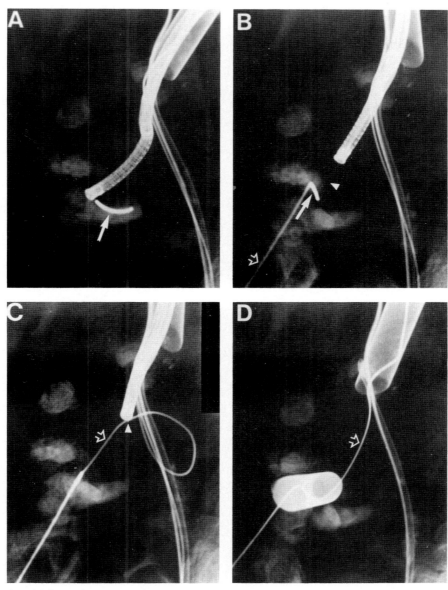

Fig. 26–11 Placement of multiple nephrostomy tubes: "stick the 'scope." A. Endoscopist has maneuvered flexible nephroscope through upper pole nephrostomy tract and into lower pole stone-containing calix. Note use of an open system and presence of safety guidewire. Tip of nephrostomy needle directly overlies tip of nephroscope. B. Nephrostomy needle is positioned so its tip and hub are aligned one over the other, hence its foreshortened appearance. Needle is advanced until endoscopist sees it just entering collecting system. Loop retrieval catheter is passed through nephroscope and opened. Once it encircles tip of needle, guidewire is advanced through needle. C. Retrieval snare is closed, thereby entrapping guidewire. As nephroscope is withdrawn, guidewire is advanced. This provides a wire that traverses both new and old nephrostomy tracts. Additional guidewires need not be introduced, because the one is sufficient to serve as both safety and working wire. D. Second Amplatz working sheath has been positioned in lower pole system. Note presence of original guidewire, which now connects the two nephrostomy tracts.

the needle, it also passes through the center of the loop retrieval catheter. The catheter is tightened against the guidewire; as the nephroscope is withdrawn through the original nephrostomy tract, the guidewire follows, thereby establishing "circle wire" nephrostomy. The tract can now be dilated rapidly without the introduction of any additional wires; likewise, the nephroscopist can con-tinue to observe the dilation to help prevent perforation of the anterior wall of the collecting system by any of the larger dilators. With this maneuver, additional nephrostomy tracts can be established, the balloon inflated to 36F, and the patient intubated with a working sheath within 5–10 min.

CONCLUSION

The realm of rigid and flexible nephroscopy in conjunction with fluoroscopy (endofluoroscopy) provides the endourologic team with the greatest opportunity for performing successful percutaneous intrarenal surgery. It is expected that as further advances in medical technology occur, and as the urologic–radiologic team concept becomes more widely accepted, most surgical procedures on the urinary tract will be transformed into closed, controlled endourologic maneuvers.

References

1. Trattner HR: Instrumental visualization of renal pelvis and its communications: proposal of a new method (preliminary report). *J Urol* 1948;61:817
2. Leadbetter WF: Instrumental visualization of renal pelvis at operation as an aid to diagnosis: presentation of a new instrument. *J Urol* 1950;63:1006
3. Alken P: Percutaneous ultrasonic destruction of renal calculi. *Urol Clin North Am* 1982;9:145
4. Miller RA, Wickham RA: Percutaneous nephrolithotomy: advances in equipment and endoscopic techniques. *Urology* 1984;23:2
5. Marshall VF: Fiberoptics in urology. *J Urol* 1964;91:110
6. Harris RD, McLaughlin AP, Harrell JH: Percutaneous nephroscopy using fiberoptic bronchoscope. *Urology* 1975;6:367
7. Clayman RV, Castañeda–Zuñiga WR: Rigid and flexible nephroscopy, in *Techniques in Endourology: A Guide to Percutaneous Removal of Renal and Ureteral Calculi.* Minneapolis, EndoPress, 1984, p 153
8. Clayman RV, Castañeda–Zuñiga WR: Instrumentation for nephrolithotomy, in *Techniques in Endourology: a Guide to Percutaneous Removal of Renal and Ureteral Calculi.* Minneapolis, EndoPress, 1984, p 185
9. Wickham JEA, Miller RA: The application of percutaneous techniques to noncalculous disease of the upper urinary tracts, in *Percutaneous Renal Surgery.* New York, Churchill–Livingstone, 1983, p 148
10. Badlani G, Eshghi M, Smith AD: Percutaneous surgery for ureteropelvic junction obstruction (endopyelotomy): technique and early results. *J Urol* 1986;135:26
11. Huffman JL, Clayman RV: Endoscopic visualization of the supravesical urinary tract: transurethral ureteropyeloscopy and percutaneous nephroscopy. *Semin Urol* 1985;3:60

27

Interventional Techniques in the Hepatobiliary System

S. MURTHY TADAVARTHY, M.D., DAVID W. HUNTER, M.D., CHRISTOPH L. ZOLLIKOFER, M.D., CAROL C. COLEMAN, M.D., WERNER BRÜEHLMAN, M.D., TONY P. SMITH, M.D., JANIS GISSEL LETOURNEAU, M.D., ANTONY T. YOUNG, M.D., MICHAEL D. DARCY, M.D., ANDREW H. CRAGG, M.D., FLAVIO CASTAÑEDA, M.D., ERICH K. SALOMONOWITZ, M.D., GUNNAR LUND, M.D., KURT AMPLATZ, M.D., AND WILFRIDO R. CASTAÑEDA-ZUÑIGA, M.D., M.Sc.

PERCUTANEOUS TRANSHEPATIC FINE-NEEDLE CHOLANGIOGRAPHY

The differential diagnosis of jaundice caused by parenchymal liver disease and that caused by extrahepatic obstruction is difficult if only the clinical and laboratory findings are considered. Nonetheless, such a distinction is critical for the institution of the proper medical or surgical therapy. The conventional radiologic studies also are of little value, because, in the patient with a serum bilirubin concentration 3 mg/dl, oral cholecystography and intravenous cholangiography are seldom successful. Fortunately, introduction of new imaging techniques, such as ultrasound (US), computed tomography (CT), and nuclear scanning, has substantially improved our capabilities in the evaluation of hepatic disease.

Ultrasonography is an accurate and sensitive method of distinguishing obstructive from nonobstructive jaundice; detection of obstruction depends on the demonstration of dilated intrahepatic or extrahepatic ducts. CT also images dilated bile ducts and, more often than US, reveals the level and cause of the obstruction. However, the demonstration of small lesions, partial obstructions, and biliary tree anatomy is beyond the capabilities of either US or CT. In addition, 10%–20% of patients with surgically correctable obstructing lesions, such as common duct stones, strictures, and tumors, will not have dilated ducts demonstrable by US or CT. In these cases, fine-needle transhepatic cholangiography (THC) is invaluable.[1,2]

HISTORY AND DEVELOPMENT

The technique of cholangiography was originally described by Burkhardt and Muller in 1921. They injected the gallbladder with contrast medium through a needle introduced through the liver under either local or general anesthesia.[3] In 1937, the technique was modified by Huard and Do-Xuan-Hop, who performed intrahepatic intraductal injections of iodized oil (Lipiodol).[4] Royer and associates injected contrast medium into the gallbladder under direct vision at the time of peritoneoscopy.[5] Despite these pioneering efforts, cholangiography was not extensively used until 1952, after the reports by Carter and Leger and their colleagues.[6,7] Even then all of these procedures were performed by surgeons, and their use was virtually restricted to the intraoperative or immediate preoperative period because of the complications attendant upon multiple liver punctures with a large needle.

In 1960, Prioton et al injected contrast medium into the biliary radicles by introducing the needle from the posterior aspect of the liver, thereby containing the leakage of bile and blood to the confines of the coronary ligament in the extraperitoneal space.[8] In 1966, Seldinger reported his experience with THC via a right subcostal approach using a sheathed-needle technique to decompress the biliary system and lower the complication rate.[9] In 1974, Okuda et al popularized THC by using a long, thin, flexible needle in 314 patients,[10] thus modifying a technique originally described by Ohto and Tsuchiya.[11,12] The fine-needle technique eliminated the need for surgical intervention immediately after the procedure. Compared with the large-needle techniques, there was a reduction in the complication rates: for intraperitoneal hemorrhage by a factor of 6, for bile leakage by a factor of 3, and for the mortality rate by a factor of 2.6.[13] Skinny-needle cholangiography is now a rapid and accurate method of differentiating intrahepatic and extrahepatic cholestasis. It is readily available, inexpensive, easy to learn, and associated with low morbidity and mortality rates.

INDICATIONS AND CONTRAINDICATIONS

Indications

At present, the accepted indications for THC are:

1. To differentiate medically treatable from surgically treatable jaundice[1,2];
2. To reveal intrahepatic calculi and extrahepatic choledocholithiasis[14,15];
3. To diagnose congenital abnormalities such as biliary atresia and choledochal cyst;
4. To evaluate biliary–enteric anastomoses postoperatively in patients with abdominal pain and jaundice[16];
5. To document intrahepatic abscesses communicating with the biliary radicles;
6. To perform pressure–flow studies in order to gain insight into the physiology and anatomy of the biliary system[17]; and
7. To study the biliary system prior to radiologic inter-

ventions such as biopsy and placement of drainage catheters.[18]

Contraindications

The contraindications to THC are:

1. Bleeding disorders that cannot be corrected by administration of vitamin K or blood products; in this situation, endoscopic retrograde cholangiopancreatography (ERCP) is the preferred procedure;
2. A history of a life-threatening reaction to iodinated contrast medium; and
3. Known hepatic vascular tumors or malformations.

Ascites and an uncooperative patient are relative contraindications.

PREPARATION OF THE PATIENT

An intravenous line is inserted before the procedure and kept open for the administration of fluids and drugs during the procedure. A coagulation profile is obtained, and any abnormality is corrected.

Intravenous broad-spectrum antibiotics are started, because the incidence of infected bile is 25%–36% in patients with malignant biliary obstruction and 71%–90% in those with choledocholithiasis.[19,20] The infecting microorganisms are gram-negative (especially *Escherichia coli* and *Enterobacter aerogenes*) in 66% of the cases and gram-positive (especially *Streptococcus faecalis*) in 21%. Therefore, the parenteral adminstration of

antibiotics such as ampicillin and gentamyicin is started 6–12 hr before the procedure and continued for 48–72 hr afterward. Other antibiotics with a similar broad spectrum of activity can be used; second- and third-generation cephalosporins, which penetrate effectively into bile, are particular favorites.

Intravenous or oral diazepam (Valium) and short-acting barbiturates or narcotics are administered as premedication. A vagolytic agent such as atropine is not given routinely but is readily available if it is needed during the procedure.

PROCEDURE

The patient is studied in the supine position, preferably with multidirectional fluoroscopy. The puncture site is selected using the fluoroscopically visible liver as a guide, and the tract is planned so that it traverses safely the maximum amount of liver substance. The usual tract, therefore, parallels the caudal edge of the liver (slight cephalad orientation of the needle tip) about a third of the way up from the caudal edge to the dome of the liver under the diaphragm. Thus, the puncture is usually made from the 7th to the 10th intercostal space, slightly anterior to the midaxillary line, and below the costophrenic angle. One should keep in mind that the pleural reflection—which in the back lies at the level of the 12th rib—laterally reaches to the level of the 10th rib (Fig. 27–1) before swinging superiorly on its anterior course (Fig. 27–2). Therefore most punctures above the 10th rib will be transpleural (across the costophrenic angle), although not necessarily transpulmonary, because the lung commonly lies at a higher level during shallow normal breathing, reaching down into the costophrenic recess only during deep inspiration (Fig. 27–3). To avoid the intercostal vessels, it is preferable to stay close to the top edge of the lower rib. Liver size and position are evaluated dur-

ing the initial fluoroscopic examination. Interposition of bowel loops should be carefully sought.

After the skin is prepared and draped in the usual fashion, the puncture site is infiltrated with 1% lidocaine down to the liver capsule. A 15-cm-long flexible 22-gauge needle with a 30° noncutting bevel is used for the puncture.[10–12] Under normal, shallow breathing, the needle is advanced under fluoroscopic control parallel to the table top until the tip reaches the midline of the vertebral body. The stylet is then removed, and a 12-ml syringe filled with dilute (1:1) contrast medium is attached to clear flexible polyethylene tubing, which is connected to the hub of the needle. Under fluoroscopic observation, contrast medium is steadily and slowly injected while the needle is slowly withdrawn. The goal is to create a thin, continuous tract of contrast behind the retreating needle. If too much contrast is injected, "puddles" will form which obscure future attempts, whereas if too little is injected, the subtle "flowing away" of contrast from the needle tip (which signifies that either a vessel or a duct has been entered) will be missed. As long as the needle tip is in parenchyma, the contrast medium will stay close to the tip and have a faint cloud-like appearance; as soon

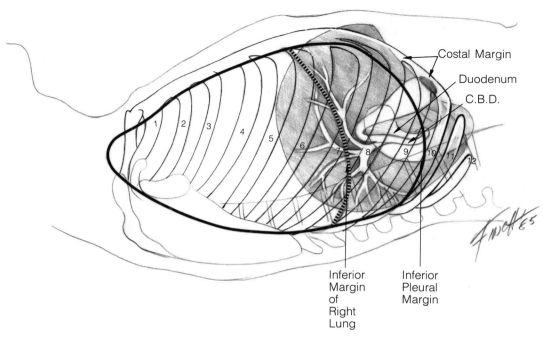

Fig. 27–1 Relation of inferior margin of lung, inferior pleural margin, liver, ribs (1–12), and intercostal spaces in respect to biliary tree in the lateral projection. C.B.D. = common bile duct.

as the tip enters a duct or vessel, the contrast will flow quickly away from the tip. Thus, injection of slightly larger amounts of contrast permits rapid, and usually easy, identification of the structure. If a duct has been entered, the contrast moves slowly at first, with a puddled appearance, toward the hilum. Branching of the ducts should quickly be obvious. If a duct is not found on the first puncture, subsequent needle passages should fan out

from the first tract, going first in a cephalad direction, then anterior, then posterior, and finally caudad (Fig. 27–4). In more caudal passages, the operator should be careful not to advance the needle too far medially, not only because of the risk of puncturing the gallbladder, porta hepatis, vena cava, or aorta, but also because inadvertent extrahepatic passage of the needle through the medial capsule and intraperitoneal injection of contrast medium

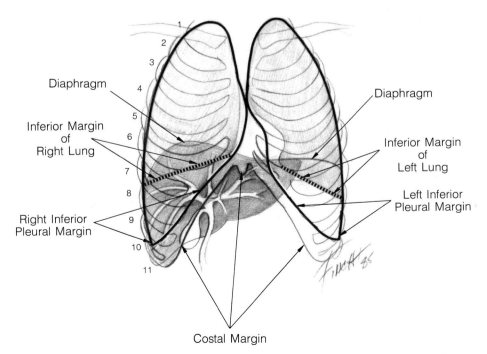

Fig. 27–2 Relations of inferior pleural margin, inferior margin of lung, diaphragms, liver, and ribs (1–11) in the anteroposterior projection. Typical entry points through eighth or ninth intercostal space are transpleural.

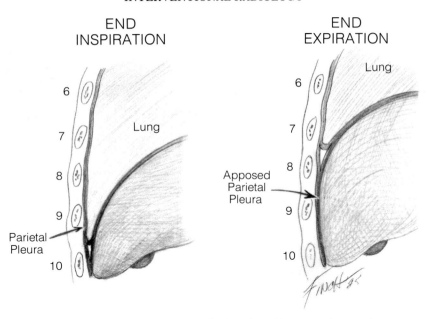

END INSPIRATION   **END EXPIRATION**

Fig. 27–3   Change in the relations between the inferior lung margin, ribs (6–10), and intercostal spaces in respect to the liver during inhalation and exhalation.

can be extremely painful for the patient. Indeed, many patients with this complication may have such severe shortness of breath and right shoulder pain, and such problems with vasovagal reactions, that the examination may have to be delayed.

In patients with dilated bile ducts, a 99%–100% success rate can be achieved with 4–6 needle passages,

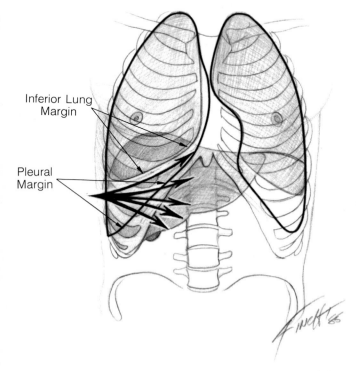

Fig. 27–4   Use of fine-needle cholangiography to localize biliary radicles with single entry point.

although as many as 14 passages have been used routinely by some authors without increasing the complication rate.[13] In patients with nondilated bile ducts, more punctures may be required. In these cases, a direct puncture of the larger extrahepatic ducts, either blindly, with the aid of bony landmarks, or under US guidance can be attempted (Fig. 27–5). No complications such as bile leak or hemorrhage have occurred as a result of this technique.

Continuous fluoroscopic monitoring, with magnification if possible, is of paramount importance during needle withdrawal and contrast injection in order to identify any structure entered by the needle. As previously mentioned, one should always be able to see a persistent tract through the liver parenchyma caused by contrast injection during needle withdrawal (Fig. 27–6).

The hepatic lymphatic channels are identified by their small size and beaded appearance and by the direction of the flow toward the porta hepatis (Fig. 27–7). The channels typically remain opacified for 5–10 min. The celiac lymph nodes also may be opacified.[21] The hepatic vein radicles are recognized by the rapid clearance of the contrast medium in the direction of the right atrium. Portal vein radicles are identified by the rapid clearance of contrast medium toward the periphery and, except for the speed of flow, may be difficult to distinguish from branches of the hepatic artery. In addition, injection into a hepatic artery seems to cause a more intense parenchymal stain. Bile ducts, as mentioned, are recognized by the slow flow of puddled contrast medium, which may flow in a peripheral direction initially but eventually will always flow toward the common hepatic duct.

With the patient supine, contrast medium, which has a higher specific gravity than bile, will flow to the most dependent posterior ducts (Fig. 27–8). Unless an anterior duct has been entered, this flow occasionally causes difficulties with opacification of the central ducts and

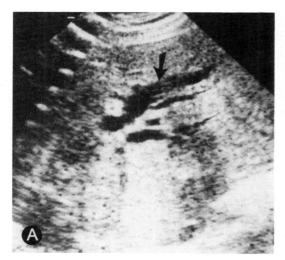
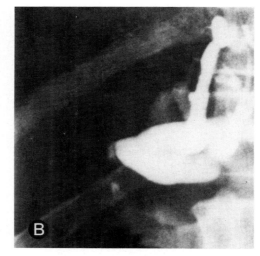

Fig. 27–5 Puncture under ultrasound guidance. A. Ultrasound shows marked dilatation of left biliary radicles (arrow). B. Puncture of left biliary radicles was performed with 22-gauge Chiba needle. Contrast medium shows marked dilatation of left biliary radicles not communicating with right biliary tree. (Reproduced from Mueller PR, et al: Fine-needle transhepatic cholangiography: reflections after 450 cases. *AJR* 1981;136:85–90 with the permission of the American Roentgen Ray Society.)

almost always causes some difficulty with opacification of the left anterior ducts, which is important if an epigastric approach is desired for drainage (Fig. 27–9). To fill the ducts completely, a variety of maneuvers may be needed, such as turning the patient into the left posterior oblique or even the prone oblique position or tilting the table.[22,23] A simpler technique, described by Young et al for opacification of the anterior biliary radicles, consists of the introduction of 30–50 ml of CO_2 through the needle. Because of its lower specific gravity, the gas will flow to the most elevated part of the biliary tree, the anterior ducts, which can then be punctured (Fig. 27–10).[23] This technique has been much less successful than in the urinary tract, because the CO_2 is difficult to see and diffuses rapidly out of the ducts. Forceful attempts to opacify the entire biliary tree with contrast medium should be avoided, inasmuch as this increases the chances of bacteremia and sepsis.

At the completion of the procedure in the presence of obstruction or partial obstruction in a patient in whom drainage will not be done, an attempt can be made to aspirate the contrast medium through the skinny needle.

Fig. 27–6 Chiba needle tract opacified with contrast medium.

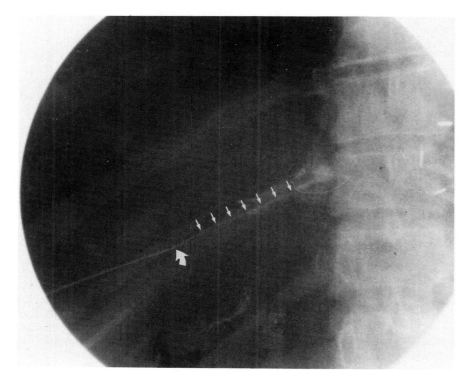

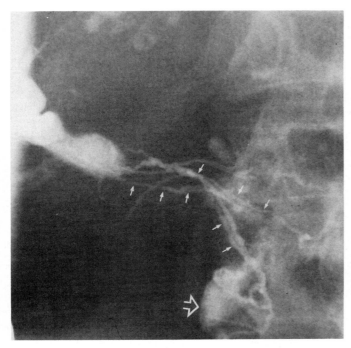

Fig. 27-7 Incidental opacification of hepatic lymphatics (small arrows) and retroperitoneal lymph node (open arrow) during fine-needle cholangiography.

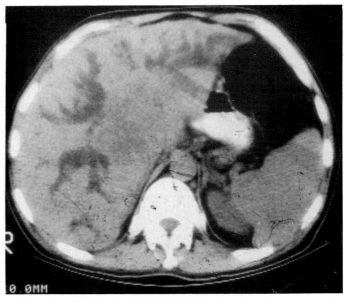

Fig. 27-9 CT scan through liver shows enormous dilatation of biliary tree due to mass at porta hepatis obstructing common hepatic duct. Observe short distance from skin to left biliary radicles because of their anterior location.

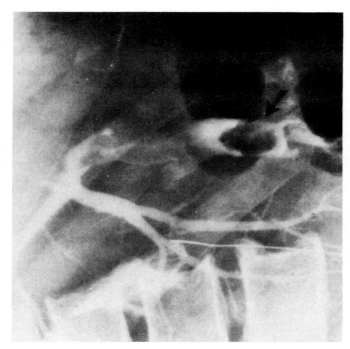

Fig. 27-8 Cross-table fine-needle cholangiogram shows accumulation of contrast medium in most dependent portions of biliary tree with no opacification of anterior biliary radicles. Large stone is seen within common bile duct (arrow). (Reproduced from Mueller PR, et al: Fine-needle transhepatic cholangiography: reflections after 450 cases. *AJR* 1981;136:85–90 with the permission of the American Roentgen Ray Society.)

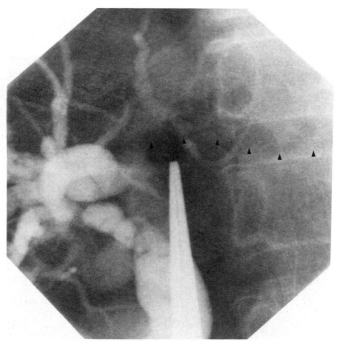

Fig. 27-10 Hemostat marks intended puncture site into left duct, which is filled with CO_2(arrowheads). (Reproduced from Young AT, Cardella JF, Castañeda–Zuñiga WR, Hunter DW, Amplatz K: The anterior approach to left biliary catheterization. *Semin Intervent Radiol* 1985;2:31–38 with the permission of Thieme, Inc.)

If successful, this maneuver decreases the distention of the biliary ducts and decompresses the system. However, it is difficult to aspirate the viscous contrast along with the thick, viscous bile through a skinny needle, and the yield is usually slight. After needle withdrawal, the patient is observed closely for complications such as sepsis and hemorrhage. Usually, bed rest for 4–6 hr is required.

TRANSHEPATIC CHOLANGIOGRAPHY VERSUS ENDOSCOPIC RETROGRADE CHOLANGIOPANCREATOGRAPHY (ERCP)

ERCP is useful when one desires to study both the biliary and pancreatic ducts as well as the pancreas. However, the 90%–99% success rate of THC in demonstrating the bile ducts compares favorably with ERCP's success rate of 70% in patients with suspected biliary obstruction.[13,22,24–28] In addition, THC is available in most health care centers and is less expensive than ERCP, which requires expensive endoscopic instruments and highly skilled endoscopists, who may not be available in smaller community hospitals. Also, the total cost of ERCP is at least four times that of THC.[29] There is no statistical difference between the THC morbidity (3%) and mortality (0.1%) rates and the ERCP morbidity (3%) and mortality (0.3%) rates.[13]

COMPLICATIONS

Harbin et al, in a study compiled from several institutions, found a complication rate of 3.28% in 3596 patients who underwent THC with a fine needle.[13] The complications of THC included:

1. Death;
2. Sepsis;
3. Hemorrhage;
4. Bile leakage;
5. Miscellaneous (pneumothorax, contrast reactions, hepatic arteriovenous fistulae, and vasovagal reactions).

Death

The five reported deaths yield a 0.14% mortality rate for the 3596 patients in the study of Harbin et al. All five of these patients had required immediate operation for complications of THC and died in the postoperative period. Therefore, some of the deaths may not have been directly related to complications of THC but rather to the operation.[13]

Sepsis

Because of the high incidence of infected bile (70%–90% in choledocholithiasis and 25%–36% in malignant obstruction), it is not surprising that sepsis occurred in 1.8% of patients after THC.[13,19,20] Sepsis is more common in patients with obstructed biliary ducts. At the time of cholangiography, bacteria are forced into hepatic veins by forceful injections.[30] Sepsis can be manifested as fever, chills, light-headedness, nausea, or malaise and is documented by the finding of hypotension or a positive blood culture. Septic shock can occur. In two-thirds of the patients, more than one type of organism is found. To minimize this complication, antibiotics effective against both gram-positive and gram-negative bacteria should be administered prior to THC.[31]

Hemorrhage

Intraperitoneal hemorrhage occurred in only 0.28% of the 3596 patients.

Bile Leakage

At operation, intraperitoneal leakage was found in 1.03% of patients after fine-needle cholangiography, compared to 3.45% after use of a larger needle.[13]

Miscellaneous Complications

Allergic contrast reactions, such as skin rash, bronchospasm, and hypotension, were seen in 0.15% of the patients. Vasovagal reactions were infrequent. If clinically indicated, such reactions can be prevented by premedication with intramuscular atropine.

Three silent hepatic arteriovenous fistulae have been demonstrated by hepatic arteriography.[32] In patients with hemobilia secondary to fistulae or hepatic artery aneurysms, transcatheter arterial embolization has been done.[33–36] Hemobilia and its management are discussed in Chapter 10.

PERCUTANEOUS BILIARY DRAINAGE PROCEDURES

Forty-three years passed after the first description of THC before the possibility of percutaneous transhepatic biliary drainage (PTBD) was recognized.[9,37] Simple external drainage using a sheathed-needle technique was reported by several authors beginning in 1974.[18,38–40] Subsequently, guidewires and catheters were developed to negotiate areas of stricture and obstruction. Now, indwelling catheters can be placed, and combined external–internal drainage with antegrade flow of bile into the bowel can be achieved.[41–46] The new techniques offer the possibility of palliative decompression of the bile ducts in either benign or malignant disease with low morbidity and mortality rates.

The traditional therapy for malignant biliary obstruction has been the surgical creation of a biliary–enteric anastomosis, but this technique has significant morbidity and carries an operative mortality rate of as much as 15%–60%, depending on the severity of the liver disease.[47–53] The factors influencing the outcome of surgical decompression are the presence of a high common hepatic duct, obstruction necessitating a high biliary–enteric anastomosis and a mass extending into the hilum producing a separate, noncommunicating obstruction of the left and right ducts. In such cases, surgical decompression should not be attempted.[43,47–56] An additional consideration is that as many as 90% of patients with obstructive jaundice who undergo exploratory laparotomy are found to have inoperable tumors.[47,50,54,57]

The principal application of PTBD has been for nonoperative drainage of malignant biliary obstruction. The criteria for determining whether a particular patient will undergo surgical or percutaneous decompression are either anatomic or physiologic. Patients with high or multiple branch obstructions and patients who are high operative risks because of cardiac, pulmonary, or renal complications are candidates for PTBD. Patients with malignant obstructions and a short life expectancy are probably also well served by the less morbid percutaneous techniques. In some cases, PTBD may be used to stabilize a patient for other procedures. Several authors have claimed a reduction in morbidity and mortality rates from 28% to 6% in patients operated on after a period of percutaneous biliary drainage,[41,42,57–60] supposedly attributable to better liver function and improved

wound healing.[47,55,56] However, current data do not support this belief,[57,61,62] and a randomized prospective trial will be needed to settle the question.

Patients with lower common duct or periampullary obstructions who present in stable hemodynamic condition earlier in the course of their disease will typically undergo surgical palliation. This preselection of less ill patients for operation has led to statements in the surgical literature that open palliation is more effective than PTBD in the management of biliary obstruction.[63–67] However, when similar groups of patients are treated, or when the data are corrected statistically for severity bias, similar morbidity and mortality rates are found.[58] Nevertheless, PTBD should not be used indiscriminately in every patient with biliary obstruction, because patients often will derive benefit from PTBD only when they are symptomatic or when their life expectancy may be shortened by recurrent cholangitis, progressive hepatic dysfunction, or nutritional deficiencies secondary to bile flow obstruction. In most patients with biliary obstruction secondary to malignancy, death occurs in 6 months to 1 year.[47–51,54,68,69] Exceptions to these grim statistics are patients with cholangiocarcinoma, who have a mean survival of 14 months,[70] and those with ampullary carcinoma, who have a survival rate of 33% at 5 years.[71] The net results of PTBD in improving the quality of life and the length of survival have to be weighed against the possible complications.

Technologic advances in instrumentation and imaging have extended the use of the percutaneous biliary tract originally designed for drainage to the management of biliary duct strictures and biliary fistulae, and to stone removal, biopsies, and intracanalicular radiation therapy with remarkable success.

INSTRUMENTATION FOR BILIARY DRAINAGE PROCEDURES

Catheters

Drainage catheters can be divided into two large groups:

1. Exteriorized drainage catheters. This group includes both those catheters that are solely for external drainage and those that have an external portion but extend past the area of obstruction and permit internal drainage.
2. Internal drainage catheters. This group includes only those stents that have no external portion.

The exteriorized drainage catheters can be further divided into two groups according to their retention characteristics:

1. "Free" catheters, which have minimal self-retaining ability; examples are the pigtail, Ring's biliary catheter, and any straight multipurpose catheter such as the universal stents; and
2. "Fixed" catheters, which have a stronger self-retaining mechanism; examples are the Sack's, Cope's, Hawkins accordion, any of the "U"-loop types, and any catheter with a retention balloon, such as a Foley.

The internal stents can be classified according to the material from which they are made, as well as according to any alterations in shape or design incorporated to inhibit migration. Materials in common use today for internal biliary stents include Teflon, C-Flex, and Silastic.

FREE CATHETERS

Pigtail Catheters

The pigtail is an angiographic catheter available in sizes of 5F–10F (Fig. 27–11). For drainage purposes, particularly for temporary internal drainage, polyethylene is used so that sideholes can be created along the catheter shaft, something that obviously is not possible with a torque control (wire mesh) pigtail catheter. The two chief disadvantages of this catheter are its lack of self-retaining capabilities and the small size of the sideholes, which is limited by the narrow diameter of the hole punches. The authors commonly use a pigtail as an initial, temporary catheter to establish drainage, because it is so easy to insert. The pigtail is usually replaced by a permanent internal–external or internal stent at a second sitting.

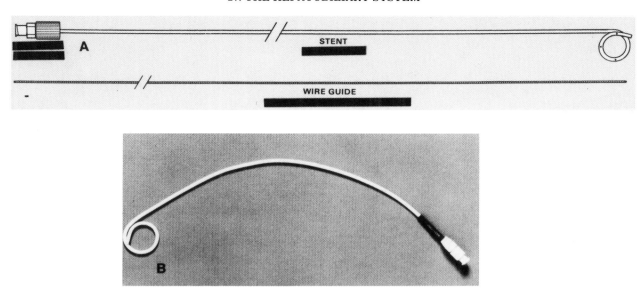

Fig. 27–11   Drainage catheters. A. Pigtail catheter. Sideholes must be made in appropriate position. (Courtesy of Cook, Inc.) B. C-Flex stent. (Courtesy of Medi–Tech, Inc.)

Ring Catheter

The Ring biliary catheter is an 8F polyethylene catheter with an outer diameter of 2.7 mm, an inner diameter of 1.8 mm, and 40 sideholes in the distal 12 cm.[72] For the drainage of thick, viscous bile, 9.6F catheters are also commercially available. A right-angle bend is present at the distal end of the catheter (Fig. 27–12); when the bend is positioned at the ampulla, catheter migration is inhibited. If the catheter is properly positioned, most of the sideholes are in the common duct and duodenum to provide antegrade drainage. For a higher obstruction, closer to or above the bifurcation, additional proximal sideholes are made with a hole punch. Although the holes in the distal 3 cm are designed to maintain antegrade drainage, they also, unfortunately, allow duodenal contents to enter the catheter, which can impede antegrade flow of bile or even completely block the catheter.

Practically speaking, the self-retaining properties of the catheter do not prevent migration in all cases. However, the stiffness of the catheter makes it easy to insert through the liver parenchyma, and good external drainage of bile can easily be maintained for 1–5 days. Later, this catheter is replaced with one of the softer and larger (10F–12F) polyethylene catheters for long-term drainage.

FIXED CATHETERS

Hawkins Catheter

The Hawkins accordion catheter is a 6.5F Teflon catheter with excellent self-retaining capabilities and probably the best long-term patency for its size because of the low encrustation coefficient of Teflon.[73] The catheter has a distal sigmoid curve with several sideholes and a distal tip tapered to 0.028 inch. A monofilament thread passes as a loop in and out through the sideholes, and the ends of the string are brought through the lumen of the catheter into the proximal hub. When the strings are pulled, the distal end folds or "accordions" on itself (Fig. 27–13). The shape is maintained by securing the strings in a Tuohy–Borst adapter (Fig. 27–14).

The catheter is mounted over a long 22-gauge flexible needle for insertion in one step. After puncture of the bile duct, an 0.018-inch mandril guidewire is advanced through the flexible needle (Fig. 27–15), which can then be advanced safely over the smooth steel section of the mandril for a few millimeters into the duct. The slippery accordion catheter is then advanced over the stiff mandril–needle combination.

To remove the catheter, the monofilament thread is

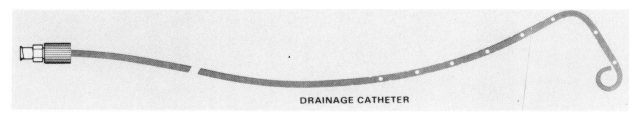

Fig. 27–12   Ring biliary drainage catheter. (Courtesy of Cook, Inc.)

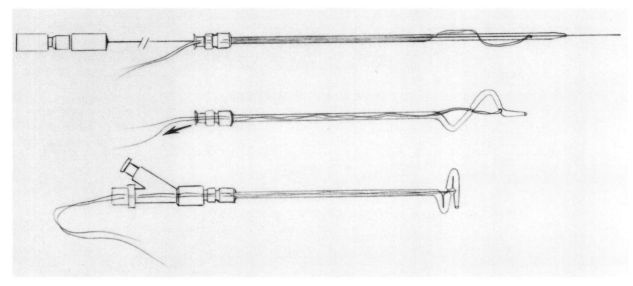

Fig. 27–13 "Accordion" catheter.

released, and a 0.025-inch guidewire is advanced through the lumen. This guidewire is small enough to pass through the distal end and under most circumstances is strong enough to straighten the distal accordion loop (Fig. 27–16). If the guidewire will not exit through the catheter tip, one can introduce a 0.035-inch guidewire, which is too large to go through the tip but will usually exit through the larger proximal sidehole. The stent is then exchanged for a similar or larger catheter. Because of the stiffness of Teflon, it is almost impossible to pull the stent out when it is properly looped within the biliary tree.

Cope Catheter

The Cope loop is an 8F or 10F pigtail catheter with several distal sideholes and a distal loop that is fixed by a thread that runs through the lumen of the catheter to the external hub, where it is tied (Fig. 27–17). However, unlike conventional pigtail catheters, which are somewhat stiff and can be withdrawn accidentally despite being sutured to the skin, the Cope catheters are usually made from a softer material such as polyvinyl chloride, Silastic, C-Flex, or rubber, and the fixed loop configura-

tion prevents accidental removal.[74] The loop is created by applying tension on the thread, the proximal end of which is knotted around the proximal portion of the catheter and is covered with rubber tubing. The loop should be tested prior to placement by gently pulling on the string; the limbs should fold across each other without undue kinking.

Although the Cope loop has excellent self-retention capabilities, the patency rate is poor because of rapid encrustation of biliary salts around the thread used to form the loop. Indeed, sometimes the encrustation is so pronounced that it is impossible to pass a wire to straighten the loop for exchange purposes. In this situation, a technique originally described by Cope is used in which the catheter hub and the thread are cut off and a sheath introducer is passed over the catheter until it reaches the loop.[75] The loop is then pulled back forcefully against the leading edge of the sheath, breaking the encrustation and allowing the loop to straighten (Fig. 27–18). The catheter is removed through the sheath, and a guidewire is passed into the biliary tree to complete the exchange.

Due to the softness and high coefficient of friction of C-Flex, introduction of these catheters is simplified by

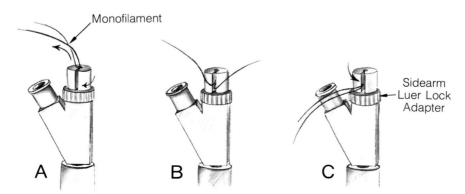

Fig. 27–14 Luer Lok adaptor used for securing monofilament in Hawkins accordion catheter.

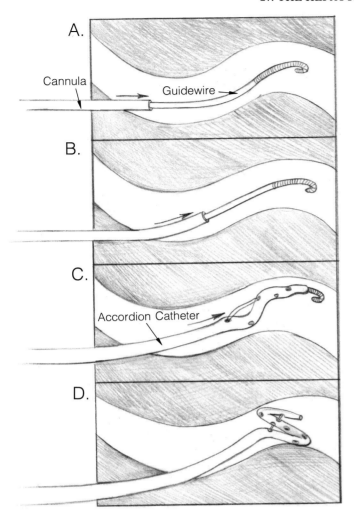

using a cannula introducer inside the catheter that fits over a 0.038-inch wire. The cannula is flexible enough to follow gentle curves, or it can be curved prior to introduction.

One disadvantage of the Cope loop is the large size of the loop, which can form only in a significantly dilated biliary radicle. However, with experience the operator can reshape the loop in moderately dilated bile ducts. For internal drainage, the loop can be reshaped in the duodenum. In this case, extra sideholes must be present in the shaft. Cope loops with extra sideholes proximal to the loop are available; alternatively, sideholes can be made with a hole punch or paper punch, taking care not to cut the thread.

Sacks–Malecot Catheters

The Sacks–Malecot catheter (Medi–Tech, Inc.) is made of Percuflex in 8F and 10.3F sizes. It has the largest lumen for its outer diameter of all the catheters now available and comes in two lengths: 35 cm for external drainage and 40 cm for combined internal–external drainage (Fig. 27–19A,B). The longer catheter is available with the large Malecot opening two different distances from the catheter tip; the level of the obstruction usually dictates which design to use. That is, in patients with a

Fig. 27–15 Insertion of accordion catheter. A. The 0.018-inch mandril guidewire is advanced through 21-gauge flexible needle. B. Needle is advanced over smooth steel section of mandril into duct. C. Teflon catheter has been advanced over stiff needle–guidewire assembly, and needle has been withdrawn. D. After removal of guidewire, monofilament is pulled to reshape the accordion, which is then fixed with Luer-Lok adapter.

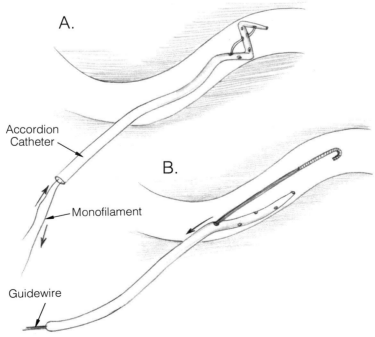

Fig. 27–16 Removal of accordion catheter. A. Hub of the accordion has been cut to allow monofilament to retract, loosen the accordion.

B. A 0.025-inch guidewire is advanced; although it commonly exits through end hole, it may also exit through a sidehole.

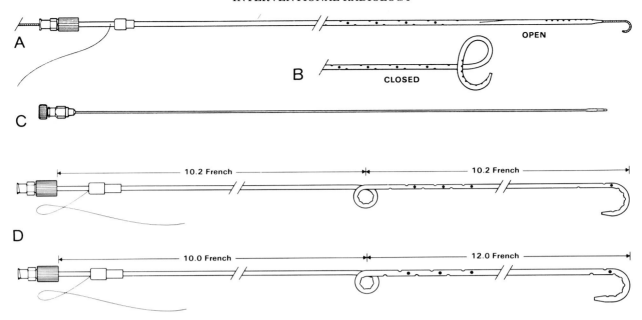

Fig. 27–17   Cope loop catheters. A. Standard biliary loop. B. Close-up of loop. C. Stiff introducer. (Courtesy of Cook, Inc.) D. Cope proximal loop. Loop in middle of catheter secures its position; terminal pigtail prevents trauma of bowel wall. Larger diameter of distal segment drains bile better. (Courtesy of Cook, Inc.)

high obstruction (near the porta hepatis), the catheter with the Malecot opening farther from the tip is used. With this design, there are no sideholes proximal to the Malecot tip, which is placed above the obstruction and serves as the primary or sole egress for the obstructed bile. The segment of catheter distal to the tip has several sideholes for internal drainage of bile into either the distal common bile duct or the duodenum. In the other design, the Malecot tip is only 2–3 cm away from the catheter tip and there are several sideholes proximal and distal to the Malecot opening. This design is more often used in common bile duct obstruction, especially that close to the ampulla. The Malecot tip is advanced beyond the ampulla into the duodenum and prevents retrograde migration of the catheter while providing good internal drainage. Depending on the clinical situation and the

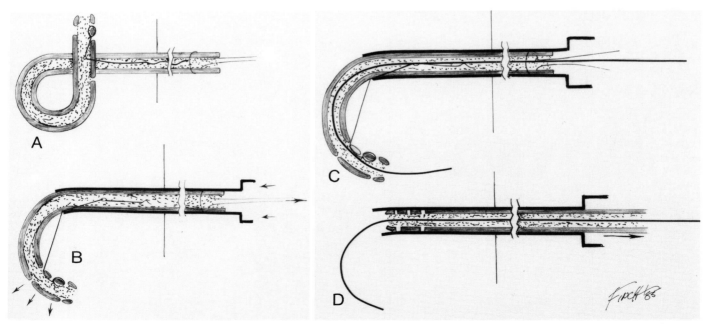

Fig. 27–18   Technique for removal of stuck Cope loop. A. After hub of catheter is cut, a suture is placed through tubing. B. A sheath is advanced over the shaft and sutured. C. Leading edge of sheath is used to straighten the stuck loop forcefully, subsequently advancing guidewire through catheter. D. Catheter is removed through sheath, keeping guidewire in place.

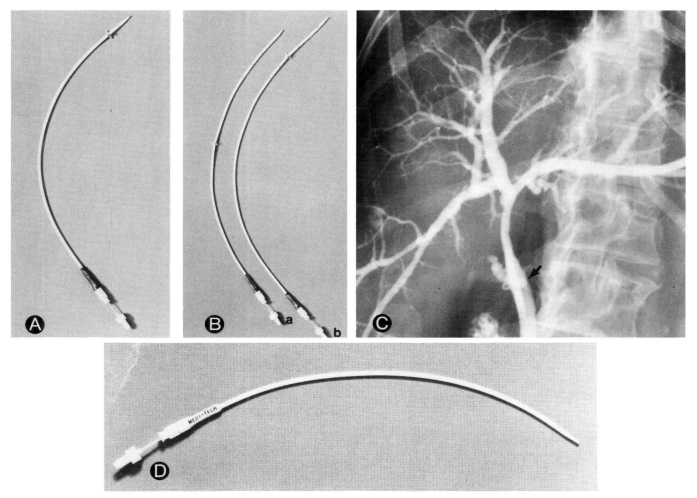

Fig. 27-19 Sacks–Malecot catheters. A. Design for external drainage. (Courtesy of Medi-Tech, Inc.) B. Design for internal–external drainage. (Courtesy of Medi-Tech, Inc.) C. Sack catheter (arrow) in patient with obstruction of common bile duct. D. Universal stent designed to accommodate differences in anatomy; sideholes are created with paper punch. (Courtesy of Medi-Tech, Inc.)

anatomic configuration of the biliary system, necessary additional holes can be made with a paper punch, which gives a very smooth edge to the hole, or, if that device is unavailable, with scissors or a blade.

Passage of a guidewire or stiffener through the catheter prior to removal or exchange may be difficult because of the sideholes. This problem can be overcome by advancing the internal stiffener inside the stent up to the difficult area and then carefully probing with a slightly curved or torque control guidewire. Occasionally, the stent must be pulled back slightly and straightened in order to negotiate the guidewire beyond a sidehole.

These catheters are soft, which is desirable for patient comfort but which makes it necessary to use an internal stiffener for introduction and removal. The stiffener is also needed to straighten the wings of the Malecot tip during introduction and, occasionally, during removal.

The use of an obtuse-angle Molnar disk (VanTech, Medi–Tech, Surgitech) is recommended to prevent kinking of the catheter at the skin level. The self-retention properties provided by the Malecot tip are, at best, mediocre, but the resistance to encrustation is excellent.

INTERNAL STENTS

There are several internal stents that can be used in the patient with biliary obstruction. Many of these are homemade, but some good stents are available commercially, each of which comes with a special introducer system.

Teflon stents are available from Cook, Inc. of Europe. These stents come in 12F or 14F sizes and in different lengths and shapes to accommodate the variable anatomy of the biliary tree. A flange at the proximal (intrahepatic) end of the stent prevents forward migration and another at the distal (common duct or duodenal) end prevents retrograde displacement (Fig. 27–20). The main disadvantage of this stent is its stiffness, which makes it almost impossible to remove endoscopically. Its main advantage is the long-term patency rate achieved by Teflon, which has one of the lowest encrustation coefficients of all the available materials.

The Carey–Coons stents from Medi–Tech are made of soft plastic (Percuflex). The 12F 15-cm-long stent has an angiographic tip tapered to fit a 0.038-inch guidewire and multiple sideholes at the proximal and distal ends (Fig.

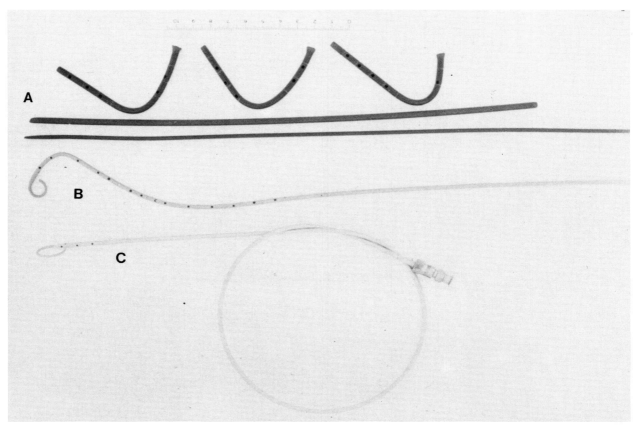

Fig. 27–20 Drainage catheters. A. Cook internal stent; different shapes and lengths to accommodate variable anatomy of bile ducts. B. Ring catheter. C. Pigtail catheter.

27–21). Attached to the stent is a monofilament nylon suture designed to pass out through the tract to an anchoring button that is left under the skin to prevent stent migration and for eventual use in case the stent gets obstructed.[76] However, because they may encourage infection, the suture and button are usually cut off and discarded. The tapered tip of the stent makes introduction simple but also impedes antegrade flow of bile and therefore tends to speed up the precipitation of biliary salts in the distal lumen. The soft texture of the stent permits easy retrieval under fluoroscopic or endoscopic control.

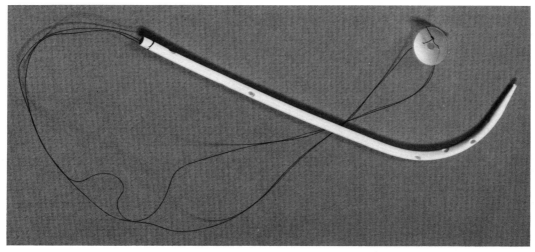

Fig. 27–21 Carey–Coons Percuflex stent; tapered tip and multiple sideholes along shaft. String at proximal end is for fixation under the skin with the help of a Silastic button.

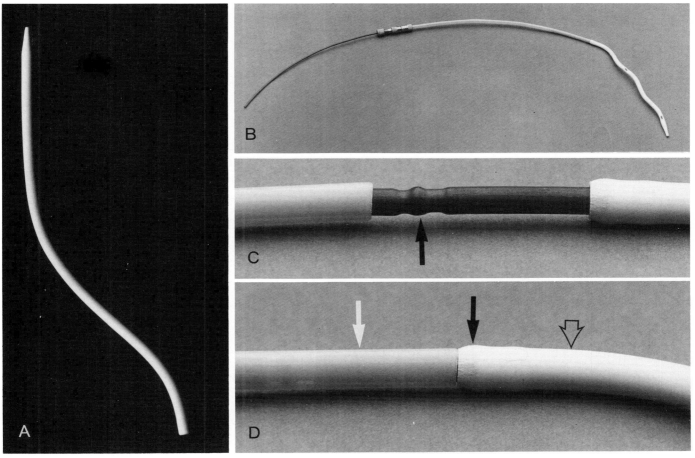

Fig. 27–22 Amplatz C-Flex biliary stent. A. Stent. B. Stent with introducer/stiffener. C. Close-up view of introducer shows position of bead (arrow) on midsegment to lock stent while it is being advanced. D. Stent (open arrow) locked over bead (black arrow); pusher (white arrow).

Cook has a new 10F–12F C-Flex stent with an introducing system that makes placement easy and accurate. Several S-shaped curves in the stent help prevent migration (Fig. 27–22).

A 12F–14F Silastic stent available from USCI has a Malecot design in the proximal (intrahepatic) end to prevent migration and radiopaque stripes along the edge of the tube to permit fluoroscopic examination (Fig. 27–23). The high coefficient of friction of Silastic makes introduction of this stent more difficult. Predilation of the tract to 2F larger than the stent is helpful even when the internal stiffener introducing system is used.

Needles

The needles commonly used for biliary interventional techniques are the Chiba (skinny) needle (22- or 23-gauge), the sheathed needle (TLA, MEC, Hawkins), and the nonsheathed 18-gauge needle.

CHIBA (SKINNY) NEEDLES

These 22- or 23-gauge needles (Fig. 27–24) are the usual choice for the preprocedure cholangiogram. The puncture can be made either under fluoroscopic control

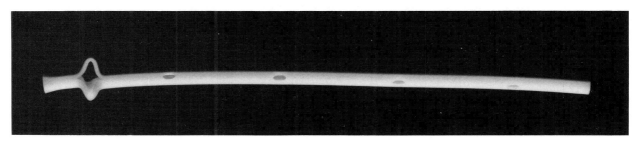

Fig. 27–23 Silastic Malecot stent.

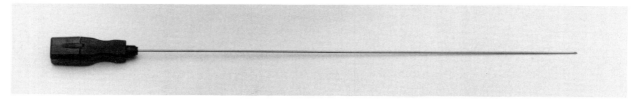

Fig. 27–24 Chiba needle (21 gauge).

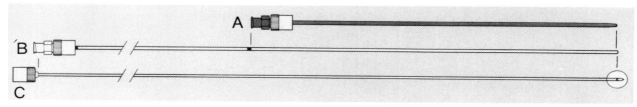

Fig. 27–25 Hawkins needle. A. Teflon catheter. B. Metal cannula; black marker indicates that tip of Teflon catheter is even with tip of cannula. C. Stylet. (Courtesy of Cook, Inc.)

through a right lateral approach or under ultrasound guidance through the epigastrium into a left biliary radicle.[10]

SHEATHED NEEDLES

The Hawkins needle is a 20-gauge, 20-inch-long needle with a Teflon accordion stent mounted on the shaft (Fig. 27–25).[73,77] A special stiff 0.018-inch wire is passed

through the needle into the collecting system for stent introduction.

The translumbar aortography needle is 18 gauge with either a diamond or a beveled tip and comes with a snugly fitted Teflon sheath.[9] A 0.038-inch guidewire fits through this needle (Fig. 27–26).

The MEC set consists of a 22-cm-long, 21-gauge needle with a 19-gauge, 15-cm-long metallic cannula over which a 16F Teflon sheath is snugly fitted. No wire is provided with this set (Fig. 27–27).

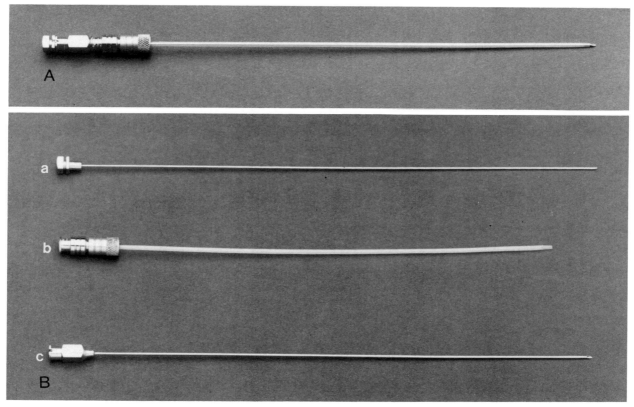

Fig. 27–26 Translumbar aortography needle. A. Assembled. B. Unassembled, showing stylet (a), Teflon sheath (b), and cannula (c).

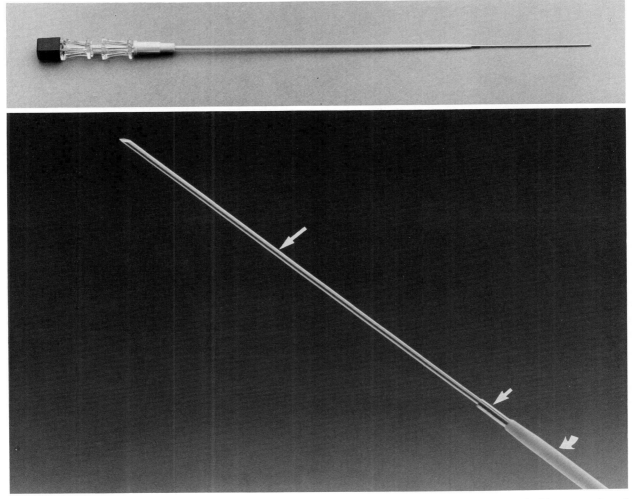

Fig. 27–27 MEC needle. A. Assembled. B. Unassembled, showing 21-gauge needle (long arrow), 18-gauge cannula (short arrow), and sheath (curved arrow).

NONSHEATHED NEEDLES

An 18-gauge diamond-tip needle that accepts a 0.038-inch guidewire is provided with all Cook nephrostomy sets.

Guidewires

A wide selection of angiographic guidewires can be used in biliary interventional procedures. The authors have found the following most useful:

0.035-inch floppy-tip Bentson wire (Cook, Inc.);
0.038-inch J-wire (Cook, Inc.);
Lunderquist wire (0.038-inch; Cook, Inc.; Surgimed);
Lunderquist–Ring torque control wire (0.038-inch; Cook);
Amplatz stiffening wire (0.035-inch, 0.038-inch; Cook, Inc.);
"Coat-hanger" wire (0.018-inch; Cook, Inc.);
Wire stiffeners (Dotter cannula).

BENTSON WIRE

A long floppy-tip, 0.035-inch, Teflonized guidewire is used with a torque control catheter to traverse dilated, tortuous bile ducts with minimal trauma. When this wire is used, the entire floppy portion should be coiled within the bile ducts before one attempts to pass dilators or catheters; if the floppy portion is even partially outside the ducts, the entire wire can easily be dislodged. If a fresh tract is lost, it is usually impossible to recanalize.

J-WIRE

These 0.038-inch Teflonized guidewires are used for dilation and catheter placement.[78] There is no advantage to a tight (3-mm) J over a wide (15-mm) J.

LUNDERQUIST WIRE

This 0.038-inch wire, available in either stainless-steel (Cook, Inc.) or Teflon-coated (Surgimed) versions, is extremely strong and consists of two parts: a longer (80-

cm) section of rigid stainless steel and a 5–10-cm-long flexible tip (Fig. 27–28A).[79] The stiff part of the wire is useful for passing drainage catheters or dilators in patients with cirrhosis, extensive metastatic disease, tight fibrotic stenoses, or ascites. The Teflonized version permits slightly smoother exchanges, especially of Silastic catheters. The weak point of the wire is the joint between the stiff and floppy segments, where the wire may bend and, occasionally, break. This sharp transition confers two other disadvantages on the wire. First, sometimes it is difficult or impossible to get the juncture point around a sharp bend. Second, the floppy part can bend back at the joint, creating a sharp, stiff leading edge that can easily perforate a duct wall.

LUNDERQUIST–RING WIRE

This torque control wire is a 0.038-inch stainless-steel wire with a short floppy tip that can be rotated to manipulate it around bends. The torque control is the result of its construction, with the spring coil soldered at intervals to the central stiff core (Fig. 27–28B); this makes it possible to shape the wire into different curves. The external segment of the guidewire is coiled into a loop which, when rotated, gives a direct one-to-one response, with the tip rotating in the same direction. The wire's stiffness also facilitates passage of catheters through fibrotic or neoplastic livers. Both the Lunderquist and the Lunderquist–Ring wires are valuable for passing catheters for internal drainage through severe, tight obstructions of the distal common bile duct.

COAT-HANGER WIRE

The coat-hanger guidewire is a 60-cm-long, 0.018-inch guidewire made of a 52.5-cm-long stainless-steel shaft attached to a 7.5-cm-long floppy tip made from a helical spring with its tip curved into a 6-mm J.[80] This wire is used through the 22-gauge Chiba needle in the Cope one-step technique.[80,81]

DOTTER STIFFENER

The wire stiffener originally described by Dotter is a semiflexible stainless-steel cannula for stiffening polyvinyl angioplasty balloon catheters. The hollow cannula fits inside the catheter and passes over the guidewire. The same cannula can be used to insert biliary stents, providing added stiffness and stability to the guidewire, particularly in patients with ascites, cirrhosis, or extensive metastatic disease, where kinking of the wire at the liver capsule is a common problem (Fig. 27–29).

NEPHROSTOMY DILATORS

With the exception of the telescoping metallic type, the same dilator systems that are used in percutaneous nephrostomy tracts can be used to dilate tracts through the liver. They can be placed in three groups depending on their mechanism of action or insertion:

1. Over-the-guidewire dilators:
   a. Angiographic Teflon;
   b. Fascial (Cook Urological);
2. Coaxial dilators:
   a. Cook biliary;
   b. Amplatz renal (Cook, Inc.; Cook Urological; VanTech);
3. Balloon dilators:
   a. Grüntzig type;
   b. Olbert type.

Over-the-Guidewire Dilators

Angiographic Teflon dilators. These range in size from 6F–24F and are tapered to fit a 0.038-inch guidewire. Because of their rigidity, they can be used to dilate tracts through fibrous livers and through liver replaced by tumor. One significant disadvantage is that they are only faintly radiopaque.

Fascial dilators. These are radiopaque, semiflexible polyurethane dilators in 8F–36F sizes with the tip tapered to fit a 0.038-inch guidewire. Each dilator in the sequence must be passed over the guidewire (Fig. 27–30).

Coaxial Dilators

Cook coaxial biliary dilators. These are constructed according to Dotter's original design. These radiopaque Teflon dilators range in size from 8F–18F. The 10F and 12F dilators fit coaxially over the 8F one, whereas the 17F and 18F fit over the 10F. The 8F dilator is tapered to fit a 0.038-inch guidewire (Fig. 27–31). These dilators are strong and have a low coefficient of friction, which makes them useful for dilation of tracts through fibrotic livers.[82]

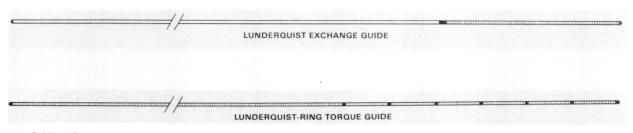

LUNDERQUIST EXCHANGE GUIDE

LUNDERQUIST-RING TORQUE GUIDE

Fig. 27–28 Stiff guidewires for manipulation and catheter introduction. A. Lunderquist guidewire. B. Lunderquist–Ring torque control wire. (Courtesy of Cook, Inc.)

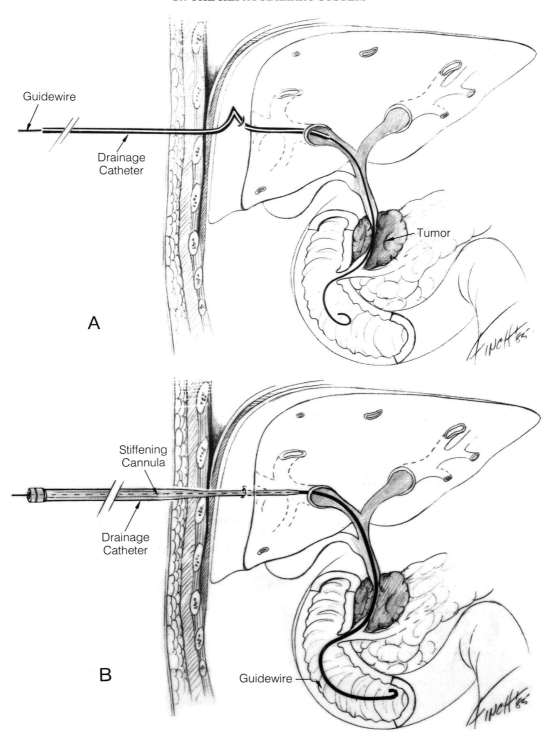

Fig. 27–29 Schematic representation of use of Sotter's stiffening cannula to overcome kinking of wire at liver capsule. A. Drainage catheter kinks at liver capsule during attempts to introduce it over guidewire. B. Metallic stiffening cannula with 8F biliary drainage catheter mounted on top has been advanced over the guidewire, placing tip of cannula within biliary radicle. C. While stiffening cannula is held in place, biliary drainage catheter is easily advanced over guidewire and across obstruction. D. Dotter stiffening cannula.

Amplatz renal dilators. These are radiopaque, semiflexible, polyurethane dilators ranging in size from 8F–30F. All of the dilators 10F and larger are tapered to fit coaxially over the 8F Teflon guiding dilator (Fig. 27–

32). The main advantage of this system is that dilation of the tract is not done over a guidewire but rather over the guidewire–8F Teflon dilator assembly, providing added safety.[83] Further, 28F, 32F, and 34F Teflon working

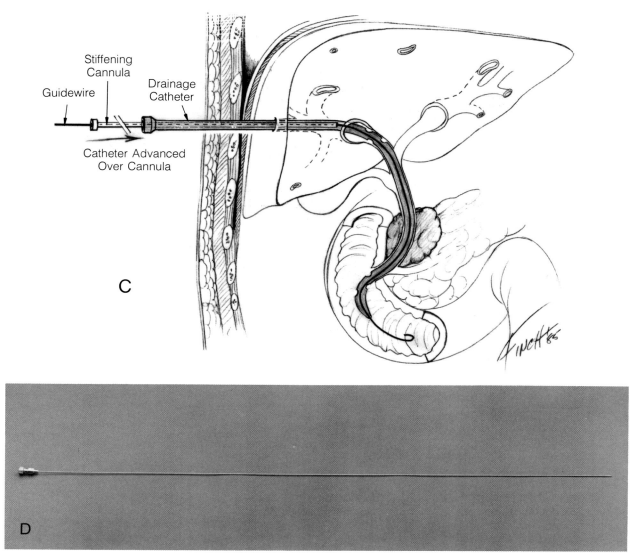

Fig. 27–29C,D

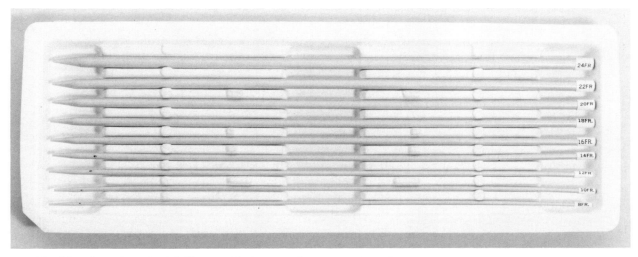

Fig. 27–30   Flexible polyurethane fascial dilators with tip tapered to 0.038-inch guidewire.

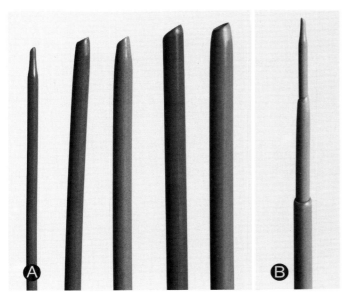

Fig. 27–31   A. Unassembled biliary coaxial dilators. B. Assembled dilators.

sheaths are provided that fit snugly over the dilator 4F smaller; these sheaths can be used for intraductal manipulations during any biliary interventional procedures that require a large tract through the liver. The sheath tamponades the tract and protects the tissues from undue trauma. When smaller tracts are needed, a nontapered Teflon dilator can be used as a conduit.[83]

Balloon Dilators

Angioplasty balloons can be used for dilation of percutaneous biliary tracts. Ideally, the balloon will be long enough to dilate the entire tract and capsule with one inflation. Balloons as large as 8–10 mm have been used without significant complications. The balloons should be able to withstand 10–12 atm of pressure, although in most cases only 4–6 atm are needed. Balloons currently available with these characteristics include the Olbert (Surgimed), the enforcer (Cook), the PE Plus (USCI), and the Blue Max (Medi–Tech).[84,85]

INDICATIONS AND CONTRAINDICATIONS FOR BILIARY DRAINAGE

Indications

The indications for percutaneous biliary drainage are:

1. Palliation for unresectable primary or metastatic malignancy;

2. Benign strictures, particularly stenotic biliary–enteric anastomoses;
3. Sepsis accompanying biliary obstruction;
4. Preoperative decompression;

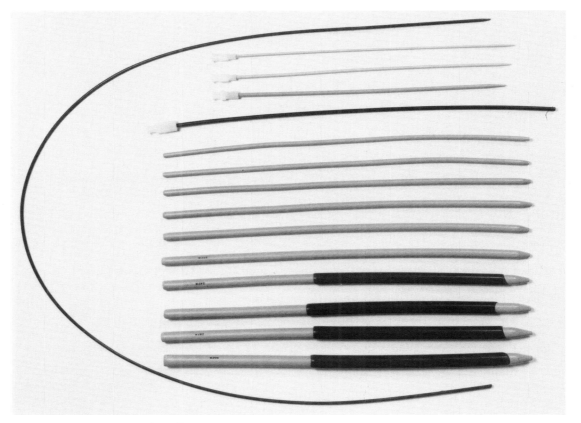

Fig. 27–32   Amplatz renal dilators tapered to 8F.

5. Prophylactic decompression after THC or ERCP;
6. Ancillary therapeutic maneuvers.

PALLIATION FOR UNRESECTABLE PRIMARY OR METASTATIC MALIGNANCY

PTBD is commonly indicated in patients with biliary duct obstruction secondary to unresectable or advanced tumor, usually of the pancreas.

At the time of diagnosis, 80%–90% of pancreatic malignancies are unresectable, and in the other cases, attempts at resection carry a mortality rate of 20%.[47,54,86] The mean survival time from the date of diagnosis of pancreatic carcinoma is 5–7 months.[47,53,54] PTBD offers a cost-effective nonoperative method to relieve jaundice, avoiding the morbidity and mortality of operation. However, surgical biliary decompression is indicated in those patients who require a gastroenterostomy for relief of concomitant duodenal obstruction.

PTBD is also indicated in cases of cholangiocarcinoma involving both the right and left intrahepatic ducts. In this type of tumor, operation is technically difficult, and microscopic tumor invasion is often present at the margin of resection.

In cases of metastases to the porta hepatis from carcinomas such as those of the colon, lung, and breast, effective palliation can be accomplished with a combination of PTBD and local tumor control with radiation.[45,87]

Certain tumors that cause biliary obstruction are sensitive to chemotherapeutic agents such as doxorubicin hydrochloride (Adriamycin) and vincristine, which are excreted into the biliary system. However, these drugs cannot be administered to patients with jaundice.[36] In this situation, PTBD is useful to relieve the obstruction and normalize the serum bilirubin concentration. As soon as tumor growth is controlled and the obstruction has been relieved by chemotherapy, radiation, or both, the catheter can be removed.

BENIGN STRICTURES

Most (95%) benign common bile duct strictures are related to previous surgery,[88] and reoperation is associated with a 30% recurrence rate.[69] In these conditions, PTBD is invaluable.[44,88–90] Antegrade drainage of bile can be established, so surgical repair of the stricture can be delayed until the patient's clinical condition becomes optimal. In this way, liver function and overall nutrition are improved, and cholangitis can be controlled. Alternatively, strictures at the choledochoenterostomy site are amenable to balloon dilation. PTBD can also be successful in many patients with sclerosing cholangitis, and on rare occasions the strictured ducts can also be dilated.[91,92]

SEPSIS ACCOMPANYING BILIARY OBSTRUCTION

In some patients, biliary obstruction is complicated by sepsis. In these cases, PTBD is not only a safe and effective treatment but also the most rapid way to achieve what can be a lifesaving therapy. PTBD as the primary therapy for biliary sepsis is associated with a 17% mortality rate[93] compared to the 50%–75% surgical mortality rate.[53,94,95]

The milder forms of biliary sepsis are manifested by fever, chills, pain in the right upper quadrant, and jaundice. Patients with severe cholangitis exhibit mental confusion, lethargy, and shock[93] and are the ones who should undergo emergency removal of the purulent material, which is usually under high pressure in the obstructed biliary system. Even though antibiotics cannot be expected to penetrate significantly into the biliary system, aggressive parenteral antibiotic treatment is instituted prior to the procedure.[94,96] If untreated, cholangitis can lead to liver abscess, septic shock, and death.

In an infected biliary system, catheter manipulation should be minimized, because excessive manipulation or transient elevation of pressure following contrast injection can precipitate retrograde flow of infected bile into the hepatic veins or lymphatics and result in a startlingly rapid development of septic shock.

PREOPERATIVE DECOMPRESSION

A surgical mortality rate of 20%–30% has been reported in jaundiced patients who undergo laparotomy.[43,47,54,57] The mortality and morbidity are significantly decreased if the serum bilirubin levels are reduced to <10 mg/dl by a percutaneous drainage procedure such as cholecystotomy or PTBD.[43,57–59] The decrease in morbidity was believed to result from better liver function, reversal of secondary portal hypertension, and improvement of wound healing.[47,54] However, recent reports suggest that there may be no significant benefit or decrease in the operative risk for randomly selected patients. The higher operative risk in previous studies is thought to have been due to the severity of the malignant disease that was treated operatively.[61,62] The most recent studies still do not give an unequivocal answer to this question of the value of preoperative PTBD.

The percutaneously introduced catheter has one clear operative benefit, which is that it can be palpated by the surgeon to assist in finding the site of obstruction during laparotomy.

Prophylactic Decompression after Skinny-Needle Transhepatic Cholangiography

In cases of high-grade obstruction of the biliary system, cholangitis and bile leakage following THC can be prevented by PTBD. Effective drainage also helps prevent septic complications by eliminating the chance for retrograde entry of infected bile into the systemic venous and lymphatic circulation. By decreasing the pressure in the biliary tree, seepage of bile through the needle track can be prevented, thereby avoiding bile peritonitis or biloma.

Contraindications

The only true and absolute contraindication to PTBD is the presence of a bleeding diathesis. However, coagulation disorders can usually be corrected by the administration of fresh-frozen plasma, vitamin K, platelets, or specific blood coagulation components. Any concurrent problem requiring surgical management, such as duo-denal–gastric outlet obstruction, is also considered a contraindication, because both problems can be dealt with by operation.

Sepsis is a relative contraindication, because PTBD is the procedure of choice for sepsis due to cholangitis. However, if a patient scheduled for elective decompression has a nonbiliary infection or sepsis, PTBD should wait for sepsis control. A patient presenting as an emergency with biliary sepsis is treated only after intravenous antibiotic coverage is started and an adequate venous access for fluid administration has been secured.

The presence of large amounts of fluid in the abdomen makes PTBD technically difficult although not impossible. Catheters and guidewires tend to buckle between the liver and abdominal wall, and the ascitic fluid that leaks out at the puncture site lubricates everything, increasing the chances for migration, buckling, or dislodgment. Cau-tion at every step of the catheter introduction is imperative. The process is greatly facilitated by the use of stiffer guidewires, such as the Lunderquist or Lunderquist–Ring designs. External leakage of ascitic fluid also tends to irritate the skin and can form a nidus for infection.

Combined extrahepatic and intrahepatic or multiple intrahepatic obstructions are also relative contraindications to PTBD. Even though extrahepatic obstruction exists, the intrahepatic ducts may not be dilated due to the multicentric mass effect of intrahepatic metastases. Also, the introduction of catheters into the biliary system invariably invites colonization by bacteria, and the stagnant bile in any nondrained segments of liver can rapidly become infected. Therefore, it is vital to perform high-quality THC to evaluate the entire biliary duct anatomy in cases of intrahepatic metastases before introducing catheters.

PATIENT EVALUATION, PREPARATION, AND MONITORING

The clinical history and physical findings should be reviewed. The indication for the procedure should be clearly stated.

Except in emergency situations, when a single, simple coagulation screening test will suffice, several laboratory tests should be obtained to provide the minimum preparatory and baseline information:

Coagulation profile (thrombin and prothrombin times, partial thromboplastin time, platelet count);
Bilirubin (total and direct);
Complete blood count; and
Blood urea nitrogen and creatinine levels.

Any coagulation abnormalities are corrected before the procedure.

Certain radiologic examinations are also of great value: an ultrasound, computed axial tomography scan of the abdomen, and a chest radiograph.

An adequate intravenous line (minimum: 18-gauge needle) should be inserted before the procedure for hydration, correction of any electrolyte imbalances, and easy delivery of medications and blood products.

The incidence of bacteriobilia in common bile duct obstructions ranges from 65%–100%,[94–101] and the reported incidence of septicemia after bile duct manipulation is 4%–10%.[93,100,102] This is an important fact for any radiologist performing interventional procedures in the biliary tract to remember. In one series, bile cultures revealed a 62% incidence of gram-positive and a 27% incidence of gram-negative organisms,[102] and the incidence of anaerobic bacteria ranges from 24%–56%.[98] Effective coverage of 84%–91% of the organisms can be obtained with a combination of one of the newer aminoglycosides and a third- or fourth-generation cephalosporin.[101]

The exact mechanism or relative importance of cholangiovenous or cholangiolymphatic regurgitation as a cause of septicemia is not known. However, higher biliary pressures seem to be significant.[102] This pressure can easily be raised as high as 80–90 cm H_2O at the time of cholangiography, and at these higher biliary pressures, bacteria can be transmitted from the bile ducts to the blood stream.[102]

Prophylactic antibiotic coverage should be instituted 24 hr prior to the procedure and continued for at least 3 days afterward.[102] The patient who already has cholangitis and septicemia is given antibiotics selected on the basis of the results of bile and blood cultures. The patient undergoing biliary stone removal is also given broad-spectrum antibiotics before and during the procedure, and in these more highly traumatized patients, coverage is continued until the last tube is taken out of the tract.

Preprocedural drugs for relaxation or sedation are helpful in most patients but are certainly not required and must be used cautiously in older patients and patients with respiratory difficulties. The drugs generally are selected according to personal preferences, and several analgesic–sedative–amnesic combinations are popular, such as meperidine–diazepam, meperidine–hydroxyzine, and secobarbital–hydroxyzine. They are usually given when the patient is called to the angiography suite. Atropine is given by some radiologists to decrease secretions and the incidence of vasovagal reactions.

For internal stent placement, difficult procedures, or dilatation of the tract for stone removal, the authors prefer stronger intraprocedureal sedation, such as intravenous narcotics, nitrous oxide by mask, or general anesthesia, because of the severe visceral pain that can be associated with these procedures. In such cases, preprocedural medications are not used.

Careful patient monitoring throughout interventional biliary procedures is critical. Vital signs (pulse, blood pressure, breathing) are monitored continuously either by a circulating nurse or by an anesthetist. Electrocardiographic (ECG) monitoring is generally recommended and is mandatory in the following circumstances:

Debilitated patients, because respiratory depression can be induced by analgesics or sedatives;
Patients requiring difficult manipulations, because deep sedation and analgesia are needed;

Septic patients;

Postoperative patients in need of biliary decompression. In the patient from the intensive care unit, it is particularly useful to have a circulating nurse or nurse anesthetist monitor all the lines and tubes.

Intraprocedural sedation and pain control are important, especially because pain is a prominent cause of severe vasovagal reactions. Most biliary interventional procedures can be performed under local anesthesia given in adequate amounts down to and including the liver capsule with the help of sedatives and analgesics. Several combinations have proved safe: diazepam with butorphanol tartrate (Stadol), meperidine (pethidine), morphine, or fentanyl. Of these, diazepam–butorphanol has proved safest in the absence of direct monitoring by the anesthesiology department. Patients who express negative feelings or even fear about the PTBD usually do so because it was painful. This is neither kind nor necessary.

VASCULAR ANATOMY OF THE LIVER

Ultrasound imaging of the liver is performed with the patient in a supine or right anterior oblique position and usually in suspended deep inhalation. Real-time scanning techniques permit direct imaging of vessels and other structures in several planes. Examinations are guided by reference to anatomic landmarks and key structures such as the hepatoduodenal ligament (Fig. 27–33), the common bile duct within the head of the pancreas, and the confluence of the splenic and superior mesenteric veins to form the portal vein dorsal to the neck of the pancreas (Fig. 27–34).

The size and form of the liver vary individually and according to body habitus, although craniocaudal diameter usually does not exceed 15 cm. The liver is a segmental organ, with well-defined internal anatomy consisting of right and left lobes. The normal left lobe is always smaller than the right lobe but the disparity differs from individual to individual. Sonographically, the normal liver is slightly more echogenic than is the adjacent normal kidney.

Portal Venous Anatomy

The portal vein approaches the porta hepatis in a characteristic position within the hepatoduodenal ligament (Fig. 27–33). This anatomic relation can be demonstrated by sonography in a high percentage of cases. The patient is scanned in a right anterior oblique position and in suspended deep inhalation.

The intrahepatic portal venous system has a highly constant course. The main portal vein divides into a larger right and a smaller left branch. These divide into anterior and posterior (right) and medial and lateral (left) divisions, as demonstrated in Figure 27–35. Note that the portal vein radicles lie within the hepatic segments, whereas the hepatic veins course between the segments.

Both the anterior and the posterior divisions of the right portal vein can be identified by sonography. The main stem of the right portal vein is an important landmark on longitudinal sections, because this vessel has a constant location centrally in the right lobe, where it is surrounded by a rim of high-amplitude reflections. Sonographically, portal vein radicles are characterized by strong marginal echoes, whereas hepatic veins are sonolucent tubular structures.

The left portal vein branch courses along the anterior surface of the caudate lobe, then characteristically turns anteriorly (Fig. 27–35), dividing into medial and lateral branches. The caudate lobe is supplied by portal vein branches of its own.

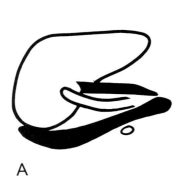

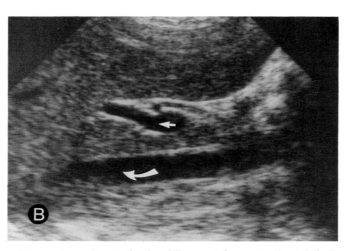

Fig. 27–33 A. Characteristic right anterior oblique view of hepatoduodenal ligament and porta hepatis. Note triad of common bile duct (black), and inferior vena cava with its typical curved appearance. Right renal artery crosses behind inferior vena cava. B. Sonogram of hepatoduodenal ligament demonstrating triad of common bile duct, portal vein (straight arrow), and inferior vena cava (curved arrow). At times, common or proper hepatic arteries can be identified by their pulsations between common bile duct and portal vein.

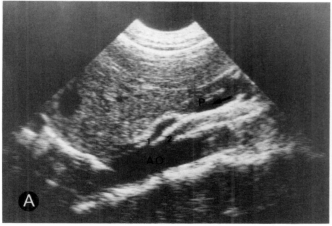

Fig. 27–34 A. Sagittal sonogram demonstrating aorta (AO) and origins of celiac trunk (1) and superior mesenteric artery (2). Note superior mesenteric vein (arrow) on its course dorsal to the pancreas (P). B. Transverse section of upper abdomen. Splenic vein (curved arrow) courses behind pancreatic body (P) and joins superior mesenteric vein to form portal vein (asterisk). Small star indicates superior mesenteric artery. D = duodenal bulb; dotted line markes duodenal sweep. Note common bile duct within pancreatic head. V = inferior vena cava; A = aorta.

Hepatic Venous Anatomy

Hepatic veins are divided into three major components, the right, middle, and left hepatic veins (Fig. 27–36). The three hepatic veins characteristically run toward the inferior vena cava and the right atrium. These veins divide the parenchyma of the liver into four segments: the ventrocaudal (anterior) and dorsocranial (posterior) segments of the right lobe and the medial and lateral segments of the left lobe. The right hepatic vein is usually single and runs along the intersegmental plane between the anterior and posterior hepatic segments and, together with the dorsal hepatic veins, drains the right lobe of the liver. The dorsal veins are numerous and of various sizes and locations, depending on the size of the right hepatic vein; they drain directly into the inferior vena cava. The middle and left hepatic veins frequently form a common trunk.

Hepatic veins can easily be distinguished from portal vein radicles by:

1. Tracing the veins upward toward the inferior vena cava and right atrium;
2. Remembering that hepatic veins course between the lobes and segments; and
3. Demonstrating the absence of a high-amplitude "collar" of the vessel, suggesting a hepatic venous structure.

Hepatic Lobar Anatomy

The main lobar fissure divides the liver into right and left lobes. Anatomists term its groove on the inferior liver surface the "gallbladder–vena cava line." The middle hepatic vein courses cranially within the main lobar fissure.

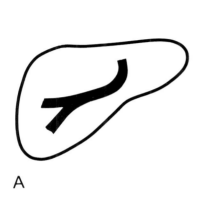
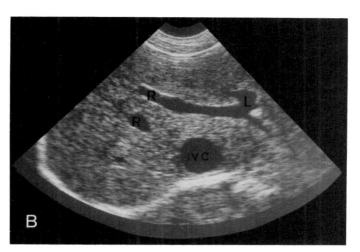

Fig. 27–35 A. Characteristic course of right and left portal veins in subcostal view. B. Subcostal sonogram of liver showing right (R) and left (L) portal vein divisions. IVC = inferior vena cava.

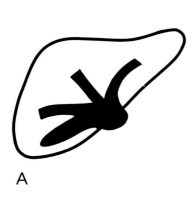

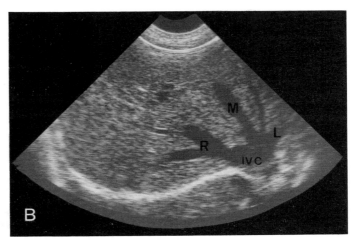

Fig. 27–36 A. Characteristic appearance of hepatic veins and their point of entry into inferior vena cava on subcostal approach. B. Subcostal veiw of hepatic venous anatomy showing right (R), middle (M), left hepatic veins (L). Dorsal hepatic veins are not demonstrated. IVC = inferior vena cava.

The right segmental fissure separates the anterior and posterior segments of the right lobe. The right hepatic vein and its major branches course within the intersegmental planes of the anterior and posterior lobes.

The left segmental fissure separates the medial and lateral segments of the left lobe. The term "quadrate lobe" refers to the dorsal aspect of the medial lobe. The falciform ligament containing the ligamentum teres hepatis is found within the fissure; this ligament represents the obliterated umbilical vein and is seen on transverse sections as an echo-dense structure.

The caudate lobe is the posterior portion of the liver, lying between the inferior vena cava and the fissure of the ligamentum venosum. It receives a portal venous and a hepatic arterial blood supply from both the right and left sides. Its blood usually drains into dorsal hepatic veins. The caudate process may project between the portal vein and the inferior vena cava.

Inferior Vena Cava

The dorsal aspect of the liver contains the inferior vena caval fossa. Infrequently, the vein takes its course inside the dorsal portion of the liver parenchyma. The vessel can always be demonstrated sonographically. In a right

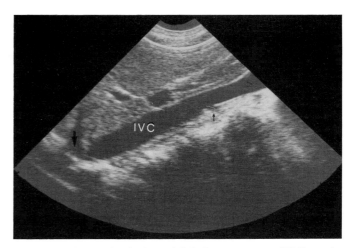

Fig. 27–37 Parasagittal view of inferior vena cava (IVC) on its course behind liver. Note entry of middle hepatic vein (large arrow). Small arrow points to right renal artery.

parasagittal section, the inferior vena cava can be seen receiving the middle hepatic vein (Fig. 27–37). It enlarges considerably with deep inhalation and has pulsatile movements on real-time sonography.

ULTRASOUND BILIARY ANATOMY

Normal peripheral bile ducts are too small for ultrasound portrayal. However, normal right and left hepatic ducts can be seen on subcostal views ventral to the main portal vein in the liver hilum (porta hepatis). In subcostal sections, incipient intrahepatic cholangiectasis may be assessed. With increasing distention, dilated ducts can be demonstrated as sonolucent tubular structures in their typical location ventral to the portal vein branches.

Extrahepatic bile ducts, specifically the proximal common bile duct, can be seen in 90% of examinations (Fig. 27–38). The common bile duct courses in front of the portal vein in the hepatoduodenal ligament. Measurements

of the common bile duct lumen can be obtained at this level and should not exceed 7 mm in the normal individual and 11 mm after cholecystectomy ("rule of 7/11"). The ultrasound examination is best performed with the patient in a right anterior oblique position and in suspended deep inhalation.

Extrahepatic cholangiectasis can be assessed in about 95% of cases (Fig. 27–39). Sonography can distinquish accurately between obstructive and hepatocellular jaundice by revealing the dilated ducts of an obstructed biliary system. The level of obstruction can be assessed in about 75% of cases. Distended bile ducts become visible

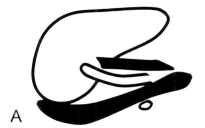

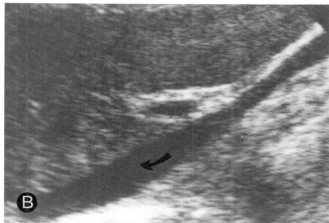

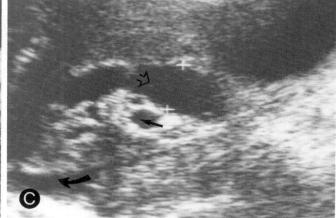

Fig. 27–38 A. Hepatoduodenal ligament, right anterior oblique view. Note classic triad of common bile duct (black), portal vein, and inferior vena cava, with its typical curved appearance. Right renal artery (avoid structure) crosses dorsal to inferior vena cava. B. Sonogram of hepatoduodenal ligament and porta hepatis, demonstrating triad of normal common bile duct, portal vein, and inferior vena cava (curved arrow). C. Sonogram showing dilated common bile duct (open arrow) on its course within hepatoduodenal ligament. Duct lumen diameter is indicated by two white crosses. Note portal vein (small arrow) and inferior vena cava (curved arrow).

in the periphery of the liver (Fig. 27–39). With real-time imaging, the ducts can be traced as they converge in the region of the porta hepatis, giving rise to the "stellate" sign (Fig. 27–39). Dilated ducts run close to the portal vein radicles and arterial branches within the portal triad and are seen sonographically in a "double-barrel shotgun," "railroad track," or "parallel-channel" appearance (Fig. 27–39). These terms refer to the typical location of the dilated ducts in front of portal vein branches, i.e., two parallel tubular structures are visible instead of one.

Ultrasound may aid in detecting, locating, measuring, and puncturing dilated bile ducts, as in Figures 27–38

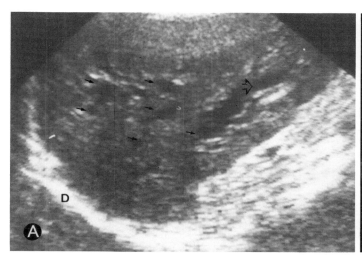

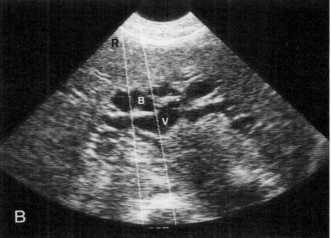

Fig. 27–39 A. Longitudinal parasagittal sonogram of right lobe of liver demonstrating dilated peripheral bile ducts (small arrows). Note "parallel channel sign." Ducts converge toward liver hilum (open arrow). D = Diaphragm. B. Subcostal sonogram demonstrating porta hepatis with portal vein (V) and distended biliary branches (B). Electronic puncture guide is displayed over right (R) bile duct for puncture using "supine approach." Note diverging "stellate" appearance of ducts.

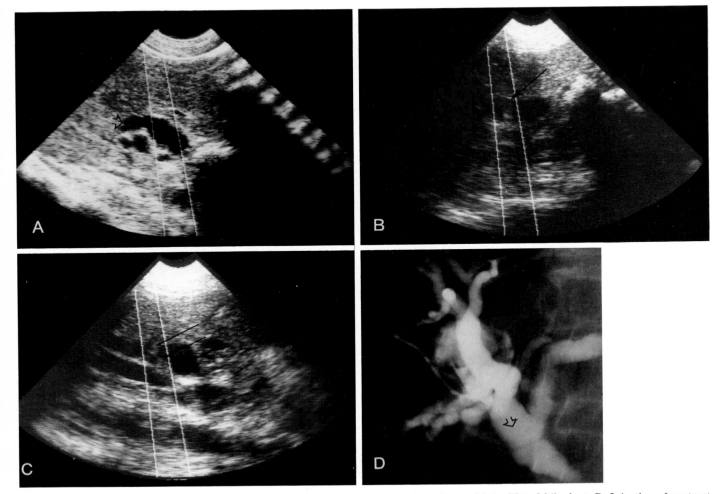

Fig. 27–40   Needle puncture of common bile duct from right anterior oblique approach. A. Common bile duct (open arrow) is located
within puncture calipers. B. Echogenic needle (arrow) is advanced
under real-time control. C. Needle is removed and Teflon sheath

(arrows) is advanced into dilated bile duct. D. Injection of contrast
medium under fluoroscopic control demonstrates distended biliary
system. Common bile duct (open arrow).

through 27–40. The authors use real-time guidance and
skinny needles. Two techniques have proved particularly
useful:

1. The anterior approach, with the patient supine and
   the needle advancing into the right (Fig. 27–39) or left
   main bile ducts; and
2. The "RAO" approach, with the patient in the right
   anterior oblique position and the needle advancing
   into the dilated common bile duct (Fig. 27–40).

However, ultrasound has technical limitations. It cannot
depict contrast medium or the guidewire inside the biliary system. Therefore, manipulation inside the biliary
tree should be controlled by fluoroscopy. Technically, a
drainage procedure can be carried out solely under ultrasound guidance, but in the authors' opinion, this is too
dangerous for clinical practice.

BILIARY DUCT DEMONSTRATION

There are several methods to demonstrate the collecting system for percutaneous procedures.

Ultrasound

A good method of observation and guidance in the
patient with obstructed bile ducts is ultrasonic demonstration of the dilated left biliary radicles using any of the

several modalities available (A, B, or real-time) to guide
the puncture with either a skinny or an 18-gauge needle.
This method accurately reveals the bile duct dimensions
and depth from the skin, particularly of the left ducts.
The principal limitation of the ultrasonic method is its
inadequate demonstration of the biliary duct anatomy,
particularly of the right ducts, due to interposition of the
ribs.

Several techniques have been used for puncture under ultrasonic guidance. In one, ultrasound is used to locate the biliary system and determine its depth. The best site of entry for the needle puncture is marked on the skin, and the needle is introduced in the direction and to the depth determined by the ultrasound study (Fig. 27–41). A more popular technique involves real-time ultrasound guidance. Two systems have been described:

1. A sidearm attachment (Fig. 27–42) for the real-time transducer that allows imaging of the needle, which is advanced in an oblique path to the bile duct, which is kept in the center of the field (Figs. 27–40A–C)[103]; and
2. Removal of the central crystal of a linear array real-time transducer to allow observation of the needle tip within the target area (Fig. 27–43). A sterilizable funnel-shaped attachment is used to fit the needle through the special transducer without the necessity of sterilizing the entire transducer.[104]

Fluoroscopy

The technique of fluoroscopic percutaneous transhepatic cholangiography (PTC) is detailed at the beginning of this chapter. Most authors advocate a right lateral approach, and this is also the present authors' initial choice. A 22-gauge Chiba needle is used, and once a duct has been located, sufficient contrast medium is injected to confirm obstruction and, if possible, to outline the underlying lesion(s). Overfilling the ducts in the presence of biliary obstruction should be avoided, because it increases the risk of septic complications. Some authors advocate percutaneous biliary drainage whenever PTC indicates obstruction in order to avoid this complication.

Imaging of the Left-Sided Ducts

Although at PTC the needle may enter a left biliary radicle, particularly if it has been directed well into the

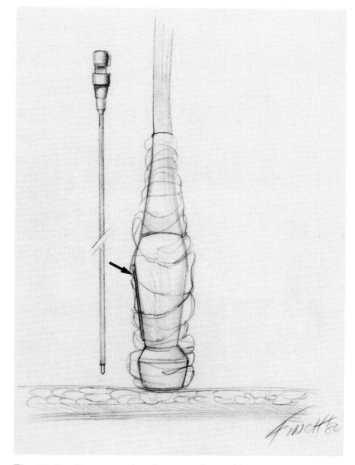

Fig. 27–41 Face array tranducer used to guide percutaneous punctures of biliary radicles. Observe that the needle should be parallel to grooves (arrow) in transducer.

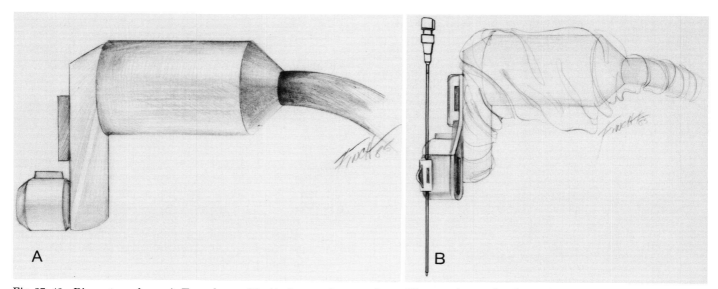

Fig. 27–42 Biopsy transducer. A. Transducer with attachment plate for needle placement. B. Sterile surgical glove covering head of transducer. The attachment has been placed on head of transducer to guide biopsy into biliary radicle.

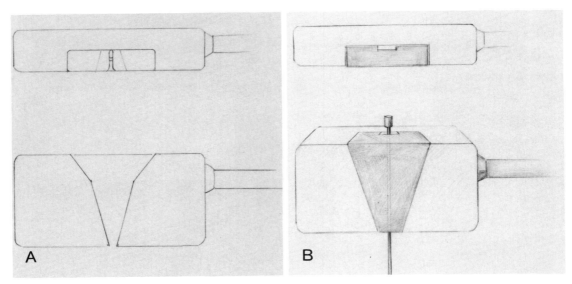

Fig. 27–43   Linear array transducer. A. Transducer with one crystal removed from its center, where an adaptor can be placed to guide introduction of needle under direct real-time imaging. B. Top view of transducer with insert in place and front view with insert assembled and needle going through insert.

left lobe, more often a right-sided duct fills. Often, the left-sided ducts do not fill because they are relatively anterior, and because conventional contrast medium is denser than bile, it flows first into the posterior ducts. Injection of large volumes of contrast may produce satisfactory opacification but at the expense of a higher risk

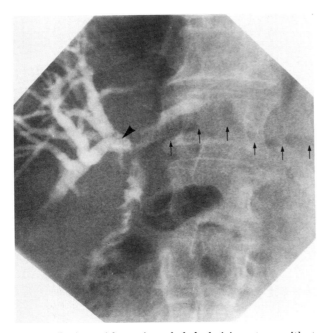

Fig. 27–44   Patient with previous choledochojejunostomy with stenoses of both hepatic ducts and small calculus in a right radicle (arrowhead). Conventional contrast medium fills right ducts, and CO_2 fills the more anterior left duct (small arrows). (Reproduced from Young AT, Cardella JF, Castañeda–Zuñiga WR, Hunter DW, Amplatz K: The anterior approach to left biliary catheterization. *Semin Intervent Radiol* 1985;2:31–38 with the permission of Thieme, Inc.)

of septic complications. Carefully rolling the patient onto the left side will usually cause the contrast medium to flow toward the dependent left ducts at the risk of dislodging the Chiba needle. Lowering the head of the table may also facilitate left ductal filling.

Another technique uses CO_2 as a "lighter-than-bile" contrast agent that preferentially fills the anterior ducts (Fig. 27–44).[23] However, CO_2 is somewhat more difficult to see in the bile ducts than in dilated renal calices, probably because of the smaller caliber of the ducts and the relatively low visibility of CO_2. Also, it has been the authors' impression that the half-life of CO_2 is much shorter in bile ducts than in the renal collecting system, perhaps because of the alkalinity of bile. If CO_2 is used, it must be injected carefully because the low viscosity of gas causes much higher flow rates through the Chiba needle than are seen with conventional liquid contrast media at a given pressure. In addition, because the CO_2 is compressed in the syringe, it is difficult to control the volume delivered through the needle. Overdistention of the biliary tree is therefore more likely with CO_2 than with conventional contrast.[23]

There are some situations in which the left ducts cannot be opacified despite use of these techniques. Most often, the cause is obstruction in the region of the porta hepatis, involving the right hepatic duct, left hepatic duct, or both and impeding free flow of contrast agent from one side to the other. If there is a compelling indication for catheterization or examination of the left ducts, another PTC must be performed directly into the left lobe (Fig. 27–45). This may be achieved from the right lateral approach as in the conventional technique but with a deeper pass of the needle, which is directed anteriorly and medially into the left lobe. Alternatively, a subxiphoid approach may be taken. A 22-gauge Chiba needle punctures the skin in the midepigastrium, just beneath the xiphoid cartilage, and is aimed in the transverse plane at an angle of 30–40° toward the patient's

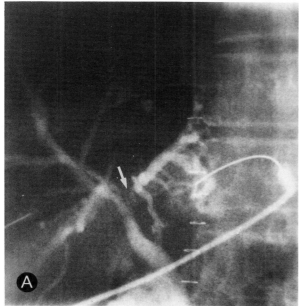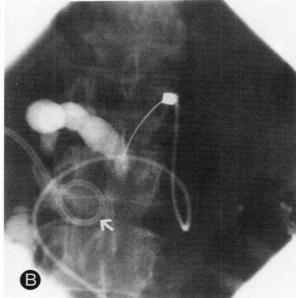

Fig. 27–45   A. Chiba needle placed under fluoroscopic control to opacify independently right and left hepatic ducts in patient with metastatic colon carcinomma. Note complete obstruction of left common hepatic duct (arrow). B. Chiba needle positioned in left hepatic duct with real-time ultrasound guidance. Patient has metastasis from carcinoma of the breast obstructing both hepatic ducts at porta hepatis. Previously placed pigtail catheter (arrow) drains right side. (Reproduced from Young AT, Cardella JF, Castañeda–Zuñiga WR, Hunter DW, Amplatz K: The anterior approach to left biliary catheterization. *Semin Intervent Radiol* 1985;2:31–38 with the permission of Thieme, Inc.)

right side (Fig. 27–46). The needle is advanced approximately 8 cm and then slowly withdrawn during continuous contrast injection in order to locate the bile duct, as in the conventional technique.

The use of real-time ultrasound greatly facilitates locating the left ducts, and the use of a needle guide transducer has allowed the authors to enter the left hepatic duct in a single pass (Fig. 27–40B,C). If a 21-gauge "single-stick" needle is used with ultrasound guidance, a drainage catheter can be inserted via this same tract; otherwise, a second puncture is performed in the manner outlined below.

PUNCTURE TECHNIQUES

The puncture techniques in use today for PTBD are variations on either the single-stick or the double-stick technique. The single-stick techniques require that the primary skinny-needle puncture of the bile ducts be appropriate both for opacification of the ducts and for placement of a catheter or stent. With the double-stick technique, this is not a consideration.

Single-Stick Techniques

Cope was one of the first to describe a single-stick technique for the placement of a biliary catheter using a 22-gauge needle for the primary puncture (Fig. 27–47).[81] After opacification of the biliary radicles, if the needle entry site is appropriate, an 0.018-inch coat-hanger wire is passed through the needle into the bile ducts, and the needle is removed (Fig. 24–48A). A specially modified 6.3F Teflon dilator mounted on a stiffening metal cannula is advanced over the guidewire until the tip of the dilator is within the biliary radicle. The dilator–cannula assembly is stiff and so must be handled with considerable caution to avoid perforating the opposite wall or kinking the narrow wire. The metal cannula is removed, and the dilator is gently manipulated into a more desirable position deeper within the bile duct. The guidewire is exchanged for a 0.038-inch Teflon-coated tight (3-mm) J guidewire. The dilator is tapered over its distal 3 cm so that the tip will permit only a 0.021-inch guidewire to pass, but 2 cm behind the tip is a slight bend and a sidehole through which a 0.038-inch guidewire can exit. (Because of the position of the sidehole in the angled portion and the distal taper, the curved 0.038-inch wire will always exit through the sidehole (Fig. 27–48B).) The 0.038-inch wire is advanced as far as possible into the bile ducts before the Teflon dilator is removed. Dilation of the tract and placement of a stent can then be performed as usual.

Hawkins described a slightly simpler single-stick technique involving a kit consisting of a 45-cm-long 22-gauge needle over which a 5F or 6.5F Teflon accordion stent is tightly fitted (Fig. 27–49A).[73,77] The initial puncture is done with the front, bare end of the skinny needle under ultrasonic or fluoroscopic guidance. If the needle enters an appropriate duct, an 0.018-inch rocket or coat-hanger wire is passed through the needle until an adequate length has been coiled within the ducts (Fig. 27–49B). With the needle hub and wire held with one hand to prevent forward movement, the operator gently advances the

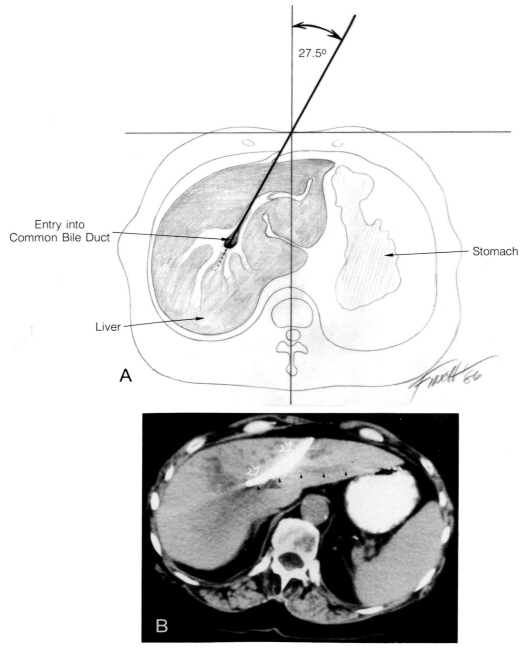

27.5⁰

Entry into
Common Bile Duct

Stomach

Liver

A

B

Fig. 27–46 A. Cross-sectional diagram across level of left hepatic lobe shows approximate angulation needed to orient path of needle with long axis of left hepatic duct. B. CT slice at level of biliary drainage catheter shows favorable angle from left hepatic duct (arrowheads) into common bile duct. Biliary drainage catheter is in place (open arrows). (Reproduced from Young AT, Cardella JF, Castañeda–Zuñiga WR, Hunter DW, Amplatz K: The anterior approach to left biliary catheterization. *Semin Intervent Radiol* 1985;2:31–38 with the permission of Thieme, Inc.)

Teflon stent over the needle–wire combination with the other hand until the folding portion of the stent is completely within the ducts (Fig. 27–49C). The needle and wire are then removed. By pulling on the monofilament string, the loops of the "accordion" stent are folded together. This maneuver, which is easily done in a dilated duct, can be more difficult in an only moderately dilated or a nondilated duct.

The greatest disadvantage of this technique is the very long skinny needle, which is cumbersome. Hawkins rec-

ommends holding the needle with both hands, one at the skin and the other 6–8 inches behind, and leaving the rest of the needle hanging loose (Fig. 27–49A).

The most serious problem with any single-stick technique is that the skinny needle may, and indeed often does, enter a duct that is not suitable for biliary drainage either because of its size, location, the angle that it makes with the needle, or the angle that it makes with the common hepatic duct.

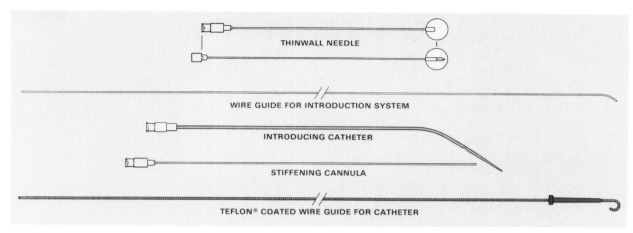

Fig. 27–47 Cope one-stick system for percutaneous drainage procedures. (Courtesy of Cook, Inc.)

Double-Stick Techniques

As its name implies, a double-stick technique requires two punctures. The first puncture, for opacification of the ducts, is done with a 22- or 23-gauge needle under ultrasonic or fluoroscopic guidance. The second, definitive, puncture is done with an 18-gauge thin-walled needle that accepts a 0.038-inch wire and over which dilation and drainage catheter placement can be performed.[41,44–46]

APPROACHES

Although PTBD has traditionally been performed through a right lateral approach, other alternatives have been described, including anterior and posterior approaches.

Right Lateral Approach

For the lateral approach, after skinny-needle opacification of the biliary ducts, a peripheral site in a right anterior duct is selected for the definitive puncture. The duct must be localized in two planes with the help of either biplane/multidirectional fluoroscopy or cross-table lateral films. The entry site should be chosen primarily with the aim of minimizing the angle between the needle tract and the duct and should be below the 10th rib to avoid perforating the pleural reflection. Ideally, a peripheral duct entry site is selected to maximize catheter purchase and to reduce the risk of damaging large vessels, which are more centrally located (Fig. 27–50). Either a skinny needle (single-stick system) or an 18-gauge needle (double-stick technique) will be used for the puncture, which is done under continuous fluoroscopy. The needle is advanced during normal shallow breathing, which usually produces a straighter pathway through the liver capsule.

The main disadvantage of the lateral approach is that the needle placement is done blindly. (Even though fluoroscopy is used during needle advancement, it is usually in only one plane (AP) and therefore provides no depth perception.) Commonly, more than one pass is needed with the 18-gauge needle to puncture the duct, and multiple passes with such large needles increase the risk of vascular complications.[56] However, the effect of the needle pressing on the bile duct can be seen and felt, and bile can be aspirated through the larger needles to confirm the position of the needle tip in the duct. Bile is difficult to aspirate through a Chiba needle in the single-stick method.

Anterior Approach

The anterior approach is technically somewhat simpler. The puncture is usually into an anterior left biliary radicle, although anterior right ducts also can be used.[105] Multidirectional fluoroscopy is needed to minimize radiation exposure of the operator's hands. After opacification of the biliary radicles through a standard right lateral approach PTC, a peripheral entry site is selected in an anterior left biliary radicle. With the patient supine, the anteriorly positioned left ducts are frequently difficult to opacify; appropriate maneuvers to deal with this problem were described earlier.

Once the ductal system has been satisfactorily opacified, the access site to the left biliary tree is chosen. In making the choice, it should be recognized that, within the liver parenchyma, each bile duct is closely related to branches of the portal vein and the hepatic artery, the hepatic veins running a separate course. Moreover, the exact anatomic relations between the duct and its two accompanying vessels are inconstant, so trauma to these vessels cannot always be avoided. Puncture of a peripheral duct minimizes the size of the vessels at risk from such inadvertent trauma and in addition places a sufficient number of drainage sideholes proximal to the stricture.

One of the principal advantages of the anterior approach under multidirectional fluoroscopy is that it is technically much easier to line up a "down-the-barrel"

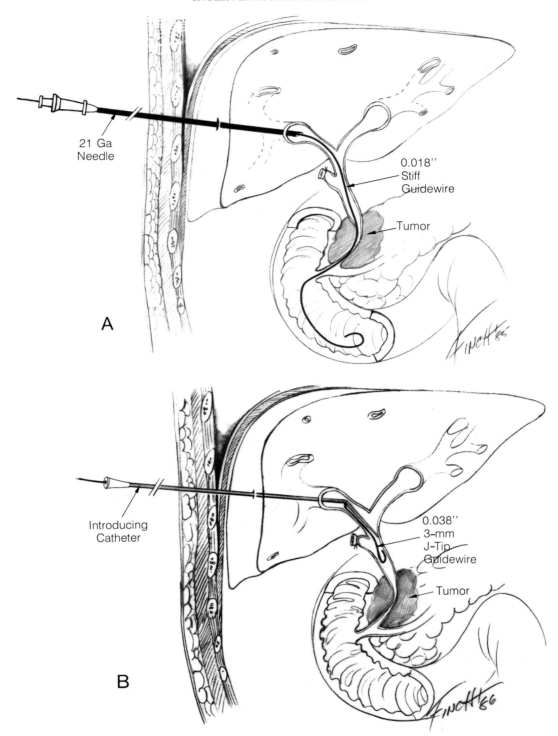

Fig. 27–48 Use of the Cope's single-stick technique to enter biliary tree. A. A 21-gauge needle has been placed in a right biliary radicle. An 0.018-inch coat-hanger guidewire has been manipulated across obstruction into duodenum. B. After removal of needle cannula, introducing catheter has been passed over 0.018-inch guidewire, which has been replaced with 0.038-inch J-tipped guidewire that has exited through the sidehole at bend in introducing catheter.

puncture, which makes accurate first-pass punctures easy even for inexperienced operators. For this puncture technique, the skin entry site is aligned with the duct entry site in the center of the fluoroscopic field (Fig. 27–51). The 18-gauge needle, supported by a radiolucent holder,[106] is advanced parallel to the x-ray beam so that the needle is seen as a dot (Figs. 27–52 and 27–53).[23,105] The needle is advanced until indentation or displacement of the bile duct is seen or until the operator feels that the appropriate depth has been reached. The multidirec-

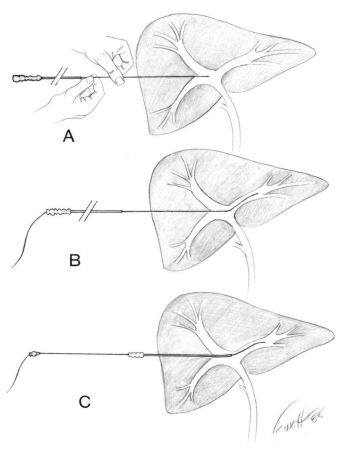

Fig. 27–49   Hawkins one-stick technique for drainage procedures. A. A 21-gauge needle has entered biliary tree. B. Coat-hanger guidewire has been passed through needle into biliary radicles. C. 6F accordion catheter has been advanced over needle cannula and guidewire, which are held in position.

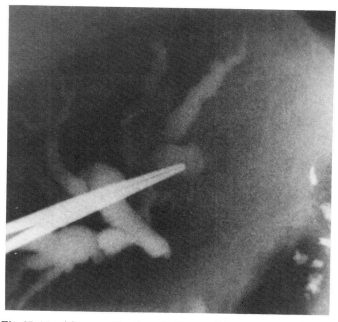

Fig. 27–51   After opacification of biliary radicles, an entry point into a biliary radicle has been selected and is marked under fluoroscopy with forceps.

tional fluoroscope is rotated away into a new projection (Fig. 27–54), and the relation of the needle tip to the biliary radicle is examined (Fig. 27–55). The goal is to make a one-wall puncture, thus avoiding extravasation of contrast medium and false passage of the guidewire through a puncture hole in the distal wall. Further manipulations

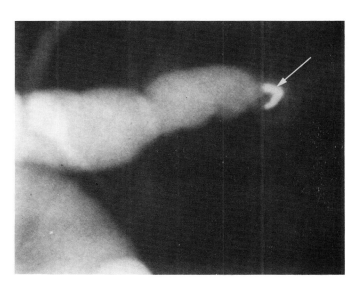

Fig. 27–50   Lateral fluoroscopy shows entrance of needle (arrow) through anterior wall of a peripheral left biliary radicle.

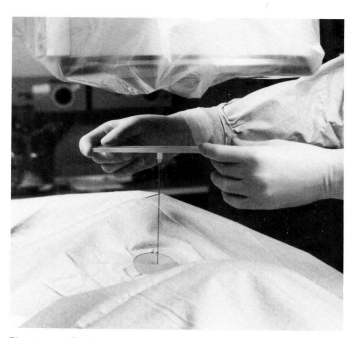

Fig. 27–52   Continuous fluoroscopy allows accurate puncture, while radiolucent handle keeps operator's hands from the primary beam. (Reproduced from Young AT, Cardella JF, Castañeda–Zuñiga WR, Hunter DW, Amplatz K: The anterior approach to left biliary catheterization. *Semin Intervent Radiol* 1985;2:31–38 with the permission of Thieme, Inc.)

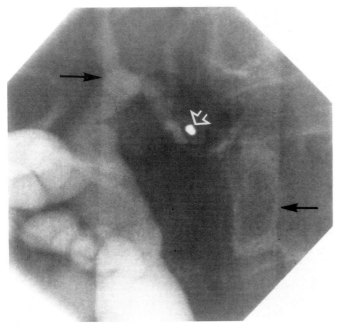

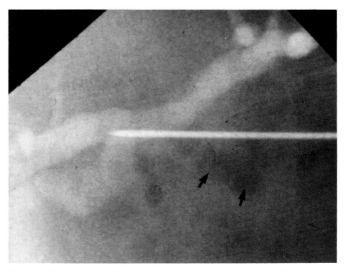

Fig. 27–55 Lateral fluoroscopy shows entrance of needle tip into biliary tree. Note gas-filled peripheral left radicles (arrows).

Fig. 27–53 Needle, seen as a dot on anteroposterior plane (open arrow), projected over duct. Amplatz radiolucent handle is barely visible (arrows). (Reproduced from Young AT, Cardella JF, Castañeda–Zuñiga WR, Hunter DW, Amplatz K: The anterior approach to left biliary catheterization. *Semin Intervent Radiol* 1985;2:31–38 with the permission of Thieme, Inc.)

are performed with the image intensifier angled 90° from the entry tract in order to minimize the radiation exposure of the operator's hands.

The tract should be angled approximately 30° from vertical toward the patient's right side (Figs. 27–54 and 27–56) in order to create a favorable angle between the parenchymal tract and the bile duct. A more vertical angle may make it difficult to pass dilators and catheters into the duct and has led to troublesome buckling in the liver, with resulting extravasation of bile. On the other hand, a more horizontal angle brings the entry point in the bile duct closer to the porta hepatis, possibly increasing the risk of vascular trauma and creating a shorter distance for the sideholes in the drainage catheter.

In most patients, the skin entry site for an anterior bile duct puncture is to the left of the midline near the costal

margin and slightly below the xiphoid cartilage. When the left lobe is small, the puncture can be made on the right side of the epigastrium, beneath the right anterior costal arch. Commonly, a puncture site is chosen beneath the xiphoid cartilage, but if the left lobe extends across the midline, then the puncture may be made beneath the left anterior costal arch.

The complications resulting from left lobe puncture are fewer than with the more popular right lobe puncture.[107]

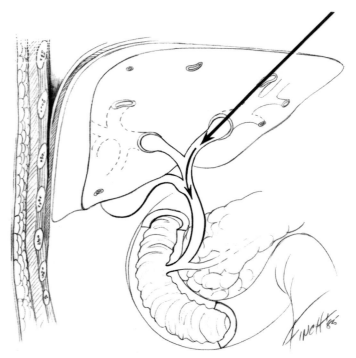

Fig. 27–56 Section through liver shows approximate angle of left hepatic duct in relation to common bile duct during epigastric approach to biliary tree.

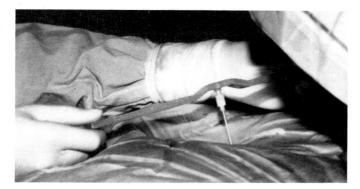

Fig. 27–54 C-arm has been rotated away to provide a lateral projection.

The left biliary duct puncture has several other advantages:

1. The left biliary duct is large, has a fairly constant anatomy, and is in a relatively horizontal position, which makes it an easier target.[108]
2. Left duct puncture avoids the pleural space, because the pleural reflection usually terminates at the level of the 10th intercostal space in the midaxillary line. In contrast, the conventional right lobe puncture can result in pneumothorax or hemothorax or even biliary–pleural fistulae.
3. Left duct puncture creates a straighter course with a shorter tract through the liver, which facilitates advancement of guidewires, stents, and balloons.[23,105,108]
4. External drainage catheters do not pass between the ribs, so there is less trouble with pain with movement or breathing. Also, the catheters are easier for the patient to manage, dress, and clean and are slightly less likely to be dislodged.
5. Conventional right lobe punctures can also be associated with referred pain to the shoulder and neck secondary to diaphragmatic irritation from either needle or catheter passage.[105] A left duct puncture cannot cause these problems, because it does not traverse the diaphragm.

Left duct puncture does have some minor disadvantages:

1. The left medial segment duct, which is often the preferred entry site because it is slightly more anterior, can make a rather sharp curve cephalad before joining the lateral segment duct and passing caudad toward the common hepatic duct. This curve can make it difficult to pass large catheters, dilators, or endoprostheses (Fig. 27–57A,B).
2. Although radiation exposure of the operator's hands during the puncture can be minimized by using the radiolucent needle handle, scatter radiation during the remainder of the procedure with the fluoroscope in the angled position can result in significant operator exposure.
3. Opacification of the left anterior ducts can be difficult with the patient supine.
4. Theoretically, the shorter tract through the liver parenchyma could mean that there is less tamponading and therefore a greater chance of bleeding or bile leak. The present authors have not found this to be a problem, however.

Left biliary duct puncture is easy to learn. Using the principles of down-the-barrel and parallax with beam rotation, needle placement is accurate and precise. The left lobe approach has been recommended by Nakayama et al,[43] Tahada et al,[46] and Mueller et al.[108]

Indeed, in certain situations, the left anterior approach to a left duct is necessary. One such situation is when there are separate right and left duct obstructions resulting from benign or malignant processes in the porta hepatis. In this case, drainage of both the right and the left lobe of the liver is necessary to ameliorate the symptoms and prevent cholangitis, which can follow drainage of only one of the obstructed lobes of the liver (Fig. 27–58).[105,107,108] Another situation in which a left anterior approach is necessary is when there is a segmental biliary duct obstruction in the left lobe alone.

Posterior Approach

A posterior approach for PTC has also been described.[8] With the patient in the prone decubitus position, the biliary tree is opacified with a Chiba needle through either a right lateral or a posterior approach. A suitable posterior duct is selected, and the puncture site is prepared. The puncture is generally made at the lower margin of

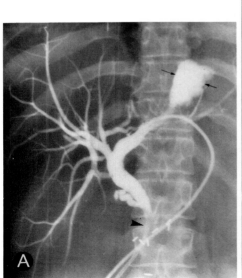

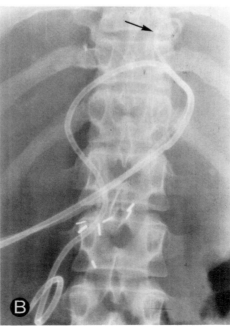

Fig. 27–57 A. Buckling of dilator within liver during attempt to traverse postoperative stricture of common bile duct (arrowhead) results in liver laceration (arrows) communicating with biliary system. Note cephalad direction of initial segment of the tract. B. This injury was treated successfully with external drainage by placing 5F catheter (arrow) into "biloma" alongside biliary drainage catheter. (Reproduced from Young AT, Cardella JF, Castañeda–Zuñiga WR, Hunter DW, Amplatz K: The anterior approach to left biliary catheterization. *Semin Intervent Radiol* 1985;2:31–38 with the permission of Thieme, Inc.)

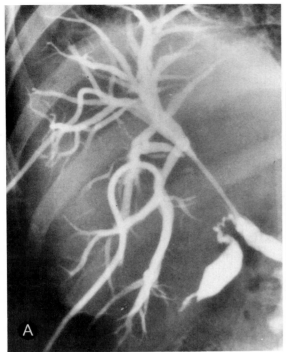
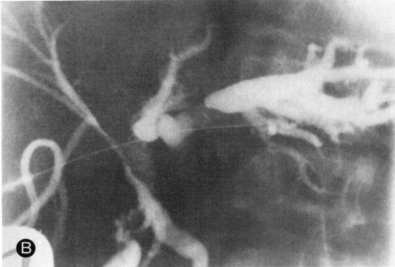

Fig. 27–58 Patient with cholangiocarcinoma involving bifurcation as well as right and left hepatic ducts. A. Two biliary drainage catheters have been placed: one through a right anterior biliary radicle across a long segment of obstruction of common hepatic duct into distal common bile duct and second to drain lower half of right lobe of liver. Observe that there is no opacification of left biliary radicles. B. Because of persistent fever and leukocytosis, attempts to drain left biliary tree were deemed necessary. Chiba needle cholangiogram shows enormous dilatation of left hepatic radicles.

the 12th rib, about 8–9 cm lateral to the spinous processes. The relation of the lung to the entry site must be determined, because passage through the pleural reflection is associated with higher morbidity and mortality rates.[8] A down-the-barrel puncture can then be performed with the help of multidirectional fluoroscopy. The posterior technique has these advantages:

1. There is no risk of bile peritonitis.
2. The posterior right biliary ducts have a fairly constant anatomy.
3. There is no risk of gallbladder or colonic puncture.

However, there also are some disadvantages:

1. A posterior approach can cause a retroperitoneal hematoma if the needle is not passed through the coronary ligament.
2. It is uncomfortable for the patient to have a posterior drain.

Discussion of the Possible Approaches

Catheterization of a left biliary duct from an epigastric approach is, in the authors' opinion, technically simpler than the conventional right lateral approach and lends itself to the tools and techniques developed for interventional approaches to the kidney. The incidence of complications has been acceptable and similar to that reported from institutions that use other methods.[107,108] The approach has been suitable not only for the estab-

lishment of external drainage, but also for the passage of catheters across strictures to allow internal drainage and to insert prosthetic stents. The technique has also been applied to biliary stone extraction, to dilation of benign strictures, and, most recently, to transcatheter placement of radioactive implants for the treatment of cholangiocarcinoma.

Accurate puncture of a right duct from a right lateral approach is technically more difficult and requires lateral fluoroscopy. This results in superimposition of the ducts and also creates a poor fluoroscopic image because of the thickness of the soft tissue, which hinders delineation of the anatomy. Therefore, in most medical centers, right lateral punctures usually are performed using fluoroscopy in the conventional posteroanterior direction, perhaps supplemented by a lateral radiograph of the ducts or by biplane fluoroscopy.

Attention has recently been drawn to the potential for pleural complications from biliary catheterization via the right lateral approach.[109] The lateral costodiaphragmatic recess of the pleural cavity commonly extends down to the 10th rib at the midaxillary line, so punctures below the 10th rib are considered safe; but sometimes, particularly in patients with small or high livers, considerable cephalad angulation of the needle is required to reach a duct from below the 10th rib. As pointed out by Jaques et al[107] this angulation may make it difficult to advance the catheter, because the vector of force is upward toward the heart rather than toward the liver hilum. Epigastric approaches to the left lobe usually create a favorable

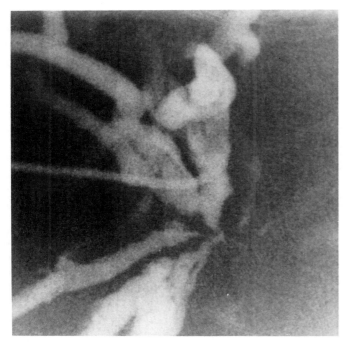

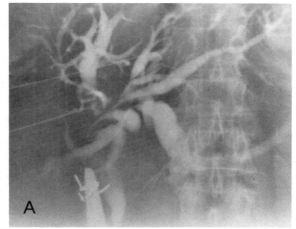

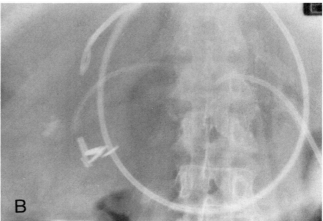

Fig. 27–59 Patient with metastatic colon carcinoma; lesions at porta hepatis obstruct several branches of right hepatic duct. Drainage catheter, introduced from right lateral approach, passes peripherally into liver. (Reproduced from Young AT, Cardella JF, Castañeda–Zuñiga WR, Hunter DW, Amplatz K: The anterior approach to left biliary catheterization. *Semin Intervent Radiol* 1985;2:31–38 with the permission of Thieme, Inc.)

Fig. 27–60 Metastatic carcinoma of the colon with mass in porta hepatis causing obstruction of biliary tree. A. Two Chiba needles have been used, one to opacify left hepatic and part of right lower lobe ducts and second to opacify superiorly located biliary radicles in right lobe. No connection between these two systems was apparent. B. An epigastric approach was used to drain left biliary radicles, extending tip of catheter into right lower lobe biliary radicles. A second catheter was placed from anterior approach to drain obstructed superior biliary radicles in right lobe.

angle down to the hilum and avoid the diaphragm and pleura entirely.[105,108]

When an obstructing lesion in the region of the porta hepatis involves both the left and the right hepatic ducts, the decision regarding where to place drainage catheters may be difficult. Drainage of both lobes reduces the risk of cholangitis secondary to persistent obstruction but leaves the patient with the morbidity of two external tubes. The right lobe is the larger, and therefore drainage of this lobe alone presumably provides better palliation than drainage of the left. Conversely, however, it has been said to be more likely that the radicles will be separately obstructed in the right lobe than in the left because of the anatomic differences between the two ductal systems, the right hepatic duct being shorter than the left with a shorter extrahepatic course.[106] Right-sided drainage may therefore leave large areas undrained within the right lobe. This problem has been observed in the authors' experience (Fig. 27–59). Commonly several catheters are

required for adequate palliation in these cases (Fig. 27–60).

The optimal management for a particular patient and the decision as to whether biliary catheterization should be attempted at all will depend on the nature of the underlying disease process, the clinical status of the patient, and the individual anatomy of the biliary tree in question.

TECHNIQUE OF CATHETERIZATION

The authors' technique for biliary catheterization starts with infiltration of the skin and subcutaneous tissues with 1% lidocaine. A small dermatotomy is then made. The C-arm fluoroscopy unit is invaluable for down-the-barrel imaging during the puncture, allowing highly accurate placement of the 18-gauge diamond-tip

nephrostomy needle. The use of the radiolucent needle holder keeps the operator's hands away from the primary radiation beam.

The position of the needle tip relative to the bile duct is checked by frequent parallax fluoroscopy, either by axial rotation of the C-arm or of the patient or, preferably, by utilizing the cephalad–caudad angulation. The proximity of the needle to the duct is determined by their relative motions as seen on the fluoroscope monitor.

When the needle tip has been shown to lie within the biliary radicles, the stylet is withdrawn, and a 0.035-inch floppy-tip guidewire is carefully passed into the ducts. It usually passes toward the porta hepatis (Fig. 27–61); rarely, it passes toward the periphery of the liver. The use of a preshaped torque control wire may allow the tip to be turned centrally toward the porta. The wire is passed as far as possible in the duct, and dilation is performed using sequential 7F, 8F, and 9F fascial dilators. These dilators are carefully rotated down as far as the entry point into the duct while constant tension is maintained on the guidewire. The operator's hands are kept out of the primary beam by angulation of the C-arm or by rotating the patient if a conventional fluoroscopic unit is used.

Once dilation is complete, a 6F–8F catheter is passed for manipulation within the biliary tree or for drainage. A preshaped catheter (e.g., a 7F Cobra-1) with the long floppy-tip guidewire will traverse most strictures, benign or malignant (Fig. 27–62), although extensive manipulations should be avoided at this first sitting to minimize septic complications. Generally, once an 8F catheter has been passed beyond the stenosis or has been parked satisfactorily above it, the procedure is terminated to allow the parenchymal tract to mature, the biliary tree to decompress, and sepsis to defervesce (Fig. 27–63). Further manipulations or passage of a larger (10F–16F) catheter for long-term drainage is usually performed at a second sitting 2–5 days later.

Samples of bile are usually aspirated and sent for culture, cytology study, or both. Transcatheter biopsy of a stricture may also be performed either during the initial procedure or subsequently (Fig. 27–64).

The catheter is secured to the skin using suture, dressings, or any of the large number of available fixation devices described below.

If a pigtail catheter is to be introduced, it is advanced until the entire pigtail loop is seen to be well within the biliary tree. The wire is removed, and the position of the loop and sideholes within the biliary tree is checked fluoroscopically by rapidly injecting 2–3 ml of contrast medium. The loop should be coiled on itself and freely rotatable within the duct to prevent duct injury by the tip. All the sideholes should lie within the biliary tree; otherwise, bleeding through the stent can be a problem, with the stent and bile ducts rapidly becoming obstructed by clots.

The Hawkins accordion catheter is placed in one step over the needle–cannula and coat-hanger 0.018-inch wire. Because of the low encrustation coefficient of Teflon, the patency rate of this catheter is said to be one of the best in spite of its small diameter.

For insertion of a Cope loop (Medi–Tech; Cook, Inc.; USCI), the 8F–10F catheter and the stiffening cannula are advanced together over the guidewire until the desired length of catheter is within the biliary tree. Making a gentle curve in the cannula helps to direct the catheter around any bends in the tract or ducts. In particular, if there is a sharp bend at the entry site into a dilated duct, one must be careful not to perforate the distal wall of the duct with the tip of the catheter–cannula combination. Once the catheter is within the ducts, the loop can be reshaped by pulling the silk or monofilament synthetic thread and rotating the stent.

In some patients with Cope loops, biliary salt encrustation on the thread blocks bile flow and prevents the loop from opening during catheter exchange. In these cases, a smaller (0.035-, 0.025-, or even 0.018-inch) wire can usually be passed through the lumen. If a guidewire cannot be passed, the catheter hub is cut, and, while the monofilament threads are held, a peel-away sheath is advanced into the bile duct over the catheter until it reaches the loop (Fig. 27–65A). The catheter can then be pulled back forcefully against the sheath or dilator, cracking the encrusted loop open at the crossover point (Fig. 27–65B). The loop is removed after advancing the

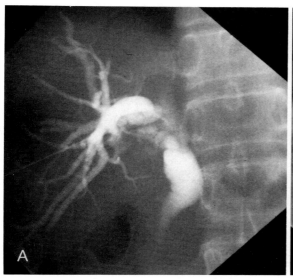
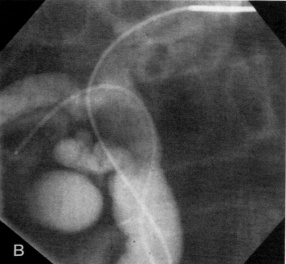

Fig. 27–61   Metastatic colon carcinoma with a large mass at porta hepatis obstructing common hepatic duct. B. Through an epigastric approach, a left biliary radicle was punctured; guidewire has been passed into distal common bile duct.

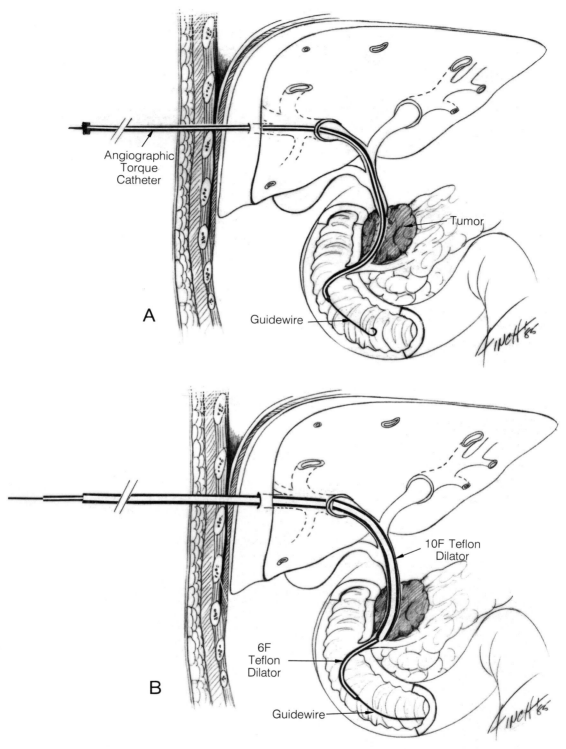

Fig. 27–62   Biliary drainage catheter placement. A. Through right biliary radicle, guidewire has been manipulated across obstruction into duodenum with the help of angiographic torque control catheter.

B. Percutaneous tract and area of obstruction are being dilated with the help of a 6/10 Amplatz Teflon stricture dilator. C. 10F Ring catheter has been placed with tip in duodenum for internal drainage.

sheath–dilator farther into the biliary tree. A new drainage catheter can then be inserted through the sheath or dilator.[75]

Malecot catheter introduction also requires a stiffening cannula, not only to counteract the softness of the C-Flex

material (Medi–Tech and Cook catheters) but also to straighten the wings of the Malecot tip. For exchange purposes, it is best if a guidewire can be passed through the end hole. If a straight wire does not pass spontaneously, the stiffener can be inserted into the catheter

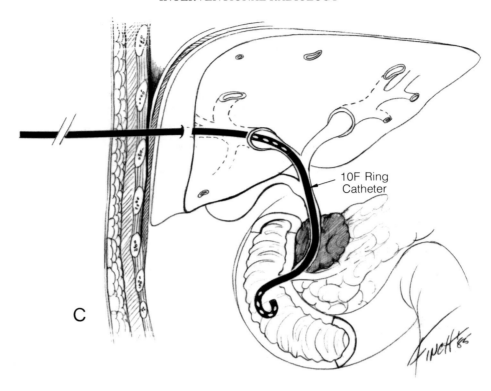

10F Ring
Catheter

Fig. 27–62C

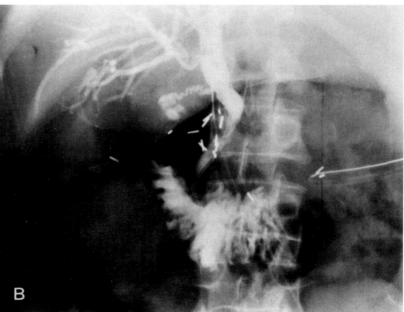

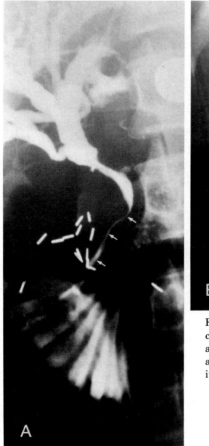

Fig. 27–63   A. Fine-needle cholangiogram in patient with carcinoma of pancreas causing obstruction of distal common bile duct (arrows). Observe displacement and narrowing of intrahepatic radicles. B. Through an anterior epigastric approach, Ring biliary drainage catheter has been placed across obstruction with its tip in duodenum for internal drainage with exteriorized catheter.

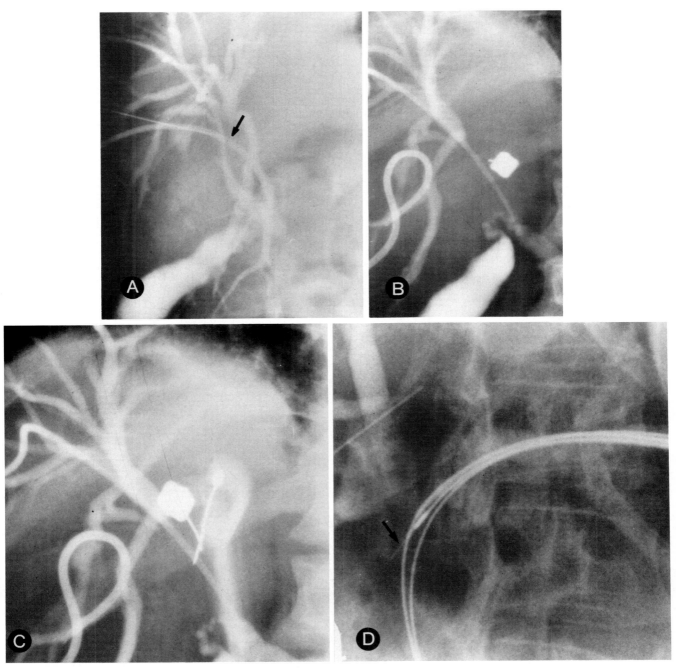

Fig. 27–64 Patient with cholangiocarcinoma involving common hepatic duct. With guidance of contrast medium injected through biliary drainage catheters, percutaneous biopsy of the mass was performed using 21-gauge Sure-Cut needle. A. Oblique view shows position of tip of needle (arrow) at level of mass obstructing common hepatic duct. B. Anteroposterior view shows needle at level of mass. C. A second needle has been placed in tandem fashion to obtain additional tissue for histologic examination. D. Prior to dilation for placement of larger external–internal biliary stent, specimen is taken using intracanalicular biopsy set (arrow).

until it reaches the Malecot opening. The catheter is then gently pulled back a short distance over the stiffener, which will partially close the wings of the Malecot tip. Once the wings are straightened, passage of a wire through the end hole is easy. If these maneuvers fail, the wire can be passed through the sideholes of the Malecot and 2–10 cm of it coiled in the biliary tree (Fig. 27–66).

The catheter is then gently pulled back under fluoroscopic control to prevent dislodgment of the wire. The wire is repositioned with a torque control catheter and the new catheter is inserted.

Circle loop tubes are a special form of external drainage for patients in whom long-term drainage is planned because of contraindications to or complications of sur-

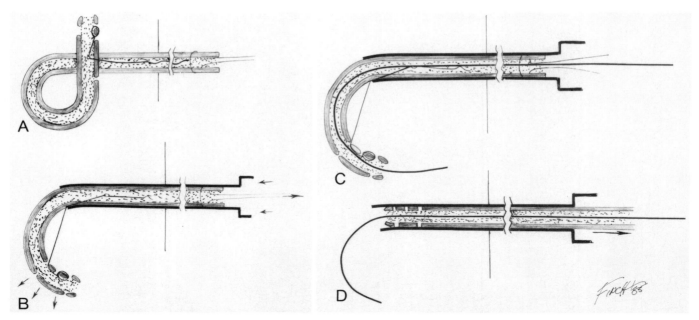

Fig. 27–65 Removal of stuck Cope loop. A. Encrustation prevents removal. B. After hub of catheter is cut, introducer sheath is advanced over shaft. C. Leading edge of sheath is used to forcefully straighten the loop. D. After straightening of loop, guidewire has been advanced through catheter, which is then withdrawn through sheath.

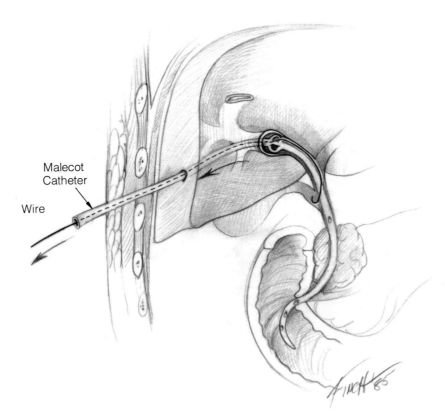

Malecot
Catheter

Wire

Fig. 27–66 Malfunctioning Malecot biliary drainage catheter is being replaced. Guidewire has been advanced through catheter, and due to inability to pass it into distal end of catheter, guidewire was passed through Malecot orifices into common hepatic duct. Catheter can then be pulled back while holding guidewire in place.

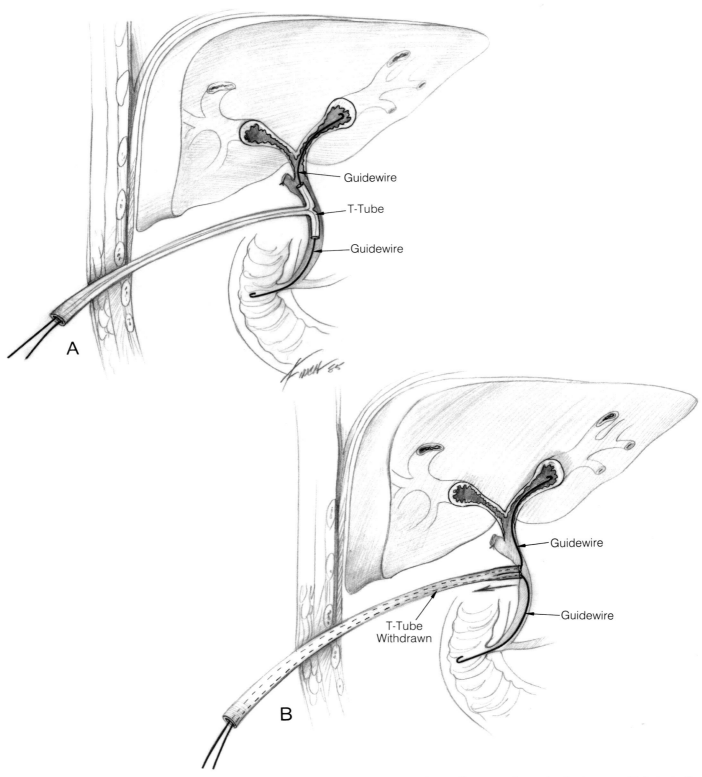

Fig. 27-67 Creation of circle loop using existing T-tube tract. A. Two guidewires have been passed through T-tube, one into common bile duct and duodenum and second into left biliary radicle. B. T-tube is withdrawn, keeping guidewire in place. C. Angiographic torque control catheter has been used to catheterize an anterior biliary radicle in right lower lobe of liver. After catheter tip has been placed as far distally as possible within biliary radicle, stiff end of the wire has been advanced and pushed across biliary radicle wall, liver parenchyma, liver capsule, and soft tissues until it tents the skin, which is then cut with scalpel. D. Through-and-through wire is now present through the T-tube tract, biliary tree, and skin. E. After dilatation of percutaneous tract into the biliary radicle with bifunnel plastic adaptor, 8F Silastic circle loop tube is being advanced, following lead of 8F Teflon dilator. F. After successful positioning of circle loop Silastic catheter, both ends have been connected to T-adaptor.

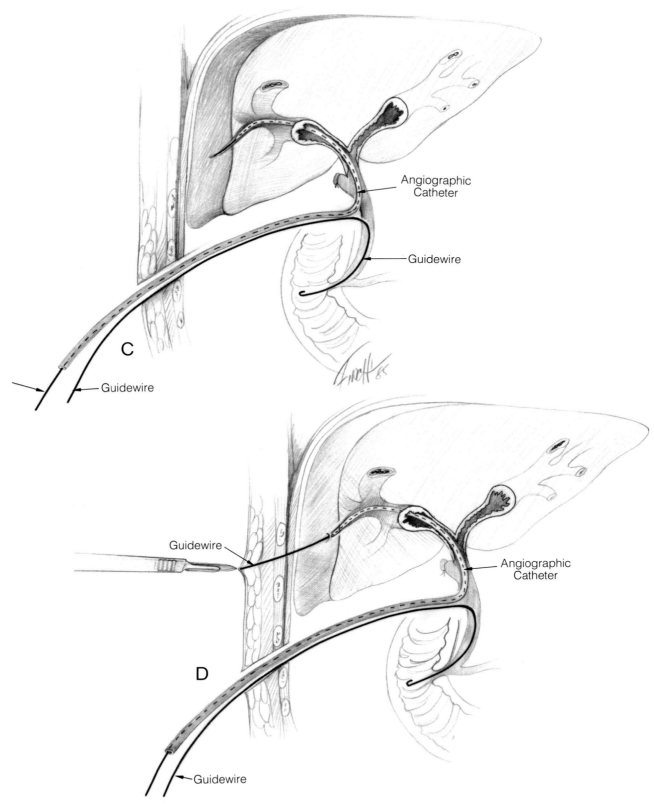

C

Angiographic
Catheter

Guidewire

Guidewire

Guidewire

D

Angiographic
Catheter

Guidewire

Fig. 27–67C,D

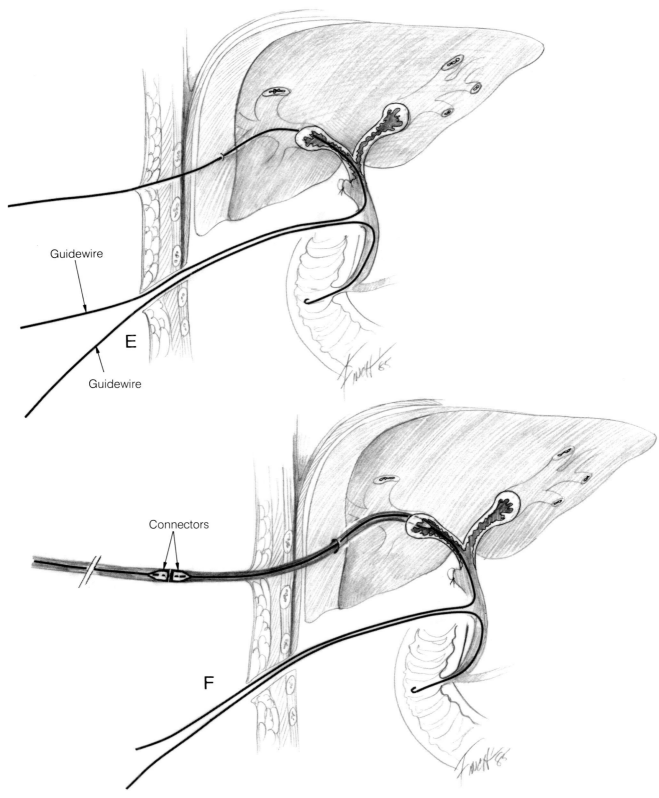

Guidewire

Guidewire

E

Connectors

F

Fig. 27–67E,F

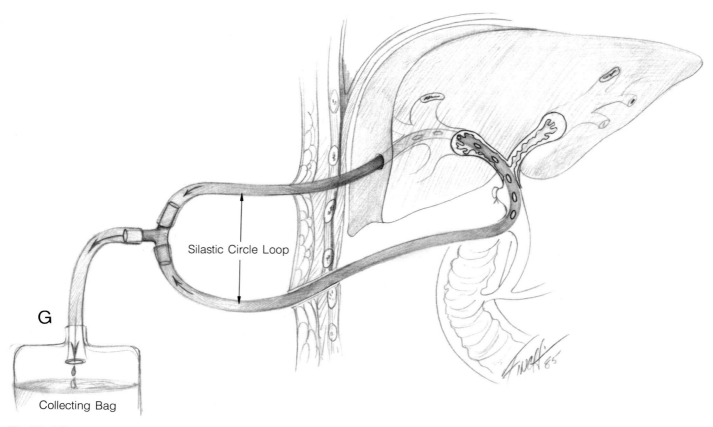

Fig. 27–67G

gery or because the patient is uncooperative about taking care of the drainage catheter. The circle loop drainage system has several advantages:

1. It is easy to replace, even without fluoroscopy.
2. Long-term patency is good, because the catheter is made of Silastic.
3. It is well tolerated by the patient because of its softness.
4. It is difficult to dislodge, because both tube ends are hooked to the drainage bag.

In order to establish circle loop drainage, two percutaneous tracts must be created. Almost always, one of these tracts is a T-tube tract.[110] Through this tract, an angiographic catheter is advanced selectively into an anteriorly directed biliary radicle (Fig. 27–67A,B). A wire is parked in the duct, and the angiographic catheter is replaced by a 9F Teflon guiding catheter, which is wedged (Fig. 27–67C). A 21-gauge needle inside a 5F Teflon sheath (the Hawkins "inside-out" nephrostomy kit) is introduced until it reaches the end of the 9F dilator, and the needle is advanced until it reaches the skin, which is tented by the needle tip (Fig. 27–67D). The skin is incised with a blade to allow the needle to exit. Alternatively a percutaneous tract can be created and the guidewire extracted through the T-tube tract (Fig. 27–68). The 5F Teflon dilator can then be advanced over the needle until it exits through the skin. The needle is replaced by a 0.038-inch exchange guidewire (Fig. 27–67E), and the tract is gradually enlarged with Teflon dilators until the desired

French size (2F larger than the stent) is reached. The Silastic stent can be attached to the end of the last dilator, which is pulled forward, bringing the stent along (Fig. 27–67F). Once the stent is traversing the tract, the dilator is detached, and the guidewire is removed. The position of the sideholes within the biliary radicles is verified by injecting contrast medium through one end of the stent while occluding the other. The position of the stent can be adjusted by pulling on either end (Fig. 27–67G).[109] With time and experience, the patient learns to adjust the loop either by using positioning marks on the catheter or by being sensitive to any sensation of discomfort that indicates that the sideholes are misplaced, thus partially blocking drainage and distending the bile ducts. If distention and pain are absent in this situation, bile will usually leak along the tract. The loop can easily be exchanged by using a bifunnel connector to attach one arm of the old loop to one arm of the new loop, which is then simply pulled into position.

If the patient does not have a T-tube tract, the circle loop can still be created utilizing the inside-out Hawkins nephrostomy kit. One percutaneous tract is made into an anterior right or left biliary radicle (Fig. 27–69A). The biliary tree is decompressed, and, in a second sitting, an anterior biliary radicle in the hepatic lobe opposite the initial puncture is selectively catheterized with the help of an angiographic catheter (Fig. 27–69B). The second tract is then created in the same inside-out fashion as before, using the 9F Teflon dilator and the 21-gauge needle inside a 5F Teflon catheter (Fig. 27–69C,D).

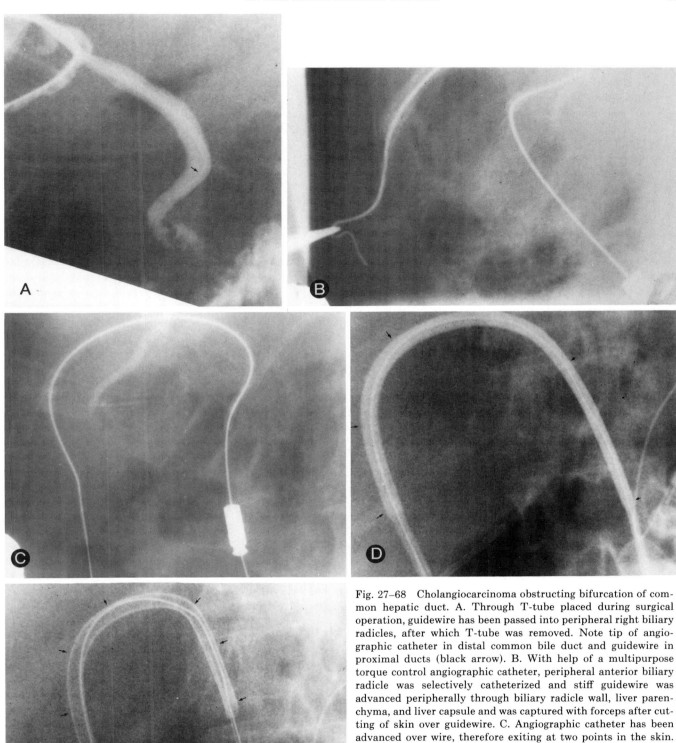

Fig. 27–68 Cholangiocarcinoma obstructing bifurcation of common hepatic duct. A. Through T-tube placed during surgical operation, guidewire has been passed into peripheral right biliary radicles, after which T-tube was removed. Note tip of angiographic catheter in distal common bile duct and guidewire in proximal ducts (black arrow). B. With help of a multipurpose torque control angiographic catheter, peripheral anterior biliary radicle was selectively catheterized and stiff guidewire was advanced peripherally through biliary radicle wall, liver parenchyma, and liver capsule and was captured with forceps after cutting of skin over guidewire. C. Angiographic catheter has been advanced over wire, therefore exiting at two points in the skin. Stiffer guidewire is passed through catheter, and catheter is removed for subsequent dilatation and stent placement. D. U-loop tract dilated with coaxial Teflon dilators (arrows). E. Silastic stent in position (arrows).

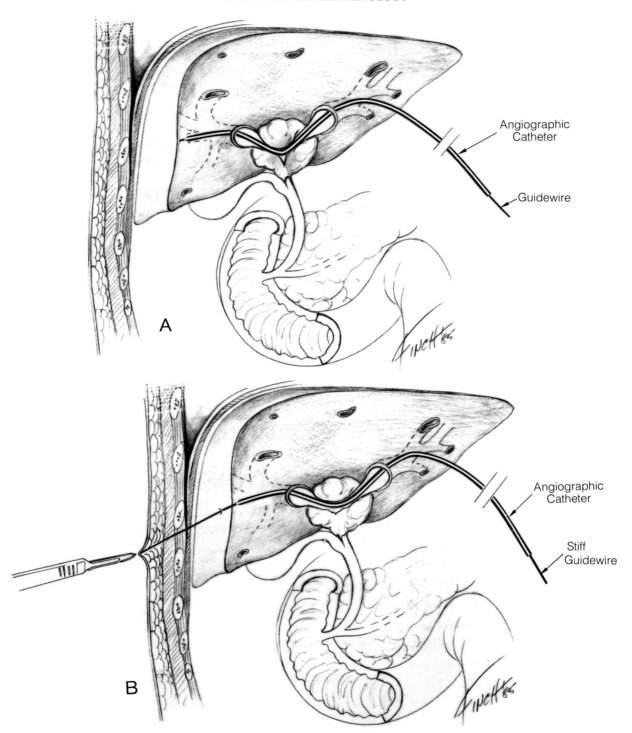

Fig. 27–69 A. Through an epigastric approach, catheter has been passed from the left into an anterior right biliary radicle. Stiff guidewire is subsequently advanced, perforating wall of bile duct. B. Guidewire has perforated wall of bile duct, liver parenchyma, and liver capsule and is seen tenting skin. A scalpel is used to cut the skin over guidewire.C. After withdrawal of guidewire across the skin, two 8F Teflon dilators are used to dilate tract into right and left biliary trees. D. After adequate dilatation of percutaneous tract; 8F Silastic circle loop catheter has been placed and is joined by T-connector to drainage bag.

CATHETER PLACEMENT FOR INTERNAL–EXTERNAL DRAINAGE

If the procedure goes smoothly, the patient remains stable, and the stenosis can be traversed without great difficulty, passage of an internal drainage catheter to the distal common bile duct or duodenum can be accomplished at the first sitting. Often, however, the attempt to pass through the stenosis into the duodenum is postponed until a second sitting, when the biliary tree has been decompressed and the patient is more stable.

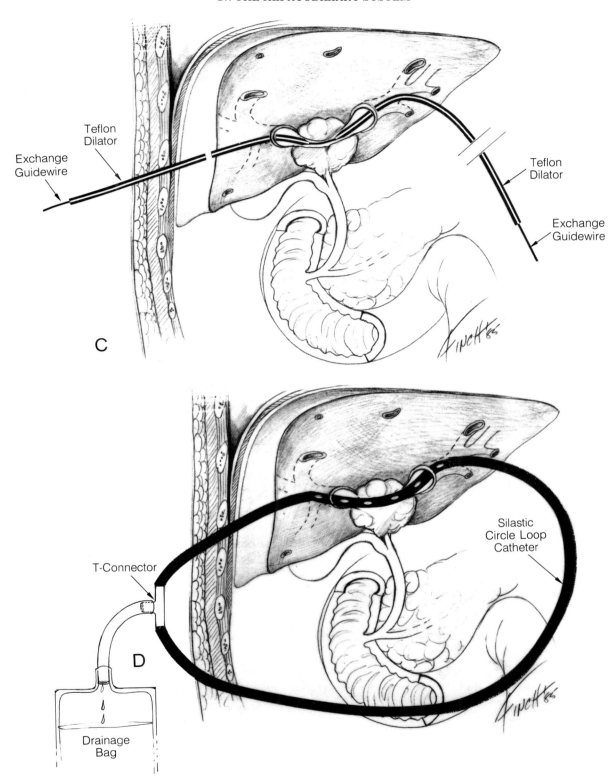

Fig. 27–69C,D

In the second sitting, the skin and the previously placed external drainage catheter are cleaned, prepared, and draped. Contrast medium is injected through the catheter to locate the stenosis and opacify the ducts. A 0.035-inch floppy-tip guidewire is passed through the catheter, which is removed.

Although a large variety of wires and catheters can be used to catheterize the biliary tree, there are two techniques the authors prefer. One technique uses a torque control Cobra (Cordis) or multipurpose (Cook, Inc.) catheter and a 0.035-inch floppy-tip wire. The catheter tip is used to direct the wire through the stenoses and around the bends in the tortuous, dilated ducts. The other technique relies for its directional control on a slightly curved Lunderquist or torque control Lunderquist–Ring wire. In this case, the wire is used to pass through stenoses and around bends in the biliary radicles into the duodenum, and the slightly curved catheter follows. One should be careful not to apply too much axial pressure to the Lunderquist wire when advancing around curves, because the joint between the soft end and the stainless-steel shaft may kink or fracture, becoming a sharp spear that can easily perforate the wall. Once the guidewire has passed across the obstruction and into the duodenum, a stent can usually be passed over the wire.

In some cases, the ducts can easily be catheterized down to the point of the obstruction, but neither a catheter nor a wire will pass through the obstruction. In such cases, it is most helpful to decompress the biliary tree for 4–5 days with an external drain and then try again to traverse the obstruction. Decompressing the dilated bile ducts allows some time for edema at the obstruction site to resolve and the ducts to return to more normal dimensions (Fig. 27–70). As a result, ductal tortuosity is decreased, which greatly facilitates catheterization.

The length of catheter in which sideholes should be made is easily determined by one of the following techniques:

1. Once the guidewire is in the duodenum, a catheter is passed over the wire into the bowel and then pulled back to the level of the ampulla. The first clamp is applied to the wire at the catheter hub (Fig. 27–71). With this clamp in place, the wire is pulled back until the tip is well above the obstruction but inside the ducts, and a second clamp is applied to the wire at the catheter hub. The wire is then removed. The length of wire between the clamps is the distance between the ampulla and the entry site into the ducts and represents the length of catheter where sideholes have to be made. Normally, for drainage purposes, sideholes are needed only proximal to the obstruction and distally in the distal common bile duct or duodenum, although a few additional ones can be made in the intermediate area, especially if some bile ducts branch off in that region.

2. A slightly simpler technique involves the use of a 0.038-inch endoruler consisting of 0.038-inch Teflon tubing inside of which radiopaque marks are placed 1 cm apart (Fig. 27–72).[111] Once an angiographic catheter is in the duodenum, the guidewire is removed, and the endoruler is introduced in the same manner as a guidewire. The exact distance from the duodenum to the duct entry site proximal to the obstruction can then be measured directly from the fluoroscope screen or from a film of the abdomen. This measurement is transferred to the drainage catheter to make the sideholes.

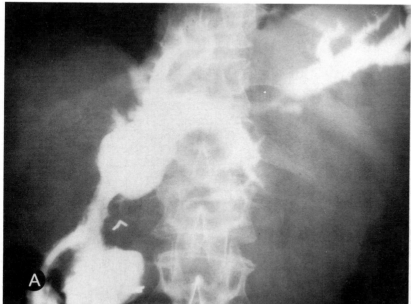
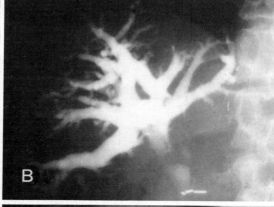
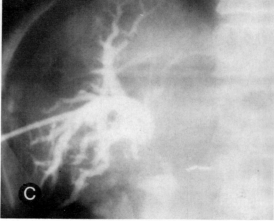
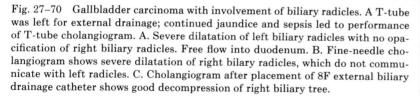

Fig. 27–70   Gallbladder carcinoma with involvement of biliary radicles. A T-tube was left for external drainage; continued jaundice and sepsis led to performance of T-tube cholangiogram. A. Severe dilatation of left biliary radicles with no opacification of right biliary radicles. Free flow into duodenum. B. Fine-needle cholangiogram shows severe dilatation of right bilary radicles, which do not communicate with left radicles. C. Cholangiogram after placement of 8F external biliary drainage catheter shows good decompression of right biliary tree.

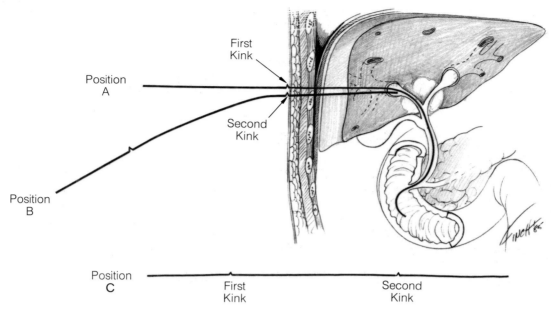

CATHETER-SECURING TECHNIQUES

The finger-trap method is a simple and useful maneuver by which accidental removal or dislodgment can be minimized.[112] A suture is knotted at the skin and then again around the catheter, leaving two ends of equal length. The suture ends are wound upward in opposite directions around the catheter for approximately 5–6 cm. At this level, a secure knot is made around the catheter.

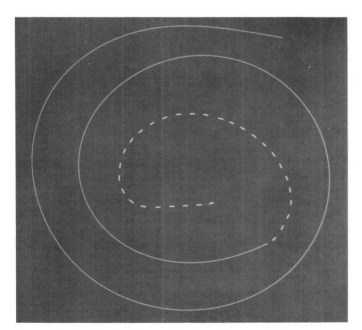

Fig. 27–72   Endoruler. (Reproduced from Herrera M, Brawerman S, Castañeda WR, et al: The endocatheter ruler: a useful device. *AJR* 1982;139:828–829 with the permission of the American Roentgen Ray Society.)

The direction is reversed, and the ends are wound back down to the skin, where another knot is made around the catheter. For added security, the suture can once more be knotted to the skin. The disadvantage of this method is that in the long term, sutures of any type tend to cut through the skin or to be cut off accidentally during cleansing. In addition, if the suture is too loose, it may slip, whereas if it is too tight, it may kink or obstruct the catheter.

Taping the catheter to the skin has the disadvantage that the adhesive properties are lost in the presence of bile leakage, diaphoresis, or bleeding, all of which are common after percutaneous biliary procedures. In addition, nurses frequently remove the unclean tape with the unclean dressings, and one will later find a nice clean wound with a partially pulled-back, untaped catheter.

Molnar discs of different shapes and sizes are available (Cook, Inc.; Cook Urological; Vantech; Medi–Tech). Molnar discs are manufactured of silicone or rubber and are tightened around the catheter with plastic serrated ties. The disc is fixed to the skin with either a suture or the Molnar disc adhesive.[89,113] This is probably one of the best ways to secure a long-term drainage catheter, but it has the disadvantage that secretions tend to collect under the disc, where cleaning is difficult.

The authors designed a variant of the Molnar disc that consists of two concentric metallic rings joined by three arms (Fig. 27–73). The catheter is passed through the central ring, to which it is stitched. The open surface allows cleaning of the puncture site, and the flat configuration makes it well tolerated.

Stoma adhesive alone is also an excellent method of securing a long-term catheter, especially those through which internal drainage has been achieved so the external

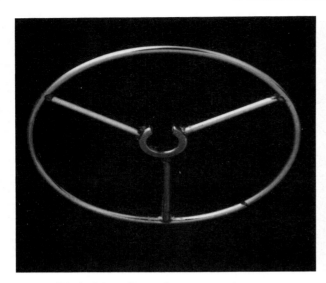
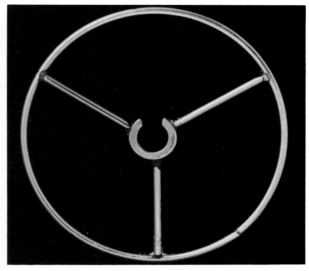

Fig. 27–73 Modified Molnar disc made of flat stainless-steel wire, allowing easy cleaning of wound around catheter entry point.

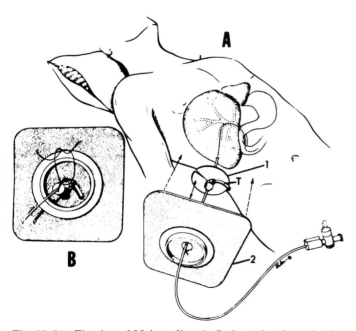

Fig. 27–74 Fixation of Molnar disc. A. Catheter has been fixed to Molnar disc (1) by tightening band (T) which has been stitched to skin. Preloaded stoma adhesive wafer (2) is subsequently advanced to cover disc. B. Disc is stitched to rim of wafer. (Reproduced from Shoenfeld RB, Lecky D, Ring EJ, McLean GK, Freiman DB: Stabilization of percutaneous catheteters. *AJR* 1982;138:972 with the permission of the American Roentgen Ray Society.)

puncture site can be kept clean and dry. To install it, the circular hole in the stoma adhesive is enlarged and slipped around the catheter (Fig. 27–74). The skin is sprayed with benzoin, which sticks the stoma wafer firmly to the skin. A silk adhesive tape is wrapped around the catheter, and several lock stitches are made through the tape and tied to the flange of the stoma adhesive.[114] Stoma adhesives need a change every 2–3 weeks; otherwise, they may become dry, loose, and crumbly. Stoma adhesive should be changed only by experienced persons, because the catheter is secured with a direct suture.

Another way of securing the catheter with stoma adhesive is first to fix the catheter with a Molnar disc and a serrated tie. A stoma wafer with a central hole is slipped over the catheter until the nipple of the Molnar disc protrudes through the hole. The stoma adhesive wafer is then secured to the skin and disc with benzoin. The stoma adhesive can be changed by the patient without help from medical personnel simply by removing the wafer and not disturbing the Molnar disc.[113]

One other catheter-securing technique uses a Tuohy–Borst adapter tightened around the catheter at the puncture site (Fig. 27–75). The Tuohy–Borst adapter is then stitched to the skin.[115]

THE DISLODGED BILIARY DRAINAGE CATHETER

Accidental dislodgment of a drainage catheter commonly requires creation of a new percutaneous tract, because attempts to catheterize the old tract, particularly a laterally placed tract, usually fail. Anterior tracts tend to be easier to recatheterize because of their straighter and shorter courses.

Two cardinal rules apply in these patients:

1. Do not attempt blind manipulations through the tract, regardless of how old and mature it is, because these

tracts are usually tortuous even if they were straight when created. Once a false passage has been created by blind manipulations, it is almost impossible to catheterize the true channel.

2. Do not infiltrate the tract with local anesthetic before attempting to catheterize it, because this can distort or disrupt it. It is preferable to administer sufficient sedation to make the patient comfortable during the manipulation. Once the tract is catheterized, local anesthesia can be given for further manipulations.

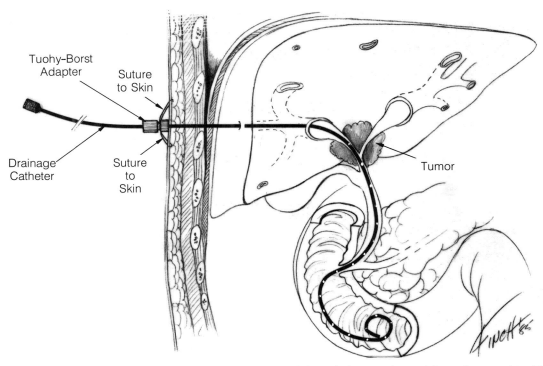

Fig. 27-75   Tuohy–Borst adapter has been used to secure internal–external biliary drainage catheter. Adapter is secured to skin, and catheter has been fixed with help of adapter.

The technique for replacing a dislodged catheter begins with the patient in the supine decubitus position. The old site of entry is prepared and draped. Under fluoroscopic control and video recording, a Christmas tree adapter is inserted into the tract opening,[116] and 50% contrast medium is instilled to opacify the tract (Fig. 27–76A). Freeze-framing on the video recorder is useful to guide the catheterization; if it is unavailable, a film of the abdomen can be obtained after the injection of contrast medium. Especially with lateral approaches, it is occasionally necessary to inject contrast during a complete and full inhalation by the patient. As the liver moves with breathing, the hole through the lateral body wall may suddenly align with the tract in the liver, allowing contrast to flow toward the bile ducts.

Once the tract is opacified, the Christmas tree adapter is removed, and a 0.035-inch floppy-tip guidewire is gently manipulated through the bends in the tract with the help of an angiographic catheter (Cobra (Cordis) or multipurpose (Cook, Inc.)) until the wire reaches the biliary tree (Fig. 27–76B). Once a guidewire reaches the bile ducts, placement of a catheter or stent proceeds in the usual fashion.

If the procedure is attempted more than 24 hr after accidental dislodgment, the tract is frequently closed, and attempts to reopen it more commonly result in false passages than in recatheterization. In these cases, and in those referred after blind manipulations have created one or more false passages, creation of a new tract will be faster and safer than attempting to manipulate in a traumatized and possibly infected old one.

TECHNIQUE OF INTERNAL STENT PLACEMENT

Teflon stents are available in 10F, 12F, and 14F sizes and with several configurations to help prevent migration.[117–124] Depending on the size of the stent, a kit consists of an 8F guiding dilator, coaxial dilators (10F, 12F, and 14F) up to the size of the stent, and the stent itself.

The 8F guiding dilator is introduced over the guidewire, which has previously been advanced well into the duodenum. The 10F dilator is passed over the 8F to dilate the tract and is withdrawn. The 10F stent is then advanced coaxially over the 8F dilator until it reaches the skin. At that point, the blunt end of the 10F dilator is used to push the stent until it is positioned across the obstruction (Fig. 27–77). The 8F dilator is removed, and a 5F catheter is advanced over the guidewire until its tip is proximal to the stent. After removal of the guidewire, contrast medium is injected through the catheter to verify the position of the stent. In order to move the stent backward, it is necessary to insert a balloon catheter into the trailing edge of the stent.[125] Once the balloon is firmly inflated inside both the stent and the pusher, retraction of the balloon catheter will bring the stent along. Contrast injection and aspiration can also be used to flush the stent and bile ducts and to make sure blood clots are cleared away. If the bile is clear and the stent in good position, everything can be removed, starting with the monofilament suture, which is removed by gently pulling on one end while applying forward pressure with the pusher.

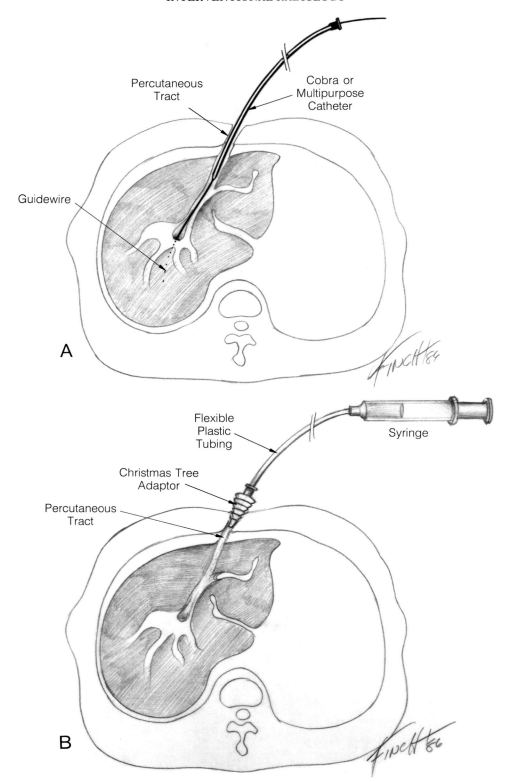

Fig. 27–76 Replacement of fallen-out biliary drainage catheter. A. Christmas tree adapter has been placed against opening of percutaneous tract; contrast medium is injected through adapter, opacifying tract and biliary tree. B. By gentle probing and with the help of angiographic torque control catheter, floppy-tipped guidewire has been manipulated into biliary tree.

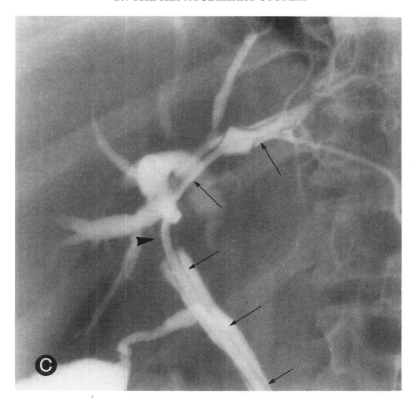

Fig. 27–79C

mal end. An introducer system is under development. Meanwhile, an elaborate technique is necessary to overcome the softness and high friction. First, the tract is dilated to 16F. A 5-mm angioplasty balloon catheter is positioned with the tip of the balloon just protruding from the leading edge of the stent, and the balloon is inflated. The balloon and stent are then advanced over the guidewire until the stent is positioned across the obstruction and the Malecot tip is completely inside the bile ducts (Fig. 27–79A). Further adjustments can be made by either pushing farther with the inflated balloon or pulling back on a monofilament suture looped through the Malecot wings. The balloon is subsequently deflated and withdrawn while a large dilator–pusher holds the stent in place (Fig. 27–79B). A smaller (5F–6F) catheter is then advanced over the guidewire until the tip lies within the stent. The guidewire is removed, and contrast medium is injected to check the position and patency of the stent. An ingenious technique was described for application in patients with Klatzke's tumor. A tract is created and dilated to pass two wires. An angiographic catheter is used to pass from the right to the left biliary radicles, while the second wire is passed to the common bile duct (Fig. 27–80A,B). One catheter is passed over each guidewire, which are then removed, and the catheters are connected, creating in this manner a U-loop which is left on internal drainage (Fig. 27–80C). Alternatively, an endoprosthesis can be placed to drain one lobe of the liver while an external catheter draws the other lobe, either externally or by capping the external catheter, internally through the endoprosthesis (Fig. 27–80D).

COMPARISON OF EXTERNAL CATHETER DRAINAGE AND INTERNAL STENTS

General Considerations

External biliary drainage with the catheter placed proximal to an obstruction is a relatively simple procedure that leads to effective biliary decompression in most patients. However, long-term external diversion of bile causes problems such as infections at the entry site, catheter dislocations or accidental removal, and bile salt depletion, resulting in malaise and loss of appetite.

Internal drainage via an internal–external catheter with the external end plugged avoids the problems of bile salt loss. Care of the catheter is easier, because no drainage bag must be carried, and access to the biliary system is preserved. If necessary, the catheter can easily be exchanged without repuncture of the liver. On the other hand, the patient is inconvenienced by the presence of a catheter in the flank and, often, by infections at the entry

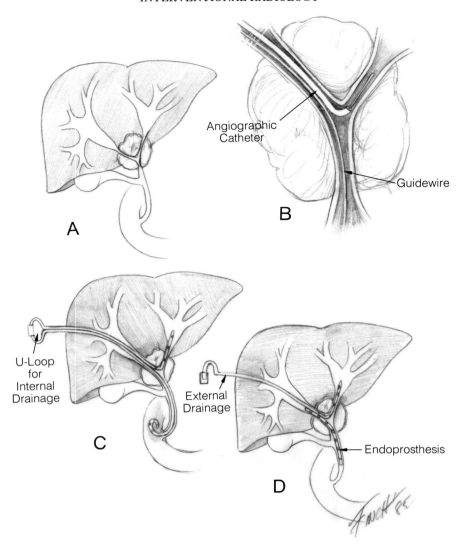

Fig. 27–80   Percutaneous tract has been dilated, and two guidewires have been passed. One wire has been parked in distal common bile duct. Over second guidewire, angiographic torque control catheter has been passed, and its tip has been manipulated into ostium of left hepatic duct. Guidewire has been passed into left biliary radicles. C. One biliary drainage catheter has been passed over each of the guidewires, and both have been connected to plastic adapter to allow internal drainage of both right and left lobes of liver into duodenum. D. Because bile can leak along tract due to presence of two catheters, an alternative is placement of internal prosthesis over one of the wires, leaving second catheter draining both right and left biliary radicles externally as an access for future needle.

site. Inadvertent pulling on the catheter may lead to complete removal from the biliary tree. Also, with a lateral approach, the parietal pleura is almost inevitably transgressed, which may lead to biliary pleuritis.[109,126] In addition, if such internal–external drainage is attempted through an 8F catheter, the size most widely used for that purpose, it is frequently complicated by recurrent cholangitis. This is probably due to insufficient drainage and bile stasis, because the rate of septic complications drops after replacement of the original catheter by a large-bore (10F–12F) catheter.[59]

Theoretically, a large-bore endoprosthesis that remained unfailingly patent would be the ideal solution for long-term biliary drainage.

Discussion

Migration of stents is a common technical problem; it occurred in 15% of the cases in the series of Mendez et al.[127] Migration used to be more common with Teflon stents because of their low friction coefficient and was partially overcome by adding retention devices such as proximal flares and distal flanges. Migration is less of a problem with the Carey–Coons stent because of its length and the higher friction coefficient of the Percuflex material. The same reasoning applies to the Tieslink (USCI) stent, which has the highest friction coefficient of all available stents.

The long-term patency of internal stents is controversial. Some authors report 100% patency in patients followed as long as a year,[76] whereas other authors report at least a 30% occlusion rate within a year.[127] The main problem in determining the patency rate of the stent lies in the fact that it frequently is difficult to determine whether a persistently elevated bilirubin concentration is caused by progressive hepatic failure or by obstruction of the internal stent. In these cases, evaluation with radioisotopes is most useful in determining whether the stent is patent.

The complications of endoprosthesis placement probably are slightly more common than after the placement of internal–external stents. They generally are related to the dilatation of the transhepatic tract. Bleeding and subcutaneous wound abscesses are the most common problems. Cholangitis occurs less commonly with internal stents than with internal–external drainage catheters. The chief objection to the placement of internal stents seems to be related to the problem of stent migration or occlusion, which requires a new percutaneous procedure to reposition or clean the stent.

Efficiency of Drainage

After the establishment of functioning biliary drainage, the serum bilirubin concentration will drop along an exponential curve. The times required to reduce bilirubin values by 50% for external and internal–external 8F catheters as well as for 12F endoprostheses (all from William Cook–Europe) are displayed in Table 27–1. If one uses the decrease in serum bilirubin concentration as the principal criterion of drainage efficiency, internal drainage via a 12F endoprosthesis is clearly better than drainage with an 8.3F catheter. Endoprostheses are twice as effective as internal–external catheters draining internally (p < 0.02).

Drainage Dysfunction

The causes of dysfunction are summarized in Table 27–2. The most common are clogging by biliary salts, blood clots, or intestinal contents or by displacement of the sideholes out of the biliary tree or below the obstruction. Dysfunction of catheters (or endoprostheses) leads to persistently high or rising bilirubin concentrations and, frequently, to cholangitis due to stasis of infected bile. An obstructed catheter can, in most cases, be easily cleaned by flushing or by passing a wire or a cytology brush through it. Alternatively, it can be replaced with the aid of a guidewire. Recalcitrant obstructions caused by inspissated bile can often be dissolved by repeated injections of mucolytic agents.

Dysfunctions of endoprostheses can be caused by migration proximal or distal to the stenosis, clogging by tumor overgrowth, or by obstruction of the duodenum. Intraductal migration, either proximal or distal, is uncommon with the newer stents and can be prevented by fitting the length and curve of the stent to the anatomic situation in each patient (Fig. 27–81). Extraductal migration, a type of dislocation not described before, has occurred twice in the authors' experience. Both patients were thought initially to have malignant biliary obstruction. Endoprostheses were correctly placed across the obstruction, with both ends within the bile ducts. After 2 and 2 ½ years, the previously normal serum bilirubin concentrations began to rise again. At operation, the stents

Table 27–1
Half-Value Time of Serum Bilirubin Concentration with Different Drainage Modalities

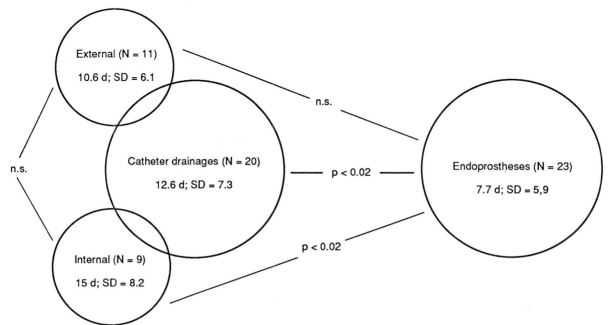

Table 27–2
Incidence of Drainage Dysfunction with Different Drainage Modalities

	Total		Follow up >1 Month	
	N	Dysfunction	N	Dysfunction
External catheter	16	3 (19%)		
Internal catheter	19	3 (16%)	6	1 (17%)
Endoprosthesis	39	10 (25%)	24	8 (33%)
Dysfunction corrected		−4		−3
Definitive dysfunction		6 (15%)		5 (19%)
Tumor patients only	35	4 (11%)	21	3 (14%)

were found to be partially dislodged from the common bile duct into the hepatoduodenal ligament (Fig. 27–82). Apparently, stents made of stiff Teflon tubing tend to erode slowly through the walls of the biliary tree during long-term drainage. Thus, for patients with benign lesions, a softer stent material such as polyurethane or Silastic might be advantageous.

Obstruction of an endoprosthesis is commonly caused by reflux of duodenal contents in addition to encrustation by biliary salts. Clogging is frequently associated with cholangitis, the stent being filled with a plug of debris and pus (Fig. 27–83). Obstruction of an endoprosthesis by debris or tumor overgrowth usually necessitates reintervention.

Tumor overgrowth has been the most frequent cause of dysfunction in the authors' series of patients. It often occurs in the preterminal stage of the disease, so that further interventions are not justified.

If signs of drainage dysfunction are accompanied by anorexia or bilious vomiting, duodenal obstruction must be suspected. In such cases, bilirubin concentrations will rise in spite of a patent endoprosthesis until the duodenum is decompressed by a nasogastric tube or by gastroenterostomy.

The dysfunction rate of endoprostheses, especially in patients surviving longer than 1 month, is higher than that of drainage catheters. These dysfunctions can be corrected by several maneuvers, which will be described later in this chapter.

Complication Rate

CHOLANGITIS

Cholangitis and biliary sepsis are the most frequent complications with any type of biliary drainage. The reported occurrence rates range from 3.3%[128] to 67%.[129] The frequency seems to depend on the diameter of the drainage catheters. According to Mueller et al, cholangitis occurred in 63% of patients after clamping of 8F catheters for internal drainage vs. 11% after replacement by 10F–12F tubing.[60] Incomplete drainage of the biliary tree with obstruction of multiple segments carries a significantly higher risk of cholangitis (64%), compared with 15% in patients with a single stenosis.[60]

The frequency of cholangitis with different drainage modalities in the authors' patients is summarized in

Fig. 27–81 Periampullary carcinoma. A. Curved endoprosthesis is inserted into stenosis with its tip through papilla. B. Dysfunction after 3 weeks. Percutaneous transhepatic cholangiography during reintervention shows proximal dislocation of stent.

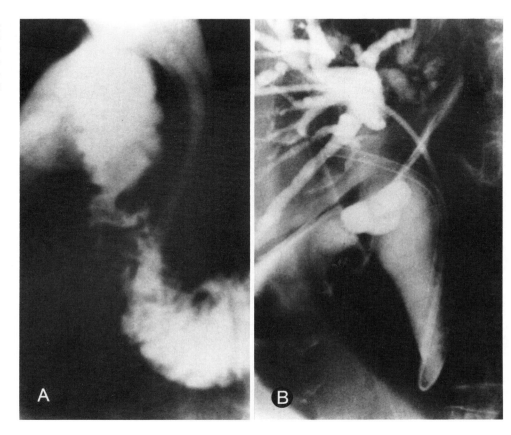

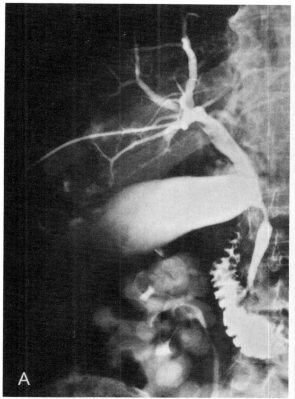

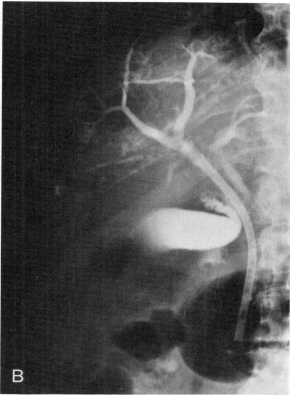

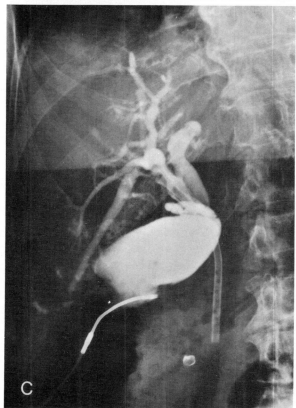

Fig. 27–82   Patient with obstructive jaundice. A. Percutaneous transhepatic cholangiography shows short, eccentric common bile duct stenosis thought to be of malignant origin. B. Endoprosthesis placed across stenosis. C. Dysfunction after 2½ years. Intraoperative cholangiogram shows extraductal position of proximal end of endoprosthesis.

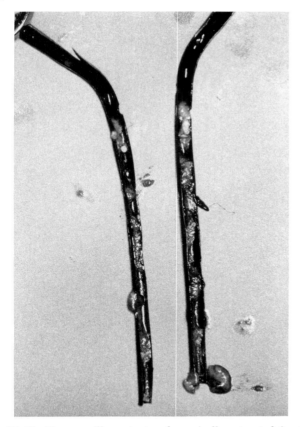

Fig. 27–83 Transpapillary stent endoscopically extracted for dysfunction after 3 1/2 months. Endoprosthesis is cut longitudinally in two halves; its lumen is filled with a plug of pus and debris.

Table 27–3. Biliary drainage with 12F endoprostheses carries a lower risk of cholangitis than does 8F catheter drainage. This difference is statistically significant if the high-risk patients with only partial drainage of multisegment obstructions are excluded. In three patients with catheter drainage who had recurrent cholangitis, infection did not recur after replacement of the catheter.

Table 27–3
Risk of Cholangitis with Different Drainage Modalities

	All Cases		"Complete" PTBD Only[a]	
	N	Cholangitis	N	Cholangitis
Catheter drainage	43	7 (16%)	36	4 (11%)
Endoprosthesis	45	2 (4%)	36	0 (0%)
Statistical significance	n.s. (0.1 > p > 0.05)		p < 0.05	

[a]"Complete" PTBD means that all obstructed segments, if multiple stenoses present, were drained.

OTHER COMPLICATIONS

Serious complications, such as severe bleeding and biliary peritonitis, occur with a frequency of 2%–5% after either catheter drainage or endoprosthesis placement.[60,65,130,131] However, there are complications intrinsic to catheter drainage alone. External drainage causes chronic loss of bile salts, with resulting malaise and anorexia. With high fluid output, especially from catheters placed through the papilla, hypovolemia and electrolyte imbalance may occur.[131,132]

In one patient with external drainage for obstruction secondary to pancreatic carcinoma, the serum bilirubin concentration failed to decrease, although about 1 liter of bile was drained per day, in spite of normalization of other liver test results. The patient complained of slight shortness of breath. A chest radiograph revealed a large right-sided pleural effusion (Fig. 27–84), which proved to be bile on thoracocentesis. The resorption of bile from the pleura had prevented a decrease of serum bilirubin. The effusion was drained and the incorrectly placed drainage catheter was replaced with an endoprosthesis. The serum bilirubin concentration promptly decreased. Pleural effusion did not recur.

SPECIAL INDICATIONS AND MANEUVERS

Retraction of Endoprostheses

If a loop of monofilament suture is threaded through the most proximal sidehole of the endoprosthesis and through the lumen of the pusher, an endoprosthesis inadvertently inserted too far can be pulled back. Another advantage of the loop retraction technique, described by Owman and Lunderquist,[133] is the possibility of positioning the trailing end of an endoprosthesis farther out in the duct than the actual entry point into the biliary tree. If the guidewire and the inner catheter are removed and the pusher is left in place with its front end just outside the entry into the duct, pulling on the thread will bring the sidehole through which the loop passes back to the level of the entry, and the trailing end of the endoprosthesis will be slightly farther out in the duct. In this way, an unfavorable stent position resulting from a puncture too close to the obstructing lesion can be corrected.

Tight rigid stenoses should be dilated by either a coaxial dilator or a balloon catheter before insertion of an endoprosthesis. Despite such precautions, an endoprosthesis can get stuck at the proximal end of a stenosis. If the device has been secured by a loop, it can be extracted together with the pusher. If there is no loop, the inner catheter of the delivery system is replaced with a balloon dilatation catheter, and the endoprosthesis is caught by inflating the balloon half within the endoprosthesis and half within the pusher catheter. Both can then be extracted, leaving the guidewire in place.[76]

Reintervention for Dysfunction of Endoprosthesis

After diagnostic PTC to establish the nature of the dysfunction, the biliary tree is entered well above the intrahepatic end of the endoprosthesis. If the aspirated

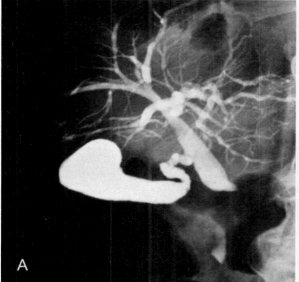
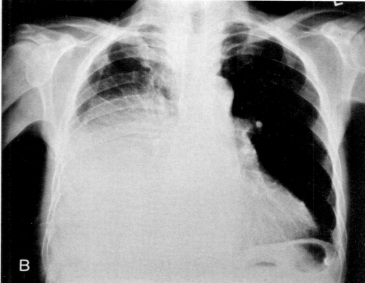
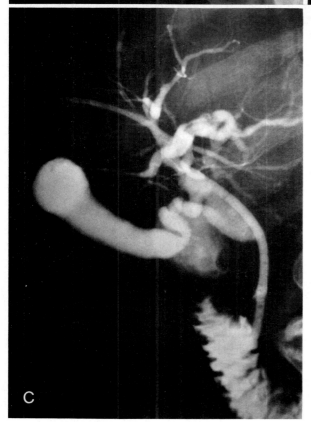

Fig. 27–84 A. External catheter drainage in patient with obstructive jaundice due to pancreatic carcinoma. Persistently high serum bilirubin level in spite of drainage of about 1 liter/day. B. Large biliary pleural effusion to the right. C. External catheter is replaced by 12F endoprosthesis. Prompt normalization of serum bilirubin, no recurrence of pleural effusion after short-term pleural drainage.

bile contains debris and pus, the biliary tree should be drained externally for about a week, until the bile has cleared. In some cases, clogging of the endoprosthesis will resolve with simple temporary external drainage and frequent irrigation, so that the external drainage device can be removed without further manipulation.

If the stent is still plugged, it can be entered by means of a special guidewire with torque control and a memory-curvable tip or a floppy-tip guidewire and torque control

catheter. It can then either be flushed clear with a multisidehole catheter inserted into its lumen or be removed if it cannot be cleared.

Tumor overgrowth occurs mostly at the intrahepatic end of the endoprosthesis. After passage of a guidewire through the tumor stenosis and the endoprosthesis, a deflector guidewire (Fig. 27–85) or a balloon catheter can be used to retract the proximal end of the stent above the upper margin of the tumor.

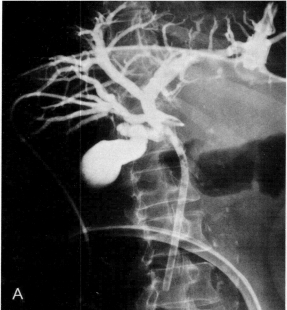

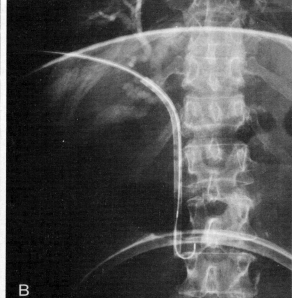

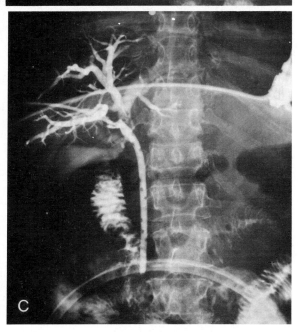

Fig. 27–85   Dysfunction 8 months after placement of endoprosthesis in patient with periportal metastases of ovarian carcinoma. A. Proximal end is occluded by tumor overgrowth. B. Retraction of stent by means of deflector guidewire. C. Upper end of stent retracted into posterocaudal branch proximal to upper tumor margin. Drainage was restored until death 2 weeks later.

Placement of Multiple Endoprostheses

As previously stated, the risk of cholangitis and biliary sepsis is significantly higher if only one segment of the liver is drained when multiple segments are obstructed. For obstructive lesions at the hepatic bifurcation, complete drainage can be accomplished by insertion of two endoprostheses, one from the lateral intercostal approach and one from the substernal approach, that will drain both hepatic ducts into the common bile duct (Fig. 27–86). Alternatively, two stents can be placed through the same tract to drain several ducts (Fig. 27–87). During insertion, both stents must be secured by a sling to prevent distal dislocation of one correctly placed endoprosthesis when the other is advanced. Alternatively, the two stents can be placed simultaneously by two operators.

Transpapillary Placement of Endoprostheses

In obstructions of the distal common bile duct, placement of stents with their distal ends at the level of the papilla may lead to early dysfunction due to distal tumor overgrowth or slight proximal dislocation. Thus, the distal end of the endoprosthesis should be inserted several centimeters into the duodenum.[76,134] Intraduodenal placement of the stent tip has an additional advantage in that the obstructed endoprosthesis can easily be extracted with a duodenoscope, obviating re-entry and percutaneous removal of the obstructed stent in the course of a reintervention. Instead, a new endoprosthesis can be placed by the usual percutaneous approach.

The sharp tip of the stiff Teflon endoprosthesis may cause ulcerations of the duodenum. Soft endoprostheses

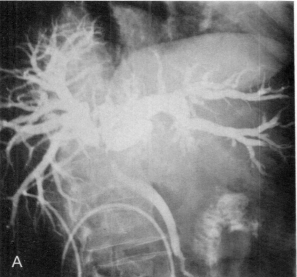

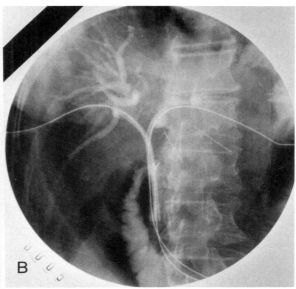

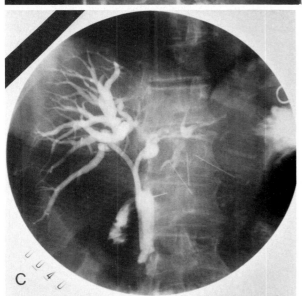

Fig. 27–86   A. Cholangiocarcinoma of the hepatic fork. B. Two endoprostheses are inserted from right and left hepatic duct through stenoses and into common bile duct. C. Final control film (catheter removed after injection) shows good drainage.

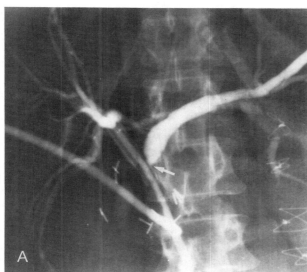

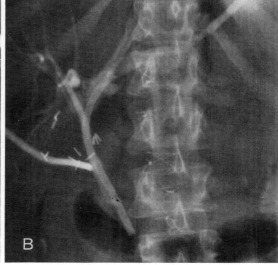

Fig. 27–87   Sixty-year-old patient with cholangiocarcinoma involving common hepatic as well as right and left hepatic ducts. A. T-tube was left in place at time of surgical exploration, with one arm in right hepatic duct and the other distally in common bile duct. Observe poor drainage from left biliary radicles due to severe stenosis at junc-tion of this duct with common hepatic duct (arrow). B. Through an anterior epigastric approach, internal stent has been placed across obstruction in left hepatic duct. T-tube is in place across right hepatic duct.

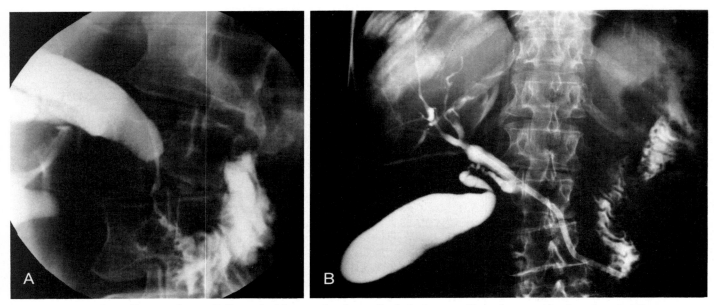

Fig. 27–88 A. Periampullary carcinoma. B. Long, double-curved endoprosthesis for transpapillary placement has been inserted. Lower curve fits into ampulla. Stent is made of soft polyurethane to avoid injuries to duodenum.

made of C-Flex are better suited for transpapillary placement (Fig. 27–88).

Primary vs. Secondary Placement of Endoprostheses

Most authors recommend insertion of endoprostheses after a short period of catheter drainage, when a tract has formed around the drainage catheter. However, this approach necessitates a hospital stay of 1–2 weeks. In the authors' series, 25 of 50 endoprostheses were placed in a one-step procedure, reducing the hospital stay to 2 or 3 days. The one-step procedure was chosen when the patient's bile was clear and free of blood after the dilation and when a dilator could easily be advanced through the stenosis. There was no significant difference between primary and secondary placment with respect to complications and dysfunction rate. However, there probably is a statistical bias in that patients with clear bile and an easily manageable stenosis might have done significantly better than other patients if both groups had been managed by the same procedure.

CONCLUSIONS

The aim of palliative PTBD is fast, efficient relief of obstructive jaundice and its symptoms with a minimum of inconvenience to the patient. Internal biliary drainage with a large-bore endoprosthesis has several advantages over internal and, especially, external catheter drainage. For example, the patient is not disturbed by the presence of an indwelling catheter, a constant reminder of the disease. Also, care of the catheter and problems with local infection are avoided. Drainage is more efficient, resulting in earlier disappearance of jaundice. Finally, the risk of cholangitis is significantly lower with drainage by a large-bore endoprosthesis than with an 8F catheter. The slightly higher rate of drainage dysfunction with endoprostheses and the attendant difficulties remain serious problems, however.

PATIENT FOLLOW-UP

All patients should be evaluated periodically. For follow-up purposes, the authors consider two groups. Patients with external or internal–external drainage catheters should be evaluated every 3 months if asymptomatic or any time there is evidence of decreased bile output, an increase in serum bilirubin or liver enzymes, leakage of bile along the tract, or bleeding. As a rule, the catheter should be replaced any time the patient is evaluated for one of these reasons. Therefore, if the patient's life expectancy is short, placement of an internal stent is recommended.

Patients with internal stents should be evaluated at the first sign of stent malfunction as manifested by jaundice, abdominal pain, bilirubin elevation, or sepsis. Evaluation can be done noninvasively by hepatobiliary nuclear scans (Fig. 27–89), which may confirm the suspicion of stent blockage, or, more invasively but more directly, by PTC, from which one can gain important anatomic information that is usually not clear from a nuclear scan. It will be clear if the stent has migrated, either distally, in which case it has to be replaced endoscopically, or proximally, in which case it must be replaced through a new percutaneous tract. It will also be clear if the stent is properly placed but is blocked. In this case, it must be replaced endoscopically or percutaneously.

In some cases, the stent is patent and the reason for the bilirubin elevation is a deterioration of liver function. These cases are probably diagnosed equally well by PTC or nuclear imaging. Nothing further needs to be done.

COMPLICATIONS

Complications can be divided into acute and delayed. The former occur in 5%–10% of patients. The most common are hemobilia and sepsis.[41–45,60,88,134,135] Less common complications are pneumothorax, bilithorax, pancreatitis, abdominal hemorrhage, and death. An unusual periprocedural hypotension secondary to high-volume biliary drainage can occur.[132]

Acute Complications

Death immediately after the procedure is usually the result of serious intra-abdominal or intrahepatic hemorrhage or sepsis. Serious intra-abdominal hemorrhage may follow repeated liver punctures with an 18-gauge needle. Death can also occur later as a result of complications such as sepsis, biliary–pleural fistulae, peritonitis, or hypersecretion of bile. The death rate following PTBD ranges from 0.5%–5.6%.[60,129,134]

Hemobilia after percutaneous transhepatic biliary drainage is not uncommon, the incidence ranging from 3.7%–13.8%.[136] It is usually transient and inconsequential but can be severe enough to be fatal. Hemobilia is often secondary to improper sidehole placement in the liver parenchyma. This is confirmed by the fluoroscopic observation of vascular opacification during contrast medium instillation through the catheter. This complication also may be due to inadvertent catheter dislocation by the patient or nursing staff. Repositioning of the catheter so that the sideholes are within the bile ducts corrects the problem.

Severe hemobilia secondary to injury of major venous or arterial branches may be associated with pseudoaneurysm formation, arterioportal or arteriohepatovenous shunting or fistulae, or vascular stenosis. The exact causal relation is unclear, inasmuch as these vascular abnormalities have been found in 19.1% of patients who have undergone percutaneous biliary drainage.[136] In most cases of hemobilia, arteriographic abnormalities are observed (see section on hemobilia). Surgical treatment of bleeding secondary to pseudoaneurysms and fistulae is difficult because of their location deep within the liver and the frequently associated tumor mass in the liver or porta hepatis. Thus, bleeding is usually treated either by placing a new catheter in a different position and removing the old one or by replacing the existing catheter with a larger one to tamponade the tract. Ideally, a self-retaining catheter is placed to avoid accidental dislodgment and subsequent severe bleeding. If the bleeding stops, the catheter should stay in the tract for 2–4 weeks before any further manipulations are attempted.

The management of severe bleeding not responsive to conservative measures usually involves selective arteriography to demonstrate the vascular abnormality followed by selective embolization. In one unusual case, the bleeding from a pseudoaneurysm was controlled by embolization through the transhepatic tract because it was impossible to achieve a selective arterial catheterization. In this case, the pseudoaneurysm was embolized with a steel coil and Gelfoam.

Bleeding that results from a communication between the portal vein and a bile duct is exceptionally difficult to manage.[36]

Acute septic shock, evidenced by both hypotension and positive blood cultures during or shortly after percutaneous biliary drainage, is uncommon, occurring in 3%–5% of patients.[60] Sepsis may occur in spite of aggressive antibiotic use before, during, and after the percutaneous procedure and probably is related to the inability of parenteral antibiotics to reach the obstructed biliary system in a concentration sufficient to combat the microorganisms before they are released into the circulation by the procedure.[93,96] To prevent this complication, catheter manipulation should be kept to a minimum in the initial procedure, especially in patients with known cholangitis.

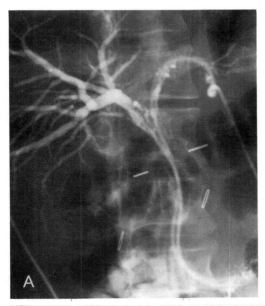

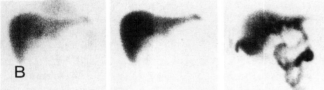

Fig. 27–89   A. Two drainage catheters have been placed, one from a right and one from a left anterior biliary radicle in a patient with a tumor at the level of the porta hepatis. B. In the same patient hepatobiliary scintigraphy shows delayed but adequate excretion of radionuclide through the stent.

In the first stage, drainage is established with an external catheter; and in a second stage, when the patient is hemodynamically stable, the catheter is converted to internal drainage. A milder form of sepsis, manifested as postprocedural fever and seen in 10.5% of cases,[60] can be controlled easily with antibiotics and intravenous fluids.

Pancreatitis is a rare postprocedural complication and may be related to catheter occlusion of the pancreatic duct.[137] It is prevented by placing the catheter tip proximal to the papilla. This placement also helps prevent cholangitis, because reflux of intestinal contents through the drainage catheter is avoided.

Pneumothorax, hemothorax, and bilithorax are infrequent complications that are encountered when a catheter crosses the pleural space, especially if the catheter inadvertently moves, so that one or more sideholes are within the pleural space. Movement of the catheter can cause bleeding from vessels that have been injured at the time of catheter placement. Retrograde propagation of blood or bile either around or through the catheter will result in bilithorax or hemothorax.[138] This complication can be prevented by choosing a puncture site in the midaxillary line several centimeters below the costophrenic sulcus. This choice often necessitates an oblique puncture of the bile ducts. The complication can be treated by replacing the external catheter with either an interior catheter or a biliary endoprosthesis and plugging the tract with compressed Gelfoam.

Hypotension secondary to high-volume biliary excretion is an infrequent complication that can cause fluid and electrolyte imbalance, especially hyponatremia. This complication is usually seen within the first few days after PTBD.[129,132] Bile secretion is usually 250–1000 ml/day. The exact pathophysiology of large-volume secretion is not known. It is not related to sepsis. Prompt recognition and treatment with intensive fluid and electrolyte replacement are essential.

Delayed Complications

The more common delayed complications include cholangitis, bile leakage, dislodgment of the catheter, and infection at the catheter site.[45,60,87,134,135] They occur in 40%–50% of patients and usually are mechanical problems related to catheter malfunction. The patient should be taught to recognize these complications and to report them immediately to the interventional radiologist for prompt correction. Less common delayed complications include peritoneal seeding of carcinoma[129] and growth of tumor along the transhepatic catheter.[58]

Cholangitis is a frequent complication and can cause significant morbidity. The reported incidence ranges from 14%[45,137] to 25%[42] in the early period, and, according to some authors, it occurs in every patient with drainage for 4 months or longer.[129] Various factors contribute to its development:

1. Trauma to the epithelium of the biliary tree at the time of catheter insertion and manipulation, making the traumatized tissues susceptible to bacterial contamination[22,139,140];
2. Poor decompression of the biliary ducts by smaller caliber stents or by improper placement of sideholes;

3. In catheters that end in the duodenum, occasional high intraduodenal pressures can cause reflux of duodenal contents, which can result in cholangitis either by clogging the catheter, with subsequent stasis, or by contaminating the biliary tree with intestinal flora.

The combination of denuded epithelium, duodenal reflux, and partial obstruction is probably present in most cases of delayed cholangitis. An incidence of cholangitis as high as 63% has been reported after tube clamping for conversion from external to internal drainage.[60] The postclamping cholangitis is simply corrected by unclamping the catheter or by exchanging it for a 10F or 12F catheter, whose tip is kept within the distal common bile duct if possible to avoid reflex of duodenal contents.

In patients with multiple duct obstructions, even though adequate partial drainage is established, cholangitis can develop in the nondrained liver segments.[60] In these cases, separate drainage of other ducts may be necessary to prevent or treat cholangitis. Another alternative is to place an internal stent at the first sitting that drains the largest possible amount of the liver.

Catheter migration and dislodgment can occur with normal breathing excursions, particularly with intercostal placements. Patients with ascites can also suffer this complication because of the unsupported segment of catheter between the liver capsule and the abdominal wall. As the liver moves with breathing, the catheter, well lubricated by ascites and bile, is pulled into the space. The displaced catheter is usually found kinked between the abdominal wall and the liver.

Migration can occur with purely external as well as with internal–external catheters if they are not secured to the skin properly with sutures or Molnar discs. External catheters, which have a shorter purchase within the biliary ducts, can be dislodged by breathing movements. This type of dislodgment can usually be prevented by advancing the catheter tip into a peripheral duct in the opposite lobe if a long segment of the common duct is not available. The longer length of catheter in the ducts both helps prevent catheter motion and gives some extra security if motion does occur.

Bile can leak around the catheter if the tract is larger than the catheter, and the tract commonly enlarges by retraction when the catheter has been in place for a long time. The problem can be corrected by replacing the catheter with one 2F larger.

Bile leakage due to an improper position of the sideholes outside the biliary tract or below the stenosis is a common problem and is corrected simply by advancing or replacing the catheter. Leakage can also be secondary to partial or complete catheter blockage by blood clots, viscous bile sludge, or duodenal contents, especially mucus. The blood clots usually lyse spontaneously or can be dislodged by saline irrigation. The viscous bile can also be dissolved by repeated irrigation with saline. Inspissated duodenal mucus frequently can be cleared by repeated injections of a mucolytic agent such as acetylcysteine.

Irrigation of the catheter with saline to maintain patency is controversial. Some authors routinely do it in the hope of retarding encrustation of biliary salts and cellular debris,[41] whereas fear of introducing infection prevents others from irrigating catheters. The latter group claims to have no higher incidence of complications.[135]

To avoid occlusion, routine catheter exchange every 3 months is recommended.[45,72] Partially obstructed catheters are usually replaced, even though drainage can be improved by reopening the lumen.[141]

Metastatic seeding of the peritoneal serosa with cholangiocarcinoma has been reported a few months after insertion of a drainage catheter. The presumed mechanism is escape of malignant cells from the catheter tract into the peritoneal cavity at the time of catheter exchange or removal.[129]

Pain after PTBD can have any of several causes. It can be due to periosteal irritation if the catheter is placed too close to a rib. Correction may require catheter relocation, although this pain usually subsides spontaneously. Pain from intercostal nerve irritation can usually be managed by local nerve block. Deeper pain associated with either right-sided or anterior catheters can be the result of fluid and blood collections around the liver or under the liver capsule. Subcapsular collections, which cause pain by distention, can require narcotics for adequate relief but fortunately usually subside within 4 or 5 days. Bile leak may result in bile peritonitis, with diffuse abdominal pain.

Skin infections, occasionally leading to abscess formation, are common with long-term external drainage. Local infections are managed by local care and antibiotics. Granulomas are managed by cauterization with silver nitrate.[36]

BILIARY STRICTURES

Most bile duct strictures are secondary to surgical trauma,[142,143] either operations on the duct itself or those performed nearby. Other types, classified by cause, are:

Malignant:
  a. Primary cancer of the bile ducts;
  b. Metastatic involvement.
Benign:
  a. Radiation fibrosis;
  b. Congenital;
  c. Infection;
  d. Sclerosing cholangitis.

Traditionally, patients with strictures of the biliary tract have been managed by operation, either by a primary repair with an end-to-end anastomosis or by creation of a biliary–enteric anastomosis. Surgical repair of biliary strictures is successful in 65%–80% of patients.[142–144]

An alternative to operation is balloon dilatation via either a transhepatic or a transendoscopic route. Recent reports from several institutions indicate that percutaneous dilation of appropriate types of benign strictures generally yields good short-term results. This kind of therapy is offered to patients in the following circumstances:

1. High surgical risk secondary to medical problems;
2. Strictures not amenable to corrective operation;
3. Previous attempt at surgical repair, which makes the second procedure extremely difficult;
4. Advanced liver disease.

Unfortunately, most published reports of this technique offer only single cases or short-term follow-up; long-term results are not available, nor are the long-term effects of balloon trauma on the biliary tree known. Important aspects of the technique, such as balloon size, inflation pressure, and the frequency and duration of inflations have not been worked out. Long-term stenting with 12F–18F catheters is highly recommended by some authors as a way to prevent recurrence, but the value is disputed by others, especially in cases of fresh postoperative strictures.[92,144]

A new technique—transhepatic electrocautery of stenotic biliary–enteric anastomoses—also has been described.[145] Even if this technique proves valuable, however, it is likely, considering the difficulty and limitations of surgical repair, that a definite place will remain for percutaneous ductal dilatation (PDD).

PREPARATION AND MONITORING OF THE PATIENT

Laboratory Studies

Candidates for PDD usually have been evaluated by the referring physician with a thorough history, a physical examination, and a medical work-up. The following laboratory examinations are the minimum needed:

Coagulation profile (prothrombin, partial thromboplastin, and thromboplastin times);
Serum bilirubin; and
Complete blood count, including platelets.

Radiologic Evaluation

THC or ERCP is used to study the anatomy of the biliary tree and any associated abnormalities, such as strictures, stones, abscesses, or biliary–enteric anastomoses. The exact location, number, and length of all strictures should be determined. Balloon size is selected on the basis of these studies.

Preoperative Preparations

An adequate intravenous line is started for administering fluids, sedatives, and analgesics. A broad-spectrum combination of antibiotics (e.g., gentamycin–ampicillin) is started 6–8 hr before and continued after the procedure until the patient leaves the hospital. Preoperative medication is usually given, the amount and type depending on operator preference and patient needs.

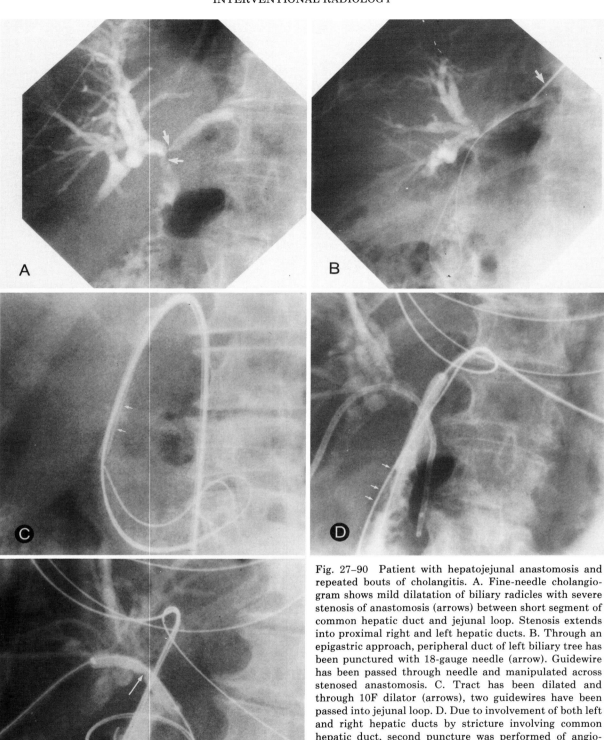

Fig. 27–90 Patient with hepatojejunal anastomosis and repeated bouts of cholangitis. A. Fine-needle cholangiogram shows mild dilatation of biliary radicles with severe stenosis of anastomosis (arrows) between short segment of common hepatic duct and jejunal loop. Stenosis extends into proximal right and left hepatic ducts. B. Through an epigastric approach, peripheral duct of left biliary tree has been punctured with 18-gauge needle (arrow). Guidewire has been passed through needle and manipulated across stenosed anastomosis. C. Tract has been dilated and through 10F dilator (arrows), two guidewires have been passed into jejunal loop. D. Due to involvement of both left and right hepatic ducts by stricture involving common hepatic duct, second puncture was performed of angiographic catheter through right biliary radicles into jejunal loop. Balloon angioplasty catheter of 6 mm diameter was passed and inflated across stricture in left hepatic and common hepatic ducts. Observe presence of safety guidewire along side (arrows). E. Balloon has been removed from left biliary tree and has now been passed through right biliary tree to dilate stricture in right hepatic duct. Note "waist" in balloon at site of stricture (arrow).

Intraoperative Care

Vital signs are closely monitored by a nurse or anesthetist. Analgesics are given intravenously by the circulating nurse or nurse anesthetist as needed and according to the cardiorespiratory status. Inhalation analgesia or general anesthesia has been used in certain cases.

TECHNIQUE

Two principal steps are involved in the dilatation of strictures: the dilatation itself and long-term stenting.

Dilatation can be performed with either semirigid or balloon dilators.[36,89-92] Because balloon dilators are easier to pass, they are preferred, and most strictures respond favorably. There are, however, a few that will require the passage of semirigid dilators.

There are many ideas about the best approach for dilation, including a single inflation without stenting, a single inflation with short-term stenting, repeated short inflations with long-term stenting, and single or repeated long inflations with long-term stenting. Which, if any, of these will prove to be best for any particular type of stenosis remains to be seen.

Just as with the drainage procedures, PDD begins with PTC, performed by a right lateral approach (Fig. 27-90A). After definitive puncture, the stricture is traversed, and the guidewire is advanced into the duodenum (Fig. 27-90B). The tract is dilated to 10F to allow the passage of a safety wire introducer, and a second wire is introduced to the duodenum (Fig. 27-90C). A 6-10-mm-diameter, 4-cm-long, high-pressure balloon catheter is passed over the working wire into the stricture, and the balloon is inflated with an inflation device (Fig. 27-90D). A simple inflation device is recommended when long balloon inflation is to be used, because adjustments have to be made by the nurses during the 10-12 hr that the balloon remains inflated.[146,147] A pressure of 4-6 atm is sufficient to dilate most strictures but fibrotic strictures require much higher pressures, which is the reason a high-pressure balloon is used. At the beginning of inflation, a "waist" is seen in the balloon at the site of the stricture (Fig. 27-90E), but it disappears as the pressure is raised.

If a short inflation is to be used, the balloon is deflated after 10-15 min and exchanged for an 8F-10F drainage catheter with sideholes proximal and distal to the dilated area. The safety wire is removed. If a long inflation is planned, the balloon is left inflated to 4-6 atm at the site of the stricture, and a drainage catheter is passed over the safety wire into the proximal biliary tree for external drainage of bile. As an alternative, a special catheter with sideholes proximal to the balloon can be used for simultaneous dilation and drainage (Fig. 27-91).

Generally, the authors leave the balloon inflated for 1 hr followed by 1 hr of deflation in sequence for 12 hr.[92] When the sequence is completed, the balloon catheter is exchanged for a 10F stent, which is left draining internally for 1-2 months, at which time the status of the dilatation site is re-evaluated. If needed, dilatation can be repeated, followed again by long-term stenting.

In some patients, the stricture is so hard that it cannot be stretched by a balloon. The Teflon coaxial dilators and the new flexible ureteral dilators (Cook Urological), which are tapered to the size of a 0.038-inch guidewire, have proved useful in these situations.

Percutaneous transhepatic internal biliary drainage is indicated after dilation of biliary strictures. Such drainage helps prevent recurrent cholangitis, bile stasis leading to formation of intrahepatic ductal stones, and biliary cirrhosis.

DISCUSSION

Primary surgical repair of biliary stricture is the traditional choice for most patients, with a success rate of 65%-80%.[142,148,149] Balloon or other forms of dilation have until recently been offered only as an alternative to surgical repair, albeit with encouraging results, particularly for dilation of choledocoenteroanastomoses.[89] Now the percutaneous procedure is used more often. Strictures following choledococholedocoanastomoses and choledochojejunoanastomoses in liver transplantation also have been dilated successfully (Fig. 27-92). In infants with liver allografts, obstruction is commonly due, not to the anastomosis narrowing, but to obstruction of the cystic duct by inspissated bile (Fig. 27-93). The management commonly involves long-term percutaneous drainage while one waits for sufficient growth of the bile ducts to permit a choledocoenteroanastomosis. In patients with sclerosing cholangitis, percutaneous dilation of strictures and long-term stenting have been extremely successful (Fig. 27-94).

In the authors' experience, multiple long inflations appear to help prevent stricture reformation, although because of the small number of cases, this cannot yet be proved.[92]

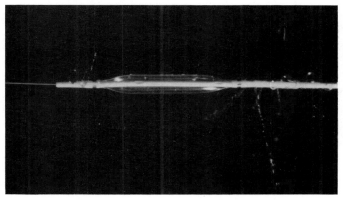

Fig. 27-91 Angioplasty balloon catheter with sideholes proximal and distal to balloon for cholangioplasty or ureteroplasty to allow decompression during long-term inflations.

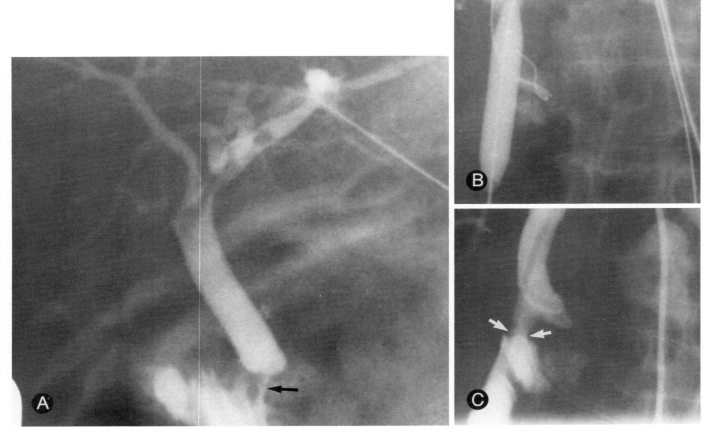

Fig. 27–92   Fever and jaundice 3 months after liver transplantation. Repeated cholangitis suspected. A. Fine-needle cholangiography reveals mild dilatation of intrahepatic radicles and severe stenosis of choledochojejunal anastomosis (arrow), although contrast medium is seen to pass into jejunal loop. B. Through left anterior epigastric approach, stenosed anastomosis has been selectively catheterized, and 10-mm angioplasty balloon catheter has been passed and inflated at site of stricture. C. Cholangiogram 2 months after dilatation prior to stent removal reveals wide open anastomosis (arrows).

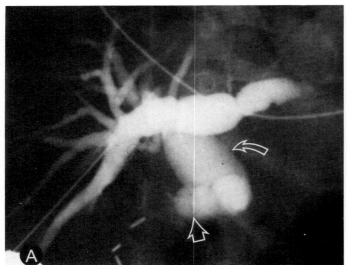

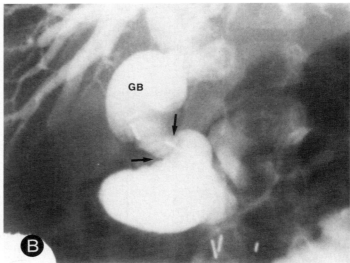

Fig. 27–93   Four-year-old patient with liver allograft with obstruction of cholecystojejunostomy in early postoperative period. A. Fine-needle cholangiogram shows dilatation of intrahepatic radicles, common hepatic duct (curved open arrow), and cystic duct (short open arrow). B. After placement of 5F biliary drainage catheter with tip in common bile duct, contrast medium is seen filling gallbladder (GB), and anastomosis between gallbladder and jejunum is seen to be widely patent (arrows).

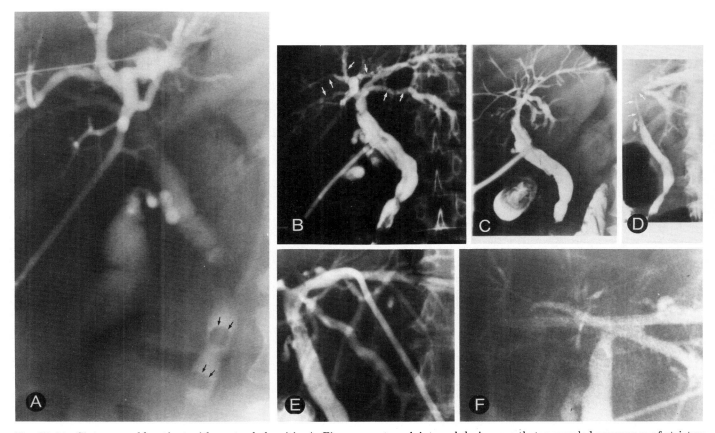

Fig. 27–94 Sixty-year-old patient with acute cholangitis. A. Fine-needle cholangiography shows moderate dilatation of intrahepatic radicles and common hepatic and common bile ducts as well as presence of two large stones within distal common bile duct (arrows). B. After cholecystectomy and surgical exploration of common bile duct, T-tube was left in place. T-tube cholangiography 2 weeks later shows marked shrinkage and irregularity of right biliary radicles and mild irregularities of left biliary radicles. Debris is seen within common bile duct. C. T-tube cholangiography 4 weeks after exploration shows marked progression of secondary sclerosing cholangitis, particularly involving right biliary tree and to a lesser extent left biliary radicles. D. After 2 years with recurrent bouts of cholangitis, the patient was admitted with severe sepsis. Fine-needle cholangiogram reveals severe obstruction of left hepatic and common hepatic ducts (arrows). Note absence of opacification of right biliary tree. E. Through an epigastric approach, left biliary tree was catheterized, and areas of stenosis in left hepatic and common hepatic ducts were dilated by inflation of 8-mm angioplasty catheter at site of stricture for 15 min. F. Only a few markedly stenosed biliary radicles were found in the right biliary tree. G. Follow-up cholangiogram through external–internal drainage catheter revealed recurrence of stricture at level of left hepatic and common hepatic ducts. Long-term dilatation was performed with 8-mm balloon catheter. Follow-up cholangiogram immediately after redilatation. A 16F internal–external stent was left in place for 6 months and then replaced with a 6F internal–external catheter, which was left for another 6 months for continuous access. H. Cholangiogram through 6F biliary drainage catheter reveals adequate lumen of common hepatic and left hepatic ducts 18 months after dilatation. I. Fine-needle cholangiogram shows severe stenosis (arrows) of anastomosis between common hepatic duct and jejunum. Observe dilatation of intrahepatic radicles and numerous filling defects representing stones retained within bile ducts. J. After successful dilatation of anastomosis, several catheters have been placed for flushing and removal of stones and debris from biliary radicles. K. Cholangiogram after several sessions reveals no evidence of filling defects within biliary radicles and wide open anastomosis (arrows). (C, D, and I reproduced from Salomonowitz E, Castañeda WR, Lund G, et al: Balloon dilatation of benign biliary strictures. *AJR* 1984;151:613 with the permission of the Radiological Society of North America, Inc.)

Percutaneous Intracanalicular Radiation Therapy

A percutaneous or T-tube tract can be used for the placement of iridium seeds for intracanalicular irradiation in patients with primary tumors of the bile ducts (Fig. 27–95A,B) with successful results and less secondary effects than extensive external radiation of the liver.

PERCUTANEOUS EXTRACTION OF RETAINED BILIARY STONES

In the United States, more than 500,000 operations are performed on the extrahepatic biliary system for stone removal each year.[150,151] The incidence of retained calculi ranges from 1.4%[152] to 8%,[152] being especially high after cholecystectomy, which, by itself, produces approximately 5,000 patients yearly with retained or recurrent

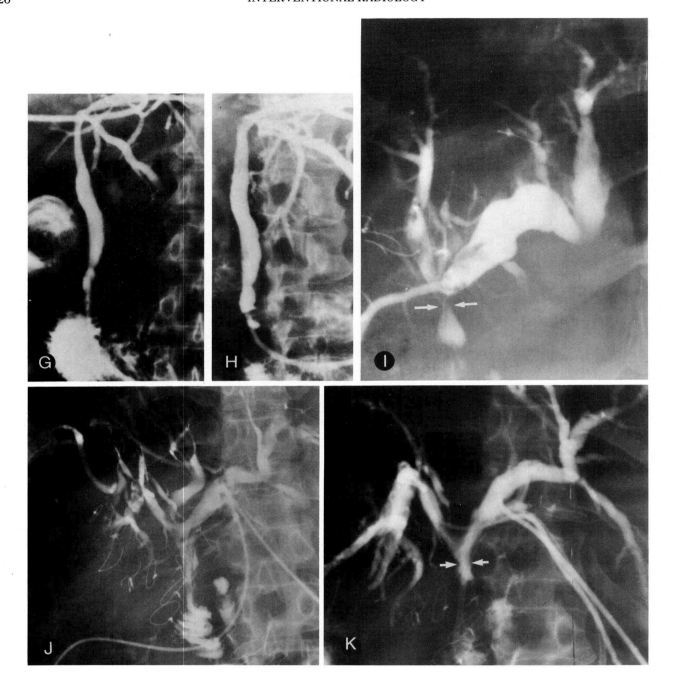

biliary calculi.[153] The routine use of intraoperative cholangiography has decreased the incidence of retained common duct stones but has not eliminated the problem. Re-
exploration for retained common duct stones is associated with increased morbidity and mortality, so a nonoperative means to remove stones is highly desirable. A
number of techniques were developed for attempting to
clear retained calculi by irrigation of the bile ducts with
saline, heparin sodium, cholic acids, and medium chain
glycerides, such as mono-octanoin. However, mechanical
methods of removing biliary stones through the T-tube
tract have proved both effective and less time consuming
than irrigation and have strikingly reduced the need for

reoperation.[153–157] The most popular technique involves
the steerable catheter developed by Burhenne and a Dormia basket; in experienced hands it has a success rate of
95%.[154] At present, a second operation for choledocholithiasis should be undertaken only if percutaneous extraction fails.

The following stone removal methods will be discussed:

1. Mechanical extraction through the T-tube tract or a
   choledochocutaneous fistula using:
   a. Burhenne catheter and Dormia basket;
   b. Mazzariello forceps;
   c. Choledochoscope and graspers;

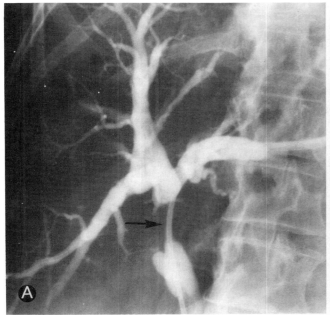

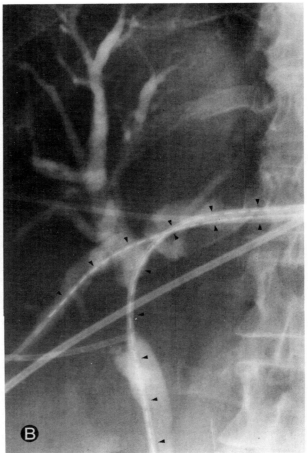

Fig. 27–95 Initial drainage catheter traverses cholangiocarcinoma obstructing common hepatic duct (arrow) and provides internal drainage. B. Two catheters were introduced via same anterior tract; one passes into right ducts, the other into common bile duct. Radiopaque markers (arrows) indicate where iridium seeds are to be placed. (Reproduced from Young AT, Cardella JF, Castañeda–Zuñiga WR, Hunter DW, Amplatz K: The anterior approach to left biliary catheterization. *Semin Intervent Radiol* 1985;2:31–38 with the permission of Thieme, Inc.)

d. Choledochoscope and an ultrasonic or electrohydraulic lithotripter.
2. Mechanical extraction via a percutaneous transhepatic approach using any of the above instruments.

3. Mechanical extraction after endoscopic papillotomy using baskets or irrigation.
4. Chemical dissolution by infusion of mono-octanoin.

MECHANICAL EXTRACTION THROUGH T-TUBE TRACT OR CHOLEDOCHOCUTANEOUS FISTULA

The mechanical extraction of retained biliary calculi with specially designed forceps by Mondet in 1962 has led to the development of other, safer techniques.[158] Mazzariello reported a 95.3% success rate using rigid forceps,[155,159] and Burhenne reported a 95% success rate using a steerable catheter and Dormia baskets under fluoroscopic guidance.[154]

Extraction of retained biliary calculi should not be attempted earlier than 4–8 weeks after the initial operation. This waiting period leads to a greater degree of fibrosis of the T-tube tract.[154,155] In the past, the waiting period was even longer in obese patients and in cases where T-tubes smaller than 14F were used because sinus tract formation in both types of patients is slower and less effective. However, at present, the use of balloon dilators and working sheaths allows safe early intervention even in these patients.

Stone removal through the T-tube tract has these component steps:

Radiologic study;
Choice of approach;
Tract anesthesia;
Tract dilatation;
Calculi extraction; and
Biliary drainage tube placement.

Radiologic Study

A T-tube cholangiogram is performed to opacify the biliary tree and establish the location and number of stones (Fig. 27–96A), because retained stones can pass spontaneously through the papilla, especially after surgical papillotomy. During the procedure, 20%–30% con-

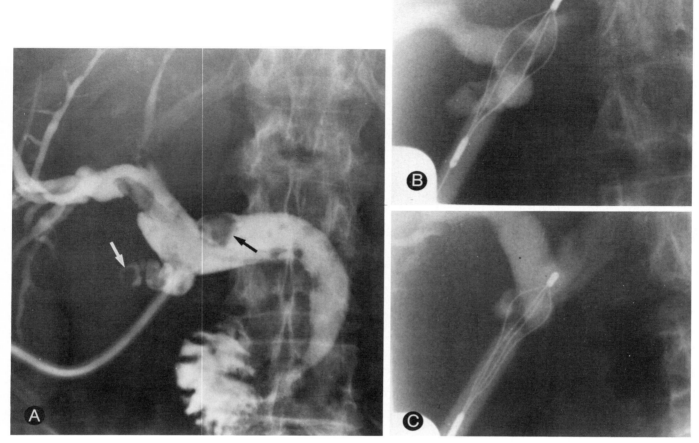

Fig. 27–96 A. T-tube cholangiogram shows retained stones (black arrow) after surgical exploration. Observe also the smaller stone within stump of cystic duct (white arrow). B. After placement of Teflon sheath through T-tube tract, large basket was inserted to entrap retained stone in common bile duct. C. Due to size of stone, traction on basket produces marked kinking of common bile duct. (A and B reproduced from Tadavarthy SM, Castañeda–Zuñiga WR, Amplatz K: Removal of small and large biliary stones. *CardioVasc Radiol* 1981;4:93–96 with permission of Thieme, Inc.)

trast medium is injected intermittently through the side port of the steerable catheter to guide the manipulation of stones under fluoroscopy.

Choice of Approach

A T-tube tract created at the time of cholecystostomy and bile duct exploration connects at a 90° angle with the common bile duct from a point in the anterior axillary line and is as straight as possible, because this will create the shortest tract and also the best access to both the upper and the lower segments of the biliary tree. A large-bore T-tube should be left in the tract for 6–8 weeks to allow maturation of a fibrous sleeve around the shaft of the T-tube, which will be the pathway from the skin to the biliary tree. The larger diameter T-tubes facilitate placement of instruments through the tract. In an analysis of 204 attempted extractions, 16 failures were attributable to technical difficulties resulting either from

smaller T-tubes or longer, tortuous tracts.[155,156] Moss et al recommend using the newly designed T-tubes with a stem 4F larger than the transverse limbs.[157]

Once the tract and biliary tree have been opacified with 20%–30% contrast medium injected through the T-tube, some authors pull out the T-tube without passing a guidewire. They then have to catheterize the tract by gently manipulating a steerable catheter and wire into the bile ducts. The present authors prefer to pass a guidewire through the T-tube and advance it through one of the limbs into the bile ducts. The T-tube is then pulled back over the guidewire, which remains within the common bile duct for further manipulations.

Generally, the T-tube can be removed easily by gently pulling it out. In some patients, however, the passage of the two limbs through the choledocotomy can be arduous, either because fibrous stenosis has narrowed the opening or because the combined size of the two limbs is too large for the opening. In these cases, one should carefully

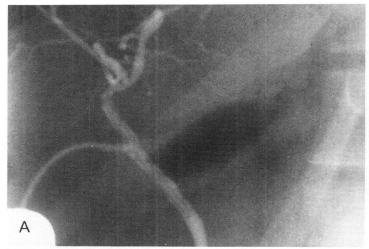

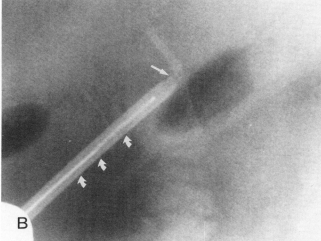

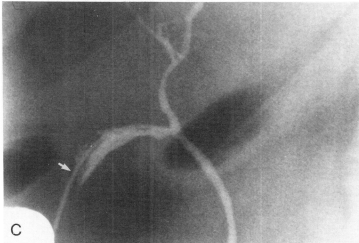

Fig. 27–97 T-tube left in place for 120 days after surgical exploration and reconstruction of common bile duct. Attempts to remove the T-tube with usual technique were unsuccessful. T-tube cholangiogram reveals decompressed biliary tree with free flow of contrast medium into distal common bile duct. B. Teflon sheath (curved arrows) has been advanced over T-tube shaft until blunt end of Teflon sleeve has reached junction of arms (straight arrow). C. With the Teflon sheath held in place, T-tube was pulled into the sheath. After removal of T-tube, 6F catheter (arrow) with multiple sideholes was placed with its tip in distal common bile duct for temporary decompression.

observe under fluoroscopy the degree of tenting of the common bile duct while pulling on the T-tube. If the tenting seems to be severe or the traction causes pain, a Teflon sheath is passed over the T-tube until it reaches the common bile duct. While the dilator is held against the common bile duct, the T-tube is pulled forcefully into the Teflon sheath (Fig. 27–97).

The authors routinely introduce a second, or safety, wire through the steerable catheter or through a safety wire introducer passed over the first wire. In difficult and complex cases, one guidewire may be inadvertently withdrawn; the presence of a safety wire assures access to the common duct. The safety wire should be "parked" away from the stone, either in an intrahepatic radicle or in the duodenum; a steerable catheter or an angiographic or multipurpose catheter can be used to manipulate the safety wire to such a site. A 5F polyethylene catheter is passed over the safety wire before being sutured to the skin to prevent slippage of the wire through the suture. Over the other, working, wire, the steerable catheter or dilators can then be introduced to dilate the tract and remove the stone.

Tract Anesthesia

The tract is anesthetized with 1% lidocaine using a 10-cm-long, 22-gauge Chiba needle. In difficult cases, a longer acting anesthetic, such as small amounts of 0.25% bupivacaine (Marcaine) can be used. Large amounts of local anesthetic should be avoided, because they may distort the tract.

Tract Dilatation

In the authors' institution, the tract is dilated either with coaxial dilators or with a balloon catheter if larger stones must be extracted intact. Historically, Mazzariello used flexible plastic sounds to dilate the T-tube tract.[155,159] Also, tracts often were dilated either by using telescoping Teflon catheters up to 14F[82] or by using modified T-tubes, and dilatation was accomplished over several days to weeks. With the coaxial or balloon method, dilation of the tract to 30F takes only a few minutes.

Tract dilatation should be performed if the T-tube was smaller than 14F or if the stone is larger than the tract.

In most cases, however, it probably is preferable to attempt to fragment the stone rather than to dilate the tract.

The types of instruments used to dilate the T-tube tract are identical to those used for percutaneous renal work. Balloons with diameters of 8 or 10 mm and 10–15 cm long can be used to dilate the tract to 24F or 30F, respectively. All of the coaxial dilators start with a long 8F Teflon dilator, which is passed over the guidewire into the common bile duct and over which successively larger dilators are passed until the desired French size is reached. The 24F, 26F, 28F, and 30F Amplatz renal dilators have fitted Teflon sheaths that can be used as a conduit in the tract (Fig. 27–96B). One should be careful to keep the tip of the sheath within the common bile duct to prevent leakage of bile and contrast medium. Graduated dilators tapered to fit a 0.038-inch guidewire are passed individually in successively larger diameters until the desired French size is reached.

Calculi Extraction

The techniques for percutaneous calculi removal can be divided into two large groups, depending on the guidance method used to control the extraction: fluoroscopic or endoscopic. Fluoroscopy is, of course, used in both methods, because it is occasionally useful during endoscopy.

The fluoroscopic techniques can be divided into three large groups: flushing, pushing, and grasping. Endoscopic techniques can be divided into two groups: grasping and fragmentation.

FLUOROSCOPIC FLUSHING TECHNIQUES

These are the simplest and least traumatic of the extraction techniques and are particularly useful for removing multiple small calculi or the fragments created by crushing or electrohydraulic lithotripsy. Adherence to the following rules permits successful flushing of calculi:

1. A papillotomy should be performed before irrigation, either at the time of biliary operation or endoscopically at the time of ERCP or percutaneously by balloon dilatation just prior to the irrigation.
2. Irrigation should be performed with a power injector under fluoroscopic control.
3. If perforation of the biliary tree has occurred during dilatation maneuvers, the flushing technique should not be used.

After fragmentation of stones with a basket[155] or forceps[155,157,159,160] or with electrohydraulic lithotripsy, an 8F or 10F catheter with several sideholes is introduced through the tract and placed proximal to the stone fragments. Flushing is then performed at 10–15 ml/sec with 20%–30% contrast medium under fluoroscopic control to observe the passage of the fluid and stone fragments into the duodenum.

If a large Teflon sheath has been inserted, the flushing can be done through it. A flexible plastic tube connected to the sheath can be used for suction and irrigation, or a catheter can be placed through or alongside the sheath for irrigation.

When the stones are lodged in the distal biliary radicles, a variant of the flushing method can be used. A 5F or 6F catheter is passed beyond the stone, and diluted contrast medium is injected at a rate of 3–5 ml/sec in an attempt to dislodge the stone into a more proximal location, from which it can be extracted mechanically.

FLUOROSCOPIC PUSHING TECHNIQUE

This technique can be used for the manipulation of stones through either a transhepatic or a T-tube tract (Figs. 27–97, 27–98). A papillotomy is a prerequisite if large stones are to pass from the common bile duct through the ampulla into the duodenum. However, small (5–6-mm) stones can be pushed gently into the duodenum without a papillotomy.

If a transhepatic approach is used, the tract is dilated to 10F. Through the 10F dilator, a balloon catheter is introduced and advanced until it is in contact with the stone. The balloon is inflated with dilute contrast medium and held in position while the 10F Teflon dilator is advanced until it is pushing on the back side of the balloon. The balloon and dilator are then pushed together against the stone (Fig. 27–99). (The dilator is needed to stiffen the soft balloon.) An alternative is the use of a rubber tube with the tip cut off (Fig. 27–100)[161,162]

If severe resistance is encountered at the ampulla, one should not push the stone forcefully, because this may result in its passage into the tissues around the sphincter or even to perforation of the common duct. Even if severe resistance is not encountered, pushing a stone through the ampulla can cause severe pain and may produce a vasovagal reaction.

After balloon or cautery papillotomy, severe spasm can occur at the sphincter. This can be counteracted by injecting 1% lidocaine through the catheter into and around the calculus.

FLUOROSCOPIC AND ENDOSCOPIC GRASPING TECHNIQUES

Grasping with Baskets

The introduction of the steerable catheter by Burhenne in 1973 greatly facilitated manipulation and stone extraction with Dormia baskets.[160] The steerable catheter is controlled by four wires embedded in the wall and attached to a control handle at the catheter hub. The catheter tip can be deflected up to 90° by rotating the knob on the handle (Fig. 27–101), permitting the catheter to advance around bends in the duct and tract. The tip control is far enough from the tip that manipulations in the common duct can be done under fluoroscopic guidance without excessive radiation exposure to the operator's hands. The steerable catheters are available in 8F, 10F, and 13F sizes (Medi–Tech).

Several designs and sizes of baskets are available:

Pfister–Schwartz, with 3-, 4-, and 6-wire helicoidal patterns and a 3-cm-long floppy tip (Fig. 27–102A);

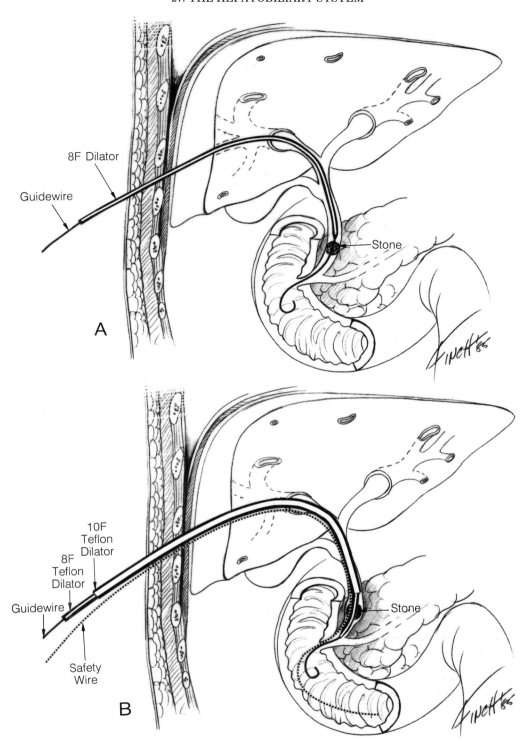

Fig. 27–98 Percutaneous transhepatic removal of retained stones in common bile duct. A. 8F dilator has been passed over guidewire. B. Tract has been dilated to 10F, and two guidewires have been placed with their tips in duodenum. Over one of the guidewires, 8F and 10F dilators have been advanced to dilate tract. C. After removal of guidewire and 8F Teflon dilator, Fogarty balloon catheter has been passed through 10F dilator and inflated behind retained stone. D. Assembled 10F dilator and Fogarty balloon catheter have been pushed forward, displacing stone across papilla. E. Stone has been passed into duodenum, and Fogarty balloon is slowly deflated. F. Teflon sheath has been placed in T-tube tract, and through it a 20F blunt-ended rubber tube has been advanced against retained stone, which is gently pushed across papilla. G. Rubber tube has pushed stone into duodenum through widely open papilla.

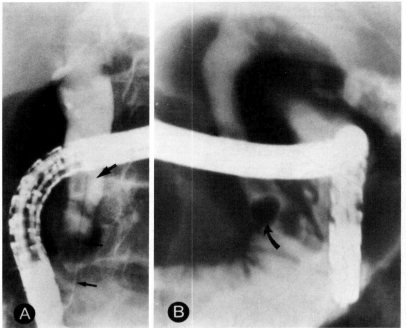

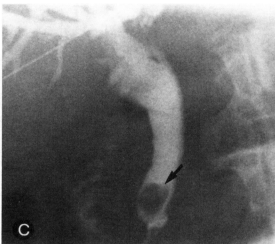

Fig. 27–99 Seventy-year-old patient with Parkinson's disease and cholangitis secondary to common bile duct stones. Attempts to remove stones endoscopically failed. A,B. Fogarty balloon used trying to remove stone (straight arrows); stone (curved arrow). C. Fine-needle cholangiography shows large calculus within distal common bile duct (arrow). D. Anterior right biliary radicle has been selected and 18-gauge needle is being advanced straight down. Note needle as a dot (arrow), indicating perpendicular down-the-barrel approach. E. Lateral view shows entrance of tip of needle into biliary radicle. F. Tract has been dilated to 10F, and two guidewires have been advanced through 10F dilator. G. Through 10F Teflon dilator, Fogarty balloon catheter (F) was passed; balloon has been inflated behind stone (arrows). H. Assembled Fogarty balloon (F) and 10F Teflon dilators are being pushed against the stone, which is being forced down through common bile duct. (Note indentation in balloon produced by the calculus (arrows).) I. Stone has been pushed into duodenum. Observe marked indentation in balloon (arrow) by stone.

the sheath. Baskets without a detachable sheath are passed through a Burhenne steerable catheter or an introducer sheath.

The technique of basketing a stone is essentially the same for all types of baskets. The basket is positioned adjacent or distal to the stone, where it is opened by withdrawing the sheath. (An open basket with a sharp tip is never advanced except within a catheter, because such a maneuver can cause significant mucosal damage or duct perforation.) The basket is rotated under fluoroscopic control first in one direction and then the other until the stone is trapped. Jiggling or back-and-forth motions with the catheter are often helpful. The stone is extracted through the working sheath or the sinus tract with a continuous, gentle pull without closing the basket. (Closing the basket will more firmly engage the stone if it is totally inside the basket but often causes the stone to slip out.) The retrieved stone is inspected. If it does not appear to be intact, the fragments are retrieved using the same technique.

The basket should be as large as the duct and the wires should touch the walls.[154] When a large stone fills the common bile duct, little space is available for complete opening of the basket. The duct dimensions may be further reduced by endothelial edema secondary to the presence of the calculus and repeated manipulations. Such space limitations are the principal reason for technical failure of the basketing technique.

Special Considerations in Fluoroscopic Basketing of Stones

Stones lodged in a cystic duct remnant. This situation creates special technical problems. Because the cystic duct is small, baskets cannot open within it, so stones usually must be dislodged with an angiographic or steerable catheter. The jet effect of contrast medium or saline injection can displace the stone into the common bile duct. Alternatively, if the cystic duct remnant is large, a Fogarty balloon catheter can be placed in the pouch, and the stone can be displaced into the common duct by withdrawing the inflated balloon under fluoroscopic guidance (Fig. 27–105).[154] Burhenne recommends doing the procedure with the patient semierect. Sometimes, the stone will then migrate spontaneously into the common duct.[154]

Impacted stones. Stones impacted in the common duct or ampulla are difficult to extract. Although baskets can be passed alongside the stone, they cannot be fully opened to entrap it. In these cases, one can simply wait, because impacted stones frequently migrate spontaneously. Alternatively, as in other cases in which space will not permit a basket to open, a 2-wire snare can be passed around the stone.

If the snare cannot engage the stone, a small Fogarty balloon can be passed through a steering catheter beyond the stone. The stone is pulled back by the inflated balloon

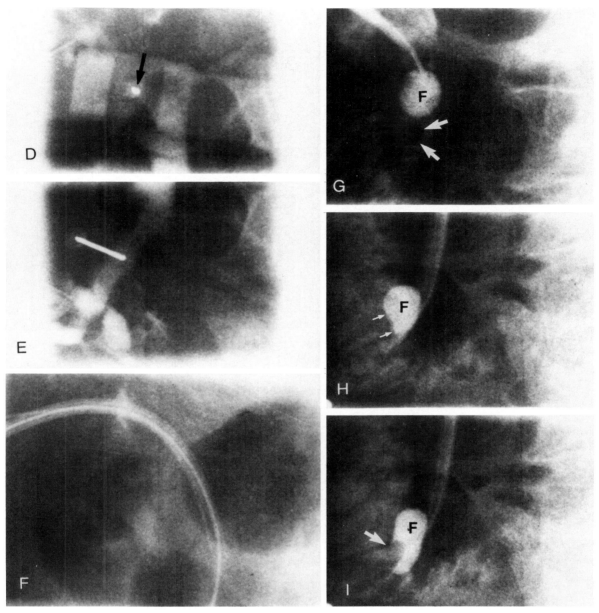

Fig. 27–99D–I

under fluoroscopic guidance. This maneuver is not always successful, because the balloon may deform and simply slide past the stone. Also, Van Way and Sawyers reported trauma to the intrahepatic biliary ducts when Fogarty balloons were used to withdraw stones intraoperatively.[163] Careful fluoroscopic manipulation is advised to avoid such damage.

Large stones. Most large stones are soft and can easily be fragmented by baskets or crushed with the Mazzariello forceps.[155] Large stones trapped in baskets are fragmented by the front end of the guiding catheter as well as by the cutting action of the basket wires. Burhenne recommends fragmenting the stone at the junction of the common duct and the sinus tract by applying steady traction on the basket.[154] If a working sheath is not used, the stone fragments in the sinus tract are removed with a basket or Fogarty balloon or by pushing them into the common duct with the steerable catheter.

In the authors' institution, 28F or 30F working sheaths are routinely placed in the T-tube tract after dilatation. Larger (1.0–1.5-cm) stones can then be withdrawn through the dilated tract without fragmentation or tearing the tract.[164]

Grasping with Flexible Forceps

Two types of flexible forceps are used for calculus removal under fluoroscopic control: 3- and 4-prong forceps (Vantech; Cook Urological) and 5F or 7F alligator forceps (Figs. 27–102D,E). The 3- and 4-prong forceps have limited use because of the small pulling force they can exert and because of the tendency of the prongs to

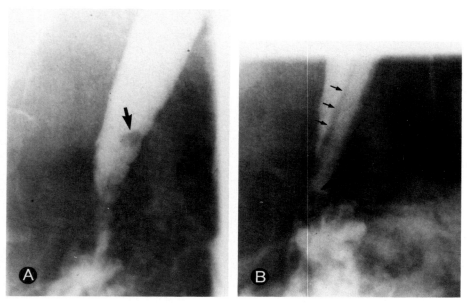

Fig. 27–100   Small stone within distal common bile duct (arrow) in patient at high surgical risk. B. Stone (large arrow) has been pushed through papilla with help of blunt-ended 20-gauge rubber tube (small arrows).

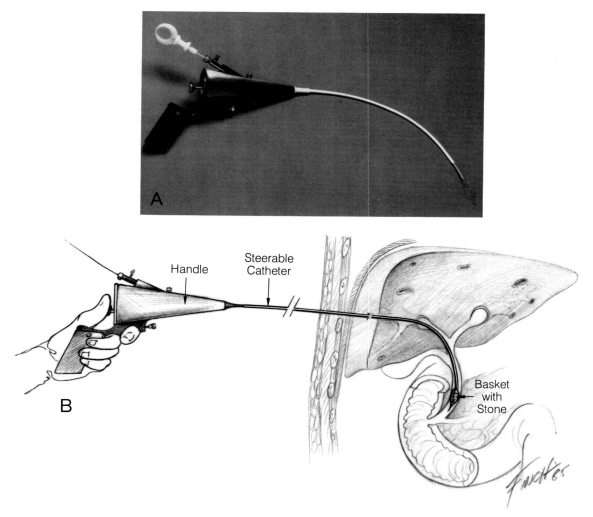

Fig. 27–101   Steerable handle with steerable catheter used for manipulation of stones in biliary tree. Through sideport, a Dormia basket has been passed. B. Use of Burhenne handle for manipulation of stone in common bile duct through percutaneous transhepatic tract. Basket has trapped stone, which will be passed into duodenum.

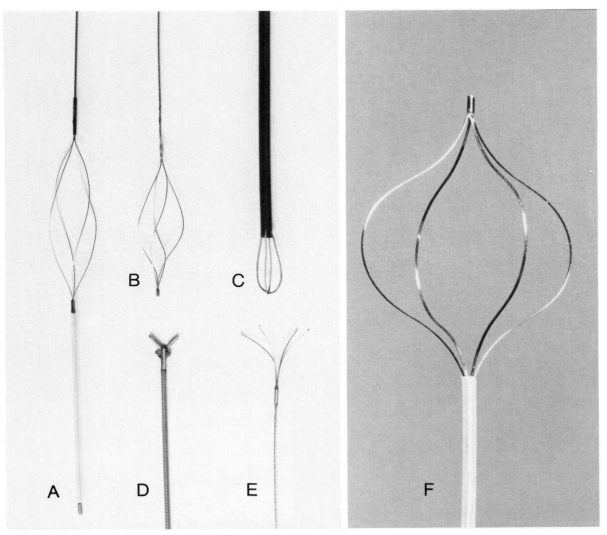

Fig. 27–102 Stone removal devices. A. Pfister-Schwartz. B. Dormia. C. Hawkins. D. Alligator forceps. E. Four-prong grasper. F. Segura.

grasp ductal endothelium as well as the stone. They are used mainly with small (2–3-mm), rough-surfaced, radiopaque calculi, preferably under direct vision. The 7F flexible alligator forceps provide a better grasp on the calculus, and the jaws can be rotated to find a better grasping point. This instrument needs a 13F Burhenne steerable catheter for introduction and guidance. The 5F alligator forceps are used via a flexible endoscope.

Grasping with Rigid Forceps

In 1960, Mazzariello routinely removed biliary tract calculi with rigid forceps shaped into one of four different curves.[155,158,159] The same technique is now used at the authors' institution with minor changes. The two types of rigid forceps that can be used are the Randall forceps, which open with a scissor motion, and the Mazzariello–Caprini forceps, which open by rotating along the axis. Both types are introduced directly through the tract without a sheath. In order to pass them along the guide-wire when they are closed, a groove must be made in the jaws.

Unskilled operators should not use rigid forceps, because severe damage can be done to the biliary system. The techniques require multidirectional fluoroscopy to facilitate manipulation and minimize trauma, as well as adequate sedation, because these maneuvers are usually painful.

FLUOROSCOPIC AND ENDOSCOPIC FRAGMENTATION TECHNIQUES

Large stones can be fragmented within the common bile duct before extraction. This technique, as previously described, is particularly important with the transhepatic approach, where attempts to extract an intact stone through the tract can cause significant trauma. Stones can be fragmented with baskets, forceps, electrohydraulic or ultrasonic lithotripsy, or, possibly, a laser.

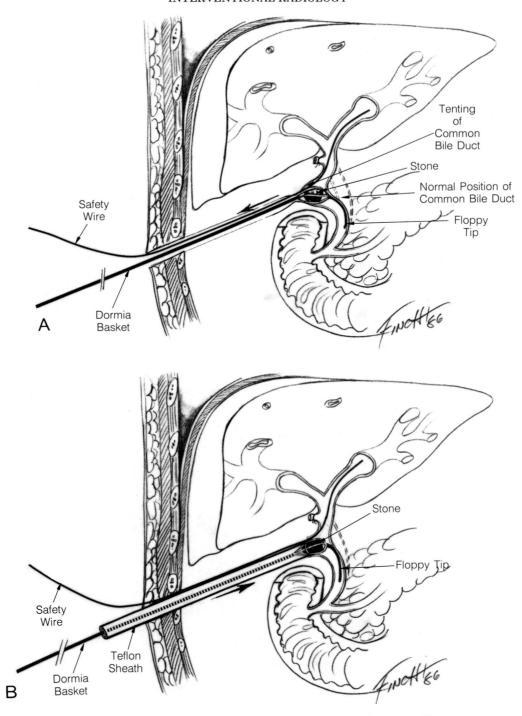

Fig. 27–103 Use of Teflon sheath during extraction of retained stones. A. Through T-tube tract, Dormia basket has been manipulated to entrap stone in distal common bile duct. Attempts to remove stone from the common bile duct through small opening of choledochotomy produced marked tenting of the duct, which has moved away from its normal position. Observe presence of safety guidewires alongside and parked within left biliary radicles. B. Teflon sheath has been passed over Dormia basket and advanced until it reaches the level of the choledochotomy. Forceful pulling of stone into sheath, which is held against the bile duct, prevents tenting of duct.

Fragmentation with Baskets

Fortunately, most retained biliary stones are soft and can be fragmented easily simply by pulling the basket against the Teflon sheath or steerable catheter. Some stones will fragment while being pulled through the choledochotomy or tract.[154] A special strong basket has been described for stone fragmentation.[160]

Electrohydraulic Lithotripter

Electrohydraulic lithotripsy was originally developed in the Soviet Union and found its greatest use in industry to fragment rocks. In 1970, Reuter reported using lithotripsy to fragment bladder stones in 50 patients,[165] and since then widespread use to fragment renal pelvic stones has been documented. Use of the lithotripter to fragment

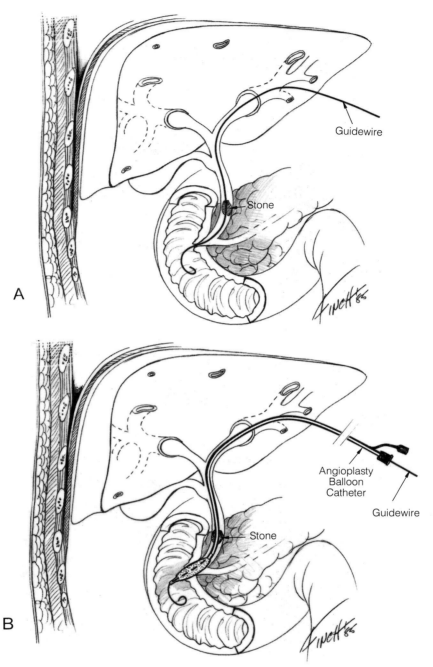

Fig. 27–104   Percutaneous transhepatic stone removal from biliary tree. A. Through a left epigastric approach, guidewire has been manipulated into duodenum. B. Angioplasty balloon catheter has been passed over guidewire and is being used to dilate papilla. C. Stone in distal common bile duct has been trapped with help of Dor- mia basket, whose long floppy tip lies within duodenum. D. Dormia basket with trapped stone has been passed across dilated papilla into duodenum. E. By gentle manipulation, stone has been released from basket into duodenum, and basket has been withdrawn into common bile duct.

biliary stones through a T-tube tract was reported by Burhenne[166] and through a transhepatic approach by Lear et al.[167]

The electrohydraulic lithotripter generates a hydraulic shockwave that shatters the stones (Fig. 27–106). The shockwave originates from the tip of a long probe that is connected to a generator. For fragmentation, the biliary stone is held in position with a basket. A ⅙ N saline solution is used to clear bile and contrast medium from the common bile duct prior to electrical discharge. The probe is introduced either through steerable Burhenne cathe- ters, other transhepatic biliary drainage catheters, or, preferably, under direct vision through a choledocho- scope. The electrode on the tip of the probe must be in contact with the stone. The discharge spark is transmit- ted through the fluid wave and fragments the stone.

Martin et al, working with dogs, were able to fragment 80% of the stones by using a pulse setting of 80 volts.[168]

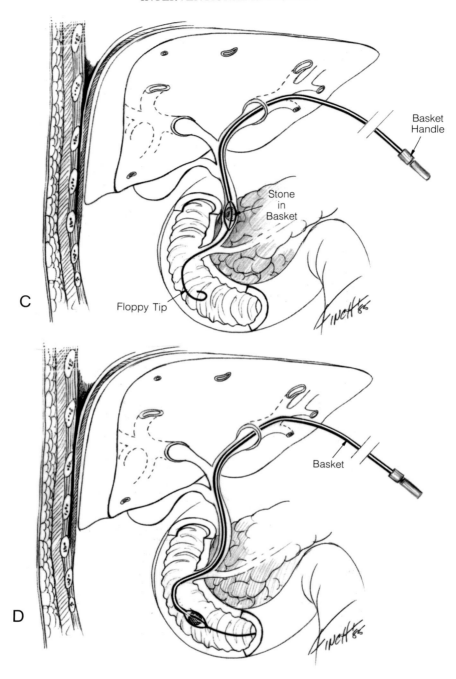

Fig. 27–104C,D

The same authors raise the possibility of late stricture formation, noting that chronic inflammatory changes and fibrin deposition occurred in the mucosa of the biliary tree in one of the seven dogs.[168]

Ultrasonic Lithotripter

The 15F, 24F, and 28F ultrasonic lithotripters can be introduced through a T-tube or transhepatic tract to fragment large, hard stones under direct vision. The chief disadvantage of the ultrasonic lithotripters is their rigidity, which prevents their use through curved tracts.

Laser

A 9F flexible endoscope has recently been described for vascular work through which a fiberoptic fiber can be passed for laser fragmentation of biliary stones. However, at present, the number of "strikes" needed makes this technique impractical.

Follow-up

At the end of the extraction procedure, a straight drainage catheter can be introduced through the Teflon

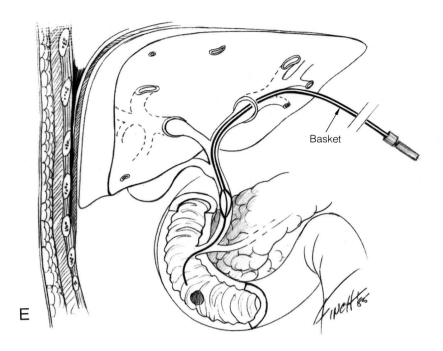

E

Fig. 27–104E

sheath, or, if a T-tube is to be reinserted, this can be done with two guidewires, one up in the proximal bile ducts and the other down in the duodenum (Fig. 27–107). Each limb of the T-tube is passed over the appropriate guide-wire, and the entire T-tube is advanced over the wires through the Teflon sheath into the bile ducts. If all goes well, each limb will follow the corresponding guidewire. The guidewires and the sheath are then removed, leaving the T-tube in position within the common bile duct.[169]

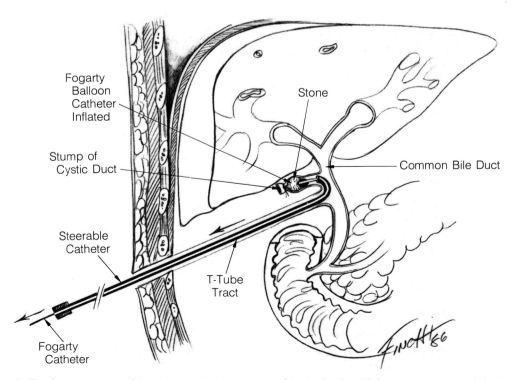

Fig. 27–105 Through T-tube tract, steerable catheter has been manipulated into stump of cystic duct, and Fogarty balloon catheter has been passed beyond the retained stone and inflated. Fogarty cathter is slowly withdrawn into common bile duct, pulling stone out of stump.

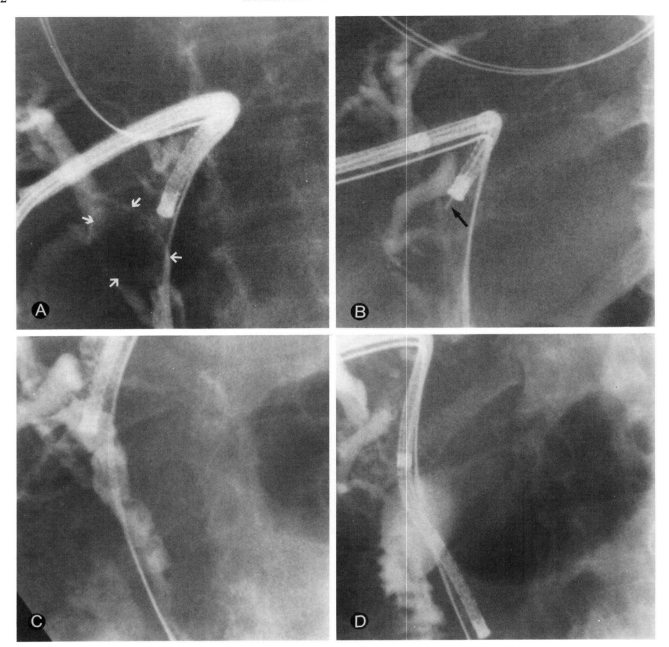

Fig. 27–106   Sixty-year-old patient with painless jaundice. A. Fine-needle cholangiography reveals large, round filling defect at level of common hepatic duct, circumferentially outlined by contrast medium and representing large bile duct stone (arrows). Flexible endoscope has been passed through Teflon sheath and is placed near stone. B. Fragmentation of calculus was performed by electrohydraulic lithotripsy under direct vision utilizing a flexible choledochoscope. Note tip of probe (arrow). C. After fragmentation, note large amount of debris in common bile duct. D. Calculus has been frag-mented. Some fragments were removed through sheath with the help of alligator forceps and baskets; other fragments were flushed down common bile duct into duodenum. After removal of all the debris and clots, choledochoscope was advanced through common bile duct to ensure that no fragments were left behind. (A reproduced from Young AT, Cardella JF, Castañeda–Zuñiga WR, Hunter DW, Amplatz K: The anterior approach to left biliary catheterization. *Semin Intervent Radiol* 1985;2:31–38 with the permission of Thieme, Inc.)

COMPLICATIONS OF EXTRACTION OF RETAINED BILIARY STONES

Death

No deaths were reported in the two largest series, 570 and 661 patients, reported by Mazzariello and Burhenne.[154,159,170] However, another author reported one death secondary to pancreatitis 10 days after the procedure.[171]

Morbidity

The morbidity rate associated with nonoperative extraction of bile duct stones is low, approximately 4%–5%.[154,170]

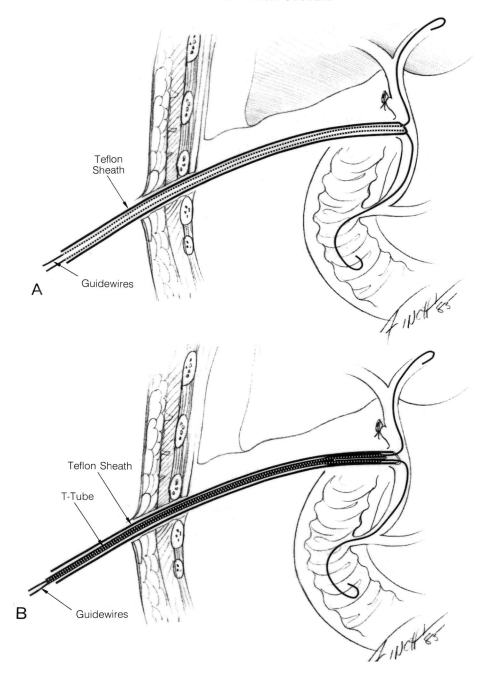

Fig. 27–107 Schematic representation of repositioning of fallen-out T-tube. A. After catheterization of T-tube tract, dilatation is performed for placement of 24F Teflon sheath with its tip within common bile duct. Two guidewires are placed, one into proximal biliary tree and a second with its tip in duodenum. B. Each arm of T-tube is fed over a guidewire, which then exit together through main shaft of T-tube. T-tube is subsequently advanced through Teflon sheath, which has been lubricated with mineral oil. C. By gentle advancement and manipulation, each of the arms of the T-tube is advanced over corresponding leading guidewire into proximal and distal common bile duct. D. Teflon sheath and guidewires have been removed, leaving T-tube in place.

TRACT PERFORATION

Perforation and contrast extravasation can be seen in T-tube tracts after removal of large stones through small tracts. Use of working sheaths, especially following dilatation of the T-tube tract, permits easy entry and exit of instruments and minimizes the chance of perforation. Remarkably, extensive tract perforation that communicates with the abdomen usually has no sequelae.[170]

VASOVAGAL REACTIONS

Advancement of stones through the ampulla and extraction of large stones through small tracts frequently

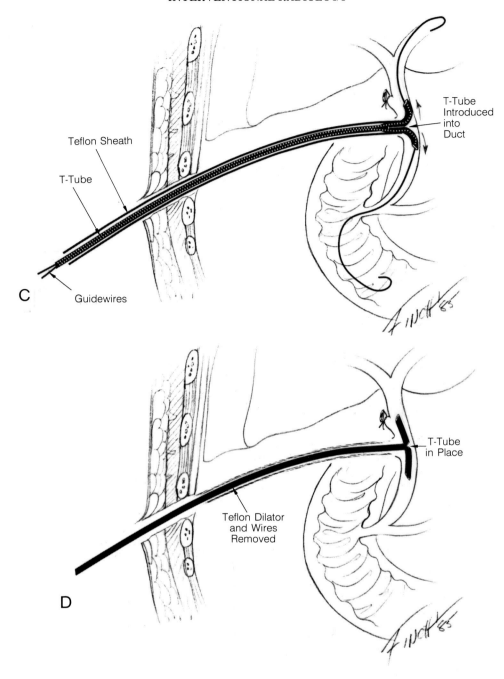

Fig. 27–107C,D

causes abdominal pain and vasovagal reactions. Appropriate treatment consists of intravenous fluids, sedation, and atropine.

FEVER AND SEPSIS

Fever occurs infrequently and can be controlled easily with antibiotics. Prolonged manipulation in complicated cases, such as those with multiple, large, or intrahepatic stones, can precipitate sepsis. Blood cultures should be obtained and appropriate antibiotics administered. In difficult cases, and in known cases of cholangitis, antibiotics that cover both gram-positive and gram-negative organisms are routinely administered starting preoperatively.

PANCREATITIS

Mild to severe pancreatitis can result from manipulation and trauma to the pancreas or duct or from reflux of contrast medium into the pancreatic duct. This is an infrequent occurrence.

SUBHEPATIC BILE COLLECTION

In a series of 661 patients, subhepatic bile collection occurred in two cases.[154] In one case, the collection caused partial common duct obstruction and necessitated operation.

In many patients with an uncomplicated single stone,

the procedure can be completed in one outpatient session. However, in 30%–40% of cases, repeated sessions and hospitalization will be required. Examples of such situations are the following.

Small or Strictured T-Tube Tracts and Mid-Size or Large Stones

In the authors' institution, the sinus tract usually is dilated by either balloon or coaxial dilators to the desired size so that the procedure can be done in a single session.

Multiple Extrahepatic Stones

Frequently, these cases require several sessions because of their complexity and the number of stones to be snared. Multiple extractions on the same day can damage the sinus tract if working sheaths are not used.

Stones Impacted in the Cystic or Common Duct

Multiple sessions may actually benefit these patients, because excessive persistence on the part of the operator in the first session might push the stones farther into the common duct wall and result in false passages and undue discomfort for the patient.[172]

Large Stones

Large stones require fragmentation, after which the larger pieces must be snared and the smaller ones either snared or flushed into the duodenum. During the manipulations, air bubbles, blood clots, or mucosal edema may interfere with satisfactory interpretation of the cholangiograms. Therefore, it is best to bring the patient back 1 or 2 days later for cholangiography and any necessary intervention.

INTRAHEPATIC STONES

Patients with intrahepatic stones commonly require more than one session for complete stone removal.

The left hepatic duct is a common site for intrahepatic lithiasis.[159,173] The anterior location and larger size of the left hepatic duct probably contribute to the stasis of bile and stone formation, but usually the most important problem is a stricture proximal to the stones at the junction of the left and common hepatic ducts.

Intrahepatic lithiasis is one of the more common complications of biliary–enteric anastomoses. As the initial procedure, any strictures should be dilated, thereby improving access to the stones and the chances for successful flushing.

Intrahepatic stones usually require a creative potpourri of techniques, such as flushing, aspiration, snaring with baskets, dislodgment by Fogarty balloons, and extraction by forceps. On occasion, the intrahepatic stones must be dissolved by infusion of chemical agents, such as monooctanoin.

PERCUTANEOUS CHOLECYSTOSTOMY

Recent articles have discussed the use of percutaneous cholecystostomy as a preoperative adjunctive measure for stabilizing critically ill patients (Fig. 27–108) before cholecystectomy tubes are placed.[174–179] The technique has also been used for the percutaneous disolution of gallbladder stones.[180–182] Mono-octanoin has been used suc-

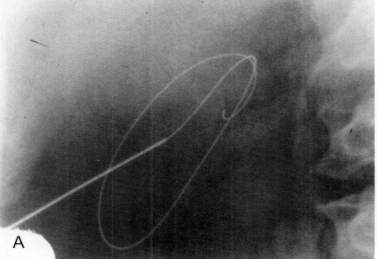
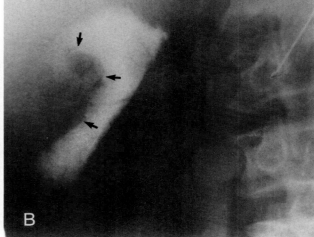

Fig. 27–108 Ultrasonically guided puncture of gallbladder with 18-gauge needle. A. A 0.035-inch guidewire has been looped in gallbladder for placement of drainage catheter in patient with acute acalculous cholecystitis. B. Cholecystogram through drainage catheter shows large amount of debris within gallbladder (arrows).

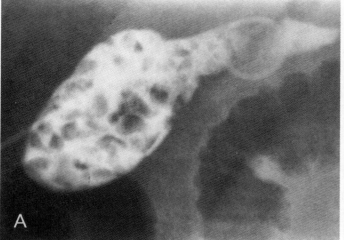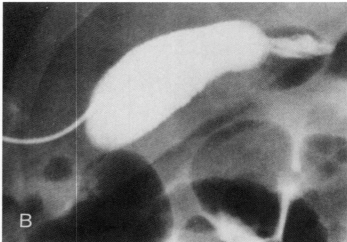

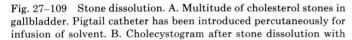

Fig. 27–109   Stone dissolution. A. Multitude of cholesterol stones in gallbladder. Pigtail catheter has been introduced percutaneously for infusion of solvent. B. Cholecystogram after stone dissolution with methyl tertiary butyl ether. (Courtesy of Dr. G. R. May, Mayo Clinic.)

cessfully, although dissolution is slow. No secondary effects of the infusion have been reported.[180,181] Stone dissolution with methyl tertiary butyl ether is, on the other hand, fast and without major secondary effects (Fig. 27–109).[182] As long as the percutaneous tract is placed through the liver, no significant complications have occurred.[174–182]

References

1. Nichols DA, et al: Cholangiographic evaluation of bile duct carcinoma. *AJR* 1983;141:1291
2. Mueller PR, et al: Fine-needle transhepatic cholangiography: reflections after 450 cases. *AJR* 1981;136:85
3. Burkhardt H, Muller W: Versuche über die Punktion der Gallenblase und ihre röntgendarstellung. *Dtsch Chirug* 1921;161:168
4. Huard P, Do-Xuan-Hop D–X: La ponction transhepatique des canaux biliares. *Bull Soc Med Chir Indoch* 1937;15:1090
5. Royer M, Solari AV, Lottero-Lanari R: La cholangiografia no quirurgica: nuevo metodo de exploracion de las vias biliares. *Arch Argent Enferm Aparato Digest Nutric* 1942;17:368
6. Carter FR, Saypol GM: Transabdominal cholangiography. *JAMA* 1952;148:253
7. Leger L, Zara M, Arvay N: Cholangiographie et drainage biliaire par ponction transhepatique. *Presse Med* 1952;60:936
8. Prioton JB, Vialla M, Pous JG: Nouvelle technique de cholangiographie transparieto-hepatique. *J Radiol Electrol* 1960;41:205
9. Seldinger SI: Percutaneous transhepatic cholangiography. *Acta Radiol* (Suppl) 1966;253:1
10. Okuda K, Tanikawa K, Emura T, et al: Nonsurgical, percutaneous transhepatic cholangiography: diagnostic significance in medical problems of the liver. *Am J Dig Dis* 1974;19:21
11. Ohto M, Tsuchiya Y: Medical cholangiography: technique and cases. *Medicina (Tokyo)* 1969;6:735
12. Tsuchiya Y: A new safer method of percutaneous transhepatic cholangiography. *Jpn J Gastroenterol* 1969;66:438
13. Harbin WP, et al: THC: complications and use patterns of the fine needle technique. *Radiology* 1980;135:15
14. Jutti Judata P, et al: Percutaneous transhepatic cholangiography with the Chiba needle in patients with biliary calculi. *Radiology* 1983;146:643
15. Smith GA: Fine needle cholangiography in post-cholecystectomy patients. *AJR* 1978;130:697
16. Gold RP, et al: Thin-needle cholangiography as the primary method for the evaluation of the biliary-enteric anastomoses. *Radiology* 1980;136:309
17. Van Sonnenberg E, et al: Biliary pressure: manometric and perfusion studies of percutaneous THC and percutaneous biliary drainage. *Radiology* 1983;148:41
18. Molnar W, Stockum AE: Relief of obstructive jaundice through percutaneous transhepatic catheter—a new therapeutic method. *AJR* 1974;122:356
19. Keighley MRB, Lister DM, Jacobs SI, et al: Hazards of surgical treatment due to microorganisms in the bile. *Surgery* 1974;75:578
20. Keighley MRB: Micro-organisms in the bile: a preventable cause of sepsis after biliary surgery. *Ann R Coll Surg Engl* 1977;59:328
21. Goldberg HI, Dodds WJ, Lawson TL, Stewart ET, Moss AA: Hepatic lymphatics demonstrated by percutaneous transhepatic cholangiography. *AJR* 1975;123:415
22. Ferrucci JT, et al: Refinements in Chiba needle transhepatic cholangiography. *AJR* 1977;129:11
23. Young AT, Cardella JF, Castañeda–Zuñiga WR, Hunter DW, Amplatz K: The anterior approach to left biliary catheterization. *Semin Intervent Radiol* 1985;2:31
24. Katon RM, Lee TG, Parent JA, Bilbao MK, Smith FW: Endoscopic retrograde cholangiopancreatography (ERCP): experience with 100 cases. *Am J Dig Dis* 1974;19:295
25. Nebel OT, Fornes MF: Endoscopic pancreatocholangiography. *Dig Dis* 1973;18:1042
26. Bilbao MK, Potter CI, Lee TG, Katon RM: Complications of endoscopic retrograde cholangiopancreatography (ERCP): a study of 10,000 cases. *Gastroenterology* 1976;70:314
27. Robbins AH, Paul RE Jr, Norton RA, Schimmel EM, Tomas JG, Sugarman HJ: Detection of malignant disease by peroral retrograde pancreatico-biliary ductography. *AJR* 1973;117:432
28. Rohrmann CA, Silvis SE, Vennes JA: Evaluation of the endoscopic pancreatogram. *Radiology* 1974;113:297
29. Ferrucci JT, et al: Fine needle THC: a new approach to obstructive jaundice. *AJR* 1976;127:403
30. Hultborn A, Jacobsson B, Rosengren B: Cholangiovenous reflux during cholangiography: an experiment and clinical study. *Acta Chir Scand* 1962;123:111
31. Flemma RJ, Schauble JF, Gardner CE Jr, et al: Percutaneous

cholangiography in the differential diagnosis of jaundice. *Surg Gynecol Obstet* 1963;116:559

32. Okuda K, Musha H, Nakajima Y, et al: Frequency of intrahepatic arteriovenous fistula as a sequela to percutaneous needle puncture of the liver. *Gastroenterology* 1978;74:1204

33. Hoevels J, Nilsson U: Intrahepatic vascular lesions following nonsurgical percutaneous transhepatic bile duct intubation. *Gastrointest Radiol* 1980;5:127

34. Druy EM: Hepatic artery-biliary fistula following percutaneous transhepatic biliary drainage. *Radiology* 1981;141:369

35. Rosen RJ, Rothberg M: Transhepatic embolization of hepatic artery pseudoaneurysm following biliary drainage. *Radiology* 1982;145:532

36. Ring EJ, Kerlan RK: Interventional biliary radiology. *AJR* 1984;142:31

37. Kaude JV, Weidenmier CH, Agee OF: Decompression of bile ducts with the percutaneous transhepatic technic. *Radiology* 1969;93:69

38. Burcharth F, Nielbo N: Percutaneous transhepatic cholangiography with selective catheterization of the common bile duct. *AJR* 1976;127:409

39. Mori K, Misumi A, Sugiyama M, et al: Percutaneous transhepatic bile drainage. *Ann Surg* 1977;185:111

40. Tylen U, Hoevels J, Vang J: Percutaneous transhepatic cholangiography with external drainage of obstructive biliary lesions. *Surg Gynecol Obstet* 1977;144:13

41. Hoevels J, Lunderquist A, Ihse I: Percutaneous transhepatic intubation of bile ducts for combined internal/external drainage in preoperative and palliative treatment of obstructive jaundice. *Gastrointest Radiol* 1978;3:23

42. Hansson JA, Hoevels J, Simert G, et al: Clinical aspects of nonsurgical percutaneous transhepatic bile drainage in obstructive lesions of the extra-hepatic bile ducts. *Ann Surg* 1979;189:58

43. Nakayama T, Ikeda A, Okuda K: Percutaneous transhepatic drainage of the biliary tract. *Gastroenterology* 1978;74:554

44. Ring EJ, Oleaga JA, Freiman DB, et al: Therapeutic applications of catheter cholangiography. *Radiology* 1978;128:333

45. Ferrucci JT Jr, Mueller PR, Harbin WP: Percutaneous transhepatic biliary drainage: technique, results and applications. *Radiology* 1980;135:1

46. Tahada T, Hanyu F, Kobayashi S, Uchida Y: Percutaneous transhepatic cholangeal drainage: direct approach under fluoroscopic control. *J Surg Oncol* 1976;8:83

47. Braasch JW, Gray BN: Considerations that lower pancreatoduodenectomy mortality. *Am J Surg* 1977;133:480

48. Buckwalter JA, Lawton RL, Tidrick RT: Bypass operations for neoplastic biliary tract obstruction. *Am J Surg* 1965;109:100

49. Nakase A, Matsumoto Y, Uchida K, Honja I: Surgical treatment of cancer of the pancreas and the periampullary region. *Ann Surg* 1977;185:52

50. Brooks JR, Culebras JM: Cancer of the pancreas: palliative operation, Whipple procedure or total pancreatectomy? *Am J Surg* 1976;131:516

51. Hertzberg J: Pancreaticoduodenal resection and bypass operation in patients with carcinoma of the head of the pancreas, ampulla, and distal end of the common duct. *Acta Chir Scand* 1974;140:523

52. Dow RW, Lindenauer SM: Acute obstructive suppurative cholangitis. *Ann Surg* 1969;169:272

53. Ferrucci JT, Mueller PR: Interventional radiology of the biliary tract. *Gastroenterology* 1982;82:974

54. Feduska NJ, Dent TL, Lindenauer SM: Results of palliative operations for carcinoma of the pancreas. *Arch Surg* 1971;103:330

55. Pitt HA, Cameron JL, Postier RG, Gadacz TR: Factors affecting mortality in biliary tract surgery. *Am J Surg* 1981;141:66

56. Wittenstein BH, Giacchino JL, Pickleman JR, et al: Obstructive jaundice: the necessity for improved management. *Am Surg* 1981;47:116

57. Maki T, Sata T, Kakizaki G, et al: Pancreaticoduodenectomy for periampullary carcinomas: appraisal of two-stage procedure. *Arch Surg* 1966;92:825

58. Clouse ME, Evans D, Costello P, Alday M, Edwards SA, McDermott WV Jr: Percutaneous transhepatic biliary drainage: complications due to multiple duct obstructions. *Ann Surg* 1983;198:25

59. Denning D, Ellison C, Carey L: Preoperative percutaneous transhepatic biliary decompression lowers operative morbidity in patients with obstructive jaundice. *Am J Surg* 1981;141:61

60. Mueller PR, VanSonnenberg E, Ferrucci JT Jr: Percutaneous biliary drainage: technical and catheter related problems—experience with 200 cases. *AJR* 1982;138:17

61. Norlander A, Kalin B, Sundblad R: Effect of percutaneous transhepatic drainage upon liver function and postoperative mortality. *Surg Gynecol Obstet* 1982;155:161

62. Hatfield ARW, Terblanche J, Fataar S, et al: Preoperative external biliary drainage in obstructive jaundice. *Lancet* 1982;2:896

63. Neff RA, Frankuchen EI, Cooperman AM, Helmrich ZV, Martin EC: The radiological management of malignant biliary obstruction. *Clin Radiol* 1983;34:143

64. McPherson GAD, Benjamin IS, Hodgson HJF, Bowley NB, Allison DJ, Blumgart LH: Pre-operative percutaneous transhepatic biliary drainage: the results of a controlled trial. *Br J Surg* 1984;71:371

65. McPherson GAD, Benjamin IS, Habib NA, Bowley NB, Blumgart LH: Percutaneous transhepatic drainage in obstructive jaundice: advantages and problems. *Br J Surg* 1982;69:261

66. Stambuk EC, Pitt HA, Pais SO, Mann LL, Lois JF, Gomes AS: Percutaneous transhepatic drainage. *Arch Surg* 1983;118:1388

67. Robison R, Madura J, Scholten D, et al: Percutaneous transhepatic drainage for malignant biliary obstruction. *Am Surg* 1984;50:329

68. Shapiro TM: Adenocarcinoma of the pancreas: statistical analysis of biliary bypass vs. Whipple resection in good risk patients. *Ann Surg* 1975;182:751

69. Crile G Jr: The advantages of bypass operations over radical pancreatoduodenectomy in the treatment of pancreatic carcinoma. *Surg Gynecol Obstet* 1970;130:1049

70. Case records of the Massachusetts General Hospital: case no. 35. *N Engl J Med* 1976;295:492

71. Ferrucci JT, et al: Advances in the radiology of jaundice: a symposium and review. *AJR* 1983;141:1

72. Ring EJ, Husted JW, Oleaga JA, Freiman DB: A multihole catheter for maintaining longterm percutaneous antegrade biliary drainage. *Radiology* 1979;132:752

73. Hawkins IF Jr: Single-step placement of a self-retaining accordion catheter. *Semin Intervent Radiol* 1984;1:15

74. Cope C: Improved anchoring of nephrostomy catheters: hook technique. *AJR* 1980;135:402

75. Cope C: Replacement of obstructed loop and pigtail nephrostomy and biliary drains. *AJR* 1982;139:1022

76. Coons HG, Carey PH: Large-bore, long biliary endoprostheses (biliary stents) for improved drainage. *Radiology* 1983;148:89

77. Andrews RC, Hawkins IF: The Hawkins needle-guide system for percutaneous catheterization: instrumentation and procedure. *AJR* 1984;142:1191

78. Harrington DP: Teflon sheath placement in the biliary tree using high-torque J guidewires. *Radiology* 1980;134:248

79. Lunderquist A, et al: Guidewire for percutaneous transhepatic cholangiography. *Radiology* 1979;132:228

80. Cope C: Stiff fine-needle guidewire for catheterization and drainage. *Radiology* 1983;147:264

81. Cope C: Conversion from small (0.018-inch) to large (0.038-inch) guidewires in percutaneous drainage procedures. *AJR* 1982;138:170

82. Bean WJ, et al: T-tube tract dilatation for removal of large biliary stones. *Radiology* 1975;115:485

83. Rusnak B, Castañeda–Zuñiga WR, Kotula F, et al: An improved dilator system for percutaneous nephrostomies. *Radiology* 1982;144:174

84. Grüntzig A, Kumpe DA: Technique of percutaneous transluminal angioplasty with the Grüntzig balloon catheter. *AJR* 1979;132:547

85. Clayman RV, Castañeda–Zuñiga WR, Hunter DW, Miller RP, Lange PH, Amplatz K: Rapid balloon dilatation of nephrostomy track for nephrostolithotomy. *Radiology* 1983;147:884

86. Gudjonsson B, Livestone EM, Spiro HM: Cancer of the pancreas: diagnostic accuracy and survival statistics. *Cancer* 1978;42:2494

87. Ferrucci JT Jr, Mueller PR, Harbin WP: Percutaneous biliary drainage, in Ferrucci JT Jr, Wittenberg J (eds): *Interventional Radiology of the Abdomen*. Baltimore, Williams & Wilkins, 1981

88. Oleaga JA, Ring EJ: Interventional biliary radiology. *Semin Roentgenol* 1981;16:116

89. Molnar W, Stockum AE: Transhepatic dilatation of choledocoenterostomy strictures. *Radiology* 1978;129:59

90. Schwarz W, Rosen RJ, Fitts WR Jr, et al: Percutaneous transhepatic drainage pre-operatively for benign biliary strictures. *Surg Gynecol Obstet* 1981;152:466

91. Martin EC, et al: Percutaneous dilatation in primary sclerosing cholangitis: two experiences. *AJR* 1981;137:603

92. Salomonowitz E, Castañeda WR, Lund G, et al: Balloon dilatation of benign biliary strictures. *AJR* 1984;151:613

93. Icadir S, et al: Percutaneous biliary drainage in the management of biliary sepsis. *AJR* 1982;138:25

94. Ostermiller W Jr, Thompson RJ Jr, Carter R, Hinshaw DB: Acute obstructive cholangitis. *Arch Surg* 1965;90:392

95. Boey JH, Way LW: Acute cholangitis. *Ann Surg* 1980;191:264

96. Lou MAS, Mandal AK, Alexander JL, Thadepalli H: Bacteriology of the human biliary tract and the duodenum. *Arch Surg* 1977;112:965

97. Andrews E, Henry LD: Bacteriology of normal and diseased gallbladders. *Arch Intern Med* 1935;56:1171

98. Nielsen ML, Justesen I: Anaerobic and aerobic bacteriological studies in biliary tract disease. *Scand J Gastroenterol* 1976;11:437

99. Walloch Y, Feigenberg Z, Zer M, Dintsman M: The influence of biliary infection on the postoperative course after biliary tract surgery. *Am J Gastroenterol* 1977;67:456

100. Pitt HA, Postier RG, Cameron JL: Postoperative T-tube cholangiography: is antibiotic coverage necessary? *Ann Surg* 1980;191:30

101. Wayne PM, Whelan JG: Susceptibility testing of biliary bacteria obtained before bile duct manipulation. *AJR* 1983;140:1185

102. Jacobsson B, Kjellander J, Rosengren B: Cholangiovenous reflux: an experimental study. *Acta Chir Scand* 1962;123:316

103. Heckemann R, Meyer–Schwickerath M, Hezel J: Percutaneous nephropyelostomy under continuous real time ultrasound guidance. *Urol Radiol* 1981;3:171

104. Ohto M, Karasawa E, Tsuchiqa Y, et al: Ultrasonically guided percutaneous contrast medium injection and aspiration biopsy using a real time puncture transducer. *Radiology* 1980;136:171

105. Castañeda–Zuñiga WR, Tadavarthy SM, Laerum F, Amplatz K: Anterior approach for biliary duct drainage. *Radiology* 1981;139:746

106. Rusnak B, Castañeda–Zuñiga WR, Kotula F, Herrera M, Amplatz K: Radiolucent handle for percutaneous puncture under continuous fluoroscopic monitoring. *Radiology* 1981;141:538

107. Jaques PF, et al: Percutaneous transhepatic biliary drainage: advantages of the left-lobe subxiphoid approach. *Radiology* 1982;145:534

108. Mueller PR, et al: Obstruction of the left hepatic duct: diagnosis and treatment by selective fine needle cholangiography and percutaneous biliary drainage. *Radiology* 1982;145:297

109. Neff C, Mueller P, Ferrucci J, et al: Serious complications following transgression of the pleural space in drainage procedures. *Radiology* 1984;152:335

110. Kerlan RK, Ring EJ, Pogany AC, Jeffrey RB: "Pull-through" method for Silastic catheter insertion. *AJR* 1984;142:103

111. Herrera M, Brawerman S, Castañeda WR, et al: The endocatheter ruler: a useful device. *AJR* 1982;139:828

112. Mitchell SE, Clark RA: Finger-trap method of suturing biliary drainage catheters to the skin. *AJR* 1981;137:628

113. Bron KM: The non-suture skin fixation of drainage catheters. *AJR* 1982;139:404

114. Shoenfeld RB, Lecky D, Ring EJ, McLean GK, Freiman DB: Stabilization of percutaneous catheters. *AJR* 1982;138:972

115. Pais SO: Simple method for skin fixation of percutaneous perfusion catheters. *AJR* 1982;139:1021

116. Gordon RL, Oleaga JA, Ring EJ, Freiman DB, Funaro AH: Replacing the "fallen out" catheter. *Radiology* 1980;134:537

117. Pereiras RV Jr, Rheingold OJ, Hutson D, et al: Relief of malignant obstructive jaundice by percutaneous insertion of a permanent prosthesis in the biliary tree. *Ann Intern Med* 1978;89 (part 1):589

118. Burcharth F: A new endoprosthesis for nonoperative intubation of the biliary tract in malignant obstructive jaundice. *Surg Gynecol Obstet* 1978;146:76

119. Burcharth F, Efsen F, Christiansen LS, et al: Nonsurgical internal biliary drainage by endoprosthesis. *Surg Gynecol Obstet* 1981;153:857

120. Lorelius LE, Jacobson G, Sawada S: Endoprosthesis as an internal biliary drainage in inoperable patients with biliary obstruction. *Acta Chir Scand* 1982;148:613

121. Gouma D, Wesdorp R, Oostenbroek R, Soeters P, Greep J: Percutaneous transhepatic drainage and insertion of an endoprosthesis for obstructive jaundice. *Am J Surg* 1983;145:763

122. Dooley S, Dick R, Irving D, Olney J, Sherlock S: Relief of bile duct obstruction by the percutaneous transhepatic insertion of an endoprosthesis. *Clin Radiol* 1981;32:163

123. Miskowiak J, Mygind T, Baden H, Burcharth F: Biliary endoprosthesis secured by a subcutaneous button to prevent dislocation. *AJR* 1982;139:1019

124. Owman T, Lunderquist A: Sling retraction for proximal placement of percutaneous transhepatic biliary endoprosthesis. *Radiology* 1983;146:228

125. Harries-Jones EP, Fataar S, Tuft RJ: Repositioning of biliary endoprosthesis with Grüntzig balloon catheters. *AJR* 1982;138:771

126. Nichols D, Cooperberg P, Golding R, Burhenne H: The safe intercostal approach? Pleural complications in abdominal interventional radiology. *AJR* 1984;141:1013

127. Mendez G, Nunez D, Yrizarry JM, Russell E, Guerra J: Uses and misuses of biliary endoprosthesis. *Semin Intervent Radiol* 1985;2:60

128. Grelet PH, Boedec R, Sabrie C, Balp V: Drainage biliaire non chirurgical. *J Radiol [Paris]* 1981;62:177

129. Carrasco C, Zornoza J, Bechtel W: Malignant biliary obstruction: complications of biliary drainage. *Radiology* 1984;152:343

130. Dooley J, Dick R, George P, Kirk R, Hobbs K, Sherlock S: Percutaneous transhepatic endoprosthesis for bile duct obstruction. *Gastroenterology* 1984;86:905

131. Zollikofer CH, Bruhlmann W, Pouliadis G, Metzger G: Interventionelle Radiologie beim Verschlussikterus. *Praxis* 1984.42

132. Taber DS, Strohlein JR, Zornoza J.: Work in progress: hypotension and high-volume biliary excretion following external PTBD. *Radiology* 1982;145:639

133. Owman T, Lunderquist A: Sling retraction for proximal placement of percutaneous transhepatic biliary endoprosthesis. *Radiology* 1982;146:228

134. Berquist TH, May GR, Johnson CM, et al: Percutaneous biliary

decompression: internal and external drainage in 50 patients. *AJR* 1981;136:901

135. Clark RA, Mitchell SE, Colley DP, Alexander E: Percutaneous catheter biliary decompression. *AJR* 1981;137:503

136. Monden M, Okamura J, Kobayashi N, et al: Hemobilia after percutaneous transhepatic biliary drainage. *Arch Surg* 1980;115:161

137. Probst P, Castañeda–Zuñiga WR, Amplatz K: Percutaneous transhepatic drainage catheter: a valuable therapeutic aid in obstructive jaundice. *RöFo* 1978;128:443

138. Dawson SL, et al: Fatal hemothorax after inadvertent transpleural biliary drainage. *AJR* 1983;161:33

139. Huang T, Bass JA, Williams RD: The significance of biliary pressure in cholangitis. *Arch Surg* 1969;98:629

140. Williams RD, Fish JC, Williams DD: The significance of biliary pressure. *Arch Surg* 1967;95:374

141. Severini A, et al: Brushing device to keep biliary drainage catheters clean. *Radiology* 1982;143:566

142. Warren KW, McDonald WM: Facts and fiction regarding strictures of the extrahepatic bile ducts. *Ann Surg* 1964;159:996

143. Glenn F: Iatrogenic injuries to the biliary duct system. *Surg Gynecol Obstet* 1978;146:430

144. Burhenne HJ: Dilatation of biliary tract strictures: a new roentgenologic technique. *Radiol Clin [Basel]* 1975;44:153

145. Guenther RW, et al: Work in progress: percutaneous transhepatic electrocutting of stenoses after hepaticojejunostomy. *Radiology* 1983;146:355

146. Cragg AH, Kotula F, Castañeda–Zuñiga WR, Amplatz K: A simple mechanical device for inflation of dilating balloons. *Radiology* 1983;147:273

147. Salomonowitz E, Kotula F, Coleman CC, et al: Balloon-inflation device: the inflation helix. *Radiology* 1984;150:587

148. Cattell RB, Braasch JW: Primary repair of benign strictures of the bile duct. *Surg Gynecol Obstet* 1959;109:531

149. Pitt HA, Miyamoto T, Parapatis SK, Tompkins RK, Longmire WP: Factors influencing outcome in patients with postoperative biliary strictures. *Am J Surg* 1982;144:14

150. Bordlet G, et al: Causes for 340 perforations of the intrahepatic bile ducts. *Ann Surg* 1979;189:662

151. Schulenburg CA: Operative cholangiography: 1000 cases. *Surgery* 1969;65:723

152. Smith SW, Engel C, Averbrook B, Longmire WP Jr: Problems of retained and recurrent common bile duct stones. *JAMA* 1957;164:231

153. Fotopoulos JP, Caprini JA: Percutaneous forceps extraction of retained biliary tract calculi. *Gastrointest Radiol* 1977;1:319

154. Burhenne HJ: Garland Lecture: Percutaneous extraction of retained biliary tract stones: 661 patients. *AJR* 1980;134:889

155. Mazzariello R: Removal of residual biliary calculi without reoperation. *Surgery* 1970;67:556

156. Mazzariello R: Tubo en T modificado para el drenage de la via biliar. *Bolet Socied Argent Cirujanos* 1968;28:31

157. Moss JP, Whelan JB, Fry DE: Unsuccessful post-operative extraction of retained common duct stones: an analysis. *Am J Surg* 1978;135:785

158. Mondet A: Tecnica de la extraccion incruenta de los calculos en la litiasis residual del coledoco. *Bol Soc Cir Buenos Aires* 1962;46:278

159. Mazzariello RM: Residual biliary tract stones: nonoperative treatment of 570 patients. *Surg Ann* 1976;8:113

160. Burhenne HJ: Nonoperative retained biliary tract stone extraction: a new roentgenologic technique. *AJR* 1973;117:388

161. Fennessy JJ, You K–D: A method for the expulsion of stones retained in the common bile duct. *AJR* 1970;110:256

162. Wendth A, Liberman RC, Aldept M: Nonsurgical removal of a retained common bile duct calculus. *Radiology* 1972;103:207

163. Van Way CW, Sawyers JJ: Damage to the intrahepatic biliary system from the use of the balloon tipped catheter. *Am J Surg* 1973;125:343

164. Tadavarthy SM, Castañeda–Zuñiga WR, Amplatz K: Removal of small and large biliary stones. *Cardiovasc Radiol* 1981;4:93

165. Reuter HJ: Electronic lithotripsy: transurethral treatment of bladder stones in 50 cases. *J Urol* 1970;104:834

166. Burhenne HJ: Electrohydrolytic fragmentation of retained common duct stones. *Radiology* 1975;117:721

167. Lear JL, Ring EA, Macoviak JA, Baum S: Percutaneous transhepatic electrohydraulic lithotripsy. *Radiology* 1984;150:589

168. Martin EC, Wolff M, Neff RA, Casarella WJ: Use of the electrohydraulic lithotriptor in the biliary tree of dogs. *Radiology* 1981;139:215

169. Herrera M, Colemann CC, Castañeda WR, Amplatz K: New T-tubes. *AJR* 1984;142:102

170. Burhenne HJ: Complications of nonoperative extraction of retained common duct stones. *Am J Surg* 1976;131:260

171. Polack EP, Fainsinger MH, Bonnano SV: A death following complications of roentgenologic nonoperative manipulation of common bile duct calculi. *Radiology* 1977;123:585

172. Smith PL, Mirza FH: Percutaneous removal of biliary stone impacted in cystic duct remnant. *Radiology* 1981;140:240

173. Clouse ME, Falchuk KR: Percutaneous transhepatic removal of common duct stones: report of ten patients. *Gastro-enterology* 1983;85:815

174. vanSonnenberg E, Wittich, GR, Cusola G, et al: Diagnostic and therapeutic percutaneous gallbladder procedures. *Radiology* 1986;160:23

175. Elyaderani MK, Gabriele OF: Percutaneous cholecystostomy and cholangiography in patients with obstructive jaundice. *Radiology* 1979;130:601

176. McGahan JP, Walter JP: Diagnostic percutaneous aspiration of the gallbladder. *Radiology* 1985;155:619

177. Brunelle F, Chaumont P: Percutaneous cholecystography in children. *Ann Radiol* 1984;27:111

178. Pearse DM, Hawkins IF, Shouer R, Vogel S: Percutaneous cholecystostomy in acute cholecystitis and common duct obstruction. *Radiology* 1984;152:365

179. Eggermont AM, Lameris JS, Jeekel J: Ultrasound guided percutaneous transhepatic cholecystostomy for acute calculus cholecystitis. *Arch Surg* 1985;120:1354

180. Shortsleeve MJ, Schafzki SC, Lee DL: Monooctanoin dissolution of gallstones via a cholecystostomy tube: *Radiology* 1984;153:547

181. Thiestle JL, Carlson GL, Hoffman AF, et al: Monooctanoin, a dissolution agent for retained cholesterol bile duct stones: physical properties and clinical application. *Gastroenterology* 1980;78:1016

182. Allen MJ, Borody TJ, Bugliosi TF, et al: Cholelitholysis using methyl tertiary butyl ether. *Gastroenterology* 1985;88:122

28

Dilation of Esophageal Strictures

MANUEL MAYNAR–MOLINAR, M.D., CARLOS GUERRA, M.D., FRANCISCO MARTINEZ, M.D., AND WILFRIDO R. CASTAÑEDA–ZUÑIGA, M.D., M.Sc.

Traditionally, esophageal strictures have been treated by the transoral blind introduction of dilators of two different types: soft mercury-weighted rubber dilators, such as the Maloney or the Hurst (bougie), and rigid dilators (Eder–Puestow).[1] The first type of dilator has been used in the management of mild (12-mm (36F)), smooth, concentric stenoses, dilation being performed gradually until the lesion reaches a diameter of 50F. In patients with severe stenosis, the treatment is usually started with metallic dilators under either endoscopic or fluoroscopic control.[2–4] Obstructions of the distal esophagus, particularly those caused by achalasia, are treated by pneumatic balloon dilation.[5] Complication rates of 0.4%–8% have been reported; the risk of complications appears to be related to the severity of the obstruction and to the number of dilations needed.[2–4]

After the development by Grüntzig[6] of nonexpandable balloon catheters for dilation of vascular stenoses, his technique was extended to the management of esophageal strictures.[7–12] Newer and larger balloons were then developed for use in the gastrointestinal (GI) tract.[7,13]

The percutaneous balloon technique has been largely limited to patients with severe stenoses or to patients in whom other methods have failed,[14] although it has been the primary approach of other investigators.[8,15] The advantage claimed for balloon dilation is the decrease in the morbidity and mortality in comparison with surgical correction or the use of other dilators such as the pneumatic ones for dilation of the cardia, which has an incidence of perforation of 1.6%–2.6%.[5,16] With the use of balloon dilators, the risk of perforation decreases significantly, particularly during the dilatation of severe (1–2-mm) stenoses, probably because of reduced shear stress and because catheter passage across the area of stenosis is performed over a guidewire and under fluoroscopic control rather than blindly (Fig. 28–1).[17,18]

Conservative treatment of esophageal strictures includes not only the dilation itself but also adequate medical treatment of the etiologic factors, such as reflux esophagitis. Conservative treatment of unresectable malignant strictures can be beneficial temporarily.[8,15]

MATERIALS AND METHODS

From May 1984 until June 1985, 137 dilations were performed in 35 patients with esophageal strictures of different etiologies (Table 28–1).

All procedures were performed under mild sedation and under fluoroscopic control, often in an outpatient setting. Angiographic torque control catheters (*e.g.*, multipurpose, cobra) were used to manipulate the guidewires across the area(s) of stenosis. Different types of guidewires were used, although the authors prefer wires with a soft floppy segment (Bentson 0.035-inch) to minimize trauma to the esophageal and gastric mucosa, and thereby decrease the chances of perforation. Esophageal dilation balloons of the Graüntzig type with diameters of 12–20 mm and lengths of 4–8 cm were used.

The patients were evaluated before dilation with a barium swallow in multiple projections to determine the severity of the narrowing, the eccentricity and length of the lesion (Fig. 28–2), and any associated problems such as esophageal diverticula or gastroesophageal reflux. Frequently, endoscopic examinations were performed to evaluate the lesion or to obtain material for cytologic and histologic examination.

Preoperative drugs include atropine and diazepam. Sedation and analgesia are commonly required during the procedure, for which several combinations have been used, including diazepam with meperidine or morphine. An intravenous line is usually established before the procedure for the administration of these drugs.

TECHNIQUE

The barium swallow films are reviewed to determine the exact location of the lesion in respect to bone or soft tissue landmarks, such as a vertebral body, trachea, bronchus, or metallic sutures. If there is any doubt about the location of the lesion, a small amount of dilute water-soluble contrast medium is administered through the angio-

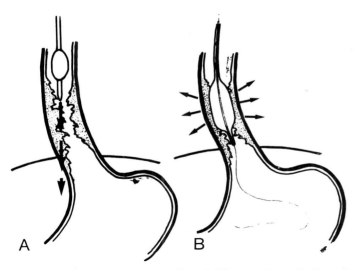

Fig. 28–1 Schematic representation of difference in mechanism of dilatation with traditional esophageal dilators (bougie)(A) and balloon dilators (B).

Table 28–1
Cause of Esophageal Stricture in 35 Patients Treated by Balloon Dilation

Cause	No. Patients
Stenosis of surgical anastomosis	16
Caustic ingestion	4
Postinfection	4
Achalasia	5
Carcinoma	3
Unknown	3

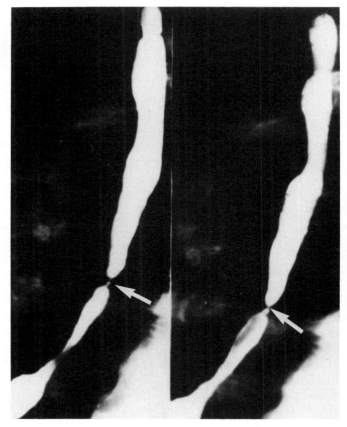

Fig. 28–2 Severe stenosis of the midesophagus caused by caustic ingestion (arrow).

graphic catheter to locate the lesion. Its location is marked on the surface of the patient by putting clamps at the proximal and distal ends.

Using a transnasal approach, an angiographic guidewire is manipulated across the stricture with the help of the angiographic catheter and, commonly, is looped within the gastric fundus. The angiographic catheter is exchanged for the balloon catheter. Under fluoroscopic control, the radiopaque marker in the balloon tip is advanced beyond the distal edge of the stricture, and the balloon is inflated under fluoroscopy to observe the indentation produced by the stricture (Fig. 28–3A). The pressure in the balloon is then gradually increased until the indentation disappears (Fig. 28–3B). Usually, a pressure of 4–6 atm is sufficient to dilate even the hardest and most resistant strictures. The balloon is commonly left inflated for 5–10 min. Several dilations have been performed by some authors during the same sitting.[14] Ideally, the largest possible balloon is introduced in the first sitting.[14]

In patients with severe, extensive narrowing of the esophagus, as is common after caustic ingestion (Fig. 28–2), after passage of a wire across the stricture, the dilation is approached in a different fashion. Initially, dilation to 5–7 mm is performed using balloon catheters (Fig. 28–4A). In subsequent dilations, the caliber of the esophagus is increased gradually (to minimize the chances of esophageal wall rupture) until a suitable diameter is reached (Fig. 28–4B).[15]

In patients with achalasia, the marked dilation of the esophagus makes catheterization of the gastroesophageal hiatus difficult unless torque control angiographic catheters are used for the manipulation.

Anastomoses following gastroesophageal or gastrointestinal (particularly gastrocolonic) interpositions are often difficult to catheterize due to the disparity in size between the esophagus and the stomach or bowel loop. Careful manipulation with angiographic catheters, torque control guidewires, or both is usually successful (Fig. 28–5).

At the completion of the procedure, a barium swallow study is performed to document the change in diameter of the dilated site. A repeat dilation has routinely been performed on the third day after the procedure.

RESULTS

Most of the patients received two or three dilations with the largest number of dilations usually being performed in patients with strictures secondary to reflux esophagitis. In these latter patients, dilation was usually

Fig. 28–3 Dilation of lesion in Figure 28–2. A. 20-mm dilating balloon inflated across stricture; note "waist" (arrow). B. After increase in intraballoon pressure, waist has disappeared.

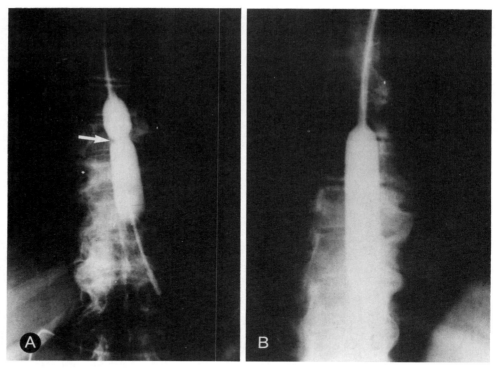

successful, but restenosis was common if the acid reflux was not corrected. In postoperative stenoses, the results of dilation were generally excellent (Figs. 28–6 and 28–7). In only one case was success not complete, and this failure was the result of the type of operation performed to correct gastroesophageal reflux. A tight Nissen fundoplication was the cause of extrinsic compression of the distal esophagus, causing obstruction. In stenosis secondary to ingestion of caustic agents, even when long segments were affected, dilation was generally successful, although a high incidence of recurrence has been observed in patients with long-segment involvement. In patients with reflux esophagitis and associated strictures, dilations were performed as a temporizing maneuver until the problem could be corrected. Usually, balloons of 20-mm diameter were used with good results in patients with achalasia (Fig. 28–8A,B), although occasionally overdilation of the stricture site with two 20-mm balloons side by side has been necessary.[13]

In malignant strictures, dilation with large (20–40-mm) balloons can open a channel for adequate feeding of the patient, although recurrence of the stricture is common with tumor growth. A channel of 20 mm is adequate for oral alimentation. These patients can be redilated without any problems, thereby maintaining alimentation by mouth.

In nine patients who underwent dilation of strictures following surgical correction of esophageal atresia, adequate results were obtained, with follow-up for as long as 2 years. Dilation was performed with balloons 7–10 mm in diameter.

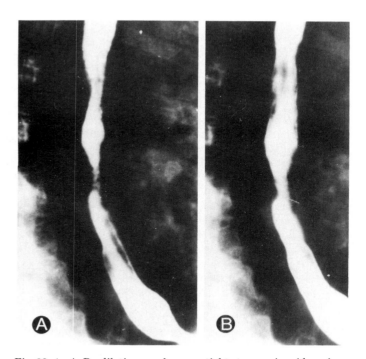

Fig. 28–4 A. Predilation esophagram: tight stenoses in midesophagus. B. Follow-up esophagram after gradual dilatation of stricture in middle third of esophagus.

COMPLICATIONS

With transnasal balloon dilations, three complications have been observed: pain, bleeding, and esophageal rupture. The pain reported by the patients at the time of maximum balloon inflation is usually more severe during

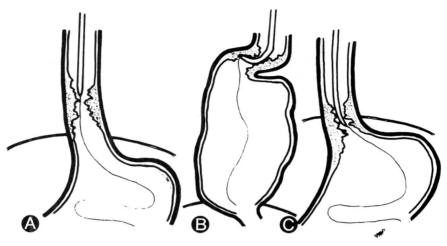

Fig. 28–5 Depending on the anatomy of esophageal stricture, different types of angiographic catheters and guidewires might be needed for manipulations across area of narrowing.

the dilation of tight stenoses and in patients with peptic strictures. Bleeding occurs in >50% of the patients as a result of trauma to the nasal mucosa or at the site of dilation, but no sequelae have been observed. Rupture of the esophagus has been observed in only one patient, in whom it occurred during the second dilation of a malignant stricture.[19] In this patient, the esophagram performed after the first dilation showed an outpouching at

the site of the tear, which should have made the authors think of localized extravasation of barium due to the absence of mucosal folds at the level of the outpouching (Fig. 28–9). In such a case, endoscopy should be performed to corroborate the existence of a tear before any further attempts to dilate the lumen. A longitudinal tear was repaired at operation, and the patient recuperated uneventfully.

DISCUSSION

Classically, dilation of esophageal strictures has been performed with the blind transoral passage of bougies or

metallic olives. Commonly, patients referred for balloon dilation have previously undergone one or more success-

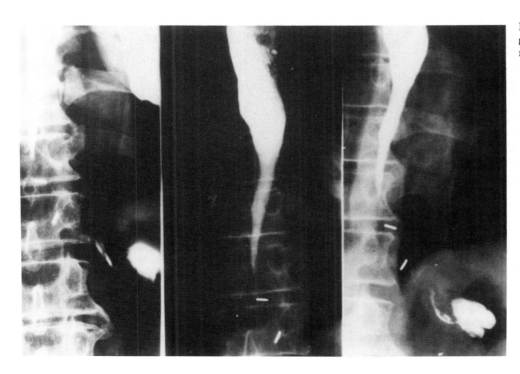

Fig. 28–6 Postsurgical stricture of gastroesophageal junction; note severe narrowing of distal esophagus.

loons and repeated dilations (an average of three per patient).

It is too early to predict the final status of these strictures following balloon dilatation, but the decreased morbidity and mortality and the ability to repeat the procedure make the technique very attractive.

References

1. Earlam R, Cunha–Melo JR: Benign oesophageal strictures: historical and technical aspects of dilatation. *Br J Surg* 1981;68:829
2. Lanza F, Graham D: Bougienage is effective therapy for most benign esophageal strictures. *JAMA* 1987;240:844
3. Patterson DJ, Graham DY: Natural history of benign esophageal strictures: follow-up study in 100 patients. *Gastroenterology* 1983;85:346
4. Wesdorp I, Bartelsman J, et al: Results of conservative treatment of benign esophageal strictures: a follow-up study in 100 patients. *Gastroenterology* 1982;82:487
5. Vantrappen JJ: To dilate or to operate. *Gut* 1983;24:1.013
6. Grüntzig A, Kump DA: Technique of percutaneous transluminal angioplasty with the Graüntzig balloon catheter. *AJR* 1979;132:547
7. London R, Trotman BW, DiMarino AJ Jr, et al: Dilatation of severe esophageal strictures by an inflatable balloon catheter. *Gastroenterology* 1981;80:173
8. McLean GK, Rosen RJ, Ring EJ: Miscellaneous interventional procedures, in Ring EJ, McLean GK: *Interventional Radiology: Principles and Techniques*. Boston, Little, Brown, 1981, p 411
9. Götberg S, Afzelius LE, Hambraeus G, et al: Balloon catheter dilatation of strictures in the upper digestive tract. *Radiology* 1982;22:479
10. Merrell N, McCray RS: Balloon catheter dilation of a severe esophageal stricture. *Gastrointest Endosc* 1982;28:254
11. Ball W, Strife J, Rosenkrantz J, Towbin R, Noseworthy J: Esophageal strictures in children: treatment by balloon dilatation. *Radiology* 1984:150;253
12. Kollath J, Sarck E, Vittorio P: Dilation of esophageal stenosis by balloon catheter. *CardioVasc Intervent Radiol* 1984;7:35
13. Owman T, Lunderquist A: Balloon catheter dilatation of esophageal strictures: a preliminary report. *Gastrointest Radiol* 1982;7:301
14. Dawson S, Mueller E, Ferrucci J Jr, et al: Severe esophageal strictures: indications for balloon catheter dilation. *Radiology* 1984;153:31
15. McLean GK, Ring EJ, Freiman DB: Applications and techniques of gastrointestinal intubation. *CardioVasc Intervent Radiol* 1982;5:108
16. Follows IW, Ogilvie AL, Atkinson M: Pneumatic dilation in achalasia. *Gut* 1983;24:1.0201
17. Goldthorn J, Ball W Jr, Wilkinson L, Seigel R, Kosloske A: Esophageal strictures in children: treatment by serial balloon catheter dilatation. *Radiology* 1984;153:655
18. Lunderquist A: Balloon catheter dilation of benign obstructions. Presented at the VIII Congress of the European Society of Cardiovascular and Interventional Radiology, Elsinore, Denmark, May 20–25, 1984
19. Maynar M, Martinez F, Facal P, et al: Esophageal dilation by balloon catheter. Presented at the Annual Postgraduate Course and Joint Meeting of the European Society of Cardiovascular and Interventional Radiology, Vienna, Austria, April 22–27, 1985
20. Starck E, Paolucci V, Herzer M, Crummy A: Esophageal stenosis: treatment with balloon catheters. *Radiology* 1984;153:637
21. Tulman A, Worth Boyce H Jr: Complications of esophageal dilation and guidelines for their prevention. *Gastrointest Endosc* 1981;27:229
22. Ferrucci JT Jr, Wittenberg J, Mueller PR, Simeone JF (eds): *Interventional Radiology of the Abdomen,* ed. 2. Baltimore, Williams & Wilkins, 1985